Urinary INCONTINENCE

Urinary INCONTINENCE

PAT D. O'DONNELL, M.D.

Professor of Urology,
University of Cincinnati College of Medicine;
Director, University of Cincinnati Center for Incontinence,
University Hospital,
Cincinnati, Ohio

Mosby

St. Louis Baltimore Boston Carlsbad Chicago Naples New York Philadelphia Portland
London Madrid Mexico City Singapore Sydney Tokyo Toronto Wiesbaden

Mosby
Dedicated to Publishing Excellence

A Times Mirror
Company

Publisher: Anne S. Patterson
Editor: Susie Baxter
Developmental Editor: Ellen Baker Geisel
Project Manager: Dana Peick
Production Editor: Cindy Deichmann
Manuscript Editor: Carl Masthay
Designer: Amy Buxton
Composition Specialist: Terri Knapp
Manufacturing Manager: Betty Mueller, Karen Boehme

Printed in the United States of America
Composition by Mosby Electronic Production, St. Louis
Lithography/color film by Accu-color, Inc.
Printing/binding by Maple-Vail

Mosby-Year Book, Inc.
11830 Westline Industrial Drive
St. Louis, Missouri 63146

International Standard Book Number 0-8151-6517-X

98 99 00 01 / 9 8 7 6 5 4 3 2

C O N T R I B U T O R S

Paul Abrams, M.D., FRCS
Clinical Senior Lecturer,
University of Bristol;
Consultant Urologist,
Bristol Urological Institute,
Southmead Hospital,
Bristol, Avon, United Kingdom
10: The Cystometrogram
57: Etiology of Urinary Incontinence

Sherif R. Aboseif, M.D.
Assistant Professor,
Department of Urology,
University of California–San Francisco,
San Francisco, California
32: Retropubic Suspension Procedures

Rodney A. Appell, M.D.
Head, Section of Voiding Dysfunction and Female Urology,
Department of Urology,
The Cleveland Clinic Foundation,
Cleveland, Ohio
24: Practical Urodynamics
31: Intraurethral Injections

Michael P. Aronson, M.D.
Assistant Professor of Obstetrics and Gynecology,
Tufts University School of Medicine;
Chief, Division of Urogynecology/Reconstructive Pelvic Surgery,
Department of Obstetrics and Gynecology,
Division of Reconstructive Pelvic Surgery,
Tufts–New England Medical Center,
Boston, Massachusetts
45: Urinary Incontinence After Pelvic Surgery

Said A. Awad, M.D.
Professor and Head,
Department of Urology,
Dalhousie University,
Halifax, Nova Scotia, Canada
26: Urge Incontinence

Gopal H. Badlani, M.D.
Professor of Urology,
Albert Einstein College of Medicine;
Associate Chairman, Department of Urology,
Long Island Jewish Medical Center,
New Hyde Park, New York
60: Surgical Management Decisions in Geriatric Incontinence

D. Duane Baldwin, M.D.
Resident Physician,
Department of Urology,
Loma Linda University School of Medicine,
Loma Linda, California
25: Stress Urinary Incontinence

Stuart B. Bauer, M.D.
Associate Professor of Surgery,
Department of Urology,
Harvard Medical School;
Senior Associate,
Department of Surgery (Urology),
The Children's Hospital,
Boston, Massachusetts
20: Urodynamics

Tamara G. Bavendam, M.D.
Associate Professor,
Director, Female Urology,
University of Washington School of Medicine;
Department of Urology,
Seattle, Washington
1: The Personal Side of Incontinence
3: Quality of Life for Those with Urinary Incontinence

Nabil K. Bissada, M.D.
Professor and Chief of Urologic Oncology,
Department of Urology,
Medical University of South Carolina;
Chief of Urologic Oncology,
Medical University of South Carolina Hospitals,
Charleston, South Carolina
41: Vesicovaginal Fistula

Jerry G. Blaivas, M.D.
Clinical Professor of Urology,
Cornell University Medical School;
Attending Surgeon, Department of Urology,
New York, New York
7: Office Evaluation of Incontinence
15: Videourodynamics

David A. Bloom, M.D.
Professor, Department of Surgery,
The University of Michigan School of Medicine;
Chief, Pediatric Urology,
University of Michigan Medical Center,
Ann Arbor, Michigan
19: Clinical Evaluation of Children

David S. Breslin, M.D.
Assistant Clinical Professor of Urology,
New York Medical College,
Valhalla, New York
48: Bladder Noncompliance

Carol A. Brink, R.N., M.P.H.
Associate Professor of Clinical Nursing,
University of Rochester School of Nursing,
Rochester, New York
61: Containment of Involuntary Urine Loss

Kathryn L. Burgio, Ph.D.
Associate Professor, Department of Medicine,
Division of Gerontology and Geriatric Medicine,
University of Alabama Medical Center,
Birmingham, Alabama
58: Behavior Therapy

Arthur L. Burnett, M.D.
Assistant Professor,
Department of Urology,
Brady Urologic Institute,
Johns Hopkins Medical Institute,
Baltimore, Maryland
4: Anatomic Aspects of Urinary Incontinence

Patricia A. Burns, M.D.
Associate Professor,
Family Nurse Practitioner Program,
State University of New York at Buffalo,
Buffalo, New York
38: Behavioral Therapy

Michael C. Carr, M.D., Ph.D.
Assistant Professor, Department of Urology,
University of Washington School of Medicine;
Attending Surgeon, Division of Pediatric Urology,
Children's Hospital & Medical Center,
Seattle, Washington
22: Anatomic Incontinence

Anthony J. Casale, M.D.
Associate Professor,
Department of Urology,
Indiana University School of Medicine,
Riley Hospital for Children,
Indianapolis, Indiana
18: Clinical Management Decisions

Jong M. Choe, M.D.
Female Urology/Urodynamics Fellow,
Beth Israel Hospital/Harvard Medical School,
Division of Urology,
Boston, Massachusetts
8: The Incontinence History and Physical Examination

Ashok Chopra, M.D.
Assistant Professor of Urology
University of Tennessee Medical Center
Knoxville, Tennessee
33: Anterior Vaginal Wall Sling

Joyce Colling, R.N., Ph.D., FAAN
Professor,
Gerontological Nursing,
Oregon Health Sciences University,
School of Nursing,
Portland, Oregon
55: Incontinence Assessment

Christos E. Constantinou, Ph.D.
Associate Professor of Urology,
Stanford University Medical School
Stanford, California
12: Urethral Pressure in the Evaluation of Female Incontinence

William C. de Groat, Ph.D.
Professor of Pharmacology and Neuroscience,
Department of Pharmacology,
University of Pittsburgh School of Medicine,
Pittsburgh, Pennsylvania
6: Central Nervous System Control of Micturition

Ananias C. Diokno, M.D.
Clinical Professor, Department of Urology,
Section of Urology,
University of Michigan;
Chief, Department of Urology,
William Beaumont Hospital,
Royal Oak, Michigan
36: Artificial Urinary Sphincter
53: Clean Intermittent Catheterization

Deborah R. Erickson, M.D.
Assistant Professor of Surgery,
Division of Urology,
Pennsylvania State University College of Medicine;
Director, Female Urology and Neurourology,
Department of Surgery, Division of Urology,
The Milton S. Hershey Medical Center,
Hershey, Pennsylvania
43: Interstitial Cystitis

Harris E. Foster, Jr., M.D.
Assistant Professor of Surgery,
Department of Surgery, Section of Urology,
Yale University School of Medicine;
Attending Physician, Department of Surgery,
Section of Urology,
Yale–New Haven Hospital,
New Haven, Connecticut
35: Urethrolysis

Jerzy B. Gajewski, M.D., FRCSC
Associate Professor,
Department of Urology,
Dalhousie University;
Active Staff, Department of Urology,
Camp Hill Medical Centre,
Halifax, Nova Scotia, Canada
26: Urge Incontinence

Cheryle B. Gartley
President and Founder,
Simon Foundation for Continence–U.S.,
Wilmette, Illinois
1: The Personal Side of Incontinence

Patricia S. Goode, M.D., M.S.N., E.T.
Assistant Professor of Medicine,
Division of Gerontology and Geriatric Medicine,
University of Alabama at Birmingham,
Birmingham, Alabama
58: Behavior Therapy

E. Ann Gormley, M.D.
Assistant Professor of Surgery (Urology),
Dartmouth Medical School;
Director of Urodynamics and Voiding Dysfunction,
Section of Urology,
Dartmouth Hitchcock Medical Center,
Lebanon, New Hampshire
34: Pubovaginal Sling Procedure

Saul P. Greenfield, M.D.
Associate Professor, Department of Urology,
State University of New York at Buffalo Medical School;
Director, Pediatric Urology,
Children's Hospital of Buffalo,
Buffalo, New York
23: Spina Bifida and Spinal Lesions

François Haab, M.D.
Assistant Professor of Urology
Tenon Hospital
Paris, France
11: Pressure-Flow Studies

Roger Hadley, M.D.
Professor and Chairman,
Division of Urology,
Loma Linda University School of Medicine,
Loma Linda, California
25: Stress Urinary Incontinence

Peter G. Hammerer, M.D.
Assistant Professor of Urology,
Department of Urology,
University Hospital Hamburg,
Hamburg, Germany
44: Postprostatectomy Incontinence

Dianne M. Heritz, M.D., FRCSC
Lecturer, Department of Surgery,
Division of Urology,
University of Toronto;
Urologist,
Women's College Hospital,
Toronto, Ontario, Canada
15: Videourodynamics

Jay B. Hollander, M.D.
Attending Physician, Department of Urology,
William Beaumont Hospital,
Royal Oak, Michigan
53: Clean Intermittent Catheterization

Hartwig Huland, M.D.
Chairman, Department of Urology,
University Hospital Hamburg,
Hamburg, Germany
44: Postprostatectomy Incontinence

Simon Jackson, M.D., MRCOG
Senior Registrar,
Department of Gynecology,
Southmead Hospital,
Bristol, Avon, United Kingdom
10: The Cystometrogram
57: Etiology of Urinary Incontinence

Katherine F. Jeter, Ed.D.
Executive Director, Help for Incontinent People, Inc.;
Clinical Assistant Professor of Urology,
Medical University of South Carolina (Spatanburg);
Adjunct Professor of Nursing,
Mary Black School of Nursing,
University of South Carolina,
Spartanburg, South Carolina
3: Quality of Life for Those with Urinary Incontinence

Mickey M. Karram, M.D.
Associate Professor of Obstetrics and Gynecology,
University of Cincinnati;
Director of Urogynecology,
Department of Obstetrics and Gynecology,
Good Samaritan Hospital,
Cincinnati, Ohio
42: Pelvic Prolapse and Lower Urinary Tract Dysfunction in Females

Michael J. Kennelly, M.D.
Clinical Instructor,
Department of Surgery School of Medicine,
The University of North Carolina at Chapel Hill,
Chapel Hill, North Carolina
28: Intrinsic Sphincter Deficiency
47: Incontinence Caused by Neurologic Diseases

Aaron Kirkemo, M.D.
Director of Urodynamics Laboratory,
Department of Urology,
Henry Ford Hospital,
Detroit, Michigan
17: Radiographic Evaluation

Robert J. Krane, M.D.
Professor and Chairman,
Department of Urology,
Boston University Medical Center,
Boston, Massachusetts
14: Electromyography in Urodynamics

Richard F. Labasky, M.D.
Assistant Professor of Surgery,
Division of Urology,
University of Utah Health Sciences Center,
Salt Lake City, Utah
16: Endoscopic Evaluation

Gary E. Leach, M.D.
Associate Clinical Professor of Urology
University of California, Los Angeles;
Chief, Department of Urology,
Kaiser Permanente Medical Center,
Los Angeles, California
37: Complications of Incontinence Surgery

Scott A. MacDiarmid, M.D.
Assistant Professor,
Department of Urology,
University of Arkansas for Medical Sciences,
Little Rock, Arkansas
59: Pharmacologic Management

Anders Mattiasson, M.D., Ph.D.
Professor, Department of Urology,
Lund University Hospital,
Lund, Sweden
5: Physiology of Continence

Edward J. McGuire, M.D.
Professor and Director, Division of Urology,
Department of Urology,
University of Texas Health Science Center,
Houston, Texas
13: Leak Point Pressure
28: Intrinsic Sphincter Deficiency
34: Pubovaginal Sling Procedure
35: Urethrolysis

John R. Miklos, M.D.
Fellow, Division of Urogynecology and Pelvic Floor Reconstruction,
Department of Obstetrics and Gynecology,
Good Samaritan Hospital–Seton Center,
Cincinnati, Ohio
42: Pelvic Prolapse and Lower Urinary Tract Dysfunction in Females

Michael E. Mitchell, M.D.
Professor and Chief of Pediatric Urology,
Department of Urology,
Children's Hospital and Medical Center,
University of Washington for School of Medicine;
Chief of Pediatric Urology,
Department of Urology, Division of Pediatric Urology,
Children's Hospital and Medical Center,
University Hospital,
Seattle, Washington
22: Anatomic Incontinence

Jacek L. Mostwin, M.D., D.Phil.
Associate Professor of Urology,
The Johns Hopkins Medical Institute,
Baltimore, Maryland
4: Anatomic Aspects of Urinary Incontinence

Denise A. Nigro, M.D.
N.I.H./A.F.U.D. Fellow,
Division of Urology,
Hospital of the University of Pennsylvania,
Philadelphia, Pennsylvania
39: Pharmacologic Therapy

Victor W. Nitti, M.D.
Assistant Professor of Urology,
Director of Neurourology and Female Urology,
New York University Medical Center,
New York, New York
52: Management of Complicated Incontinence in Women

Helen E. O'Connell, M.B.B.S., FRACS
Senior Lecturer,
University of Melbourne,
Royal Melbourne Hospital,
Parkville, Australia
13: Leak Point Pressure
19: Clinical Evaluation of Children

Pat D. O'Donnell, M.D.
Professor of Urology,
University of Cincinnati College of Medicine;
Director, University of Cincinnati Center for Incontinence,
University Hospital,
Cincinnati, Ohio
27: Mixed Urinary Incontinence
29: Raz Suspension Procedure
38: Behavioral Therapy
55: Incontinence Assessment

Joseph G. Ouslander, M.D.
Professor of Medicine,
Director, Division of Geriatric Medicine and Gerontology;
Chief of Medicine,
Wesley Woods Geriatric Center at Emory University;
Director, Rehabilitation Research and Development Center,
Atlanta, Georgia
56: Management of Incontinence in Long-Term Care

Christopher K. Payne, M.D.
Assistant Professor of Urology,
Director, Center for Neurourology,
Stanford University,
Stanford Medical Center,
Stanford, California
40: Electrostimulation

Mark W. Plawker, M.D.
Resident, Department of Urology,
State University of New York,
Health Science Center at Brooklyn,
Brooklyn, New York
52: Management of Complicated Incontinence in Women

Kevin Pranikoff, M.D.
Associate Professor of Urology and Rehabilitation Medicine,
Vice-Chairman, Department Of Urology,
State University of New York at Buffalo;
Clinical Director of Urology,
Erie County Medical Center,
Buffalo, New York
54: Clinical Management Decisions

Ross A. Rames, M.D.
Assistant Professor of Urology,
Attending Urologist, Department of Urology,
Medical University of South Carolina,
Charleston, South Carolina
30: Nondissected Needle Suspension Procedures

Shlomo Raz, M.D.
Professor of Surgery/Urology,
University of California, Los Angeles,
Los Angeles, California
33: Anterior Vaginal Wall Sling

Michael Rentzepis, M.D.
Fellow,
Department of Surgery,
Division of Urology,
Memorial Sloan-Kettering Cancer Center,
New York, New York
51: Augmentation Cystoplasty

Richard C. Rink, M.D.
Associate Professor, Urology,
Indiana University School of Medicine;
Chief, Pediatric Urology,
James Whitcomb Riley Hospital for Children,
Indianapolis, Indiana
18: Clinical Management Decisions

Michael L. Ritchey, M.D.
Associate Professor of Surgery and Pediatrics,
University of Texas;
Chief of Pediatric Urology,
Hermann Children's Hospital
Houston, Texas
19: Clinical Evaluation of Children

Jessie F. Rohner, Dr.P.H., M.D., B.S.N., R.N.
Executive Administer,
Penna Nurses Association,
Harrisburg, Pennsylvania
2: Urinary Incontinence in America: the Social Significance

Thomas J. Rohner, Jr., M.D.
Professor of Surgery (Urology),
Chief, Division of Urology,
Department of Surgery (Urology),
The Pennsylvania State University College of Medicine;
Chief, Division of Urology,
Department of Surgery (Urology),
The Milton Hershey Medicine Center,
University Hospital,
Children's Hospital,
Hershey, Pennsylvania
2: Urinary Incontinence in America: the Social Significance

Lauri J. Romanzi, M.D.
Assistant Professor,
Department of Obstetrics and Gynecology;
Director, Division of Urogynecology,
New York Hospital,
New York, New York
7: Office Evaluation of Incontinence

Randall G. Rowland, M.D., Ph.D.
Professor and Acting Chairman,
Department of Urology,
Indiana University School of Medicine,
Indiana University Hospital,
Indianapolis, Indiana
49: Continent Diversion

Delbert C. Rudy, M.D.
Associate Professor of Surgery (Urology),
Department of Surgery/Division of Urology,
University of Texas Health Sciences Center at Houston;
Director of Urology,
Urodynamics Laboratory,
The Institute for Rehabilitation and Research,
Houston, Texas
46: Spinal Cord Injuries
47: Incontinence Caused by Neurologic Diseases

Grannum R. Sant, M.D.
Professor and Chairman Ad Interim,
Department of Urology,
Tufts University School of Medicine,
Boston, Massachusetts
45: Urinary Incontinence After Pelvic Surgery

John F. Schnelle, Ph.D.
Director, Anna & Harry Borun Center for Gerontological Research,
Professor in Residence,
Department of Medicine,
University of California, Los Angeles;
Director of Research and Quality Assurance,
Los Angeles Jewish Home for the Aging,
Reseda, California
56: Management of Incontinence in Long-Term Care

Curtis A. Sheldon, M.D.
Associate Professor of Surgery,
Director, Pediatric Urology,
Children's Hospital Medical Center,
Cincinnati, Ohio
21: Enuresis

Larry T. Sirls, M.D.
Co-Director, Urodynamics Laboratory,
Department of Urology,
Henry Ford Hospital,
Detroit, Michigan
8: The Incontinence History and Physical Examination

Mike B. Siroky, M.D.
Professor of Urology,
Boston University School of Medicine;
Chief of Urology,
Boston Veterans Affairs Medical Center,
Boston, Massachusetts
14: Electromyography in Urodynamics

David R. Staskin, M.D.
Assistant Professor of Surgery/Urology,
Harvard Medical School;
Director, Continence Center,
Beth Israel Hospital,
Boston, Massachusetts
48: Bladder Noncompliance

Anthony R. Stone, M.B., FRCS, Ed
Associate Professor, Department of Urology,
University of California, Davis
University of California, Davis Medical Center,
Sacramento, California
51: Augmentation Cystoplasty

Kevin T. Stone, M.D.
Chief Resident, Department of Urology,
William Beaumont Hospital,
Royal Oak, Michigan
36: Artificial Urinary Sphincter

Lynn Stothers, M.D., M.H.Sc., FRCSC
Assistant Professor of Urology,
University of British Columbia;
St. Paul's Hospital,
Vancouver, British Columbia, Canada
33: Anterior Vaginal Wall Sling

Eddie H.M. Sze, M.D.
Assistant Professor of Ob/Gyn,
Director of Undergraduate Medical Education,
Medical Center of Central Georgia,
Mercer University School of Medicine,
Macon, Georgia
42: Pelvic Prolapse and Lower Urinary Tract Dysfunction in Females

Emil A. Tanagho, M.D.
Department of Urology,
University of California School of Medicine,
San Francisco, California
32: Retropubic Suspension Procedures

Brett A. Trockman, M.D.
Fellow, Female Urology and Urodynamics,
Kaiser Permanente Medical Center,
Los Angeles, California
37: Complications of Incontinence Surgery

Jeffrey Wacksman, M.D.
Associate Professor of Clinical Surgery,
Department of Surgery, Division of Urology,
University of Cincinnati College of Medicine;
Associate Director, Pediatric Urology Department,
Children's Hospital Medical Center,
Cincinnati, Ohio
21: Enuresis

Todd Wagner, B.A.
Cost and Outcomes Assessment Team,
Department of Urology,
University of Washington Medical Center,
Seattle, Washington
3: Quality of Life for Those with Urinary Incontinence

Gregory R. Wahle, M.D.
Assistant Professor of Urology,
Indiana University School of Medicine,
Indianapolis, Indiana
9: The Urinary Flow Rate

Julian Wan, M.D.
Assistant Professor of Urology,
Department of Urology,
State University of New York at Buffalo;
Attending Urologist, Department of Pediatric Urology,
Children's Hospital of Buffalo,
Buffalo, New York
23: Spina Bifida and Spinal Lesions

George D. Webster, M.B., FRSC
Professor of Urology,
Department of Surgery,
Duke University Medical Center,
Durham, North Carolina
50: Neobladder

Alan J. Wein, M.D.
Professor and Chair, Division of Urology,
University of Pennsylvania School of Medicine;
Chief of Urology,
Hospital of the University of Pennsylvania,
Philadelphia, Pennsylvania
39: Pharmacologic Therapy

Thelma J. Wells, R.N., Ph.D.
Helen Denne Schulte Professor of Nursing,
University of Wisconsin, Madison;
Nurse Researcher,
Department of Geriatric Research, Education, and Clinical Center,
William S. Middleton Veterans Hospital,
Madison, Wisconsin
62: Nursing Management

Jack Christian Winters, M.D.
Clinical Associate Professor of Urology,
Louisiana State University Medical Center,
New Orleans, Louisiana
24: Practical Urodynamics
31: Intraurethral Injections

Jean F. Wyman, Ph.D., R.N.
Professor, Department of Adult Health Nursing,
School Of Nursing,
Virginia Commonwealth University,
Richmond, Virginia
55: Incontinence Assessment

Philipe E. Zimmern, M.D.
Associate Professor,
Division of Urology,
University of Texas Southwestern Medical School at Dallas,
Dallas, Texas
11: Pressure-Flow Studies

To my mother, Elsie O'Donnell, my brother, Everett O'Donnell, and in memory of my father, Howard O'Donnell, for the enduring love that has been the source of strength and courage throughout my life.

FOREWORD

You will find that this book is truly comprehensive. It covers the whole of that important and expanding field, incontinence. It includes areas not usually seen in texts, such as how incontinence places personal and social burdens on our population and what can be done about it educationally, medically, and surgically.

This is only supplemental to the latest information on anatomy and physiology, including neurophysiology, basic areas that are described in detail by four of the country's recognized authorities. The practical aspects of diagnosis include the latest clinically useful information on urodynamic techniques and other methods of evaluation.

Especially valuable is an extensive section on incontinence in children, collected information that is otherwise scattered and inaccessible. Each form of incontinence is discussed in one informative chapter after another. Those describing the surgical and medical techniques of each of the current methods of treatment follow, again written by experts. Postsurgical incontinence is also discussed, as well as continent diversion and bladder augmentation and replacement.

As you can see, this volume contains the whole of present knowledge on incontinence placed in a usable form by the leaders in the field. It will be valuable to students and residents as they acquire grounding and will be a boon to the urologist, nurse, and health worker in their everyday practices.

Frank Hinman, Jr., M.D.

PREFACE

This book was written as a comprehensive desk reference for all health care professionals involved in the care of patients who have urinary incontinence. An immense effort was made with this book to place the clinical management decisions about the incontinent patient at the fingertips of the health care professional. As a desk reference for the management of urinary incontinence, both surgical and nonsurgical management of all types of incontinence in children, adults, and the elderly are included. From the uncomplicated incontinent patient to the most complex incontinence problem, each clinical management decision is described as clearly as possible with current treatment options that can be readily applied by the health care professional to the immediate clinical management problem.

This book strongly emphasizes clinical evaluation of the incontinent patient. The clinical basis for successful therapy in almost every patient is an adequate assessment. The importance of the clinical history and physical examination cannot be overemphasized. The subsequent diagnostic urodynamic studies often can be confusing to the patient as well as to the practicing health care professional. For this reason, separate chapters are devoted to each study in the urodynamic evaluation of the patient with a complete explanation of how the patient assessment is done and what it means.

Also, the personal side of incontinence is emphasized throughout this book. Just as every aspect of the life of the patient is affected by urinary incontinence, so is every aspect of that life a consideration in the evaluation and treatment of urinary incontinence. The effect of urinary incontinence on the quality of life of every patient is the most important consideration that determines the complexity of the evaluation and the invasiveness of treatment. The personal side of incontinence is integrated with the most current technology in both the evaluation and treatment of incontinence to emphasize a requirement for sensitivity to the patient needs and quality of life without compromising the clinical management.

Urinary incontinence is a devastating problem that affects almost 20 million Americans. The annual health care costs of urinary incontinence are more than the combined cost of all coronary artery bypass surgery and all renal dialysis in the United States. Moreover, the financial costs are small compared with the personal cost to the individual in self-imposed social isolation and loss of self-esteem. Many patients with urinary incontinence suffer in silence because they are ashamed to discuss the problem with their physician or feel that nothing can be done for them. It is important for every health care professional to realize that almost everyone with urinary incontinence can be treated successfully.

Pat D. O'Donnell

ACKNOWLEDGMENTS

It is with the deepest respect and appreciation that I thank the many contributors for the outstanding effort and immense commitment that resulted in this textbook. To be involved in bringing together in one textbook the excellent work of so many outstanding people has been the greatest privilege of my life. Also, I will always be grateful to Shlomo Raz, M.D., for being a great teacher and clinician during my fellowship as well as a close friend throughout my career. In addition, it has been a unique privilege for me to work with Edward McGuire, M.D., who has taught me so much during my career.

CONTENTS

PART SIX

INCONTINENCE IN OLDER PEOPLE

APPENDIXES

PART ONE URINARY INCONTINENCE

Chapter 1 The Personal Side of Incontinence

Tamara G. Bavendam, Cheryle B. Gartley

It took 3 cups of coffee to hang in there, but the meeting is finally over. My next appointment is across town in 30 minutes—manageable if there are no delays. I need to "go," but time is tight—no big deal—I'll go when I get there.

Traffic is unbearably slow and then comes to an abrupt standstill just before the bridge. I'll be late for my appointment—thank goodness for my cellular phone. If I had only known there was going to be a delay, I would have stayed and used the bathroom. The urge is increasing. Is there any way of getting out of traffic and finding a bathroom? No!

Thinking of other things helps. Concentrate on the radio—it's not so bad. . . . Fifteen minutes later the traffic is thankfully moving. Where is the nearest bathroom? Just thinking about a bathroom makes the urge become overwhelming, almost painful. "What if I don't get to the bathroom soon? Will my bladder rupture? Will I wet my pants? Don't think about it; just drive!"

A gas station ahead on the right. Great! Just cross the three lanes of traffic and I'm home free. The urge and spasms are building every second. There's a constant throbbing sensation I can't ignore.

Screech! Slam on the brakes! Where did that idiot come from? At least I didn't get hit! Wait, why am I feeling warm? ***I WET MYSELF—#X@!X%Z@!!*** *Now what am I going to do?*

Given the appropriate circumstances, involuntary loss of urine can happen to anyone. We are all at risk. Many adults have vivid childhood memories of a particular episode of urinary incontinence that still brings back the feelings of embarrassment and humiliation—being sent home from school or not being invited back to a friend's for a slumber party.

The mechanisms that promote voluntary control of our lower urinary tract function—the storage and evacuation of urine from the bladder—are a complex, delicate balance of the autonomic and somatic nervous systems and are subject to intense conscious facilitory and inhibitory influences. The storage and evacuation of urine are complex and very delicately balanced between the autonomic and somatic nervous systems and subject to intense conscious facilitatory and inhibitory influences. When everything is working normally, lower urinary function is taken for granted. We often are in the position to push our bladders to their limits and expect them to comply with our needs. When we push too hard and expect too much, the consequences can be devastating. No matter how uncontrollable the circumstances precipitating urinary incontinence may be, loss of bladder control is viewed by oneself and by others as a significant personal failure.

The scenario described above is not a personal failure, nor does it mean anything is malfunctioning with the lower urinary tract. The involuntary loss of urine was the expected outcome of that particular set of circumstances where the limits of the bladder and the bladder-outlet mechanism were reached and exceeded. The sudden distraction of the "near accident" and "slamming" on the brakes allowed the developing bladder contraction to overcome the forces of the sphincter mechanism.

Such an episode may change this person's behavior forever. The appointment had to be canceled. The rest of the day was missed to go home, take a bath, and take the suit to the cleaners. What do you say to the cleaners about the urine odor? "My newborn grandson urinated on me while I was changing his diaper"—a modern grandfather for sure. He certainly will never pass up the opportunity to go to the bathroom before he decides to drive across town. In fact, he will stop putting off the urge to go to the bathroom—*ever!* He certainly does not ever want to go through that again. In fact, he may even trade in his car to get rid of the reminder of his failure. One episode can be a life-changing event.

Millions of people face the sudden involuntary loss of urine several times a day. No matter how many times it happens, it is not something you "get used to" and "don't mind." You always mind; there is always the "Ohhhh!—where is the bathroom?" "Did I put a pad on today? When did I last change it? Will I make it to the bathroom before I leak through the pad? Did I bring an extra pad—a change of clothes?" This litany of questions can happen with each and every episode of urinary incontinence. You never know what may happen between now and the bathroom; you may leak again.

Imagine the time it takes to plan a day, or the rest of your life for that matter. Decisions have to be made about what to wear that is washable and will not "look wet." How much fluid can be taken and when to drink it to minimize the risk. How to discreetly carry enough pads just in case it is a bad day. Should I go on this trip? What happens if the bathrooms are hard to find? New jobs can be a nightmare. Not only do you have to decide if the position and people are compatible with your professional capabilities and desires, you also have to make sure your work location is readily accessible to a bathroom, and you can never be put in a position to be alone at the cash register. What happens if the urge hits when a customer walks in?

The consequences for each person as an individual can be significant, but the great effect on each individual's family can also be devastating. Incontinence sufferers who have contacted the Simon Foundation for Continence claim that breakup of their marriages can be attributed to incontinence. When a relationship is based on physical activities such as camping, hiking, biking, or soccer and the incontinent individual no longer feels comfortable participating in those activities, the relationship must be able to adapt. Some people become reclusive and feel they are no longer physically attractive. They must change their style of dress to loose or baggy clothes that are dark colors in order to hide the external protection they must wear and the inevitable leakage.

Incontinence in the family can be similar to alcoholism. For a period of time, the problem may be hidden from other family members. However, the family usually senses the changes in behaviors and wonders what they may have done to contribute to the behavioral changes. After the first episode of urinary incontinence, most sufferers react in extreme fear of public exposure of their "shameful" problem. They often choose to isolate themselves at home rather that take any risks. Isolation can quickly lead to depression, and depression contributes to loss of coping skills. This can result in an emotional downward spiral that ends with loss of self-esteem.

Public and professional education campaigns are vitally important to raise the level of recognition that not only is urinary incontinence a common occurrence but it can also have devastating effects on an individual's behavior and self-esteem even at degrees that would not seem significant to most health care professionals. We need to prepare ourselves to identify the problem early and work toward solutions before the vicious downhill cycle toward isolation, depression, and loss of self-esteem results. We must educate our patients and ourselves to understand that there are many viable treatment options and that the belief that "nothing can be done" or "I am too old" or "my problem is not bad enough for surgery" are misconceptions.

A Health Professional's Story

As a woman and a practicing urologist, I have listened to thousands of stories of men and women over the past decade. The great effect of urinary incontinence on an individual's life and perception of self was difficult to imagine until I had my first sudden sneezing episode with a full bladder in the middle of a busy clinic. Wait a minute, I believe in empathy, but not like this. Fortunately, the scrub clothes were just around the corner and my patients are used to seeing surgeons in scrubs.

I was able to remain anonymous and pretend it didn't happen until it happened again. Now I am altering my own behavior because of my bladder. It is no longer safe to put off going to the bathroom; what happens if I cough or sneeze? Damp or wet underwear, even when not visible to others, is a very distracting, "icky" feeling.

Am I *now* motivated *enough* to take steps to correct my own pelvic muscle weakness and be in a position to prevent repeat occurrences next winter when bronchitis hits again? *No!* Out of sight, out of mind. What will motivate me to begin rehabilitation of my weakened pelvic floor muscles? I wish I knew the answer to that question. I am surprised by my own reluctance to take the time and energy to work with pelvic muscle rehabilitation now, because I have no intention of having an operation to fix the "pelvic muscle weakness." I at least have the advantage of knowing what my options are and what the risk-to-benefit ratio is for each of the surgical and nonsurgical options. I can make an informed decision. I will know what my threshold for "motivation" is when I get there. I will also be able to get the kind of treatment I desire if I am not able to get motivated for pelvic muscle rehabilitation.

I sometimes fear that the perception of incontinence as a behavioral issue that seems to be so deeply ingrained in all of us will unnecessarily "force" patients who are not good candidates for behavioral treatments into a required pathway of behavioral treatment mandated by practice guidelines. Failure to comply with these behavioral recommendations may be viewed by health care professionals as an indication that the problem "must not be very bad" and therefore not warrant further treatment. We must guard against judging our patients negatively for lack of compliance with potentially effective but demanding behavioral treatments. Urinary incontinence is a medical condition like diabetes and coronary artery disease. We do not withhold treatment for diabetes if someone is not totally compliant with dietary changes or withhold treatment for coronary artery disease if the patient does not quit smoking. Urinary incontinence should be no different.

Much of the stigma surrounding urinary incontinence is a result of lack of knowledge that begins with "toilet training." My experience lecturing worldwide confirms that tremendous value is assigned to "being trained," and the occurrence of "accidents" often results in the admonishment of "bad boy" or "bad girl." This pervasive regard of urinary incontinence as a behavioral issue is carried throughout childhood into adulthood. One 14-year-old girl with spina bifida was made to write "I will not wet my pants" 100 times with each episode of loss of bladder control. Despite having an underlying reason, it was still viewed by her parents as behavioral. The effect of the urinary incontinence on her family had been profound. She had become so embarrassed about her problem that she refused to go to school and face the ridicule and teasing. Her father therefore gave up his job, the family was forced to move, and the whole family lived in fear that her "problem" would be exposed in their new location.

Unfortunately the shame and embarrassment surrounding bladder control are carried into adulthood. Although it is easy to tell people that there is no shame in loss of bladder control and that embarrassment is unnecessary, it is impossible to get anyone to believe that this is true. We are all capable of handling embarrassment, and in fact do so on a daily basis without becoming a recluse. Who hasn't spilled his or her coffee, stumbled up stairs, spilled the contents of his or her briefcase? Aside from a chagrined look, we learn to accept our momentary "clumsiness" and get on with the day. We do not suffer the unrelenting shame experienced by those who experience loss of bladder control. This shame is what usually keeps persons from reporting the problem and seeking evaluation and treatment. Instead, these people go through life feeling as though they have a red stamp on their forehead reading "THE INCONTINENT."

How can we change these attitudes? We can start by changing our language. Going to the bathroom is a part of life. However, we have developed many euphemisms to help make sure we do not have to say *bathroom* or *toilet.* "I have to see a man about a dog," "spend a penny," and "powder my nose" are commonly used. Rarely do we use the term *toilet.* Common slang expressions for toilet are "the john," "the head," and "the ladies' room" or "the men's room." What is wrong with "excusing ourselves to go to the toilet?" Being willing to change our vocabulary will help us to change our perceptions. What if the health care professionals wore a button that simply said, "Urine is beautiful"? It would likely communicate to patients that they will not be embarrassed to talk about bladder problems. Once the problem is mentioned, it must be addressed openly—at least to the extent of determining its significance to the patient and deciding whether it is something that can be addressed or it requires a specialty referral. It is not realistic to expect that all primary care professionals will become expert in the evaluation and treatment of UI (urinary incontinence), but it is reasonable to expect that health care professionals have an awareness of the full range of treatment options so that, when called upon to authorize evaluation and treatment recommendations, they can act as an informed advocate for patients. If the specialist usually referred to has only one or two options for treatment, other resources need to be sought. Urinary incontinence is multifactorial in cause, and rarely is one treatment strategy good for all patients. The treatment should fit the patient, rather than trying as we often do to make the patient fit the treatment.

A Health Advocate's Story

Looking for help today can be just as difficult and frustrating as it was when I became incontinent many years ago. In my *early* twenties, I had a sudden onset of severe urinary tract infections and concomitant incontinence. Although I didn't know the word "incontinence" at the time, I was able to communicate to my physician and nurses, though with some embarrassment, that I had to dehydrate myself to be able to make it to their office. Thus, when I arrived in the office, I would not be able to give a urine specimen. If I did not dehydrate myself, I would arrive in their office in all likelihood having had a bladder-control accident. Although it was understandable that they were concerned and wanted to treat the urinary tract infection before reflux into the kidneys or any other problems happened, it was my incontinence that was ruining my life. I quit my job, stopped my MBA work at the University of Chicago, and became a recluse in my own home! Even going to the grocery store was a traumatic event, because not only did they have no public washroom, but the checkout lines were often very long. Like many people with incontinence, I took to going to the store at odd hours to avoid the lines.

No health professional spoke to me about treatment options, absorbent products, clean intermittent catheterization . . . nothing. Yet, located in the city of Chicago, I was seeing leading authorities in urology to try to find an answer to my problem. Not until many years later, when I was working for the cause of incontinence sufferers at the Simon Foundation, did I receive a correct diagnosis of my condition—a lipoma at the L4-L5 level, tethering the spinal cord and affecting the nerves to the bladder.

I was lecturing to the meningomyelocele team at Children's Memorial Hospital in Chicago when David McClone, M.D., a pediatric neurosurgeon who was in the audience, correctly suspected what was causing my incontinence. David came to his diagnosis not only by observing my gait but also by listening to my personal story about the sudden onset of urinary tract infections (UTI) and incontinence. Because of both his diagnostic and his surgical skills, I am able to walk today. I'd still be playing championship tennis had someone looked beyond my UTI and my incontinence for the underlying cause years earlier.

Today thousands of people have heard the message that incontinence can be cured, treated, and managed successfully so that they can go on about their daily lives normally. Equally important, Americans are learning that incontinence is a symptom of something else happening in the body. Whether that something else is of minor consequence medically, such as loss of estrogen or the natural enlargement of the prostate gland, or it is the first indication of a serious medical problem, it is not to be ignored. Sadly, now that more and more individuals are motivated to seek treatment, they often cannot locate expert help in their communities. A symptom that influences so many lives so harshly certainly deserves far more attention.

Through our professional experiences, it has become obvious that urinary incontinence is a very individual experience, both in what is "tolerable" and in what people are willing to do to correct the problem. The threshold for seeking treatment is variable. For some persons, the loss of one drop of urine with a strong cough on a full bladder is enough of a trigger; for others, wearing heavy pads full time may be perceived as a minor inconvenience while they continue to travel the world with an extra suitcase full of pads for the trip.

There is also extreme variability in each person's willingness to work with behavioral techniques such as bladder training, dietary changes, and pelvic muscle exercise programs. Lack of ability or willingness to comply with a behavioral treatment should not be viewed as an "uncooperative patient" who does not warrant more aggressive therapy any more than persons who are unable to stop smoking are denied treatment for their emphysema or coronary artery disease.

The full range of nonsurgical and surgical options should be available to each person. The health care professional needs to help each patient work through the options from least aggressive to most aggressive at the pace that is appropriate for the individual.

It is crucial that health care professionals recognize the magnitude of the problem of urinary incontinence and understand the effect this problem can have on each person's sense of well-being. It is not easy to admit that this is a problem, and so health care professionals need to be comfortable asking questions about urinary control just as they ask questions about shortness of breath while climbing stairs.

Health care professionals can also help each person understand the effect of incontinence on their life, by asking questions such as, "What have you done to minimize your episodes of urinary incontinence?" and, "What physical and social activities are you no longer comfortable doing?" People may give up activities gradually enough that they do not even realize the effect on themselves until they are forced to think back about life before pads, extra laundry, and so forth.

Although we do not know if urinary incontinence is preventable or can be lessened with aggressive preemptive pelvic floor rehabilitation strategies, common sense and knowledge about skeletal muscle physiology would indicate that it should be preventable in many if not most cases. Common sense would also indicate that the problem is more likely to be correctable or reversible when it is identified early. It is never appropriate to say, "What do you expect at your age?" "That's what all women experience after having kids!" "What's the big deal about wearing a small pad? You're used to it." "Come back when the problem is really bad, like when you're in diapers, and we'll see what we can do." "You're cured of your prostate cancer. Be thankful and wear a pad when you play golf."

Having a personal experience with loss of bladder control or watching a loved one struggle with the condition can serve to lower the threshold of concern and make it a routine part of practice. We hope that this chapter can serve to raise your level of awareness and lower your threshold of concern for all of your patients. At least open the door and let them tell you about their reality. You can then choose to initiate evaluation and treatment as appropriate for your level of knowledge or to refer to a specialist. The information in this book should help you feel more comfortable in all aspects of the evaluation and treatment of urinary incontinence.

Chapter 2 Urinary Incontinence in America: The Social Significance

Thomas J. Rohner, Jr., Jessie F. Rohner

Urinary incontinence (UI) is defined by the International Continence Society as "the involuntary loss of urine that represents a hygienic or social problem to the individual."[1] In addition to the individual, there is significant evidence that UI represents a condition that has immense social, economic, and stress implications for caregivers and society as well.[2]

It is clear that UI is common and profoundly alters the daily lives of a large number of Americans. Despite significant federal, medical, and popular press focus on this condition in recent years, including clinical practice guidelines,[3] in most cases UI remains a personal unreported matter and is managed privately by individuals without benefit of medical evaluation or therapy.

PREVALENCE AND INCIDENCE

The prevalence of UI is defined as the number of incontinent persons divided by the total number of persons included in the study. Published prevalence estimates[4-7] vary widely and are significantly dependent on the age, sex type, mental and functional status, definition and severity of incontinence used, and general health of the population studied. Randomly selected community-based surveys would reasonably be assumed to give more reliable prevalence estimates than those based on a clinic or patient group. Two early studies by Nemir and Middleton[8] and Middleton and Wolin[9] evaluated young nulliparous women and found some degree of stress urinary incontinence in 52.4% and 50.7% respectively, with daily loss of urine reported in 12% without history of urinary tract infection.

Prevalence estimates of UI for women in the 15 to 64 years of age group ranges from 2% to 46%, with 10% to 20% a reasonable estimate. For men in this age range, the prevalence is 1.5% to 5%. Studies of elderly persons defined as over 60 years of age living in the community show an approximate doubling of prevalence, with 30% to 40% of women considered incontinent and approximately half that number, or 15%, of men reporting incontinence.[10,11] The prevalence of UI in institutionalized elderly is over 50%, with half of those also experiencing fecal incontinence.[12]

Although adults have generally been the subject of incontinence studies,[13] it is important to recognize that urinary incontinence represents an important and special social concern for individuals in all age groups. Enuresis, especially the nocturnal type, or "bed-wetting," in boys accounts for 90% of incontinence in the 19% of boys 5 to 14 years of age reporting incontinence.[10] One study found nocturnal enuresis occurred in 7.4% of children at 8 years of age with 3.3% never having achieved nighttime continence.[14]

The important urologic care provided to spina bifida and spinal cord–injured patients is devoted to both the preservation of renal function and the management of UI. In the older male, physician-patient discussions of treatment choices for benign prostatic hyperplasia (BPH), and especially radical prostatectomy or radiotherapy for prostate cancer, importantly include continence expectations for the patient considering radical prostatectomy or radiation therapy as an acceptable treatment. These decision-making discussions involve not only what may represent the best therapy for the disease, but also the possible risks and complications of the treatment modality chosen.

The incidence of incontinence is defined as the probability of a person becoming incontinent over a given period of time.[4] Fewer studies of incidence have been done, but a general estimate is that 10% of older men and 20% of women become incontinent over a 1-year period. A 10% incidence rate over 3 years has been reported for younger community-dwelling individuals.

Economic Costs

The general economic costs related to UI have not been systematically studied and are largely unknown except for the elderly in nursing homes. Hu[15,16] has written most extensively on the effect of UI on health care costs. For the year 1987, he estimated that there were 4.6 million incontinent individuals in the United States, with this number including 2.6 million elderly living in the community, 1.2 million individuals 25 to 64 years of age living in the community, and 800,000 incontinent elderly living in nursing homes.

The total economic costs for the 4.6 million incontinent individuals was estimated to be $10.6 billion, with $3.26 billion expended on the 800,000 nursing home residents. This represents $4,104 per year for each incontinent nursing home patient and 10% of total nursing home costs. Cella and Ouslander[17,18] found lower contributions of UI to nursing home costs (3% to 8%). Direct costs, including caregivers' time, supplies (pads, diapers, and catheters), and laundry accounted for the majority of the expenses (58.4%, or $1.9 billion), with the other major area of expense (33%, or $1.1 billion) representing the 5% of nursing home patients who required admission to nursing homes because their incontinence could not be managed at home.

The costs incurred by the incontinent 2.6 million elderly community-dwelling persons were estimated at 4.8 billion dollars, with 2.2 billion dollars spent by the 1.2 million incontinent persons between 25 to 64 years of age. The majority of expense (60%) for the nonnursing home incontinent was for incontinent supplies, including pads, briefs, and added laundry costs. The average cost per incontinent individual living in the community was estimated to be $1,848 per year. Estimates of sales of disposable diapers have increased significantly over the past 5 years, from $492 million in 1989 to over $1 billion in 1994.[19] The cost of diagnostic studies and treatment, including surgical and pharmacologic modalities, was estimated to cost only 0.26% ($7.9 million) in nursing homes and 0.5% ($35 million) for individuals living in the community. Urinary incontinence–related morbidities including care of skin irritation (1.6%), urinary tract infections (2%), falls (1%), and longer hospital stays (35%) consume significantly more dollars ($2.8 billion) than diagnostic and treatment costs ($35 million) in the community. Hu estimates that only 5% of incontinent persons in the community and 2% in nursing homes receive appropriate medical evaluation and diagnostic studies for their incontinence.

The cost of managing UI in nursing homes can be reduced by the use of indwelling urethral catheters. Hu has estimated the cost of managing UI in nursing homes without catheters is $6 per day per patient but only $3 per day per patient using urethral catheters. Ouslander and Kane[18] also found the lowest first-order costs were obtained by the use of a catheter ($2.90 versus $5.11 per day), when compared with diapers or bed pads ($3.77 versus $11.09). They pointed out, however, that the complications related to indwelling catheters including urinary tract infection and urosepsis with high mortality requiring hospitalization in acute care settings make urethral catheters at least as expensive as other care methods. From the standpoint of nursing home economics, catheter use clearly represents a cost-saving measure, since transfer to an acute care setting is reimbursed by other private or federal insurance sources.

In recent years, the rapidly increasing number of elderly and recognition of the high cost of institutionalized care has resulted in an increased emphasis on home care. Baker[20] has evaluated the effect of UI on home care services and found that costs of caring for the incontinent home-bound patient are 25% greater than care of the continent home-bound. She noted that Medicare expenditures for home health care grew from $141 million in 1974 to $3.7 billion in 1990, an annual increase of 23%. Medicaid expenditures grew even more during the same period, from $70 million in 1974 to $4.1 billion in 1990, an average annual rate of change of 29%. Vetter[21] found that 25% of the home-bound requiring care are incontinent of urine.

Efforts to evaluate and improve incontinence in elderly nursing home patients has not been shown to be a successful strategy from the purely economic standpoint. Hu et al.[22] carried out a 3-month behavioral program in elderly females and were successful in reducing incontinent episodes by 0.6% wet episodes per day, a 26% improvement, which was a durable response over the next 22 weeks of follow-up study. The program consisted of hourly prompting and toileting during waking hours and was very labor intensive. The modest improvement resulted in a savings of only $0.57 per patient per day. It was estimated that, given this level of improvement, it would require 2.5 years to recover the expenses related to the 13-week bladder-training program. Schnelle et al.[23] also concluded that a bladder-training program was not cost effective when compared to the usual patterns of nursing care. The lower cost of usual nursing care, however, could be largely attributed to the fact that patients were not checked or changed with each incontinent episode but only 1.34 times per day. Thus even modest success with toilet training programs cannot compete economically with usual nursing home practice patterns, which limit changes and are less expensive than labor-intensive and supply-expensive ideal care. Toileting programs are generally considered to improve patients' self-esteem, sense of well-being, and perineal skin integrity but cannot easily be shown to be economically worthwhile.

The disposable diaper or brief has been shown to be the least expensive method of managing incontinence, depending on laundry costs.[24] Disposable diapers also have the advantage of maintaining or improving skin care. Although indwelling urethral catheters may initially have cost advantages, the costs of morbidity associated with catheters, especially sepsis, make catheters a less attractive option.

Psychosocial Considerations

Numerous studies[25-27] have documented the negative effect of urinary incontinence on an individual's social interactions, feelings of self-esteem, and daily activities. There is also evidence that successful treatment of urinary stress incontinence can improve psychosocial effects.[28] Despite the negative aspects of incontinence there is evidence that a majority of women do not actively seek help or even mention it to their physicians.[29] Although the exact reasons for each individual may vary, there is general agreement that reasons include the belief that UI is a normal aspect of aging, that personal embarrassment and esteem are involved, and that treatment may include surgery that is, at the least, threatening and, at worst, unlikely to be successful. These perceptions regarding a condition that is common, not immediately life threatening, and manageable by the individual albeit at personal, economic, social, and psychic expense tend to confuse estimates of the magnitude of incontinence and the adequate allocation of resources.

Conclusions

It is recognized that UI represents a common but often underreported and undertreated disabling condition that has important social and economic implications both for the affected individual and for society. The aging of the population indicates that UI will become more prevalent in the coming decade and will require substantial additional funding for appropriate care. Although behavioral, surgical, and pharmacologic treatment programs have been shown to be successful in subsets of incontinent individuals, the long-term outcomes and expenses associated with them have not been well studied.

Current concern with the increasing cost of health care and expanded role of managed care plans in caring for patients may well present a new challenge for incontinent patients and their physician and nurse advocates. Innovative, cost-effective therapies with positive outcomes will be needed to convince health care organizations that attention and resources should be allocated for the evaluation and treatment or management of UI.

References

1. International Continence Society committee for the standardization of terminology of the lower tract function, *Br J Obstet Gynaecol* Suppl 6:1-16, 1990.
2. Yu LC, Kaltreider DL: Stressed nurses dealing with incontinent patients, *J Gerontol* Nurs 13:27-30, 1987.
3. *Urinary incontinence in adults: clinical practice guidelines,* AHCPR Pub. #92-0038, Rockville, Md., March 1992, Agency for Health Care Policy and Research, US Public Health Service, US Department of Health and Human Services.
4. Herzog AR, Fultz NH: Prevalence and incidence in community-dwelling population, *J Am Geriatr Soc* 38:273-281, 1990.
5. Brocklethurst JC: Urinary incontinence in the community—analysis of a MORI poll, *Br Med J*306:832-834, 1993.
6. Burgio KL, Matthews KA, Engel BT: Prevalence, incidence and correlates of urinary incontinence in healthy middle-aged women, *J Urol* 146:1255-1259, 1991.
7. Diokno AC, Brock BM, Brown MB, et al: Prevalence of urinary incontinence and other urological symptoms in the noninstitutionalized elderly, *J Urol* 136:1022-1025, 1986.
8. Nemir A, Middleton RP: Stress incontinence in young nulliparous women, *Am J Obstet Gynecol* 68:1166-1168, 1954.
9. Wolin LH: Stress incontinence in young healthy nulliparous female subjects, *J Urol* 101:545-549, 1969.
10. Thomas TM, Plymat KR, Blannin J, et al: Prevalence of urinary incontinence, *Br Med J* 281:1243-1245, 1980.
11. Elving LB, Foldspang A, Lam GW, Mommsen S: Description epidemiology of urinary incontinence in 3100 women, age 30-59, *Scand J Urol Nephrol* 125(Suppl):37-43, 1989.
12. Ouslander JG: Urinary incontinence in nursing homes, *J Am Geriatr Soc* 38:289-291, 1990.
13. Urinary incontinence in adults NIH consensus development conference, *JAMA* 261:2685-2690, 1989.
14. Fergusson DM, Horwood LJ, Shannon FT: Factors related to the age of attainment of nocturnal bladder control: an 8-year longitudinal study, *Pediatrics* 78:884-890, 1986.
15. Hu TW: Impact of urinary incontinence on health-care costs, *J Am Geriatr Soc* 38:292-295, 1990.
16. Hu TW: The economic impact of urinary incontinence, *Clin Geriatr Med* 2:673-687, 1986.
17. Cella M: The nursing costs of urinary incontinence in a nursing home population, *Nurs Clin North Am* 23:159-168, 1988.
18. Ouslander JG, Kane RL: The costs of urinary incontinence in nursing homes, *Med Care* 22:69-79, 1984.
19. Greg Adamson, Ph.D., Personal communication, Proctor and Gamble, Cincinnati, Ohio.
20. Baker DI, Bice TW: The influence of urinary incontinence on publicly financed home care services to low-income elderly people, *The Gerontologist* 35:360-369, 1995.
21. Vetter N, Jones DA, Victor CR: Urinary incontinence in the elderly at home, *Lancet* 2:1275-1277, 1981.
22. Hu TW: Cost effectiveness of training incontinent elderly in nursing homes: a randomized clinical trial, *Health Serv Res* 25:455-477, 1990.
23. Schnelle JF, Sowell VA, Hu TW, Traughber B: Reduction of urinary incontinence in nursing homes: does it reduce or increase costs? *J Am Geriatr Soc* 36:34-39, 1988.
24. Hu TW: The cost-effectiveness of disposable vs. reusable diapers: a controlled experiment in a nursing home, *J Gerontol Nurs* 16:19-24, 1990.
25. Wyman JF, et al: Psychosocial impact of urinary incontinence in the community-dwelling population, *J Am Geriatri Soc* 38:282-288, 1990.
26. Hunsakaar S, Vinsues A: The quality of life in women with urinary incontinence as measured by the sickness impact profile, *J Am Geriatr Soc* 39:378-382, 1991.
27. Mitteness LS: Knowledge and beliefs about urinary incontinence in adulthood and old age, *J Am Geriatr Soc* 38:374-378, 1990.
28. Rosenzweig BA, Hischke D, Thomas S, et al: Stress incontinence in women: psychological status before and after treatment, *J Reprod Med* 36:835-838, 1991.
29. Norton PA, MacDonald LD, Sedgewick PM, Stanton SL: Distress and delay associated with urinary incontinence, frequency, and urgency in women, *Br Med J* 297:1187-1189, 1988.

Chapter 3

Quality of Life for Those with Urinary Incontinence

Katherine F. Jeter, Todd Wagner, Tamara G. Bavendam

The deleterious psychologic, social, and economic sequelae of urinary incontinence have been widely researched, conjectured, and frequently reported in recent years.[1-15] These patient issues are usually not considered in published articles regarding the treatment of urinary incontinence (UI). Reports of treatment outcome traditionally are concerned with success or failure, dry or wet, ignoring that UI is a condition that is particularly subject to individual interpretation. One person may not feel that resolution of stress urinary incontinence in exchange for frequency of urgency of urination is a positive outcome in his or her life, whereas another person may consider it a total success.

To provide better care for our patients with urinary incontinence, it is imperative that we gain an understanding of all the issues that are involved in the individual interpretation of quality of life, and adapt our way of thinking about treatment success or failure to what meets the patient needs.

Quality of life (QOL) refers to *individuals' perceptions* of *their* position in life in the context of the culture and value systems in which *they live* in relation to *their* goals, expectations, standards, and concerns.[16] Over the past 20 years, the concept of QOL and the importance of its measurement have gained support among clinicians. This increasing interest in QOL measurement is in part based on the realization that therapeutic success is determined by more than objective measures. For example, is a blood pressure of 120/85 a desirable outcome if the patient cannot drive a car or feel comfortable leaving home because of the dizziness resulting from an antihypertensive medication?

Unlike many medical markers of health and well-being, quality of life can be interpreted by both clinicians and patients; however, interpretations of the same objective "data" may be vastly different. Ultimately, having a method to give credence to the patient's interpretation and following the patient's assessment of QOL over time may be a very important determination in outcome studies and cost-effective treatment.

The "Achilles tendon" of QOL research is that sample-based norms are often established to make comparisons between people, even though quality of life is inherently individualistic. This is particularly true when we relate quality of life in persons with urinary incontinence. Further complexities arise because there is no uniform definition of what UI is or agreement on how to quantify UI. The many causative and contributing factors make comparisons between groups difficult. The misconceptions and cultural taboos surrounding issues of bladder control make it difficult for persons to talk openly about this condition. We are therefore hampered in our ability to gather the data necessary to establish baselines for comparison.

In this chapter, we explore the complex issues surrounding UI that limit our ability to define QOL. We discuss work that has been done to quantify QOL and provide some suggestions for practitioners who truly want to be effective in identifying UI in patients and to understand the great effect of incontinence on each person as an individual. The majority of people affected by incontinence are women, and much of what we know is about women; this chapter will therefore be biased toward the experience of women. We will discuss the implications for future research and suggestions to improve current clinical practices in the management of incontinent females.

The Problem of Defining Incontinence

The first limitation in defining QOL in persons with UI is that urinary incontinence still eludes definition. Currently there are three commonly used definitions and numerous others that are used occasionally. The International Continence Society (ICS) defines incontinence as "involuntary loss of urine which is a social or hygienic problem and which is objectively demonstrable."[17] The Clinical Practice Guideline on Urinary Incontinence in Adults chose instead "the involuntary loss of urine which is sufficient to be a problem."[15] They eliminated the need to be objectively demonstrated as a part of the definition but left a value judgment as part of the definition—"sufficient to be a problem." In lay publications a common explanation of incontinence is "the unexpected loss of urine in any amount, on a regular basis, in an inconvenient place...."[1,18] This definition would indicate that if the involuntary loss of urine happened only once or twice and in the confines of your own bathroom where the "damage" was slight, you should not consider yourself incontinent and thus not seek treatment.

Since previous studies have not shown an association between the amount or frequency of urine loss and the degree of emotional distress associated with any particular episode, still other definitions must be considered: "Incontinence is the inability to choose when and where you will empty your bladder." A person with dementia may not have emotional distress over episodes of incontinence, yet family members and caretakers will likely feel the distress for themselves and for their loved one. Urinary incontinence is a leading cause of admission to nursing homes when families find it too taxing to care for an incontinent relative. Therefore the simplest and most accurate definition of UI may be "the uncontrolled passage of urine," which requires no objective observation, or threshold of frequency or distress.

Social Influences Across the Life Span

Evaluating the social effect of incontinence requires scrutiny of the social milieu as well as the cultural and historical attitudes of patients and health providers. Early definitions of the term "incontinence" refer to it as the inability to suppress sexual appetite.[5] By 1976, English dictionaries added urine and fecal loss to the earlier definition, but incontinence was still defined primarily in terms of sexual promiscuity and bad temper. Thus, from the beginning, incontinence was defined with value-laden terms—lack of restraint and control.

Furthermore, time, place, and method of urination are culturally proscribed. The age of expected continence (toilet training) and the point at which incontinence is no longer tolerated varies between cultures, within cultures, and between generations. In the 1950s and 1960s in the United States, early toilet training was the mode. Children in most states, even as late as the 1970s, were not allowed to attend public schools until they had achieved continence. Social attitudes and laws have changed remarkably in the past three to four decades. In the 1990s, young parents are less likely to attempt toilet training as early as their parents did and are less likely to be punitive toward preschoolers who have not achieved bladder control. Incontinent children, by virtue of legislation ensuring that all children have equal access to education in the least restrictive environment, now are assured entry into public schools. The popular press, however, continues to refer to the subject of incontinence as a "closet issue" and the "last taboo," reinforcing the social stigma that continues to be associated with lack of bladder control.

In the past, efforts have been made to discover a psychogenic component.[2,4,19,20] Although several studies have shown that neuroticism and psychologic factors may coexist with incontinence, there probably is not a cause-and-effect relationship.[2,4,19-26] Even though there is no cause-and-effect relationship, it is understandable that a reduction of sensory urgency and urine leakage have been shown to reduce psychologic symptoms and improve quality of life.[2,27-28] Practically speaking, elimination of the "fear of accidents," while one regains the comfort and confidence of being able to toilet predictably every 2 to 3 hours rather than unpredictably every 30 to 90 minutes, would certainly seem to enhance psychologic well-being and facilitate the opportunity to participate in social activities.

Psychologic and social influences have a powerful influence on attitudes toward toileting and loss of bladder control, and these influences are different at different stages of life. Bowel and bladder control are highly prized beginning in early childhood because they connote maturity, intelligence, and discipline. Lack of total bladder control can of course mean only immaturity, with a lack of intelligence and discipline.

Childhood and Adolescence

Children with nocturnal enuresis usually will not sleep at friends' homes or go away to camp because of fear of ostracism or taunting. During adolescence, girls report unwillingness to use toilets at school because there are no doors on the stalls to give them privacy during urination. Schools explain that there are no such doors because they must be able to maintain surveillance for drug use and cigarette smoking in the bathrooms. There is often inadequate time for girls to use the toilet between classes. Students report being censured when their use of the bathroom between classes causes them to be late for the next class. School officials say they cannot allow pupils unrestricted access to bathrooms between and during classes because this would be disruptive and most students would abuse the privilege. It is not uncommon for female middle school and high school students to void only before and after school. Such common practices do not engender healthy attitudes toward appropriate timely elimination or reasonable bladder habits in adulthood. This can certainly be a contributing factor to incontinence and urinary tract infections. Careful questioning regarding what each patient considers "normal" habits is very important.

Adulthood

In adult females there are more environmental and occupational impediments to good bladder habits. Although several states have introduced "potty parity" laws to increase the number of female toilets in public places, it is not unusual to see long lines in and from ladies' restrooms at cultural and sporting events, airports, and meeting sites where predominantly female audiences are gathered. Some women report restricting the amount and types of fluids they consume in anticipation of particular activities. If they have a problem with UI, they may have no choice but to eliminate all activities that might put them at risk for "being too far" from the bathroom or facing a long line.

Some employers restrict access to toilets. Assembly line workers, stenographers, and teachers may be required to urinate by the job's schedule rather than their bladder capacity. Even without published policy and procedure governing toilet use, nurses, waitresses, and secretaries may find it difficult to urinate at reasonable intervals. Symptoms of sensory urgency, frequency, and incontinence may preclude a female from taking or keeping certain jobs. A recent tongue-in-cheek article in a popular women's magazine describes the inadequacy of female restrooms in office and government buildings and asserts that "the American economy is not going to appreciate the importance of a decent restroom to the average female worker until the American economy is run by women."[29]

Later Life

Among the ever-increasing elderly population there are myriad social influences on bladder habits and serious repercussions for women who become incontinent or whose continence is marginal. Many public facilities and churches do not have accessible bathrooms. A female with precarious bladder control or irritable voiding symptoms will soon determine "safe environments" in which she can get to the bathroom. Consciously or subconsciously she will eliminate places and programs where toileting would be difficult. Buses and vans that transport senior citizens to social functions and medical appointments usually do not have toilets. Older women report being unable to take advantage of lower-cost transportation services because of this lack of toilets.

Incontinence should be taken seriously not only because it is a leading cause of admission to nursing homes, but also because it may affect the living arrangements of tens of thousands of other older women. In the burgeoning retirement community industry, in which there are usually three levels of care—independent living, personal care, and skilled care—loss of bladder or bowel control usually results in a resident being moved from an independent living arrangement to a unit that provides more personal services. This loss of independence with enforced and increased professional assistance is an expensive and demeaning consequence of urinary incontinence. This is especially troublesome when urinary incontinence can often be treated and improved with simple interventions, thus preventing the need for the move to a personal care environment with the loss of personal freedoms. Early identification demands that practitioners ask each and every patient about his or her bladder control in the same manner that each is asked about chest pain and shortness of breath.

RESEARCH

Descriptive Reports: Identifying the Issues and Feelings

In 1983, a year after Help for Incontinent People (HIP),* a national nonprofit advocacy organization, was founded, the popular advice columnist for "Dear Abby" discussed incontinence and advised her readers to write HIP for more information. Nearly 50,000 people wrote for help. They complained of embarrassment, loneliness, isolation, and frustration with the medical profession. In 1986 HIP developed a six-page 34-item questionnaire, which was mailed to 33,500 people. Completed surveys were returned by 10,427 individuals.[10] The majority were reasonably healthy females, 60 years of age or older, living at home. The average length of time they had been incontinent was 9 years. Many of their management or coping strategies were self-devised. Modifying drinking habits and toileting practices were the two methods most commonly used to control urine loss. Feminine hygiene products and paper towels were the products most often used.

Incontinence was described as a major problem with important social implications by 17.3%. This is consistent with the findings of Bayliss, Wyman, and others.[28,30,31] However, the fact that most women say that they are not severely burdened by incontinence does not mean that all patients should not be carefully assessed to determine the great effect incontinence is having on their health and their quality of life.[32-35] There were several worrisome findings in the 1986 HIP survey. Nearly 40% of the respondents believed that they were incontinent because they were old; another 20% said they did not know why they were incontinent, and only 25% to 50% of the women had consulted a physician. The misconceptions that UI is a natural consequence of getting old or being a woman or having borne children may account for some women's failure to report their incontinence to a physician or to articulate their symptoms during an office visit.

The medical profession received poor marks from this sample population. Half of the respondents described doctors or nurses as not helpful or too busy; 37.5% did not believe that the health provider was informative or knowledgeable. Nearly one fourth (24.4%) believed that doctors were embarrassed or unsympathetic. Only 9.7% said they were helped very much by their doctor, and 56.5% reported that their treatment was "no help at all." Findings from this survey cannot be generalized because the population represented a unique group. The majority of those surveyed were readers of an advice column and recipients of a quarterly newsletter about incontinence. However, it gave valuable insight into the lived experience of women with incontinence.

In 1992 a similar survey was sent to 115,000 people.[36] Half of them were members of Help for Incontinent People, and half had made one request for information from the organization but had not sustained contact with the organization. Analyses of 3986 (4%) completed surveys were tabulated. The survey population was again predominantly healthy older women living in the community. Some attitudes and behaviors had changed noticeably since the 1986 survey. More than 86% of the women had seen a physician about their incontinence, a number that is a sharp increase from previous studies, which reported only 25% to 50% of women had consulted a physician.[11,14,37,38] As in the earlier HIP survey, incontinence was perceived quite differently within the group. Women whose incontinence was characterized by urgency and frequency were most likely to consider it a major problem.

Dissatisfaction with the medical profession was high but not so high as in the earlier survey. More people who sought treatment got worse (6%) than were improved (3.2%) by it. Women who elected to have surgery had both the highest levels of success and the highest levels of treatment failure. This is consistent with Diokno's study of 51 women in which it was reported that only 39% of those who had surgery to correct urine loss had achieved absolute continence for a median follow-up exam of 12 years. Diokno and his colleagues also found that urologic symptoms were reported more frequently by respondents who had had surgery than by nonoperated respondents, suggesting that symptoms may have been induced by the operation. HIP's 1992 survey supported this finding, though it was impossible to determine whether the bothersome symptoms of frequency and urgency were caused by the operation or simply became more noticeable once symptoms of stress incontinence were alleviated.

Respondents to HIP's 1992 survey were asked to rate their bladder control problems on a scale of 1 to 5, with 5 being the greatest and 1 being the least of their concerns. Embarrassment was ranked highest, and odor ranked second. Isolation from friends and family was the *least* worrisome to the respondents. These data refute earlier reports that isolation from friends and family is common among incontinent people, and it may reflect an attitudinal change resulting from a decade of public education and, perhaps, improved management options.[11,15] In their daily lives, 55% of the respondents termed their loss of bladder control as "always bothersome but manageable." Only 13.5% described it as a major problem, and 26% described it as an occasional nuisance. More than twice as many respondents in 1992 had been taught to do Kegel exercises than had been taught in the earlier questionnaire, an indication of a probable shift toward behavioral interventions.

A New Tool

As indicated earlier, one weakness of QOL research is that norms are often established to compare people. In other words, based on responses to a standardized questionnaire, a person may be

*In 1996 HIP became the National Association for Incontinence (NAFC).

judged as having poor quality of life as compared to others, and this judgment may not always be fair. One may address this measurement issue by making comparisons within the same patients over time; however, QOL measures can be sensitive to exogenous factors and placebo effects.[39,40] This should not be seen as a fault of QOL but rather a testament to the enigmatic nature of humans—a person's quality of life can be influenced by a wide array of factors, many of which cannot be controlled for during measurement. As a result, interpreting QOL scores in the same individual over time can be difficult because the changes may be attributable to influences unrelated to the treatment.

Recently the number of "disease-specific" QOL questionnaires has substantially grown. Disease-specific, as it implies, refers to asking questions with respect to how a single disease or condition influences one's feelings about himself or herself. In part, this boom has been fueled by the desire to assess meaningful changes that are not captured by more traditional outcome measures, such as morbidity and mortality, or by general QOL questionnaires. One of the benefits from using disease-specific QOL measures is that they are more likely to detect minimally significant changes.[41,42]

In many clinical specialties, researchers have raced to develop the first disease-specific QOL measure. As a result there are numerous medical conditions, including urinary incontinence, for which more than one measure exists. Whether the tools are equal in their ability to reflect QOL is not clear. The reported quality of life effects of urinary incontinence are problems with social, domestic, physical, occupational, and leisure activities.[43-47] Many people report giving up or restricting household chores, church attendance, shopping, traveling, vacations, physical recreation, and hobbies. Along with these restrictions, many people worry about being embarrassed,[31] and some individuals cope with embarrassment by decreasing their social contacts.[34] In addition, relationships with spouses, other family members, and close friends may be affected, making the person feel alone.[31,43,48]

Given the limitations of measuring quality of life across populations, as discussed above, one should be careful when interpreting results. Nonetheless, research has shown that quality of life is related to type of incontinence and its severity. Hunskaar and Visnes,[49,50] Sandvik et al.,[51] and Grimby et al.[52] noted that urge symptoms were associated with a higher distress score than symptoms of stress incontinence. Similarly, Lagro-Janssen et al.[53] found that those with genuine stress incontinence reported the smallest effect on quality of life.

Previous studies have also investigated the relationship between the severity of incontinence and the resulting effect on quality of life. This relationship, however, is obscured by the difficulty in defining severity. Frequency and amount of urine leakage have both been used as proxies, and, in general, quality of life worsens as severity increases.[31,51,53]

There is little information comparing the QOL differences between men and women. Urinary incontinence occurs less frequently in men than in women and is generally assumed to be associated with an obstructing prostate gland, which can be surgically treated with resolution of the UI, or related to neurologic processes such as cerebrovascular accident and Parkinsonism. Men may be much less likely than women to report persistent incontinence after treatment, yet be more devastated by its consequences. This is particularly true in the men who have had radical prostatectomies for prostate cancer. UI is far more common than we have thought, and we as urologists are finally asking the questions in a way that allow men to express what the real incidence of UI is. Wearing pads or any sort of protection is totally foreign to men and may represent one reason why seemingly "minor" degrees of UI may cause more significant QOL changes. This perception is based on clinical experience, but with our increased awareness of the prevalence of postprostatectomy incontinence and the development of QOL assessment tools, we will have the ability to begin to answer some of these questions.

Hunskaar and Sandvik[54] interviewed 150 men and found that severity was negatively related with quality of life, and that younger men were more "handicapped" than older men. Most of the recent research for males has pertained to the treatment effects from prostate cancer.[55-59]

In the past decade, a handful of questionnaires have evolved to measure QOL for people with urinary incontinence.* As part of a study funded by Eli Lilly and Company, a review of urinary incontinence–specific quality of life questionnaires that were publicly available as of 1993 was conducted.

In the study, we interviewed 20 people to determine how urinary incontinence affects their QOL. The interviews were also used to determine if the existing QOL questionnaires were complete in covering all the pertinent issues. After learning that the study participants, especially the men, believed that none of the existing questionnaires adequately covered their areas of most frequent concern, we decided to develop our own urinary incontinence QOL measure based on the interviews.

Following standardized methods developed by Hunt and McKenna,[62] we created a 22-item urinary incontinence quality of life questionnaire (I-QOL) (Appendix 3-A). We then tested the I-QOL's statistical properties on a group of incontinent individuals from the University of Washington Department of Urology and the general population. Like physiologic measures, desired characteristics are validity (that is, accuracy) and reliability. Our results indicated that the I-QOL had a high test-retest reliability ($r2=.93$) and that it was accurate in discriminating between people of different severity. An article describing our findings was published in the December 1995 issue of *Urology.*

During the course of our study, we learned a significant amount about how urinary incontinence affects people. We interviewed both young and old, as well as women and men. In the 20 interviews, when asked about how their incontinence makes them feel, all 20 said they feel embarrassed, 16 (80%) said it is important to know where a bathroom is, 14 (70%) said they avoid going places, worry about leaking, and worry about having sex, 10 (50%) said they plan everything in advance, and 9 (45%) expressed feeling depressed. For example, one man said, "I have to plan everything well in advance. This doesn't mean that I don't do things spontaneously, but I think about where a bathroom might be." When asked about how it affects his social life, he said, "I would see only a woman with the same

*References 31,34,43,47,53,60,61.

condition. I would be too embarrassed otherwise. I think of myself as socially unacceptable."

In a small focus group with three women, one expressed, "I don't have a social life—I'm too embarrassed." Another woman responded shortly thereafter to a discussion of depression, "I don't get depressed, but I'm very fearful of the future. You sort of feel like your body is failing."

When asked about their experiences seeking medical care for their incontinence, a frequent response was that they had difficulty because of the embarrassment, which is consistent with past findings.[63,64] Moreover, most participants thought that the information they received from health professionals was lacking and perceived that this was something they would have to learn to live with. For example, one woman said, "Doctors never really tell you anything; they don't know what causes it. It seems like this is something a lot of people have and there's not much information on it."

We also interviewed one woman who had found an effective medical therapy. It was clear that the medicine improved her quality of life, even though she was taking less than the prescribed amount. About the medication, she said, "My prescription says to take one pill three times daily, and I take one [pill a day]. It works just beautifully. I can go any place now." Clearly, some people have found an effective treatment, but based on our interviews the pervasive feeling is that this condition is something that most people feel they will have to hide for the rest of their lives.

How can it be that a condition that is so common and so clearly affects the quality of life in profound ways is so poorly cared for by the medical profession? One of the reasons is the lack of importance assigned by health professionals, both primary and as specialists in this debilitating medical condition. There are many reasons UI is given far less attention than it warrants. The first is lack of professional education during medical school, residency, and postresidency educational programs. This lack of education makes it likely that the problem will be discounted or ignored when the problem is brought up by patients because we all tend to ignore or minimize what is outside of our "comfort zone of knowledge." It would be highly unlikely that health professionals would actively seek to identify a problem that they were not comfortable evaluating and treating. Another reason is the lack of understanding by health professionals that "fact of UI" is much different from "lived experience of UI." Wearing a pad to play a round a golf may not seem like it should be such a big deal until you begin to understand that the pad is just the tip of the iceberg. Not only is there the pad to contend with, there is controlling the amount and type of fluid ingested before playing golf, being hesitant to play on new courses because of lack of knowledge about toilet facilities, concern that the pad may not contain the urine loss if you swing one time just a little bit "too hard," and how to carry discreetly an extra pad on the course. Most people do not take their golf bags into the bathroom with them. Managing the details of UI can become a fulltime job when you desire to stay active—which is the reason many individuals ultimately become physical and social recluses. Finally, specialists charged with caring for urinary incontinence have a tendency to keep the useful information "shrouded in jargon" and secrecy, increasing the likelihood that primary care physicians will not feel comfortable with the evaluation and treatment and subsequently need to refer the patients to the specialists.

Relating Social Implications of Urinary Incontinence to Clinical Practice

As previously indicated, to interpret the social implications of UI and apply them to current clinical practices to improve care for persons with this pervasive condition, the lived experience of urine leakage must be separated from the fact of urine loss. This is especially true for women, who suffer from this condition more often than men. The fact and the lived experience may be quite dissimilar within groups, and it certainly varies between age groups.[37,65] Urine leakage during intercourse in a 25-year-old, newly married woman cannot be equated with urine leakage in a 19-year-old paraplegic in her work setting; an 84-year-old woman who wants to travel with a church group; and a severely cognitively impaired 78-year-old nursing home resident. However, despite individual differences, varying urinary symptoms, and changing social norms, incontinent women currently share several unique burdens:

1. They do not report the onset of incontinence promptly and may "put up with it" for 6 to 9 years before seeking medical treatment for this condition.[7,10,37,28,34]
2. Women are accustomed to using feminine hygiene products and choose them in many instances instead of products specifically designed for urine absorption.[10,37]
3. Women are likely to have their incontinence symptoms dismissed and to be dissatisfied with the results of their treatment. When their symptoms cannot be verified objectively by pad tests or urodynamically, they may be referred for psychologic counseling or labeled as neurotic.[20]
4. Despite mounting evidence that behavioral intervention promises improvement and even cure in many women with voiding dysfunction and urinary incontinence, American females are rarely offered this therapy.[36,33,28,66-68]

The reason or reasons that women tolerate incontinence for many years before seeking medical care remain unclear. Norton and Bayliss found embarrassment as a major factor for the delay.[28,34] Both of these study populations were British, and the majority (79%) of general practitioners in England are male. Since embarrassment is acutely felt among incontinent American women and 81.9% of physicians in the United States are male, this may explain the similar delay in seeking treatment among American women. Norton found that elderly women waited twice as long to get treatment as younger women do because they feared that surgery would be required and they were too old to have surgery. Other studies indicate that many women believe that their urine leakage is nominal and not a condition that warrants medical treatment.[28] Others believe it to be or are told that it is an expected part of getting old. It is possible that some do not deem their incontinence troublesome enough to spend money or time for medical care. This latter attitude merits future research. These various attitudes have important implications for health providers.

Clinical Implications for Health Care Providers

Evaluation

A sensitive approach to the subject of urine leakage is required from the very beginning—by seeking to identify the problem, taking the history and physical exam, and gaining an understanding of the effect on this particular patient before one makes treatment decisions. It is helpful to send history forms and voiding diaries before the initial office visit. This will imply that incontinence is common and may put patients at ease with the subject. It may also help them distill their own urinary history better when they are given adequate time to think about it and be spared the embarrassment of having to describe it in a face-to-face encounter with a health professional of the opposite sex. A prescreening intake or incontinence history might best be taken by another woman. Patients may be more comfortable with an office or clinic nurse, a physical therapist, or even a medical social worker whom they may perceive as an ally.

Continuing public information and patient education is essential to empower women to recognize incontinence as a treatable symptom and to aggressively seek solutions for it. Consumers need to be taught how to access a health provider with special interest in the diagnosis and treatment of incontinence and to request a second opinion when their primary physician does not take the complaint seriously or dismisses it as part of being female or as an expected complaint of aging.

Treatment

Once urinary incontinence has been identified after a patient's history and physical examination, the cause and the effect on quality of life merit equal attention. Symptoms that are not secondary to anatomic displacement, concomitant medical conditions, or pharmacologic therapy required by another illness may be minimized or eliminated completely by modification of toileting behavior, daily activities, diet, and lifestyle.[68] The patient's active participation in the treatment plan is required. Women are most likely to become involved, to be compliant, and to be successful in treatment if their bladder symptoms interfere with social, intimate, or occupational activities and when a therapeutic relationship is developed between caregiver and patient.[27,31,45] Psychotherapy has been shown to improve bladder symptoms even in the absence of cystometric changes. Might the sympathetic and proactive attitude of a physician or nurse be equally therapeutic? Various types of behavioral interventions have been shown to be effective in reducing incontinence in women.[28,33,36,66,69] Although cost-comparison data are not yet available, it seems obvious that two to six sessions with a patient conducted by a nurse or licensed allied health professional to teach toileting procedures, describe dietary influences on bladder habits, teach pelvic muscle exercises, monitor progress, and reinforce desired outcomes would be less expensive than medication for a lifetime or surgery, especially given the potential adverse effects.[26,68-70] Other obvious advantages are that many of these interventions might have an additive effect with pharmacologic therapy or surgery.

Rosenzweig and colleagues attempted to evaluate psychologic status before and after surgery for stress incontinence.[36] They concluded that women who continued to experience urinary symptoms and psychologic distress after surgery that was deemed curative by urodynamic measures should be considered for psychologic evaluation. Perhaps those women would have benefited by a therapeutic relationship with a health provider who could help them improve their bladder habits with behavioral therapy before surgery was undertaken. Experiences in programs that offer *only* behavioral therapy suggest that patients are not so frustrated when behavioral therapy yields only partial success as they are when expensive medications or surgical procedures do not result in complete resolution of symptoms.[27,28,69]

A caveat to primary care providers and specialty providers (urologists and gynecologists) is that they must be enthusiastic proponents of behavioral interventions as first-line therapy. This will reassure their patients that initiating behavioral treatment is the best initial treatment for them, rather than drugs or surgery, and does not imply that their symptoms are unimportant or "not bad enough for medicine or surgery."

Because symptoms of frequency and urgency have been shown to be so troubling to patients, bladder training to increase intervals between toileting coupled with dietary modification to minimize irritative voiding symptoms should improve a patient's psychologic well-being.[26,27,33,36,68] Several factors have been identified as impediments to successful outcome of behavioral interventions: duration of incontinence, poor compliance, and obesity.[2,33] Addressing each of these issues with patients and assisting them with printed materials and record-keeping forms, having office personnel to monitor progress and reward success, and encouraging a weight-control program may improve treatment outcome. Reaching women who are just beginning to have problems with incontinence, in health clubs, beauty salons, and health education forums, may be the key to improving success of behavioral therapies. Bavendam, in a study of women who used the weighted vaginal cones, found that those who self-referred for cone use had the most successful outcome.[71] In a recent survey of women who completed a 4-hour educational program about the course, treatments, and management alternatives of urinary incontinence, 24 of 40 women who completed the course were interviewed. One participant (5.8%) was cured, 47% rated their improvement between 20% and 90%, two (11.6%) elected to have surgery, and one patient (5.8%) rated her incontinence as worse after the class. Five women (29%) had no change in their symptoms but also admitted they had made none of the recommended changes in their daily activities or bladder habits.[69] All women expressed satisfaction with the program and said they would recommend it to a friend. The cost to the hospital to conduct the classes, including simple refreshments, was $34.00 per person. Such classes warrant investigation, refinement, and pilot programs to investigate efficacy.

Preparing Health Professionals for This Challenge

Primary care providers should be encouraged to include a sensitive and thorough evaluation of bladder symptoms in their routine patient assessment.[8,32,35] Nurse practitioners, nurse specialists, and some physical therapists are in clinical settings where a detailed and thorough incontinence evaluation could be performed once the problem is identified. With some advanced training, these health professionals should be able to evaluate patients' bladder control problems and recognize those for whom behavioral intervention would be appropriate and those for whom referral to a specialist would be essential. Women who are admitted to the hospital for other conditions should be screened for UI and have a thorough continence evaluation as soon as it is appropriate.

Discussing healthy bladder habits should be a part of maintenance health visits particularly in young girls who are prone to urinary tract infections as they enter middle school or junior high school. Fluid restriction and infrequent voiding are unhealthy habits. When we are young, we can often push our bodies to tremendous limits and get by with it. At some point, we can't get by anymore. This may happen in the twenties after the first child, in the thirties after three children and a hysterectomy, in the forties associated with perimenopause, in the fifties associated with early prostatic enlargement or after prostate surgery, in the sixties after starting the "water pill" for high blood pressure, or in the seventies after arthritis starts to limit mobility and thereby increases the time it takes to get to the bathroom. With each decade, the number of contributing factors to the potential loss of total bladder control increases; the later these multiple factors are recognized, the harder it may be to return things to a state where one can assume total bladder control under all circumstances.

How much of the depression, inadequate exercise, weight gain, constipation, or social isolation reported in any primary care practice may be, to some degree, related to loss of bladder control? How much bladder control loss could be prevented if all women were instructed in pelvic muscle exercises with their first pelvic exam, and would their ability to do these exercises to strengthen their muscles increase if they were checked with each yearly pelvic exam?

Questions about bladder habits and control need to be assimilated into every standard physical exam, with the patients being invited to talk about their concerns. Each provider should be comfortable helping each patient identify what the level of significance is to them and understand the great influence their problem may be having on their quality of life and other health concerns. A strategy for evaluation should be immediately presented. All primary providers should be able to assess for infection, atrophic changes, significant anatomic prolapse in women, lax anal tone suggestive of neuropathy, and appropriate referral whenever their comfort level with the evaluation and treatment of UI is exceeded. Primary care providers do not all have to be experts in treating UI, but they must be experts in identifying the problem, understanding its significance to the patient, and making sure that the problem is evaluated and treated as aggressively as the patient desires. They should be responsible for knowing whether the experts they commonly refer to treat UI as a serious problem and work with the patients to work out the treatment strategy that will work best for them. In a condition that has multiple etiologic factors, it make sense that treatment strategies may require behavioral, pharmacologic, and rehabilitative therapies as well as potential surgery. If specialists only present two options—pill or surgery—they are neglecting many other feasible options, and patients should seek other specialists.

It is also important that the primary physician understand that QOL can be improved significantly without "cure" of incontinence, and for many people such improvement may be enough. Everyone's tolerance of episodes of UI is different. Assuming everyone must be continent under all circumstances or the treatment has been a failure is just as inappropriate as assuming all incontinence is secondary to growing old and "nothing can be done." The desire for "cure" that we have all been trained to strive for as the only appropriate successful outcome will cause us all to underestimate the importance and good influence of simple instructions about behavioral changes to patients. It is quite possible that a primary care physician recommending the simple noninvasive behavioral treatment regimen (appropriate fluid intake, timed voiding, and bladder training with pelvic muscle exercises) would have patients that were equally if not more satisfied with treatment outcome and improved quality of life than patients going to a specialist who only does medication or surgery.

Implications for Future Research

Regardless of the difficulties inherent in defining the social effect of urinary incontinence on the lives of incontinence sufferers of all ages, it is obvious that loss of bladder control results in restricted activities and other physical and social limitations. However, fewer than 20% of women describe incontinence as a major problem. There is no explanation for why women tolerate incontinence for an average of 7 to 9 years before seeking treatment. Are they resigned to their "female lot"?[72] Have they felt rebuffed by health professionals? Are they unaware that treatments may improve or cure their symptoms? Do they fear that the cure would be worse than the disease? Why are tens of thousands of women responding to nonprofit advocacy organizations and government agency numbers for help? Why are so many women dissatisfied with their treatment outcome and the care that they receive? What accounts for the difference between a study conducted by medical researchers, which showed that consumers believed that physicians could help them with their incontinence even after failed surgery, and studies conducted by nonmedical groups in which women perceived physicians as "not helpful"?[10,36,72,73]

Prospective studies to identify strategies to maintain continence and prevent incontinence are urgently needed. Efforts must be sustained to destigmatize incontinence and to develop more reasonable attitudes toward healthy bladder function and understand the dysfunctions across the life span. Now that behavioral interventions have proved effective, future research should be directed toward comparing the relative effects of different treatments and toward identifying factors associated with treatment failure.[5] It is time to change the focus from research studies that select subjects by age or symptoms to research that addresses how the experience of urinary incontinence varies across the life span and how treatment choices—surgical, pharmacologic, and behavioral—influence the quality of life.

References

1. Gartley CB: *Managing incontinence,* Ottawa, Ill., 1985, Jameson Books, p. 11.
2. Oldenburg B, Millard RJ: Predictors of longterm outcome following a bladder retraining program, *J Psychosom Res* 30(6):691-698, 1986.
3. Mohide EA: The prevalence and scope of urinary incontinence, *Clin Geriatr Med* 2(4):639-654, 1986.
4. Morrison M, Morrison LM, McAlister A, Glen FS: Visual analog scores and urinary incontinence, *Br Med J* 295:854, 1987.
5. Smith PS, Smith U: *Continence and incontinence,* London, 1987, Croom Helm Ltd., p. 27.
6. Breakwell SL, Walker SN: Differences in physical health, social interaction, and personal adjustment between continent and incontinent homebound aged women, *J Comm Health Nurs* 5(l):19-31, 1988.
7. National Institutes of Health: Urinary Incontinence in Adults, Consensus Conference, *JAMA* 261:2685-2690, 1989.
8. Jolleys JV: Reported prevalence of urinary incontinence in a general practice, *Br Med J* 296:1300-1302, 1988.
9. Teasdale TA, Taffet GE, Luchi RJ, et al: Urinary incontinence in a community residing elderly population, *J Am Geriatr Soc* 36(7):600-606, 1988.
10. Jeter KF, Wagner DB: Incontinence in the American home a survey of 36,500 people, *J Am Geriatr Soc* 38(3):379-383, 1990.
11. Muteness LS: Knowledge and beliefs about urinary incontinence in adulthood and old age, *J Am Geriatr Soc* 38(3):374-378, 1990.
12. Wyman JF, Fantl JA: Bladder training in ambulatory care management of urinary incontinence, *Urolog Nurs* 11(3):11-17, 1991.
13. Sommer P, Bauer T, Nielsen KK, et al: Voiding patterns in prevalence of incontinence in women, *Br J Urol* 66:12-15, 1990.
14. Thiede HA: Prevalence of pelvic floor dysfunction in women. In *Conference on pelvic floor dysfunction: an initiative for curriculum enhancement in residency education,* Chicago, 1992, The American Board of Obstetrics and Gynecology.
15. Urinary Incontinence Guideline Panel: *Urinary incontinence in adults: clinical practice guideline,* AHCPR Publ. No. 92-0038, Rockville, Md., 1992, Agency for Health Care Policy and Research, Public Health Service, U.S. Department of Health and Human Services.
16. WHOQOL Group: Study protocol for the World Health Organization project to develop a quality of life instrument, *Qual Life Res* 2:153-159, 1993.
17. Abrams P, Blaivas JG, Stanton SL, Andersen JT: The standardization of terminology of lower urinary tract dysfunction, *Scand J Urol Nephrol* 114(suppl):5-19, 1988.
18. Chalker R, Whitmore KE: *Overcoming bladder disorders,* New York, 1990, Harper-Collins, p.62.
19. Norton KR, Bhat AV, Stanton SL: Psychiatric aspects of urinary incontinence in women attending an outpatient urodynamic clinic, *Br Med J* 301(6746):271-272, 1990.
20. Rosenzweig BA, Hirschke D, Thomas S, et al: Stress incontinence in women, psychological status before and after treatment, *J Reprod Med* 36(12):835-838, 1991.
21. Hafner RJ, Stanton SL, Guy J: A psychiatric study of women with urgency and urge incontinence, *Br J Urol* 49:211-214, 1977.
22. Frewen WK: An objective assessment of the unstable bladder of psychosomatic origin, *Br J Urol* 50:246-249, 1978.
23. Stone CB, Judd GE: Psychogenic aspects of urinary incontinence in women, *Clin Obstet Gynecol* 21(3):807-815, 1978.
24. Crisp A, Sutherst J: Psychological factors in women with urinary incontinence, *Proc International Continence Society and Urodynamic Soc* 1:174-176, 1983.
25. Morrison LM, Eadie AS, McAlister A, et al: Personality testing in 226 patients with urinary incontinence, *Br J Urol* 58:387-389, 1986.
26. Macaulay AJ, Stem RS, Holmes DM, Stanton SL: Micturition and the mind: psychological factors in the etiology and treatment of urinary symptoms in women, *Br Med J* 294:540-543, 1987.
27. Fantl JA, Wyman JF, McClish DK, et al: Efficacy of bladder training in older women with urinary incontinence, *JAMA* 265(5):609-613, 1991.
28. Bayliss V: Female incontinence: "the Basing stroke-project," *J R Soc Health* 6:207-208, 1988.
29. Collins G: Potty politics: the gender gap, Working Woman, p. 93, March 1993.
30. Lagro-Janssen ALM, Debruyne FMJ, Van Weel C: Psychologic aspects of female urinary incontinence in general practice, *Br J Urology* 70:499-502, 1992.
31. Wyman JF, Harkins SW, Choi SC, et al: Psycho-social impact of urinary incontinence in women, *Obstet Gynecol* 70(3):378-381, 1987.
32. Burgio KL, Matthews KA, Bernard TE: Prevalence, incidence and correlates of urinary incontinence in healthy middle-aged women, *J Urol* 146:1255-1259, 1991.
33. Woodruff J, Thomas S: Behavioral medicine and the treatment of urinary symptoms, *AUGS Q Rep* 11(l):1-5, 1993.
34. Norton PA, MacDonald LD, Sedgwick PM, Stanton SL: The stress and delay associated with urinary incontinence, frequency, and urgency in women, *Br Med J* 297:1187-1189, 1988.
35. Ouslander JG: Urinary incontinence: out of the closet, *JAMA* 261(18):2695-2696, 1989.
36. Jeter KF, Verdell LL: Consumer focus '93 a survey of community-dwelling incontinent people, Union, S.C., 1993, Help for Incontinent People.
37. Burgio KL, Matthews KA, Engel BT: Prevalence, incidence and correlates of urinary and primary care, *Med J Austr* 157:537-542, 1992.
38. Norton PA: Non-surgical management. In *Conference on pelvic floor dysfunction: an initiative for curriculum enhancement in residency education,* Chicago, 1992, The American Board of Obstetrics and Gynecology.
39. Norton P, Karram M, Wall LL, et al: Randomized double-blind trial of terodiline in the treatment of urge incontinence in women, *Obstet Gynecol* 84:386-391, 1994.
40. Amir M, Cristal N, Bar OD, Liodl A: Does the combination of the ACE inhibitor and calcium antagonist control hypertension and improve quality of life? The LOMIR-MCT-IL study experience, *Blood Press Suppl* 1:40-42, 1994.
41. Patrick DL, Erikson P: *Health status and health policy: allocating resources to health care,* New York, 1993, Oxford University Press.
42. Guyatt GH, Feeny DH, Patrick DL: Measuring health-related quality of life, *Ann Intern Med* 118:622-629, 1993.
43. Norton P: The effects of urinary incontinence in women, *Int Rehabil Med* 4:9-14, 1982.
44. Ouslander JG, Abelson S: Perceptions of urinary incontinence among elderly outpatients, *The Gerontologist* 30(3):369-372, 1990.
45. Wyman JF, Harkins SW, Fantl JA: Psychosocial impact of urinary incontinence in the community-dwelling population, *J Am Geriatr Soc* 38:282, 1990.
46. Gardner J, Fonda D: Urinary incontinence in the elderly, *Disabil Rehabil* 16(3):140-8, 1994.
47. Shumaker SA, Wyman JF, Uebersax JS, et al: Health-related quality of life measures for women with urinary incontinence: the Incontinence Impact Questionnaire and the Urogenital Distress Inventory, *Qual Life Res* 3(5):291-306, 1994.
48. Harris T: Aging in the eighties: prevalence and impact of urinary problems in individuals age 65 years and over (advance data no. 121), Washington, D.C., 1986, National Center for Health Statistics.
49. Hunskaar S, Visnes A: The quality of life in women with urinary incontinence as measured by the Sickness Impact Profile, *J Am Geriatr Soc* 39(4):378-382, 1991.
50. Hunskaar S, Visnes A: The quality of life in women with urinary incontinence as measured by the Sickness Impact Profile, Erratum, *J Am Geriatr Soc* 40(9):976-997, 1992.
51. Sandvik H, Kveine E, Hunskaar S: Female urinary incontinence—psychosocial impact, self care, and consultations, *Scand J Caring Sci* 7(1):53-56, 1993.

52. Grimby A, Milsom I, Molander U, et al: The influence of urinary incontinence on the quality of life of elderly women, *Age and Aging* 22(2):82-89, 1993.
53. Lagro-Janssen T, Smits A, Van Weel C: Urinary incontinence in women and the effects on their lives, *Scand J Prim Health Care* 10:211-216, 1992.
54. Hunskaar S, Sandvik H: One hundred and fifty men with urinary incontinence. III. Psychosocial consequences, *Scand J Prim Health Care* 11(3):193-196, 1993.
55. Leandri P, Rossignol G, Gautier JR, Ramon J: Radical retropubic prostatectomy: morbidity and quality of life; experience with 620 consecutive cases, *J Urol* 147(3 Pt 2):883-887, 1992.
56. Walsh PC, Fartin AW, Epstein JI: Cancer control and quality of life following anatomical radical retropubic prostatectomy: results at 10 years, *J Urol* 152(5 Pt 2):1831-1836, 1994.
57. Herr HW: Quality of life of incontinent men after radical prostatectomy, *J Urol* 151(3):652-654, 1994.
58. Jonler M, Ritter MA, Brinkmann R, et al: Sequelae of definitive radiation therapy for prostate cancer localized to the pelvis, *Urol* 44(6):876-882, 1994.
59. Braslis KG, Santa Cruz C, Brickman AL, Soloway MS: Quality of life 12 months after radical prostatectomy, *Br J Urol* 75(1):48-53, 1995.
60. Yu L: Incontinence stress index: measuring psychological impact, *J Gerontol Nurs* 13(7):18-25, 1984.
61. Reilly MC, Clark TT: Methodological issues in assessing quality of life in patients with urinary incontinence: a preliminary report, *J Res in Pharm Economics* 2(4):3-15, 1990.
62. Hunt S, McKenna SP: The QLDS: a scale for the measurement of quality of life in depression, *Health Policy* 22:307-319, 1992.
63. Cotton P: Physicians hear about incontinence, *JAMA* 264(18):2361-2362, 1990.
64. Ashworth PD, Hagan MT. The meaning of incontinence: a qualitative study of non-geriatric urinary incontinence sufferers, *J Adv Nurs* 18(9):1415-23, 1993.
65. Klemm LW, Creason NS: Self-care practices of women with urinary incontinence—a preliminary study, *Health Care for Women International* 12:199-209, 1991.
66. Jeter K: Pelvic muscle exercises with and without biofeedback for the treatment of urinary incontinence. In Leach GE, editor: *Problems in urology,* 5(l):72-83, Philadelphia, 1991, Lippincott.
67. Newman DK, Smith DA: Pelvic muscle re-education as a nursing treatment for incontinence, *Urol Nurs* 12(l):9-15, 1992.
68. Bavendam TG: Geriatric female incontinence. In Leach GE, editor: *Problems in urology,* Philadelphia, 1991, Lippincott, 1991, pp. 42-71.
69. Jeter KF, Tintle TE: *Behavioral therapy in a group setting to promote continence in women: a test of efficacy and economy,* research poster, American Urological Association Allied (Richmond, Va.) 25th annual meeting, San Antonio, Texas, May 16-20, 1993.
70. Forneret E, Leach GE: Cost-effective treatment of female stress urinary incontinence: modified Pereyra bladder neck suspension, *Urol* 25:365-367, 1985.
71. Bavendam TG, Kallhoff JM, Gibbs, CJ: *Femina vaginal cones for the treatment of stress urinary incontinence,* poster, AUGS 13th annual meeting, Boston, Mass., August 27-30, 1992.
72. Glew J: A woman's lot? *Nursing Times* pp. 69-71, April 9, 1986.
73. Diokno AC, Brown MB, Brock BM, et al: Prevalence and outcome of surgery for female incontinence, *Urol* 33(4):285-290, 1989.

Chapter 4

Anatomic Aspects of Urinary Incontinence

Jacek L. Mostwin, Arthur L. Burnett

Urinary incontinence, often thought of as a single entity, is but a single symptom of many different entities affecting the lower urinary tract or the nervous system. The two most common of these conditions, bladder dysfunction (or "neurogenic bladder") and genuine stress urinary incontinence, attributable either to lack of urethral support or intrinsic urethral dysfunction, are the ones that must be considered in any differential diagnosis of incontinence and the ones that are commonly discussed in most references. To introduce the other chapters that follow in this book, we have provided what we consider to be the most relevant anatomic features of these common conditions, in the following manner:

1. The neuroanatomic pathways and structure of the bladder; the effects of diseases and injuries at selected locations along these various pathways and ways in which they may affect urinary storage and emptying. These are the structures that most commonly affect conscious sensation of the stages of the bladder cycle, bladder stability, compliance, and sphincteric coordination. These are the ones most commonly altered in "neurogenic bladder" conditions. These subjects are usually treated in much greater depths in textbooks of neurourology,[1-4] on which much of the discussion here is based. If one is to approach incontinence in a complete and methodical way, there must be some understanding of these structures and pathways.
2. The anatomy of the urogenital diaphragm; the location, composition, innervation, and function of the urinary sphincters; the similarities and differences in men and women; the ways in which they are affected by age, by childbirth and menopause in women, and by pelvic surgery and prostatectomy in men.
3. The role of vaginal support in maintaining continence in women; why vaginal prolapse contributes to incontinence; and how our concepts of stress incontinence in women are changing.

The first of these areas requires familiarity with classic neuroanatomy and neurophysiology; the second two require familiarity with pelvic surgical anatomy. Taken together, they form a general anatomic framework for day-to-day work with incontinent patients.

NEUROANATOMIC PATHWAYS

Despite the long distance from bladder to cerebral cortex, the normal adult is aware of bladder filling and can willfully initiate or delay voiding until a convenient time and location to void are found. Involvement of any of the essential neuranatomic pathways by degenerative or traumatic diseases of the nervous system is the cause of much of the incontinence that is ascribed to "neurogenic bladder" and often confounds much of the discussion regarding evaluation and treatment of genuine stress incontinence.

The bladder is supplied by autonomic visceral afferent and efferent fibers arising from sacral segments 2, 3, and 4 of the spinal cord to form the pelvic nerve. The voluntary sphincter is supplied by somatic visceral afferent and efferent fibers arising from the same sacral segments but traveling in the pudendal nerve. Integration of these autonomic and somatic activities takes place at both spinal and brainstem level. The master control center, or "voiding center," is located in the pons of the brainstem.[5] A schema of these pathways is presented in Fig. 4-1.

There are two type of sensation under autonomic regulation. Normally, only proprioception giving rise to the sensation of bladder filling and fullness is experienced.[6] Proprioceptive signals are carried by long latency fibers traveling directly along dorsal column pathways to the brainstem. Nociceptors (pain, touch, and temperature) are also present in the bladder and may be activated in states such as cystitis and bladder stone, but they do not normally give rise to sensation from the lower urinary tract and do not normally influence the awareness of bladder filling. Chronic abnormalities in nociception can develop, but hypotheses are just beginning to emerge from research into sensory mechanisms. It has been suggested that nerve growth factor (NGF) released from injured bladder nerves or muscle cells may play a role.[7] Abnormal nociception can give rise to short latency

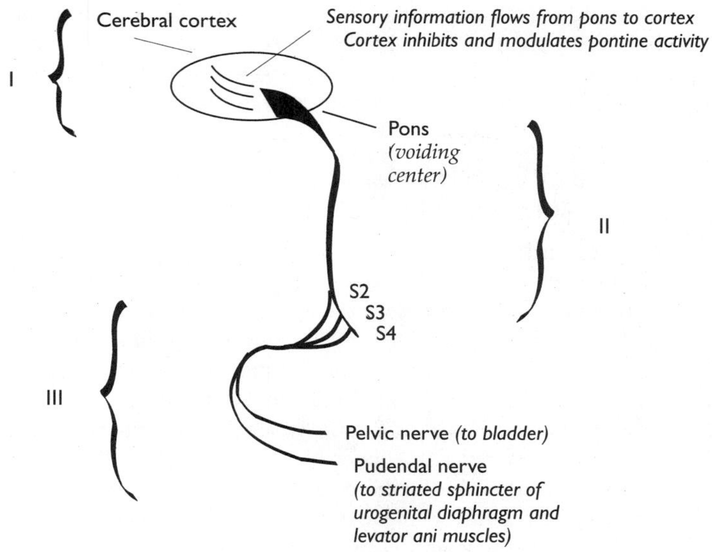

FIG. 4-1 *Neuroanatomic pathways. I, Corticopontine axis. The cerebral cortex receives sensory information from the pons and modulates and inhibits voiding by signaling the pons or initiating voluntary contraction of the striated sphincter. II, Corticospinal axis. Long-latency sensory information travels to the pons via dorsal columns. Cell bodies of autonomic and voluntary motor neurons arise within sacral segments S2, 3, and 4. Spinal interneurons provide coordination between voluntary sphincter innervation and autonomic bladder and urethral innervation. III, Peripheral axis. Sacral segments S2, 3, and 4 provide afferent and efferent innervation to two final peripheral nerves. The pelvic nerve travels in the plane between the rectum and the bladder in men and between the vagina and the bladder in women. It is vulnerable to surgical injury in these areas. The pudendal nerve enters the pelvis via Alcock's canal, traveling beneath the levator ani muscles, carrying sensory and motor supply for these muscles as well as the rhabdosphincter of the urethra. In women the pudendal nerve is vulnerable to injury from childbirth or repeat episodes of traction during prolapse.*

spinal reflexes as can be seen in experimental animal models of urethral obstruction,[8] or spinal cord transection,[9,10] which result in frequent voiding.

The voiding reflex is coordinated at the level of the pons, as are other autonomic visceral functions such as ventilation, blood pressure, and body temperature. Afferent and efferent pathways arise from this voiding center to supply conscious sensations associated with bladder activity to the cerebral cortex. In an experimental animal preparation, normal reflex voiding will take place as long as the nervous system is not injured below this critical level. This is analogous to the situation for humans with cortical degeneration such as Alzheimer's disease. If an injury occurs below this level, reflex voiding is disturbed. In addition to incontinence, more serious voiding disorders, such as detrusor-sphincter dyssynergia, may develop.

Some familiarity with neurologic pathways to and from the bladder permits generalization about how neurologic diseases and injuries affect bladder function.[11] Lesions above the pons leave the reflexes of the lower tract intact while dissociating the affected individual from any awareness of the events. This is a typical situation in Alzheimer's disease, in which a perfectly complacent individual is voiding physiologically whenever reflex voiding is initiated by bladder distension. Awareness of filling and desire and ability to control voiding are diminished or completely absent. Usually the family or the caregivers of such a person are the ones presenting with the complaint.

Diseases and injuries of the spinal cord from the level of the pons to sacral segments 2, 3, and 4, however, are associated with significant abnormalities in bladder storage, emptying, and sphincteric coordination, which then either cause or are associated with abnormalities of compliance (hypertonicity) and stability (hyperreflexia or instability). Multiple sclerosis and spinal cord transection resulting in paraplegia or quadriplegia are examples of these injuries.[12]

Selected motor injuries distal to the sacral cord (such as lower cord myelodysplasia or pelvic crush injuries) are associated with a loss of compliance (stiffness), loss of sensation, and a loss of sphincteric closure with overflow incontinence, which may occur whenever the intravesical pressure exceeds a critical level. This level, the leak point pressure, may be the result of progressive passive distention of the bladder by urine coming from the kidneys, or a transient increase in intra-abdominal pressure that may be transmitted to the bladder, or a combination of both.[13-14]

Selected sensory lesions such as tabes dorsalis, affecting the dorsal columns of the spinal cord, or diabetes mellitus, affecting the peripheral innervation of the bladder, may give rise to silent painless distention of the bladder with eventual retention or overflow incontinence depending on the strength of the sphincters.

Although there is a general relationship of neurologic disorders with certain neurourologic patterns, it is not precise enough to guide treatment for the individual. Urodynamic studies are usually required. Nevertheless, a general knowledge of the major pathways from the brain to the bladder does improve the understanding and classification of many voiding disorders associated with neurologic illness or injury.

THE BLADDER

The bladder is a hollow muscular viscus capable of storing urine for prolonged periods of time at continuously low pressure until evacuation can be conveniently initiated. The bladder is mostly composed of interdigitating fibers of smooth muscle.[16] In contrast to the gut, these smooth muscles are not organized as distinct inner longitudinal and outer circular layers except at the urethra. It helps to think of these interdigitating bundles of smooth muscle as interlacing slings of muscle originating near the urethra, traversing the spherical dimensions of the bladder, and then coursing back to the urethra. The narrow portion of the internal urethral meatus (the bladder neck) contributes to sphincteric closure of the urethra by its very muscular arrangement. At the proximal urethra, which is the region of highest intraluminal pressure and hence continence at rest, one finds an inner longitudinal arrangement of muscular fibers, representing direct continuation of these detrusor muscle bundles and a sleeve of outer circular muscle. In addition, there is a sleeve of circular striated muscle surrounding the urethra at this point, forming the external sphincter (or rhabdosphincter), which is discussed in the next section.

The arrangement of smooth muscles at the internal urethral meatus, or proximal urethra, favors tonic closure at rest.[16,17] Although it is known that a fall in urethral pressure and radiographic signs of opening of the proximal urethra are the earliest signs of the initiation of normal micturition,[2] there is no general agreement on whether this takes place because the urethra is "pulled open"—that is, the longitudinal fibers extending into the urethra from the bladder shorten, pulling apart the circular fibers while the sphincter relaxes— or whether the periurethral muscles themselves cease tonic activity, a hypothesis favored by evidence indicating that nitric oxide may play a role in urethral relaxation.[18]

Thickness and suppleness of myofibrils and interstitial connective tissue also affect compliance. Obstruction and neuropathic conditions such as myelodysplasia are associated with increased collagen deposition in the interstitium, most likely secreted by the smooth muscle cells themselves in response to injury or obstruction.[19,20] The increasing presence of collagen may affect the distensibility of the bladder at higher filling volumes and may account for a loss of compliance and higher intravesical pressures during end-filling states. This can threaten an already compromised sphincter (as in myelodysplasia), produce vesicoureteral reflux, lead to increased urgency, or trigger unstable contractions.

Muscle thickness increases in lower cord myelodysplasia and after infravesical obstruction. Thicker muscle bundles are less distensible and less compliant and may lead to the same difficulties as stiffness from collagen deposition.

Urgency remains a debilitating symptom in obstructive and neurogenic states. Two hypotheses have been proposed for its development. The earlier hypothesis is that urgency is the companion symptom of unstable contractions: as the pressure rises in the bladder, the patient experiences an impending need to void, sometimes with expulsion of urine, so-called urge incontinence. This hypothesis is based on earlier clinical observations associating prostatic obstruction with urgency and urodynamic evidence of bladder instability, which can resolve in up to 75% of affected patients after prostatectomy.[21] Additional evidence in support of this hypothesis has come from animal experiments in which partial urethral obstruction, mimicking the human condition of prostatic hyperplasia, has resulted in bladder muscle hypertrophy and unstable contractions found during in vivo cystometry.[22]

A more recent hypothesis to explain the development of urgency has come from evidence that obstruction in animal models produces new neurologic reflexes with increased frequency of voiding and evidence of unstable contractions on cystometry. In a rat model, partial obstruction increases the number of sensory nerve cell bodies in the dorsal ganglia with an increase in the neurologic events associated with reflex voiding.[8] In this model, nerve growth factor (NGF) secreted by the smooth muscle cells of the bladder may initiate the proliferation of sensory and sympathetic neurons and the development of the increased reflexes.[23] Whether the muscle cells release the NGF in response to injury, such as high pressure or ischemia, or this represents a maladaptation to increased growth requirements remains an important research question for the future.

THE UROGENITAL DIAPHRAGM AND THE STRIATED SPHINCTERS

Understanding the surgical anatomy of the urogenital diaphragm and the striated sphincters requires mastery of some of the most difficult three-dimensional anatomic concepts in urology or gynecology. The structures contained in this region are critical for the maintenance of continence in men and women. This area is directly affected by all forms of radical prostatectomy and is also involved in almost all surgical repairs of stress incontinence in women. An understanding of the true anatomy of the striated sphincters and their relationship to the smooth musculature of the lower urinary tract is therefore crucial for successful diagnosis and surgery in this area.

Two important aspects of the striated musculature of the lower tract sphincters are:

1. It is anatomically distinct from the smooth muscle of any sphincteric unit which is continuous with the intrinsic bladder musculature.
2. It is under voluntary control and is critical for many lower urinary tract activities because its contraction interrupts the stream and reflexly inhibits further bladder contraction. This is the basis for most biofeedback and behavioral modification exercises used to rehabilitate the lower tract.

Because they are anatomically and physiologically distinct, the bladder and the sphincter are often treated as two distinct units. This has given rise to an oversimplified anatomic description of the two structures over the years. Although this may be helpful in very simple descriptions of the neurologic function of the lower tract, it has held back our surgical understanding of the system with respect to both the repair of stress incontinence in women and progress in radical pelvic surgery in men.

In the anatomic position, the external sphincter in both men and women represents the most superior part of the urogenital diaphragm. Comparing the male and female urogenital diaphragms side by side and considering the different effects of male and female hormones on the common elements of the structure provide a unified view of the urogenital diaphragm within the human pelvis and offer a richer three-dimensional understanding of the structure for surgeons working in this area.

Consider first the female urogenital diaphragm. This is the unmodified result of human embryogenesis resulting from absence of intrauterine testosterone and the presence of Müllerian-inhibitory factor. The details of this structure in the adult were studied and drawn very carefully in 1912 by the anatomist and illustrator Max Brodel.[24] Brodel's drawings depict the urogenital diaphragm as a series of transversely oriented muscular slings lying across the urethra and surrounding it to varying degrees depending on the cross-sectional level of the urethra (Fig. 4-2). At the most superior point, near the proximal urethra, the muscles completely surround the urethra,

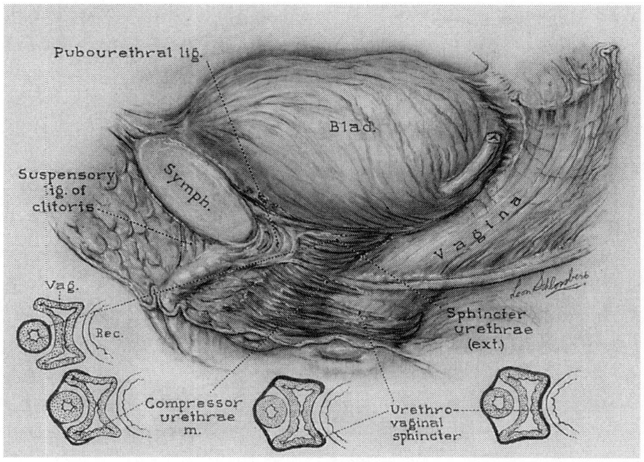

FIG. 4-2 *Relationship of the muscles of the urogenital diaphragm to the bladder and urethra (after Brodel). The muscles of the urogenital diaphragm ascend from the vaginal introitus to the proximal part of the urethra, encircling the urethra and vagina to varying degrees, depending on the level of transverse section. At the level of the proximal part of the urethra, they form a circumferential urethral sphincter. The subpubic fascial condensations of the endopelvic fascia cover the proximal urethra binding the anterior portions firmly to the pubis.*

providing a true rhabdosphincter around the proximal urethra. As the muscular sheet is followed inferiorly toward the lower portion of the vagina, the muscles inserts progressively farther and farther around the vagina until they encircle it completely near the vaginal introitus where they become confluent with the bulbospongiosus. The more modern work of Oelrich[25] and DeLancey[26] has confirmed these observations using both gross and histological techniques.

In the male, consider what would happen if there were an involution of the female structures in utero. The vagina would shrink to its analog structure in the male, the utricle. The circumferential muscles would fuse posteriorly as the vagina decreased in size, becoming confluent as one structure, the bulbospongiosus. The actual apex of the urogenital diaphragm would be in the same location and about the same relationship to the bladder neck and the proximal urethra in both the male and female (Fig. 4-3). Oelrich's descriptions support this view.[27]

Now consider the effect of hormonal stimulation on these structures in men at various stages of life. The periurethral glands in the female are the analog of the male prostate. As the normal prostate grows, it lengthens the prostatic urethra and displaces the periurethral sphincter around the proximal urethra distally and displaces the bladder neck into a more superior position. Under the further influence of hormonal changes in middle and later life giving rise to benign prostatic hyperplasia, this distance is further increased, so that the prostatic urethra becomes a definable structure in its own right, while the bladder and trigone are displaced farther superiorly. The proximal sphincteric urethra remains in the same position as it would in the female. Examination of Myers' descriptions of the variability of the prostatic apex and proximal urethra supports these descriptions.[28]

The location of the sphincteric urethra can be found by observing its relationship to the fascial coverings seen on the floor of the space of Retzius in either a cadaver dissection or a surgically exposed field such as that for Burch colposuspension or radical retropubic prostatectomy (Fig. 4-4). The pubourethral ligaments represent paired condensations of the endopelvic fascia, which cover the obturator internus muscle on either side of

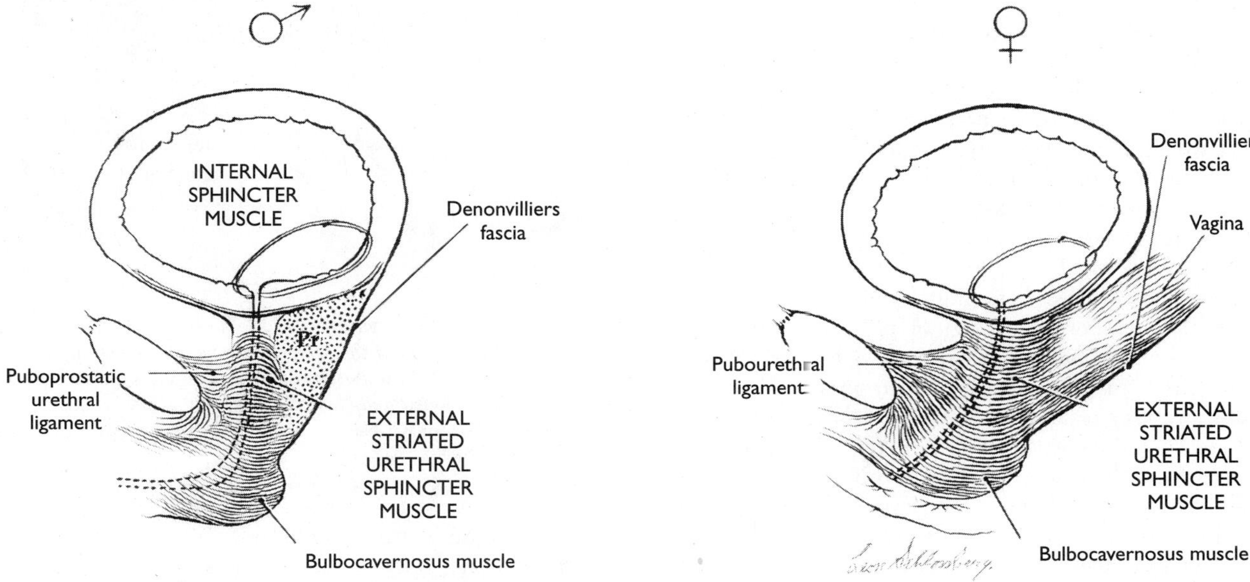

FIG. 4-3 *Comparison of the muscles of the urogenital diaphragm in a normal adult male (left) and female (right) illustrating common features. In men the sphincter is closed circumferentially as it progresses from the bladder to the bulbar urethra, flaring and merging with the bulbocavernosus muscle. In women, the muscle separates in the posterior midline to accommodate the vagina (compare transverse sections in Fig. 4-2).*

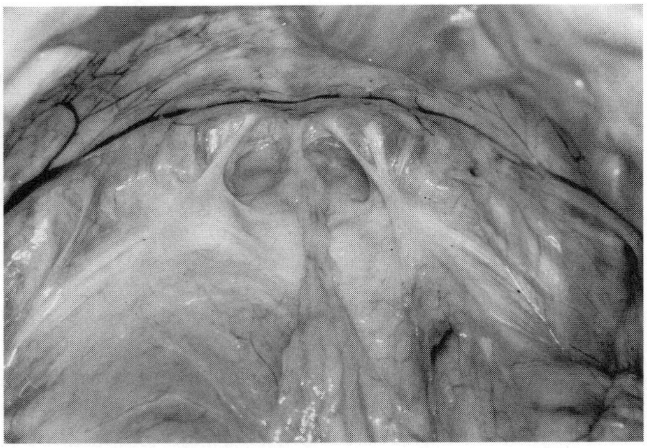

FIG. 4-4 *View of floor of space of Retzius in fresh elderly female cadaver specimen. This floor is also the roof of the urogenital diaphragm. Traction has been applied to the empty bladder to expose the symphysis pubis, seen at top center. The well-defined pubourethral ligaments can be seen as paired condensations of the endopelvic fascia, which itself forms a continuous covering of the posterior pubis, the obturator internus muscles on both sides of the pelvis, and the bladder itself. The fascia is densest over the urethrovesical junction, just beneath the thin portions of the superficial branch of the deep dorsal vein.*

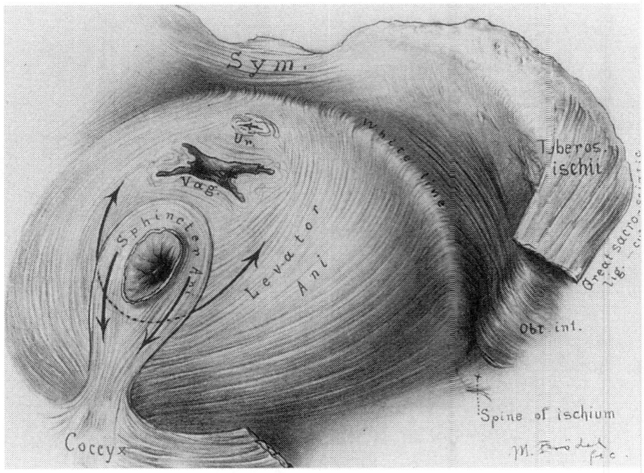

FIG. 4-5 *Origin and insertion of the fibers of the levator ani muscle, as seen from below. The sphincter ani, the lower part of the vagina, and the extremity of the urethra have been cut off on a level with the attachments of this muscle. The line of origin of the levator ani is well shown, stretching from the inner surface of the pubic arch and gently curving to the spine of the ischium. The direction of the fibers of this muscle changes from the anterior to the posterior part to such an extent that the fibers from the pelvis form almost a right angle with the posterior sides of the rectum. They have a lifting power upon these structures, which are efficient in closing the vaginal outlet.* (Courtesy the Brodel Archives: *Art as applied to medicine*, the Johns Hopkins School of Medicine, with permission. Text from Kelly HA: *Operative gynecology*, vol. I, New York, 1898, Appleton & Co., pp 77-78.)

the anterior pelvis and sweep downwards to cover the floor of the space of Retzius, crossing the midline to produce a dense covering over the prostatourethral junction in men, and the proximal urethra in women [29] The pubourethral ligaments are virtually identical in men and women. The apex of the urogenital diaphragm is located just below the point of origin of the pubourethral ligaments as they arch upwards from the sheet of endopelvic fascia to insert on the intrapelvic inferior surface of the pubis. This is a valuable surgical landmark.

The urogenital diaphragm can be imagined as a tapered sleeve sliding from below over the intrinsic muscles of the urethra and bladder neck in their customary retropubic positions (see Fig. 4-2). The sleeve is quite narrow at the apex and wider at the base, partially open posteriorly in women to permit passage of the vagina but completely closed in men. This overlap of urogenital diaphragm and urethra-bladder takes place through a defect in the other major muscular diaphragm of the pelvis, the levator diaphragm, which consists of the pubococcygeus, coccygeus, and ileococcygeus. These muscles line the pelvic bowl, running in an anteroposterior direction, providing support for pelvic viscera by drawing them toward the pubis and allowing them, particularly in the female, to remain positioned posteriorly over the levator plate, towards the back of the pelvis. The levator hiatus is a midline defect for the egress of the pelvic viscera (Fig. 4-5). It is through this hiatus that the urogenital diaphragm and the urethra meet. The levator diaphragm, particularly the pubococcygeus, gives off slips of muscle to the viscera, which pass through the diaphragm. In the female these slips are loosely attached to the superior lateral sulcus of the vagina (Fig. 4-6), and in the male they are attached to the lateral surfaces of the prostate. In both, there are slips of pubococcygeus given off to the edges of the rhabdosphincter.

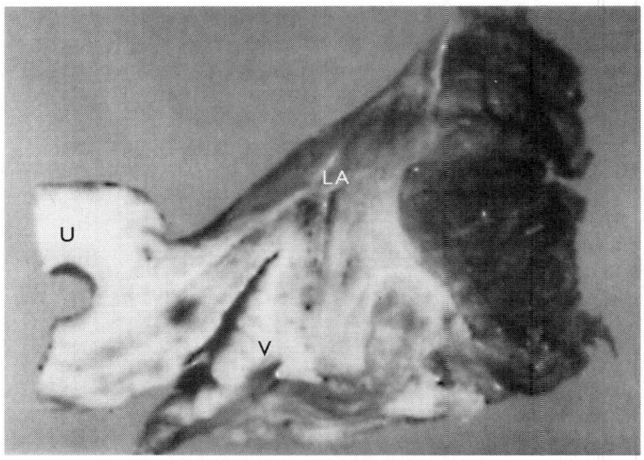

FIG. 4-6 *Transverse section through the urethra in a young Chinese woman at the junction of the upper third and lower two thirds. Urethral suspension by a musculoaponeurotic sling from the lateral pelvic wall is demonstrated clearly. LA, levator ani, U, urethra, V, vagina.* (From Zacharin RF: *Pelvic floor anatomy and the surgery of pulsion enterocele*, New York, 1985, Springer-Verlag.)

This is a difficult but very significant anatomic concept to grasp. Contrary to many popular and schematic depictions, the levator diaphragm does not form a complete transverse barrier through which the urethra passes in either male or female. It does not form a flat plane on which the bladder sits like a spinning top, balanced on a proximal urethra that penetrates the plane below. Rather, the levator diaphragm forms a gap (the levator hiatus) through which the urogenital diaphragmatic apex reaches up through the hiatus and encircles the proximal intrinsic smooth musculature of the proximal urethra.

During voluntary contraction, it is possible to imagine how these muscles might work together when one examines the orientation of their fibers. The levators are responsible for elevating and elongating the urethra along the undersurface of the pubis. No one is really sure how the periurethral muscles of the urethra function because there is no exact depiction of their orientation or the direction of fiber contraction. It is possible that they close in an irislike manner, shutting the urethra, but it makes more sense that these fibers elongate the urethra and facilitate an upward movement which draws it up along the inner undersurface of the pubis[30] (Fig. 4-7).

These two groups of muscle, the levator ani and the urethral rhabdosphincter, are composed of different types of striated muscle. Levators are fast twitch, type II, metabolically designed to contract forcefully, rapidly, and for a short duration, whereas the periurethral striated muscles are type I, slow twitch, designed to contract more slowly and provide sustained tone.[31] This is the reason it is possible to interrupt the stream voluntarily after radical prostatectomy when the levator fibers reinsert on the proximal urethral anastomosis yet have continuous sphincteric incompetence because of deficiency of the periurethral rhabdosphincter.

The urogenital diaphragm is covered by the endopelvic fascia, which fuses with it at various points and anchors it to the lower portion of the pubis, continuing beneath the pubis to anchor the clitoris in the female and the corpora cavernosa in the male (Fig. 4-8). When looking into the pelvis during retropubic exposure, the fascial surface forming the floor of the space of Retzius is exactly this "roof" of fascia covering the apex of the urogenital diaphragm (see Fig. 4-4).

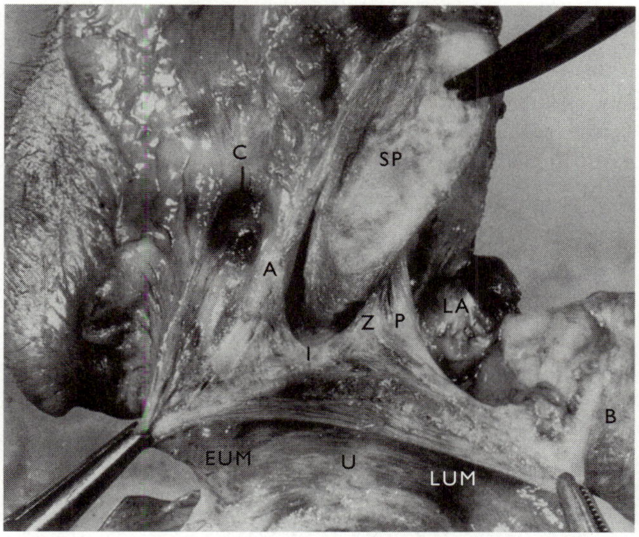

FIG. 4-8 *Sagittal section through the symphysis pubis* (SP), *urethra* (U), *and bladder* (B) *shows the suspensory mechanism of the urethra on tension. Continuity between the anterior ligament* (A) *and the posterior ligament* (P) *is shown. The levator ani* (LA), *clitoris* (C), *and external urethral meatus* (EUM) *are shown.* (From Zacharin RF: *J Anat* 91:423, 1963.)

The pubourethral complex stabilizes the urethra and permits the bladder to expand away from this retropubic point and contract toward it during storage and elimination of urine. Our own speculations regarding the major function of urethral stabilization, however, provide an alternative explanation based more on the primacy of reproduction in evolution. Considering all the possible roles for these structures in men and women, it seems likely that stabilization and accurate positioning of the

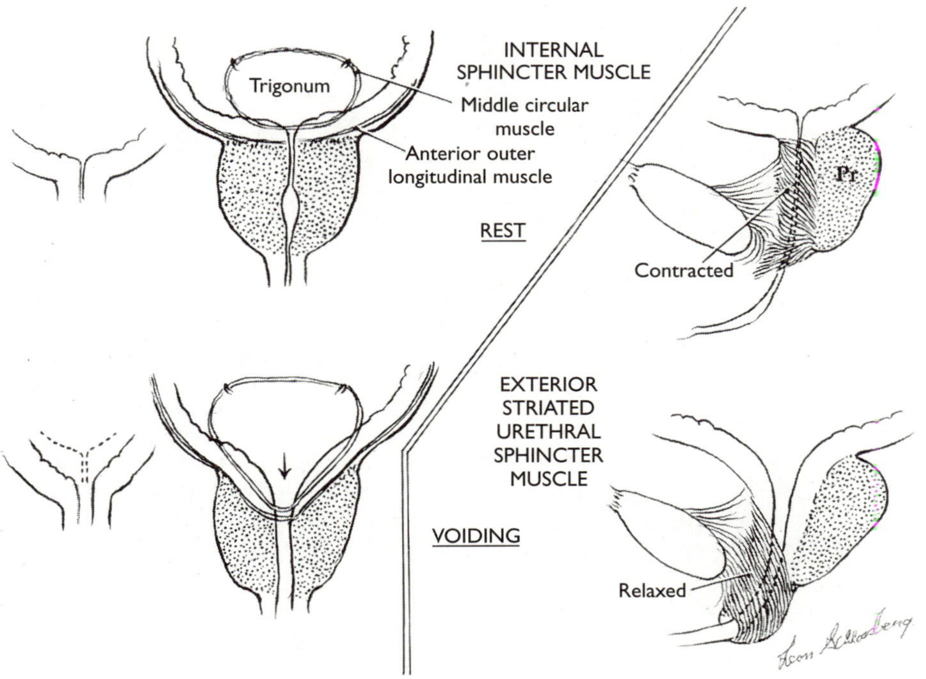

FIG. 4-7 *Hypothetical depiction of sphincteric contraction and relaxation in the male during normal voiding may give rise to the funneling and descent usually seen in voiding fluoroscopic studies.*

male urethra and the ejaculatory ducts during vaginal penetration and seminal emission would seem to be critical for successful reproduction and might represent the primary role of these structures. Their presence in the female may be incidental, much as the mammary gland is in the male, or, relying again on the theoretical primacy of reproduction, the entire complex might be important in introital stabilization for uterine contraction during parturition. In contrast to previous suggestions that the pubourethral ligaments provide stabilization of the female urethra and assist in maintaining continence,[32, 33] we believe that these structures are not critical to normal support of the female urethra and, as we discuss below, may actually contribute to the mechanical deformity of the urethra that develops during increases in intra-abdominal pressure and give rise to stress incontinence.

THE ROLE OF VAGINAL SUPPORT IN MAINTAINING URETHRAL CLOSURE IN WOMEN

To understand the role of vaginal support in urinary continence in women, one must first understand why the vagina is subject to deterioration and then consider what role this has on urethral closure.

In the healthy, nulliparous female, the vagina is a resilient muscular sheath attached firmly at several points along the intrapelvic surface of the pubis. Near the cervix, at the vaginal fornices, the vagina is supported by parametria forming cardinal and uterosacral ligaments. As the vagina continues distally towards the pubis, looser lateral connections are formed by the endopelvic fascial coverings, the arcus tendineus fasciae pelvis, which can be seen on the floor of the space of Retzius (see Fig. 4-4). As the pubis is approached, these fascial coverings become much stronger and form the pubourethral ligaments with pubococcygeus inserting immediately below onto the vaginal wall. The vagina is tethered into a high position at these two lateral superior vaginal sulci, known as the *plis du chat* (cat's corner). It is at this level that familiar transverse sections show the vagina forming a hammock passing beneath the sphincteric urethra from one side of the pelvis to the other (see Fig. 4-6). This part of the vagina produces stabilization of the urethra during increases in intra-abdominal pressure and facilitates prevention of stress incontinence.[34] Inferior to this level, the vagina is attached firmly to the medial surfaces of the pubic rami where it ends at the introitus. These three levels of support, mesenchymal, arcus tendineus, and pubourethral create the characteristic H-shape of the vagina when viewed in transverse section.[35] The lower third ascends almost vertically from the introitus to the superior lateral sulcus; the upper two thirds continue in a more horizontal direction toward the cervix.

The levator diaphragm muscles contribute greatly to the position, course, and shape of the vaginal canal. The pubococcygeus, the most medial of the levator slings, passes posterior to the rectum as the puborectalis and gives off slips to the urogenital diaphragm beneath the endopelvic fascia as can be seen in many standard transverse sections. The anterior placement of the openings of the pelvic viscera are thus maintained by a combination of countertraction between the direction of pull of the puborectalis anteriorly and the direction of support of the parametria posteriorly and superiorly. This reduces the gravitational stresses on all mesenchymal supports of the vagina and is further helped by the short anteroposterior diameter of the vaginal introitus in the nullipara (Fig. 4-9).

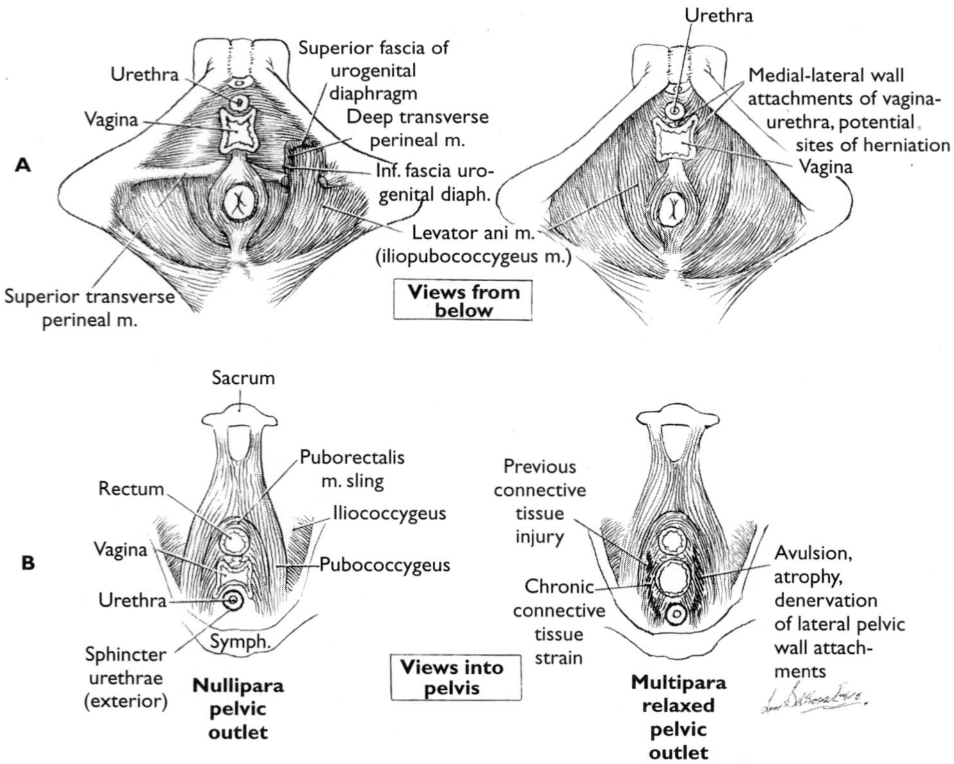

FIG. 4-9 *Comparison of levator hiatus in nulliparous and multiparous female: effects of age, childbirth, and gravitational stress. The nullipara has a shorter anteroposterior diameter of the levator hiatus, providing greater muscular support beneath the pelvic viscera, contributing to a posterior location with respect to the introitus. The multiparous female has an elongated anteroposterior hiatus diameter and may lose lateral pelvic wall attachments, contributing to reduced support beneath the pelvic viscera and increased strain on the connective tissue supports of these structures. With prolonged strain, structures may prolapse as mesenchymal support is lost.*

With time, several things happen to alter this arrangement. Childbirth produces widening and elongation of the introitus, thus lengthening and posteriorly displacing the back of the puborectalis sling and reducing its mechanical advantage in drawing the perineum forward. Pubococcygeal attachments to the vagina near the pubis may be stretched or simply avulsed. The result is the beginning of increased gravitational stresses on the mesenchymal supports of the vaginal wall.

The vagina itself can become stretched circumferentially during labor and may never recover its preparous dimensions and strength. The result can be a longer suburethral hammock stretched between the two lateral pelvic sidewalls at the level of the superior vaginal sulcus. Menopausal changes may produce involution of the mesenchymal supports and also have direct effects on the urethra.

In addition to these problems of support, there can be two direct effects on the urethral sphincter. First, menopausal changes may produce involution of the estrogen-sensitive smooth muscle and mucosa of the proximal urethra. Second, pudendal nerve injury during childbirth and with repeated episodes of pelvic prolapse can impair normal tonic and reflex contraction of the periurethral rhabdosphincter during cough, sneeze, or prolapse.[36,37]

When the anterior vaginal wall begins to show attenuation and stretching beneath the urethra, or separation from its lateral attachments, or both, the result may be clinically recognized as a cystocele, which may be more properly defined as a hernia of the vaginal wall and derives its name from the structure prolapsing through it. Applying this approach to inguinal anatomy in men, a hernia would be called an "enterocele." The underlying pathologic condition in men and women is essentially the same: increased intra-abdominal pressure and chronic gravitational stresses have led to failure at the weakest point in the system of supporting structures resisting those increases in intra-abdominal pressure.

Cystocele is such a general term that it can be confusing when one tries to decide whether a woman's incontinence is attributable to one or not. As a general rule, cystocele results in stress urinary incontinence when and only when it affects the portion of the vaginal wall that is in direct contact with the urethra. Real-time sonographic studies of women with stress urinary incontinence have shown that when the urethra rotates away from the pubis, it begins to rotate as a single unit. It then reaches a point at which the two surfaces of the urethra stop rotating together. The anterior portion of the proximal urethra is then prevented from further movement by the dense suspensory ligaments that are found immediately beneath the pubis, while the posterior portion of the urethra continues to rotate away, having lost its critical vaginal support. The point at which the two urethral walls separate may be called the "continence threshold." It has been suggested that the mechanical deformity of the urethra produced by this anatomic arrangement is one of the events responsible for stress incontinence in women[38] (Fig. 4-10). If there is lateral detachment of the vaginal wall, the urethra may rotate away from its normal position at rest within the pelvis. If there is general weakness of the vaginal wall, with stretching of the suburethral portion, there can be rotation away from the pubis even though the lateral attachments are well preserved (Fig. 4-11).

With use of this approach, it becomes clearer why cystoceles that involve only higher portions of the bladder near the cervix or the cervical cuff, often with enterocele and with loss of parametrial support, may produce significant prolapsing structures without causing incontinence, simply because the defect does not permit the urethra to reach the continence threshold.

The patterns of cystocele and pelvic prolapse are many and diverse. Only some are associated with stress incontinence. The clinician treating patients with stress incontinence must be familiar with all of them. In patients with significant prolapse or cystocele, a considerable amount of incontinence may be caused

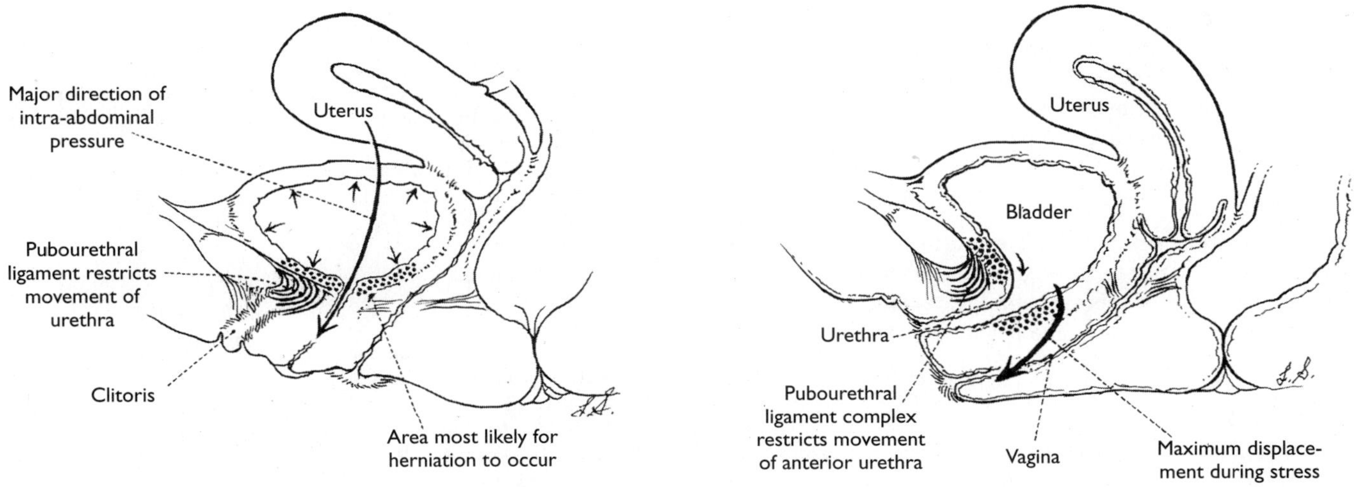

FIG. 4-10 *Relationship of vaginal mobility to urethral closure. During vaginal descent, the anterior portions of the proximal urethral wall are arrested in their rotational movement by the strength of the pubourethral complex. The posterior side of the wall continues to travel with the prolapsing vaginal wall. A shearing effect occurs at the continence threshold when the urethral walls are separated and incontinence occurs.*

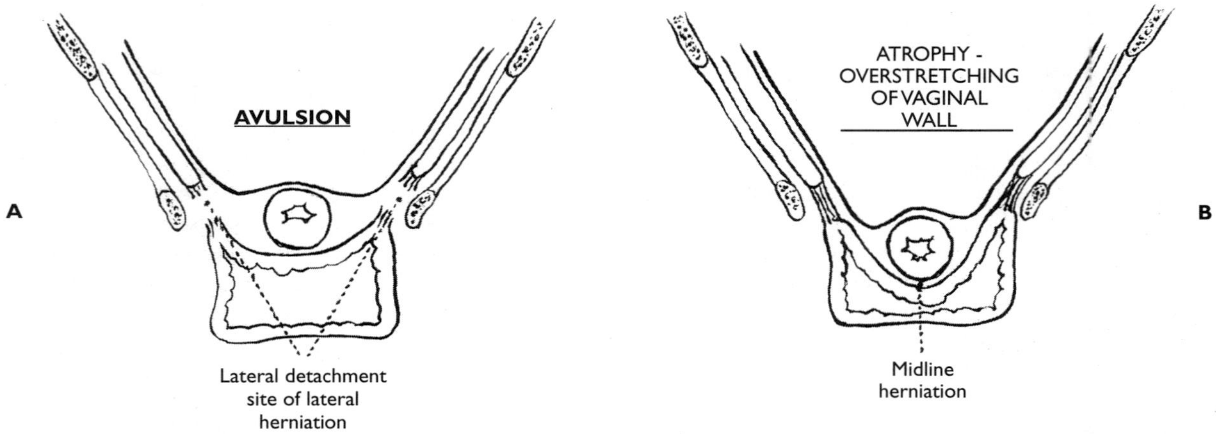

FIG. 4-11 *Relationship of site of vaginal weakness to urethral descent.* ***A,*** *Avulsion of the superior vaginal sulcus with preservation of vaginal rugae permits urethral displacement during vaginal descent. This kind of defect is well suited for suspensory operations.* ***B,*** *Midline weakness of the vagina wall with adequate preservation of the lateral attachments may result in radiographically similar urethral descent, but the attenuated vaginal wall may not hold for long if used in a suspensory operation. Such defects may require direct support such as suburethral slings.*

by concomitant intrinsic sphincteric deficiency. The overlap of pelvic prolapse and stress incontinence is complex and requires a good understanding of urethral function as well as pelvic dynamic anatomy. Interested readers should consult some of the many excellent gynecologic sources to acquaint themselves with the known range of pelvic prolapse and relate it to their own experience with stress incontinence.[35,39,40]

SUMMARY

Urinary continence depends on the integrity of structural and functional aspects of the lower urinary tract, the pelvis, and the nervous system.

1. The neurologic connections of the bladder and sphincters must be intact to permit normal storage, emptying, and sphincteric coordination.
2. The muscular strength and integrity of the rhabdosphincter must be sufficient to permit it to withstand urine escape by tonic closure and to voluntarily contract to prevent escaping urine.
3. Changes in the active and passive components of vaginal support in women can result in loss of support of the urethra, which results in stress incontinence.

The practitioner dealing with incontinence as a presenting symptom will be aided by understanding the three main features that have been outlined above: neurologic bladder function, urethral integrity and function, and pelvic support.

REFERENCES

1. Bors E, Comarr, AE: *Neurological urology: physiology of micturition, its neurological disorders and sequelae,* Baltimore, 1971, University Park Press, p. 454.
2. McGuire EJ: *Clinical evaluation and treatment of neurogenic vesical dysfunction,* vol 11, Baltimore, 1984, Williams and Wilkins, p. 162.
3. Torrens M, Morrison JFB: *The physiology of the lower urinary tract,* London, 1987, Springer-Verlag, p. 355.
4. Yalla SV, McGuire EJ, Elbadawi A, Blaivas JG: *Neurourology and urodynamics: principles and practice,* New York, 1988, MacMillan, p. 533.
5. Steers WD: Physiology of the urinary bladder. In Walsh PC, Retik AB, Stamey TA, Vaughan ED, editors: *Campbell's urology,* vol 1, ed 6, Philadelphia, 1992, Saunders, pp. 142-176.
6. George NJR, Dixon JS: Normal sensation of the lower urinary tract. In George NJR, Gosling JA, editors: *Sensory disorders of the bladder and urethra,* Berlin, 1986, Springer-Verlag.
7. Levi-Montalcini R: The nerve growth factor 35 years later, *Science* 237(4819):1154-1162, 1987 [review].
8. Steers WD, De Groat WC: Effect of bladder outlet obstruction on micturition reflex pathways in the rat, *J Urol* 140(4):864-871, 1988.
9. Kruse MN, Belton AL, de Groat WC: Changes in bladder and external urethral sphincter function following spinal cord injury in the rat, *Am J Physiol* 264:R1157-R1163, 1993.
10. Kruse MN, de Groat WC: Changes in lower urinary tract function following spinal cord injury, *J Rest Neurol Neurosci* 5:79-80, 1993.
11. Wein AJ: Neuromuscular dysfunction of the lower urinary tract. In Walsh PC, Retik AB, Stamey TA, Vaughan ED, editors: *Campbell's urology,* vol 1, ed 6, Philadelphia, 1992, Saunders, pp. 573-642.
12. Mostwin JL: Urinary problems in multiple sclerosis and other spinal cord diseases. In Johnson R, editor: *Current neurological diagnosis and treatment,* St Louis, 1990, Mosby, pp. 164-168.
13. McGuire EJ: Diagnosis and treatment of intrinsic sphincter deficiency, *Int J Urol* 2(suppl 1):7-10; discussion 16-18, 1995.
14. McGuire EJ: Urodynamic evaluation of stress incontinence, *Urol Clin N Am* 22(3):551-555, 1995.
15. Wan J, McGuire EJ, Bloom DA, Ritchey ML: Stress leak point pressure: a diagnostic tool for incontinent children, *J Urol* 150(2 Pt 2):700-702, 1993.
16. Tanagho EA: Surgical anatomy of the genitourinary tract: anatomy of the lower urinary tract. In Walsh PC, Retik AB, Stamey TA, Vaughan ED, editors: *Campbell's urology,* vol 1, ed 6, Philadelphia, 1992, Saunders, pp. 40-68.
17. Hutch JA, Amar AA: *Vesicoureteral reflux and pyelonephritis,* New York, 1972, Appleton-Century-Crofts, p. 236.
18. Lee JG, Wein AJ, Levin RM: Comparative pharmacology of the male and female rabbit bladder neck and urethra: involvement of nitric oxide, *Pharmacology* 48(4):250-259, 1994.

19. Murakumo M, Ushiki T, Abe K, et al: Three-dimensional arrangement of collagen and elastin fibers in the human urinary bladder: a scanning electron microscopic study, *J Urol* 154(1):251-256, 1995.
20. Murakumo M, Ushiki T, Koyanagi T, Abe K: Scanning electron microscopic studies of smooth muscle cells and their collagen fibrillar sheaths in empty, distended and contracted urinary bladders of the guinea pig, *Arch Histol Cytol* 56(4):441-449, 1993.
21. Turner-Warwick R: Benign enlargement of the prostate, *Trans Med Soc London* 86:41-54, 1970.
22. Speakman MJ, Brading AF, Gilpin CJ, et al: Bladder outflow obstruction—a cause of denervation supersensitivity, *J Urol* 138(6):1461-1466, 1987.
23. Steers WD, Kolbeck S, Creedon D, Tuttle JB: Nerve growth factor in the urinary bladder of the adult regulates neuronal form and function, *J Clin Invest* 88(5):1709-1715, 1991.
24. Kelly HA, Burnam CF: *Disease of the kidneys, ureters and bladder: with special reference to the diseases in women*, New York, 1922, Appleton & Co., 1922.
25. Oelrich TM: The striated urogenital sphincter muscle in the female, *Anat Rec* 205(2):223-232, 1983.
26. DeLancey JO: Structural aspects of the extrinsic continence mechanism, *Obstet Gynecol* 72(3 Pt 1):296-301, 1988.
27. Oelrich TM: The urethral sphincter muscle in the male, *Am J Anat* 158:229, 1980.
28. Myers RP, Goellner JR, Cahill DR: Prostate shape, external striated urethral sphincter and radical prostatectomy: the apical dissection, *J Urol* 138(3):543-550, 1987.
29. Mostwin JL: Current concepts of female pelvic anatomy and physiology, *Urol Clin N Am* 18(2):175-195, 1991.
30. Mostwin JL, Burnett AL, Cisek L, et al: In situ anatomical and histological study of the male subpubic urethral sphincter mechanism, *J Urol* 155:(to be presented at 1996 American Urological Association meeting, Orlando, Florida), 1996.
31. Gosling JA, Dixon JS, Critchley HO, Thompson SA: A comparative study of the human external sphincter and periurethral levator ani muscles, *Br J Urol* 53(1):35-41, 1981.
32. Milley PS, Nichols DH: The relationship between the pubo-urethral ligaments and the urogenital diaphragm in the human female, *Anat Rec* 170:281, 1971.
33. Zacharin RA: The suspensory mechanism of the female urethra, *J Anatom* 97:423, 1961.
34. DeLancey JO: Structural support of the urethra as it relates to stress urinary incontinence: the hammock hypothesis, *Am J Obstet Gynecol* 170(6):1713-1720, 1994.
35. Nichols DH, Randall CL: *Vaginal surgery*, Baltimore, 1989, Williams & Wilkins, p. 463.
36. Benson JT: Electrodiagnosis. In Benson JT, editor: *Female pelvic floor disorders: investigation and management*, New York, 1992, Norton Medical Books, pp. 157-165.
37. Snooks SJ, Barnes PR, Swash M: Damage to the innervation of the voluntary anal and periurethral sphincter musculature in incontinence: an electrophysiological study, *J Neurol Neurosurg Psychiatry* 47(12):1269-1273, 1984.
38. Sanders RC, Genadry R, Yang A, Mostwin JL: Imaging the female urethra, *Ultrasound Q* 12(3):167-183, 1994.
39. Benson JT, editor: *Female pelvic floor disorders: investigation and management*, New York, 1992, Norton & Co., p. 494.
40. Hurt WG: *Urogynecologic surgery*, Gaithersberg, Md., 1992, Aspen Publishers, p. 204.

Chapter 5

Physiology of Continence

Anders Mattiasson

Symptoms of lower urinary tract dysfunction that patients experience result from alterations in the normal function of the lower urinary tract and represent the reason that patients consult with a physician. All the clinical information available to the clinician needs to be interpreted on the basis of what is known about the function of the lower urinary tract for the symptoms to have clinical meaning and to allow the physician to approach to the management of the patient in a meaningful way.

The bladder and the urethra are two parts of a functional unit. To this unit should probably be added the pelvic floor, the vaginal musculature, and the prostate, since these structures also are of critical importance for the normal function of the lower urinary tract. A normal function means the ability on command and on socially proper occasions to empty the bladder completely with only a low resistance to the passage of urine. In the periods in between it must be guaranteed that the detrusor muscle of the bladder remains inactive and that the structures that at micturition are responsible for the outflow now instead make it possible to maintain continence. Other structures of importance are the ones that help to anchor the bladder and the urethra in their normal positions in the pelvis such as ligaments and other supporting structures.

The most remarkable thing with the lower urinary tract and its helping structures is probably that the functions are autonomically conducted but at the same time completely governed by the will. Even after paralysis of the skeletal muscles in healthy volunteers these persons still can start and stop micturition on command.[1] Our knowledge of the normal function of the lower urinary tract is limited. It might seem odd, but volumes, pressures, flows, and electrical activities are not so well defined that we in individual cases, and hardly ever in groups of individuals, always know when the limit for what might be normal is passed. Also the most well-characterized functions such as pressure and flow at micturition have a considerable gray zone between what is normal and what is pathologic.[2] We also lack a substantial amount of information about the normal nervous control of the lower urinary tract, about the hormonal dependence, and about the effect of aging. Yet we have learned a lot in recent years, not at least thanks to experimental animal studies but also thanks to new and improved clinical urodynamic measuring techniques.[3] Simple measurements that patients and volunteers easily can perform in their daily life have improved our understanding further. It is, however, still uncommon with large and well-performed investigations in normal individuals. The physiologic functions of the bladder and urethra have therefore to a considerable extent been defined indirectly through investigations in patients. A questioning of "established knowledge" has also increased the speed of progress in this field.

That a normal function of the lower urinary tract among other things means continence during the filling phase of the bladder is unnecessary to mention, but what about the emptying phase? How often is it normal to empty the bladder and how large are the volumes voided? The bladder capacity that we measure urodynamically and the maximum capacity of the bladder that can be measured under anesthesia are usually not equal to the normally voided volume in daily life. The one and a half liters of urine that we excrete in a 24-hour period is emptied in portions of 2 to 3 dl, which is considerably less than the 4 to 5 dl that often are said to be the range for the normal bladder capacity. Therefore we usually can accept eight micturitions per 24 hours as normal.

The control of the lower urinary tract function is in itself a complicated neurologic and neuromuscular process with several excitatory and inhibitory neuronal systems in reciprocal cooperation. It is the inborn, opposite functions in both the bladder and the urethra of alternating relaxation and contraction that with necessity make the nervous control so complicated. Against this background it is not difficult to understand that the normal function of the bladder and the urethra easily can be subjected to disturbances caused by processes of virtually any kind at all levels of the nervous system and in the end organs themselves. The reestablishment of a normalized situation, or at least a regained balance between the bladder and the urethra in our patients makes it necessary not only to understand the pathophysiology, but of course also the normal function of the lower urinary tract. In our clinical work we should ideally be able to consider the integrated function of all parts of the lower urinary tract, that is, the whole micturition cycle. To do this, it is necessary to be familiar with the most important neuromuscular functions, on both the central and the peripheral level.

Central Nervous Control

The central nervous engagement for the control of the bladder and the urethra is extensive and represented virtually at all levels of the nervous system. It is not meaningful to describe all events and all routes of information in the central and the peripheral parts of the nervous system taking part in lower urinary tract control. It makes more sense to summarize the net results of all events. These results can be expressed as vectors or as loops. Bradley has suggested a system with four such loops.[4]

The first of these is the one that represents the cerebral, conscious, control of the pontine micturition center. It is inhibitory in nature and thus responsible for the inactivation of the micturition reflex. The interaction of a variety of excitatory and inhibitory neuronal systems is the function of the pontine micturition center. The triggering and the inhibition of the micturition reflex can be described as an on-off mechanism. It is possible that the pontine micturition center should be regarded as a functional center more than a concise morphologic structure. The development of cerebral control of the pontine micturition center is part of the social training that children undergo, often strongly encouraged by their parents. The loss of this function fully or in part after, for example, cerebral lesions or diseases as stroke or dementia explains why some patients become incontinent. They have a loss of cerebral inhibition of the micturition reflex. The pontine micturition center is under influence of the limbic system and thus also affected by emotions. This might explain the physiologic frequency that is seen during psychogenic stress. This should of course also be remembered in the contact with patients. The second loop is the one that is identical to the micturition reflex pathway all the way from the lower urinary tract via the pontine center and back to the bladder and urethra again. The micturition reflex is characterized by its inborn excitatory nature. If not inhibited, the micturition reflex will be triggered. Once the micturition reflex has been activated it will under normal conditions be established because of a positive feedback mechanism and thus lead to complete emptying of the bladder. The third loop expresses the coordination of the bladder and the urethra during filling and emptying of the bladder. This important coordination of the detrusor, the urethra, and the pelvic floor is partly obtained through cerebellar influence. The fourth and last loop is the one representing our ability to govern the urethral sphincter function with our will so as to stop the micturition on command.

The spinal control of the lower urinary tract is only partly known. Several neuronal systems such as the cholinergic, adrenergic, gaba-ergic, and dopaminergic ones are involved. A series of other substances are probably also of importance as neuromodulators for the regulation of thresholds and possibly also as neurotransmitters. Among them we find several neuropeptides. Substance P and vasoactive intestinal polypeptide are richly represented in the dorsal sacral roots and in the sacral spinal cord. Stimulation and inhibition of both opioid and neurokinin receptors at the level of the sacral spinal cord have pronounced effects on the bladder function. Of the different spinal neuronal systems it is still only the knowledge on the gaba-ergic innervation that has been used systematically for treatment of patients. Patients with spasticity of the lower limbs and also detrusor hyperactivity have been treated successfully in small series with continuous intrathecal administration of a GABA-analog, baclofen.[5] This is probably a field that will become increasingly important when our knowledge of the spinal control of the bladder and urethra advances.

Peripheral Innervation and Receptor Functions

The peripheral innervation of the lower urinary tract is traditionally described as cholinergic, adrenergic, and somatic conveyed through the pelvic nerves (S2-4), the hypogastric nerves (Th10-L2), and the pudendal nerves (S2-4) respectively. These nerves carry not only motor but also sensory fibers. In this model of the innervation, which has been dominating for decades,[6] the excitatory cholinergic innervation of the bladder mediated by means of acetylcholine released from the nerve terminals and acting on postjunctional muscarinic receptors are considered to be the quantitatively and functionally dominating component. It is also on these muscarinic receptors that the anticholinergic drugs we offer patients with detrusor hyperactivity or urgency are supposed to exert their effects.

The dominating innervation of the urethra is adrenergic. A relatively rich occurrence of adrenergic nerve fibers are also found in the bladder base. Alpha-adrenergic receptors that are activated by the release of norepinephrine mediate contraction of smooth muscle in the urethra thereby contributing to the closure during bladder filling. Beta-adrenergic receptors in the detrusor muscle with its sparse adrenergic innervation might be of some importance for relaxation of the detrusor during filling.[7] This relatively simple model of the innervation of the bladder and urethra has become more and more questioned in recent years. There are several reasons. One important reason is that nonadrenergic noncholinergic (NANC) functions have been identified both in the bladder and in the urethra.[5,8] Neuropeptides and nitric oxide (NO) seem to be both richly represented and also of functional importance in the lower urinary tract.[9,10,11] Another reason is that the distribution of the cholinergic and adrenergic nerve fibers in fact might be different from that in the described model. There is, for example, a relatively rich cholinergic innervation also in the urethra.[12,13] A third reason might be that a representation in quantitative terms not always must correspond to the functional importance.

The role of the sensory innervation and its importance for normal function is only known to a very limited extent. It seems however to be just as important as the motor innervation. A communication between the sensory and the motor innervation, not only at central relay stations but also in the periphery, is probably of vital importance for the normal control of bladder filling and emptying.[13,14] In the same way that every part of a circle is of importance for the figure are the different components composing the micturition reflex pathway of importance for the normal function of the lower urinary tract.

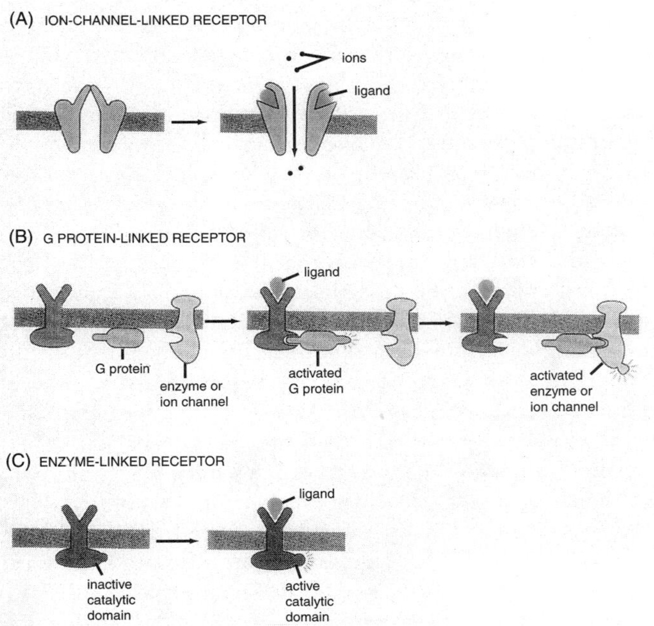

FIG. 5-1 *Three classes of cell-surface receptors of importance for the activation of lower urinary tract muscle cells.* (From Alberts B, Bray D, Lewis J, et al, editors: *The cell,* ed 3, Hamden, Conn., 1994, Garland.)

Cholinergic Innervation

The dominating innervation of the detrusor muscle is cholinergic. These nerves reach the bladder after their signals are relayed in the pelvic ganglia. During the filling phase of the bladder, impulses from the central nervous system reaching the pelvic ganglia are filtered here through a special gating mechanism.[15]

A very rich innervation of the bladder musculature can be visualized with, for example, acetylcholine esterase staining, and each individual detrusor muscle cell can be regarded as individually innervated. That a simultaneous activation of the whole bladder via the pelvic nerves easily can be achieved is not difficult to understand against this background. Of the five different types of muscarinic-receptor subtypes, M_2 and M_3 are the ones dominating in the bladder musculature. The cholinergic receptors at the ganglionic level are normally of the nicotinic type.

Muscarinic receptors on the detrusor muscle cells are the targets for acetylcholine released from cholinergic neurons. There is a very rich cholinergic innervation. This makes a simultaneous activation of the whole detrusor possible. The bladder will therefore act as one functional unit and will contract in all parts simultaneously. Transmitters other than acetylcholine might be of importance.[8] The nerve-mediated contraction cannot always be blocked completely with atropine, and an atropine-resistant component is said to be present. Such a component is found in almost all investigated animal species. The presence of such an atropine-resistant component might also depend on the nerve-stimulation pattern used. For practical reasons it seems reasonable to consider the activation of the normal human bladder as completely cholinergic. The muscarinic receptors in the detrusor are mainly of the M_2 and M_3 types. Knowledge about these subtypes of receptors is of importance for the development of drugs with selective actions on the lower urinary tract.

The contraction of the detrusor muscle cells is a process that is Ca^{++}-dependent.[16] Ca^{++} can enter the cytoplasm at the activation of smooth muscle cells either through the opening of Ca^{++} channels in the cell membrane, that is, the entrance of extracellular Ca^{++} into the cell, or by mobilization of intracellular depots in the endoplasmatic reticulum. The dominating Ca^{++} source for human bladder muscle cells is extracellular Ca^{++} and thus an entrance into the cell by Ca^{++}channels. The interaction between actin and myosin is of course energy consuming. The energy is supplied by ATP. The whole process from the activation of structures on the cell surface by mobilization of second messengers intracellularly and the activation and sliding of the contractile proteins is usually called the "excitation-contraction coupling."

As stated above also the urethra has a relatively rich cholinergic innervation. Its role is not yet clear. It is however easy to speculate that an activation of the cholinergic urethral nerves could contribute to the opening of the outflow region and the urethra.

Adrenergic Innervation

The adrenergic innervation is more dense in the urethra than in the bladder.[17] Several authors more precisely mean that the adrenergic nerve fibers are more abundant in the proximal than in the distal part of the urethra. Others question the concept of a rich adrenergic innervation of the urethral wall. During the filling phase of the bladder, activity in the hypogastric nerves contributes to the closure of the urethra through the action of norepinephrine on contraction-mediating alpha-adrenergic receptors in the urethral smooth musculature. As already mentioned, the adrenergic influence on the bladder is relaxant and is mediated through the action of beta-adrenergic receptors. This might seem as a suitable arrangement from a functional point of view, but the real importance of the adrenergic innervation for normal bladder function is unclear.[18] Considerable doses of beta-adrenergic receptor–stimulating agents are needed to influence the bladder capacity only slightly in young healthy volunteers.[7] Side effects from the lower urinary tract are seldom reported from patients on beta-receptor active drugs.

The alpha receptors in the urethra are mainly of the $alpha_1$ type. There are also $alpha_2$ receptors, but they seem to be located mainly prejunctionally on the nerve terminals, thus participating in the feedback regulation of transmitter release. An $alpha_1$-receptor agonist or antagonist will thus frequently have the opposite effect on the intraurethral pressure than what would be expected with an $alpha_2$-receptor agonist or antagonist.

The adrenergic innervation of the bladder neck region and the internal urethral sphincter in the male seems to be of functional importance, since retrograde ejaculation often is noted after retroperitoneal surgery and damage to the hypogastric nerves. It has also been well known for a long time that stimulation of the hypogastric nerves results in contraction of the bladder neck area.[6,8]

Also the smooth muscle component of the prostate has an adrenergic innervation. The dominating receptor subtype is $alpha_{1a}$ (previously called $alpha_{1c}$). $Alpha_2$-adrenergic receptors are also found, but they seem to be of less importance.

Sensory Innervation

Our knowledge about the sensory innervation of the bladder and the urethra is slowly increasing. Two types of sensory nerve fibers, myelinized A delta (AΔ) and unmyelinized C fibers, are found in the nerves supplying the lower urinary tract. The sensations of bladder filling and touch are conveyed by mechanoreceptors to the A-delta fibers. A normal sensory innervation is essential for the normal function of both the bladder and the urethra.[14] The micturition reflex is driven by a continuous afferent impulse flow from the bladder wall and is thus of a positive feedback nature. This afferent impulse flow during the emptying phase is obviously necessary for a normal bladder emptying. The C fibers are nociceptive and can be assumed to be nonfunctional under normal circumstances. They can however be activated in different pathologic situations and then play an active role in the pathophysiologic process. The C fibers can be emptied of their content of active substances by exposure to capsaicin, which is a toxic agent extracted from Spanish pepper and chilies (Maggi et al., 1989). This mechanism cannot only be used to study the role of the sensory innervation for the normal bladder function, but also to treat patients with hyperactivity and urgency. These capsaicin-sensitive, unmyelinized afferent nerve fibers contain various tachykinins such as substance P and neurokinin A and B. The effects seem to be exerted mainly by an action on neurokinin-1 receptors in the bladder. It is possible that the tachykinins in the bladder have a protective function. Irritative stimuli of various kinds most probably release these substances, which in turn will induce a response with increased permeability of fluid through the bladder wall and an increased local blood flow. These mechanisms might also play a pathophysiologic role, as in inflammatory processes of the bladder wall. If so, a new class of pharmacologic agents should be possible to develop.

Of special interest is that the most superficial layer of cells in the bladder, the urothelium, is richly innervated by a population of delicate nerve fibers. The presence of a nervous regulation of the urothelial barrier function of the bladder mucosa therefore seems probable. The afferent neurons innervating the bladder wall are probably not only sensory in function. Antidromal axons from the afferent neurons are acting as efferent neurons and seem to be of importance also in the normal bladder.[14] These axons could be of importance for the conditioning of triggering levels, that is, the regulation of thresholds for the afferent impulse flow. Even though results from animal experiments speak in favor for this kind of function, one has to be clear over the speculative nature of these data.

Nonadrenergic Noncholinergic (NANC) Innervation

Numerous investigations support the presence of transmitters other than the classical norepinephrine and acetylcholine (ACh) in nerves supplying the lower urinary tract.[10,13] The existence of any type of nerves other than adrenergic or cholinergic ones has not convincingly been demonstrated so far. A coexistence of several substances within the same nerve fibers, whether adrenergic, cholinergic or somatic, motor or sensory, seems more probable. A series of neuropeptides are of great interest in this context, but also of course the L-arginine–nitric oxide system as well as to a certain extent also a possible purinergic innervation. To classify a substance as a neurotransmitter, several criteria have to be fulfilled. One of them, and often the most critical one, is that the effect of the putative transmitter should be possible to block with an appropriate antagonist. It is only recently that some good blockers, having a nonpeptide nature, have appeared. The development of this field is very rapid, and we can expect a substantial amount of information in the near future. None of the neuropeptides, whose presence in the nerves of the lower urinary tract has been proved, has yet been demonstrated to be a transmitter in the nervous regulation of the bladder or the urethra. They might also act as neuromodulators or have trophic effects as well. The most well-recognized ones are vasoactive intestinal polypeptide (VIP), substance P (SP), neuropeptide Y (NPY), calcitonin gene-related polypeptide (CGRP), enkephalin, and somatostatin.[9,10] Drugs acting on peptide receptors can be expected to play an important role in future treatment of lower urinary tract disorders.

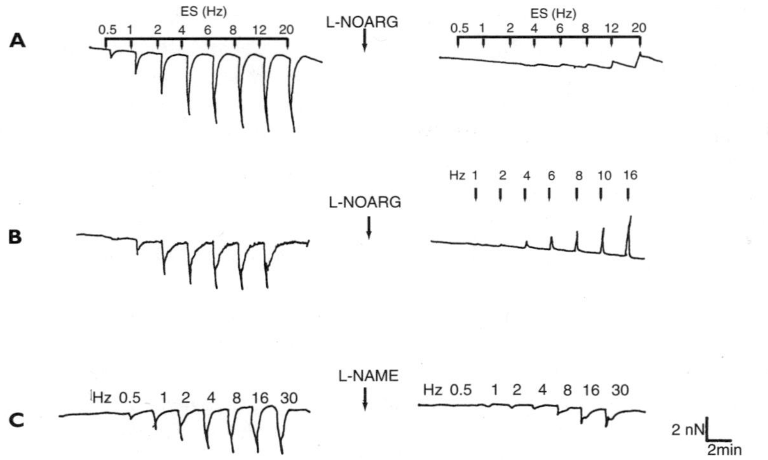

FIG. 5-2 *The nerve-mediated, electrically induced, nonadrenergic noncholinergic relaxant response in the rabbit, pig, and rat urethra. The response could be blocked with agents that block the action of nitric oxide (NO).* (From Persson K: *The* L-arginine/nitric oxide system in the lower urinary tract, doctoral thesis, University of Lund, Sweden, 1995.)

Nitric Oxide (NO)

Even though the nonadrenergically noncholinergically mediated relaxation of the urethra was described more than a decade ago,[19] it is only in recent years that the knowledge about the importance of the L-arginine–nitric oxide system in the lower urinary tract has been known and thus also contributed to our understanding of some of the probable physiologic functions in the regulation of the lower urinary tract.[8,11] NO seems to be released from cholinergic nerves. When the parasympathetic, pelvic gangions are removed in animal experiments a pronounced reduction of the NO synthase (NOS) activity is obtained in the bladder and the urethra. NO seems to be colocalized with certain neuropeptides, such as VIP in nonadrenergic ganglionic cells.[20] Chemical sympathectomy does not affect NO-mediated functions. NO has a very short half-life, counted in seconds, and it is therefore not probable that NO itself can be responsible for the relaxation in the urethra during the whole emptying phase. Other possible supporting relaxant mechanisms are still unknown. That NO plays a physiologic role for the efferent motor functions in the lower urinary tract seems obvious. It is probable that it also is of importance for sensory, afferent functions.

Neuropeptides

The presence of many neuropeptides in the lower urinary tract have been demonstrated using immunohistochemical technique.[9,10] There is an uneven distribution between different neuron populations and between the bladder and the urethra. Considerable differences are found also between various parts of the same organ, such as the bladder dome and the bladder base. Neuropeptides are found in efferent as well as afferent, in adrenergic as well as cholinergic neurons.

Substance P (SP) is relatively richly represented in afferent neurons in the bladder wall and especially abundant in the subepithelial layer. SP belongs to the family of tachykinins, to which neurokinin A and B also belong. SP is believed to be a mediator in the neurogenically initiated inflammatory reaction. It can also be a mediator of pain in the thin, unmyelinized C fibers. Whether SP is involved in inflammatory bladder disease is unknown. The occurrence of SP at the sacral level of the spinal cord is richer than at other levels. SP coexists with VIP in 25% of the dorsal sacral nerve roots.

Vasoactive intestinal polypeptide (VIP) has been supposed to participate in the relaxation of both bladder and urethral musculature. Such effects can be demonstrated at in vitro investigations, especially pronounced in urethral preparations. The occurrence of VIP in the bladder is richest in the outflow region. The physiologic importance has not been clarified. With immunohistochemical technique VIP cannot seldom be demonstrated in cholinergic neurons. There is, for example, a rich occurrence in pelvic ganglionic cells, which are supposed to be mainly cholinergic in nature. VIP is here found to coexist with NOS. It might be speculated that ACh, VIP, and NO cooperate in a cascade-like fashion for the initiation and effectuation of micturition.

Neuropeptide Y (NPY) can be found in both adrenergic and cholinergic neurons. In the nerves supplying the lower urinary tract this peptide is mainly found in the efferent adrenergic neurons. NPY has in basic investigations been shown to have multiple motor effects, and any clear-cut functional pattern does not yet exist for this peptide.

Other neuropeptides of probable functional importance are also present in the bladder and the urethra. One of these is *calcitonin gene related peptide (CGRP)*. This substance has been demonstrated to relax the bladder neck region in certain species. It could thus also be of importance for bladder emptying.[21] We also know that peptides with effects on *opioid-receptors* located spinally, but also in the periphery, affect the bladder capacity and the micturition threshold. If morphine, for example, is given intrathecally, these effects are very obvious. In the same way the bladder capacity can be decreased and urgency provoked when an antagonist, such as naloxone, is given. A considerable number of neuropeptides have thus been demonstrated to be present in the nerves of the lower urinary tract. There is quite a discrepancy between the rather detailed morphologic knowledge and the scarce information about the functional, physiologic role of the peptides. One of the main reasons is the lack of specific and selective blockers.

The Detrusor

The bladder is characterized by its motor functions, that is, contraction and relaxation, but also by the biologic barrier function in the urothelium, which makes storage of the highly osmolar urine possible. Even though this barrier function is important and interesting from a physiologic point of view, it seems appropriate here to focus on the motor functions of the bladder and thus on the detrusor.

The detrusor is, from an anatomic point of view, a syncytium. No specific layers can be identified. The muscle bundles are interdigitating as in a functional unit. All muscle cells in the bladder wall are activated simultaneously at micturition. This is probably not the result of intercellular muscle cell communication, at least not in the normal bladder.

There seems to be no electrical low resistance pathways in the human bladder between the muscle cells as has been described for certain animal species.[22] This kind of junction is relatively common in other types of smooth muscle, also in man. It seems more reasonable to explain the uniform behavior of the bladder muscle cells with a rich excitatory innervation, and it might even be that every muscle cell is innervated. When the detrusor muscle is stretched quickly, it contracts, a stretch-induced activation. The possible physiologic importance of this phenomenon is not clear.

The detrusor muscle cells are characterized by their ability to change length without any change in tension.[23] Each detrusor muscle cell can in fact be stretched to four times its original length. The relation between the volume of the bladder and the pressure increase, the compliance, can be expressed in the amount of milliliters that can be filled per centimeter-of-water pressure increase. The compliance should normally be 15 ml/cm H_2O. The bladder can thus be filled to its capacity without any real increase in intravesical pressure.[2] The small pressure increase we usually observe is partly the result of hydrostatic pressure attributable to the filling itself. Such a successive adaptation to the increased content is essential, and these viscoelastic properties are unique to the detrusor.

The small or absent increase of the intravesical pressure during filling is also the result of inhibitory nervous activity. During normal circumstances the activation mechanisms of the detrusor are suppressed completely. We learn already early in life to inhibit voluntarily the micturition reflex. As already mentioned, the micturition reflex is in itself excitatory and permanently ready to be activated, and needs to be inhibited during the filling phase of the bladder.

There is of course a limit for how much the bladder can be filled before it becomes overdistended. There is a rather pronounced protective toughness intracellularly and extracellularly that gives the bladder its necessary stabilizing and protective passive properties. A relatively good correlation exists between the passive properties and the amount of collagen in the bladder wall. The detrusor cells themselves seem to contribute to the synthesis of collagen. Another interesting observation is that fibrocytes in the bladder wall in response to increased functional demands can be transformed into myocytes and muscle cells, thereby, when needed, increasing the muscle mass of the bladder wall.[24]

There are functional differences between various parts of the bladder wall. The trigone has a structure and function in addition to that of the bladder dome. The musculature here is arranged in layers, and a part of it continues into the longitudinal urethral smooth muscle layer, and another part is a direct continuation of the smooth muscle sheath that surrounds the ureter at its passage through the bladder wall. During the emptying phase of the bladder the trigonal plate descends, thereby participating in the funneling of the outflow region. This remodulation of the trigone is the result of active muscle contraction. If the trigone and the smooth muscle of the urethra are regarded not only as a functional unit, but also as parts of a common structure, it might be called the "lissosphincter" according to Elbadawi.[13,22] Gosling, on the other hand, believes that they are separate structures and prefers to divide the trigone into layers, the superficial trigone and the deep trigone.[25]

The combination of absent excitatory stimuli and the presence of inhibitory mechanisms explain the bladder behavior during filling. The activity in the pelvic nerves is strikingly low during bladder filling.[5,15] The gating phenomenon at the ganglionic level was mentioned earlier. The electrical properties of the detrusor muscle cells themselves are probably of critical importance for both phases of the micturition cycle.

When the detrusor once has been activated, the contraction will be sustained until the bladder is emptied. This positive feedback behavior corresponds to a continuous and intense flow of impulses in the pelvic parasympathetic nerves. The bladder muscle cells are characterized by their ability to develop continuously a high and even force over a wide span at contraction. A sustained detrusor contraction at a relatively constant and normal pressure level is thus characteristic for the bladder function in the normal individual. Activation of the bladder can normally be initiated voluntarily at any degree of filling. Unlike other smooth muscle the detrusor is normally active only a few minutes per 24 hours.

The Urethral Sphincter

The coordination of the bladder and the urethra is of paramount importance both for continence during the filling phase and for an effective opening with emptying against the lowest possible resistance during micturition. The external urethral mechanism is of course of critical importance for a normal urethral function. To understand the urethral sphincter function one needs to be familiar with its structure.

Structure of the External Urethral Sphincter

The main urethral sphincteric mechanism, usually called the "distal," or "external," sphincter, is built up by smooth and striated muscles, a rich vasularization, and a thick mucosa. The exact contribution from each one of these is not known, but roughly speaking they can be said to represent one third each of the maximum urethral pressure.[26] The pressure along the urethra can be represented as a profile, and the highest pressure is found in the part where the striated muscle component of the external sphincter is located.

The *striated muscle* is rather prominent in the urethral wall, and in the female urethra it is located with its main part in the middle third of the organ and with the dominating portion anteriorly. In the male a similar structure is found, but with the whole external sphincter located directly beneath the prostate corresponding to the membranous part of the urethra. Morphologic investigations of the muscle fibers in the urethral sphincter and in the pelvic floor have demonstrated a dominance of slow-twitch over fast-twitch fibers.[25] This distribution is probably reflecting the functional roles of the different components. It means that they are fatigue resistant and thus also suitable for continuous contraction. In the female this striated musculature should be regarded as a part of a larger complex of striated muscle surrounding the distal parts of both the urethra and the vagina.

The *smooth muscle* of the urethral wall is organized into two different layers, one inner longitudinal and one outer circular. In the human urethra the circular layer seems to be more discrete than the longitudinal one. It cannot be excluded that the contraction of urethral smooth muscle is of importance not only for closure, but also for the opening of the outflow region through a contraction of longitudinal musculature in the urethral wall.

A morphologically important component, which in the female urethra represents almost half of the surface of a transverse section of the organ, is the *mucosa* and the *submucosa* (lamina propria). The importance of these structures in the urethra is not fully clarified, but it can be assumed that the sealing function has been underestimated. The submucosa is a complex structure with a very rich vascularization. Large, thin-walled veins occupy most of the submucosa. Muscle cells of smaller size than in the circular or longitudinal layers are found in the submucosa. The importance of the sealing function of the mucosa and the submucosa was described as "the inner urethral softness" by Zinner.[27]

Urethral Closure

Continence during rest can roughly be said to depend on structures and functions within the urethral wall itself, and maintenance of continence during stress or strain also needs the support from ligaments, the pelvic floor, and so forth. Therefore not only active muscle forces but also passive and supporting forces contribute to the maintenance of continence.[28] During stress or strain both active and passive forces are acting very fast and very effectively on the urethra for closure. This is possible partly because of the positioning of the urethra in the pelvis. When the intra-abdominal pressure rises, the urethra will be compressed, perhaps also kinked. The closure function of the urethra thus also depends on a normal support of the organ. The pubourethral ligament contains muscle fibers, and having such fibers makes it probable that these structures play an even more important role for maintenance of continence than we previously have assumed.

When there is a sudden intra-abdominal pressure increase, it is important that the urethral pressure can be quickly increased to a level above the bladder pressure that will develop during, for example, a Valsalva maneuver. The mechanical transmission of pressure from the abdominal cavity to the proximal part of the urethra that takes place in these situations of strain was described by Enhörning.[29] We still believe that this is an important passive mechanism but not the only factor of importance. There is also a very fast mechanism for contraction of the striated muscle around the urethra with a rapid intraurethral pressure increase that starts already 200 msec before the intra-abdominal pressure increase. These observations have been done by Constantinou et al.[30] and others. The role of the striated muscle therefore seems to be both tonic-static and, when necessary, phasic-dynamic.

Urinary continence is normally guaranteed at the level of the bladder neck, though the pressure here is substantially lower than in any part of the urethra. There is no well-defined sphincter in the bladder neck region in the female. In males such a sphincter can be identified, but here it has a sexual function by preventing retrograde ejaculation. The difference between the pressure in the urethra and that in the bladder is the so-called closure pressure, which is a calculated entity. Under normal circumstances the pressure in the urethra is much higher than that in the bladder, and the closure pressure is consequently also high. In young persons the closure pressure can approach and even exceed 100 cm H2O, whereas the closure pressure in elderly people and especially in women decreases and is usually less than 50 cm H2O. All parts of the female urethra are influenced by estrogen. When estrogen is given to a postmenopausal woman with urogenital mucosal atrophy as part of the urogenital aging process, the mucosa and musculature will grow and the vascularization becomes richer.

The mechanical properties of the urethra are not completely understood. It is difficult to describe the urethral functions for closure also with the use of sophisticated urodynamic technique. Regular urethral pressure measurements with profiles of the pressure distribution along the urethra will be sufficient only in certain patient groups, since it is a static way of describing the urethral function. With the use of more dynamic methods, both active and passive properties in the urethral wall during rest as well as under stress can be expressed. These properties, expressed in terms of hysteresis and elasticity, as well as the work performed by the urethral muscles, can be calculated by use of modern techniques. The urethral function also in normal individuals has been described carefully by Colstrup, Lose, and Thind.[31,32,33]

Urethral Opening

Since the bladder base and the pelvic floor participate in the act of bladder emptying, it is probably more correct to discuss the bladder outflow region or function instead of focusing only on the urethra. Both the urethra and the bladder base are remodeled during micturition in comparison to the situation during bladder filling. The opening of the urethra is probably the result of not only a relaxation of different components of the urethral wall, but also contraction of others. This will result in a funneling of the outflow region. Because of the efficient opening of the urethra, the intravesical pressure increase is sometimes very low. This is especially true for women. Quite low detrusor pressures at normal flow is therefore not seldom a normal urodynamic finding.

As mentioned above, the micturition starts with a urethral pressure fall preceding the bladder pressure increase. This urethral pressure fall, as well as the sequence of the events, is probably very important for a normal function of the lower urinary tract. The presence of this mechanism can be demonstrated at sacral nerve root stimulation, such as intraoperatively.[34] The importance of this function can probably best be described by the situation when the function is lost. This is seen at decentralization of the lower urinary tract. Despite the lowered urethral pressure that usually occurs after decentralization, a functional outflow obstruction will occur because of the lost ability to further decrease the urethral pressure as on normal initiation of voiding.

To what degree the initiation of micturition and the continued activation of the micturition reflex is initiated and maintained from the urethra and the outflow region has not been clarified. It seems however reasonable to assume that the rich and complex innervation of these structures reflect their importance for the emptying process. The activity of the striated musculature is inhibited effectively, and such inhibition can be demonstrated with electromyography.

Several mechanisms have been suggested to be of importance for the relaxation of the urethral musulature.[11,14] Several relaxation-mediating mechanisms are probably important to accomplish the urethral pressure fall. Since the contraction of urethral smooth muscle is mediated by alpha-adrenergic receptors it seems reasonable that a decreased influence of adrenergic nervous activity would be one of the mechanisms of urethral relaxation. A cholinergic activation leading to bladder contraction and urethral opening would also be logical but still unproved. The smooth and circular muscle of the urethra can, after contraction with, for example, norepinephrine, easily be relaxed by means of electrical nerve stimulation. This relaxant response is very pronounced and mediated by means of the L-arginine–NO system.[11] Other factors than NO probably participate, since the half-life of NO is very short, only a few seconds. NO seems to be necessary for the initiation of the response, since the whole relaxant response can be blocked by use of antagonists.

The physiologic role of this type of nonadrenergic noncholinergic mechanism in man is not known. This type of response can however be induced in vivo in the human by stimulation of the ventral sacral nerve root S3 or S4 in curarized patients treated with atropine. It is therefore reasonable to assume that the described kind of nonadrenergic noncholinergic mechanism has an important physiologic role in man.

Normal Versus Pathologic Function and Aging

The organs and tissues of the lower urinary tract are quickly responding to changed functional demands with structural, biochemical, and functional changes in muscle as well as in nerves. This is seen both in the presence of obstruction and neurogenic disturbances and perhaps in patients with so-called functional disorders. This also means that it is important to differ the normal, physiologic functions from the abnormal, pathophysiologic ones. In the pathophysiologic situation the mechanisms that should be used for treatment of a patient might be quite different from the ones normally occurring.

Many symptoms that are assumed to be caused by diseases should perhaps instead be interpreted as an expression for aging. When the lower urinary tract symptoms that elderly men often have and that have been assumed to reflect prostatic disease are compared with the corresponding symptoms in elderly women, there are striking similarities. We can of course not exclude established or incipient disease processes such as prostatic hyperplasia and estrogen deficiency as the explanations for these findings, but it might serve as a reminder for us that aging and disease should be separated from each other. This does not mean that the presence of age-induced changes in itself should imply acceptance. Women with hormonal deficiency often have what might be called urogenital aging. These women might benefit from treatment just as much as a patient with a disease process. Aging is irreversible (!), but this is also the case with many disease processes that we try to treat. We are therefore not allowed to resign to what aging has caused in us. To regain a lost balance in order to reduce or eliminate the urgency, the incontinence, or the pain will continue to be one of the most important things we can do for our patients whether they have a disease or they only happen to belong to the group of "elderly."

To understand the function of the lower urinary tract, it is not sufficient to focus only on one single component at a time. It is important to evaluate the simultaneous function of the bladder, the urethra, the pelvic floor, and other structures of importance for the normal function of the micturition cycle. This attitude is especially rewarding in daily clinical practice when the possible presence of deviations from normality shall be determined.

References

1. Lapides J, Sweet RB, Lewis LW: Role of striated muscle in urination, *J Urol* 77:247-250, 1957
2. Schäfer W: Detrusor muscle mechanics in clinical urodynamics. In *Clinical urology,* ed 2, Boston, 1991, Little, Brown.
3. Mundy AR, Stephenson TP, Wein AJ, editors: *Urodynamics—principles, practice and application,*, New York, 1994, Churchill Livingstone.
4. Bradley WE: Physiology of the urinary bladder. In Walsh PC, Gittes R, Perlmutter A, Stamey T, editors: *Campbell's urology,* ed 5, Philadelphia, 1986, Saunders.
5. Steers W: Physiology of the urinary bladder. In Walsh PC, Retik AB, Stamey TA, Vaughan ED, editors: *Campbell's urology,* Philadelphia, 1992, Saunders.
6. Learmoth JR: A contribution to the neurophysiology of the urinary bladder in man, *Brain* 54:147-176, 1931
7. Norlén L: Influence of the sympathetic nervous system on lower urinary tract and its clinical implications, *Neurourol Urodyn* 1:129-148, 1982.
8. Andersson K-E: Pharmacology of lower urinary tract smooth muscles and penile erectile tissues, *Pharmacol Rev* 45:253, 1993
9. Gu J, Blank MA, Huang WM, et al: Peptide-containing nerves in human urinary bladder, *Urol* 24:353-357, 1984
10. Maggi CA: The role of peptides in the regulation of the micturition reflex: an update, *Gen Pharmacol* 22(1):1-24, 1991.
11. Persson K: The L-arginine/nitric oxide system in the lower urinary tract, doctoral thesis, Lund University, Sweden, 1994.
12. Gosling JA, Dixon JS, Lendon RG: The autonomic innervation of the human male and female bladder neck and proximal urethra, *J Urol* 118:302, 1977
13. Elbadawi A: Neuromorphologic basis of vesicourethral function: I. Histochemistry, ultrastructure and function of intrinsic nerves in the bladder and urethra, *Neurourol Urodyn* 1:3-50, 1982
14. Maggi CA, Meli A: The sensory-efferent function of capsicin-sensitive sensory neurons, *Gen Pharmacol* 19(1):1-43, 1988.
15. DeGroat WC, Booth AM: Inhibition and facilitation in parasympathetic ganglia of the urinary bladder, *Fed Proc* 39:2990, 1980

16. Brading A: Physiology of bladder smooth muscle. In Torrens M,Morrison JFB, editors: *The physiology of the lower urinary tract,* New York, 1987, Springer-Verlag.
17. Gosling JA: The distribution of noradrenergic nerves in the human lower urinary tract, *Clin Sci* 70(suppl 14):3s-6s, 1986.
18. Nordling J: Influence of the sympathetic nervous system on lower urinary tract in man, *Neurourol Urodyn* 2:3, 1983.
19. Mattiasson A: Bladder and urethral physiology and pathophysiology. In Krane RJ, Siroky MB, Fitzpatrick JM, editors: *Clinical urology,* Philadelphia, 1994, Lippincott.
20. Uvelius B, Larsson B, Andersson K-E, Alm P: Nitric oxide synthase-containing neurons in rat major pelvic ganglia: comparison to other autonomic ganglia, *Neurourol Urodyn* 13:398, 1994.
21. Stief CG, Benard F, Bosch RJLH, et al: A possible role for calcitonin-gene-related peptide in the regulation of the smooth muscle tone of the bladder and penis, *J Urol* 143:392-397, 1990.
22. Elbadawi A: Anatomy and innervation of the vesicourethral muscular unit of micturition, In *Clinical neurourology,* ed 2, Boston, 1991, Little, Brown.
23. Uvelius B, Gabella G: Relation between cell length and force production in urinary bladder smooth muscle, *Acta Physiol Scand* 110:357, 1980.
24. Roelofs M: Plasticity of mesenchymal cells within the rabbit bladder wall in normal and pathologic conditions, doctoral thesis, University of Padova, Italy, 1995.
25. Gosling JA: The structure of the female lower urinary tract and pelvic floor, *Urol Clin North Am* 12:2, 207-214, 1985.
26. Rud T, Andersson K-E, Asmussen M, et al: Factors maintaining the intraurethral pressure in women, *Invest Urol* 17:343-347, 1980.
27. Zinner NR, Sterling AM, Ritter RC: Role of inner urethral softness in urinary continence, *Urol* 16:115, 1980.
28. Hilton P: Mechanism of continence. In Stanton SL, Tanagho E, editors: *Surgery of female incontinence,* ed 2, New York, 1986, Springer Verlag.
29. Enhörning G: Simultaneous recording of intravesical and intraurethral pressure, *Acta Chir Scand,* suppl 276, 1961.
30. Constantinou CE: Urethrometry: considerations of static, dynamic and stability characteristics of the female urethra, *Neurourol Urodyn* 7:521-539, 1988.
31. Colstrup H: Closure mechanism of the female urethra, *Neurourol Urodyn* 6: 271, 1987.
32. Lose G: Mechanical properties of the urethra in healthy female volunteers, *Neurourol Urodyn* 8:451-459, 1989.
33. Thind P: An analysis of urethral viscoelasticity with particular reference to the sphincter function in healthy women, doctoral thesis, University of Copenhagen, Denmark, 1995.
34. Torrens MJ, Morrison JFB, editors: *The physiology of the lower urinary tract, New York, 1987, Springer-Verlag.*

Chapter 6 Central Nervous System Control of Micturition

William C. de Groat

Micturition is controlled by neural circuits in the brain and spinal cord that coordinate the activity of visceral smooth muscle in the urinary bladder and urethra with the activity of striated muscle in the external urethral sphincter.[1-4] These circuits act as on-off switches to shift the lower urinary tract between two modes of operation: storage and elimination. In infants these switching mechanisms function purely in a reflex manner to produce involuntary voiding; however in adults urine storage and release are subject to voluntary control presumably mediated by the cerebral cortex. Thus the neural control of the urinary tract is distinct from that of other visceral organs such as the heart, blood vessels, and intestine, which are regulated exclusively by involuntary (autonomic) reflex mechanisms.

Injuries or diseases of the nervous system in adults can disrupt the voluntary control of micturition causing the reemergence of reflex micturition, which can result in bladder hyperactivity and incontinence.[3,4] Because of the complexity of the central nervous control of the lower urinary tract, incontinence can occur as a result of a variety of neurologic disorders. This chapter is a review of studies in animals and humans that have provided insights into the central nervous control of the lower urinary tract and how disruption of this control can alter the storage and elimination of urine.

Reflex Mechanisms Controlling the Lower Urinary Tract

As indicated in Fig. 6-1 and discussed in detail in this chapter, the lower urinary tract is innervated by three sets of peripheral nerves: (1) pelvic parasympathetic nerves, which arise in the sacral spinal cord, excite the bladder and relax the urethra; (2) lumbar sympathetic nerves, inhibit the bladder body and excite the bladder base and urethra; (3) the pudendal nerves excite the external urethral sphincter. These nerves also contain afferent (sensory) pathways. The most important afferents that are contained in the pelvic nerves trigger the sensation of bladder fullness and initiate reflex micturition.[5]

The central pathways controlling lower urinary tract function are organized as simple on-off switching circuits (Fig. 6-2) that maintain a reciprocal relationship between the urinary bladder and the urethral outlet.[1,2] The principal reflex components of these switching circuits are listed in Table 6-1 and illustrated in Fig. 6-3. Intravesical pressure measurements during bladder filling in both humans and animals reveal low and relatively constant bladder pressures when bladder volume is below the threshold for inducing voiding (Fig. 6-3, *A*). The accommodation of the bladder to increasing volumes of urine is primarily a passive phenomenon dependent on the intrinsic properties of the vesical

Table 6-1 Reflexes to the Lower Urinary Tract

Afferent pathway	Efferent pathway	Central pathway
URINE STORAGE Low-level vesical afferent activity (pelvic nerve)	1. External sphincter contraction (somatic nerves) 2. Internal sphincter contraction (sympathetic nerves) 3. Detrusor inhibition (sympathetic nerves) 4. Ganglionic inhibition (sympathetic nerves) 5. Sacral parasympathetic outflow inactive	Spinal reflexes
MICTURITION High-level vesical afferent activity (pelvic nerve)	1. Inhibition of external sphincter activity 2. Inhibition of sympathetic outflow 3. Activation of parasympathetic outflow to the bladder	Spinobulbospinal reflexes
	4. Activation of parasympathetic outflow to the urethra	Spinal reflex

smooth muscle and quiescence of the parasympathetic efferent pathway.[1,3,4] In addition, in some species urine storage is also facilitated by sympathetic reflexes that mediate an inhibition of bladder activity, closure of the bladder neck, and contraction of the proximal part of urethra (Table 6-1; Fig. 6-4). During bladder filling the activity of the sphincter electromyogram (EMG) also increases (Fig. 6-3, *B*), reflecting an increase in efferent firing in the pudendal nerve and an increase in outlet resistance, which contributes to the maintenance of urinary continence.

The storage phase of the urinary bladder can be switched to the voiding phase either involuntarily (reflexively) or voluntarily (Fig. 6-3, *B*). The former is readily demonstrated in the human infant (Fig. 6-3, *A*) or in the anesthetized animal when the volume of urine exceeds the micturition threshold. At this point, increased afferent firing from tension receptors in the bladder reverses the pattern of efferent outflow, producing firing in the sacral parasympathetic pathways and inhibition of sympathetic and somatic pathways. The expulsion phase consists of an initial relaxation of the urethral sphincter (Fig. 6-3, *A*) followed in a few seconds by a contraction of the bladder, an increase in bladder pressure, and the flow of urine. Relaxation of the urethral outlet is mediated by activation of a parasympathetic reflex pathway to the urethra[6] that triggers the release of nitric oxide, an inhibitory transmitter,[7] and by removal of adrenergic and somatic cholinergic excitatory inputs to the urethra. Secondary reflexes elicited by flow of urine through the urethra facilitate bladder emptying.[4,8]

These reflexes require the integrative action of neuronal populations at various levels of the neuraxis (Figs. 6-4 and 6-5). Certain reflexes, such as those mediating the excitatory outflow

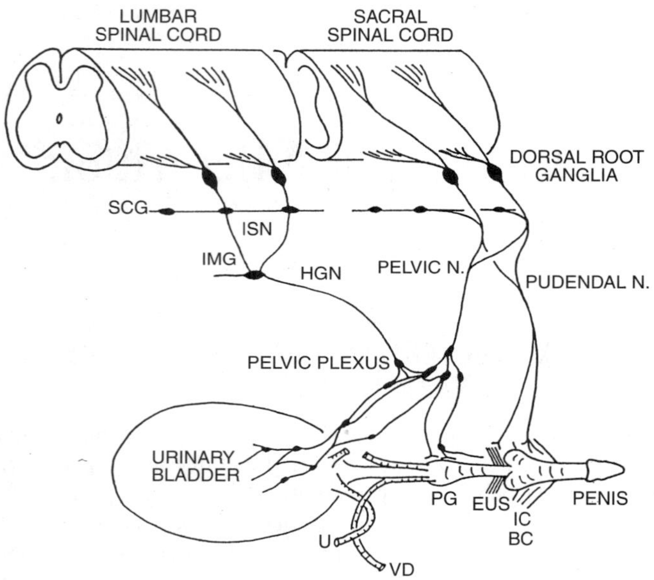

FIG. 6-1 *Diagram showing the sympathetic, parasympathetic, and somatic innervation of the urogenital tract of the male cat. Sympathetic preganglionic axons emerge from the lumbar spinal cord and pass to the sympathetic chain ganglia (SCG) and then in the inferior splanchnic nerves (ISN) to the inferior mesenteric ganglia (IMG). Preganglionic and postganglionic sympathetic axons then travel in the hypogastric nerve (HGN) to the pelvic plexus and the urogenital organs. Parasympathetic preganglionic axons that originate in the sacral spinal cord pass in the pelvic nerve to ganglion cells in the pelvic plexus and to distal ganglia in the organs. Sacral somatic axons are contained in the pudendal nerve, which provides an innervation to the penis, the ischiocavernosus (IC), bulbocavernosus (BC), and external urethral sphincter (EUS) muscles. The pudendal and pelvic nerves also receive postganglionic axons from the caudal sympathetic chain ganglia. These three sets of nerves contain afferent axons from the lumbosacral dorsal root ganglia. PG, prostate gland; U, ureter; VD, vas deferens.* (From de Groat WC: The neural control of urinary bladder and sexual function. In Bannister R, Mathias CJ, editors: *Autonomic failure,* ed 3, Oxford, 1992, Oxford University Press.)

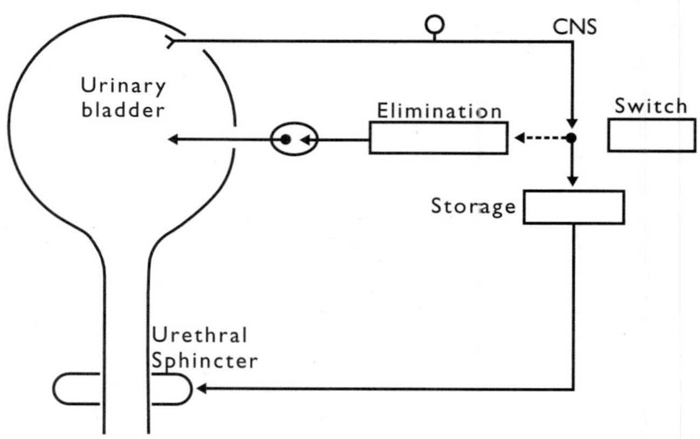

FIG. 6-2 *Diagram of the anatomy of the lower urinary tract and the switchlike function of the micturition reflex pathway. During urine storage, a low level of afferent activity activates efferent input to the urethral sphincter. A high level of afferent activity induced by bladder distension activates the switching circuit in the central nervous system (CNS), producing firing in the efferent pathways to the bladder, inhibition of the efferent outflow to the sphincter, and urine elimination.*

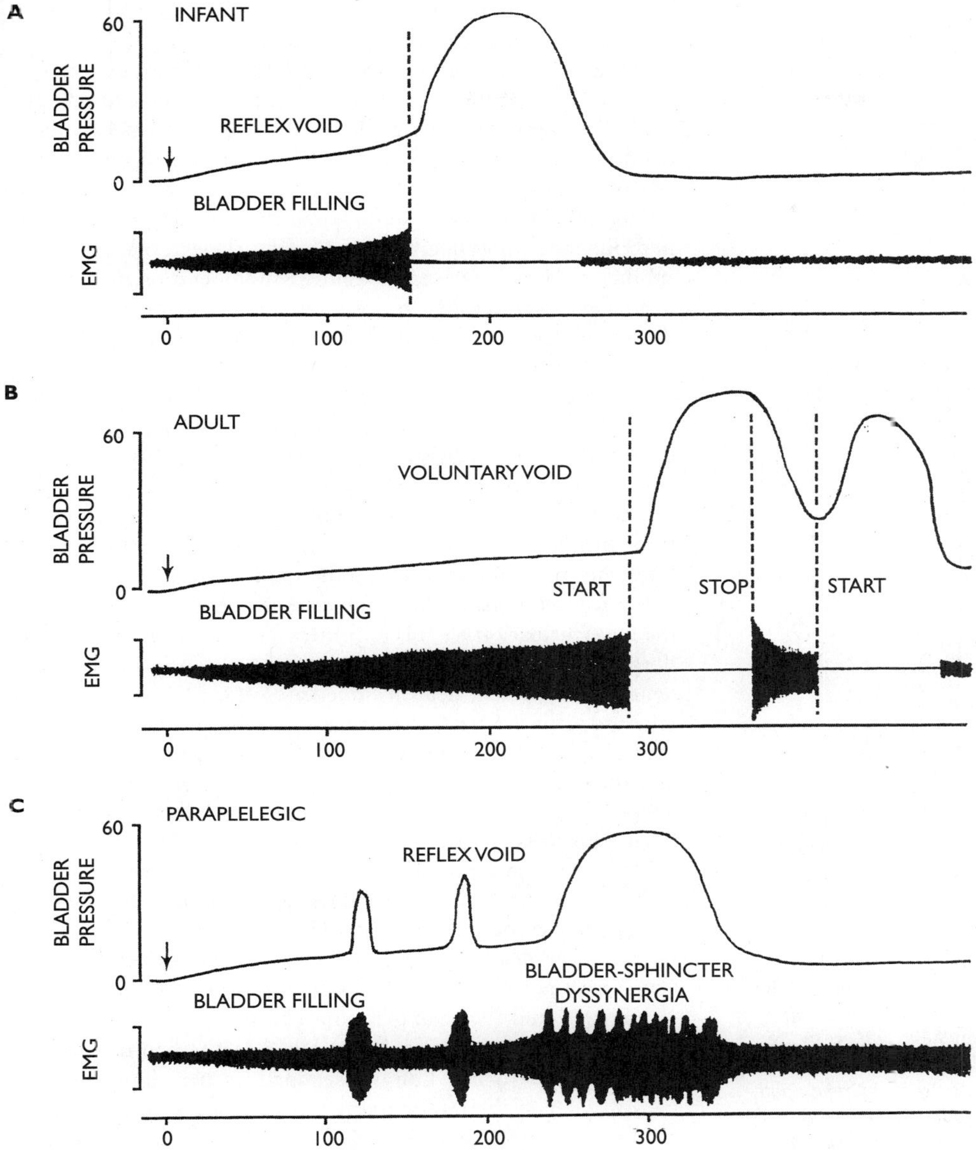

FIG. 6-3 *Combined cystometrograms and sphincter electromyograms (EMG) comparing reflex voiding responses in an infant,* ***A,*** *and in a paraplegic patient,* ***C,*** *with a voluntary voiding response in an adult,* ***B.*** *The abscissa in all records represents bladder volume in milliliters, and the ordinates represent bladder pressure in centimeters of water (cm H_2O) and electrical activity of the EMG recording. On the left side of each trace the arrows indicate the start of a slow infusion of fluid into the bladder (bladder filling). Vertical dashed lines indicate the start of sphincter relaxation, which precedes by a few seconds the bladder contraction in* ***A*** *and* ***B.*** *In* ***B*** *notice that a voluntary cessation of voiding (stop) is associated with an initial increase in sphincter EMG activity followed by a reciprocal relaxation of the bladder. A resumption of voiding is again associated with sphincter relaxation and a delayed increase in bladder pressure. On the other hand, in the paraplegic patient,* ***C,*** *the reciprocal relationship between bladder and sphincter is abolished. During bladder filling, transient uninhibited bladder contractions occur in association with sphincter activity. Further filling leads to more prolonged and simultaneous contractions of the bladder and sphincter (bladder-sphincter dyssynergia). Loss of the reciprocal relationship between bladder and sphincter in paraplegic patients interferes with bladder emptying.* (From de Groat WC, Steers WD: Autonomic regulation of the urinary bladder and sex organs. In Loewy AD, Spyer KM, editors: *Central control of autonomic functions,* Oxford, 1990, Oxford University Press.)

to the sphincters and the sympathetic inhibitory outflow to the bladder, are organized at the spinal level (Fig. 6-4), whereas the parasympathetic outflow to the detrusor has a more complicated central organization involving spinal and spinobulbospinal pathways (Fig. 6-5).

Anatomy of Central Nervous Pathways

The reflex circuitry controlling micturition has four basic components: spinal efferent neurons (autonomic preganglionic neurons and sphincter motoneurons), spinal interneurons, primary afferent neurons, and neurons in the brain that modulate spinal reflex pathways. New research methodology including transneuronal virus tracing,[8-12] intracellular labeling,[13] measurements of gene expression,[14,15] and patch clamp recording in spinal cord slice preparations[16-18] have recently provided many new insights into the morphologic and electrophysiologic properties of these reflex components. Neurotropic viruses, such as pseudorabies virus (PRV), have been particularly useful, since they can be injected into a target organ (urinary bladder, urethra, urethral sphincter) and then move intra-axonally from the periphery to the central nervous system where they replicate and then pass retrogradely across synapses to infect second- and third-order neurons in the neural pathways. Since PRV can be transported across many synapses, it could sequentially infect all the neurons that connect directly or indirectly to the lower urinary tract (Fig. 6-6). PRV has been used in the rat to identify neurons in the spinal cord and the brain involved in the control of the lower urinary tract.[8-11]

Pathways in the Spinal Cord

The spinal cord gray matter is divided into three general regions: (1) the dorsal horn, which contains interneurons that process sensory input (2) the ventral horn, which contains motoneurons; and (3) the intermediate region which is located between the dorsal and ventral horns and which contains interneurons

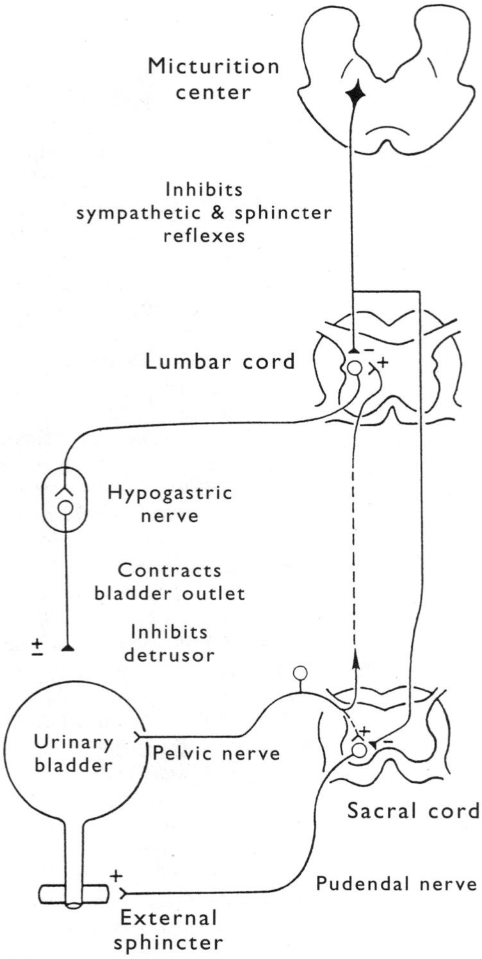

FIG. 6-4 *Diagram showing detrusor-sphincter reflexes. During the storage of urine, distension of the bladder produces low-level vesical afferent firing, which in turn stimulates (1) the sympathetic outflow to the bladder outlet (base and urethra) and (2) pudendal outflow to the external urethral sphincter. These responses occur by spinal reflex pathways and represent "guarding reflexes," which promote continence. Sympathetic firing also inhibits detrusor muscle and transmission in bladder ganglia. At the initiation of micturition, intense vesical afferent activity activates the brainstem micturition center, which inhibits the spinal guarding reflexes.* (From de Groat WC, Booth AM. Autonomic systems to urinary bladder and sexual organs, In Dyck PJ, Thomas PK, editors: *Peripheral neuropathy,* ed 3, Philadelphia, 1993, Saunders.)

and autonomic preganglionic neurons. These regions are further subdivided into layers, or laminae, which are numbered starting with the superficial layer of the dorsal horn (lamina I) and extend into the ventral horn (lamina IX) and to the commissure connecting the two sides of the spinal cord (lamina X) (see Fig. 6-8).

Preganglionic neurons. Parasympathetic preganglionic neurons innervating the lower urinary tract are located in the intermediolateral gray matter (laminae V to VII) in the sacral segments of the spinal cord[1,8,10] whereas sympathetic preganglionic neurons are located in both medial (lamina X) and lateral sites (laminae V to VII) in the intermediate gray matter of the rostral lumbar spinal cord. As shown in Fig. 6-7, parasympathetic preganglionic neurons send dendrites to discrete regions of the spinal cord including (1) the lateral and dorsal lateral funiculus, (2) lamina I on the lateral edge of the dorsal horn, (3) the dorsal gray commissure (lamina X), and (4) gray matter and lateral funiculus ventral to the autonomic nucleus.[1,13] As discussed below, this dendritic structure very likely indicates the origin of important synaptic inputs to these cells.

Sphincter motoneurons. Retrograde axonal tracing has identified pudendal motoneurons innervating the external urethral sphincter (EUS).[1,4,19-22] In the cat EUS motoneurons are located in the ventrolateral division of Onuf's nucleus and send dendritic projections into (1) the lateral funiculus, (2) lamina X, (3) intermediolateral gray matter, and (4) rostrocaudally within the nucleus (Fig. 6-7). The dendrites occur in bundles passing through restricted regions of the spinal cord. Thus the dendritic distribution of sphincter motoneurons (that is, lateral, dorsolateral, and dorsomedial) is similar to that of sacral preganglionic neurons, and such a similarity indicates that these two populations of neurons may receive synaptic inputs from the same interneuronal and fiber tracts in the spinal cord.

Afferent projections in the spinal cord. Afferent pathways from the lower urinary tract (LUT) project to discrete regions of the dorsal horn that contain the interneurons as well as the soma or dendrites of efferent neurons innervating the LUT. Pelvic nerve afferent pathways from the urinary bladder of the cat[1,23] and rat[24] project into Lissauer's tract at the apex of the dorsal horn and then pass rostrocaudally giving off collaterals that extend laterally and medially through the superficial layer of the dorsal horn (lamina I) into the deeper layers (laminae V to VII and X) at the base of the dorsal horn (Fig. 6-8). The lateral pathway that is the most prominent projection terminates in the region of the sacral parasympathetic nucleus (SPN) and also sends some axons to the dorsal commissure (Fig. 6-8). Bladder afferent axons have not been detected in the center of the dorsal horn (laminae III and IV) or in the ventral horn.

Spinal interneurons. As shown in Fig. 6-6, interneurons retrogradely labeled by injection of pseudorabies virus into the urinary bladder of the rat are located in the regions of the spinal cord receiving afferent input from the bladder, that is, autonomic nucleus, the dorsal commissure, and the superficial laminae of the dorsal horn.[8,9,22] Interneuronal locations also overlap in many respects with the dendritic distribution of the efferent neurons. A similar distribution of labeled interneurons has been noted after injections of virus into the urethra[10] or the external urethral sphincter,[11] indicating a prominent overlap of the interneuronal pathways controlling the various target organs of the lower urinary tract.

The spinal neurons involved in processing afferent input from the lower urinary tract have been identified by the expression of the immediate early gene, c-*fos*[14,15] (Fig. 6-2). The protein product of the c-*fos* gene can be detected immunocytochemically in the nuclei of neurons within 30 to 60 minutes after synaptic activation. In the rat, noxious[14] or nonnoxious[15] stimulation of the bladder and urethra and electrical stimulation of the pelvic nerves[25] increase the levels of *fos* protein primarily in the dorsal commissure, the superficial dorsal horn and the area of the sacral parasympathetic nucleus, the major sites of termination of afferents from the lower urinary tract (Fig. 6-8).

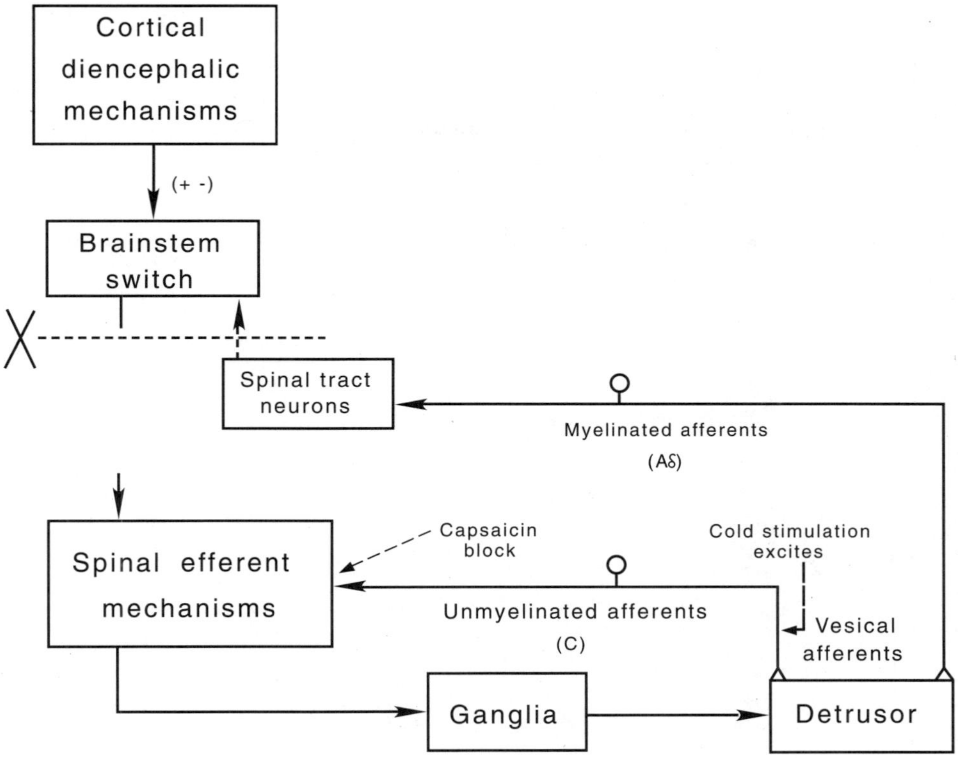

FIG. 6-5 *Diagram of the central reflex pathways that regulate micturition in the cat. In an animal with an intact neuraxis, micturition is initiated by a supraspinal reflex pathway passing through a center in the brainstem. The pathway is triggered by myelinated afferents (Aδ) connected to tension receptors in the bladder wall. In spinal animals, connections between the brainstem and the sacral spinal cord are interrupted (X) and micturition is initially blocked. In chronic spinal cord–transected animals, however, there emerges a spinal reflex mechanism that is triggered by unmyelinated (C-fiber) vesical afferents. The C-fiber reflex pathway is usually weak or undetectable in animals with an intact nervous system. Capsaicin (20 to 30 mg/kg, subcutaneously) blocks the C-fiber reflex in chronic spinal cord–transected cats but does not block micturition reflexes in intact cats. Infusion of cold water into the bladder excites C-fiber afferents and induces a voiding reflex in spinal cord–injured patients exhibiting automatic micturition.* (From de Groat WC, Kawatani M, Hisamitsu T, et al: *J Auton Nerv Syst* 30[suppl]:S71-S77, 1990.)

Pathways in the Brain

The neurons in the brain that control the lower urinary tract have been studied with a variety of anatomic tracing techniques in several species. In the rat, transneuronal virus–tracing methods have identified many populations of central neurons that are involved in the control of the bladder,[8,9] urethra,[10] and the urethral sphincter.[11] As illustrated in Fig. 6-6, injection of PRV into the bladder labeled several areas of the brainstem, including the laterodorsal tegmental nucleus (also known as Barrington's nucleus, or the pontine micturition center, PMC); medullary raphe nucleus, which contains serotonergic neurons; the locus ceruleus which contains noradrenergic neurons, periaqueductal gray, and the A5 noradrenergic cell group[8,9,22] Several regions in the hypothalamus and the cerebral cortex also exhibited virus-infected cells. Neurons in the cortex were located primarily in the medial frontal cortex. Similar brain areas were labeled after injection of virus into the urethra[10] and urethral sphincter,[11] and such labeling indicated that coordination between different parts of the lower urinary tract is mediated by diverse populations of neurons in the brain.

Other anatomic studies[27] in which anterograde tracer substances were injected into brain areas and then identified in terminals in the spinal cord (Fig. 6-9) are consistent with the virus-tracing data. Tracer injected into the paraventricular nucleus of the hypothalamus labeled terminals in the sacral parasympathetic nucleus as well as the sphincter motor nucleus. On the other hand, neurons in the anterior hypothalamus project to the pontine micturition center (PMC). Neurons in the PMC in turn project primarily to the sacral parasympathetic nucleus and the lateral edge of the dorsal horn and the dorsal commissure, areas containing dendritic projections from the preganglionic neurons, sphincter motoneurons, and afferent inputs from the bladder. Conversely, projections from neurons in the lateral pons terminate rather selectively in the sphincter motor nucleus (Fig. 6-9). Thus the sites of termination of descending projections from the pontine micturition center are optimally located to regulate reflex mechanisms at the spinal level.

Organization of Urine Storage and Voiding Reflexes

Storage Reflexes

Sympathetic pathways. Studies in animals indicate that sympathetic input to the lower urinary tract is tonically active during bladder filling.[1,2] Surgical or pharmacologic blockade of the sympathetic pathways can reduce urethral resistance, reduce bladder capacity, reduce bladder wall compliance, and increase the frequency and amplitude of bladder contractions.[1]

Sympathetic firing is initiated at least in part by a sacrolumbar intersegmental spinal reflex pathway which is triggered by vesical afferent activity in the pelvic nerves[1,27] (Fig. 6-4). This vesicosympathetic reflex represents a negative feedback mechanism whereby an increase in bladder pressure triggers an increase in inhibitory input to the bladder thus allowing the bladder to accommodate larger volumes of urine. The reflex pathway is inhibited during micturition, and this inhibition is in turn abolished by transection of the spinal cord at the thoracic level indicating that it originates at a supraspinal site, possibly the pontine micturition center (see Fig. 6-4).

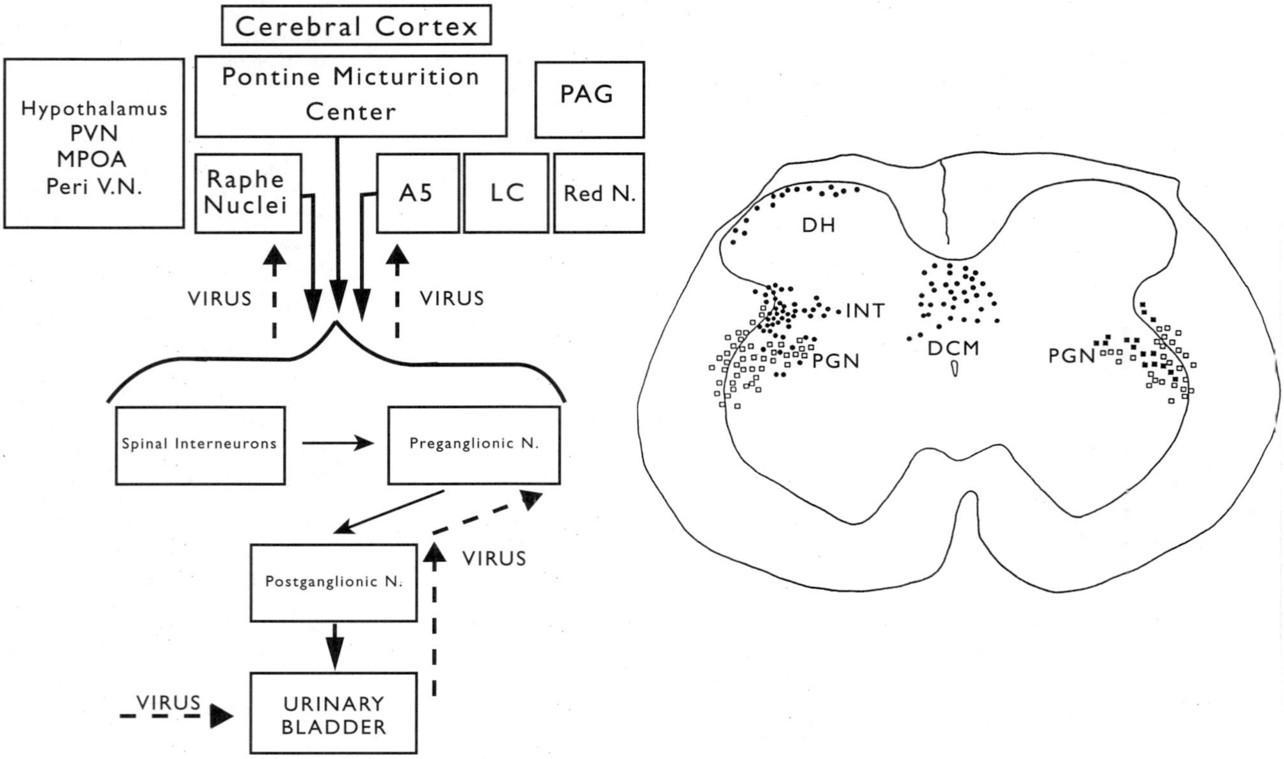

FIG. 6-6 *Transneuronal virus tracing of the central pathways controlling the urinary bladder of the rat. Injection of pseudorabies virus into the wall of the urinary bladder leads to retrograde transport of virus* (dashed arrows) *and sequential infection of postganglionic neurons, preganglionic neurons, and then various central neural circuits synaptically linked to the preganglionic neurons. Normal synaptic connections are indicated by* solid arrows. *At long survival times virus can be detected with immunocytochemical techniques in neurons at specific sites throughout the spinal cord and brain extending to the pontine micturition center in the pons (that is, Barrington's nucleus or the laterodorsal tegmental nucleus) and to the cerebral cortex. Other sites in the brain labeled by virus are (1) the paraventricular nucleus* (PVN), *medial preoptic area* (MPOA), *and periventricular nucleus* (PeriV.N.) *of the hypothalamus, (2) periaqueductal gray* (PAG), *(3) locus ceruleus* (LC) *and subceruleus, (4) red nucleus* (RN), *(5) medullary raphe nucleus, and (6) the noradrenergic cell group designated* A5. *L6 spinal cord section showing on the left side the distribution of virus-labeled parasympathetic preganglionic neurons (❑) and interneurons (●) in the region of the parasympathetic nucleus, the dorsal commissure* (DCM), *and the superficial laminae of the dorsal horn* (DH), *72 hours after injection of the virus into the bladder.* The left side *shows the entire population of preganglionic neurons (PGN) labeled by axonal tracing with the fluorescent dye fluorogold, injected into the pelvic ganglia.* The right side *shows the distribution of virus-labeled bladder PGN (■) among the entire population of PGN (❑). Composite diagram of neurons in 12 spinal sections (42 μm).* (From de Groat WC: Mechanisms underlying the recovery of lower urinary tract function following spinal cord injury, *Paraplegia* 33:493-505, 1995.)

Somatic efferent pathways to the urethral sphincter. The reflex control of the striated urethral sphincter is similar to the control of the sympathetic outflow to the lower urinary tract (Fig. 6-4). During bladder filling pudendal motoneurons are activated by vesical afferent input, whereas during micturition the motoneurons are reciprocally inhibited. The inhibition is dependent in part on supraspinal mechanisms, since in chronic spinal cord–transected animals and paraplegic patients it is weak or absent. In paraplegics the uninhibited spinal vesicosphincter excitatory reflex pathway commonly initiates a striated sphincter contraction in concert with a contraction of the bladder (bladder-sphincter dyssynergia)[3-4] (Fig. 6-3). This reflex interferes with bladder emptying.

Electrophysiologic studies in animals have revealed that sphincter motoneurons receive short-latency excitatory synaptic inputs from afferent axons in the pelvic and pudendal nerves as well as excitatory and inhibitory inputs from supraspinal pathways.[73] Electrical stimulation in the lateral pontine reticular formation, an area designated the "urine storage center" elicits an increase in sphincter electromyographic (EMG) activity and also inhibits bladder activity. On the other hand, stimulation in the medial pontine micturition center inhibits sphincter EMG activity.[26,30] These findings indicate that spinal reflex pathways that mediate urine storage are strongly modulated by descending input from the brain.

Voiding Reflexes

Spinobulbospinal micturition reflex pathway. Micturition is mediated by activation of the sacral parasympathetic efferent

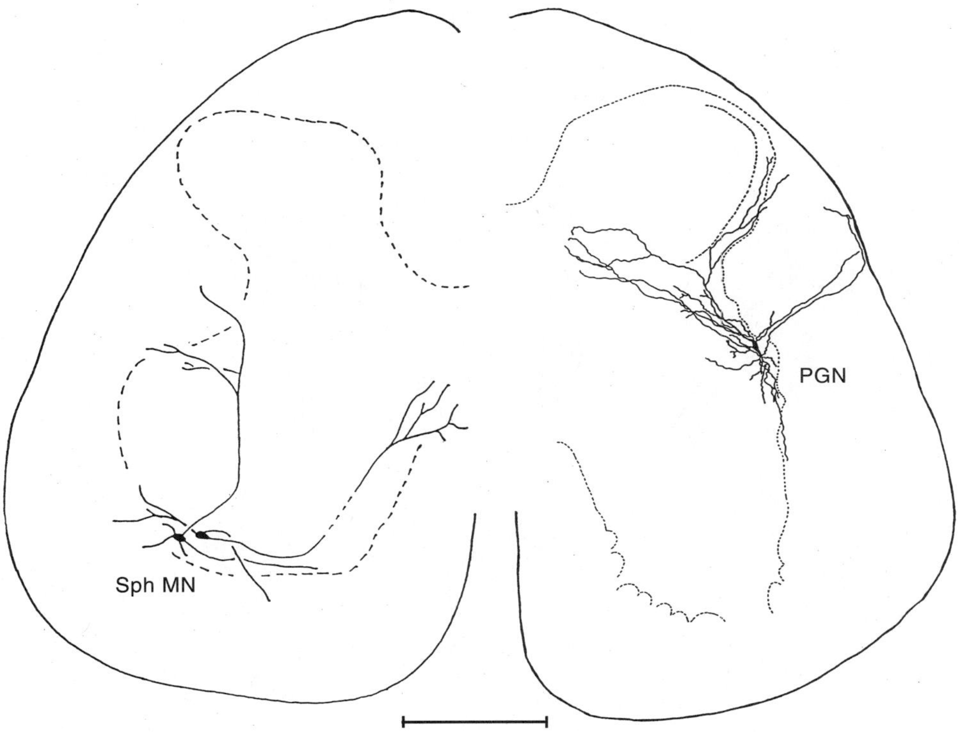

FIG. 6-7 *Comparison of the dendritic distributions of external urethral sphincter motoneurons* (Sph MN, left side) *and a sacral parasympathetic preganglionic neuron* (PGN, right side) *in the cat. The sacral preganglionic neuron that was filled intracellularly with neurobiotin exhibits dendrites that extend into (1) the lateral funiculus, (2) the lateral lamina I, (3) the dorsal commissure, and (4) the sacral autonomic nucleus. Dendrites were reconstructed from serial sections extending 500 μm rostral and caudal to the cell body. Two sphincter motoneurons* (left side) *were labeled by retrograde axonal transport after injections of cholera toxin–HRP (horseradish peroxidase) into the external urethral sphincter. Although the dendritic distributions are incomplete, they show prominent dendritic projections of one cell to lamina X around the central canal and projections of another cell to the intermediolateral region. Right and left sides are at sightly different rostrocaudal levels. Calibration represents 500 μm.* (From de Groat WC, Booth AM, Yoshimura N: Neurophysiology of micturition and its modification in animal models of human disease. In Maggi CA, editor: *The autonomic nervous system,* vol 3, *Nervous control of the urogenital system,* London, 1993, Harwood Academic Publishers.)

pathway to the bladder and the urethra as well as reciprocal inhibition of the somatic pathway to the urethral sphincter (Table 6-1) (Fig. 6-3, *B*). Studies in cats using brain-lesioning techniques revealed that neurons in the brainstem at the level of the inferior colliculus have an essential role in the control of the parasympathetic component of micturition[1,4,28,29] (Fig. 6-10). Removal of areas of the brain above the inferior colliculus by intercollicular decerebration usually facilitates micturition by elimination of inhibitory inputs from more rostral centers Fig. 6-10.[1,4,28,29] However, transections at any point below the colliculi abolish micturition. Bilateral lesions in the rostral pons in the region of the locus ceruleus in cats or the laterodorsal tegmental nucleus in rats also abolishes micturition, whereas electrical or chemical stimulation at these sites triggers bladder contractions and micturition.[1,4,28,30-32] These observations led to the concept of a spinobulbospinal micturition reflex pathway that passes through a center in the rostral brainstem (the pontine micturition center) (Fig. 6-5). The pathway functions as an on-off switch (Figs. 6-2 and 6-5) that is activated by a critical level of afferent activity arising from tension receptors in the bladder and is in turn modulated by inhibitory and excitatory influences from areas of the brain rostral to the pons (such as the diencephalon and cerebral cortex) (Figs. 6-5 and 6-10).

In contrast to the reflex control of the bladder, the parasympathetic control of the urethra in the rat appears to be dependent on pathways organized in the spinal cord[6,33] that are modulated by input from the brain. Nitric oxide–mediated relaxation of the urethra[7] that occurs in response to bladder distension is reduced but not eliminated by transection of the spinal cord. The reflex relaxation of the urethra is also very prominent in chronic spinal cord–transected rats.

Electrophysiologic studies in cats and rats have confirmed that the parasympathetic efferent outflow to the urinary bladder is activated by a long-latency supraspinal reflex pathway.[1,2,34-36] In cats, recordings from sacral parasympathetic preganglionic neurons innervating the urinary bladder show that reflex firing occurs with a long latency (65 to 100 msec) following stimulation of myelinated (Aδ) vesical afferents in the pelvic nerve.[1,3,34,36] Afferent stimulation also evokes negative field potentials in the rostral pons at latencies of 30 to 40 msec, whereas electrical stim-

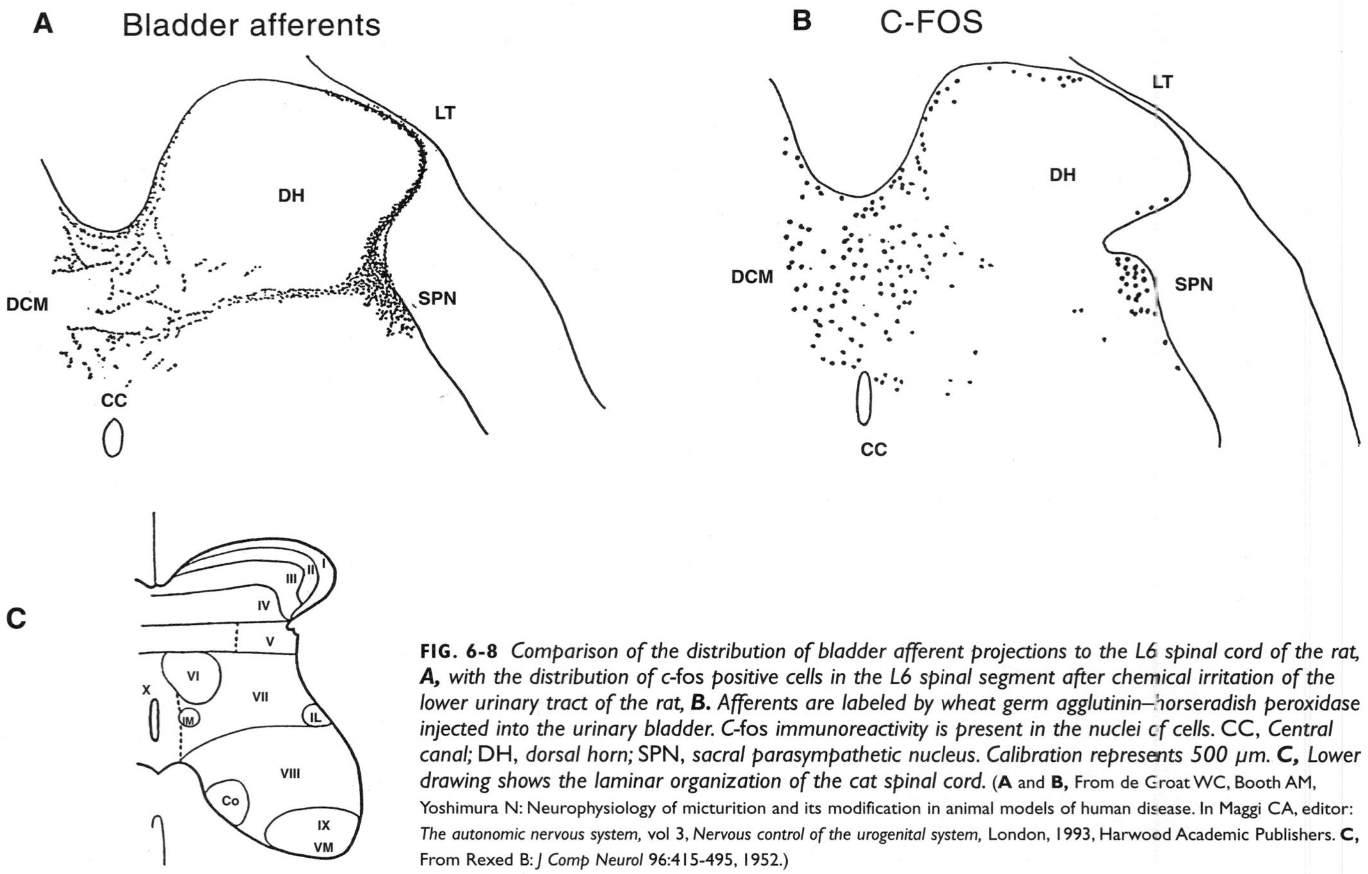

FIG. 6-8 *Comparison of the distribution of bladder afferent projections to the L6 spinal cord of the rat,* ***A,*** *with the distribution of c-fos positive cells in the L6 spinal segment after chemical irritation of the lower urinary tract of the rat,* ***B.*** *Afferents are labeled by wheat germ agglutinin–horseradish peroxidase injected into the urinary bladder. C-fos immunoreactivity is present in the nuclei of cells.* CC, *Central canal;* DH, *dorsal horn;* SPN, *sacral parasympathetic nucleus. Calibration represents 500 μm.* ***C,*** *Lower drawing shows the laminar organization of the cat spinal cord.* (**A** and **B,** From de Groat WC, Booth AM, Yoshimura N: Neurophysiology of micturition and its modification in animal models of human disease. In Maggi CA, editor: *The autonomic nervous system,* vol 3, *Nervous control of the urogenital system,* London, 1993, Harwood Academic Publishers. **C,** From Rexed B: *J Comp Neurol* 96:415-495, 1952.)

ulation in the pons excites sacral preganglionic neurons at latencies of 45 to 60 msec.[2] The sum of the latencies for the spinobulbar and bulbospinal components of the reflex pathway approximate the latency for the entire reflex.

Pontine micturition center (PMC) Physiologic and anatomic experiments have provided substantial support for the concept that neuronal circuitry in the PMC functions as a switch in the micturition reflex pathway. The switch seems to regulate bladder capacity and also coordinate the activity of the bladder and external urethral sphincter.[1,35] Electrical or chemical stimulation in the PMC of the rat, cat, and dog induces (1) a suppression of urethral sphincter EMG activity (2) firing of sacral preganglionic neurons, (3) bladder contractions, and (4) release of urine.[1,4,30,32,40] On the other hand, microinjections of putative inhibitory transmitters into the PMC of the cat can increase the volume threshold for inducing micturition and in high doses can completely block reflex voiding, two indications that synapses in this region are important for regulating the set point for reflex voiding and also are an essential link in the reflex pathway.[30] In addition, administration of antagonists for certain inhibitory transmitters (such as the GABA antagonist bicuculline or the opioid antagonist naloxone) can reduce the micturition volume threshold, and such a reduction indicates that the setpoint is under tonic inhibitory modulation.

Virus-tracing studies in the rat have revealed extensive labeling in the PMC (Fig. 6-6) after injections of virus into the bladder, urethra, and the external urethral sphincter.[8-11] These data are consistent with the view that neurons in this region coordinate the activity of all the major organs involved in voiding.

Spinal micturition reflex pathway Spinal cord injury rostral to the lumbosacral level eliminates voluntary and supraspinal control of voiding, leading initially to an areflexic bladder and complete urinary retention followed by a slow development of automatic micturition and bladder hyperactivity mediated by spinal reflex pathways.[1,3,4,37-39] However, voiding is commonly inefficient because of simultaneous contractions of the bladder and urethral sphincter (bladder-sphincter dyssynergia).

Electrophysiologic studies in rats and cats have shown that the reflex pathways in intact and chronic spinal cord–transected animals are considerably different. In both species, the central delay for the micturition reflex in chronic spinal cord–transected animals is considerably shorter (< 5 msec in rats; 15 to 40 msec in cats) than in intact animals (60 to 75 msec).[1,2,35,36] In addition, in chronic spinal cord–transected cats the afferent limb of the micturition reflex consists of unmyelinated (C-fiber) afferents, whereas in intact cats it consists of myelinated (Aδ) afferents[40] (Fig. 6-5). This was not only demonstrated with electrophysiologic recording but also by administering capsaicin,[40] a

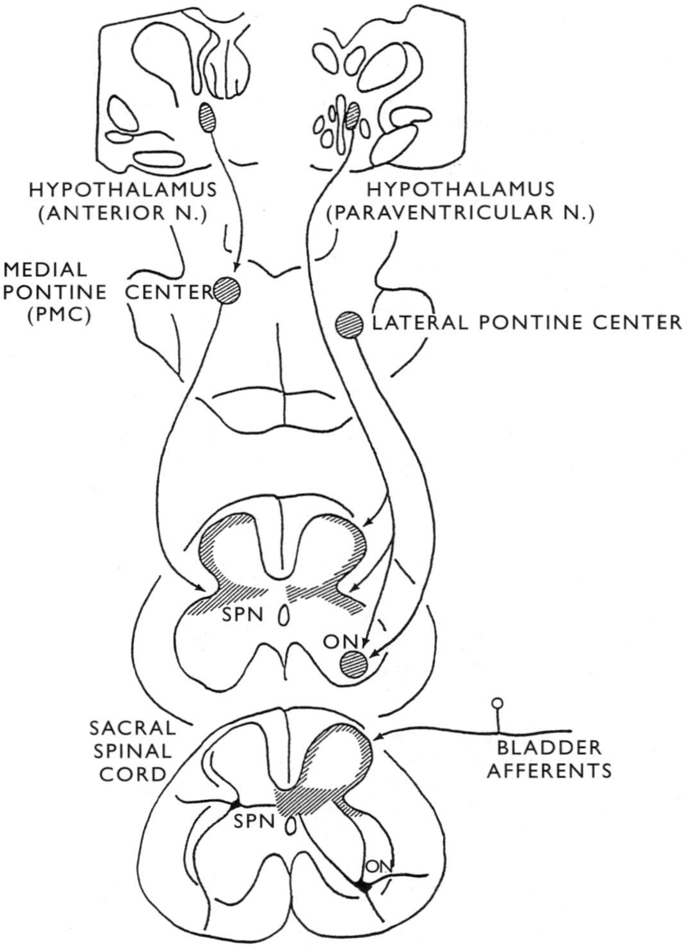

FIG. 6-9 *Neural connections between the brain and the sacral spinal cord that may be involved in the regulation of the lower urinary tract in the cat. Lower section of spinal cord shows location and morphology of (1) a preganglionic neuron in the sacral parasympathetic nucleus* (SPN), *(2) a sphincter motoneuron in Onuf's nucleus* (ON), *and (3) the sites of central termination of afferent projections from the urinary bladder. Upper section of spinal cord shows the sites of termination of descending pathways arising in the pontine micturition center (medial), the pontine sphincter or urine storage center (lateral), and the paraventricular nuclei of the hypothalamus. Section through the pons shows projection for anterior hypothalamic nuclei to the pontine micturition center.* (Based on studies of Holstege G et al.[26]) (From de Groat WC: Neural control of urinary bladder and sexual organs. In Bannister R, Mathias CJ, editors: *Autonomic failure,* ed 3, Oxford, 1992, Oxford University Press.)

neurotoxin that is known to disrupt the function of C-fiber afferents.[41] In normal cats, capsaicin injected systemically in large doses (30 to 45 mg subcutaneously) did not block reflex contractions of the bladder or the Aδ fiber–evoked bladder reflex. However, in chronic spinal cord–transected cats (3 to 6 weeks after spinal transection), capsaicin (20 to 30 mg/kg subcutaneously) completely blocked the rhythmic bladder contractions induced by bladder distension and blocked the C-fiber–evoked reflex firing recorded on bladder postganglionic nerves.[36,40] Thus there seems to be a considerable reorganization of reflex connections in the spinal cord after the interruption of descending pathways from the brain. C fiber afferent–evoked reflexes that are weak and occur in only 60% of cats with an intact neuraxis[36] are facilitated, whereas Aδ fiber afferent–evoked reflexes are completely eliminated in chronic spinal cord–transected animals. These data indicate that two distinct central pathways (supraspinal and spinal) utilizing different peripheral afferent limbs (A and C fiber) can mediate detrusor to detrusor reflexes in the cat (Fig. 6-5). The properties of the peripheral C-fiber afferent receptors also appear to be changed in the spinally injured cat. C-fiber bladder afferents in the cat usually do not respond to the bladder distension (that is, silent C fibers).[42] However, in chronic spinal cord–transected cats bladder distension initiates automatic micturition by activating C-fiber afferent neurons[12, 40] Thus a spinal injury must change the properties of these afferent receptors in the bladder. The mechanisms that may contribute to the emergence of C fiber–mediated bladder reflexes have been discussed in several recent papers.[1,12,40]

Other reflexes that are unmasked after spinal cord injury also appear to be mediated by C-fiber afferents. For example, it is known that instillation of cold water into the bladder of patients with upper motoneuron lesions induces reflex voiding (the Bors Ice water test).[43] This reflex does not occur in normal patients. Recently it has been shown in the cat that C-fiber bladder afferents are responsible for cold-induced bladder reflexes[44] (Fig. 6-5). Intravesical administration of a capsaicin solution to spinal cord injured patients blocks the ice water reflex, and such blocking indicates that it is mediated by C-fiber afferents in humans as well.[45,46] The ice water test is also positive in patients with multiple sclerosis, cerebrovascular disease, and Parkinson's disease, as well as in normal infants.[47-51] These observations indicate that cold-evoked bladder reflexes are mediated by a primitive spinal pathway that is present in the immature nervous system and then is suppressed during postnatal development as supraspinal mechanisms assume the dominant role in controlling micturition. However, when supraspinal controls are eliminated by spinal cord injury[43,46,50] or neurologic diseases, such as multiple sclerosis, that damage central pathways,[47] it appears that the spinal reflexes reemerge.

It is noteworthy that the cold-induced bladder reflex also has been detected in elderly patients who have uninhibited overactive bladders and an impaired perception of bladder fullness.[48] Since these patients did not exhibit other neurologic problems, it is possible that subtle cerebral dysfunctions that selectively affect micturition pathways eliminate supraspinal input to the spinal cord and allow the emergence of primitive bladder reflexes that can trigger bladder hyperactivity and incontinence.

Similar developmental and injury-induced changes are exhibited by a somatovesical excitatory reflex pathway that is activated by stimulation of perineal afferents in the pudendal nerve. This reflex, which is organized in the spinal cord, can be triggered in neonatal animals and human infants by tactile stimulation of the penis, vagina, and the surrounding perineum.[1,36,52-54] In many species of animals the perineal-bladder reflex is the principal mechanism for voiding until the spinobulbospinal micturition reflex becomes functional several weeks after birth. The reflex is activated when the mother licks the per-

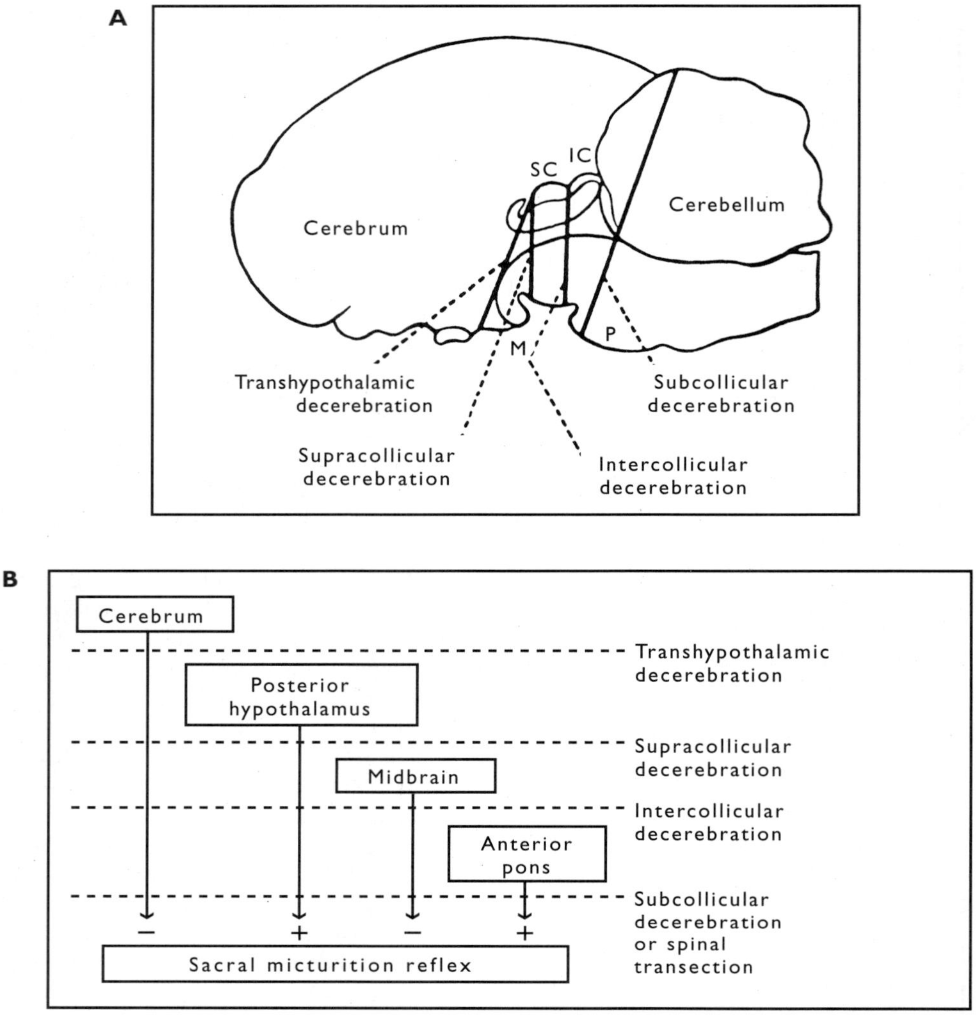

FIG. 6-10 *A, Drawing of sagittal section of the cat brain showing various levels of brain transections made in the study of the supraspinal control of micturition. SC, IC, Superior and inferior colliculi, respectively; M, midbrain; P, pons. B, Diagram indicating the net facilitatory and inhibitory actions of the various levels of the brain identified by the transection procedures shown in A.* (From Tang PC: Levels of the brain stem and diencephalon controlling the micturition reflex, *J Neurophysiol* 18:583, 1955.)

ineum. Thus separation of neonatal animals (such as rats and cats) from their mother leads to complete urinary retention.[53,55] As the brain control of voiding develops, the perineal-bladder reflex is suppressed; however it reappears after spinal cord injury in mature animals and humans.[1,36] In humans this spinal reflex is not essential, since the micturition pathways in the brain are functioning at the time of birth.

Other reflexes also emerge after spinal cord injury. For example, arterial pressor responses induced by bladder distension occur in spinal cord–injured patients and animals.[3,4,56] In normal and spinal cord–injured rats the increase in blood pressure induced by isometric bladder contractions or distension is suppressed by capsaicin, the C-fiber neurotoxin.[56,57] This is suggestive that C-fiber afferents mediate bladder-vascular reflexes in this species. Similar capsaicin-sensitive afferents may be responsible for autonomic dysreflexia in quadriplegic patients.

Capsaicin has also been evaluated clinically for the treatment of various types of neurogenic disorders of the lower urinary tract.[45,46,58-61] When administered intravesically in concentrations between 100 μM and 2 mM, capsaicin increases bladder capacity and reduces irritative symptoms in patients with hypersensitive bladders[41,58] and similarly increases bladder capacity and reduces the frequency of incontinence in patients with multiple sclerosis.[59,60] The effects of high concentrations of capsaicin in patients with multiple sclerosis persist for weeks to months after treatment, presumably because of degeneration of the bladder C-fiber afferents.

In preliminary studies on a small population of spinal cord–injured patients with detrusor hyperreflexia and autonomic dysreflexia, intravesical capsaicin treatment increased bladder capacity, depressed the micturition-contraction pressure, decreased autonomic dysreflexia, decreased urge incontinence and blocked the bladder-cooling reflex in some patients.[45,46,61] These observations indicate that capsaicin-sensitive, C-fiber bladder afferents may be involved in several pathologic conditions associated with neurogenic bladder hyperactivity.

Brain Modulation of Voiding

Cerebral cortex and diencephalon. Studies in humans indicate that the voluntary control of micturition is dependent on (1) connections between the frontal cortex and the septal-preoptic region of the hypothalamus and (2) connections between the paracentral lobule and the brainstem and spinal cord.[1,62] Lesions to these areas of cortex resulting from tumors, aneurysms, or cerebrovascular disease appear to indirectly increase bladder activity by removing cortical inhibitory control over the anterior hypothalamic area, which normally provides an excitatory input to micturition centers in the brainstem.[4]

In cats, lesion studies also revealed an inhibitory role of the cerebral cortex. For example, removal of the motor cortex on one side reduced bladder capacity (Fig. 6-10), and removal of the contralateral cortex further decreased capacity.[63] Subsequent decerebration did not elicit any additional change in bladder function. This indicates that the prominent facilitatory effect of decerebration observed in animals with an intact neuraxis[1,28,29] may be attributable in large part to the removal of tonic inhibition originating at the cortical level (Fig. 6-10). Cortical influences may be mediated by several projections to subcortical sites (the hypothalamus and pons), by extrapyramidal pathways to the brainstem, and by the corticospinal system as well.

The literature concerning the hypothalamic influences on lower urinary tract function is extensive (see reviews in references 1 and 4). Electrical stimulation of the anterior or the lateral area of hypothalamus of animals activates the sacral parasympathetic excitatory pathway to the bladder and induces bladder contractions and voiding. In the cat the effects of hypothalamic stimulation are probably mediated by actions in the brainstem as well as direct projections to the spinal cord. In addition to the anterior hypothalamic projections to the pontine micturition center[64-65] (Fig. 6-9), the lateral hypothalamic area projects to the parabrachial nucleus,[65] which reportedly has facilitatory effects on micturition.[4] The anterior, medial and paraventricular areas of the hypothalamus project to the central gray matter and medullary raphe nuclei. Electrical stimulation of the latter areas and adjacent reticular formation (such as the nucleus reticularis intermedius gigantocellularis) has been shown to exert prominent modulatory effects on bladder and urethral sphincter activity.[4,32,66] Thus hypothalamic control may be mediated by direct inputs to pontine and sacral micturition centers or by indirect mechanisms through other brainstem regions.

The influence of the hypothalamus on bladder function may in turn be modulated by afferent input from the bladder. Tracing studies in rats have identified a spinohypothalamic pathway arising from neurons in the region of the sacral parasympathetic nucleus.[67,68] Studies of c-*fos* gene expression showed that a large percentage of these neurons receive afferent input from the lower urinary tract.[68] This spinohypothalamic pathway may provide one means by which changes in bladder pressure modulate the firing of hypothalamic neurons.[69] This pathway also provides the anatomic substrate for putative spinohypothalamospinal and spinohypothalamopontine loops that could provide important modulatory control over micturition.

Midbrain. Lesion studies[29] indicated that the predominant effect of midbrain circuitry on bladder function is inhibition (Fig. 6-10). However electrical stimulation in the midbrain can produce excitatory as well as inhibitory effects.[1,28,31,70] One area of the midbrain that has attracted attention as a possible facilitatory micturition center is the periaqueductal gray (PAG). Electrical or chemical stimulation in the dorsolateral portion of the PAG and in the adjacent tegmental reticular formation produced bladder contractions in the cat[30] and also reduced the volume threshold for inducing micturition in the rat.[70] Since the PAG receives afferent input from the bladder[31] via spinal tract neurons in the intermediolateral region of the lumbosacral cord[1,71] and since it also receives prominent inputs from the hypothalamus, it may play a pivotal role in processing information before it is received by the PMC. Neurons in the ventrolateral PAG project to the PMC, raising the possibility that PAG neurons may be an important link in the micturition reflex pathway.

Medulla. Medullary centers have been implicated in both inhibitory and facilitatory modulation of the micturition reflex pathway. The two most prominent modulatory mechanisms are mediated by descending bulbospinal projections from the nucleus reticularis gigantocellularis (NRG) and from the caudal raphe nuclei.[4,8-10,72] Electrical stimulation in the NRG: (1) inhibits bladder motility, (2) reduces reflex firing in the pelvic nerve efferent pathways,[72] and (3) elicits both excitatory postsynaptic potentials and inhibitory postsynaptic potentials in sphincter motoneurons.[73]

Electrical or chemical stimulation of the nucleus raphae magnus (NRM), which is the origin of descending serotonergic projections to the spinal cord inhibits reflex bladder contractions and reflex firing in the sacral efferent pathways to the bladder of the cat.[32,72] Stimulation of the NRM also inhibits the firing of spinal dorsal horn neurons activated by afferents in the pelvic nerve.[74] Thus descending raphe spinal pathways may modulate bladder sensory mechanisms in the spinal cord, and this in turn may account for the inhibitory effect of raphe stimulation on bladder reflexes. In the rat and cat, raphe neurons are activated by bladder distension.[24,25] This raises the possibility that afferent input from the bladder may trigger a reflex loop resulting in activation of a raphe-spinal inhibitory pathway that could suppress the micturition reflex pathway at the spinal level.

Neurotransmitters in Micturition Reflex Pathways

Since the sacral parasympathetic reflex pathway to the bladder is essentially a positive-feedback circuit, it requires tonic inhibitory modulation to store urine properly and to prevent voiding at low bladder volumes. Damage to central inhibitory mechanisms after disease or injury to the nervous system leads to failure of urine storage and bladder hyperactivity and incontinence. Animal studies indicate that multiple transmitters may be involved in regulating transmission in the PMC (Fig. 6-11) and in the spinal cord (see references 1 and 72 for detailed summary).

Inhibitory Neurotransmitters

Several types of inhibitory transmitters, including (1) opioid peptides (enkephalins), (2) inhibitory amino acids (GABA, glycine), (3) 5-hydroxytryptamine (serotonin), (4) acetylcholine, (5) dopamine, and (6) nonopioid peptides (corticotropin-releasing factor, motilin, and neuropeptide Y) can inhibit the micturition reflex when applied to the central nervous system. Experimental evidence in anesthetized animals indicates that GABA and enkephalins exert a tonic inhibitory control in the PMC and regulate bladder capacity. The inhibitory effects are mediated by GABA-A and mu opioid receptors, respectively.[1,30,77] Administration of GABA-A or opioid receptor antagonists into the PMC reduced the micturition volume threshold, and such reduction indicates that the setpoint for reflex voiding is regulated by inhibitory mechanisms in the brain (Fig. 6-11).

GABA and enkephalins also have inhibitory actions in the spinal cord.[1,16,77] Baclofen, a GABA-B agonist that mimicks the inhibitory effect of GABA, has been used clinically by intrathecal administration in patients with hyperactive bladders to suppress bladder activity and to promote urine storage.[78]

Intrathecal administration of corticotropin-releasing factor (CRF), which is a peptide contained in PMC neurons and in descending pathways from the PMC to the lumbosacral parasympathetic nucleus in the rat, inhibits the micturition reflex in the rat,[1,79] This raises the possibility that CRF may be an inhibitory cotransmitter in the descending limb of the micturition reflex pathway.

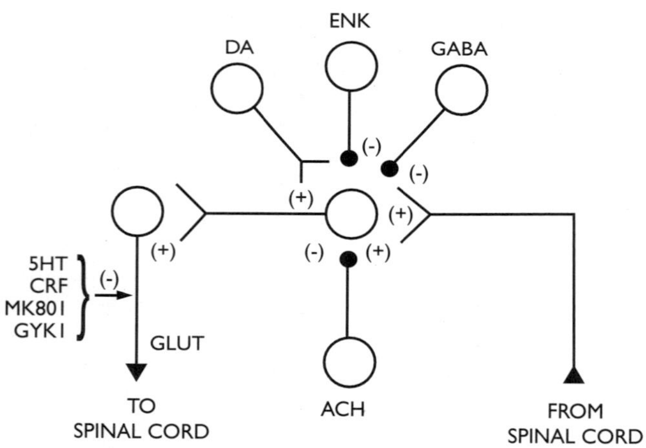

FIG. 6-11 *Diagram showing the variety of neurotransmitters that may regulate transmission in the pontine micturition center and in the descending limb of the micturition reflex pathway.* ACH, *acetylcholine;* CRF, *corticotropin releasing factor;* DA, *dopamine;* ENK, *enkephalins;* GABA, *γ-aminobutyric acid;* GLUT, *glutamic acid;* GYKI, *a non-NMDA glutamate receptor antagonist;* 5-HT, *5-hydroxytryptamine;* MK-801, *a noncompetitive NMDA (N-methyl-D-aspartate) glutamate receptor antagonist; (+), excitatory; (-), inhibitory synapse (indicated by filled circles). ACH has both excitatory and inhibitory effects in the pontine micturition center. Descending limb of the reflex can be depressed by 5-HT agonists, CRF, MK-801, and GYKI.* (From de Groat WC, Booth, AM, Yoshimura N: Neurophysiology of micturition and its modification in animal models of human disease. In Maggi CA, editor: *The autonomic nervous system,* vol 3, *Nervous control of the urogenital system,* London, 1993, Harwood Academic Publishers.)

5-Hydroxytryptamine (5-HT), which is present in a dense collection of terminals in the lumbosacral spinal autonomic nuclei and the sphincter motor nucleus,[80,81] is likely to have a complex role in the regulation of lower urinary tract function. The 5-HT–containing terminals are part of an extensive bulbospinal projection system that arises in the medullary raphe nuclei. Pharmacologic studies in animals indicate that this system may promote urine storage by exciting sympathetic and sphincter efferent pathways and inhibiting parasympathetic excitatory outflow to the bladder.[1]

Interest in the role of dopamine in the control of bladder function arises from the clinical observation that patients with idiopathic Parkinson's disease often exhibit bladder hyperactivity. Parkinson's disease is a disorder of basal ganglionic function caused by degeneration of dopamine-containing neurons. An animal model for Parkinson's disease has been developed in monkeys by administration of a neurotoxin (1-methyl-4-phenyl-1,2,36-tetrahydropyridine, MPTP) that destroys dopamine neurons.[76] Animals treated with MPTP show motor symptoms typical of Parkinson's disease and also have hyperactive bladders. Pharmacologic studies[76] in MPTP-treated monkeys revealed that the bladder hyperactivity was attributable to the loss of dopaminergic inhibition mediated by D1 dopaminergic receptors. On the other hand, D2 dopaminergic receptors can mediate a facilitation of micturition. The functional significance of these receptors is not known.

Excitatory Neurotransmitters

Excitatory transmission in the central pathways to the lower urinary tract may depend on several types of transmitters including (1) glutamic acid, (2) neuropeptides (substance P, vasoactive intestinal polypeptide), (3) norepinephrine, (4) acetylcholine, and (5) nitric oxide.

Glutamic acid[83] and norepinephrine[84] have been implicated as transmitters in bulbospinal excitatory pathways arising in the region of the PMC. Glutamic acid has attracted the most interest, since it is the major excitatory transmitter in the central nervous system. Experiments in rats indicate that glutamatergic transmission in the spinal cord is essential for bladder and urethral sphincter reflexes and for the spinal processing of afferent input from the urinary bladder.[85-89] Both *N*-methyl-D-aspartate (NMDA) and non-NMDA glutamatergic receptors have been implicated in transmission between the brain micturition center and the spinal preganglionic neurons[86,87] (Fig. 6-11). These receptors also mediate excitatory transmission between interneurons and preganglionic neurons.[17] Glutamic acid has also been identified as a mediator of a spinal micturition reflex pathway triggered by perineal afferents in neonatal rats[90] and by bladder distension in adult paraplegic rats.[91] Non-NMDA receptors are involved in these pathways. Thus glutamate is likely to be involved at various sites in the micturition reflex pathway.

Neuropeptides, such as substance P and vasoactive intestinal polypeptide (VIP), which are contained in a considerable percentage of bladder afferents[41,92,93] can modulate the micturition reflex when injected intrathecally. Intrathecal administration of substance P antagonists in rats suppresses reflex bladder activity induced by distension or chemical irritation of the bladder indicating that the peptide may be involved in several types of bladder reflexes in this species.[94,95] In the cat, VIP has been implicated as a C-fiber afferent transmitter that mediates automatic micturition in chronic paraplegic animals.[1,40]

Nitric oxide, which is present in nerve fibers and neurons in the spinal autonomic nuclei and at interneuronal sites in the spinal cord,[96-98] does not appear to function as a spinal transmitter in the normal micturition reflex in the rat.[99,100] However, intrathecal administration of an inhibitor of nitric oxide synthesis suppressed the bladder hyperactivity induced by chemical irritation of the bladder in rats.[99,100] This indicates that nitric oxide has a role in the spinal cord in the initiation of bladder hyperreflexia. Chronic chemically induced cystitis and damage to the pelvic nerves can also increase the expression of nitric oxide synthase in bladder afferent neurons,[101,102] raising the possibility that nitric oxide may have a more prominent transmitter function in afferent pathways in chronic inflammatory conditions affecting the lower urinary tract.

Summary

The lower urinary tract has two main functions: storage and periodic elimination of urine. These functions are regulated by a complex neural control system located in the brain and the spinal cord. This control system performs like a simple switching circuit to maintain a reciprocal relationship between the reservoir (bladder) and the outlet components (urethra and urethral sphincter) of the urinary tract. The switching circuit is modulated by various neurotransmitters and is therefore sensitive to a variety of drugs. Many neurologic diseases can disrupt voluntary control of micturition and unmask primitive voiding reflexes, which can induce urinary incontinence. A more complete understanding of the neurohumoral mechanisms involved in bladder and urethral control will no doubt facilitate the development of new diagnostic methods and therapies for incontinence.

References

1. de Groat WC, Booth AM, Yoshimura N: Neurophysiology of micturition and its modification in animal models of human disease. In Maggi CA, editor: *The autonomic nervous system,* vol 3, *Nervous control of the urogenital system,* London, 1993, Harwood Academic Publishers.
2. de Groat WC: Nervous control of the urinary bladder of the cat, *Brain Res* 87:201-211, 1975.
3. Van Arsdalen K, Wein AJ: Physiology of micturition and continence. In Krane RJ, Siroky M, eds: *Clinical Neuro-Urology,* ed 2, New York, 1991, Little Brown.
4. Torrens M, Morrison JFB: *The physiology of the lower urinary tract,* Berlin, 1987, Springer-Verlag.
5. Jänig W, Morrison JFB: Functional properties of spinal visceral afferents supplying abdominal and pelvic organs, with special emphasis on visceral nociception, *Prog Brain Res* 67:87-114, 1986.
6. Bennett BC, Kruse MN, Roppolo JR, et al: Neural control of urethral outlet activity in vivo: role of nitric oxide, *J Urol* 153:2004-2009, 1995.
7. Andersson K-E: Pharmacology of lower urinary tract smooth muscles and penile erectile tissues, *Pharmacol Rev* 45:253-308, 1993.
8. Nadelhaft I, Vera PL, Card JP, et al: Central nervous system neurons labelled following injection of pseudorabies virus into the rat urinary bladder, *Neurosci Lett* 143:271-274, 1992.
9. de Groat WC, Roppolo JR, Yoshimura N, et al: Neural control of the urinary bladder and colon. In Taché Y, Wingate D, Burks T, editors: *Proceedings of the Second International Symposium on Brain-Gut Interactions,* Boca Raton, Fl., 1993, CRC Press, pp. 167-190.
10. Vizzard MA, Erickson VL, Card JP, et al: Transneuronal labeling of neurons in the adult rat brainstem and spinal cord after injection of pseudorabies virus into the urethra, *J Comp Neurol* 355:629-640, 1995.
11. Erickson VL, Erdman SL, Vizzard MA, et al: The distribution of pseudorabies virus (PRV) labeled neurons in the central nervous system (CNS) following injection into external urethral sphincter (EUS), *Soc Neurosci Abstr* 20(1):115, 1994.
12. de Groat WC: Mechanisms underlying the recovery of lower urinary tract function following spinal cord injury, *Paraplegia* 33:493-505, 1995.
13. Morgan CW, de Groat WC, Felkins LA, et al: Dendritic morphology indicates separate types of lateral band preganglionic neurons in the sacral spinal cord of the cat, *J Comp Neurol* 331:161-182, 1993.
14. Birder LA, de Groat WC: Increased c-*fos* expression in spinal neurons after chemical irritation of the lower urinary tract of the rat, *J Neurosci* 12:4878-4889, 1992.
15. Birder LA, de Groat WC: Induction of c-*fos* gene expression in spinal neurons in the rat by nociceptive and non-nociceptive stimulation of the lower urinary tract, *Am J Physiol* 265:R643-R648, 1993.
16. Araki I: Inhibitory postsynaptic currents and the effects of GABA on visually identified sacral parasympathetic preganglionic neurons in neonatal rats, *J Neurophysiol* 72:2903-2910, 1994.
17. Araki I, de Groat WC: Glutamatergic excitatory postsynaptic currents evoked in preganglionic neurones by stimulating internuncial neurones in neonatal rat sacral parasympathetic nucleus, *J Neurolphysiol* 76:215-226, 1996.
18. de Groat WC, Vizzard MA, Araki I, et al: Spinal interneurons and preganglionic neurons in sacral autonomic reflex pathways. In Holstege G, Bandler R, Saper C, eds: *The emotional motor system: progress in brain research,* Amsterdam, 1996, Elsevier Science Publishers, pp. 97-111.
19. Thor KB, Morgan C, Nadelhaft I, et al: Organization of afferent and efferent pathways in the pudendal nerve of the female cat, *J Comp Neurol* 288:263-279, 1989.
20. Sasaki M: Morphological analysis of external urethral and external anal sphincter motoneurons of cat, *J Comp Neurol* 349:269-287, 1994.
21. Beattie MS, Li Q, Leedy MG, et al: Motoneurons innervating the external anal and urethral sphincters of the female cat have different patterns of dendritic arborization, *Neurosci Lett* 111:69-74, 1990.
22. de Groat WC, Yoshimura N, Roppolo JR, et al: Identification of bladder preganglionic (PGN) and interneurons (INTs) in the L6-S1 spinal cord of the adult rat using pseudorabies (PRV) and fluorogold (FG) dye tracing techniques, *Soc Neurosci Abstr* 20:114, 1994.
23. de Groat WC: Spinal cord projections and neuropeptides in visceral afferent neurons, *Prog Brain Res* 67:165-187, 1986.
24. Steers WD, Ciambotti J, Etzel B, et al: Alterations in afferent pathways from the urinary bladder of the rat in response to partial urethral obstruction, *J Comp Neurol* 310:401-410, 1991.
25. Birder LA, Roppolo JR, Iadarola MJ, et al: Electrical stimulation of visceral afferent pathways in the pelvic nerve increases c-*fos* in the rat lumbosacral spinal cord, *Neurosci Lett* 129:193-196, 1991.
26. Holstege G, Griffiths D, De Wall H, et al: Anatomical and physiological observations on supraspinal control of bladder and urethral sphincter muscles in the cat, *J Comp Neurol* 250:449-461, 1986.
27. de Groat WC, Lalley PM: Reflex firing in the lumbar sympathetic outflow to activation of vesical afferent fibres, *J Physiol (Lond)* 226:289-309, 1972.
28. Kuru M: Nervous control of micturition, *Physiol Rev* 45:425-494, 1965.

29. Tang PC: Levels of the brain stem and diencephalon controlling the micturition reflex, *J Neurophysiol* 18:583-595, 1955.
30. Mallory BS, Roppolo JR, de Groat WC: Pharmacological modulation of the pontine micturition center, *Brain Res* 546:310-320, 1991.
31. Noto H, Roppolo JR, Steers WD, et al: Excitatory and inhibitory influences on bladder activity elicited by electrical stimulation in the pontine micturition center in rat, *Brain Res* 492:99-115, 1989.
32. Chen SY, Wang SD, Cheng C-L, et al: Glutamate activation of neurons in cardiovascular reactive areas of the cat brain stem affects urinary bladder motility, *Am J Physiol* 265:F520-F529, 1993.
33. Fraser MO, Flood HD, de Groat WC: Urethral smooth muscle relaxation is mediated by nitric oxide (NO) released from parasympathetic postganglionic neurons, *J Urol* 153:461A, 1995.
34. de Groat WC, Ryall RW: Reflexes to sacral parasympathetic neurones concerned with micturition in the cat, *J Physiol (Lond)* 200:87-108, 1969.
35. Mallory B, Steers WD, de Groat WC: Electrophysiological study of micturition reflexes in rats, *Am J Physiol* 257:R410-R421, 1989.
36. de Groat WC, Nadelhaft I, Milne RJ, et al: Organization of the sacral parasympathetic reflex pathways to the urinary bladder and large intestine, *J Auton Nerv Syst* 3:135-160, 1981.
37. Kruse MN, Belton, AL, de Groat WC: Changes in bladder and external urethral sphincter function after spinal cord injury in the rat, *Am J Physiol* 264:R1157-R1163, 1993.
38. Kruse MN, de Groat WC: Spinal pathways mediate coordinated bladder/urethral sphincter activity during reflex micturition in normal and spinal cord injured neonatal rats, *Neurosci Lett* 152:141-144, 1993.
39. Kruse MN, de Groat WC: Consequences of spinal cord injury during the neonatal period on micturition reflexes in the rat, *Exp Neurol* 125:87-92, 1994.
40. de Groat WC, Kawatani M, Hisamitsu T, et al: Mechanisms underlying the recovery of urinary bladder function following spinal cord injury, *J Auton Nerv Syst* 30(suppl):S71-S77, 1990.
41. Maggi CA: The dual, sensory and efferent function of the capsaicin-sensitive primary sensory nerves in the bladder and urethra. In Maggi CA, editor: *The autonomic nervous system,* vol 3, *Nervous control of the urogenital system,* London, 1993, Harwood Academic Publishers.
42. Häbler HJ, Jänig W, Koltzenburg M: Activation of unmyelinated afferent fibres by mechanical stimuli and inflammation of the urinary bladder in the cat, *J Physiol (Lond)* 425:545-562, 1990.
43. Bors E, Comarr AE: *Neurological urology, physiology of micturition, its neurological disorders and sequelae,* Baltimore, 1971, University Park Press.
44. Fall M, Lindström S, Mazieres L: A bladder-to-bladder cooling reflex in the cat, *J Physiol (Lond)* 427:281-300, 1990.
45. Geirsson G, Fall M, Sullivan L: Effect of intravesical capsaicin treatment on postraumatic spinal detrusor hyperreflexia and bladder cooling reflex, *Neurourol Urodyn* 13:346-347, 1994.
46. Geirsson G, Fall M, Sullivan L: Clinical and urodynamic effects of intravesical capsaicin treatment in patients with chronic traumatic spinal detrusor hyperreflexia, *J Urol* 154:1825-1829, 1995.
47. Geirsson G, Fall M, Lindström S: Effect of menthol on the bladder cooling reflex in man, *Neurourol Urodyn* 10:374-375, 1991.
48. Geirsson G, Fall M, Lindström S: Cystometric subtypes of bladder overactivity: a retrospective analysis of 501 patients, *Int Urogynecol J* 4:1-8, 1993.
49. Geirsson G, Lindström S, Fall M, et al: Positive bladder cooling test in neurologically normal young children, *J Urol* 151:446-448, 1994.
50. Geirsson G, Lindström S, Fall M: The bladder cooling reflex in man: characteristics and sensitivity to temperature, *Br J Urol* 71:675-680, 1993.
51. Geirsson G, Fall M, Lindström S: The ice-water test: a simple and valuable supplement to routine cystometry, *Br J Urol* 71:681-685, 1993.
52. Thor K, Kawatani M, de Groat WC: Plasticity in the reflex pathways to the lower urinary tract of the cat during postnatal development and following spinal cord injury. In Goldberger ME, Gorio A, Murray M, editors: *Development and plasticity of the mammalian spinal cord,* Fidia Research Series, vol III, Padova, 1986, Liviana Press, pp. 65-80.
53. Thor KB, Blais DP, de Groat WC: Behavioral analysis of the postnatal development of micturition in kittens, *Dev Brain Res* 46:137-144, 1989.
54. de Groat WC, Douglas JW, Glass J, et al: Changes in somato-vesical reflexes during postnatal development in the kitten, *Brain Res* 94:150-154, 1975.
55. Capek K, Jelinek J: The development of the control of water metabolism, I. The excretion of urine in young rats, *Physiol Bohemoslov* 5:91-96, 1956.
56. Giuliani S, Maggi CA, Meli A: Capsaicin-sensitive afferents in the rat urinary bladder activate a spinal sympathetic cardiovascular reflex, *Naunyn-Schmiedebergs Arch Pharmacol* 338:411-416, 1988.
57. Cheng C-L, Ma C-P, de Groat WC: Effects of capsaicin on micturition and associated reflexes in the rat, *Am J Physiol* 265:R132-R138, 1993.
58. Maggi CA, Barbanti G, Santicioli P, et al: Cystometric evidence that capsaicin-sensitive nerves modulate the afferent branch of micturition reflex in humans, *J Urol* 142:150-154, 1989.
59. Fowler CJ, Jewkes D, McDonald WI, et al: Intravesical capsaicin for neurogenic bladder dysfunction, *Lancet* 339:1239, 1992.
60. Fowler CJ, Beck RO, Gerard S, et al: Intravesical capsaicin for treatment of detrusor hyperreflexia, *J Neurol Neurosurg Psychiatry* 57:169-173, 1994.
61. Sendor JF, Chancellor MB, Rivas DA, et al: Intravesical capsaicin in neurologic impaired patients with detrusor hyperreflexia, *J Urol* 155:592A, 1996.
62. Nathan PW: The central nervous connections of the bladder. In Williams DI, Chisholm GD, editors: *Scientific foundations of urology,* vol II, St Louis, 1976, Mosby.
63. Langworthy OR, Kolb LC: The encephalic control of tone in the musculature of the urinary bladder, *Brain* 56:371-382, 1933.
64. Holstege G: Some anatomical observations on the projections from the hypothalamus to brainstem and spinal cord: an HRP and autoradiographic tracing study in the cat, *J Comp Neurol* 260:98-126, 1987.
65. Moga MM, Herbert H, Hurley KM, et al: Organization of cortical, basal forebrain, and hypothalamic afferents to the parabrachial nucleus in the rat, *J Comp Neurol* 295:624-661, 1990.
66. McMahon SB, Spillane K: Brain stem influences on the parasympathetic supply to the urinary bladder of the cat, *Brain Res* 234:237-249, 1982.
67. Burstein R, Wang JL, Elde RP, Giesler GJ Jr: Neurons in the sacral parasympathetic nucleus that project to the hypothalamus do not also project through the pelvic nerve—a double labeling study combining Fluoro-gold and cholera toxin B in the rat, *Brain Res* 506:159-165, 1990.
68. Birder LA, Roppolo JR, Iadarola MJ, et al: C-*fos* as a marker for subsets of visceral second order neurons in the rat lumbosacral spinal cord, *Soc Neurosci Abstr* 16:703, 1990.
69. Stuart DG, Porter RW, Adey WR, et al: Hypothalamic unit activity. I. Visceral and somatic influences, *Electroencephalogr Clin Neurophysiol* 16:237-247, 1964.
70. Kruse MN, Noto H, Roppolo JR, et al: Pontine control of the urinary bladder and external urethral sphincter in the rat, *Brain Res* 532:182-190, 1990.
71. van der Horst VGJM, Holstege G: Afferent projections from the spinal cord to the periaqueductal gray in the cat, *Soc Neurosci Abstr* 18(1):311, 1993.
72. Morrison JFB, Spillane K: Neuropharmacological studies on descending inhibitory controls over the micturition reflex, *J Auton Nerv Syst Suppl* 393-397, 1986.

73. Mackel R: Segmental and descending control of the external urethral and anal sphincters in the cat, *J Physiol (Lond)* 294:105-122, 1979.
74. Lumb BM: Brainstem control of visceral afferent pathways in the spinal cord, *Prog Brain Res* 67:279-293, 1986.
75. Chandler MJ, Oh UT, Hobbs SF, et al: Responses of feline raphe-spinal neurons to urinary bladder distension, *J Auton Nerv Syst* 47:213-224, 1994.
76. de Groat WC, Steers WD: Autonomic regulation of the urinary bladder and sex organs. In Loewy AD, Spyer KM, editors: *Central regulation of autonomic functions,* Oxford, 1990, Oxford University Press.
77. Hisamitsu T, de Groat WC: The inhibitory effect of opioid peptides and morphine applied intrathecally and intracerebroventricularly on the micturition reflex in the cat, *Brain Res* 298:51-65, 1984.
78. Nanninga JB, Frost F, Penn R: Effect of intrathecal baclofen on bladder and sphincter function, *J Urol* 142:101-105, 1989.
79. Suzuki T, Kawatani M, Erdman S, et al: Role of CRF and 5-HT in central pathways controlling micturition in the rat, *Soc Neurosci Abstr* 16:1064, 1990.
80. Dahlström A, Fuxe K: The distribution of monoamine terminals in the central nervous system. II. Experimentally induced changes in the interneuronal amine levels of the bulbospinal neuron systems, *Acta Physiol Scand* 64(suppl 274):1-36, 1965.
81. Tashiro T, Satoda T, Matsushima R, et al: Convergence of serotonin, enkephalin- and substance P-like immunoreactive afferent fibers on single pudendal motoneurons in Onuf's nucleus of the cat: a light microscope study combining the triple immunocytochemical staining technique with the retrograde HRP-tracing method, *Brain Res* 481:392-398, 1989.
82. Yoshimura N, Mizuta E, Kuno S, et al: The dopamine D_1 receptor agonist SKF 38393 suppresses detrusor hyperreflexia in the monkey with parkinsonism induced by 1-methyl-4-phenyl-1,2,3,6-tetrahydropyridine (MPTP), *Neuropharmacol* 32:315-321, 1993.
83. Yoshiyama M, Roppolo JR, de Groat WC: Effects of MK-801 on the micturition reflex in the rat: possible sites of action, *J Pharmacol Exp Ther* 265:844-850, 1993.
84. Yoshimura N, Sasa M, Yoshida O, et al: α_1-Adrenergic receptor–mediated excitation from the locus coeruleus of the sacral parasympathetic preganglionic neuron, *Life Sci* 47:789-797, 1990.
85. Yoshiyama M, Roppolo JR, de Groat WC: Effects of MK-801 and CNQX, glutamate receptor antagonists, on the micturition reflex: comparison between unanesthetized decerebrate and urethane-anesthetized intact rats, *Eur J Pharmacol* 264:417-425, 1994.
86. Matsumoto G, Hisamitsu T, de Groat WC: Role of glutamate and NMDA receptors in the descending limb of the spinobulbospinal micturition reflex pathway of the rat, *Neurosci Lett* 183:58-61, 1995.
87. Matsumoto G, Hisamitsu T, de Groat WC: Non-NMDA glutamatergic excitatory transmission in the descending limb of the spinobulbospinal micturition pathway in the rat, *Brain Res,* 693:246-250, 1995.
88. Birder LA, de Groat WC: The effect of glutamate antagonists on c-fos expression induced in spinal neurons by irritation of the lower urinary tract, *Brain Res* 580:115-120, 1992.
89. Kakizaki H, Yoshiyama, M, de Groat WC: C-*fos* expression in spinal neurons after irritation of the lower urinary tract depends on synergistic interactions between NMDA and AMPA glutamatergic transmission, *Am J Physiol* 270:R990-R996, 1996.
90. Sugaya K, de Groat WC: Effects of MK-801 and CNQX, glutamate receptor antagonists on bladder activity in neonatal rats, *Brain Res* 640:1-10, 1994.
91. Yoshiyama M, Roppolo JR, Thor KB, et al: Effects of AMPA/kainate (LY215490) and metabotropic (MCPG) glutamatergic receptor antagonists, on the micturition reflex in rats, *Soc Neurosci Abstr* 21:1873, 1995.
92. de Groat WC: Neuropeptides in pelvic afferent pathways, *Experientia* 43:801-812, 1987.
93. Keast JR, de Groat WC: Segmental distribution and peptide content of primary afferent neurons innervating the urogenital organs and colon of male rats, *J Comp Neurol* 319:615-623, 1992.
94. Lecci A, Giuliani S, Maggi CA: Effect of the NK-1 receptor antagonist GR 82,334 on reflexly-induced bladder contractions, *Life Sci* 51:277-280, 1992.
95. Kawatani M, Matsumoto G, Birder LA, et al: Intrathecal administration of NK1 receptor antagonist, CP96345, inhibits the micturition reflex in the rat, *Regulatory Peptides* 46:392-395, 1993.
96. Vizzard MA, Erdman SL, Forstermann U, et al: Ontogeny of nitric oxide synthase in the lumbosacral spinal cord of the neonatal rat, *Devel Brain Res* 81:201-217, 1994.
97. Vizzard MA, Erdman SL, de Groat WC: The effect of rhizotomy on NADPH diaphorase staining in the lumbar spinal cord of the rat, *Neurosci Lett* 152:77-80, 1993.
98. Dun NJ, Dun SL, Wu U, et al: Nitric oxide synthase immunoreactivity in the rat, mouse, cat and squirrel monkey spinal cord, *Neurosci* 54:845-857, 1993.
99. Kakizaki H, de Groat WC: Role of spinal nitric oxide in the facilitation of the micturition reflex by bladder irritation, *J Urol* 155:355-360, 1996.
100. Rice ASC: Topical spinal administration of a nitric oxide synthase inhibitor prevents the hyper-reflexia associated with a rat model of persistent visceral pain, *Neurosci Lett* 187:111-114, 1995.
101. Vizzard MA, Erdman SL, de Groat WC: Increased expression of neuronal nitric oxide synthase (NOS) in visceral neurons after nerve injury, *J Neurosci* 15:4033-4045, 1995.
102. Vizzard MA, Erdman SL, de Groat WC: Increased expression of neuronal nitric oxide synthase (NOS) and Fos proteins in neural pathways following acute and chronic irritation of the urinary tract, *J Comp Neurol,* 370:191-202, 1996.

PART THREE · EVALUATION OF URINARY INCONTINENCE

Chapter 7 Office Evaluation of Incontinence

Lauri J. Romanzi, Jerry G. Blaivas

Many patients who have urinary incontinence delay consulting with a physician until the severity of incontinence interferes with their daily activities to an extent that their lives become restricted in what they can do. In an office evaluation of incontinence, it is the objective of the physician to provide the patient with as much information about their problem as possible and what the choices and solutions are that can resolve the problem. The various categories of incontinence have been reviewed elsewhere in this text and are briefly reviewed here in Table 7-1. Assessment of urinary incontinence begins with a thorough history and physical examination. The goals of the initial assessment for incontinence are to determine (1) the nature of the incontinence, (2) how long it has been present and to what degree it interferes with his or her lifestyle and activities, (3) whether there are any predisposing medical or surgical conditions, (4) whether there has been any prior surgical or medical therapy and the degree to which these therapies were successful, and (5) whether there is pelvic floor relaxation or other associated conditions (in women).

The nature and severity of the incontinence can be assessed with subjective, semiobjective, and objective data obtained from the history, supplemented by questionnaires, voiding diaries and pad tests, physical examination, cystourethroscopy, and urodynamic evaluation as delineated below.

INCONTINENCE HISTORY

The history begins with a detailed account of the precise nature of the patient's symptoms. Each symptom should be characterized and quantified as accurately as possible. When more than one symptom is present, the patient's own assessment of the relative severity of each should be noted. The patient should be asked how often he or she urinates during the day and night, how long he or she can comfortably go between urinations, and how long micturition can be postponed once he or she gets the urge. If frequency is a complaint, it should be determined why the patient voids as often as he or she does. Is it because of a severe urge or is it merely out of convenience or an attempt to prevent incontinence? The nuances of this issue were well illustrated in our recent review of 132 patients with detrusor overactivity. We found that 63% of patients with a primary complaint of frequency or urgency without incontinence actually did experience incontinence during involuntary detrusor contractions demonstrated at the time of urodynamic evaluation.[1] We believe that these patients have consciously or subconsciously altered their voiding habits so that they void frequently to avoid incontinence.

The severity of incontinence should be graded. Does stress incontinence occur during coughing, sneezing, rising from a sitting to standing position, or only during heavy physical exercise? If the incontinence is associated with stress, is urine lost only for an instant during the stress or is there uncontrollable voiding? Is the incontinence positional? Does it ever occur in the lying or sitting positions? Is there a sense of urgency first? Does urge incontinence occur? Is the patient aware of the act of incontinence or does he or she just find himself or herself wet (unaware incontinence)? Is there continuous involuntary loss of urine? Does the patient lose a few drops or saturate his or her outer clothing? Does he or she have postvoid dribbling or enuresis? Are protective pads worn? Do they become saturated? How often are they changed?

Is there difficulty initiating the stream, requiring pushing or straining to start? Is the stream weak or interrupted? Is there postvoid dribbling? Has the patient ever been in urinary retention? Is there incontinence or other bladder symptoms during sexual activity? In a subjective review of 54 women with stress, urge, or mixed incontinence, Clark and Romm found that 56% reported incontinence during vaginal intercourse, most frequently during penetration and orgasm.[2] The most common adaptive mechanism reported was precoital and postcoital voiding. There was no statistically significant difference between the diagnostic groups in this study, nor did results vary with age, parity, or estrogen status. Other investigators have found a higher incidence of sexual dysfunction among women with an element of detrusor instability.[3]

Table 7-1 Symptoms, conditions, and medicosurgical causes of urinary incontinence

SYMPTOM	CONDITION	MEDICOSURGICAL CAUSES
Urge incontinence	Detrusor overactivity	1. Idiopathic 2. Neurogenic 3. Urinary tract infection 4. Bladder cancer 5. Outlet obstruction
Stress incontinence	1. Sphincter hypermobility 2. Intrinsic sphincter deficiency	1. Pelvic floor relaxation 2. Prior urethral, bladder, or pelvic surgery 3. Neurogenic
Unaware incontinence	1. Detrusor overactivity 2. Sphincter abnormality 3. Extraurethral incontinence	1. Idiopathic 2. Neurogenic 3. Prior urethral, bladder, or pelvic surgery 4. Vesico-, Uretero-, or urethrovaginal fistula 5. Ectopic ureter
Continuous leakage	1. Sphincter abnormality 2. Extraurethral incontinence	1. Neurogenic 2. Prior urethral, bladder, or pelvic surgery 3. Ectopic ureter 4. Urinary tract–vaginal fistula
Nocturnal enuresis	1. Sphincter abnormality 2. Detrusor overactivity	1. Idiopathic 2. Neurogenic 3. Outlet obstruction
Postvoid dribble	Postsphincteric collection of urine	1. Idiopathic 2. Urethral diverticulum
Extraurethral incontinence	1. Vesico-, uretero-, or urethrovaginal fistula 2. Ectopic ureter	1. Trauma: surgical, obstetrical, other 2. Congenital

In women, symptoms of uterine or vaginal vault prolapse include pressure in the groin, sacral backache that resolves when the patient is lying down, and perineal wetness or bleeding from vaginal ulceration. In addition, many patients complain of a sensation of fullness or a "ball" protruding at the introitus, particularly when the bladder is full or when they exert themselves in the upright position. The patient may report difficulty voiding and a dribbling urine flow if the prolapse is severe (procidentia). They may also have concomitant sexual dysfunction or incontinence of feces or flatus caused by the underlying pelvic floor relaxation.

Women with cystocele may present with symptoms ranging from urinary retention to overt stress incontinence. Between the two extremes of this range fall symptoms of urgency and urge incontinence, frequency, straining to void, and a dribbling stream. The intensity of voiding symptoms do not directly correspond to the size of a cystocele. Some women with cystocele may be less symptomatic when supine when the cystocele is reduced. Others may enhance voiding by applying pressure on the anterior wall of the vagina. Symptoms of obstructive voiding may be replaced by stress incontinence when a pessary is inserted (Fig. 7-1).

Symptoms caused by a rectocele include the sensation of inability to empty the rectum of stool, or having to apply pressure on the posterior vaginal wall to evacuate. Constipation is not usually attributable to a rectocele alone. Sudden changes in bowel movements may require colon and rectal examination to rule out carcinoma.

PAST MEDICAL HISTORY

The patient should be specifically queried about neurologic conditions that are known to affect bladder and sphincteric function such as multiple sclerosis, spinal cord injury, lumbar disk disease, myelodysplasia, diabetes, stroke, or Parkinson's disease. If the patient does not have a previously diagnosed neurologic disease, it is important to ask about double vision, muscular weakness, paralysis or poor coordination, tremor, numbness, and tingling. A history of prostate or vaginal surgery or an operation for incontinence should indicate the possibility of sphincteric injury. Abdominoperineal resection of the rectum or radical hysterectomy may be associated with neurologic injury to the bladder and sphincter. Radiation therapy may cause a small-capacity, low-compliance bladder or radiation cystitis.

Medications may also exacerbate or, less commonly, cause incontinence. Sympatholytic alpha-adrenergic receptor blocking agents such as terazosin hydrochloride (Hytrin) and prazosin hydrochloride (Minipres) may cause stress incontinence by relaxing the intrinsic smooth muscle sphincter of the bladder. Beta-adrenergic receptor blocking agents such as propranolol (Inderal) and nadolol (Corgard) may enhance smooth muscle activity in

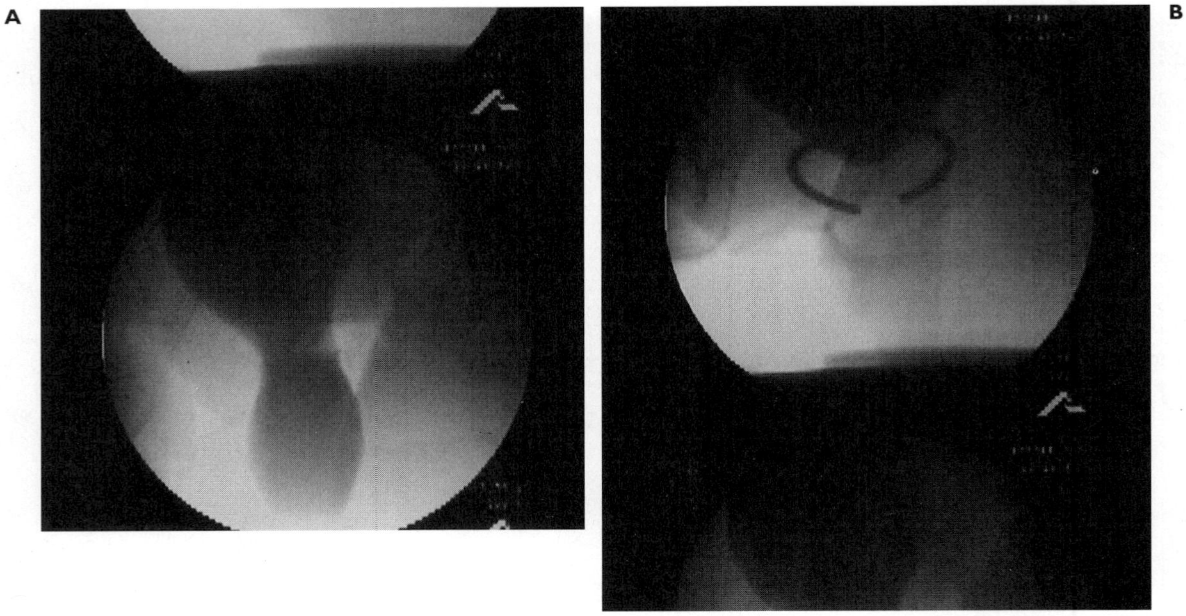

FIG. 7-1 ***A,*** *Cystogram of a woman with uterine procidentia and grade 4 cystocele. Notice the typical hourglass configuration.* ***B,*** *Placement of a ring pessary demonstrates reduction of the anatomic defect. Pessary insertions can be utilized both during physical assessment and cystometrics and may unmask stress incontinence in women with severe cystocele.*

the bladder dome, where the density of beta receptors is highest, and may exacerbate detrusor instability. On the other hand, sympathomimetic alpha-adrenergic receptor agonists such as ephedrine, pseudoephedrine, and phenylpropanolamine stimulate the smooth muscle of the vesical neck where alpha-adrenergic receptors predominate and may cause urinary retention or decrease stress incontinence. Parasympathomimetics such as bethanechol (Urecholine) or neostigmine (Prostigmin) may cause the symptoms of frequency and urgency by lowering the threshold for detrusor contractions. Parasympatholytics, or anticholinergics, such as dicyclomine (Bentyl), hyoscyamine (Levsin), and oxybutynin (Ditropan) block neuromuscular transmission and thereby inhibit detrusor contractions. These agents are common causes of urinary retention but may also result in overflow incontinence. Calcium-channel blockers such as nifedipine (Procardia) and verapamil (Calan) are utilized in the treatment of angina, arrhythmia, and hypertension and also may inhibit detrusor contractility. Tricyclic antidepressants such as imipramine (Tofranil) may induce tonic contraction of the smooth muscle of the intrinsic sphincter, causing bladder-outlet obstruction, urinary retention, and overflow incontinence. Benzodiazepines (Valium, Centrax, Ativan, and so forth) are powerful central striated-muscle relaxants and theoretically may exacerbate stress incontinence, though our practical experience has not reflected this effect.

In women, the hormonal status should be categorized as either premenopausal, menopausal, or postmenopausal. If postmenopausal, it should be noted whether she is receiving hormone replacement therapy, since hypoestrogenic atrophy of the urethral mucosa can have a negative effect on urethral coaptation. Obstetric history should include total number of live births, birth weights, delivery modes, and, if possible, length of second stage (the period between full dilatation and delivery). Heavier birth weight and long second stage of labor have been correlated with electromyographic evidence of pelvic floor nerve damage.[4] The patient should be asked whether the onset of incontinence was associated with pregnancy, childbirth, menopause, or surgery, becasue this can lend insight into the pathophysiology of her symptoms.

Bladder Questionnaire

We have found that a questionnaire can expedite the retrieval of all the above information. We have fashioned two questionnaires, one directed toward bladder symptoms and another addressing past medical history, medications, and allergies. These questionnaires may be sent to the patient before the office visit. The patient has the opportunity to ponder the questions and to acquire information, such as the names of medications and the dates of previous surgeries, before the office visit. The incontinence questionnaire (Appendix 7-A) is a section of the bladder questionnaire. The incontinence questionnaire is a one-page series of 11 questions, with a selection of five graded responses. Questions relate to urge and stress incontinence, number of pads used, amount of leakage, and a visual analog "bothersome score." The reproducibility (or test-retest) and accuracy of this questionnaire were validated at our institution.

Voiding Diary

To document the nature and severity of urinary incontinence a voiding diary and pad test are indispensable.[5] As long ago as 1979, Turner Warwick advised that the voiding chart is a "more useful guide to bladder function than endoscopy."[6] Information obtained from a voiding diary includes (1) total voided volume, (2) frequency of micturition, (3) mean voided volume, (4) largest single volume, (5) diurnal distribution, and (6) nature and severity of incontinence episodes. The International Continence Society (ICS) advised the inclusion of a frequency and volume chart in the patient's clinical assessment. The definition of functional bladder capacity by the ICS is the largest voided volume written in the patient's voiding diary.[7]

Can the voiding diary actually give you more data than a patient's history? We retrospectively reviewed randomly selected charts of 50 male and female patients presenting with a history of voiding dysfunction, focusing on nocturia. These 50 patients had completed a bladder questionnaire, and a history was taken before each patient had completed a 24-hour voiding diary. The recorded episodes of nocturia was compared to the reported number of times on the patient questionnaire. There was poor correlation of nocturia based on these two instruments even though both had been validated using test-retest data ($r = 0.29$, $p = 0.038$). This study obviously has implications for the accuracy of a patient's reporting on symptoms alone, without objective or semiobjective validation.

The patient is asked to complete a printed voiding diary for a single representative 24-hour period (Appendix 7-B). In the first column the time that the patient gets the first urge to void is recorded. In the second column the severity of the urge is subjectively graded on a scale from zero to 10. The actual time of urination is recorded in the third column. The fourth column records the measured voided volume, and in the fifth column the time and estimated amount of urinary leakage are recorded.

Pad Tests

Conceptually, a pad test will provide a semiobjective measurement of urine loss over a given period. Several pad tests have been described[7,8]; none has met with widespread approval, mainly because of poor test-retest validation.[9,10] The simplest pad test can be done when one has the patient change his or her pads every 6 hours for one representative 24-hour period while he or she is taking phenazopyridine Hcl (Pyridium) (200 mg tid). The amount of staining on the pads is a rough estimate of the severity of the incontinence. Alternatively the pads can be weighed and the total weight, minus the weight of an unused pad, recorded in the patient's record as an estimate of the volume of urine loss (1 g approximately equals 1 ml of urine). We believe that the pad test is very useful and recommend that, once it is completed, the patient simply be asked to state whether it was representative of his or her expected degree of incontinence or was better or worse than usual. If the patient states that the urinary loss was unusually large or small, that information is recorded and, if appropriate, the pad test is repeated.

Physical Examination

The physical examination begins by observing the patient's gait and demeanor as he or she first enters the office. A slight limp or lack of coordination, an abnormal speech pattern, facial asymmetry, or other abnormalities may be subtle signs of a neurologic condition. The abdomen and flanks should be examined for masses, hernias, and signs of a distended bladder. The lower extremities are then evaluated for gross motor coordination and strength. Patellar and Achilles deep tendon reflexes, bulbocavernosus and perianal reflexes, and sensation in dermatomes L1 to S5 are evaluated. Findings consistent with a sacral neurologic lesion included absent or diminished anal sphincter tone and control, absent bulbocavernosus reflex, and absent or diminished perianal sensation. Patients with suprasacral spinal neurologic lesions usually have characteristic changes below the level of the lesion including spastic paralysis, loss of sensation, hyperactive somatic reflexes, and abnormal Babinski reflexes.

In men, the prostate is examined. Hardness of the prostate is suggestive of prostate cancer, whereas an enlarged gland of normal or rubbery consistency is suggestive of benign prostatic hyperplasia. One assesses the bulbocavernosus reflex by suddenly squeezing the glans penis or pulling the balloon of a Foley catheter against the vesical neck. A visible or palpable contraction of the anal sphincter is the normal reflex response. The patient is then asked to cough and strain in the Valsalva maneuver, and the presence or absence of urinary incontinence is noted. If incontinence is not reproduced in the supine or lithotomy position, the examination is repeated in the standing position with a full bladder.

In women, a pelvic examination is performed with the bladder comfortably full in the lithotomy position. The patient is asked to cough or strain in an attempt to reproduce the symptom of incontinence. The degree of urethral hypermobility is assessed by Q-tip test. The Q-tip test is performed by insertion of a well-lubricated, sterile cotton-tipped applicator gently into and through the urethra into the bladder, or, alternatively, a rigid straight catheter such as those used for self-catheterization may be utilized. Once in the bladder, the Q-tip is then withdrawn to the point of resistance, which is at the level of the urethrovesical junction. The resting angle is assessed and recorded. The patient is then requested to strain as if constipated, and the degree of rotation is assessed and recorded. Hypermobility is defined as a resting or straining angle of more than 35 degrees from the horizontal. One then examines the anterior vaginal wall by applying gentle pressure on the posterior vaginal wall with the posterior blade from a split vaginal speculum. The blade, if metal, should be warmed with water and inserted into the vagina so that it depresses the posterior wall. While the patient is straining, the presence of a cystocele and cervical mobility are assessed. Women with cystoceles require careful examination in both lithotomy and sitting or standing positions. The design of our urodynamic chair allows the perineum to be visualized and examined while the patient is sitting. We have found incontinence present while the patient is sitting and not in a lithotomy position and vice versa. Careful reduction of the cystocele (either manually or with a pessary) in both positions may be necessary to demonstrate stress incontinence. The cervix is normally mobile, but descent to the hymenal ring is abnormal. After the anterior vaginal wall has been examined, the blade is then rotated and the anterior wall of the vagina is gently supported. The posterior vaginal wall and vault are examined for the presence of a rectocele or enterocele. As the speculum is slowly withdrawn, a transverse groove separating an enterocele from a rectocele below may be visible, and a finger inserted into the rectum can "tent up" a rectocele but not an enterocele.[11]

Pelvic floor strength is assessed by use of a clinical rating scale[12] as outlined in Table 7-2. With two fingers in the vagina, the patient is instructed regarding contraction of the pelvic floor. A properly performed contraction will displace the anterior vaginal wall in a caudal-ventral direction as the levator ani muscle contracts. The contraction is then rated for pressure generated, duration of palpable contraction, and vaginal wall displacement. Rectal sphincter tone and control are also assessed by rectal exam. The patient is asked to contract the anal sphincter around the examining finger as if she were trying to contain flatus or stop the urinary stream. A lax introitus or anal sphincter or the inability to actively contract either orifice may be signs of neurologic damage, but some women simply don't know or don't understand how to contract these muscles, whereas others may be too embarrassed to comply with the instructions. The bulbocavernosus reflex assesses the second through fourth sacral reflex arc. One can demonstrate it by tapping or squeezing the clitoris or tugging the inflated Foley balloon against the vesical neck. The absence of this reflex in men is almost always associated with a neurologic lesion, but the reflex is not detectable in up to 30% of otherwise normal women.[13]

If incontinence is not demonstrated in lithotomy or sitting positions, the examination is repeated in the standing position. The standing position also facilitates the diagnosis of prolapse in women and is particularly useful for distinguishing between an enterocele and a rectocele. The female patient should be positioned standing in front of the examiner with one foot elevated on a short stool. An enterocele will be palpable between the forefinger (in the rectum) and the thumb (in the vagina). If bowel is not palpable between the index finger and thumb, any posterior protrusion is a high rectocele. The perineal body and vaginal rectal septum are examined by palpation of the septum through the vagina and rectum.

The patient is then asked to void, and urowflometry is performed. If a uroflometer is not available at the time, the voided volume should be measured, so that a preliminary assessment of the approximate range of the patient's functional capacity can be provided. Thereafter, postvoid residual volume is assessed sonographically. Alternatively, straight catheterization can be utilized to both measure postvoid residual volume and obtain a specimen for urinalysis and culture. It is essential to diagnose and treat urinary tract infection when present because such infection can cause or exacerbate urinary incontinence. If urinalysis results and culture were previously obtained, sonographic assessment of bladder volume can be utilized to measure postvoid residual volume.

Women who present for evaluation with a pessary in place should be examined both with and without the pessary in the vagina. With the pessary in place, she should be checked for stress incontinence with a full bladder; without the pessary, the degree of prolapse should be assessed. The pessary is removed, and the patient should be upright and ambulatory for a minimum of 30 minutes before examination to allow an accurate assessment of the degree of prolapse. Not infrequently, patients with significant prolapse have seemingly good support even after many hours without pessary support, and maneuvers other than

Table 7-2 Pelvic muscle rating scale

	0	1	2	3
Pressure	none	weak	moderate	strong
Duration	none	<1 sec	1-5 sec	>5 sec
Displacement	none	slightly anterior	wholly anterior	gripped

ambulation may be necessary to demonstrate the defect after pessary removal. Alternatively the patient may leave the office without the pessary in place and return after the prolapse descends in the course of her daily activities. The vagina should be examined for any erosions or pudendal nerve injury from an ill-fitted pessary. Pudendal nerve injury is associated with paravaginal anesthesia, incontinence, worsening prolapse, and decreased anal sphincter tone.[14]

When evaluating the incontinent patient, one must bear in mind that more than one cause for involuntary urine loss may be present. Sphincteric incontinence commonly coexists with detrusor instability; vesicovaginal fistula may be associated with either or both of these conditions. In most instances vesicovaginal and urethrovaginal fistulas can be diagnosed on examination with a full bladder, but ectopic ureter, ureterovaginal, or vesicouterine fistula are usually not apparent and require intravenous pyelography, retrograde pyelography, cystography, or hysterosalpingography. A vesicovaginal fistula may be detected by instillation of indigo carmine or methylene blue into the bladder after insertion of a tampon into the vagina. The tampon is removed and assessed for discoloration after approximately half an hour. Cystoscopic examination of the bladder is almost always definitive and further delineates the location, size, and degree of inflammation of the fistula.

ROUTINE UROLOGIC ASSESSMENT

Routine laboratory studies include urinalysis, urine culture, and serum blood urea nitrogen (BUN) and creatinine (to evaluate renal function). Positive urine cultures should be treated with culture-specific antibiotics, but patients with persistent bacteriuria or recurrent infections may require invasive testing while receiving antibiotics. Hematuria should be evaluated by urinary cytologic methods, upper tract imaging studies, and cystourethroscopy.

CYSTOURETHROSCOPY

Although not necessary in all patients with incontinence, we find the cystoscopic examination to be quite useful for reasons that defy simple logic. In women with classic stress incontinence, the cystoscopic appearance of the bladder and urethra adds little to diagnosis but offers a degree of intimacy with the patient that helps more with the art than the science of medicine. It's nice to know the number and anatomic location of the ureteral orifices and their proximity to the vesical neck, the patient's reaction to passage of the cystoscope, and her pain threshold. Her reaction to bladder filling, bladder capacity, and reexamination and confirmation of the type of incontinence are all useful pieces of information. Finally, in some patients, incontinence may be demonstrated by reexamination with a full bladder after cystoscopy even though it was not reproduced during prior clinical and urodynamic examinations.

In a retrospective review of 99 incontinent female patients who had undergone both urethrocystoscopy and urodynamic testing, Scotti et al. found dynamic urethroscopy (evaluation of the urethra and bladder neck under direct endoscopic visualization at rest and during cough and straining) to have a sensitivity and specificity of 60% and 79% for the diagnosis of stress incontinence, as opposed to the urodynamic evaluation, which had a sensitivity and specificity of 95% and 100%.[15] Despite these findings, we continue to find cystoscopy quite useful, and, in patients who have previously undergone bladder or urethral surgery, it is important to exclude sutures and stones, whereas in those with urgency and urge incontinence, bladder tumor must be excluded.

To evaluate the urethra, one introduces a 0- to 30-degree lens after sterile preparation and urethral injection of lidocaine jelly. Despite recent studies to the contrary, we believe that local anesthesia provides a significant degree of comfort. Urethritis may appear as a shaggy, deeply erythematous, painful mucosal lining. An extremely pale appearance is consistent with postmenopausal atrophy of the urethral mucosa. It is also possible to visualize the orifice of a urethral diverticulum. If a urethral diverticulum is suspected, occlusion of the vesical neck by digital compression of the anterior vaginal wall may aid in distending the urethral lumen and allowing a greater possibility of visualizing a diverticular orifice.[16] Inflammatory polyps are common near the vesical neck. These are edematous, cystlike structures on a small stalk and do not appear to be of any great significance. Rarely, a benign fibroepithelial urethral polyp may be visualized on a long stalk. In patients who have undergone previous incontinence procedures or other pelvic or vaginal surgery, sutures that have damaged the integrity of the lower urinary tract by erosion or unrecognized misplacement at the time of operation can be visualized with the 0- or 30-degree lens. Patients with intrinsic sphincter deficiency (type III stress incontinence) may have obvious lack of closure of the vesical neck, and this observation will lend support to the diagnosis.

Once inside the vesical neck, a wide-angle 30- to 70-degree lens is used to inspect the interior of the bladder and to visualize the ureteral orifices. The flexible cystoscope is especially useful for detecting sutures just inside the vesical neck. In premenopausal women the trigone is frequently coated with a shaggy gray epithelium. Embryologically the trigone is of mesodermal origin, whereas the remainder of the bladder is endodermal, which may be a factor in the presence of this anatomic finding. Histologically this shaggy layer is a squamous metaplasia and is not pathologic by itself. Attention is then turned to the remainder of the bladder wall, which is systematically inspected in a circumferential fashion. Observations are made as to the presence and degree of trabeculation and any mucosal lesions or stones. If found, bladder diverticula are inspected for intraluminal stones and tumors. Careful inspection for the orifice of an ectopic ureter or urinary fistula should be carried out when suspected. Finally the cystoscopic bladder capacity is assessed and recorded.

In men with incontinence after prostatectomy, the cystoscopic view is extremely important to assess for the presence of scars, strictures, retained sutures, and stones. In addition, the pliability of the urethral wall is important for determining whether it is feasible to consider injectable agents such as collagen.

"Eyeball Urodynamics"

Urodynamic technique varies from "eyeball urodynamics" to sophisticated multichannel synchronous video/pressure/flow/EMG studies. We believe that synchronous multichannel videourodynamics (which is reviewed elsewhere in this book) offers the most comprehensive, artifact-free means of arriving at a precise diagnosis, and we perform them routinely when urodynamics are indicated. When multichannel studies are not routinely performed, they should be considered under the following circumstances: (1) when simpler diagnostic tests have been inconclusive, (2) when the patient complains of incontinence, but it cannot be demonstrated clinically, (3) in patients who have previously undergone corrective surgery for incontinence, (4) in patients who have previously undergone radical pelvic surgery, such as abdominoperineal resection of the rectum or radical hysterectomy, (5) in patients with known or suspected neurologic disorder that might interfere with bladder or sphincter function, that is, myelodysplasia, spinal cord injury, multiple sclerosis, herniated disk, cerebrovascular accident, Parkinson's disease, and Shy-Drager syndrome, and (6) in most men with incontinence. With these categories in mind, simple, or "eyeball," urodynamics can be a very useful, convenient, low-cost method, particularly when one is assessing women with an uncomplicated history of stress incontinence, findings of pelvic floor relaxation, and no history of prior vaginal or incontinence operations.

"Eyeball urodynamics" is performed with the patient in the lithotomy position. A Foley catheter is inserted, and the postvoid residual urine is measured. A 60-ml catheter-tipped syringe is connected to the Foley catheter after the barrel has been removed. Water or saline solution is then poured in through the open end of the syringe and allowed to drip into the bladder by gravity. As the water level in the syringe falls, its meniscus represents the intravesical pressure, which can be estimated in centimeters of water above the symphysis pubis. When the water level in the syringe falls to the level of the catheter tip, it is refilled.

During bladder filling the patient is told to neither void nor try to inhibit micturition but to simply report his or her sensations to the examiner. When the patient perceives the urge to void, he or she is asked if that is the usual feeling that is experienced when the need to urinate is felt. Changes in intravesical pressure are demonstrated by a slowing down in the rate of fall or a rise in the level of the fluid meniscus. A change in pressure may be caused by a detrusor contraction, an increase in abdominal pressure, or by low bladder wall compliance. As soon as a change in pressure is noted, the examiner should attempt to determine the cause. Visual inspection will usually belie abdominal straining, but in doubtful cases the abdomen should be palpated. In most instances the cause of the rise in intravesical pressure will be obvious, but when in doubt, formal cystometry with rectal pressure monitoring is necessary.

Any sudden rise in pressure that is accompanied by an urge to void or by incontinence is an involuntary detrusor contraction. In some instances the cause of the patient's incontinence is easily discernible as uncontrollable voiding around the catheter during an involuntary detrusor contraction. If involuntary detrusor contractions do not occur, the bladder is filled until a normal urge to void is experienced. The bladder is left full, and the catheter is removed. The presence or absence of gravitational urinary loss is noted. The patient is asked to cough and bear down with gradually increasing force to determine the ease with which incontinence may be produced. In women, the introitus is observed for signs of cystourethrocele, rectocele, enterocele, and uterine or vaginal vault prolapse, as outlined under physical examination.

If the patient complains of urinary incontinence, but it has not been demonstrated, the examination should be repeated in the standing position. In women, it is best performed by having the patient stand with one foot on a small stool. The examiner sits beside her and performs a vaginal exam while she coughs and strains. If the examiner is still unable to detect the incontinence, the patient is given a prescription for a urinary dye, such as Pyridium, and asked to complete a pad test as outlined above.

Conclusion

The collection of subjective, semiobjective, and objective data, as outlined above, allows for comprehensive evaluation of the incontinent woman. These results will serve to direct further evaluation and the treatment plan in an efficient, effective manner.

References

1. Blaivas JG, Romanzi LJ, Heritz DM: *Characterization of detrusor overactivity* [Abstract], annual meeting, Baltimore, 1995, American Urological Association.
2. Clark A, Romm J: Effect of urinary incontinence on sexual activity in women, *J Repro Med* 38:679, 1993.
3. Hilton P: Urinary incontinence during sexual intercourse: a common, but rarely volunteered, symptom, *Br J Obstet Gynaecol* 95:377, 1989.
4. Allen RE, Hosker GL, Smith ARB, Warrell DW: Pelvic floor damage and childbirth: a neurophysiological study, *Br J Obstet Gynaecol* 97:770, 1990.
5. Larsson G, Victor A: Micturition patterns in a healthy female population studied with a frequency/volume chart, *Scand J Urol Nephrol* 114:53, 1988.
6. Turner Warwick R, Milroy E: A reappraisal of the value of routine urological procedures in the assessment of urodynamic process in the assessment of urodynamic function, *Urol Clin North Am* 6:163, 1979.
7. Abrams P, Blaivas JG, Stanton SL, Andersen JT: The standardization of terminology of lower urinary tract function, *Scand J Urol Nephrol* 114(suppl):5, 1988.
8. Hahn I, Fall M: Objective quantification of stress urinary incontinence: a short, reproducible, provocative pad-weighing test, *Neurourol Urodyn* 10:475, 1991.
9. Christensen SJ, Colstrup H, Hertz JB, et al: Inter- and intra-departmental variations of the perineal pad-weighing test, *Neurourol Urodyn* 5:23, 1986.
10. Lose G, Gammelgaard J, Jørgensen TJ: The one-hour pad-weighing test: reproducibility and the correlation between the test result, start volume in the bladder and the diuresis, *Neurourol Urodyn* 5:17, 1986.
11. Zacharin RF: *Pelvic floor anatomy and the surgery of pulsion enterocoele,* Vienna, 1985, Springer-Verlag, p 77.
12. Worth AM, Dougherty MC, McKey PL: Development and testing of the circumvaginal muscles rating scale, *Nurs Res* 35:166, 1986.
13. Blaivas JG: The bulbocavernosus reflex in urology: a prospective study of 299 patients, *J Urol* 126:197, 1981.
14. Bruskewitz R: Female incontinence: signs and symptoms. In Raz S, editor: *Female urology,* Philadelphia, 1983, Saunders.
15. Scotti RJ, Ostergard DR, Guillaume AA, Kohatsu KE: Predictive value of urethroscopy as compared to urodynamics in the diagnosis of genuine stress incontinence, *J Repro Med* 35:772, 1990
16. Boyd SD, Raz S: Female urethral diverticula. In Raz S: *Female urology,* Philadelphia, 1983, Saunders.

Chapter 8 The Incontinence History and Physical Examination

Larry T. Sirls, Jong M. Choe

On a daily basis, a clinician may encounter a child with enuresis, a woman with stress incontinence, a man with postprostatectomy incontinence, or a geriatric patient with functional incontinence. This range of varying pathologic processes demands a consistent thoughtful approach, one that guides the clinician to the appropriate therapy or determines the need for additional diagnostic tests. The intial guidance toward appropriate diagnostic evaluation and subsequent treatment is provided by the urologic history and physical examination.

Nomenclature

Incontinence is defined as any involuntary loss of urine. Further descriptive terms are used to characterize urinary incontinence based on symptoms relayed by the patient. *Total incontinence* occurs at all times, day and night, regardless of stress maneuvers or positional change. *Urge incontinence* describes the patient with the urge to urinate yet cannot postpone voiding. Urge incontinence is usually but not always associated with an overactive bladder. There are two types of urge incontinence, motor urgency and sensory urgency. Although important conceptually, the differentiation can be made only with urodynamic testing. Motor urgency is present when the patient has the urge to urinate that is accompanied by a urodynamically documented uninhibited (involuntary) bladder contraction. An uninhibited detrusor contraction is called *detrusor hyperreflexia* in the patient with documented neurologic disease (such as stroke or multiple sclerosis) and *detrusor instability* in the patient without a known neurologic lesion. Sensory urgency is present when the patient feels a strong urge to urinate but there is no demonstrable detrusor contraction on a cystometrogram (CMG). In our experience, sensory urgency rarely causes incontinence (but may cause severe frequency) and should alert the investigator to another potential cause such as stone, cystitis, or bladder tumor. *Stress incontinence* is suggested by the loss of urine with activities that increase abdominal pressure such as laughing, coughing, or sneezing, or with positional changes. Stress incontinence by definition implies some functional disorder of the urethral sphincteric mechanism. *Overflow incontinence* reflects a bladder that is full to capacity and cannot accommodate more volume, and so further urine production results in frequent, obligatory low-volume urine loss across the outlet. An example of overflow incontinence is the man with bladder outlet obstruction and urinary retention from benign prostatic hyperplasia. *Functional incontinence* implies a situational incontinence that is not related to the bladder or outlet itself, but instead reflects a patient's immobility or mental incapacitation. A simple example would be an immobile arthritic patient who cannot make it to the toilet and subsequently is incontinent. *Mixed incontinence* is the combination of stress and urge incontinence and is common in both men and women. Examples of mixed incontinence are men with postprostatectomy incontinence, where up to 50% have bladder dysfunction (poor compliance or instability),[1] and women with stress urinary incontinence, where up to 60% have symptoms of urgency and urge incontinence. Although mixed incontinence is common, to properly manage these patients it is important to quantify the separate stress and urge components and their relative contribution to the patient's chief complaint.

HISTORY

The history and physical examination remain the cornerstone on which a urologic diagnosis is made. However, the incontinence history may be difficult to obtain if the patient is embarrassed or anxious, is hard of hearing, or has difficulty with verbal communication. In these cases, or with geriatric patients, it may be helpful to have a family member present during the interview. The interviewing physician must be patient, understanding, and reassuring and proceed in a confident stepwise fashion. A detailed history is used to survey for an overt cause or less obvious causes of incontinence and to help one decide whether additional tests are necessary.[2]

Urinary incontinence may be caused by pathologic, anatomic, or physiologic processes affecting the lower urinary tract or other organ systems. Many factors may be transient and reversible such as infection, atrophic vaginitis, acute confusional states, immobility, stool impaction, medical conditions that cause polyuria or nocturia, and medication side effects. In older people, the problem of incontinence is occasionally transient. The transient causes of incontinence are listed in in the box below and can be recalled using the mnemonic DIAPPERS.[3] A voiding diary (see Appendix 7-B) may provide useful information on urinary frequency, nocturia, and the number of episodes of urine loss in the incontinent patient. In the absence of diuretics, the volume of urine output is a good indication of the patient's fluid intake.

Voiding Symptoms

When evaluating the incontinent patient, one needs to establish baseline voiding symptoms. Urgency is described as an intense desire to void secondary to an abrupt sensation of bladder discomfort, or as a conditioned response from the fear of urine leakage. Urgency symptoms must be probed carefully, since they are not sensitive or specific for detrusor overactivity. One must consider functional factors such as patient mentation, mobility, motivation, and access to a toilet. The symptom of urgency that immediately precedes an abrupt gush of urine must be differentiated from the sense of urgency arising from the patient's *fear* of incontinence.

Frequency of urination (more than 7 diurnal voids) is common and may simply reflect excessive fluid intake, diuretic medication, or dietary stimulants such as caffeine. Many patients choose to void frequently to avoid incontinence of any cause. Urinary frequency may indicate pain with low volume bladder filling (inflammation), detrusor overactivity, reduced bladder capacity, noncompliance (a "stiff" bladder), incomplete bladder emptying, or even complete urinary retention with overflow incontinence. Again, bladder irritation secondary to infection, stone, malignancy, or external mass must be considered. Nocturia may be secondary to detrusor overactivity, reduced detrusor capacity, excessive urine output, or a primary sleep-related disorder. A voiding diary may assist in differentiating these processes. Daytime frequency without nocturia may be suggestive of a psychogenic component, increased fluid intake, timing of diuretic medications, or dietary stimulants such as caffeine.

One must not ignore bladder outlet obstructive symptoms (decreased force of urinary stream, hesitancy, sensation of incomplete bladder emptying, and postvoid dribbling) in the patient with urinary incontinence. These symptoms may be present in patients with a poorly contractile bladder from diabetes mellitus or from various neurologic disorders. Although women with a large cystocele may complain of bladder outlet obstruc-

Transient causes of urinary incontinence may be easily recalled using the mnemonic DIAPPERS

D	Delirium/confusional state
I	Infection-urinary (symptomatic)
A	Atrophic urethritis/vaginitis
P	Pharmaceuticals
P	Psychologic, especially in the form of depression
E	Endocrine (hypercalcemia, hyperglycemia)
R	Restricted mobility
S	Stool impaction

Modified from Pannil FC, Williams TF, Davis R: *J Amer Geriatr Soc* 36:902-910, 1988.

tive symptoms (secondary to urethral hyperangulation), men are far more likely to have obstructive symptoms associated with urinary incontinence. Incontinence associated with benign prostatic hyperplasia (BPH) usually reflects detrusor overactivity secondary to bladder outlet obstruction.

Urinary Incontinence

In both males and females, urinary incontinence may be approached conceptually as a problem with detrusor overactivity, a problem with urethral sphincteric function, or a combination of the two. After listening to the chief complaint, directed questions identify whether the incontinence is related to urgency symptoms suggestive of bladder overactivity or provocative maneuvers suggestive of stress incontinence and some degree of urethral dysfunction. Simple processes such as vaginal voiding in the female or more complex pathologic conditions such as ectopic ureter or urinary fistula may be suggested by a detailed history.

Focused questions to evaluate and preliminarily classify urinary incontinence are listed in the boxed material below. Basic questions for all patients include the duration and characterization of incontinence, precipitating events, and previous incontinence treatments and their effect. What is the frequency and severity of incontinent episodes (daily, weekly, or rarely)? What types of physical activity typically result in urine loss (aerobic exercises versus quiet walking)? Are protective pads used (panty liners, maxipads, or diapers)? If so, how many pads are used daily, and when changed are the pads wet, damp, or dry (changed by habit)? Other factors that influence continence include daily fluid intake and dietary stimulants such as caffeine.

Important historical factors in the evaluation and preliminary characterization of urinary incontinence

- Duration and characteristics of incontinence (stress, urge, mixed, total, others)
- Frequency, timing, and amount of continent and incontinent voids
- Other lower urinary tract symptoms
- Precipitants and associated symptoms of incontinence (such as cough, surgery, medication)
- Use of pads, briefs, or other protective garments
- Fluid intake including dietary stimulants such as caffeine
- Alteration in bowel or sexual habits
- Previous treatment and effect on urinary incontinence

Important historical risk factors for women with severe urinary incontinence that may be suggestive of the presence of intrinsic sphincteric dysfunction (ISD)

- Prior bladder neck suspension
- Neurologic lesion or injury
- Radiation therapy
- Radical pelvic surgery
- Pelvic trauma

Female Stress Incontinence

Female stress incontinence represents a range of urethral sphincteric dysfunction but can conceptually be subdivided into anatomic stress incontinence (also called "simple stress incontinence") or intrinsic sphincteric dysfunction (ISD). By definition, ISD implies some functional damage to the urethral sphincteric mechanism, and these patients will almost always have some historical risk factor for urethral sphincteric damage. The risk factors for ISD, listed in the box at bottom left, must be probed in every patient with urinary incontinence. Identifying the patient with ISD is critical, since they require different treatment from that of patients with "simple" anatomic stress incontinence. Usually patients with simple anatomic incontinence will have mild or moderate urine loss, and patients with a damaged urethral sphincteric mechanism will have severe urine loss. Although additional urodynamic testing is required to make this differentiation, history can help determine whether additional testing is required.[3] The severity of urethral sphincteric dysfunction may be estimated by history alone. Stamey presented a grading system of stress urinary incontinence based on the degree of physical activity required to cause urine loss (see the box below).[4] McGuire demonstrated that the Stamey grading system for stress urinary incontinence correlated with the severity of urethral sphincteric dysfunction.[5] Furthermore, Raz showed that women with severe incontinence preoperatively had a greater risk of failure after a standard bladder neck suspension procedure.[6] Clearly, when one is interviewing the female patient with stress incontinence, the severity of incontinence is critical and may be suggestive of the presence of ISD.

The patient with mild to moderate urine loss associated with provocative maneuvers (coughing, laughing, or sneezing) will most commonly have bladder neck and proximal urethral hypermobility, often with an associated cystocele. Therefore, additional questions probe for the presence of a cystocele. Symptoms of pelvic pressure, the sensation of a mass or bulge in the vagina, or dyspareunia may be suggestive of a cystocele or other vaginal vault prolapse. Occasionally a large cystocele or other vaginal prolapse may be described as a mass protruding from the vagina. These clues may be supported by information in the past medical history such as multiple vaginal deliveries, a difficult vaginal delivery requiring the use of forceps, or previous hysterectomy (all of which may weaken the pelvic supporting structures).

Patients with a large cystocele may not complain of significant incontinence but may instead have bladder outlet obstructive symptoms such as weak force of urinary stream, hesitancy, and sensation of incomplete bladder emptying. Bladder outlet

The Stamey incontinence scoring system based on the severity of incontinence by history

Grade 0	No incontinence
Grade 1	Incontinence with coughing or straining
Grade 2	Incontinence with change in position or walking
Grade 3	Total incontinence at all times of day

From Stamey TA: *Ann Surg* 192:465, 1980.

obstruction in this setting is typically secondary to urethral obstruction from the prolapsing cystocele. Rarely a large prolapsing cystocele may cause hyperangulation of the ureters and cause obstructive renal impairment and even renal failure.[7]

Urge Incontinence

Urge incontinence is the sudden desire to void with the inability to voluntarily postpone voiding until one reaches the toilet. As mentioned, urgency may reflect detrusor overactivity or may be secondary to sensory instability. Another cause of UI is bladder *noncompliance,* in which the detrusor cannot accommodate increasing volumes of urine at a normal, low pressure (that is, it is a "stiff" bladder). A focused interview probing neurologic symptoms is critical in all incontinent patients, but particularly in patients with urgency and urge incontinence. Specific questions about radicular pain, paresthesias, muscle weakness, or altered vaginal or penile sensation with sexual activities are important clues to possible radiculopathy or other spinal cord disorders. A history of ocular symptoms may indicate multiple sclerosis; in fact, up to 10% of patients with multiple sclerosis may first be diagnosed by the urologist.[8] Finally, symptomatic bowel dysfunction may be informative, and in our opinion fecal incontinence in the absence of known gastrointestinal disease is abnormal and warrants further neurologic evaluation.

Male Urinary Incontinence

Urinary incontinence may occur in men with bladder-outlet obstruction from benign prostatic hyperplasia, from neurologic injury affecting urethral sphincteric dysfunction, or from physically induced injury to the sphincteric mechanism. However, the most common cause of male incontinence in our experience is postprostatectomy incontinence. The major differential diagnosis in men with postprostatectomy incontinence is detrusor overactivity versus stress urinary incontinence from urethral sphincter damage. This differentiation is difficult and requires additional urodynamic testing to identify the cause of incontinence. However, symptoms of frequency, urgency, urge incontinence, and nocturnal incontinence are suggestive of detrusor hyperactivity. If the incontinence is related to exertional maneuvers and the patient is not incontinent at night, urethral sphincteric dysfunction may be more strongly considered. *One cannot assume that the incontinent man after prostatectomy automatically has sphincteric damage.* It is important to recognize that up to 50% of men will have both detrusor hyperactivity and sphincteric dysfunction, and additional urodynamic testing is required for diagnosis.[1]

Men with urgency and urge incontinence but without pertinent history or risk factors for urethral sphincteric denervation or damage may have detrusor instability from bladder outlet obstruction secondary to BPH. These patients should be carefully questioned about obstructive and irritative voiding symptoms and may be assessed with the American Urologic Association symptom 7 index.[9] One still must consider other sources of detrusor overactivity such as infection, tumor, stone, or neurologic lesion.

Past Medical History

The past medical history provides relevant information on past and present medical disease, past surgical history, obstetric and gynecologic history, current medication use, alcohol and drug use (that is, tobacco and caffeine), and drug allergies (including Latex). Knowledge of medication use is particularly relevant in the geriatric patient. Specific medications of importance include diuretics, alpha-adrenergic agents (agonists or antagonists that may affect bladder neck tone), and estrogens in the postmenopausal woman. Additional focused questions are used to probe for factors other than lower urinary tract dysfunction that may contribute to the development of incontinence. This is also more evident in the elderly, as the prevalence of concurrent disease processes increases with age. One example is the diurnal variation in urine production seen with congestive heart failure (mobilization of peripheral edema when supine) and diuretic use, as well as the polyuria seen with poorly controlled diabetes. Significant improvements may result from simple recommendations like bedside commode, timing of diuretic use, or encouraging better management of peripheral edema or diabetes mellitus.

Past surgical history of radical pelvic surgery (radical hysterectomy, abdominoperineal resection), prostatectomy (for benign or malignant disease), bladder-neck suspension procedures, or spinal surgery are critical. As discussed, women with severe incontinence must be probed for risk factors of intrinsic sphincteric dysfunction (ISD) (see the box, p. 56). Rarely, an elderly woman will have severe incontinence without a risk factor for ISD, which may reflect a severe low estrogen state atrophy. The temporal relationship of incontinence or new voiding symptoms to past surgical procedures may be helpful. New onset urinary frequency and urgency (with or without urge incontinence) after a bladder suspension procedure may be found to have new detrusor instability from bladder outlet obstruction.[10] Severe incontinence after multiple bladder suspension procedures is strongly suggestive of ISD. Finally, a woman with new-onset severe incontinence (usually total incontinence) after hysterectomy may be suspected of having a urovaginal fistula.

Often, from the history alone one can *preliminarily* classify the type of urinary incontinence. The physical examination may then permit one to identify specific findings that support or contradict the diagnosis suspected from history. Caution should be exercised when one is definitively classifying a type of incontinence based on clinical evaluation alone because it will be misleading in nearly 50% of cases.[11,12] Further radiologic or urodynamic evaluation is often needed.

Physical Examination

The focused urologic examination of the incontinent patient must be performed in a stepwise fashion. First, a methodical abdominal examination is performed, and any abnormalities of the back are noted. Second, a directed pelvic examination, either female (vaginal, associated vaginal disorder, bimanual) or male (genitalia, rectal, prostatic, bimanual) is performed. Third, a focused examination is performed to assess for a gross neurologic lesion.

Initial Evaluation

The initial evaluation involves abdominal inspection for obesity, a previous surgical scar, or an abdominal or inguinal hernia. Skin lesions that are known to be associated with neurologic disease (such as neurofibromatosis and café au lait spots) are noted. The abdomen is palpated to assess for pain or for a suprapubic mass (such as a distended bladder or a pelvic tumor). Suprapubic percussion is usually better than palpation for detection of a distended bladder.

The back and spine are inspected for skeletal deformities, scars from trauma, or scars from previous surgery. The presence of a subcutaneous lipoma, cutaneous vascular malformation, tuft of hair, or skin dimple on the lower back may indicate an occult spinal dysraphism, warranting further neurologic evaluation. A low, short gluteal cleft and flattened buttocks may indicate sacral agenesis (in children born to insulin-dependent diabetic mothers). Palpation of the coccyx or a lateral film of the lower spine may confirm sacral absence.

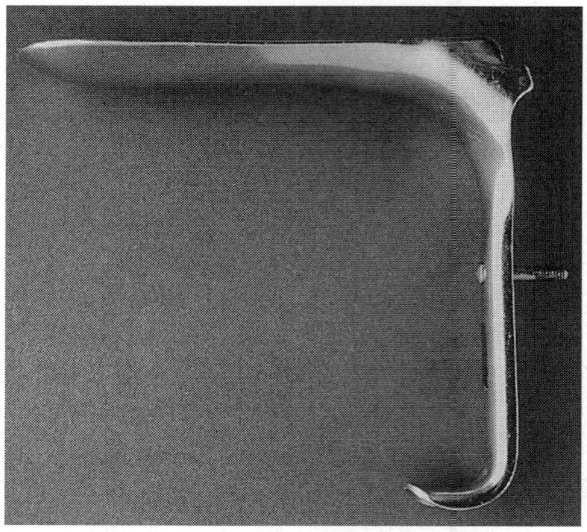

FIG. 8-1 *The posterior half of a Graves speculum is used to expose the anterior and then posterior vaginal walls. A second posterior half is used to expose the vaginal apex.*

Female Pelvic Examination

Remember that the severity of incontinence and other historical information may help us preliminarily characterize the type of incontinence. The history will provide some insight into the cause of the incontinence, and the focused pelvic examination provides objective evidence that may support the working diagnosis or be suggestive of an alternative disorder. For example, a history of severe incontinence after a previous bladder neck suspension is suspicious for ISD. The finding of a well-supported, fixed, and scarred anterior vaginal wall further supports the diagnosis of ISD. Alternatively a history of mild incontinence precipitated by stress maneuvers may imply an anatomic problem that is supported by the finding of bladder-neck and proximal urethral hypermobility.

The female pelvic examination is performed with the patient in the lithotomy position. The labia majora and minora, introitus, and perineum are inspected. The vaginal introitus is inspected for atrophy or stenosis. Labia minora that are widely separated inferiorly or an anus that is displaced posteriorly may indicate a weakened or denervated perineal body.

Speculum Examination

Proper lighting is mandatory for a speculum examination. Two posterior halves of a Graves speculum (Fig. 8-1) are used sequentially for exposure. This methodical vaginal examination should address three distinct areas in a systematic fashion: the anterior vaginal wall, the vaginal apex, and the posterior vaginal wall.

Anterior vaginal wall. A single Graves speculum is placed along the posterior vaginal wall (vaginal floor) and gentle retraction exposes the anterior vaginal wall. An associated vaginal wall disorder such as urethral caruncle, paraurethral cyst, urethral prolapse, or an inflamed Skene's gland may be noted. Urethral induration may be a sign of chronic inflammation, urethral diverticulum, or tumor. Milking a urethral diverticulum may elicit a purulent urethral discharge. Pale, thin, shining vaginal mucosa or loss of rugation may indicate atrophic vaginitis secondary to a low estrogen state. This is important because atrophic vaginitis is a potentially reversible cause of urinary incontinence in elderly women.[13] A fixed and scarred anterior vaginal wall in the setting of severe incontinence supports the diagnosis of ISD.

Bulging of the anterior vaginal wall at rest when the posterior wall is stabilized usually indicates the presence of a cystocele. The extent of the cystocele may be assessed when one asks the patient to do a Valsalva maneuver or strain. Blaivas described the degrees of anatomic defect and a clinical grading of cystoceles in the presence of stress urinary incontinence.[14] A commonly used clinical grading system for cystocele is presented in the box on p. 59 and is important, since cystocele size determines the surgical procedure necessary for repair. A small, or grade 1, cystocele (Fig. 8-2) may be amenable to simple bladder neck suspension. A medium, or grade 2, cystocele (Fig. 8-3) may require a four-corner bladder neck suspension, whereas a large cystocele (Fig. 8-4) will require a formal cystocele repair.

Vaginal apex. A second posterior half of a Graves speculum is placed along the anterior vaginal wall, and the vaginal apex is inspected. The position of the cervix or, in posthysterectomy patients, the apical vaginal cuff is noted. Cervical descent with straining indicates some degree of uterine descensus. If uterine or vaginal vault descensus is suspected, the patient must be reexamined in the standing position (Fig. 8-5). Any suspicious vaginal mucosal findings or cervical abnormalities are referred for gynecologic evaluation.

Posterior vaginal wall. In posthysterectomy patients, vaginal apical descent with coughing or straining may indicate the presence of an enterocele or vaginal vault prolapse. This distinction may be aided by examination of the posterior vaginal wall length. If there is vaginal vault prolapse, the posterior vaginal wall is usually shortened. If the apical bulge is an enterocele, the posterior vaginal wall length is usually preserved (Fig. 8-6). When one is assessing for an enterocele, a simultaneous rectal and vaginal examination is essential. With coughing or straining, the impulse of the prolapsing enterocele sac (peritoneal pouch of Douglas) may be felt between the two examining fingers, and examination in the standing position may greatly aid in differentiating these apical herniations (see Fig. 8-5).

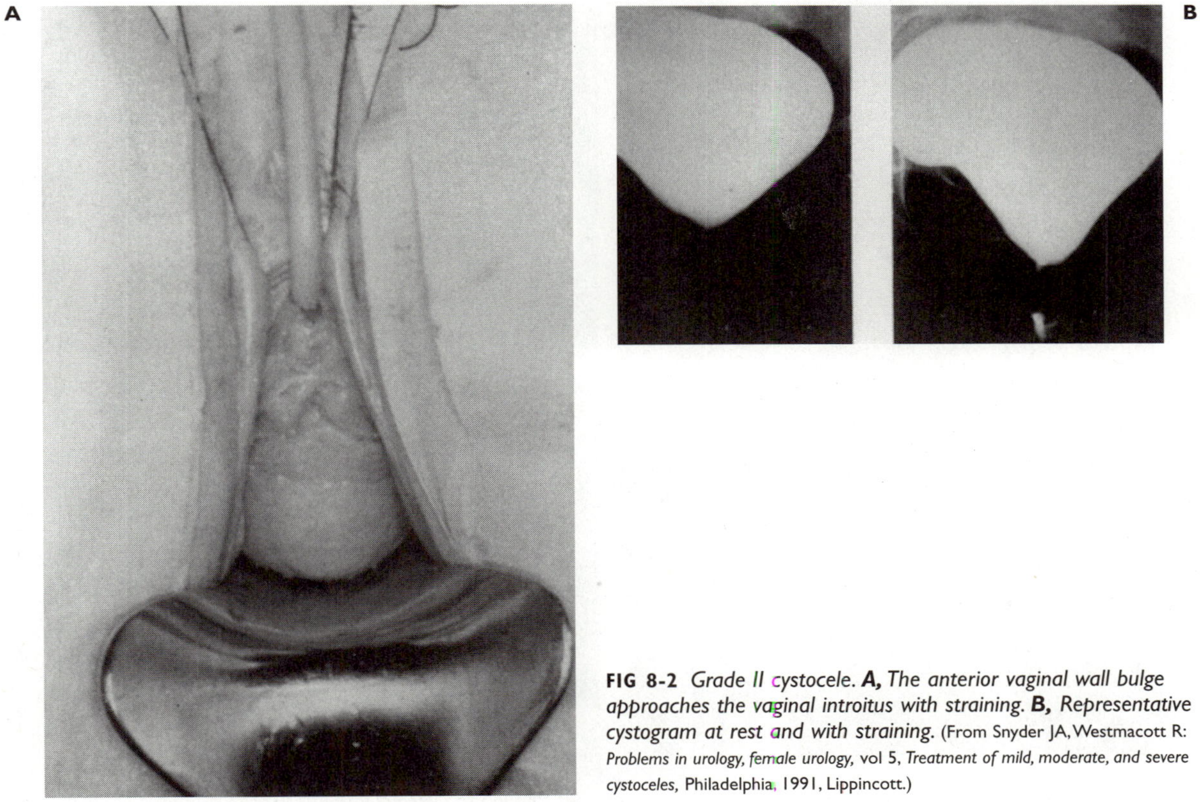

FIG 8-2 *Grade II cystocele.* ***A,*** *The anterior vaginal wall bulge approaches the vaginal introitus with straining.* ***B,*** *Representative cystogram at rest and with straining.* (From Snyder JA, Westmacott R: *Problems in urology, female urology,* vol 5, *Treatment of mild, moderate, and severe cystoceles,* Philadelphia, 1991, Lippincott.)

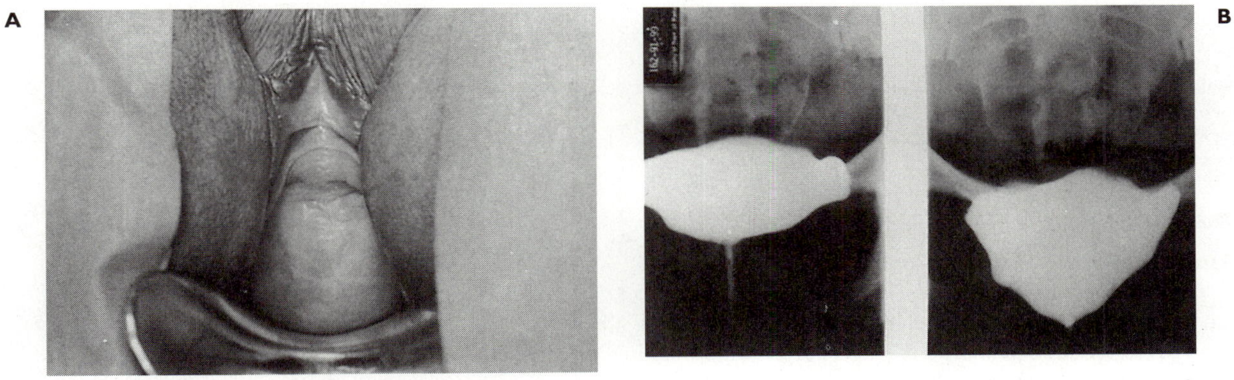

FIG. 8-3 *Grade III cystocele.* ***A,*** *The anterior vaginal wall reaches the vaginal introitus at rest but does not protrude out of the introitus.* ***B,*** *Representative cystogram at rest and at straining. Notice the significant descent of the base of the bladder below the level of the pubic symphysis.* (From Snyder JA, Westmacott R: *Problems in urology, female urology,* vol 5, *Treatment of mild, moderate, and severe cystoceles,* Philadelphia, 1991, Lippincott.)

Commonly used clinical grading system of cystoceles

Grade I	Minimal bladder descensus
Grade II	Bladder descensus to vaginal introitus with straining
Grade III	Bladder descensus to vaginal introitus at rest
Grade IV	Bladder prolapse through the labia at rest or with straining, or both

From Snyder JA, Westmacott R: *Problems in urology: female urology,* vol 5, *Treatment of mild, moderate, and severe cystoceles,* Philadelphia, 1991, Lippincott.

When a posterior vaginal wall bulge is seen after the anterior vaginal wall is stabilized, a rectocele or an enterocele may be present. A rectocele is usually represented by a bulge closer to the vaginal introitus and may be separate from the apical vaginal bulges already discussed (Fig. 8-7). However, if the posterior vaginal floor bulge is high in the vaginal apex, differentiation between an enterocele and high rectocele may be difficult. Occasionally this differentiation can be made only at the time of surgical repair. When addressing a rectocele, one should assess

A B C

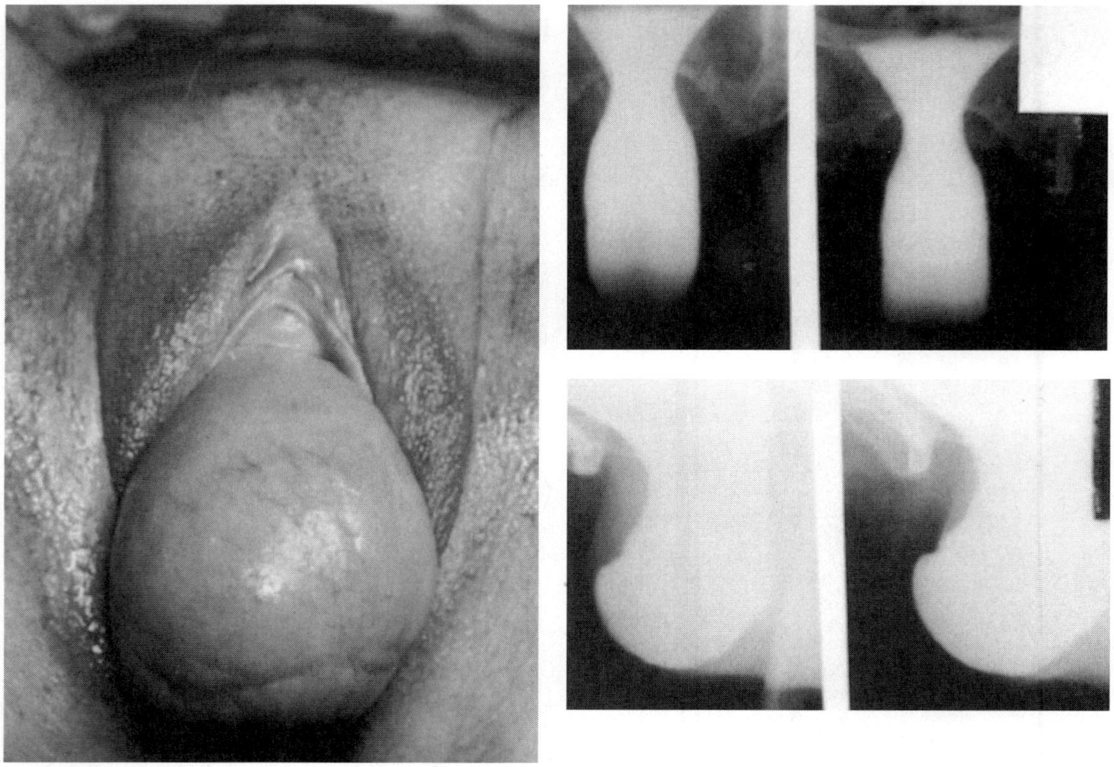

FIG. 8-4 *Grade IV cystocele.* ***A,*** *The anterior vaginal wall protrudes through the vaginal introitus.* ***B,*** *The dramatic prolapse is well demonstrated on the anterior posterior and lateral cystogram films.* (From Snyder JA, Westmacott R: *Problems in urology, female urology,* vol 5, *Treatment of mild, moderate, and severe cystoceles,* Philadelphia, 1991, Lippincott.)

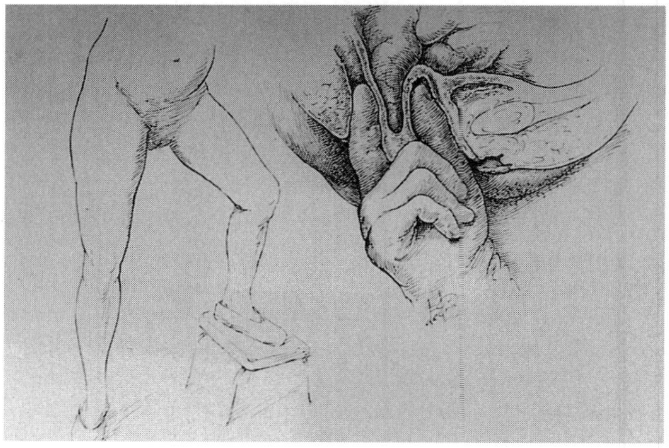

FIG. 8-5 *Simultaneous rectal and vaginal examination with the patient in the standing position helps identify and characterize apical vaginal bulges such as an enterocele.* (From Foote JE, Zimmern PE, Leach GE: *Reconstructive urology,* Cambridge, Mass., 1993, Blackwell Scientific Publications.)

perineal integrity and tone by examining the central tendon and the perineal musculature. This support is believed to represent a critical "backboard" of vaginal support.

Bimanual Examination

The female pelvic examination is concluded with a bimanual examination to detect any mass or tenderness of the vaginal wall, bladder, uterus, adnexa, or other pelvic structure. One hand is placed on the lower abdomen and two fingers of the other hand are placed in the vagina. The bladder, uterus, and adnexa are palpated between the abdomen and the vagina. Any abnormal findings on the pelvic examination may require radiologic evaluation. During the rectal examination, a note is made for gluteal asymmetry, sphincter tone, fecal impaction, and rectal masses.

Other Physical Findings

The Q-tip test is a simple means of estimating the degree of proximal urethral and bladder neck hypermobility. With the patient in the lithotomy position, a well-lubricated, sterile Q-tip is inserted 1 to 2 cm into the cleansed urethra. The patient is asked to strain at a Valsalva maneuver. Exaggerated movement of the Q-tip (usually described as greater than 35 degrees) is felt to represent proximal urethral and bladder neck hypermobility. However this test is subjective, adds little to visual inspection of bladder neck and proximal urethral hypermobility and is not specific for stress urinary incontinence.[15,16]

As part of a complete speculum examination, the patient is asked to do a Valsalva maneuver or cough with a full bladder in an attempt to demonstrate urine leakage, the so-called "stress

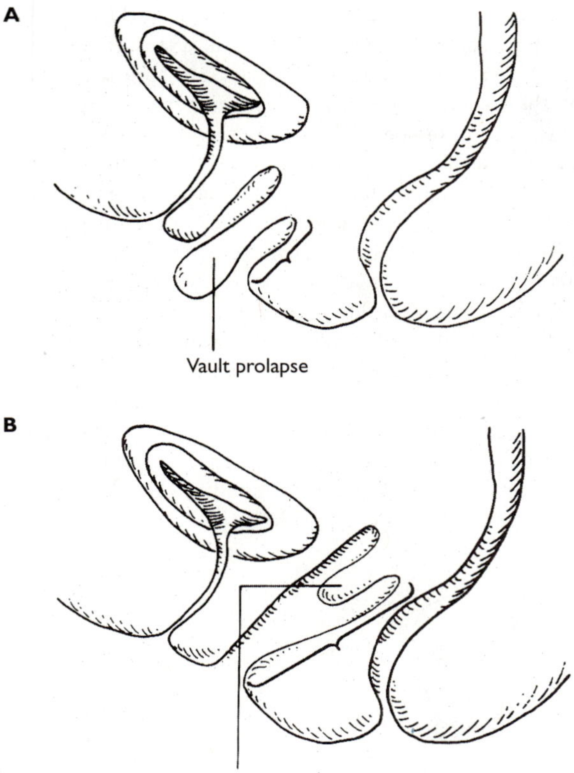

FIG. 8-6 *The length of the posterior vaginal wall is shortened with vaginal vault prolapse yet is usually preserved with an enterocele.* (From Foote JE, Zimmern PE, Leach GE: *Reconstructive urology,* Cambridge, Mass., 1993, Blackwell Scientific Publications.)

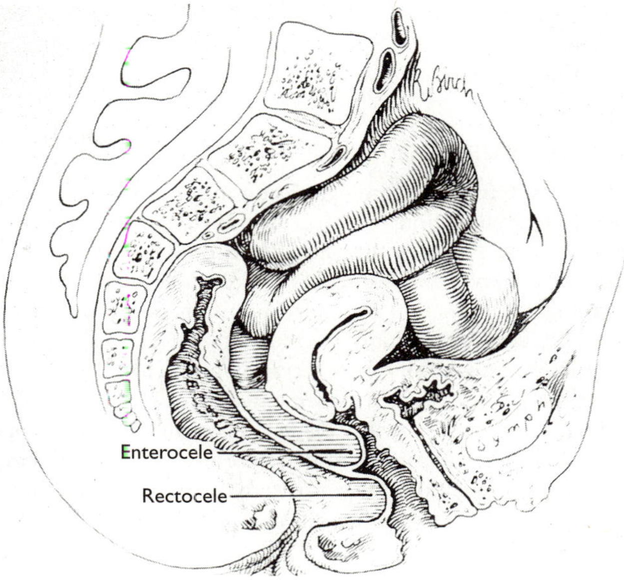

FIG. 8-7 *The bulge from an enterocele is usually located near the vaginal apex compared to the rectocele, which is closer to the vaginal introitus.*

test." If leakage occurs coincident with the cough, it is probably secondary to incompetent bladder outlet. This test is important because federal guidelines on the evaluation of urinary incontinence indicate that women with "simple" stress incontinence by history (no risk factors of ISD, no symptoms of detrusor overactivity, and a normal postvoid residual urine volume) may be treated without further urodynamic testing.[2] Incontinence that occurs a few seconds after the cough may be secondary to an uninhibited detrusor contraction (triggered by the cough) rather than bladder outlet incompetence[17] and may indicate the need for further urodynamic testing.

One performs the bladder neck elevation test of Bonney by placing two fingers in the lateral vaginal fornices and asking the patient to cough. This technique is used to stabilize (not occlude) the bladder neck and prevent proximal urethral and bladder neck hypermobility. If urine leakage is prevented by this technique, urethral hypermobility is considered to be present. However, this test may be limited secondary to the potential for iatrogenic urethral occlusion resulting in a false-positive test.[18]

Total Incontinence

Total incontinence may be attributable to overflow from a distended bladder, fistula (urethrovaginal, vesicovaginal, and ureterovaginal), or an ectopic ureter. Occasionally, severe ISD may mimic total incontinence. A postvoid residual urine volume is essential to rule out overflow incontinence. The most common site of an ectopic ureter in the female is the posterior wall of the urethra, followed by vaginal vestibule, vaginal wall, and the uterus or cervix. Depending on the clinical suspicion, further evaluation of total incontinence may include vaginoscopy, cystoscopy, intravenous pyelography, retrograde pyelography, and intravesical methylene blue or indigo carmine.

Male Pelvic Examination

A focused male pelvic examination includes assessment of the external genitalia and perineum, a digital rectal examination (DRE), and a neurologic examination (discussed later in this chapter). The DRE should assess the size of the prostate and the likelihood of bladder outlet obstruction and abnormalities suspicious for prostate cancer. Normally the prostate is about the size of a chestnut, feels rubbery, and has a consistency of a contracted thenar eminence. One must keep in mind that the DRE cannot assess the median lobe or the intravesical extension of an enlarged prostate. Subsequently there is little correlation between the estimated prostate size and voiding symptoms. Finally, during the rectal examination the anal sphincter tone and integrity of sacral innervation is tested (discussed below).

Postvoid Residual Volume

The postvoid residual (PVR) urine volume is essential for all incontinent patients. Methods to obtain a PVR volume include urethral catheterization or office ultrasonography. The postvoid residual volume provides additional information on voiding efficiency and bladder capacity. In an alert patient, a true PVR volume is determined immediately after voiding. In the demented patient a PVR volume may be determined after an incontinent episode.

Neurologic Examination

Incontinence from a neurologic lesion may present as urethral sphincteric dysfunction and stress incontinence, bladder overactivity (hyperreflexia) with urgency and urge incontinence, or detrusor denervation and overflow incontinence. The focused neurologic examination is divided into four parts: (1) mental status, (2) sensory function, (3) motor function, and (4) reflex integrity. Begin with simple observation of the patient for signs of neurologic disease such as dementia, paresis, plegia, tremor, and the degree of immobility (cane, walker, wheelchair). Mental status is assessed by observation of the patient's level of consciousness, orientation, speech pattern, memory, and comprehension. Voiding disorders may be associated with mental status changes from dementia, stroke, brain tumor, Parkinson's disease, or multiple sclerosis. Sensory deficits at a specific dermatomal level are suggestive of a localized lesion either at the spinal cord or at the nerve root level. A focused sensory examination includes testing of specific dermatomes for position, vibration, pinprick, light touch, and temperature. Important sensory dermatomes to remember for a focused neurourologic examination are T4-5 (nipples), T10 (umbilicus), L1 (base of penis, upper scrotum, labia majora), L1-2 (midscrotum, labia minora), L3 (front of knee), S1 (sole and lateral area of foot), and S3-5 (perineum and circumanal skin) (Fig. 8-8).

When assessing motor function, first inspect the muscle bulk for atrophy. Incomplete loss of motor strength is termed "paresis," and complete loss is termed "-plegia." Important muscles to remember are the tibialis anterior (L4-S1), the gastrocnemius (L5-S2), and the toe extensors (L4-S1). The motor strength of these individual muscles may be tested by dorsiflexion, plantar flexion, and toe extension.

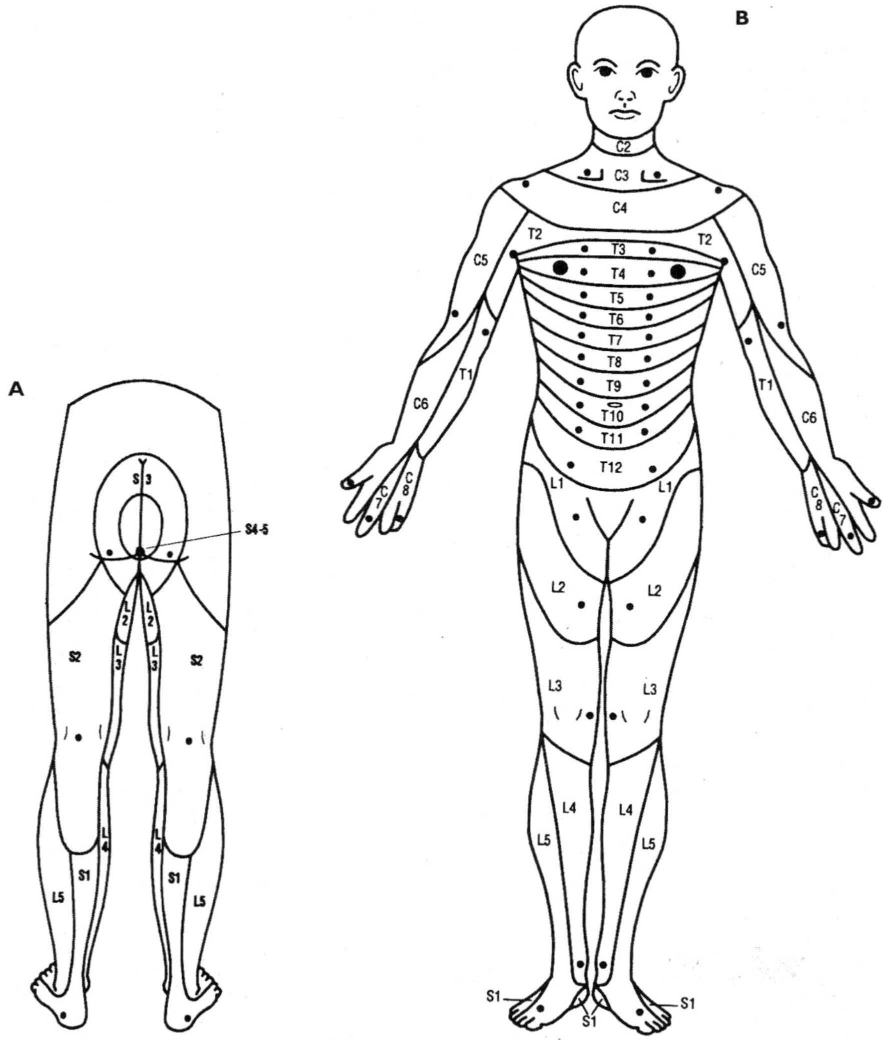

FIG. 8-8 *Topographic representation of sensory dermatomes. Important dermatomes for a focused urologic examination are listed in the text.* (From Gutierrez PA, Young RR, Vulpe M: *Urol Clin North Am* 20:3, 376.)

The focused sensory evaluation is also used to assess the cutaneous sacral reflexes. The sacral nerve roots (S2-4) innervate both the external urethral and the anal sphincters. The external anal sphincter is believed to clinically represent all perineal striated muscles and may be used to predict urethral sphincteric function. Stimulation of the anal reflex (S2-5) by light stroking of the mucocutaneous junction of the circumanal skin causes a visible contraction of the external anal sphincter (anal wink). Absence of the anal wink reflex usually is suggestive of sacral nerve disease except in the elderly patient, where absence of the anal wink is not always pathologic.[19] A finger is then placed in the rectum to assess sphincter tone and volitional contraction. The presence of voluntary contraction of the external anal sphincter usually indicates normal integrity of pelvic floor innervation and of the conus medullaris. Absence of or a decrease in the sphincter tone or of voluntary anal contraction may reflect a sacral or peripheral nerve lesion and usually indicates absent conal activity. The presence of anal sphincter tone in the absence of a voluntary anal contraction indicates a suprasacral lesion.

The bulbocavernosus reflex (BCR) refers specifically to the contraction of the bulbocavernosus muscle; however, this reflex is often used to test the innervation of all perineal striated muscles. The BCR is a local sacral spinal cord reflex arc reflecting activity in S2-4. In men, the BCR is elicited by squeezing the glans penis, which causes a reflex contraction of the external anal sphincter. In women, the glans clitoris is used. Pulling on an indwelling Foley catheter against the bladder neck may stimulate a BCR. Absence of the BCR after any of these maneuvers may indicate sacral nerve damage (the BCR should be absent in all patients with a complete lower motor neuron lesion). However, it should be remembered that the BCR may be absent in up to 20% of neurologically normal females.[20]

Finally, muscle stretch reflexes (deep tendon reflexes) reflect the integrity of upper motor neuron (UMN) and lower motor neuron (LMN) function. Upper motor neuron lesions usually are associated with detrusor overactivity (hyperreflexia), whereas LMN lesions usually result in an acontractile bladder. Hyperactive deep tendon reflexes are suggestive of a UMN lesion, whereas hypoactive deep tendon reflexes are suggestive of an LMN lesion. The deep tendon reflexes important in neurourology are the quadriceps (L3-4) and the Achilles tendon (L5, S1-2). Patients with complete spinal cord lesions above the conus medullaris (UMN/suprasacral/suprasegmental) may have hyperactive deep tendon reflexes, hyperreflexic bladder, skeletal spasticity, pathologic toe sign (Babinski), ankle clonus, and absent skin sensation below the level of the lesion. Complete spinal cord lesions at or below the conus medullaris (LMN/sacral/segmental) may demonstrate absent deep tendon reflexes, areflexic bladder, skeletal flaccidity, absent Babinski's sign, absent ankle clonus, and absent skin sensation below the level of the lesion.

REFERENCES

1. Leach GE, Yun S: Post prostatectomy incontinence: part 1. The urodynamic findings in 107 men, *Neurourol Urodyn* 11:91-97, 1992.
2. Urinary Incontinence Guideline Panel: *Urinary incontinence in adults: clinical practice guideline*, ACHPR Pub No 92-0038, Rockville, Md., 1992, Agency for Health Care Policy and Research, Public Health Service, United States Department of Health and Human Services.
3. Pannil FC, Williams TF, Davis R: Evaluation and treatment of urinary incontinence in long-term care, *J Am Geriatr Soc* 36:902-910, 1988.
4. Stamey TA: Endoscopic suspension of the vesical neck for urinary incontinence in females, *Ann Surg* 192:465, 1980.
5. McGuire EJ, Fitzpatrick CC, Wan J, Bloom D: Clinical assessment of urethral sphincter function, *J Urol* 150: 1452-1454, 1993.
6. Raz S, Erickson DR: SEAPI QMM Incontinence Classification System, *Neurourol Urodyn* 11:187-199, 1992.
7. Miles BJ, Melser M: Chronic renal failure secondary to post hysterectomy vaginal prolapse, *Urology* 38(4):361-363, 1991.
8. Sirls LT, Zimmern PE, Leach GE: Efficacy of limited evaluation and aggressive medical management in multiple sclerosis: review of 113 patients, *J Urol* 151:946, 1994.
9. Barry MJ, Fowler FJ, O'Leary MP, et al: The American Urological Association symptom index for benign prostatic hyperplasia, *J Urol* 148:1549-1557, 1992.
10. Nitti VW, Raz S: Obstruction following anti-incontinence procedures: diagnosis and treatment with transvaginal urethrolysis, *J Urol* 152:93-98, 1994.
11. Katz GP, Blaivas JG: A diagnostic dilemma: when urodynamic findings differ from the clinical impression, *J Urol* 129:1170, 1983.
12. Wise BG, Cutner A, Cardozo LD, et al: Do detailed symptom questionnaires negate the need for urodynamic investigation? *Neurourol Urodyn* 11:353, 1992.
13. Resnick NM, Yalla SV: Management of urinary incontinence in the elderly, *N Engl J Med* 313:800, 1985.
14. Blaivas JG, Olsson CA: Stress incontinence: classification and surgical approach, *J Urol* 139:727, 1988.
15. Montz FJ, Stanton SL: Q-tip test in female urinary incontinence, *Obstet Gynecol* 67:258, 1986.
16. Walters MD, Diaz K: Q-tip test: a study of continent and incontinent women, *Obstet Gynecol* 70:208, 1987.
17. Kader N: The value of bladder filling in the clinical detection of urine loss and selection of patients for urodynamic testing, *Br J Obstet Gynecol* 95(7):698-704, 1988.
18. Bhatia NN, Bergman A, Gunning JE: Urodynamic effects of a vaginal pessary in women with stress urinary incontinence, *Am J Obstet Gynecol* 147:876, 1983.
19. Resnick NM, Yalla SV: Chapter 14 in Walsh PC, Retik AB, Tamey TA, Vaughn ED, editors: *Campbell's urology,* vol 1, ed 6, Philadelphia, 1992, Saunders.
20. Blaivas JG, Zayed AAH, Labib KB: The bulbocavernosus reflex in urology: a prospective study of 299 patients, *J Urol* 126:197, 1981.

Chapter 9

The Urinary Flow Rate

Gregory R. Wahle

The urinary flow rate is an extremely important measurement of voiding function that can be done in the physician's office without significant inconvenience to the patient. Also, the urinary flow rate is inexpensive and relatively easy to interpret, though correct interpretation is essential for the study to be clinically useful.

Normal lower urinary tract function may be thought of as having two phases; low-pressure insensate filling and storage of urine and efficient evacuation under voluntary control. The rate of urinary flow reflects the result of the second phase (the micturition process), which normally consists in integrated activity between detrusor motor function and both bladder neck and striated sphincter opening and unimpeded conduction of urine through the bladder outlet and urethra. Uroflowmetry is generally used to evaluate for the presence of bladder outlet obstruction (usually prostatism) and therefore may be valuable in the assessment of a patient with overflow incontinence. Although urine flow studies are usually not diagnostic by themselves, they are inexpensive and simple and are frequently helpful in the evaluation of voiding symptoms when done in conjunction with a careful history and physical examination and the judicious use of other tests including measurement of residual urine, cystometry, and cystoscopy.

Definition of Urinary Flow

As with any fluid, the flow rate of urine is defined as the volume conveyed per unit time interval and is usually measured in milliliters (ml) per second. Although information regarding urine flow may be gained using techniques as simple as observation of the stream or stop-watch timing of a collected voiding event, clinical testing of urinary flow is generally obtained by use of electronic collection equipment and is expressed as a graphic representation of the instantaneous flow rate as a function of time (Fig. 9-1).

Uroflow Testing

To obtain meaningful information regarding uroflow, the patient is asked to produce a flow curve that he believes is typical of his usual voiding behavior. Anxiety may inhibit or even prevent a patient from voiding. A cooperative patient, wishing to provide a "good" test, may require instruction to avoid straining or pushing during urination. Several voids may be required to produce a representative voiding curve. Occasionally a patient will require fluid loading, diuresis, or bladder filling by means of catheterization to obtain a usable flow curve. This information and the fluid used to fill the bladder and the position of the patient during the collected void (supine, sitting, or standing) should be specified to allow for standardization and permit comparison of results.[1]

Uroflow Parameters

The uroflow graph can be scrutinized with varying degrees of intensity to obtain clinically relevant information concerning lower urinary tract function. As mentioned previously, uroflow studies are usually obtained in the evaluation of suspected bladder outlet obstruction. Uroflow curves are most commonly analyzed by use of parameters and nomenclature recommended by the International Continence Society.[11]

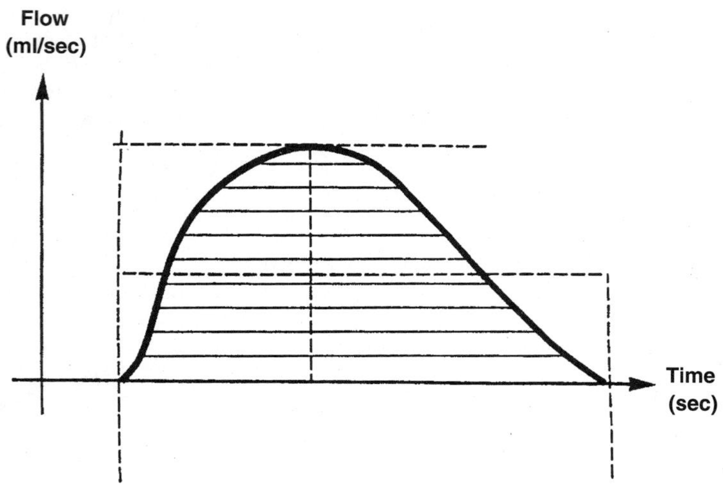

FIG. 9-1 *Schema of a normal, continuous flow curve expressed as instantaneous flow as a function of time.* (From International Continence Society second report on the standardisation of terminology of lower urinary tract function, *Br J Urol* 49:207, 1977.)

Voiding Time

Total voiding time is defined as the interval over which measurable urinary flow occurs and is therefore related to the volume of the voiding event (Fig. 9-2). Although this parameter is easily measured, voiding time is equivalent to actual urinary flow time only in the setting of continuous voiding. Voiding time may be overrepresentative of obstructive dysfunction in the case of intermittent voiding behavior, hesitancy in the initiation of the usual urine stream, or terminal dribbling. Inclusion of only the middle 90% of the voided volume in the consideration of voiding time may partially correct for artifacts in the initiation or termination of voiding. Normal voiding times vary between 10 seconds for a voided volume of 100 ml to 23 seconds for a volume of 400 ml.[1]

Time to Peak Flow

Time to peak flow is the period from the onset of urine flow until the maximal flow rate is achieved (Fig. 9-2). The absolute value, like voiding time, is related to the volume of the voided event, but the time to peak flow is generally around one third of voiding time in unobstructed patients. At least 45% of the total voided volume is produced during the time to peak flow in normal individuals.[3]

Mean Flow Rate

Mean flow rate is obtained when the total voided volume is divided by the voiding time (Fig. 9-2) and therefore is subject to the same inaccuracies of artifacts in the initiation or termination of urination or intermittent flow. This parameter can be measured without sophisticated urodynamic equipment simply by timing a collected voiding event and in continuous urine flow provides useful data in evaluating voiding function.

Peak Flow Rate

Peak flow rate is the maximum value of flow during an adequate void (Fig. 9-2) and is generally obtained through visual review of

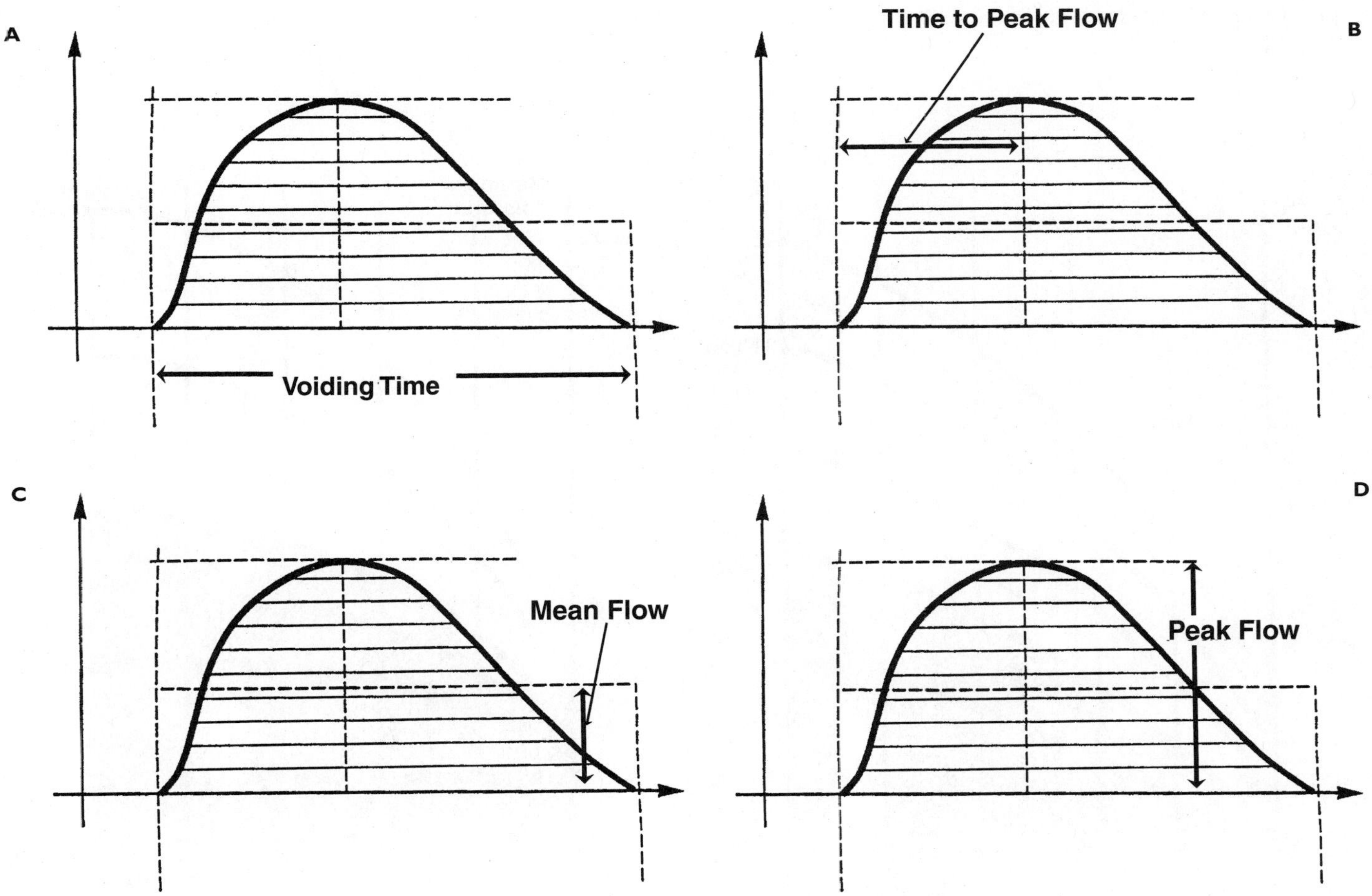

FIG. 9-2 *Uroflow parameters.* ***A,*** *Total voiding time, the period during which measurable flow occurs.* ***B,*** *Time to peak flow rate, the interval between the onset of voiding and the moment of peak flow.* ***C,*** *Mean flow rate, calculated by dividing total voided volume by total voiding time.* ***D,*** *Peak flow rate, the maximum flow rate achieved during a representative voiding event.*

the flow curve. It may be somewhat difficult to determine the most relevant peak flow rate in patients with intermittent voiding patterns or if abdominal straining produces "spikes" of elevated flow rates above the curve generated by the detrusor musculature of the bladder (Fig. 9-3). Peak flow rate is the most widely used flow parameter in the evaluation of patients with suspected bladder outlet obstruction and in the comparison of the efficacy of treatments for benign prostatic hyperplasia.

Normal Uroflow Rates

Normal uroflow parameters vary widely according to characteristics within a given patient and between individuals of different sex or age. The most important variable that must be controlled for between each in any given patient is some measure of bladder volume. It has long been recognized that urinary flow rates are dependent on the degree of bladder distension over a physiologic range. Peak flow rates are the highest and most consistent in the voided volume range between 200 and 400 ml and may actually decrease in a given individual if the voided volume exceeds 500 ml (Fig. 9-4). Nomograms for peak and mean urinary flow rates in young unobstructed males over a range of physiologic bladder volumes (bladder volume is equivalent to voided volume in the setting of complete emp-

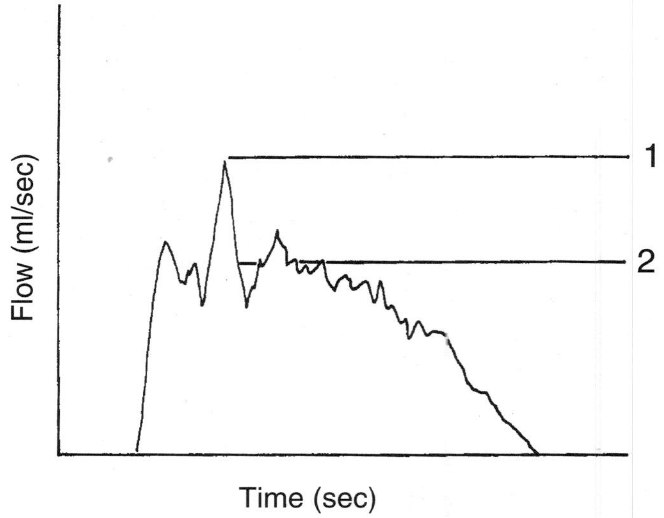

FIG. 9-3 *A uroflow trace during which abdominal straining occurred. Use of the true maximum flow rate, 1, results in an overestimation of the actual peak flow resulting from detrusor function, approximated by visual inspection as 2.* (From Stott M, Abrams PH: Technique and theory of uroflowmetry. In O'Reilly PH, George NJR, Weiss RM, editors: *Diagnostic techniques in urology*, Philadelphia, 1990, Saunders.)

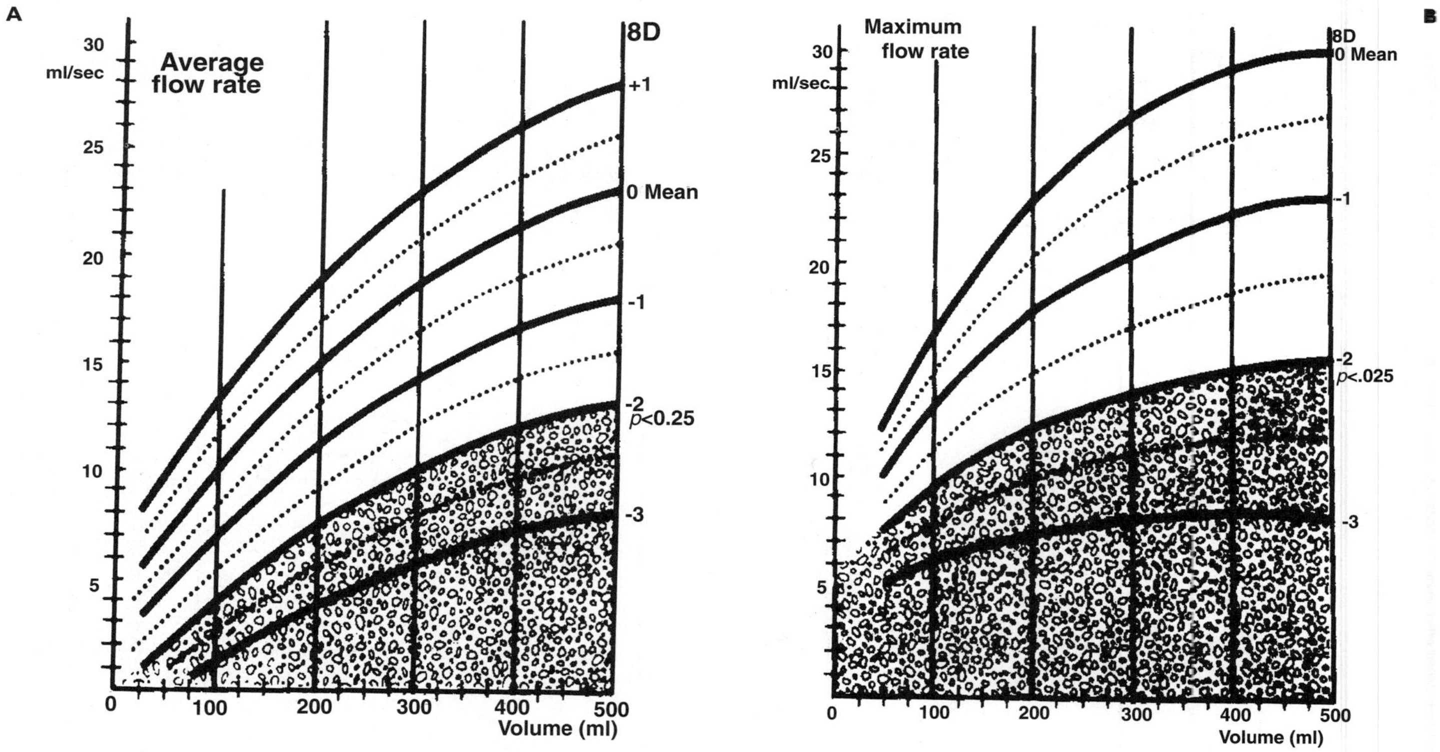

FIG. 9-4 *Uroflow nomograms for average and maximum flow rates over a range of bladder volumes, obtained from flow studies of young male subjects.* Shaded area, *Values less than 2 standard deviations below the mean.* (From Siroky MB, Olsson CA, Krane RJ: *J Urol* 122:665, 1979.)

tying during micturition) have been described1 and are often used as "normal" values (Fig. 9-5).

With growth, urinary flow rates increase throughout childhood to reach a maximum value in early adulthood (Table 9-1). Normal flow rates then decrease as a function of age, particularly in males. Some authors have argued that the decline in normal flow rates in females is too small (0.3 ml/sec per decade) to justify adjusting normal values for age in women.[5] Drach has described a peak flow rate nomogram controlling for both age and voided volume that may be used to investigate the possibility of obstructive dysfunction.[6]

Abnormal Uroflow Rates

Normal urinary flow varies as a function of voided volume, age, sex, patient anxiety, and other factors. As is emphasized below, visual inspection of a flow curve from a representative voiding event gives more accurate information regarding a given patient's voiding function than consideration of isolated flow rates will. Nevertheless, George has listed several observations regarding peak urinary flow rates in men that may be of some use to a clinician concerned about the possible presence of bladder outlet obstruction.[7]

Table 9-1 Minimum acceptable peak uroflow rates for males and females of various ages (Each value represents one standard deviation below the mean).

Age	Minimum volume (ml)	Male (ml/sec)	Female (ml/sec)
4-7	100	10	10
8-13	100	12	15
14-45	200	21	18
46-65	200	12	15
66-80	200	9	10

From Abrams PH, Feneley RCL, Torrens M: Urodynamic investigations. In Abrams PH, Feneley RCL, Torrens M, editors: *Urodynamics*, New York, 1983, Springer-Verlag.

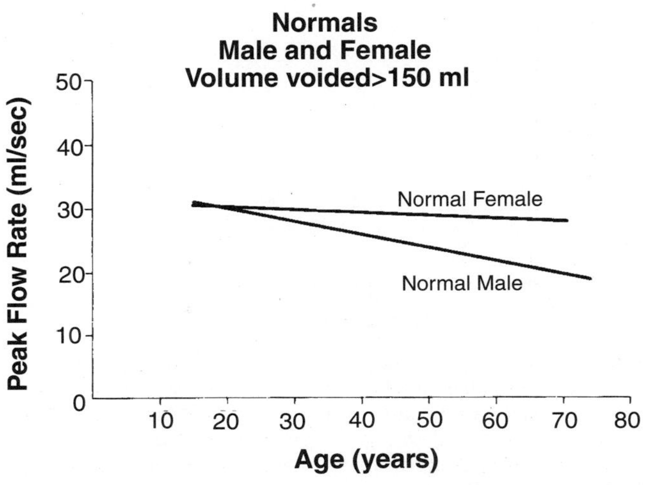

FIG. 9-5 *Normal peak uroflow rate versus age in normal subjects.* (From Drach GW, Ignatoff J, Layton T: *J Urol* 122:215, 1979.)

Rates over 20 ml/sec

The incidence of bladder outlet obstruction is low in people who have a peak flow rate greater than 20 ml/sec. Normal young men void with peak flow rates of up to 40 ml/sec, and so a value in the low 20s in an otherwise normal man might warrant periodic follow-up study and repeated flow rates.

Rates between 15 and 20 ml/sec

Peak flow rates in this range also are associated with a low incidence of outlet obstruction. In the setting of bladder neck obstruction in young men, unusually strong detrusor function may produce peak flow rates well above 15 ml/sec. Symptomatic young men with flow rates in this range should therefore be considered for more sophisticated urodynamic evaluation.[8]

Rates between 10 and 15 ml/sec

Peak flow rates between 10 and 15 ml/sec are equivocal in evaluating for suspected obstruction and generally mandate further investigation.

Rates less than 10 ml/sec

Although the possibility of poor detrusor function as a cause or contributing factor to this range of peak flow rate exists and must always be considered, peak uroflow less than 10 ml/sec is often the result of obstructive voiding.

Flow Curves

Although examination of the numerical uroflow data is valuable, visual inspection of flow curves from multiple representative voiding events of adequate volume will give much more accurate information regarding a given patient's voiding function than consideration of the peak or mean uroflow rate will. In normal unobstructed individuals, the flow curve is smooth, continuous, and nearly bell shaped, with a rapid ascent to peak flow within the first third of eventual total voiding time, after which there is a somewhat slower decline to a relatively abrupt termination of flow. Mean flow rate is slightly greater than half of the peak flow rate (see Figs. 9-1 and 9-2).

Patients with uninhibited detrusor activity often complain of urinary frequency and urgency with voiding of small volumes of urine, which may be accompanied by incontinence of urine during the intense desire to void associated with an uninhibited bladder contraction. These patients often try to suppress voiding during the involuntary bladder activity through voluntary contraction of pelvic floor musculature and may generate high bladder pressures before the release of the pelvic floor activity, resulting in an explosive void of small volume and duration with supranormal peak and average uroflow rates. Some patients exhibit voiding behavior in which the uroflow curves waver during micturition. This is usually the result of abdominal straining on the part of a patient attempting to compensate for inadequate detrusor contractility or outlet obstruction (or both). Patients with neurologic impairment affecting the lower urinary tract, including those with a loss of coordination between detrusor contractility and outlet relaxation (detrusor-sphincter dyssynergia) or fluctuation in the strength of detrusor contractions may also generate intermittent flow curves (Fig. 9-6).

Patients with outlet obstruction from benign enlargement of the prostate typically demonstrate low peak and mean uroflow rates with preservation of the prompt rise to maximum flow rates and prolongation of the descending limb of flow rates at the terminal portion of the flow curve. Obstructive voiding resulting from scarring of the urethra or bladder neck leads to a flow curve with a "flat top," or plateau, of diminished peak uroflow from the fixed, noncompliant resistance to flow.[2] Uroflow curves in patients with loss of detrusor motor function also show low peak and mean flow rates, but tend to achieve maximum flow rates toward the middle of the voiding event (Fig. 9-7). Because the difference between the flow curves of patients with outlet obstruction and detrusor impairment is nonspecific and may be quite subtle, it is impossible to differentiate between the two when one is comparing uroflow data without simultaneous measurement and consideration of bladder pressure during voiding.

Pressure-Flow Studies

Uroflow studies alone do not provide the necessary information to establish bladder outlet obstruction, and pressure-flow studies are required to make the diagnosis. However, measurements of uroflow rates and examinations of uroflow curves are commonly used as the initial studies to evaluate patients with voiding dysfunction, particularly when obstruction is suspected.

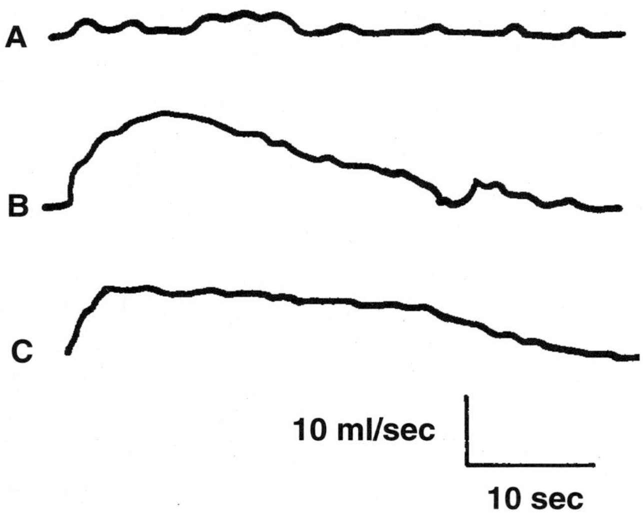

FIG. 9-6 *Uroflow tracings in three obstructed patients.* ***A,*** *Urinary retention with a minimal, dribbling stream.* ***B,*** *Benign prostatic hyperplasia, with decreased peak and mean flow rates and prolongation of the descending limb of the curve.* ***C,*** *Urethral stricture, with decreased peak and mean flow rates and a plateau, or "flat top," appearance from noncompliant obstructive tissue.* (From Siroky MB: *Urol Clin North Am* 17(3):537, 1990.)

Subnormal flow rates and abnormal curves may be the result of outlet obstruction, impaired detrusor motor function, or both. On the other hand, patients presenting with symptoms suggestive of obstruction who generate relatively normal curves with reasonable flow rates may in fact be voiding against a significant degree of resistance but with considerably elevated bladder pressures, which may have deleterious effects.

Urine flow is determined not only by outlet resistance, but also by the magnitude of the detrusor contraction during voiding. From a viewpoint of pure fluid dynamics, the most accurate definition of bladder outlet obstruction is low uroflow in the presence of a detrusor contraction of adequate force, duration, and speed.[9] Simultaneous measurement of intravesical pressure during uroflow studies will therefore lead to a more meaningful evaluation regarding the presence of outlet obstruction.

Many investigators have described means by which a simultaneous expression of bladder pressure and uroflow can be used to determine the degree and significance of obstruction during voiding.[10-12] Currently the most widely used clinical tool incorporating simultaneous consideration of detrusor pressure and uroflow was described by Abrams and Griffiths.[13] Using the

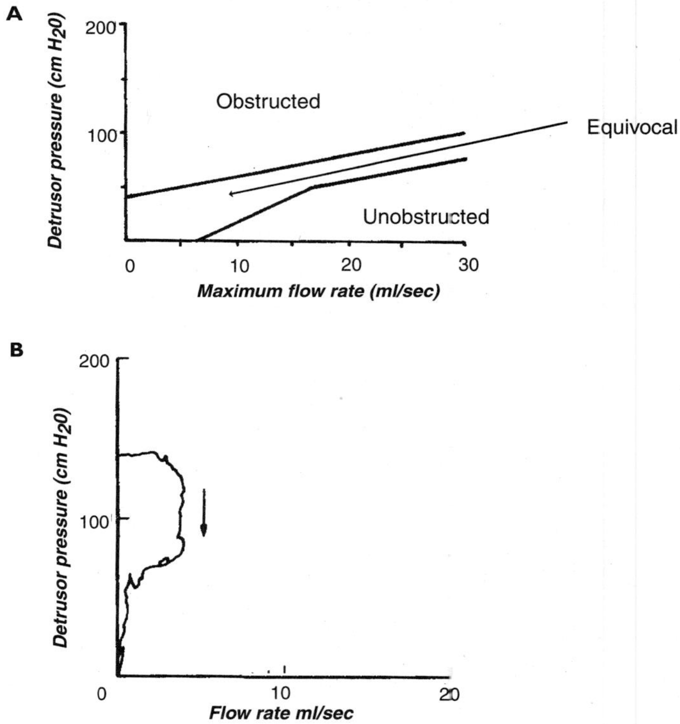

FIG. 9-7 *Pressure-flow nomogram, originally developed by Abrams and Griffith.* ***A,*** *Three zones are established, and a comparison of peak flow versus detrusor pressure at peak flow is used to further delineate the presence of obstruction. Diagnostic accuracy is increased from 50% to 66% over isolated peak flow rates.* ***B,*** *In the remaining 33% of patients in the equivocal zone, an x-y plot of flow rate versus detrusor pressure is used to distinguish between obstruction (present in this patient) and detrusor impairment.* (Modified from Abrams PH, Griffiths DJ: *Br J Urol* 51:129, 1979.)

detrusor pressure observed at the peak uroflow rate, they were able to increase accuracy in the diagnosis of outlet obstruction from 50% to 66% as compared to the peak uroflow rate alone. In the remaining 33% of patients, a graphical plot of pressure versus flow throughout the voiding event was used to distinguish between obstruction and detrusor impairment (see Fig. 9-7). There are some data that indicate that patients classified as "obstructed" using this technique may have a higher rate of subjective improvement from surgical relief of the obstruction than symptomatic patients who are "unobstructed."[14] However, as Kaplan and Te have recently stated, "The relationship between a urodynamic diagnosis of prostatic obstruction and both symptoms and progression of disease in treated and untreated patients remains to be defined."[15]

Conclusions

Although complete urodynamic testing is essential in the evaluation of most lower urinary tract dysfunctions, uroflowmetry as an initial study gives reliable, objective information that can indicate problems in detrusor function, neuromuscular events of micturition, and the presence of possible bladder outlet obstruction. When the interpretation of the urinary flow rate is guided by the voiding history and clinical presentation of the patient, the study is extremely useful as an office diagnostic test. Also, if a noninvasive residual urine can be measured after voiding using an office ultrasonic unit, very important additional clinical information can be obtained quickly in the physician's office without inconvenience to the patient. The clinical application of the results of the urinary flow rate is dependent on the ability of the clinician to interpret the results of the studies and to integrate the information with the voiding history and residual urine volume. In the clinical evaluation of bladder outlet obstruction, it is important to recognize that the urinary flow studies are not a substitute or even an acceptable compromise for pressure-flow studies in establishing the diagnosis of bladder outlet obstruction in either men or women. However, the uroflow evaluation is perhaps the most valuable initial study in both the office and the laboratory assessment of patients who present to any physician's office with symptoms related to micturition.

References

1. International Continence Society second report on the standardisation of terminology of lower urinary tract function, *Br J Urol* 49:207, 1977.
2. Siroky MB: Interpretation of urinary flow rates, *Urol Clin North Am* 17(3):537, 1990.
3. Barrett DM Wein A J: Voiding dysfunction: diagnosis, classification, and management. In Gillenwater JY, Grayhack JT, Howards SS, Duckett JW, editors: *Adult and pediatric urology,* ed 2, St. Louis, 1991, Mosby.
4. Siroky MB, Olsson CA, Krane RJ: The flow rate nomogram I: development, *J Urol* 122:665, 1979.
5. Drach GW, gnatoff J, Layton T: Peak urinary flow rate: observations in female subjects and comparison to male subjects, *J Urol* 122:215, 1979.
6. Drach GW, Layton T, Bottaccini MR: A method of adjustment of male peak urinary flow rate for varying age and volume voided, *J Urol* 128:960, 1982.
7. George NJR: Clinical uroflowmetry. In O'Reilly PH, George NJR, Weiss RM, editor: *Diagnostic techniques in urology,* Philadelphia, 1990, Saunders.
8. Norlen LJ, Blaivas JG: Unsuspected proximal urethral obstruction in young and middle-aged men, *J Urol* 135:972, 1986.
9. Blaivas JG: Multichannel urodynamic studies in men with benign prostatic hyperplasia: indications and interpretation, *Urol Clin North Am* 17(3):543, 1990.
10. Gleason DM, Lattimer JK: The pressure flow study: a method for measuring bladder neck resistance, *J Urol* 87:844, 1962.
11. Coolsaet BRLA, Blok A: Detrusor properties related to prostatism, *Neurourol Urodyn* 5:435, 1986.
12. Schafer W, Rubben H, Nopepeney R, et al: Obstructed and unobstructed prostatic obstruction: a plea for urodynamic objectivation of bladder outflow obstruction in benign prostatic hyperplasia, *World J Urol* 6:198, 1989.
13. Abrams PH Griffiths DJ: The assessment of prostatic obstruction from urodynamic measurements and from residual urine, *Br J Urol* 51:129, 1979.
14. Jensen KME Clinical evaluation of routine urodynamic investigations in prostatism, *Neurourol Urodyn* 8:545, 1989.
15. Kaplan SA, Te AE: Uroflowmetry and urodynamics, *Urol Clin North Am* 22(2):309, 1995.

Chapter 10

The Cystometrogram

Simon Jackson, Paul Abrams

When presented with lower urinary tract symptoms, the clinician must decide if the patient has a functional bladder disorder. The goal of cystometry is to understand a clinical problem in pathophysiologic terms by recording bladder pressure during filling and voiding. If therapeutic decisions are based on symptoms alone, more than 25% of patients may be treated by inappropriate and potentially harmful therapy, since there is often a poor correlation between symptoms and pathophysiologic features.[1-4]

The aim of cystometry is to reproduce the patient's symptoms as accurately as possible and provide a pathophysiologic explanation of the patient's problem. There are three important facets to this:

1. A technically sound recording should be produced.
2. The patients subjected to the investigation must be appropriate.
3. The interpretation of the study should result in an accurate diagnosis.

The cystometrogram (CMG) is used to measure the following features of bladder behavior:

Capacity
Sensation
Compliance
Contractility
Urethral function

During cystometry the following measurements are required:

1. *Intravesical pressure* (P_{ves}), which is usually measured with a urethral or a suprapubic catheter.
2. *Intra-abdominal pressure* (P_{abd}), which is taken to be the pressure surrounding the bladder. It is usually estimated from rectal or vaginal pressure.
3. *Detrusor pressure* (P_{det}), which is the component of intravesical pressure created by the active and passive forces in the bladder wall. It is derived from electronic subtraction of P_{abd} from P_{ves}.
4. *Urine flow rate,* so that leakage during filling and flow during voiding can be recorded.
5. *Volume infused,* so that bladder volume is known at any instant.

In addition, optional measurements and observations include the following:

Urethral closure pressure (P_{ura}), which is derived from urethral pressure profilometry.
Electromyography (EMG) of pelvic floor or intraurethral striated sphincter.
Videocystourethrography (VCU). If VCU is combined with pressure flow recordings it is known as videourodynamics.

Early interest focused on the assessment of voiding function, but since the 1970s emphasis has been placed on defining bladder function during the filling phase, and filling cystometry has now been refined into a more standard technique. Initial efforts aimed to unmask detrusor instability, often using extreme methods such as gas cystometry, ice-cold filling solutions, or fast-fill at 150 ml per minute. The early popularity of gas cystometry owed much to its cleanliness, making it suitable for use in the "office." However, because the gas is compressible, highly soluble, and irritative and infusion rates are rapid, the test has little to recommend it clinically. The International Continence Society (ICS) has done much over the years to standardize the methodology and interpretation of cystometry.[5] In general the patient should not be taking drugs that affect bladder function before cystometry unless specified, and variable factors that may affect results should be noted. These include whether a transurethral or percutaneous catheter was used for filling, whether the filling medium was liquid or gas, what the temperature of the filling medium was, whether the patient was supine, sitting, or standing during the test, and the rate of artificial bladder filling.

That these parameters can affect the nature of the CMG is well established. The characteristics of the filling medium can influence the function of the bladder. Cold solutions are provocative, forming the basis of the "ice water test,"[6] and ideally one should warm the fluid to body temperature before instillation, though we find that fluid at warm room temperature is adequate. The pH of the filling solution also has an effect, such that alkaline solutions (pH 8.5) increase bladder capacity in approximately one third of patients,[7] whereas acid solutions (pH 3.3) provoke instability in one third of previously stable patients.[8] Fast bladder filling may produce significant urodynamic artifacts, particularly in neurologic patients, and in its report the ICS has defined bladder filling as fast (when it is 100 ml/min), medium (10 to 100 ml/min), or slow (up to 10 ml/min). It should, however, be remembered that the average physiologic filling rate of the bladder is only 1 ml/min, and therefore even the ICS slow fill rate is unphysiologic except under extreme diuretic conditions. However, for the nonneurologic patient a filling rate of 50 to 60 ml/min while a conventional CMG is being performed appears to be a reasonable compromise, allowing realistic filling times and an apparent low incidence of artifacts.

TECHNIQUE

Pressure Measurement

There are two basic techniques; pressure can be measured by external transducers, connected to the patient by fluid-filled catheters or by solid-state transducer catheters. We use an epidural catheter connected to manometer tubing to measure P_{ves} and manometer tubing alone (with the tip protected from fecal occlusion by a finger stall) for measuring P_{abd} (Fig. 10-1). Alternatively 6 French gauge catheter-tip transducers may be used to measure P_{ves} and P_{abd} (Fig. 10-2). Urethral catheters distort the normal anatomy and may change the urine flow characteristics[9]; therefore suprapubic catheters have been suggested as a superior alternative.[10] However, because this is invasive, most units rely on urethral catheters, since there is no convincing evi-

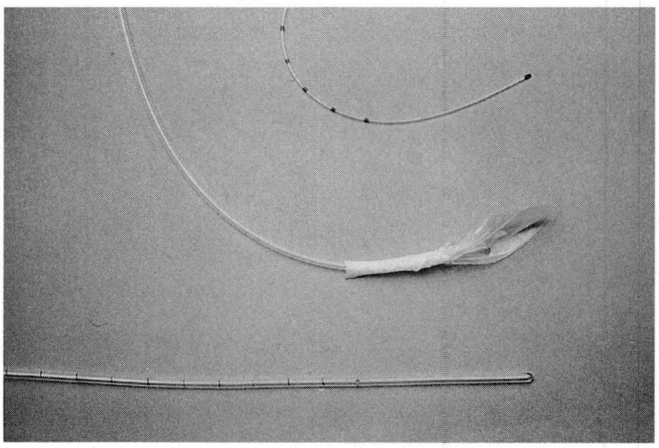

FIG. 10-1 ***A,*** *Epidural catheter manometer tubing used to measure P_{ves}.* ***B,*** *Manometer tubing, with the tip protected from fecal occlusion by a finger stall, for measuring P_{abd}.* ***C,*** *8 Fr gauge intravesical filling catheter.*

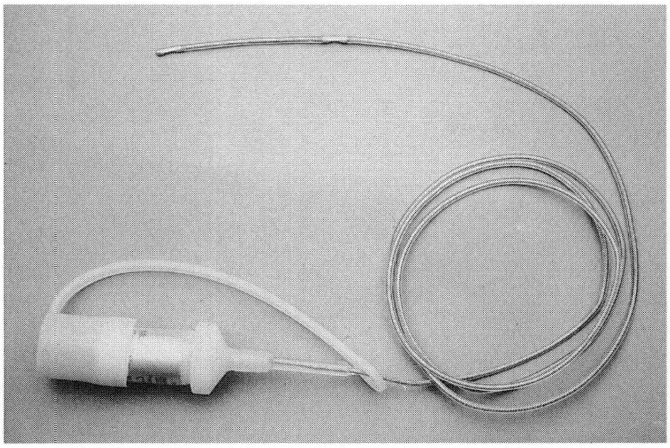

FIG. 10-2 *Catheter-tip transducers can be used as an alternative to manometric tubing for measuring P_{ves} and P_{abd}. This 6 Fr catheter has two transducers 6 cm apart at the tip, allowing the additional measurement of urethral pressure profiles.*

dence that a fine catheter (8 Fr or less) has a significant influence on outlet mechanics. To avoid unnecessary artifact, before one performs the voiding cystogram, the larger diameter filling catheter (8 Fr) can be removed, with only the smaller pressure measuring catheter in situ being left.

Proper placement of catheters is imperative. The P_{ves} catheter should be advanced so that it coils in the bladder. The P_{abd} catheter needs to be advanced well beyond the anal sphincter. Alternatively, in women, the vagina can be used, provided that the tip of the catheter is advanced into the upper two thirds of the vagina, above the level of the pelvic floor.[11] In addition, to prevent catheter movement, the catheters must be carefully taped close to the external urethral meatus and the anal verge respectively.

To produce a technically sound CMG a few points need to be carefully addressed:

1. All systems are zeroed at atmospheric pressure. For external transducers the reference point is the level of the superior edge of the symphysis pubis. For catheter-mounted transducers the reference point is the transducer itself. Failure to correctly zero the transducers will result in an unreliable determination of detrusor pressure.
2. If P_{ves} and P_{abd} are being recorded by fluid-filled manometric catheters, it is imperative that all air bubbles are thoroughly flushed out of the system before recording is begun. If this is not done, pressure transmission will be defective (Fig. 10-3, *A*).
3. At the beginning of the study it is essential to get the patient to cough, demonstrating a rise in both intravesical and rectal pressure. The rise in rectal and intravesical pressure should be identical, with the electronically subtracted P_{det} line remaining flat, though an artifactual background "blip" on the P_{det} line can be impossible to eradicate because of the delayed response inherent in the system; this need not be a cause for concern (Fig. 10-3, *B*). Furthermore, to ensure that the pressure response recording in both bladder and rectal lines continues to be satisfactory throughout the test, with adequate subtraction for P_{det}, one should continually check throughout filling by asking the patient to cough at regular intervals; we advocate every 1 minute. Similarly, after completion of the voiding CMG, before removal of the manometric catheters, it is essential to ensure that they have not been dislodged during the void and are still recording pressure changes reliably by asking the patient to cough once more.

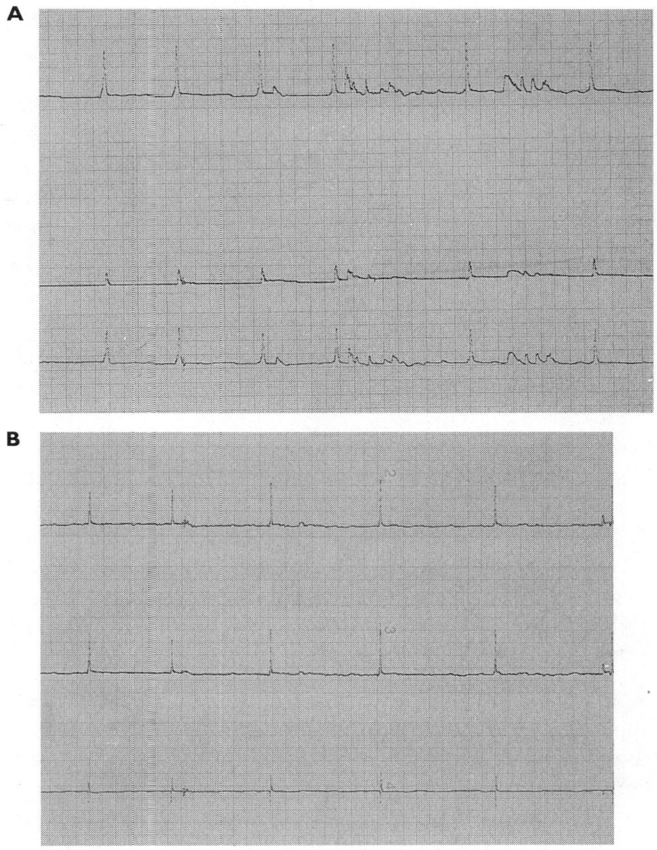

FIG. 10-3 ***A,*** *In this recording, there is an air within the abdominal manometric tubing. As a result, recorded P_{abd} is artificially low, in this case falling below the 0 cm H_2O reference line obtained when the system is initially zeroed at atmospheric pressure. Coughing results in intravesical pressure rises of 80 cm H_2O, but there is defective transmission of abdominal pressure through the rectal line; consequently an artifact is present on the electronically subtracted P_{det} line.* ***B,*** *This figure should be compared to* ***A.*** *Both manometric lines are now flushed free of air bubbles and are recording satisfactorily, resulting in identical pressure rises of up to 80 cm H_2O on coughing. The electronically subtracted P_{det} line therefore remains flat. However, there is a background "blip" on the P_{det} each time we ask the patient to cough. This can be impossible to eradicate because of delayed response times inherent in the system and need not be a cause for concern.*

Filling Cystometry

During filling CMG the following observations are made:

Capacity. The volume infused during filling and hence the calculated bladder volume are measured, either by timing the infusion time at a known filling rate, or by using a weight transducer to measure loss of weight from the filling bag. If one assumes a normal rate of diuresis, a natural filling should have a negligible contribution over the time span of a medium-filled CMG.

Sensation. The patient is asked to comment upon bladder sensation during filling. Terminology that can be used during the filling phase of the CMG and have been defined by the ICS include the following:

> **First desire to void.** This is usually felt at approximately half capacity (150 to 200 ml).
>
> **Normal desire to void.** This is defined as *the feeling that leads the patient to pass urine at the next convenient moment, but voiding can be delayed if necessary.* It commonly occurs at 75% of capacity.
>
> **Strong desire to void.** This is defined as *a persistent desire to void without fear of leakage* and is felt at capacity (300 to 600 ml).
>
> **Urgency.** This is defined as *a strong desire to void accompanied by fear of leakage or pain* and may be described particularly by patients with detrusor instability.
>
> **Maximum cystometric capacity.** This is *the volume at which the patient feels unable to delay micturition.*

In practice, maximum cystometric capacity has little clinical application. We ask all patients attending for a CMG study to complete a frequency and volume chart in the preceding week. From this and the residual volume, measured at the beginning of the CMG study, the *functional bladder capacity* can be calculated, which is 300 to 600 ml in most adults. Functional capacity is of much greater clinical relevance than maximum capacity, and we would not recommend filling beyond functional capacity during the CMG study; overfilling yields no useful clinical data, and there is a risk of precipitating poor voiding or even acute urinary retention because of overdistension of the bladder.

Although of a subjective nature, *sensation can be described as normal, reduced (hyposensitive), increased (hypersensitive), or absent.* If the sensation is hypersensitive, the volumes at first desire, normal desire to void, and cystometric capacity are all reduced. Hyposensitivity may coexist with a bladder of large capacity and poor contractility caused by autonomic neuropathy or chronic retention secondary to outflow obstruction, though hyposensitivity is commonly idiopathic.

Compliance

Compliance indicates *the change in volume for a change in pressure.* It is expressed as milliliters per centimeter of water and may be reduced if an underlying disorder exists. *During normal bladder filling little or no pressure change occurs; this is termed "normal compliance."* Rapid filling rates may alter this. At present there are insufficient data to define normal, high, and low compliance, but *an increase of 40 ml in bladder volume for a rise of 1 cm H_2O* in detrusor pressure may represent the upper limit of normal compliance.[12] When one is reporting compliance, the rate of bladder filling should be noted as well as the volume increment and the part of the cystometrogram curve used for the calculation because bladder compliance may be reduced near bladder capacity.

Contractility

If during the filling phase the bladder volume increases without a significant rise in pressure and with no involuntary contractions despite provocation, the detrusor function is normal (stable). *Detrusor instability is characterized by involuntary contractions during the filling phase,* which may be spontaneous or provoked and cannot be completely suppressed. *Any associated urinary leakage is called "urge incontinence"* (Fig. 10-4). Provocation may include rapid filling, alterations in posture and movement, coughing, tap running, and other triggering procedures. Detrusor instability results in phasic contractions, which should be contrasted with altered compliance, where the detrusor pressure rises gradually. Originally it was suggested that clinical judgment should be exercised regarding the significance of phasic contractions of less than 15 cm H_2O in amplitude,[13] but currently no lower limit is specified,[5] since the relation to symptoms is more important than any arbitrary lower amplitude limit. If detrusor instability is present and there is objective evidence of a relevant neurologic disorder, the instability may be termed "detrusor hyperreflexia."

Urethral Function

The involuntary loss of urine during filling cystometry is genuine stress incontinence (GSI) if it occurs in the absence of a detrusor contraction. To examine for this we ask the patient to cough during the filling phase. Typically, such provocation will result in an instantaneous loss of urine, and examination of the subtracted P_{det} should confirm that there is no associated cough-induced instability before the diagnosis of GSI is made (Fig. 10-5).

Once the functional bladder capacity is reached, if GSI has not been clearly demonstrated during the filling phase and the clinical history is suggestive of stress incontinence, the larger-diameter filling catheter is removed, with the epidural manometric tubing or electronic pressure-sensing catheter being left in situ. We then examine for urinary loss using a variety of provocative maneuvers that can include coughing, squatting, heel bouncing, and jumping. If urinary loss is observed, reference to the simultaneous P_{det} will elucidate whether GSI, or activity-provoked detrusor instability and its subsequent urge incontinence, is the cause.

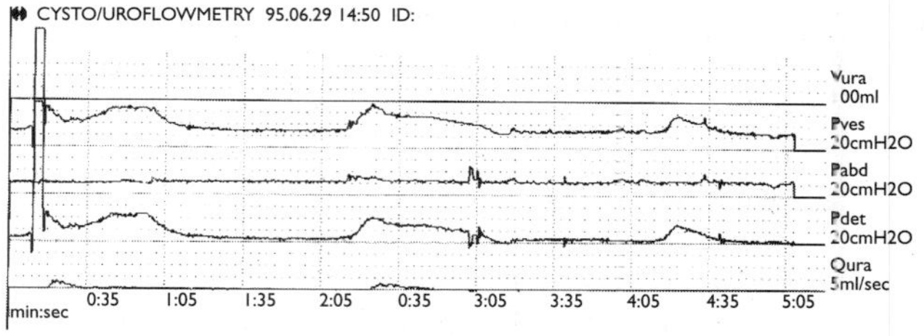

FIG. 10-4 *Cystometrogram showing detrusor instability and urge incontinence. The rise in pressure of 40 cm H_2O seen on the P_{ves} and subtracted P_{det} lines represents involuntary detrusor activity. There is urinary leakage sufficient to register on the flowmeter at 2 to 3 ml/sec (represented by Q_{ura}). Because this leakage occurred in association with detrusor contractions, it represents urge incontinence.*

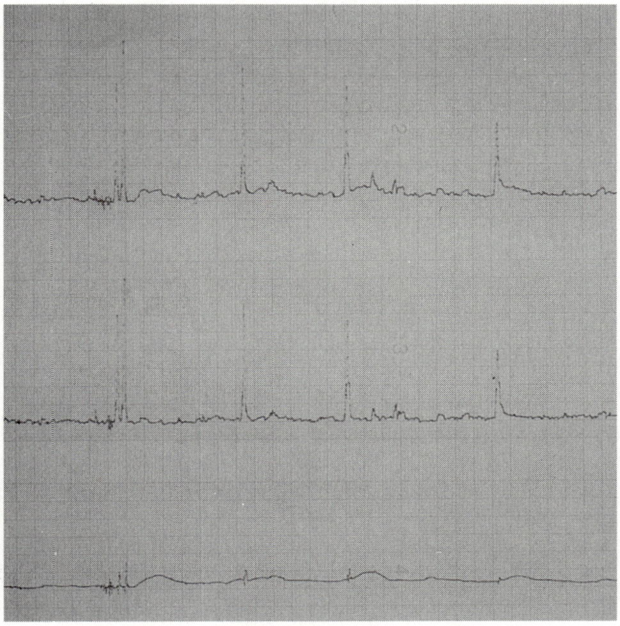

FIG. 10-5 *Cystometrogram showing spike rises in pressure on both P_{ves} and P_{det} lines, associated with the patient's coughing when asked. The subtracted P_{det} line show low-amplitude pressure rises after each cough, representing cough-provoked detrusor instability. In this case leakage did occur upon coughing, registering as flow on the Q_{ura} line. However, the leakage was observed immediately on coughing, and on close examination of the cystometrogram (as one remembers that there is a 0.5- to 1-second delay from actual urinary leakage to urine reaching the flowmeter) the leakage can be seen to be occurring before the cough-provoked detrusor activity. It therefore represents genuine stress incontinence.*

Voiding Cystometry

Having performed filling cystometry, one completes the CMG by performing a voiding study. As previously discussed the filling catheter is removed before voiding to avoid unnecessary artifact through urethral obstruction. The intravesical and rectal pressure recording lines are left in situ, so as to allow the simultaneous measurement of detrusor pressure along with the urine flow rate.

Normal voiding is achieved by voluntary initiation of a detrusor contraction that is sustained until the bladder is empty. The magnitude of the pressure rise depends on the degree of outlet resistance and on the detrusor contraction itself. The normal male voids with a detrusor pressure of 20 to 40 cm H_2O, but women have considerably lower pressures (10 to 25 cm H_2O), some voiding with excellent flows but little or no rise in pressure. This does not imply inadequate detrusor function but simply that the contraction is isotonic in the presence of low outlet resistance. The lower urethral resistance is reflected in the greater flow rates achieved by women. As part of the voiding study one can ask the patient to interrupt the stream when maximum flow is reached. The resulting isometric contraction is termed "$P_{det.iso}$." This gives some idea of detrusor contractility and may indicate the likelihood of poor voiding after bladder neck stress incontinence surgery. However, we do not routinely use this test because it impairs other voiding parameters. Detrusor activity is defined as inadequate if contractions are of insufficient magnitude or duration to effect bladder emptying in a normal time span in patients without significant outlet obstruction. *If the detrusor pressure during voiding is low with low flow rates, the detrusor is termed "underactive" (impaired contractility)* and there may or may not be residual urine. *If the detrusor shows no evidence of activity, it is "contractile." If there is an associated neurologic abnormality, this is called "detrusor areflexia." Abdominal straining should not be required if the detrusor is functioning normally.*

The urinary flow recorded during voiding cystometry should be correlated with the detrusor activity: it may be remembered that there is a 0.5- to 1-second delay because of the time it takes for urine to reach the flowmeter. In most circumstances in adults a voided volume of less than 100 ml cannot be interpreted reliably, whereas flow rates obtained above a 500 ml cystometric capacity may also be low, perhaps because of bladder decompensation.[14] Outlet obstruction should cause a low to normal flow with raised detrusor pressure when compared with normal controls. However, unrepresentative micturitions and underactive detrusor function can complicate the issue. Most patients will be able to void during the study, but inability to do so does not in itself indicate a functional abnormality if subsequent free flow rates with residual urine assessment indicates normality.

Postmicturition Events

Postmicturition events such as *persistent detrusor activity (after contraction) after the completed void* are not well understood and are of doubtful significance; we will not therefore discuss them further here.

It should be remembered that urodynamic studies are invasive, and, although relatively free of complications, exceptions such as knotting of the epidural catheter and urinary tract infections rarely occur.[15-17] Therefore, to avoid unnecessary morbidity and expense it is important to select patients appropriately for cystometry, and such selection requires an understanding of the test's clinical indications.

Indications for Cystometry

Storage Problems

Symptoms suggestive of urinary stress incontinence. Genuine stress incontinence (GSI) is the most common cause of urinary leakage in women, and bladder neck surgery is the definitive treatment for such cases. However, even women presenting with symptoms suggestive of pure stress incontinence will have underlying detrusor instability (DI) as the cause of incontinence detected on subsequent urodynamic assessment 11% to 16% of the time.[3,4,18] It follows that surgery planned on the basis of symptoms alone will not infrequently result in inappropriate treatment. This point is contested by some investigators who claim that history alone is adequate assessment in patients presenting with pure stress incontinence symptoms.[19,20] Others, however, claim that surgery performed on the basis of symptoms alone will result in inappropriate treatment up to 27% of the time,[21] and we would advocate urodynamic assessment before bladder neck surgery to ensure the presence of GSI. Furthermore, surgery for stress incontinence can result in detrusor instability[22] and assessment of detrusor function before surgery may be medicolegally prudent. A final reason for performing a urodynamic assessment in this group of patients is that postoperative voiding difficulties can sometimes be predicted in those who void by straining and or have poor detrusor contractility.

Symptoms suggestive of detrusor instability. The likeliest disorder underlying urinary frequency and urgency is detrusor instability, which may be strongly suspected from the patient's frequency and volume chart.[23] However, there is conflicting evidence regarding the specificity of the symptoms associated with DI; the incidence of urodynamically proved DI varying from 43% to 100% in patients with such symptoms,[3,4] whereas up to 22% will actually prove to have pure GSI without DI.[21] The primary treatment for DI is by bladder training with or without pharmacologic therapy (anticholinergic medication). Anticholinergic drugs may cause unpleasant side effects but are essentially safe and have a rapid onset of action. Therefore, because inappropriate treatment does not expose the patient to risk, it would seem reasonable clinical practice to commence a short course of empirical treatment with anticholinergic medication in such cases, provided that a midstream urine specimen and cytologic results are negative. DI should respond rapidly to such treatment. Urodynamic investigation can be reserved for unresponsive cases where confirmation of the diagnosis of DI is essential, both to avoid unnecessary continuation on unpleasant drugs and to exclude other pathologic states such as sensory urgency and stress incontinence where a different intervention will be required.

Voiding Problems

Symptoms suggestive of outlet obstruction. Outlet obstruction and voiding disorders in women are uncommon and if suspected require urodynamic investigation. Symptoms associated with prostatic obstruction can be mimicked by poor detrusor contractility, by bladder hypersensitivity, or by DI, the last being found in up to 60% of such patients.[24] DI can lead to frequency, urgency, and urge incontinence, whereas hypersensitivity is characterized by decreased functional bladder capacity and leads to symptoms of frequency and sensory urgency.

Although hesitancy, poor stream, intermittent stream, and terminal dribbling are often thought of as typical of outlet obstruction and the symptoms of frequency, nocturia, urgency, and urge incontinence as typical of DI, the correlation between symptoms and urodynamic diagnosis are very weak. If a definitive diagnosis is required, pressure-flow studies are essential. Men with poor outcome after prostatectomy seem to fall into two groups, those with storage symptoms who are more likely to have detrusor instability and those with low flow and low voiding pressures caused by detrusor underactivity with a nonobstructed bladder outlet.[25,26] The objective results of prostatectomy have been improved from 72% to 88%[27,28] by inclusion of urodynamic studies in the preoperative assessment of patients, reducing failure rate to less than 10%.[29]

Neuropathic Bladder

Anyone with neurologic disease and lower urinary tract symptoms should be investigated with videourodynamics. Such patients are at risk of detrusor hyperreflexia, low compliance, and detrusor and sphincter dyssynergia. Of particular concern is the risk of upper tract damage when raised intravesical pressure results in upper tract dilatation and subsequent renal impairment. In these patients a simultaneous assessment of anatomy (by videocystourethrography) and function (by pressure-flow studies) is essential. It is known as videourodynamics.

Ambulatory Studies

The controversy surrounding artificial filling rates has led to a reevaluation of the pioneering work of Douglas James,[30] who was the first urodynamicist to realize the importance of natural-fill cystometry and to perform long-term ambulatory monitoring (LTAM).

The systems use microtip pressure transducers to record rectal and bladder pressure, and the signals are digitized and transferred to solid-state memory (Fig. 10-6). If the machine incorporates an integrated voiding channel, data from a flowmeter can be stored in the memory to allow simultaneous recordings of urinary flow and detrusor activity. First desire to void, urgency, micturition, and subjective leakage can be

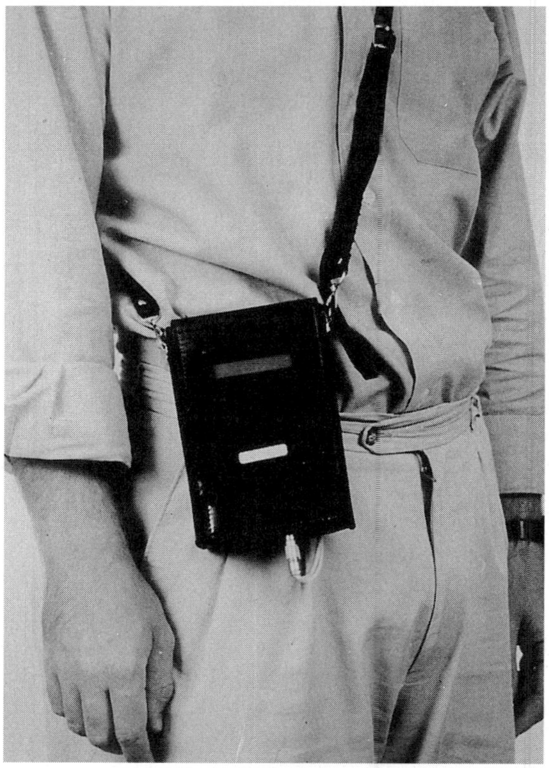

FIG. 10-6 *Ambulatory recording monitor. Data are subsequently downloaded to a PC for visual display.*

recorded by the patient in the memory by use of coded event-marker buttons. Studies may last up to 24 or even 48 hours, if required, depending on the portable memory capacity. During the course of the study the patient can perform tasks that normally provoke symptoms such as hand washing, running, and carrying heavy bags.

Simultaneous recording of urinary incontinence is more difficult than during conventional CMG, where direct inspection of the urethral meatus is possible. Currently the favored method of detecting leakage is with the "Urilos" system pioneered by James[31] in which an interweaving electrode meshwork detects the presence of salt-containing fluids. Although initially bulky, the pad can now be reduced in size sufficiently to insert into a sanitary towel[32]; however, it is not specific for urinary loss or for detecting any salt-containing fluid such as sweat, vaginal discharge, or menstrual fluid. In Bristol we have developed a pad that specifically and sensitively detects, using diode sensors, the temperature rise associated with the loss of urine.[33]

LTAM may prove to be the most significant development of the past 20 years, because it is becoming increasingly apparent that there are fundamental differences between values obtained from conventional and ambulatory studies. Data derived from artificial filling cystometry may be unreliable for several reasons; the filling rate is nonphysiologic, the test requires catheterization, it is of a relatively short duration, and it is performed in a physically confined clinical setting, often in full view of strangers. Ambulatory monitoring, using solid-state transducers with portable data-storage devices,[34,35] overcome some of these limitations. Results obtained from physiologic filling and recording of bladder pressure are leading us to reassess our views on DI and bladder compliance during the filling phase and detrusor contractility during the voiding phase. Areas where there is considerable discrepancy between conventional and ambulatory studies include the following: incidence of DI, compliance, and detrusor contractility.

Incidence of Detrusor Instability

Uninhibited detrusor contractions occur in 38% to 69% of asymptomatic volunteers.[36,37] By comparison, conventional urodynamic studies revealed an incidence of instability in up to 25% of asymptomatic volunteers,[36,37,38] with faster filling rates demonstrating significantly less instability. It is difficult to continue to regard uninhibited detrusor activity, taken in isolation, as abnormal; CMG findings must be interpreted along with the clinical picture. Neal[39] reports that although ambulatory monitoring is more sensitive than conventional CMG, reported instability in "control" subjects can often be predicted if a careful history is taken.

Compliance

High-pressure chronic retention seen in elderly men with bladder outlet obstruction,[40] initially believed to be caused by abnormally low bladder compliance now appears to be caused by DI. The very high intravesical pressures shown in conventional studies were artifactual and masked the underlying DI shown by long-term ambulatory monitoring.[41]

Detrusor Contractility

Reports by Webb et al.[42] and work from our unit in Southmead (unpublished observations) in two very different groups of patients has shown that physiologic filling appears to have a dramatic effect on voiding function. The voiding pressures during LTAM are significantly higher than those recorded during conventional voicing phase CMG. The explanation for this is not clear; possibly fast filling causes incomplete repolarization of detrusor muscle, making the ultimate contraction less efficient.

In the light of these discrepancies, the clinical role of ambulatory studies remains to be fully defined. However, it does appear more sensitive in the detection of detrusor instability and incontinence than conventional cystometry.[43,44] In elderly incontinent men, ambulatory monitoring has provided information related to the characteristics of bladder activity in this group.[45] In women with incontinence not seen on conventional CMG, LTAM with recording done over two or three micturition cycles, coupled with the use of a perineal urine leakage detection pad, will allow correlation of the patient's symptoms (recorded by a coded event marker), changes in detrusor pressure, and episodes of urinary leakage. Using this technique, we find LTAM particularly useful for defining whether leakage is attributable to DI or sphincter weakness in women with objective loss on pad testing and a normal conventional CMG study. It is also of considerable help in those patients with symptoms of frequency, urgency, and urge incontinence and a normal conventional CMG.

In summary, ambulatory studies are more physiologic than conventional CMG and have an important part to play in the investigation of lower urinary tract dysfunction where conventional CMG has failed to confirm a clinical suspicion of detrusor instability or stress incontinence. However, as it appears that instability may occur in over 50% of asymptomatic controls, the results of any ambulatory study must be treated with caution and closely correlated with the symptomatic complaints of the patient.

CONCLUSION

The International Continence Society has done much over the years to standardize the methodology and interpretation of cystometry. Urodynamic studies have matured from being a research investigation in a few centers to being an integral part of the routine assessment of patients with lower urinary tract dysfunction. We would advocate the routine use of urodynamic studies in:

1. All women for whom bladder neck surgery is being considered
2. Bladder symptoms that are unresponsive to appropriate doses of anticholinergic medication
3. Men with lower urinary tract symptoms and urinary flows above 10 ml/sec
4. All complicated cases, such as neuropathic patients with lower urinary tract symptoms and women with suspected outlet obstruction

Conventional cystometry is adequate for the majority of cases, with videourodynamics reserved for appropriate patients. Although ambulatory studies are more physiologic and may gradually replace much conventional cystometry, their interpretation and place within the field of urodynamics needs further clarification in view of the discrepancies that exist between ambulatory and conventional studies. We would currently recommend that ambulatory studies are used clinically in patients where conventional CMG has failed to confirm a history of incontinence caused by either detrusor instability or GSI, when urinary leakage has been objectively demonstrated on pad testing.

Further areas of uncertainty also exist within the field of conventional cystometry. We need a clearer definition of bladder compliance and the effects of filling speed on this. Objective parameters for investigating stress incontinence need to be accepted; at present the degree of physical provocation varies. There is no accepted method for quantifying the degree of instability by either the strength or frequency of detrusor contractions, and it is unclear what the effects of posture and filling speed on the detection of detrusor instability are. Although a clinically essential tool, the areas of controversy should be remembered when one is performing cystometry, and results are interpreted with this in mind.[46]

References

1. Bates CP, Whiteside CG, Turner-Warwick R: Synchronous cine-pressure-flow cystourethrography with special reference to stress and urge incontinence, *Br J Urol* 42:714-723, 1970.
2. Cardozo LD, Stanton SL: Genuine stress incontinence and detrusor instability—a review of 200 patients, *Br J Obstet Gynaecol* 87:184-190, 1980.
3. Shepherd AM, Powell PH, Ball AJ: The place of urodynamic studies in the investigation and treatment of female urinary tract symptoms, *J Obstet Gynaecol* 3:123-125, 1982.
4. Lagro-Janssen FM, Debruyne FMJ, Van Weel C: Value of the patient's case history in diagnosing urinary incontinence in general practice, *Br J Urol* 67:569-572, 1991.
5. Abrams P, Blaivas JG, Stanton SL, et al: The International Continence Society Committee on Standardisation of Terminology; the standardisation of terminology of lower urinary tract function, *Scand J Urol Nephrol* 114(suppl): 5-19, 1988.
6. Bors E: Neurogenic bladder, *Urological Survey* 7:177-250, 1957.
7. Sethia KK, Smith JC: The effect of pH and lignocaine on detrusor instability, *Br J Urol* 60:516-518, 1987.
8. Aslund K, Rentzhogh L, Sandströmb G: Effects of ice cold saline and acid solution in urodynamics, *Proc 18th Annual Meeting of the International Continence Society,* pp. 1-2, Oslo, Norway, 1988.
9. Tessier J, Schick E: Does urethral instrumentation affect uroflowmetry measurements? *Br J Urol* 65:261-263, 1990.
10. Rollema HJ, van Mastrigt R, Ambergen AW, et al: Detrusor instability in benign prostatic hypertrophy (BPH); low incidence by suprapubic filling cystometry, *Neurourol Urodyn* 9:422-423, 1990.
11. James ED: The vagina as an alternative to the rectum in measuring abdominal pressure during urodynamic investigations, *Br J Urol* 60:212-216, 1987.
12. Stott MA, Abrams P: Bladder compliance in patients with spina bifida, *Neurourol Urodyn* 6(3):232-233, 1987.
13. ICS Third report on the standardisation of terminology of lower urinary tract function, *Scand J Urol Nephrol* 12:191-193, 1978.
14. Abrams P, Feneley R, Torrens M: Urodynamic investigations. In *Urodynamics,* Berlin, 1983, Springer-Verlag, pp 35-39.
15. Edwards LE, Powell CS: Urodynamic studies: an unusual complication, *Br J Urol* 58:461-462, 1986.
16. McInerney PD, Stephenson TP: Knotting of the pressure line during urodynamics, *Neurourol Urodyn* 8:243-244, 1989.
17. Carter PL, Lewis P, Abrams P: Urodynamic morbidity and dysuria prophylaxis, *Br J Urol* 67:40-41, 1991.
18. Byrne DJ, Hamilton Stewart PA, Gray BK: The role of urodynamics in female urinary stress incontinence, *Br J Urol* 59:228-229, 1987.
19. Kaufman JM: Urodynamics in stress incontinence, *J Urol* 122:778-782, 1979.
20. Hastie KJ, Moisey CU: Are urodynamics necessary in female patients presenting with stress incontinence? *Br J Urol* 63:155-156, 1989.
21. Jarvis GJ, Hall S, Stamp S, et al: An assessment of urodynamic examination in incontinent women, *Br J Obstet Gynaecol* 87:893-896, 1980.
22. Cardozo LD, Stanton SL, Williams JE: Detrusor instability following surgery for genuine stress incontinence, *Br J Urol* 51:204-207, 1979.
23. Turner-Warwick RT, Milroy EJ: A re-appraisal of the value of routine urological procedures in the assessment of urodynamic function, Symposium on Clinical Urodynamics, *Urol Clin North Am* 6:63-70, 1979.
24. Abrams P, Griffiths DJ: The assessment of prostatic obstruction from urodynamic measurements and from residual urine, *Br J Urol* 51:129-134, 1979.
25. Jensen KM-E, Jørgensen JB, Morgensen P: Urodynamics in prostatism, *Scand J Urol Nephrol* 114(suppl):63-86, 1988.
26. Neal DE, Ramsden PD, Sharples L, et al: Outcome of elective prostatectomy, *Br Med J* 299:762-767, 1989.
27. Abrams PH: Prostatism and prostatectomy: the value of urine flow rate measurement in the preoperative assessment for operation, *J Urol* 117:70, 1977.
28. Abrams PH, Farrar DJ, Turner-Warwick RT, et al: The results of prostatectomy: a symptomatic and urodynamic analysis of 152 patients, *J Urol* 12:640-642, 1979.
29. Jensen KM-E, Andersen JT: Urodynamic implications of benign prostatic hyperplasia, *Urologe A* 29:1-4, 1990.
30. James D: Continuous monitoring in clinical urodynamics, *Urol Clin North Am* 6:125-135, 1979.
31. James D, Flack F, Caldwell KPS, et al: Continuous measurement of urine loss and frequency in incontinent patients, *Br J Urol* 43:233-237, 1971.
32. German K, MacLachlan D, Johnson S, et al: Improvements in the design of equipment used for ambulatory urodynamics, *Br J Urol* 74:377-378, 1994.
33. Eckford SD, Abrams PH: A new temperature sensitive device to detect incontinent episodes during ambulatory monitoring, *Neurourol Urodyn* 11:448-450, 1992.
34. Bhatia NN, Bradley WE, Haldeman S: Urodynamics: continuous monitoring, *J Urol* 128:963-968, 1982.
35. Griffiths CJ, Assi MS, Styles RA, et al: Ambulatory longterm monitoring of bladder and detrusor pressure, *Neurol Urodynam* 6:161-162, 1987.
36. Robertson AS, Griffiths CJ, Ramsden PD, et al: Bladder function in healthy volunteers: ambulatory monitoring and conventional urodynamic studies, *Br J Urol* 73:242-249, 1994.
37. van Waalwijk van Doorn ESC, Remmers A, Janknegt RA: Conventional and extramural ambulatory urodynamic testing of the lower urinary tract in female volunteers, *J Urol* 147:1319-1326, 1992.
38. Jensen KM-E, Bruskewitz RC, Madsen PO: Urodynamic findings in elderly males without prostatic complaints, *Urology* 24:211-213, 1984.
39. Neal DE: Ambulatory urodynamics. In Muncy AR, Stephenson TP, Wein AF, editors: *Urodynamics, principles, practice and application,* ed 2, Edinburgh, 1994, Churchill Livingstone.
40. Abrams PH, Dunn M, George NJR: The urodynamic findings in chronic retention of urine and the relevance to the results of surgery, *Br Med J* 2:1258-1260, 1978.
41. Styles RA, Neal DE, Ramsden PD: Comparison of long-term monitoring and standard cystometry in chronic retention of urine, *Br J Urol* 58:652-656, 1986.

42. Webb RJ, Griffiths CJ, Ramsden PD, et al: Measurement of voiding pressures on ambulatory monitoring: comparison with conventional cystometry, *Br J Urol* 65:152-154, 1990.
43. van Waalwijk van Doorn ESC, Remmers A, Janknegt RA: Extramural ambulatory urodynamic monitoring during natural filling and normal daily activities: evaluation of 100 patients, *J Urol* 146:124-131, 1991.
44. Webb RJ, Ramsden PD, Neal DE: Ambulatory monitoring and electronic measurement of urinary leakage in the diagnosis of detrusor instability and incontinence, *Br J Urol* 68:148-152, 1991.
45. O'Donnell PD, Hannish H: Telemetric electromyographic monitoring in elderly inpatient men, *Neurol Urodyn* 11(2):115-121, 1992.
46. O'Donnell PD: Pitfalls of urodynamic testing, *Urol Clin North Am* 18(2):257-263, 1991.

Chapter 11 Pressure-Flow Studies

François Haab, Philippe E. Zimmern

Pressure-flow measurement is one of the most important studies in the evaluation of patients with urinary incontinence, and pressure-flow measurement is one of the most difficult procedures in the urodynamic studies to perform and interpret accurately. Pressure-flow studies measure the voiding phase of bladder function. Although urinary incontinence represents a failure of the bladder to store urine properly, many patients with urinary incontinence have coexisting problems that involve an abnormal voiding phase of bladder function that can be a major contributing factor to incontinence, and it will not be identified without pressure-flow studies. For example, bladder outlet obstruction is a major contributing factor to bladder hyperactivity in both men and women. Patients with bladder outlet obstruction who void with a high detrusor pressure may have a low residual urine and a maximum urinary flow rate that does not indicate the degree of obstruction that exists. Women who have failed previous incontinence surgery may have renewed urge incontinence after surgery with associated recurrent symptoms of stress incontinence. Since the normal urethra has dynamic pressure responses to changes in abdominal pressure, in a woman a fixed outlet obstruction of the urethra after incontinence surgery can result in both stress incontinence and bladder outlet obstruction, which can cause bladder hyperactivity and symptoms of urge incontinence. Therefore pressure-flow studies are essential in understanding the pathophysiology of many of the patients who present with urinary incontinence.

Women who are considering surgery for treatment of stress incontinence usually express concern about the risk and duration of transient urinary retention after surgery. Patients who void with a low detrusor pressure and a low urinary flow rate preoperatively may be more likely to experience transient voiding problems after surgery than the patient with normal voiding. Pressure-flow studies are extremely important in the preoperative assessment of women who are considering surgery for incontinence both from a diagnostic standpoint and for counseling the patient about postoperative voiding problems.

Stress urinary incontinence in men is extremely rare in patients who have not had previous pelvic surgery or prostate surgery. Therefore incontinence in men usually is associated with bladder hyperactivity. When incontinence in men occurs because of bladder hyperactivity, it is important to determine if bladder outlet obstruction is a contributing factor to the bladder problem. In these patients, a pressure-flow study is essential to determine the degree of outflow obstruction. Study of an office flow rate and a residual urine can be very helpful, but these studies do not provide the information about bladder function that is obtained with the pressure-flow study. A majority of men over 60 years of age experience lower urinary tract symptoms (LUTS) such as frequency, nocturia, urgency, weak stream, or hesitancy.[1] For many years these symptoms have been attributed to the enlargement of the prostate gland also termed "benign prostatic hyperplasia" (BPH). In the last 20 years, the treatment of BPH has become less and less invasive, and most men who experience moderate to severe LUTS are offered a "prostate" operation.[1] However, since postoperative results are variable, there is a need to better define the optimal candidate for BPH treatment. But since neither history alone nor validated prostatic symptom scores were found to correlate with the diagnosis of outflow obstruction caused by BPH, a prevalent approach to improve the outcome of prostate surgery has been to demonstrate prostatic obstruction objectively.[2-4] Since the association of high voiding pressure with low flow is characteristic for obstruction, a logical emphasis has been to study these urodynamic parameters.[5]

Basic Hydrodynamics

As an example of a common clinical problem, a typical patient is presented: "Mr. Jones," a 69-year-old man came to your office for moderate LUTS. On examination, his prostate was enlarged, and his neurologic exam was normal. He has had no prior prostate surgery. Peak uroflow was 9.5 ml/sec for a 350 ml voided volume. Is Mr Jones obstructed from BPH or having a weak detrusor contraction during voiding? If Mr Jones is obstructed, he is very likely to benefit from a relief of his obstruction by medication or surgery. However, if he is not obstructed, he is at risk of side effects from any form of therapeutic intervention, and his symptoms may or may not improve much on treatment. To answer the "obstruction or no obstruction" question it has become clear that only the simultaneous measurement of pressure and flow can provide objective information.[5]

But what are the urodynamic characteristics of the urethra and bladder that participate in the pressure flow measurement ?

The male urethra, as viewed by urodynamicists, is not a rigid conduit but an elastic collapsible tube with a flow-controlling zone located in the membranous urethra.[6,7] The detrusor, like other muscles, is governed by the Hill equation. This equation relates the force of the muscular contraction to the speed of muscle shortening. The application to the bladder of this general equation translates into a relation between detrusor pressure and flow rate: the bladder-output relation (BOR). The BOR is a hyperbolic function that relates detrusor pressure to flow rate for a given micturition (Fig. 11-1). According to the BOR, a normal detrusor contraction during voiding will generate a high flow rate. On the other hand, in the presence of outlet obstruction, a high detrusor pressure will be needed to produce some flow.[7]

The relationship between detrusor (driving pressure) and urethra (resistance factor) during micturition can be divided into three sections. At rest, the urethra is closed to prevent leakage. When micturition is attempted, an isovolumetric contraction is initiated. The intravesical pressure rises to overcome the urethral resistance pressure (isovolumetric detrusor pressure). Once voiding starts, the urethra stays open and the flow stabilizes at its maximum value. At the end of micturition, the urethral lumen passively reduces its caliber as the flow decreases. The urethral opening pressure is defined as the intravesical pressure that keeps the urethra open.[7]

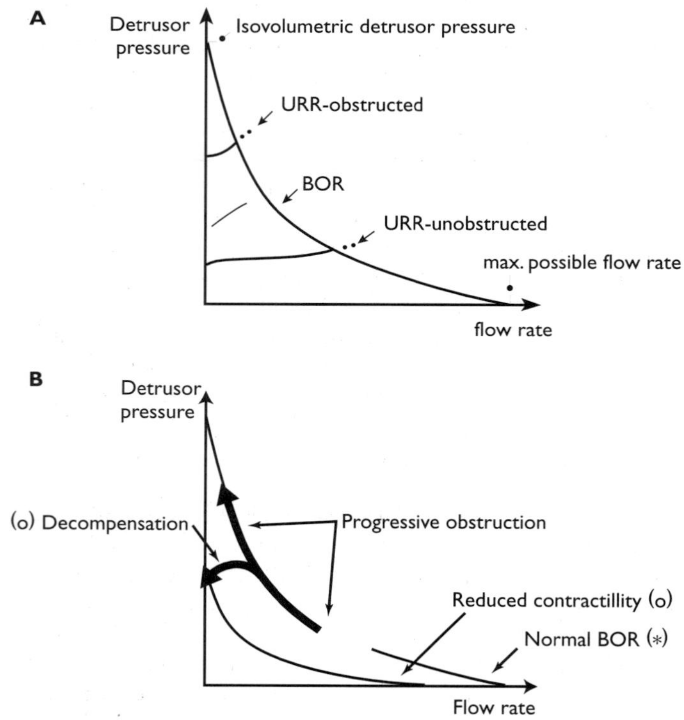

FIG. 11-1 ***A,*** *The bladder output relation (BOR) defines detrusor contraction. When there is no outlet obstruction, the detrusor pressure is low. However, with an obstructed outlet, a high detrusor pressure must be generated to produce a flow.* ***B,*** *Impact of obstruction on voiding. Initially, progressive obstruction is determined by elevation of detrusor pressure and reduction in flow (*). Decompensation is represented by a reduction in contractility (◦). URR, Urethral resistance relation.*

Technique for Pressure-Flow Studies

Urinalysis (to exclude infection)
Noninvasive uroflow
Placement of a 7 Fr dual-lumen urethral catheter
Measurement of postvoid residual
Placement of an 8 Fr rectal catheter
Patient stands up
Zeroing of transducers at level of symphysis pubis
Bladder filling (water 25 to 50 ml/min)
Pressure-flow recording when strong desire to void

Before entering the field of "curve interpretation," we'll go with Mr Jones to his urodynamic appointment to understand how the procedure is performed.

TECHNICAL ASPECTS

From a practical standpoint, our routine urodynamic testing is described (see the box above): A noninvasive uroflow (free flow) is initially performed. Intravesical pressure recording and infusion is obtained with a 7 French dual-lumen urethral catheter. Once in place, the urethral catheter is left indwelling to measure the postvoid residual. Then an 8 Fr rectal catheter is placed to record intra-abdominal pressure. The urodynamic machine automatically subtracts the intravesical pressure from the abdominal pressure to produce the "true detrusor pressure." All transducers are zeroed at the level of the symphysis pubis. Next, the bladder is filled with water at a slow-to-medium fill rate (25 to 50 ml/sec) with the patient in a standing position. When the patient has a strong desire to void, he is asked to urinate around the small catheter into the uroflowmeter.

At the end of the study, the very astute Mr. Jones might ask the following questions:

- *What is the influence of the urethral catheter size on the measurements?*

Vesical pressure can be recorded by means of a suprapubic tube or a urethral catheter. The suprapubic tube is more invasive to introduce than the urethral catheter but allows a more physiologic micturition. However, there is sufficient evidence that a small catheter (less than 10 French gauge) in the urethra does not influence pressure-flow recordings.[3,8] Nevertheless, if the variation between the noninvasive uroflow and the flow during testing is important—two features implying that the urethral catheter induced the obstruction—the pressure flow study should be repeated.[3]

- *Is it necessary to use a rectal tube?*

It is strongly recommended to use a rectal catheter to record the abdominal pressure during voiding. The computer included in the urodynamic machine automatically subtracts abdominal pressure from intravesical pressure, yielding the "true detrusor pressure." Thus the true detrusor pressure reflects only the pressure generated by the bladder contraction and is free of straining artifacts.[3]

- *Is it necessary to repeat the study to confirm the reproducibility of the measurements?*

Pressure-flow studies have good reproducibility. In 12 healthy female volunteers tested 2 months apart, the coefficients of variation for detrusor pressure at maximum flow and for maximum flow rate were 24% to 31% and 18% respectively. Repeat measurements during the same session also appear highly reproducible.[3,9]

The most common errors in the measurement of the vesical pressure result from failure in zeroing the transducers, or mechanical kinking of the tubing or urethral catheter during voiding.[3]

- *Are there other methods to demonstrate obstruction by urodynamics?*

Yalla et al. have published a technique called "elastic jump."[10,11] This technique consists in identifying the site and degree of the hydraulic jump by simultaneous measurements of the vesical pressure and the urethral pressure distal to the prostate during voiding. A pressure gradient above 25 cm H_2O is suggestive of obstruction. From a technical standpoint, this procedure necessitates a specially designed triple-lumen 10 Fr graduated urethral catheter with continuous fluoroscopic monitoring.

- *Is it possible to assess the pressure-to-flow relationship without insertion of catheters?*

A noninvasive technique that measures maximum bladder pressure in the absence of flow has recently been reported but has not yet been validated.[12]

Interpretation of the Studies

Since the consensus conference of the International Continence Society (ICS) in 1980, it has been widely accepted that the data coming from pressure-flow studies should be interpreted from an *x/y* plot showing flow on the *x*-axis and detrusor pressure on the *y*-axis.[13] Numerous methods have been described to analyze the relationship between detrusor pressure and flow rate, with various levels of data processing and sophistication involved.[14-18] The nomogram published in 1979 by Abrams and Griffiths is used by most (Fig. 11-2). When plotting the maximum uroflow (Q_{max}) and the detrusor pressure at Q_{max} (P_{det} at Q_{max}) on this nomogram, the patient can be categorized in the obstructed, nonobstructed, or equivocal zones [14] For example, a Q_{max} above 15 ml/sec with a low P_{det} at Q_{max} would be plotted in the nonobstructed zone, whereas a Q_{max} below 10 ml/sec with a P_{det} at Q_{max} above 100 cm H_2O would end up unequivocally in the obstructed area. Similarly, Mr. Jones, who has a weak stream (9.5 ml/sec), could have a high voiding pressure (above 100 cm H_2O: obstructed) or a normal to weak pressure (below 40 cm H_2O: not obstructed).

What about the equivocal zone, where more than 50% of the patients undergoing pressure-flow studies fall?

In an attempt to "narrow" this equivocal zone, Abrams recently proposed the "Abrams-Griffiths number" (AG number).[19] The AG number is easily calculated by the formula:

$$\text{AG number} = P_{det} \cdot Q_{max} - 2Q_{max}$$

An AG number above 40 is suggestive of bladder outlet obstruction. Patients who are in the equivocal zone but whose AG number is below 15 are considered not obstructed. The AG number provides a numerical variable that facilitates statistical analysis and could also serve as a quantitative evaluation criteria in pharmaceutical trials on benign prostatic hypertrophy.

Other Nomograms

Numerous other methods, such as Schaffer's model and the computer program called CLIM, have been described to interpret the pressure-flow curves.[20,21] However, despite their sophistication, none of these computerized models has so far received wide acceptance.

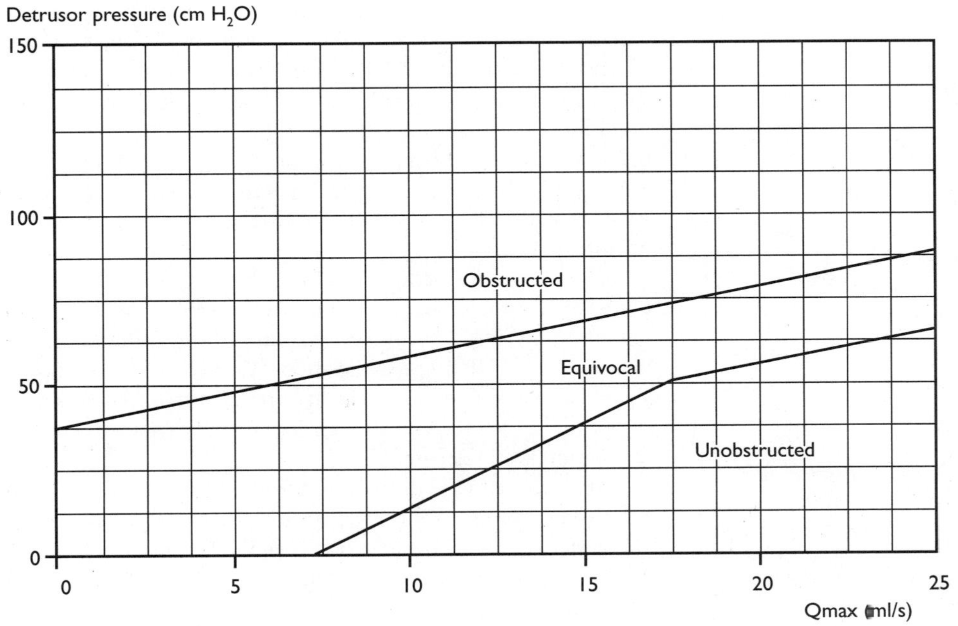

FIG. 11-2 *The Abrams-Griffiths nomogram depicting three pressure-flow zones: obstructed, nonobstructed, and equivocal.*

The most important information is that these different methods of interpretation lead to fairly similar conclusions. Abrams et al. recently reviewed the pressure-flow data of 279 consecutive men over 50 years of age with LUTS but no previous treatment or neurologic disease.[19] Disagreement between CLIM and AG nomogram was encountered in only 10% of the patients: 7% were in the equivocal zone with the AG nomogram and classified obstructed with the CLIM, and 3% were classified obstructed with the AG nomogram and not obstructed with the CLIM. In addition, this methodology article also indicates that the AG and Schaffer's nomograms compare well (Fig. 11-3).

Clinical Implications of Pressure-Flow Studies on BPH Management

Historically the objective demonstration of infravesical obstruction was first attempted using uroflow studies.[3] A classification of obstructed and nonobstructed patients based on uroflow findings was proposed with Q_{max} <10 ml/sec as obstructed, Q_{max} >15 ml/sec as not obstructed, and Q_{max} 10 to 15 ml/sec as equivocal. This noninvasive testing was widely accepted initially because of its simplicity.[3] However, this uroflow classification did not take into account bladder function. In fact, in two well-designed studies, 7% to 25% of patients referred with prostatism had high flow–high pressure obstruction.[22,23] Schaffer also reported that 25% of men with low flow were not obstructed and had impaired detrusor contractility.[24] Recently the international conference on BPH addressed the role of sophisticated urodynamic testing (pressure-flow studies) to reduce the number of patients who do not experience symptomatic relief after surgical removal of their enlarged gland.[3]

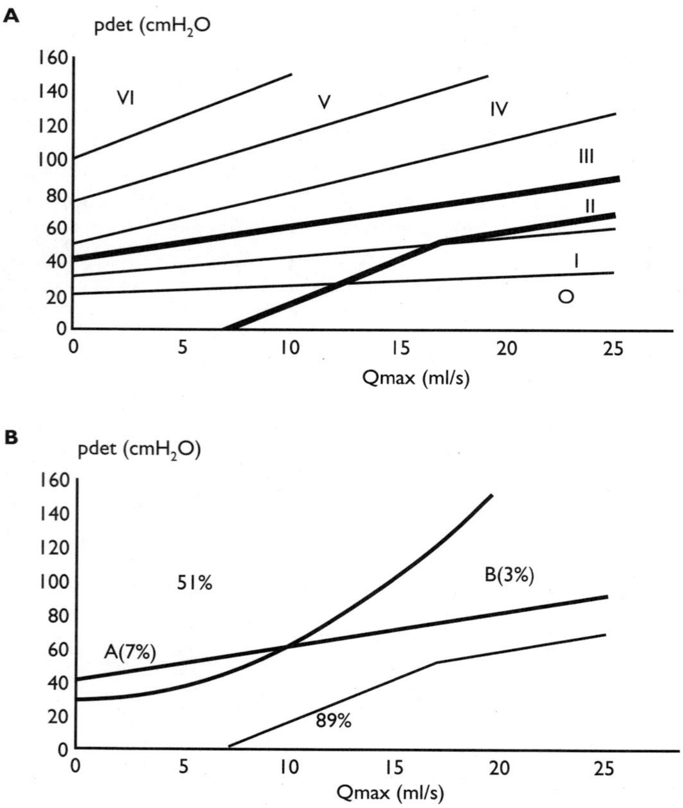

FIG. 11-3 *Comparison between the Abrams-Griffiths nomogram and Schaffer's nomogram (linPURR),* ***A,*** *and between the Abrams-Griffiths nomogram and CLIM program,* **B.** *There is a good overlap between the Abrams-Griffiths nomogram and the CLIM or linPURR techniques for differentiating between obstruction and nonobstruction.* linPURR, *Linear passive urethral resistance relation.*

Abrams reported that inclusion of pressure-flow data in the preoperative evaluation reduced the subjective failure of transurethral resection of the prostate (TURP) from 28% to 12%.[25] Moreover, the same group found that an obstructive pressure flow pattern was the best preoperative factor to allow one to predict the outcome after surgery.[26] Jensen et al. confirmed those findings in a prospective study and clearly established that all patients classified as obstructed preoperatively according to the Abrams-Griffith nomogram were unobstructed postoperatively.[27] As a correlate, postoperative subjective improvement was significantly higher in the preoperatively obstructed group.

Van Mastrigt et al. performed urodynamic evaluation before and after TURP in 29 consecutive patients.[28] The decision to perform surgery was based upon symptom severity, rectal examination, and residual urine. The operative decision was not based on the pressure-flow data. After TURP, the retrospective analysis of the curves revealed that 10 of the 29 patients were not obstructed. Subjective and objective improvements were noted in the 19 obstructed patients, whereas 30% of the nonobstructed patients remained symptomatic postoperatively.

However, contradictory findings were published by Bruskewitz.[29] A prospective study was conducted to determine if the minimum urethral resistance (as defined by P/Q^2, pressure divided by flow squared) was useful to discriminate between patients who would or would not benefit from TURP. Forty-six males referred for prostatism were divided into two groups according to the urethral resistance index. This prospective blinded evaluation found that the minimal urethral resistance was not useful to predict which patients would benefit from TURP. Of the patients, 88.9% in the nonobstructed group and 91.7% in the obstructed group stated that they had overall voiding improvement after TURP. The conclusion of that study was that for most of the patients with prostatism, symptoms represent a sufficient predictor of postoperative outcome, since even patients with a low minimum urethral resistance had a good operative outcome.

In summary, the pathophysiologic characteristics of symptomatic BPH remains largely unknown. It seems that the use of pressure-flow studies in the evaluation of BPH could lower the failure rate of TURP. The International Conference on BPH considered pressure-flow studies as an optional test for patients with symptoms of prostatism, though for research trial this recommendation is still debated.[3,30]

Quantitative methods to assess the severity of the obstruction such as the Abrams-Griffths number and the urethral resistance parameter (in the CLIM program) need to be further evaluated. These parameters might be relevant to evaluate the results of BPH treatments.

Primary Bladder Neck Obstruction (BNO)

The diagnosis of primary BNO should be considered in males under 50 years of age presenting with a long history of LUTS. Primary BNO is best diagnosed by videourodynamic studies, revealing both high voiding pressure–low flow rate and limited opening of the bladder neck during voiding. In our experience of 32 patients, voiding pressure was high in all cases (mean 94 cm H_2O; range 50 to 150), and the diagnosis of obstruction at the bladder neck was obvious on videourodynamics.[31] When patients were plotted on the Abrams-Griffiths nomogram, all were in the obstructed zone.

Diagnosis of Obstruction with Neurogenic Bladder

Patients with neurogenic bladder (such as those with diabetes, Parkinson's disease, or abdominoperineal resection) may have LUTS similar to patients with BPH.[32] However, these neurologic conditions can also alter urethral sphincteric function, an obvious risk factor for incontinence after prostatectomy.[33] In these patients with a neurologic condition, pressure-flow studies can confirm bladder outlet obstruction, therefore guiding therapeutic intervention.

Pressure-Flow Studies in the Female

Obstruction in females has been less studied than that in males, and its incidence has been estimated around 5% to 10%.[34] Physiologically the normal voiding pressure is lower in women than in men, and many women void with pelvic floor relaxation and minimal to no elevation of detrusor pressure. Moreover, women usually respond to obstruction by reducing their flow rate rather than raising detrusor pressure. The methods to get a pressure-flow relationship in women is the same as in men, but the interpretation of pressure-flow data is more questionable, since nomograms have not been validated for women.

Obstruction in the female can result from urethral angulation or deviation after surgery to correct stress urinary incontinence, especially Marshall-Marchetti-Krantz (MMK) or sling procedures, or can be associated with a moderate to large cystocele.[35,36,37] In one study, patients presented with stress incontinence alone or combined with irritative symptoms after an MMK procedure. Complete urinary retention was infrequent. Urodynamic findings were consistent with an obstructive pattern of high true detrusor voiding pressure (range 45 to 65 cm H_2O) with a simultaneous low flow rate of less than 12 ml/sec (range 3.5 to 11.5 ml/sec). Postvoid residuals were consistently increased (range 100 to 1200 ml). The site of obstruction at bladder neck and proximal urethra levels was confirmed either by a voiding cystourethrogram or videourodynamics.[36] Relief of obstruction by urethrolysis with or without resuspension benefited a majority of patients.[36] Such a positive outcome has been since documented in other studies.[38,39] We therefore recommend to perform a pressure-flow study in women with persistent LUTS after prior anti-incontinence or prolapse repair procedures.

Conclusion

Pressure-flow studies have an essential role to document bladder outlet obstruction and play an important role in the evaluation of selected patients with LUTS. Although minimally invasive, the current technique as outlined here is easy to perform and reliable. The interpretation of pressure-flow data has benefited from the Abrams-Griffiths nomogram. Many other analytical techniques have recently surfaced to enhance the diagnostic acumen of pressure-flow studies. In the absence of accepted standards, pressure-flow studies must be interpreted in light of the patient's symptoms and not as an independent parameter.

References

1. Nielsen KK, Nordling J, Hald T: Critical review of the diagnosis of prostatic obstruction, *Neurourol Urodyn* 13:201-217, 1994.
2. Reynard JM, Abrams P: Bladder outlet obstruction: assessment of symptoms, *World J Urol* 13:3-8, 1995.
3. Abrams P, Blaivas J, Nordling J, et al: The objective evaluation of bladder outflow obstruction. In Cockett ATK et al, editors: *Second International Consultation on Benign Prostatic Hypertrophy,* Jersey, 1993, Scientific Communication International Ltd, pp 153-223.
4. Sirls LT, Jay J, Kirkemo A: Does the AUA-7 symptom score correlate with urodynamic obstruction? *J Urol* 153:275A, 1995.
5. Abrams P: In support of pressure flow studies for evaluating men with lower urinary tract symptoms, *Urology* 44:153-155, 1994.
6. Bates CP, Arnold EP, Griffiths DJ: The nature of the abnormality in bladder neck obstruction, *Br J Urol* 47:651-656, 1975.
7. Griffiths D: Basics of pressure flow studies, *World J Urol* 13:30-33, 1995.
8. Reynard J, Lim C, Abrams P: Pressure flow studies in men: the obstructive effect of a urethral catheter, *J Urol* 153:453A, 1995.
9. Tan HK, Hofner K, Krah H, et al: Reproducibility of pressure flow analysis in the diagnosis of BPH obstruction, *J Urol* 153:452A, 1995.
10. Yalla SV, Sharma GVRK, Barsamian EM: Micturitional static urethral pressure profile: a method of recording urethral pressure profile during voiding and the implication, *J Urol* 124:649-653, 1980.
11. Yalla SV, Cravalho E, Resnick N, et al: Elastic jump in male urethra during voiding: clinical observations in male subjects and experimental studies in dog, *J Urol* 134:907-913, 1985.
12. McRae LP, Bottaccini MR, Gleason DM: Noninvasive quantitative method for measuring isovolumetric bladder pressure and urethral resistance in the male, *Neurourol Urodyn* 14:101-114, 1995.
13. Bates CP, Bradley WE, Glen ES, et al: Third report on the standardisation of terminology of lower urinary tract function, *Br J Urol* 52:348-350, 1980.
14. Abrams PH, Griffiths DJ: The assessment of prostatic obstruction from urodynamic measurements and from residual urine, *Br J Urol* 51:129-134, 1979.
15. Rollema HJ, van Mastrigt R: Objective analysis of prostatism: a clinical application of the computer program CLIM, *Neurourol Urodyn* 10:71-76, 1991.
16. Shaffer W: Urethral resistance? Urodynamic concepts of physiological and pathological bladder outlet function during voiding, *Neurourol Urodyn* 4:161-201, 1985.
17. Spangberg A, Teriö H, Engberg A, Ask P: Quantification of urethral function based on Griffiths' model of flow through elastic tubes, *Neurourol Urodyn* 8:29-52, 1989.
18. Höfner K, Kramer AEJL, Tan HK, et al: Chess classification of bladder outflow obstruction, *World J Urol* 13:59-64, 1995.
19. Lin CS, Abrams P: The Abrams-Griffiths nomogram, *World J Urol* 13:34-39, 1995.

20. van Mastrigt R, Krause M: Analysis of pressure flow data in terms of computer derived urethral resistance parameters, *World J Urol* 13:40-46, 1995.
21. Schaffer W: Analysis of bladder outlet function with the linearized passive urethral resistance relation, linPURR, and a disease-specific approach for grading obstruction: from complex to simple, *World J Urol* 13:47-58, 1995.
22. Gerstenberg TC, Andersen JT, Klarskov P, et al: High flow infravesical obstruction in men: symptomatology, urodynamics and the results of surgery, *J Urol* 127:943-945, 1982.
23. Iversen P, Bruskewitz RC, Jensen KME, Madsen PO: Transurethral prostatic resection in the treatment of prostatism with urinary flow, *J Urol* 129:995-997, 1983.
24. Schaffer W, Noppeney R, Rubben H, Lutzeyer W: The value of free flow rate and pressure flow studies in the routine investigation of BPH patients, *Neurourol Urodyn* 7:219-220, 1988.
25. Abrams P: Prostatism and prostatectomy: the value of urine flow rate measurement in the preoperative assessment for operation, *J Urol* 117:70-71, 1977.
26. Abrams P: The urodynamic changes following prostatectomy, *Urol Int* 33:181-186, 1978.
27. Jensen KME, Bruskewitz RC, Iversen P, Madsen PO: Predictive value of voiding pressure in benign prostatic hyperplasia, *Neurourol Urodyn* 2:117-125, 1983.
28. Rollema HJ, van Mastrigt R: Improved indication and follow up in transurethral resection of the prostate using the computer program CLIM: a prospective study, *J Urol* 148:111-116, 1992.
29. Bruskewitz R, Jensen KME, Iversen P, Madsen PO: The relevance of minimum urethral resistance in prostatism, *J Urol* 129:769-771, 1983.
30. McConnell JD: Why pressure flow studies should be optional and not mandatory studies for evaluating men with benign prostatic hyperplasia, *Urology* 44:156-158, 1994.
31. Trockman B, van Overbeke M, Zimmern PE, et al: Primary bladder neck obstruction: evaluation and treatment results in 32 men, *J Urol* 153:190A, 1995.
32. Sotolongo JR: Voiding dysfunction in Parkinson's disease, *Sem Urol* 8:166-169, 1988.
33. Staskin DS, Vardi Y, Siroky MB: Post prostatectomy continence in the Parkinsonian patient: the significance of poor voluntary sphincter control, *J Urol* 140:117-118, 1988.
34. Massey JA, Abrams PH: Obstructed voiding in the female, *Br J Urol* 61:36-39, 1988.
35. Dmochowski R, Zimmern PE, Leach GE: Female distal urethral obstruction presenting as interstitial cystitis. (Submitted.)
36. Zimmern P, Hadley HR, Leach GE, Raz S: Female urethral obstruction after Marshall-Marchetti-Krantz operation, *J Urol* 138:517-520, 1987.
37. Bass JS, Leach GE: Bladder outlet obstruction in women, *Probl Urol* 5:141-154, 1991.
38. McGuire EJ, Letson W, Wang S: Transvaginal urethrolysis after obstructing urethral suspension procedures. *J Urol* 142:1037-1039, 1989.
39. Webster GD, Kreder KJ: Voiding dysfunction following cystourethropexy: its evaluation and management, *J Urol* 144:670-673, 1990.

Chapter 12 Urethral Pressure in the Evaluation of Female Incontinence

Christos E. Constantinou

Measurement of the pressure in the urethra and the dynamic responses of urethral pressure have been used clinically more than any other objective measurement of urethral function to provide a basis for treatment of patients who have urinary incontinence. Clinical measurement of urethral pressures has provided a better understanding of the role of both intrinsic and extrinsic mechanisms of the urethra in female incontinence. The contribution of blood flow and the action of hormones on urethral closure pressure and associated biomechanics that constitute the intrinsic mechanisms of urethral closure have been studied extensively using urethral pressure measurements. The basis for understanding the mechanisms of continence require a basic understanding of urethral function. This is especially important in the clinical evaluation of patients who have symptoms of stress incontinence.

Physiologic Principles of Urethral Pressures

The International Continence Society (ICS) defines urethral closure pressure as the "subtraction of intravesical pressure from the intraluminal urethral pressure." In this ICS definition, it is implicit that the intraluminal pressure in the urethra is considered in the context and in the terms of intravesical pressure. This is a very important statement because by incorporating intravesical pressure it explicitly defines and emphasizes the importance of the intravesical pressure component and its contribution to urethral closure. Furthermore, it is essential to recognize that changes in intravesical pressures, as these may occur with changes in intra-abdominal pressures, consequently influence urethral closure pressures. The reason is that the urethra, as it traverses between the symphysis and vagina, is under the influence of intra-abdominal pressure as are many of the paraurethral structures that exert different closure forces along its length. Such urethral pressures are not directly related to intravesical pressure, but can be passively proportional to it or actively stimulated by stress.

Closure forces produced by paraurethral structures can be passive or active and not necessarily equal to intravesical pressure. What is common among paraurethral structures is that they are extrinsic to the urethra and invariably are acting in different directions. In addition to the extrinsic forces maintaining a closed urethra, there are those of the urethra itself, such as smooth muscle tone, sphincter, and blood supply, that constitute the intrinsic mechanism. The superimposition of the extrinsic forces on intraluminal pressure is far too complex to be accounted by the simple subtraction of intravesical pressure, as the ICS definition suggests. For this reason, consideration of urethral pressures in the study of female incontinence should therefore be focused on the totality of forces that act to maintain urethral closure. In view of the variety of structures involved and the degree of overlap between them, it has been proved to be practically impossible to assess continence on the basis of urethral closure alone. The reason is that there are no current diagnostic tests that are sufficiently sophisticated to assess the continence function of urethra and localize the cause of leakage with precision.

Application of Urethral Pressure Measurements

One of the first diagnostic tests introduced into the field of urodynamics for the evaluation of urethral competence was the resting urethral pressure profile (UPP). The UPP is a topographic curve representative of pressures along the length of the urethra and is at best the most urostatic measurement in the field of urodynamics. The UPP does not represent urethral function in many dynamic cases, where incontinence is likely to occur, and contrary to the expectations it has been of limited practical value in considerations of continence. This is a predictable outcome, given the fact that the UPP is inclusive of so many variables incorporated in a single recording, often done under unrealistic clinical conditions. Indeed, appreciation of the anatomy of the pelvic floor and associated paraurethral structures indicates that a primitive measurement such as the UPP alone would predictably provide only the most rudimentary parameters of urethral closure. On the other hand, if associated dynamic measurements are incorporated together with the static measurements of the UPP, a better understanding of the mechanism of urethral forces emerges.

Correlates Between Anatomic and Physiologic Considerations in Urethral Support Mechanisms

The structural support of the urethra as it relates to stress incontinence is receiving continued attention and has generated several hypotheses to explain the mechanical basis for urethral pressure generation. One of the most recent reports by DeLancey, "the hammock hypothesis," considered the anatomic structures contributing to urethral closure and divided these into two main groups: (1) structures forming the urethral sphincter and (2) its attachments, or hammock.[2] The interpretation of DeLancey's results is based primarily on the observation that the urethra lies on a supportive layer that is composed of the endopelvic fascia and the anterior vaginal wall. This layer is structurally stable because of its attachment as a hammock on the arcus tendineus fasciae pelvis and the levator ani. Pressures from above compress the urethra to close its lumen. Thus urethral closure pressure during stress arises because the urethra is compressed. This is an anatomic perspective that should be carefully considered, but the reader should be also aware that this may not be the only mechanism involved in preventing stress incontinence. Indeed the urethra is in possession of several different mechanisms composed of at least three elements that contribute approximately one third each: striated muscle, smooth muscle, and vascular elements.[3]

The term "urethral sphincter" is used to define the striated intrinsic urethral sphincter, but the smooth muscle and vessels are included here because these structures participate in maintaining the urethral closure pressure. Fig. 12-1 illustrates the anatomic correlates of a UPP together with the terminology used to define the significant parameters. It also shows a sagittal view of a magnetic resonance image enhanced to identify the outline of the urethra with a catheter within its lumen. It is understood that the urethral sphincter refers to the intrinsic external urethral sphincter and not the extrinsic periurethral musculature. Along the middle portion of the urethra the striated muscle fibers are thickest, and in that area they completely surround it.[4] The portion located between urethra and vagina is found to be relatively thin. The striated muscle fibers extend into the anterior wall of the proximal and distal thirds of the urethra but are missing laterally and posteriorly at these levels.[5] At the level of the distal third, some of the striated muscle fibers leave the confines of the

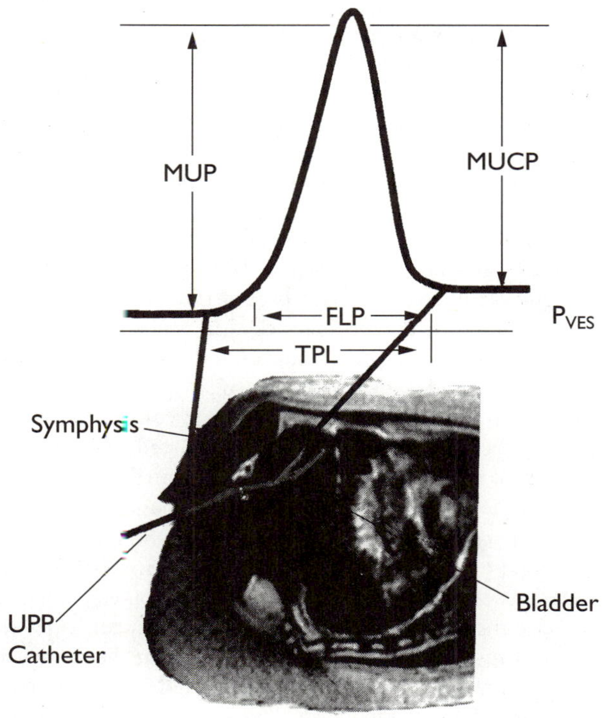

FIG. 12-1 *Schema showing the relationship between resting urethral pressures and their anatomic correlates. Bottom, Position of the catheter within the urethra. This sagittal magnetic resonance image was enhanced to show the relative position of the catheter with respect to the surrounding periurethral structures. The patient is placed supine, a position that is frequently used to produce a urethral pressure profile. FPL, Functional profile length; MUCP, maximum urethral closure pressure; MUP, maximum urethral pressure;* P_{ves}, *intravesical pressure; TPL, total profile length; UPP, urethral pressure profile.*

urethra and merge at the lateral aspect of the urethra with striated muscle fibers originating respectively near the pubic rami and the vaginal wall forming a single muscle band arching over the anterior part of urethra.[4] The part of the muscle fibers originating near the pubic rami is referred to as the "compressor urethrae." The other part, originating from the vaginal wall, is named the "urethrovaginal sphincter." The magnitude of urethra pressure that can develop within the lumen depends to a large extent on the constituents and type of muscle fibers that form this lumen. A focused study of muscle fibers present in the urethra was made by Gosling et al., who divided these into two groups: type I (slow-twitch) fibers, and type II (fast-twitch) fibers.[6] Type I fibers contract slowly but keep a sustained contraction over a long period, and type II fibers contract quickly but only over a short time. The muscle fibers in the striated urogenital sphincter can be functionally classified as slow-twitch fibers, reflecting their ability to keep a long-lasting constant tone.[6]

Studies of the periurethral part of the striated levator ani muscle have shown that this muscle, in contrast to the external sphincter, consists of a mixture of large-diameter type I and type II fibers. These observations provide evidence to support the concept that the levator ani assists the external urethral sphincter in urethral closure to ensure continence and also produce a rapid occlusion during a rise in intra-abdominal pressure and voluntary contraction.[6]

This concept is in accord with the "hammock hypothesis" described above. In addition to the skeletal constituents of the urethra and its support structures, the urethra is also made up of smooth muscle, The major part of the smooth muscles are arranged longitudinally or obliquely surrounding the submucosa. They extend from the bladder neck to the external meatus. In the periphery of this smooth muscle layer, a thin layer of muscle fibers is arranged circularly. In contrast to the intrinsic striated urethral sphincter with the type I (slow-twitch) muscle fibers, the levator ani muscle primarily consists of type II (fast-twitch) muscle fibers, except for part of the muscle adjacent to the proximal urethra and bladder neck.[7] In that region, the fibers are of the slow-twitch type, an indication that the muscle in that region is specialized in maintaining a constant tone.

Clearly on the basis of these anatomic considerations the female urethra is made up of and supported by a complex framework of muscles and structures that contribute to the balance of forces that maintain closure. In balance these forces combine the contribution of somatic innervation, periurethral muscles, and pelvic floor to play an important role in the maintenance of continence. Although there is still some debate as to the precise distribution of somatic muscle control to passive mechanical support, it is generally accepted that the levator ani muscle is supplied by somatic fibers carried in the pudendal nerve.[8] These fibers originate from the second, third, and fourth sacral segment of the spinal cord. Innervation of the external intrinsic urethral striated sphincter is described in several different ways. One opinion is that branches of the pelvic (splanchnic) nerve carry some somatic motor fibers to the sphincter.[8] Juenemann et al. have found the pudendal nerve to be responsible for innervation of both the levator ani muscle and the striated urethral sphincter, thereby inferring that fibers from the pudendal nerve to the sphincter separates before the pudendal nerve becomes easily identifiable on dissection.[9] Composed of somatic innervation that serves primarily as a controlling mechanism for continence and reflex contraction, the autonomic nervous system is represented by both parasympathetic (cholinergic) and sympathetic (adrenergic) innervation to the bladder-neck and urethra region. The bladder-neck and urethral smooth muscles are richly innervated by cholinergic nerves. Gosling has shown that in the female the number of adrenergic nerves are very few.[8] As is discussed later, urethra closure pressure is influenced directly by the urethral blood flow, supplied by the urethral artery coming from the internal pudendal artery, which again is fed by the internal iliac artery.[10]

Dynamic Imaging of Pelvic Floor Contractions

As indicated, the influence of paraurethral muscles may be voluntarily activated, thereby compressing the region of the bladder neck and urethra. Such voluntary contractions are produced by recruitment of skeletal muscle activation of the pelvic floor, and their effect can be considered as analogous to the Kegel type of exercise. By extrapolation these muscles are also recruited when stress-induced phenomena such as coughing or sneezing occur. Such responses therefore facilitate the guarding reflex, recruited to activate all pelvic floor structures to prevent urine or fecal incontinence. Using magnetic resonance imaging, Christensen et al. examined the three-dimensional configuration of structures surrounding the normal female urethra.[2,11]

Clinical Evaluation of the Urethra Using Urodynamics

The resting urethral pressure profile (UPP), composed of the contribution of the sphincteric and supporting structures of the urethra, can be measured using the principles embodied in UPP methodology. This measure gives a graph incorporating all closure forces to compress the urethral lumen. There are several methods to obtain a profile of the urethral pressures. The intraurethral pressure is measured along the urethral length when one pulls a pressure sensor from the bladder and out through the urethra. Withdrawal of the catheter can be done manually in steps or mechanically at a fixed rate.

Several types of catheter pressure systems have been used.[12,13] Either the pressure can be measured with a fluid-filled system having a fluid column connected to an external transducer, or a catheter with a small microtip transducer mounted on the catheter itself can be used. The side facing the measuring unit on a tip catheter has provided information about directional differences in profilometry. Such information is a reflection of the structures acting in different directions; thus in the lateral plane the pressures are symmetric.[14] In healthy female volunteers, the anteriorly and posteriorly oriented pressures were found to be equal, but the posterior functional length exceeds the anterior.[15] The maximum urethral closure pressure (MUCP) of women with detrusor-originating incontinence and no urethral incontinence shows that in women with proved stress incontinence there was a significantly lower posterior pressure compared to the anterior one.

Vascular, skeletal, and smooth muscle components of urethral closure play an important role in forming the shape of the UPP as measured clinically. A systematic study to characterize the contribution of striated and smooth muscles within the urethra with special focus on the influence of systemic blood pressure was undertaken by Rud et al.[3] In this study, urethral pressure profile measurements were made before, during, and after curarization, as well as clamping of the common iliac artery bilaterally. The response of urethral closure pressure as a result of these rather invasive interventions has provided a better understanding of the contributory factors that make up urethral pressures. On the basis of such observations, it has been concluded that the striated muscle in the urethra, including the pelvic floor, is responsible for approximately one third of the total intraurethral pressure. The other third of urethral closure is contributed by blood flow. The remaining third is contributed by connective and periurethral tissue. Furthermore, it was found that curarization caused a drop in maximum urethral pressure (MUP) of approximately 33%. Clamping of the common iliac artery caused another 28% drop in the MUP. Confirmatory studies have been reported recently by Bump et al.,[16] who, in an effort to evaluate both the passive function and the dynamics of urethral pressure, examined the influence of paralyzed muscles on the passive urethral function in continent and incontinent patients. Analysis of the results shows that there are highly significant anesthetic effects on all parameters and indicates that the sphincter may be involved. Thus skeletal muscle activity occurring reflexively is important in closing the urethra. Passive urethral closure is less affected by the loss of consciousness and paralysis. The data made available by Rud et al. and by Bump et al. gives further credence to our observations of an active, anticipatory neuromuscular component.[17,18] The location of this neuromuscular component and its mechanism of action has not been fully defined, though existing evidence indicates that it may be extrinsic to the urethra and may indeed involve the pelvic floor and its attachment to the urethra.

Hormonal Influences of the Biomechanical Properties of the Urethra

It is becoming increasing evident that hormones have a very important role to play in modifying the softness of the urethra, which makes it amenable to skeletal muscle compression. Such hormonal biomechanical changes of the constituent components of the urethra and surrounding structures inevitably modulate the magnitude of the UPP. In particular, estrogen has been found to increase the sensitivity and number of the adrenergic receptors[14,20] that have been demonstrated in the female urethra.[21] Furthermore, progesterone has been found to facilitate the beta-adrenergic receptor sensitivity, and also specific progesterone receptors have been demonstrated.[22] The epithelium of the urethra is similar to that of the vagina, a nonkeratinized, squamous epithelium sensitive to hormonal stimulation. To act selectively on the tissue, female sex hormones can interact with receptors. The presence of specific estrogen receptors has been detected in the urinary bladder and urethra,[21] and only a few years ago there was published histochemical evidence[22] indicating the presence of progesterone receptors in the same region. Both receptor types are found in the vagina and have the same embryologic origin as the urethra and the trigone. Theoretically, another way for gonadal hormones to influence the urinary tract is by modifying the effect of adrenergic or cholinergic stimulation, as has been shown by animal studies.[23] As indicated in the studies of Rud et al.,[3] urethral vasculature affects closure. Since the vascularity of the urethra is also affected by estrogen, the magnitude of pulsations are greatest during periods of estrogen dominance and decrease with postmenopausal age. In considering the role of hormones on the components of urethral closure, one should bear in mind that estrogen treatment improves the transmission of the intra-abdominal pressure to the urethra. Although there are few, definitive, controlled human studies identifying the role of sex hormones on urethral function, there are many recent experimental observations that merit consideration. Indeed, Iosif et al.[21] have shown that estrogen deficiency could be the cause of incontinence. Whether this estrogen effect is secondary to the reorganization (or upregulation and downregulation) of urethral receptors remains to be seen. There is sufficient clinical evidence, however, from Sørensen's studies to show that symptomatic urodynamic changes occur in the urethra relative to age, menstrual cycle, and menopause.[24] In particular, sex hormones exert additional influence on the pelvic floor, which indirectly affects urethral closure. The specific role of hormones on female urinary tract has been examined by Miodrag et al.,[23] who review their role on urethral mucosal changes, urethral blood supply, connective tissue, pelvic floor, and urethral smooth muscle.

Hormones are known to affect most components that contribute toward urethral closure in many ways such as biomechanically softening the tissues, interaction with estrogen receptors, modification of adrenergic receptors density and innervation, changes in electrophysiologic properties of smooth muscle, inhibition of extraneuronal uptake of catecholamines, modification of cholinergic responses, and interaction with prostaglandins. Clinically, however, the reported effects of estrogen treatment have been reported in very conflicting terms regarding cure rates (between 44% and 100%) and urethral pressure measurements.[25-29] Patients have reported subjective improvement of frequency, urgency, and detrusor incontinence after treatment, but attempts to show such improvement using more objective urodynamic methods were inconclusive.[25] In one study the urethral pressure and the functional and absolute urethral lengths were found to increase after estrogen therapy. However, there was no significant correlation between the improvement of these parameters and what was subjectively reported from the patients.[26] The correlation between high cure rates and estrogen and alpha-adrenergic receptor agonists (such as phenylpropanolamine) has shown promising results[30,31] that might be based on the ability of estrogen but not progesterone to increase the number of alpha-adrenergic receptors in the urethra.[19,20]

Urethral and Abdominal Pressure Transmission

The transmission of abdominal pressure to the urethra, which may occur as a result of coughing, sneezing, or other dynamic causes of changes in abdominal pressure, has been considered to be an important parameter in urodynamic studies designed to better understand the mechanisms of continence. Such pressure-transmission studies, defined as the increase in urethral pressure in proportion to the increase in bladder pressure, were conceived in an effort to develop a better clinical diagnostic test for the evaluation of urethral function in stress urinary incontinence. Such tests attempt to emulate the dynamic conditions present when the patient coughs and there is urine leakage. There are basically two ways of representing transmission studies. In one, the magnitude of pressure elevation from the baseline value is measured in the urethra. This pressure rise is divided by the pressure rise in the bladder. This type of measurement is normally performed manually and excludes the resting urethral pressure. By making many such measurements when patients cough, one can construct a plot of transmission relative to the position in the urethra. The other form of transmission measurement is made by subtraction of the abdominal or bladder pressure from the urethral pressure, thus representing the total intraluminal pressure. The results are plotted against urethral length while the subject is asked to cough repeatedly. One of the most critical aspects of transmission studies is to elicit sufficient coughing from the subjects so that the characteristics of the response are faithfully mapped out. The most critical region where this needs to be done is in the vicinity of the external sphincter, particularly in a region of about 7 mm from the sphincter to the external meatus. This can easily be missed by withdrawal of the catheter. Enhörning was one of the first to use this method of monitoring the ability of the urethra to close under such conditions when a small balloon catheter is used. Because of the size of the balloon, it was not possible to accurately localize the rise in pressure at different anatomic locations of the urethra. Enhörning[32] has shown, however, a relationship between urethral pressure rise and bladder pressure rise, which became a model on which subsequent investigations were based. Careful examination of Enhörning's recordings, but not his conclusions, shows evidence of urethral pressure rise, when the patient coughs, that is higher than the abdominal pressure rise. This finding indicates that an external active component of compression of the recording balloon is involved. The implication is that there is an active component of urethral closure. The fundamental disadvantage of the balloon was overcome by the use of the perfusion method of Brown and Wickham resulting in better resolution of measurement (a few millimeters as compared to a centimeter) that can be calibrated in hydrostatic terms.

Using this method, several studies have been reported, and in particular a systematic study of the transmission of cough pressures along the length of the urethra in a variety of subjects has been carried out using asymptomatic volunteers. Fig. 12-2 illustrates the methodology used specifically for the measurement of urethral pressures simultaneously at different locations in the lumen. It is useful in considering the role of the extrinsic and intrinsic mechanisms of urethral closure to analyze the response of the urethra to stress in the intact subject. Fig. 12-3 shows the results of cough pressure transmission values measured in young, asymptomatic volunteers, who show higher pressure increments in the urethra than expected. Such transmission studies provide supporting evidence of active urethral closure pressures based on the fact that the increment of urethral pressure increase is higher than the increment of cough pressure increase in the bladder. Transmitted pressure is shown to approach well over 100% of the cough pressure, an indication that this is an active phenomenon and not a passive transmission. The anatomic location of the maximum rise in pressure is distal to the region of maximum urethral closure pressure[17,18] in the resting UPP.

Fig. 12-3 also shows in a composite the transmission versus distance responses relative to position, summarizing the average response from many asymptomatic subjects.[17] Observations of more than a 100% rise in urethral pressure, compared to abdominal pressure, have been made by use of the perfusion

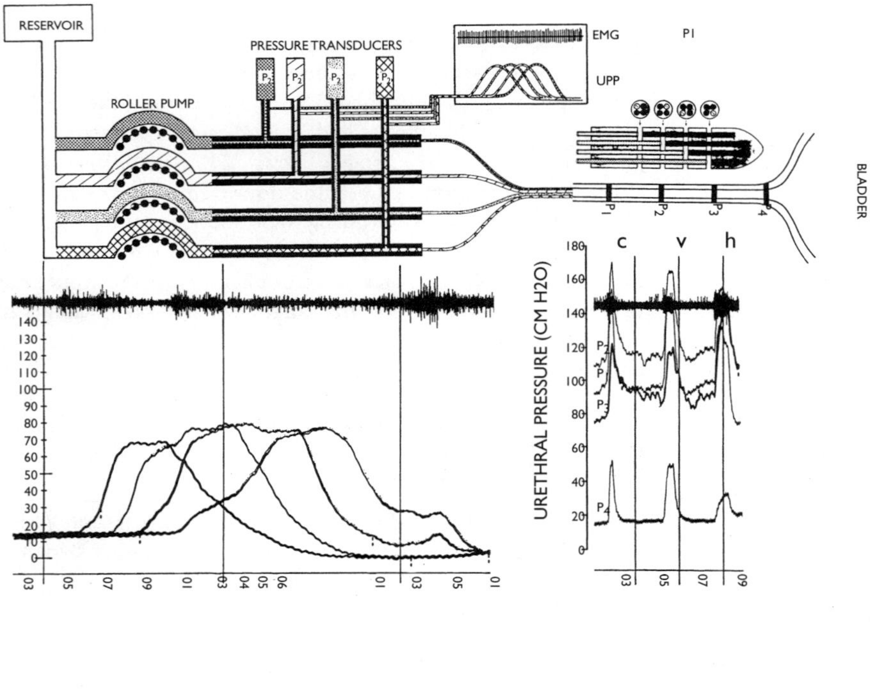

FIG. 12-2 *Methodologic approach for the dynamic measurement of resting and dynamic urethral closure pressures using the gap catheter configuration used in evaluating pressure in asymptomatic volunteers. The fluid-perfused catheter system is shown together with a typical recording of the pattern of urethral pressures during constant withdraw.* Bottom right, *dynamic pressure measurement indicating urethral responses to coughs (c), Valsalva (v), and hold (h). As indicated, coughing produced the highest increase in urethral closure at a region that is distal to the external sphincter. Holding, the equivalent to pelvic floor contraction, also produces high urethral pressures but does not increase bladder pressure to the same extent.* (From Constantinou et al: 1984).

methods of Brown and Wickham, as well as by use of microtip transducers. In the same group of volunteers careful measurements of the timing of pressure rise in the urethra compared to that in the bladder show that the urethral pressure increases first, and such an increase indicates that the guarding reflex may be faster in producing closure than the transmitted abdominal pressure and further indicates that such a mechanism ensures that the likelihood of incontinence is minimized.

Clinical studies done on patients, selected on the basis of demonstrable stress urinary incontinence observed during physical examination, show a qualitative transmission characteristic that is similar to that of controls,[32] though quantitatively the trend toward maximally developed transmission pressures in these patients does not reach the kind of values seen in controls. It is interesting that after endoscopic bladder neck suspension the characteristic trend seen in controls reappears immediately after surgery, and such a reappearance indicates that repositioning of the urethra is sufficient to bring it into the sphere of influence of the pelvic floor. This trend produces a maximum closure that is again above 150%, a value suggestive that the urethra is brought within the region where the supporting action provided by the "hammock" is more effective.

In stress incontinence such a dynamic response is greatly attenuated. Fig. 12-4 typically shows the transmission pressures characterizing patients with demonstrable stress incontinence. The comparative transmission response between the controls and incontinent women both preoperatively and postoperatively is given by Fig. 12-5. The reduced transmission evident in stress-incontinent women is evident at any position. This is illustrated by Fig. 12-5, which shows the normalized transmission characteristics of stress-incontinent women in the supine, sitting, and standing positions. This concept is further substantiated from studies by Bump et al. that evaluated the relative influence of anesthesia on pressure transmission.[16] In these careful studies Bump et al. analyzed the influence of skeletal muscle on urethral pressure-transmission ratios and reported on the role of the distal urethral compensatory mechanisms in a large number of patients. Furthermore, Versi et al., using urethral stress pro-

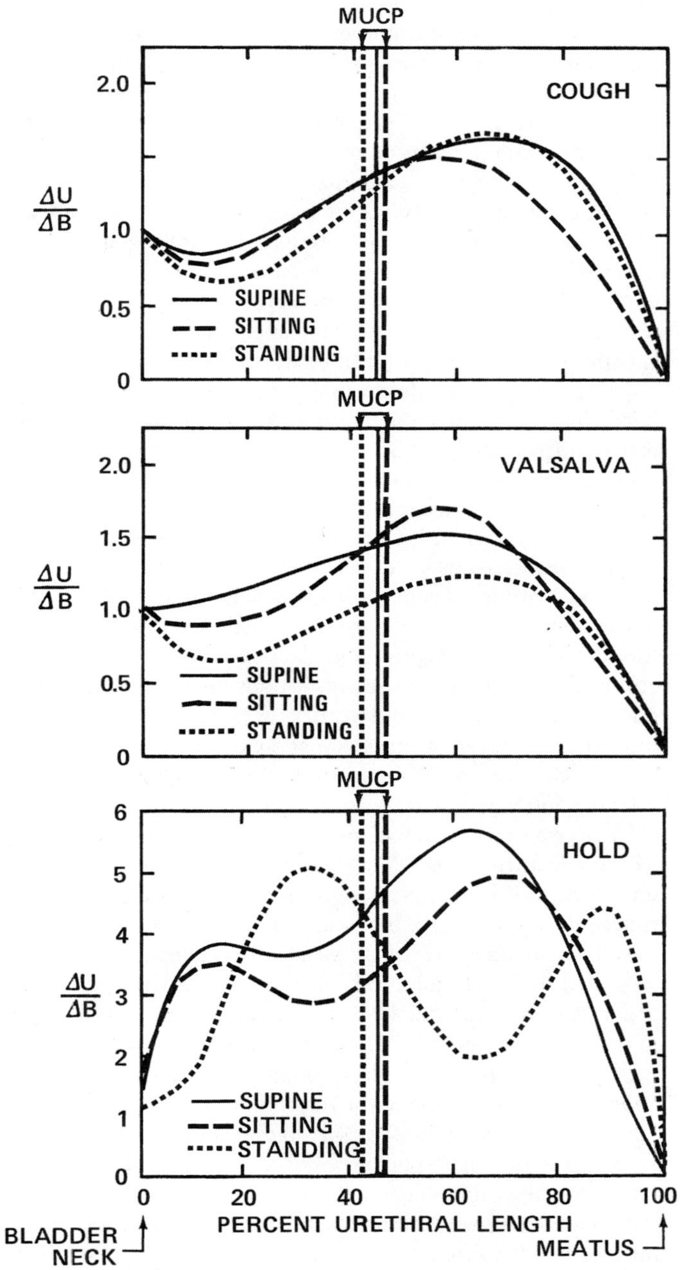

FIG. 12-3 *Ratio of change of urethral,* u, *to bladder,* b, *pressure during coughing, Valsalva maneuver, and holding in controls. This ratio is shown as a function of urethral length starting at the bladder neck to the meatus. The position of the maximal urethral closure pressure (MUCP) is shown. Controls are defined for the purposes of this study as normal, healthy volunteers with no symptoms of urinary incontinence.* (From Constantinou et al: 1984.)

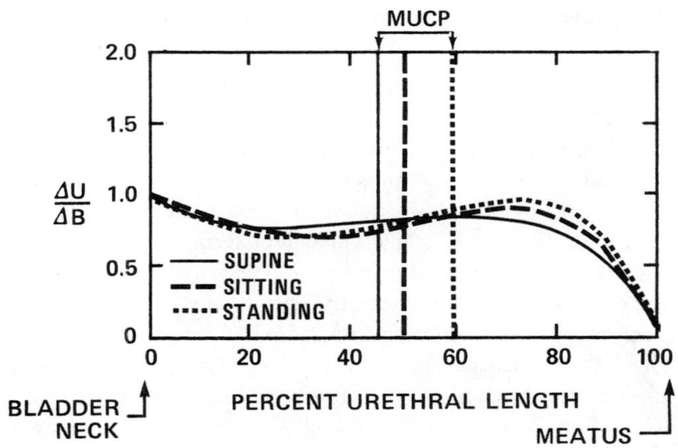

FIG. 12-4 *Urethral pressure transmission between bladder and urethra in the standing, supine, and sitting positions obtained from patients with demonstrable stress urinary incontinence. Representation of axis and units are identical to those in Fig. 12-3. Notice that in comparison to controls the point of maximum urethral closure pressure (MUCP) in incontinent patients has shifted toward the external meatus, particularly in the standing position, whereas in the controls there is comparatively a low variation in the position of MUCP along the urethra.* (From Constantinou et al: 1984)

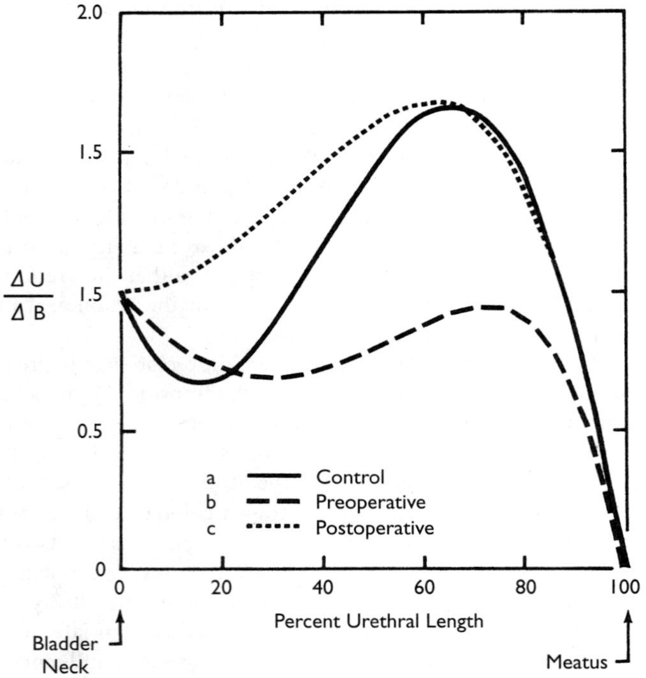

FIG. 12-5 *Comparative influence of the position in the transmission of cough pressures to the urethra relative to continence measured in the standing position. Data from **A,** asymptomatic controls; **B,** stress incontinent patients; **C,** postendoscopic bladder neck suspension. The transmission characteristics were obtained preoperatively from patients with demonstrable stress incontinence and from the same patients 1 week postoperatively after endoscopic bladder neck suspension. As indicated, the transmission of cough pressures in the postoperative state increased to approximate those of the controls.* (From Constantinou et al: 1984.)

files,[33] showed that both the transmission ratios and the subtraction of urethral pressures from abdominal pressures is relevant in the relationship between the bladder neck and the sphincter. Versi et al. suggest that female incontinence can be maintained in the presence of an incompetent bladder neck if the distal sphincter is competent. They have shown that bladder neck incompetence results in proximal shortening of the urethral stress profile while maintaining the functional length under stress by decreased distal shortening of the stress profile. This observation is interpreted by Versi et al. as a better use of the distal portion of the urethra by augmentation of the distal transmission ratio. In light of our visual observation and our own transmission studies, I interpret these results in a similar way and in addition suggest that the distal sphincter mechanism includes both the pelvic floor and other extrinsic forces as well as the intrinsic mechanisms of the urethra.

On this basis and by use of different methods of measurement, transmission studies have shown that a competent bladder neck is not absolutely essential for the maintenance of continence, since there is considerable redundancy of a competent pelvic floor and sphincter function.

The introduction of microtip transducers provided a more convenient way of measuring pressure in the bladder or urethra. However, along with the relative ease of use of the microtip transducer, several confounding considerations have emerged. Principal among these is the problem of what is being measured and how the measurement is affected by local forces. In view of the fact that some of the earlier microtip transducers were mechanically rigid, the additional factor of distortion of the curvature of the urethra has arisen.[34,35] Furthermore, although hydrostatic pressure is used to calibrate the sensitivity of the microtip transducer ex vivo, the calibration inside a tube that is flexible, like the urethra, is subject to interpretation in terms of absolute pressure values. The sensitivity of the microtip transducer to directional compression, which may be extraurethral, renders the transducer as a sensor of local forces useful as an exploratory research tool. Investigators using microtip transducers avoided the local confounding problems of anterior or posterior urethral measurements by orienting the transducer in the lateral plane. This orientation is less subject to variations and ostensibly more reproducible but may in fact mask important information. In the long run, when it is critically analyzed, the orientation of the transducers may provide the basis for better understanding of the mechanisms involved in urethral closure and may be found to be useful in the diagnosis of urethral incontinence. A sophisticated system for urethral pressure measurement was devised by Kauppila et al., who used a 6 French microtransducer catheter to evaluate the transmission of continent and incontinent patients.[36] The advantages of this system is that it obviates the need to move the transducer catheter multiple times. By using the single-cough urethrocystometry, Penttinen observed significant improvements in transmission after surgery.[37] It is evident that more careful work needs to be done to resolve the mode of action of intraurethral and extraurethral structures before such measurements are reliable. It is also important to consider that intraurethral pressure is a dynamic parameter[32] and the MUP decreases with changes in vascularization that are inevitable with the increasing age[38,39] of the patient. At the point of maximum urethral closure, pressures can vary with pulsation of the vessels, and the amplitude of vascular pulsation also decreases with age. Since no large arteries are situated in the urethral wall, it is suggested that such pulsation can be caused by changes in the abdominal pressure by direct pressure transmission,[17] in addition to abdominal pressures by arterioles, capillaries, and tissues in the urethral submucosa. Changing position also causes pressure variations[40] with an increase in the maximum urethral pressure and maximum urethral closure pressure in the standing position compared to pressure in the supine position.

Before the initiation of micturition, intraurethral pressure is reduced, whereupon the intravesical pressure increases and voiding begins.[41,42] Using combined urethrocystometry and urethrocystography it has been shown that the opening of the bladder neck and the drop in the premicturition pressure in the urethra occur simultaneously,[43] whereas during rest and sleeping a significant decrease in the maximum urethral pressure (MUP) and the maximum urethral closure pressure (MUCP) has been observed.[44] Continuous long-term recordings of intraurethral pressures show pressure variations in the MUCP.[24] Systematic studies of urethral pressure variations have been carried out by Sørensen in a variety of incontinent women. It was found that, in patients with detrusor incontinence, sudden pressure drops occur that could not be distinguished from the pressure drop seen in normal individuals at the onset of micturition.[24] In addition, it was shown in the study that no differences in pressure variations during long-term observation distinguish this group and normal fertile volunteers. The term "urethral instability" has been used to describe variations in the urethral pressure greater than 15 cm H_2O (positive or negative).[45] Three types of urethral instability are recognized and are graded from small fluctuations to large variations in pressure. No significant differences in patients with pressure variations were found between stress incontinent and healthy postmenopausal individuals during long-term pressure recording.[24] As one changes from supine to standing position, the MUCP seems to decrease because the vesical pressure increases more than the urethral pressure.[46]

New Methods of Evaluation of Urethral Function

The urethral pressure transmission studies described have inherent limitations in terms of interpretation, artifacts, and precise definition of parameters. In recent years, new methods have been introduced for the study of both static and dynamic action of the urethra in maintaining continence.[47-49] The purpose of such methods is to make possible the description of the mechanical properties of the urethra in terms of compliance, hysteresis, and power created by the urethral closure apparatus during voluntary contraction of the pelvic floor and coughing. Of particular interest is the attempt by Lose to measure the uninstrumented closure pressure using the field-gradient method.[50] In static measurements done at rest in asymptomatic volunteers and patients with stress incontinence, he showed differences in the relationship between urethral pressure and cross-sectional area at the bladder neck and the middle and distal portions of the urethra.[51,52] In comparing these differences between stress incontinent persons and controls, it was shown that, in comparison to normal women, elastance was significantly lower at the bladder neck in patients with stress incontinence, an indication that the supporting structures around the bladder neck may have been weakened. Although measurement of the urethral function using the pressure versus area methods described above have not been widely used, they have provided a reliable and quantitative way of diagnosis and have focused attention on the mechanism of continence and the role of the urethra. At first glance, it may be intuitively difficult to rationalize how the urethra can be evaluated by such tests that are based on dilatation. Reflection on the process of micturition indicates that sudden urethral dilatation of the urethra occurs during coughing. Such dilatation simulates the entry of urine into the proximal part of the urethra and thereby mimics the conditions of incontinence. Finally, an emerging new method of measuring total urethral compliance in stress incontinence based on measurements of bladder pressure and urine flow has been described by Walter et al.[53] It was shown that total urethral compliance increased in stress incontinence, and that fact may be of diagnostic value. The principal advantage of this approach is that compliance can be used as an absolute physical quantity to compare patients having different voiding pressures.

The concept of leak-point pressure has been promoted by many as a supplementary way of evaluating the competence of the urethra in resting-pressure and transmission-pressure studies. A formulation embodying these concepts has emerged on the basis of the the theoretical analysis of Kim.[54] This is a new and novel way of investigating and representing the function of the urethra and, as introduced by Kim,[54] provides a significant advance in urethral pressure methodology. In this representation Kim formulated the concept of a vesicourethral pressuregram, the purpose of which is to quantify the zero continence margin and global transmission ratio. Fig. 12-6 illustrates the basic elements of the vesicourethral pressuregram for continent and incontinent women. Results of the pressuregram using are illustrated by Fig. 12-7. Kim's pressuregrams, although reminiscent

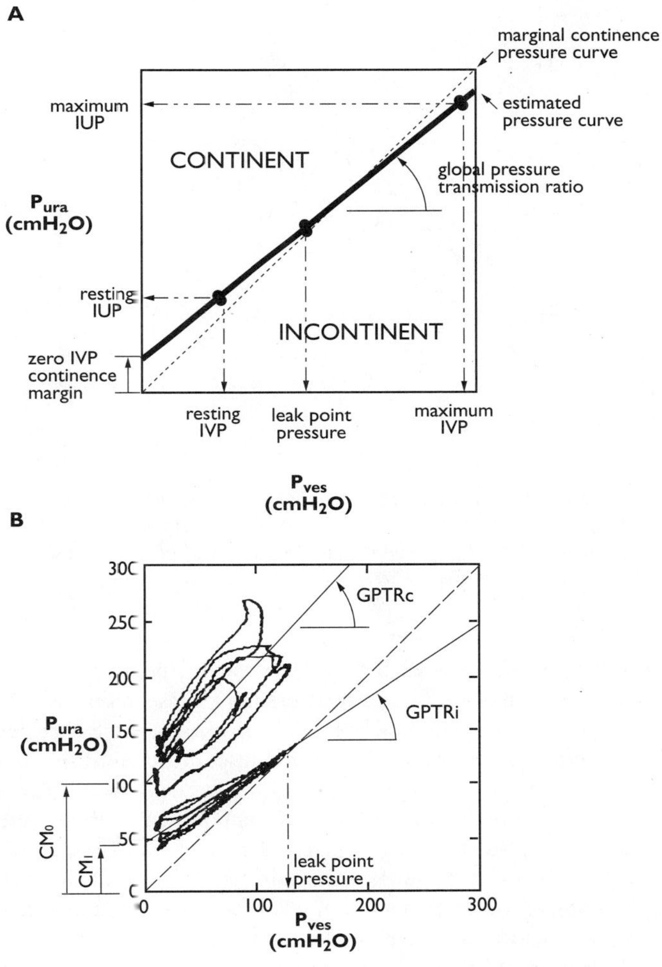

FIG. 12-6 *Representation of the vesicourethral pressuregram.* ***A,*** *Relevant physiologic parameters relating the line between continent and incontinent patients is shown defining the position of leak-point pressure and global-pressure transmission ratio.* ***B,*** *Pressuregrams from a continent woman and an incontinent woman are shown together, clearly illustrating the discriminating characteristic of the representation.* (From Kim AC, Lindskog M: *Urology* 32:273, 1988.)

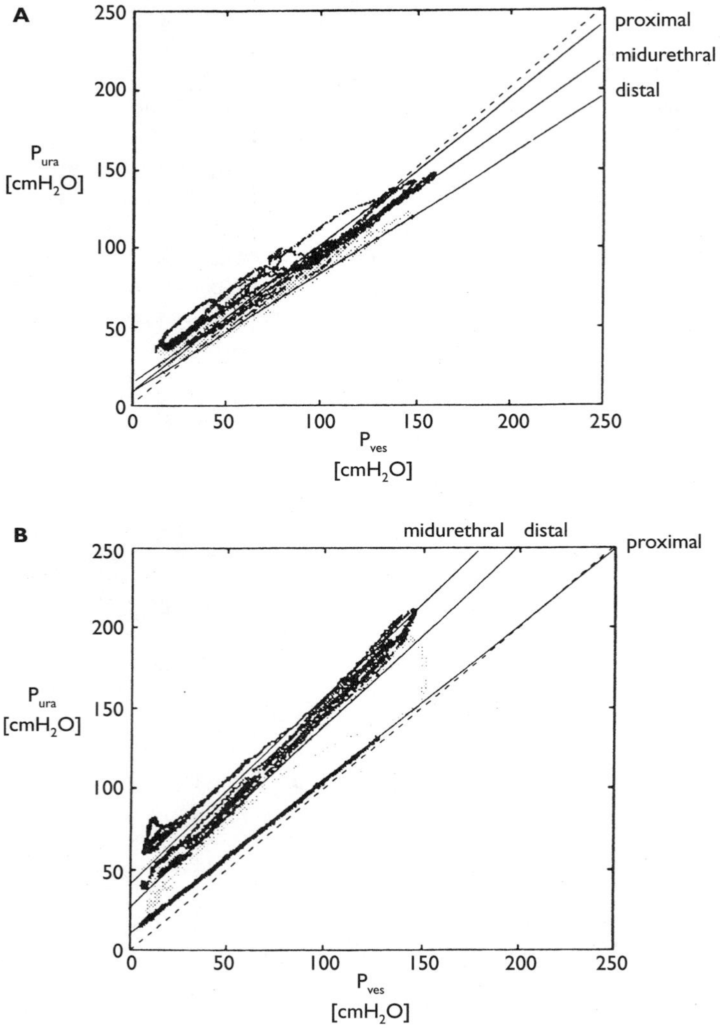

FIG. 12-7 *Kim pressuregrams obtained relative to urethral position illustrating the overlap in response in incontinent subjects shown on the top,* ***A,*** *and separation seen in continent subjects shown below,* ***B.*** (From Kim AC, Linskog M: *Urology* 32:273, 1988.)

of the pressure-flow studies used to evaluate micturition characteristics in males, differ greatly in that a representation of bladder pressure and urethral pressure is made. For a measurement of urethral pressure the pressuregram uses the full informational content of the data. One estimates the key parameter of leak-point pressure by locating the crossing point between marginal continence and and the estimated pressure curve. These studies have shown that the increase in proximal stress results from the bending of the urethra and not from the sphincter and demonstrates that the active role of the urethra in terms of stress plays the most significant role in continence.

EFFECT OF SURGICAL TREATMENT ON THE URETHRA

Surgical procedures such as endoscopic bladder neck suspension influence urethral function and urodynamic parameters measured following such procedures were examined by Leach et al., who observed an alteration from negative to positive of the transmission ratio of the abdominal pressure to the proximal urethral pressure during stress.[55] Urethral resistance, MUP and MUCP, and functional urethral length remained unchanged. Stamey bladder neck suspension was shown to increase functional urethral length in the standing position (no significant change in sitting position), and the transmission ratio of abdominal pressure to urethral pressure was also significantly increased.[56, 57] In the diagnosis of the cause of incontinence, there are basically two factors that are worth careful consideration: When urinary incontinence occurs during the breakdown of the physiologic function of the detrusor, such incontinence is termed "detrusor incontinence." The degree of incontinence that occurs depends on the physiologic factors that are recruited to suppress the detrusor and close the urethra to prevent leakage. When incontinence occurs in the absence of bladder contraction but is attributable to pressures exerted outside the bladder, this type of incontinence is dependent on the competence of the urethral closure mechanisms. Incontinence occurring because of incompetence of the urethral structures is termed "urethral incontinence." There are instances in which patients exhibit both detrusor and urethral incontinence. Localization of the origin and extent of the incontinence (urethra or detrusor) is of crucial significance in deciding whether the course of treatment is surgical or nonsurgical. In the urethra or the detrusor, or with mixed incontinence, the stimulus precipitating the loss of urine may be intrinsic to the bladder or the urethral structures or may be extrinsic (cough, sneeze, movement). Under such provocation, complex physiologic and anatomic mechanisms will be brought into play. Their response will then affect both the forces acting directly on the bladder and urethra and on the anatomic structures around them. Coughing, for example, will result in a pressure pulse applied to the bladder and urethra from all directions. The reflexes involved, guarding, will in turn activate the pelvic floor skeletal musculature to increase closure pressure of the sphincters to counteract the elevation of abdominal pressure. As shown earlier in this chapter, the urethra will be influenced by activation of surrounding structures such as the levator ani pubourethral ligaments, especially by their anatomic juxtaposition to the symphysis pubis and the pelvis and the position of the vesical neck.

Detrusor stability, urgency, and previous surgery are considered here as the principal determinants of cure. Analysis of these parameters is limited to the extent that stability is not readily quantified, and urgency is also an unmeasurable quantity by urodynamic testing. Previous surgery encompasses a wide range of anatomic and functional changes. For these reasons, these parameters were used in the simplified form of their presence or absence with no effort to quantify the degree of their severity. In patients where there is evidence of detrusor incontinence from urodynamic studies, a pharmacologic option is frequently considered first, since the ability of the urethra to overcome a high-pressure bladder contraction is limited, particularly in older patients. The pharmacologic suppression of detrusor incontinence requires a careful evaluation of each of the specific drugs frequently encountered, thereby limiting this mode of therapy.

In patients with mixed detrusor and urethral incontinence, the temptation is often overwhelming to treat urethral incontinence first, especially with surgery. There are some indications that, under such conditions, detrusor incontinence is also suppressed. The distribution of detrusor incontinence relative to urethral incontinence was systematically investigated.[58] Thus demonstrability of urethral incontinence in 151 consecutive unselected patients complaining of incontinence was 56%. This indicates that a large proportion of patients who complain of incontinence cannot be diagnosed by physical examination alone. Thus the physical examination in itself has failed to localize and reliably identify the cause of the patient's complaints. Among these patients with urethral incontinence, urodynamic evaluation has shown that approximately two thirds have stable detrusor function whereas the remaining have some evidence of instability, an indication that a significant number of patients with urethral incontinence may also have detrusor instability. In about half of the patients with a stable bladder function, physical examination failed to identify the cause of incontinence. Thus approximately half of the patients who do not demonstrate incontinence at the physical examination are likely to be incontinent because of dysfunction of the bladder. One factor that should be considered in establishing detrusor stability in diagnostic tests such as filling cystometry are the inherent limitations of the urodynamic methods of measurement. Because of such limitations in urodynamics, newer ambulatory monitoring techniques have been developed to uncover the presence of instability that can only be provoked in many cases. Filling cystometry in addition to profilometry provides some basis upon which patients with demonstrable stress incontinence may be distinguished from those with instability of the detrusor. The most significant associated parameter that can be of value in the interpretation of the UPP is detrusor contraction during voiding. The reason is that the pressure generated during voiding is partly dependent on the resistance of the urethra. Thus a low-resistance urethra will not be able to resist the contractility of the bladder, and flow will be produced at lower pressures.

Urethral incompetence can be substantiated and verified by the urethral pressure profile in most cases but not all. The posterior urethral closure pressure shows a significant difference between patients with and without demonstrable stress incontinence. The interpretation of urethral closure pressure requires correction for the patient's age before a decision on urethral competence can be made. However, even with uncorrected values, patients with urethral incontinence have significantly lower posterior urethral pressures; hence the numerical values obtained from urodynamic recordings provide the physician with reliable information as to the type of incontinence present in any particular patient.

Effect of Endoscopic Suspension on the Urethra

As shown in Fig. 12-3, transmission studies provide further useful information in the evaluation of continence. The advantage of transmission tests is that they allow one to evaluate the urethra at the very condition when it is likely to fail. It is generally regarded that successful surgical correction of urethrally incontinent women dependent on the relocation of the *proximal* portion of the urethra to a position that more completely transmits intra-abdominal pressures. However, it has been shown that this may not be the major factor involved. High transmission occurs actively, an indication of the existence of a fast mechanism to close the distal portion of the urethra. Patients with urethral incontinence do not possess high transmission pressures, and such a lack is suggestive of reduction in the effectiveness of the distal active closure mechanism. After endoscopic bladder neck suspension, high-transmission pressures are recorded, and their presence indicates that the relative position of the distal urethral mechanism to the levator ani or other periurethral structures has been realigned. As discussed above, postoperatively the transmission of cough pressures is enhanced both proximally and distally, and such enhancement explains why pure urethral incontinence is readily corrected with an endoscopic bladder neck suspension. In addition to the enhancement of transmission pressures on the urethra, endoscopic bladder neck suspension has an obstructive effect on the urethra. Obstructive pressures after endoscopic suspension approach those of isometric tests on healthy subjects.

Thus the evaluation of detrusor instability is crucial to any urodynamic study because, when there is mixed urethra and detrusor incontinence, detrusor stability becomes a parameter that determines the success or failure of incontinence therapy. If the bladder starts acting as a pump when it is in the reservoir phase, detrusor incontinence is likely to occur. In patients with a stable bladder, the cure rate is almost double that of women with detrusor instability. In consideration of the influence of previous surgery and urgency on the cure rate it was found that improvement was reported among the patients with detrusor instability, though close examination of the surgical history of the patients indicates that previous surgery is also an important parameter in predicting the success rate of the endoscopic suspension. Evidently patients with no previous surgery and with a stable detrusor function are most likely to be cured of urethral incontinence.

Conclusions

Aspects of urethral function can be reliably evaluated with pressure measurements, particularly with the functional contribution of anatomy of the pelvic floor. The reason is that the associated large structures around the urethra contribute to the dynamics of the extrinsic mechanism of urethral pressures. Evidently the anatomic contribution of the pelvic floor is most critical for the understanding of transmission studies, in that the reflex activation of skeletal muscles is important in the timing of urethra closure in response to stress-induced forces.

Urethral pressures cannot be viewed in isolation because bladder function is central in the ability of the urethra to retain its contents. The reason is that an unstable bladder can generate pressures to open the urethra and induce incontinence. Urodynamics can be used to evaluate detrusor instability; however, urgency, a sensory aspect of urethral dysfunction, cannot be measured with the current state of urodynamic instrumentation.

On a diagnostic basis, it is suggested that the combination of pelvic floor integrity, detrusor stability, and absence of urgency are the primary factors that are predictive of the optimum treatment of patients with low urethral pressures and incontinence. Based on the considerations made above, it is evident that the resting urethral pressure profile alone does not reflect the functional potential of the urethra to maintain continence.

References

1. DeLancey JOL: Structural support of the urethra as it relates to stress urinary incontinence: the hammock hypothesis, *Am J Obstet Gynecol* 170:1713-1723, 1994.
2. Christensen LL, Djurhuus JC, Constantinou CE: Imaging of pelvic floor contractions using MRI, *Neurourol Urodyn* 14(3):209-216, 1995.
3. Rud T, Anderson KE, Asmussen M, et al: Factors maintaining the intraurethral pressure in women, *Invest Urol* 17:343, 1980.
4. DeLancey JOL: Anatomy and physiology of the urinary continence, *Clin Obstet Gynecol* 33:298, 1990.
5. DeLancey JOL: Correlative study of paraurethral anatomy, *Obstet Gynecol* 68:91, 1986.
6. Gosling JA, Dixon JS, Critchley HOD, et al: A comparative study of the human external sphincter and periurethral levator ani muscles, *Br J Urol* 53:35, 1981.
7. Chritchley HOD, Dixon JS, Gosling JA: Comparative study of the periurethral and perianal parts of the levator ani muscle, *Urol Int* 35:226, 1980.
8. Gosling J: Structure of the bladder and urethra in relation to function, *Urol Clin North Am* 6:31, 1979.
9. Juenemann K-P, Lue TF, Schmidt RA, et al: Clinical significance of sacral and pudendal nerve anatomy, *J Urol* 139:74, 1988.
10. Staubesand H, Staubesand J, editors: *Sobotta Atlas of human anatomy,* ed 10, Munich and Baltimore, 1982, Urban & Schwartzenberg.
11. Christensen LL, Djurhuus JC, Constantinou PS, Constantinou CE: *Int Urogynecol J* 1995.
12. Morita T, Tsuchida S: Stereographic urethral pressure profile, *Urol Int* 39:199-206, 1984.
13. Brown M, Wickham JEA: The urethral pressure profile, *Br J Urol* 41:211, 1969.
14. Anderson RB, Shephert AM, Feneley RCL: Microtransducer urethral profile methodology: variations caused by transducer orientation, *J Urol* 130:727, 1983.
15. Constantinou C: Resting and stress urethral pressures as a clinical guide to the mechanism of continence in the female patient, *Urol Clin North Am* 12:247, 1985.
16. Bump RC, Huang KC, McClish DK, et al: Effect of narcotic anesthesia and skeletal muscle paralysis on passive and dynamic urethral function of stress continent and incontinent women, *Neurourol Urodyn* 10:523, 1991.
17. Constantinou CE, Govan DE: Spatial distribution of transmitted and reflexly generated urethral pressures in healthy women, *J Urol* 127:964, 1982.
18. Constantinou CE: Urethrometry: considerations of static dynamic and stability characteristics of the female urethra, *Neurourol Urodyn* 7:521, 1988.
19. Schreiter F, Fuchs P, Stockam K: Estrogenic sensitivity of alpha-receptors in the urethral musculature, *Urol Int* 31:13, 1976.
20. Caine M, Raz S: Some clinical implications of adrenergic receptors in the urinary tract, *Arch Surg* 110:247, 1975.
21. Iosif SC, Batra S, Ek A, et al: Estrogen receptors in the human female lower urinary tract, *Am J Obstet Gynecol* 141:817, 1981.
22. Gosling JA, Dixon JS, Lendon RG: The autonomic innervation of the human male and female bladder neck and proximal urethra, *J Urol* 118:302, 1977.
23. Miodrag A, Castleden CE, Vallance TR: Sex hormones and the female urinary tract, *Drugs* 36:491, 1988.
24. Sørensen S: Urethral pressure variations in healthy and incontinent women, doctoral thesis, *Neurourol Urodyn* 11:549, 1992.
25. Walter S, Wolf H, Barlebo H, et al: Urinary incontinence in postmenopausal women treated with estrogens: a double-blind clinical trial, *Urol Int* 33:135, 1978.
25. Wolf H, Wandt H, Jonat W: Immunohistochemical evidence of estrogen and progesterone receptors in the female lower urinary tract and comparison with the vagina, *Gyncol Obstet Invest* 32:227, 1991.
26. Rud T: The effect of estrogens and gestagens on the urethral pressure profile in urinary continent and stress incontinent women, *Acta Obstet Gynecol Scand* 59:265, 1980.
27. Schreiter F, Fuchs P, Stockamp K: Estrogen sensitivity of alfa-receptors in the urethra musculature, *Urol Int* 31:13, 1976.
28. Iosif CS: Effects of protrated administration of estriol on the lower genito urinary tract in postmenopausal women, *Arch Gynecol Obstet* 251:115, 1992.
29. Wilson PD, Faragher B, Butler B, et al: Treatment with oral piperazine oestrogene sulphate for genuine stress incontinence in postmenopausal women, *Br J Obstet Gynaecol* 94:568, 1987.
30. Kinn AC, Lindskog M: Estrogens and phenylpropanolamine in combination for stress urinary incontinence in postmenopausal women, *Urology* 32:273, 1988.
31. Henriksson L, Ulmsten U, Andersson K-E: The effect of changes of posture on the urethral closure pressure in healthy women, *Scand J Urol* 11:201, 1977.
31. Non-surgical treatment of stress incontinence (Editorial), *Lancet* 340:643, 1992.
32. Enhörning G: Simultaneous recording of the intravesical and intraurethral pressure, *Acta Chir Scand* 276(suppl) 1, 1961.
33. Versi E, Cardozo L: Distal urethral compensatory mechanisms in women with incompetent bladder neck who remain continent, and the effect of menopause, *Neurourol Urodyn* 90:574, 1990.
34. Plevnik S, Janez J, Vrtacnik P, et al: Directional differences in urethral pressure recordings: contributions from the stiffness and weight of the recording catheter, *Neurourol Urodyn* 5:117, 1984.
35. Schaffer W (letter to the editor): Directional differences in urethral pressure recordings: contributions from the stiffness and weight of the recording catheter, *Neurourol Urodyn* 5:114, 1984.
35. Ulmsten U, Andersson K-E, Persson CGA: Diagnostic and therapeutic aspects of urge urinary incontinence in women, *Urol Int* 32:88, 1977.
36. Kauppila A, Pettinen J, Haggman V: Six-microtransducer catheter connected to computer evaluation of urethral closure function of women, *Urology* 23:159, 1989.
37. Penttinen J, Käär K, Kauppila A: Effect of suprapubic operation on urethral closure: evaluation by single cough urethrocystometry, *Br J Urol* 63:384, 1989.
38. Rud T: Urethral pressure profile in continent women from childhood to old age, *Acta Obstet Gynecol Scand* 59:331, 1980.
39. Henriksson L, Ulmsten U, Andersson K-E: The effect of changes of posture on the urethral closure pressure in healthy women, *Scand J Urol* 11:201, 1977.
40. Ulmsten U, Andersson K-E, Persson CGA: Diagnostic and therapeutic aspects of urge urinary incontinence in women, *Urol Int* 32:88, 1977.
41. Rud T, Andersson K-E, Ulmsten U: Initiation of voiding in healthy and stress in continent women, *Acta Obstet Gynecol Scand* 57:457, 1978.
43. Rud T, Ulmsten U, Westby M: Initiation of micturition: a study of combined urethrocystometry and urethrocystography in healthy and stress incontinent females, *Scand J Urol Nephrol* 13:259, 1979.
44. Politano VA, Small MP, Harper JM, et al: Periurethral teflon injection for urinary incontinence, *J Urol* 111:180, 1974.
45. Ulmsten U, Henrikson L, Iosif S: The unstable female urethra, *Am J Obstet Gynecol* 144:93, 1982.
46. Henriksson L, Ulmsten U, Andersson K-E: The effect of changes of posture on the urethral closure pressure in stress-incontinent women, *Scand J Urol Nephrol* 11:207, 1977.
47. Colstrup H, Mortensen SO, Kristensen JK: A new method for investigation of closure function of resting female urethra, *J Urol* 130:507, 1983.

48. Reignier CH, Susset JG, Ghoniem GM, et al: A new catheter to measure urethral compliance in females: normal values, *J Urol* 124:1060, 1983.
49. Harada T: Experimental study on measurements of compliance and cross-sectional area in the urethra through the field gradient principle, *Jpn J Urol* 76:360, 1985.
50. Lose G: Mechanical properties of the urethra in healthy female volunteers: static measurements in resting urethra, *Neurourol Urodyn* 8:451, 1989.
51. Blute ML, Tomera KM, Hellerstein DK, et al: Transurethral microwave thermotherapy for management of benign prostatic hyperplasia: results of the united states prostatron cooperative study, *J Urol* 150:1591, 1993.
52. Lose G: Simultaneous recording of pressure and cross-sectional area in female urethra: a study of urethral closure function in healthy and stress incontinent women, *Neurourol Urodyn* 11:550, 1992.
53. Walter JS, Wheeler JS, Morgan C, et al: Measurement of total urethral compliance in females with stress incontinence, *Neurourol Urodyn* 12:2‑3, 1993.
54. Leach GE, Yip CM, Donovan BJ: Mechanism of continence after modified Pereyra bladder-neck suspension, *Urology* 24:328, 1987.
56. Constantinou CE, Faysal MH, Rother L, et al: The impact of bladder neck suspension on the mode of distribution of abdominal pressure along the female urethra. In *Female incontinence*, New York, 1981, Alan Liss.
57. Stamey TA: Urinary incontinence in the female. In Walsh PC, Gittes R, Perlmutter A, Stamey T, editors: *Campbell's urology*, New Jersey, 1992, Saunders.
58. Constantinou CE: Determinants of cure by endoscopic suspension of the bladder-neck in the incontinent female patient, *World J Urol* 4:10-15, 1986.

Chapter

13

Leak Point Pressures

Helen E. O'Connell, Edward J. McGuire

Abdominal and bladder leak point pressures determine urethral resistance to two different expulsive forces. As far as the urethra is concerned, these two forces, abdominal and detrusor pressure, constitute the sum total of the forces acting on the urethra to cause leakage. An abdominal (or stress) leak point pressure (ALPP) is a measure of stress competence of the urethra, or a measure of the ability of the urethra to resist the expulsive force of abdominal pressure. A detrusor (or bladder) leak point pressure (BLPP), however, is a measurement of the resistance of the urethra to detrusor pressure as an expulsive force. These two measurements have no relationship to each other. The BLPP has a relationship to upper tract function in that a "high" bladder leak point pressure is associated with the propensity to upper tract deterioration. BLPP incorporates a measure of bladder compliance during filling and the detrusor pressure required to overcome outlet resistance at the time of "voiding" or leaking. Leak point pressures, abdominal and bladder, actually reflect outlet resistance at the time these forces individually induce leakage. Neither leak point pressure reflects the strength or character of the detrusor contraction. Griffiths and others have demonstrated that detrusor pressure (P_{det}) at the time of leakage (or voiding) (BLPP) reflects only outlet resistance.[1]

Bladder Leak Point Pressures

Evolution

Original description of bladder leak point pressures. In 1981, McGuire et al.,[2] studying a population of myelodysplastic children, noted a relationship between detrusor pressure at the time of leakage (BLPP) and the development of upper tract deterioration. Of 42 myelodysplastic patients, 22 patients were found to have urethral leakage at a detrusor pressure of more than 40 cm H_2O. In the high pressure group, vesicoureteral reflux and ureteral dilatation occurred in 68% and 81% respectively. When this group was followed longitudinally, there was a 100% development of upper tract deterioration or vesicoureteral reflux. In the group of 20 patients in whom detrusor pressure at the time of leakage was less than 40 cm H_2O, no patient developed vesicoureteral reflux or ureteral dilatation. The importance of the detrusor pressure required to overcome urethral sphincter resistance or the bladder leak point pressure was thus demonstrated, and a hypothesis that high detrusor pressures were responsible for upper tract deterioration was formed.

The relationship between high bladder leakage and storage pressures and upper tract deterioration was then confirmed by other workers.[3,4] Sidi et al.,[3] for example, showed that neonates with abnormal upper tract radiographic changes had high associated detrusor pressures (and high BLPP). When these were reduced by anticholinergic medication and intermittent catheterization (or vesicostomy), resolution of the upper tract changes occurred.

Bladder pressure management system. A "bladder pressure management system" was developed as a result of these observations regarding BLPP and bladder compliance.[5] This consisted in a program of detecting elevated bladder pressure and lowering those pressures before upper tract dysfunction became apparent. Bladder leak point pressures were lowered by treatment designed to improve bladder function or by ablation of outlet resistance, the latter simply permitting leakage at a lower pressure.

Techniques for lowering detrusor pressure and improving storage function include anticholinergic agents and intermittent catheterization or, in more extreme circumstances, myomectomy or augmentation cystoplasty. Reduction in outlet resistance can be accomplished by sphincterotomy, urethral dilatation, or vesicostomy. Thus a variety of techniques to lower BLPP have been shown to both protect upper tract function and improve it where upper tract deterioration has already occurred. Use of the bladder pressure management system by Wang et al.[5] has been demonstrated to dramatically reduce the development of upper tract changes in children with high leak point pressures who are identified early before those changes become apparent, and resultant resolution of upper tract changes occurred in those children whose high leak point pressures were detected after upper tract changes were noted.

Ghoniem et al.[6] noted that all myelodysplastic patients with upper tract problems had poor to very poor bladder compliance. A later observation by Bloom et al. in regard to children with high leak point pressures and poor compliance is perhaps one of the most important urodynamic findings in recent years.[7] These workers performed urethral dilatation to reduce the detrusor pressure required to induce leakage and created a situation where low-pressure leakage resulted after dilatation in children who had not responded to conservative treatment, that is, intermittent catheterization and drugs. The authors of this report were trading "continence" by reducing outlet resistance for upper tract protection. They were surprised to find that the effect of a decrease in outlet resistance was a dramatic and sustained improvement in bladder compliance and no detrimental effect on continence. As a result of these observations, it became clear that elevated outlet resistance induces a change in detrusor behavior that results in a gradual progressive loss of bladder compliance. That process can result in a situation where ambient detrusor pressures reach 40 cm H_2O, which appears to be the limit of ureteral reserve pumping power.

Concept of detrusor pressure at working (typical) capacity. In the testing situation, leakage may occur as a result of bladder filling to a volume that a given bladder never reaches in day-to-day life. For example, in a myelodysplastic patient, a BLPP of 70 cm H_2O is recorded at 700 ml of bladder filling. In no circumstance does the bladder ever reach 700 ml or the 70 cm H_2O because an appropriate catheterization interval is maintained. The determination of whether a treatment is safe is made at the "typical maximum bladder capacity," which in this case was 300 ml of filling. If the bladder pressure at the time of intermittent catheterization at a maximum volume of 300 ml is less than 20 cm H_2O, it is a safe system with a definite margin of safety. This concept is referred to as the "pressure at typical capacity."[8] The volume at which high pressure occurs is critically important to whether a given bladder and its outlet are safe with respect to upper tract function and a given treatment regimen.

Control of bladder leak point pressure and incontinence. Despite a 50% propensity in myelodysplastic patients to developing upper tract deterioration and the associated high outlet resistance as measured by high BLPP, most such patients are incontinent between intermittent catheterizations. Myelodysplastic patients with high BLPP have both an areflex bladder and an open nonfunctional internal sphincter mechanism. In these patients, despite sufficiently high bladder pressures and elevated outlet resistance to induce upper tract changes, incontinence associated with poor urethral function, wherein abdominal pressure is the driving force, is extremely common. The original observation by Wang and co-workers was that control of bladder pressure did not imply incontinence, and they suggested that poor outlet closing pressure was responsible for the inability of the urethra to resist abdominal pressure as an expulsive force. This apparent paradox, that is, urethral resistance sufficient to cause upper tract changes but poor urethral resistance to abdominal pressure, seems to be associated with the difficulty that clinicians have had in understanding the difference between abdominal and bladder leak point pressures.

Technique and Interpretation of BLPP Testing

A BLPP may be measured with a simple manometer or more complex electronic equipment. In infants, a 5 French gauge feeding tube or 8 Fr urodynamic catheter may be used to introduce fluid and determine pressure responses. In older patients a 10 Fr catheter may be used.[10]

A cystometrogram is performed at a filling rate of 25 to 50 ml/min determined by the size of the patient. The patient is typically supine for this study. As filling occurs, the point at which leakage occurs is identified either by direct observation or fluoroscopically. The total bladder pressure, the largest component of which is detrusor pressure, at the time of leakage is measured and recorded. This is the BLPP (Fig. 13-1). In some patients the BLPP may occur at very large volumes and high pressures. Once a bladder pressure over 40 cm H_2O is reached, there is no value in continuing the study, and ongoing filling above these pressures known to be dangerous is not useful. In any situation where leak point pressure testing is important, it is the volume at which pressure reaches a dangerous level, that is, 40 cm H_2O, that is the critical observation. If "typical capacity" is a volume substantially less than that volume at which dangerous pressures occur, that bladder does not pose a risk to upper tract function. If the bladder is reliably emptied by intermittent catheterization at volumes and pressures that are much lower than the bladder volume recorded

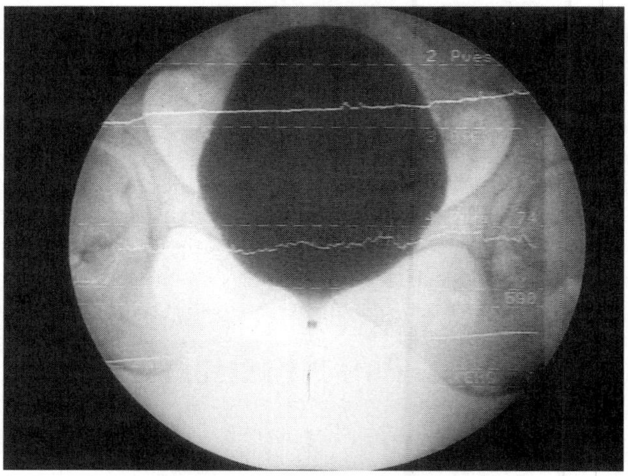

FIG. 13-1 *Demonstration of a bladder leak point pressure (BLPP). At a bladder pressure of 70 cm H_2O and volume of 590 ml, leakage (voiding) occurs. A distal urethral stricture is apparent in this 65-year-old woman obstructed after anterior vaginal repair evidenced by high voiding pressure and poor distal urethral opening.*

when the pressure reaches 40 cm H_2O, the bladder is regarded as safe, though it is intrinsically dangerous if it is not emptied completely intermittently.

Compliance. Another way of looking at the evaluation of pressure in relation to the typical capacity is to focus, during the cystometrogram, on the initial part of the curve rather than at terminal compliance, that is, compliance at the very end of filling. Patients with good initial compliance have better upper tract outcomes than patients with poor initial compliance have.[6] This observation further supports the concept that every bladder does not need to be filled to absolute capacity to gain meaningful information. The initial compliance limb of the filling cystometrogram appears to be critical information with respect to the assessment of upper tract risk posed by a given bladder.

Bladder leak point pressures were first used to measure relatively static situations where an areflex bladder is resisted by an equally areflex fixed sphincter mechanism, chiefly in the area of the membranous urethra or the external sphincter integrated by the pudendal nerve. That measurement simply required filling of the reservoir and observation of the urethral meatus for the accurate detection of a leak point pressure. This kind of testing was later applied to patients with neurogenic voiding dysfunction associated with reflex contractility of the bladder, particularly that encountered in spinal cord–injured patients with reflex-related detrusor-sphincter dyssynergia. In patients managed by intermittent catheterization with or without drugs the information sought is the bladder pressure at the maximum bladder volume achieved by that patient's bladder. In other patients treated by external sphincterotomy, ileovesicostomy, or simple vesicostomy the information sought in leak point pressure testing is the detrusor pressure required to induce leakage from the urethra or stoma.

Any bladder pressures above 40 cm H_2O with abnormal initial compliance require treatment because the risk of upper tract deterioration is 100%. Detrusor pressures at the time of leakage by the urethra or by a stoma are equally important, since it is control of bladder pressure that is the objective of sphincterotomy or ileovesicostomy. Via a stoma, the BLPP should be 10 cm H_2O or less; via the urethra, 25 cm H_2O or less. Some latitude for these values is permissible, but a "normal" bladder does not gain 20 cm H_2O pressure at capacity, and voiding pressure in normal adults and normal adults or children is always less than 30 cm H_2O.

BLPP testing in neurogenic conditions is reliable and reproducible because volitional and subconscious influences do not interfere with testing. In patients with a normal neuraxis suspected of obstructive uropathy, various artifacts can impair the accuracy of BLPP testing. These artifacts include external sphincter activity during voiding and subconscious inhibition of the voiding reflex. These problems usually require that some direct or indirect measure of urethral activity be made during BLPP testing. This can be a flow rate, a fluoroscopic observation, an electromyogram, or direct urethral pressure measurements.

Pitfalls in BLPP Testing

Catheter related. Catheter size and infusion rate can affect leak point pressure measurements. Catheter size and infusion rates need to be standardized and recorded at the time of the study so as to permit useful interpretation of results and comparative data. The effect of varying catheter size on the measurement of BLPP has been studied.[9] In 23 patients with neurogenic bladders, the BLPP was found to be higher when larger catheters were used. Children, tested with a 10 Fr catheter had higher BLPPs than when tested with a 7 Fr catheter. This difference particularly applied to children of 6 years or less. For children in that age group a 5 Fr catheter or infant feeding tube is more appropriate. In seven patients under 6 years of age, the BLPPs were less than 40 cm H_2O with a 5 Fr catheter and higher than 40 cm H_2O with the 7 Fr or 10 Fr catheters. In the original descriptions of the BLPP a 5 Fr and 8 Fr catheter was used.[2,10]

Infusion related. When a transduced pressure with a known height of a column of water was compared, the correlation between the two measures in centimeters of water was found to deteriorate as infusion rates rose.[9] This particularly applied to the 5 Fr catheter, but with larger catheters there was still a discrepancy at higher infusion rates.

Presence of severe sphincter dysfunction or vesicoureteral reflux. When intrinsic sphincter deficiency is very severe so as not to provide any resistance to detrusor pressure, the detection of abnormal compliance may be difficult. The occlusion of the bladder neck when the urethral sphincter is severely dysfunctional can result in a more accurate determination of compliance.[11] Practically speaking, abnormal compliance in the face of a urethra that does not work is important only when reconstruction is anticipated, since abnormal compliance is not a factor in upper tract deterioration if urethral function is so poor that detrusor pressures cannot reach dangerous levels.

Vesicoureteral reflux, on the other hand, is a very significant cause of misleading compliance testing. If vesicoureteral reflux is known to occur and the determined BLPP or maximum urethral closing pressure is greater than 40 cm H_2O, one can make the reasonable assumption that the vesicoureteral reflux is in fact related to poor bladder compliance. Despite that fact, it may be difficult to accurately measure bladder compliance in the presence of vesicoureteral reflux, since the compliance measured reflects the volume in both the bladder and the ureter. Woodside and Borden[12] described some years ago a technique of balloon occlusion of the ureteral orifices to prevent reflux during testing and thereby permit accurate determination of bladder compliance in that circumstance. When poor compliance is suspected but the BLPP on testing is normal, fluoroscopic urodynamics will demonstrate the presence of vesicoureteral reflux as evidence that bladder compliance is in fact impaired even if bladder pressure is not elevated. In that circumstance, vesicoureteral reflux is likely to be attributable to poor compliance, and treatment to improve compliance ("bladder pressure management") is likely to stop the vesicoureteral reflux.

Abdominal Leak Point Pressures

Evolution

A "stress," or abdominal leak point pressure (ALPP), determines the lowest total bladder pressure at a known volume at which leakage occurs during prompted increases in abdominal pressure.[10] Total bladder pressure is equal to the sum of the detrusor pressure and the abdominal pressure measured in the bladder.

"Stress" leak point pressure was first used to evaluate urethral function vis-à-vis abdominal pressure in children. Subsequently the measurement was applied to the evaluation of stress incontinence in adults.[13]

Critical to understanding why the ALPP is useful in the evaluation of stress incontinence but why, by contrast, a measure such as the maximum urethral pressure is not so useful is an understanding of the difference between the internal intrinsic closing forces and the external sphincter or extrinsic striated urethral sphincter. Three bodies of compelling evidence led to the recognition that the internal sphincter is the primary zone for resistance to abdominal pressure as an expulsive force, that is, the primary zone in the prevention of the condition of stress incontinence. The first was the observation that in myelodysplastic patients the internal sphincter is nonfunctional, whereas the external sphincter usually functions or is even overactive and yet these patients as a group are the most incontinent of any class of patients with neurogenic vesical dysfunction.[14] That incontinence, when subjected to videourodynamic testing, can seem to be the result of both expulsive forces, abdominal pressure and bladder pressure, acting on the urethra. By contrast, spinal cord–injured patients generally maintain normal proximal urethral closing function, and abdominal pressure is not an expulsive force in these patients who develop incontinence related almost exclusively to the lack of control of detrusor pressure as an expulsive force.

The second piece of compelling evidence resulted from the observation of urethral function after sacral rhizotomy in young women with midthoracic spinal cord injuries. This procedure was done to control spasticity and resulted in a decentralized bladder and external urethral sphincter but preservation of the internal sphincter function. In these patients, stress incontinence did not occur, and the urethra continued to resist the expulsive force of abdominal pressure.

In addition, fluoroscopic urodynamic testing provides compelling evidence for the role of the internal sphincter and resistance to abdominal pressure as well as a demonstration of the lack of correlation between the urethral pressure profile parameters, maximum urethral pressure, and functional urethral length and the absolute resistance to abdominal pressure as an expulsive force.[15] This situation is exemplified by the videourodynamic study of patients with incontinence after prostatectomy, especially radical prostatectomy. These individuals demonstrate maximum urethral pressures in the normal range with observable normal volitional closure of the external sphincter. The residual internal sphincter is limited to approximately 1 cm of urethra located between the anastomotic ring, or vesicourethral junction, and the external sphincter or pelvic floor. In these patients, the abdominal pressure required to cause leakage is low to very low despite measurably normal external sphincter function.

Before the development of ALPP testing, internal sphincter function could be evaluated only by use of urethral pressure profilometry. To use urethral pressure profilometry accurately in the very proximal urethra requires very sophisticated urodynamic equipment so that the measurements of pressure reflect the exact segment being recorded. Such measures were used successfully to define urethral dysfunction[16] before the development of the ALPP and are still used by some investigators.[17] By contrast, the ALPP can be reliably performed using simple equipment.[8] The test is simple to do, is reproducible, and quantitates the ability of a given urethra to resist abdominal pressure. As such it provides an accurate means of determining the presence of stress incontinence and response to treatment of that condition.

The ALPP was first validated in 15 incontinent children, 11 of whom had neurogenic vesical dysfunction or extrophy. There was a clear difference between the detrusor pressure required to cause leakage or the BLPP and the abdominal pressure required to cause leakage, that is, the ALPP.[10] The ALPP was then used to evaluate stress incontinence in women,[13] as well as men incontinent after prostatectomy.[18]

In the study of stress-incontinent women[9] the ALPP was correlated with the existing classification system (types I, II, and III) for stress incontinence[17] and to some extent the clinical grade of incontinence. Patients with type I stress incontinence typically had ALPPs of greater than 120 cm H_2O; those with type II had typically greater than 60 and less than 120 cm H_2O (Fig. 13-2); those with type III typically had an ALPP of 0 to 60 cm H_2O (Fig. 13-3). From these data it was clear that there was some incongruity in the relationship between abdominal leak point pressures and the degree of the urethral hypermobility. Although the majority of patients with gross urethral hypermobility had moderately high ALPP, a small group (9 of 86) had a very low ALPP (0 to 60 cm H_2O). These patients appeared to have a combined deficiency of urethral sphincter function, that is, leakage related to both hypermobility and poor closure of the proximal urethra.

This testing thus identified a new subtype of stress incontinence with stress incontinence that consisted of type II urethral hypermobility and some degree of intrinsic sphincter deficiency (Fig. 13-4). This refinement in the classification helps to select appropriate therapy for individual patients. For example, intrinsic sphincter deficiency tends to respond best to a procedure that

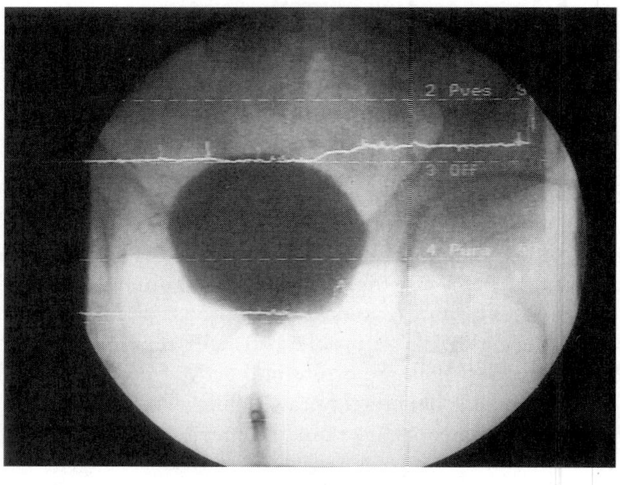

FIG. 13-2 *Cystometrogram demonstrating the abdominal leak point pressure typically associated with type II stress urinary incontinence. A value of 90 cm H_2O in the absence of any significant degree of genital prolapse is evidence that urethral hypermobility and not intrinsic sphincter deficiency is the cause of the incontinence.*

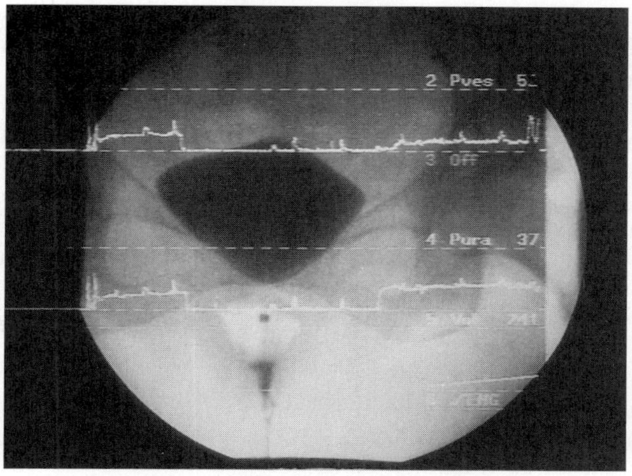

FIG. 13-3 *This 64-year-old woman has an abdominal leak point pressure (ALPP) of 55 cm H_2O with no urethral hypermobility, has an intrinsic sphincter deficiency, and is an ideal candidate for injectable treatment as with collagen.*

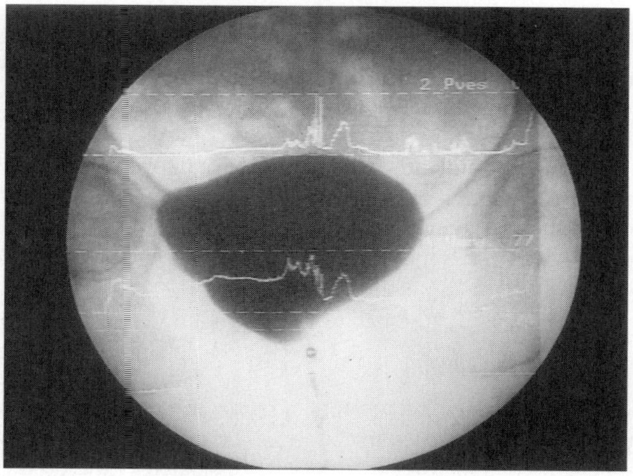

FIG. 13-4 *The combination of urethral hypermobility and intrinsic sphincter deficiency is illustrated by this study. The patient has type II hypermobility with an ALPP of 67 cm H_2O in the presence of a grade II (or III) cystocele.*

closes or coapts the proximal urethra as can be accomplished by an injectable agent, pubovaginal sling, or artificial urinary sphincter. When urethral hypermobility exists alone, a standard urethropexy or suspension procedure will be effective. In those few patients who have both urethral hypermobility and a low ALPP, the most appropriate single therapy is a sling that addresses the problem of both poor closure function and urethral hypermobility, a result that cannot be achieved either by an injectable agent or standard urethral suspension in most instances.

Technique and Interpretation of ALPP

Ideally, the technique should be standardized and done in exactly the same way each time to allow comparison between patients and to make posttreatment studies meaningful. Although very simple methods may be used for ALPP testing, the description here is based on the initial description of the technique.[9] For ALPP determination in adults a 10 Fr triple-lumen urodynamic catheter is used, and in children a 5 Fr or 7 Fr feeding tube or urodynamic catheter respectively. One channel is filled with 20% iodinated contrast solution and is infused at 60 ml/min. Bladder pressures are measured constantly through a nonfilling channel by infusion of 1 ml/min from a pump. Pressures are transduced (as between a P23 Statham transducer with a frequency response of 0.2 sec/100 cm H_2O). Urethral pressures are measured by use of an additional perfusion channel through lateral apertures located 6 cm proximal to the bladder aperture. Both urethral and bladder apertures on the catheter are marked by a radiographic marker. The transducers are zeroed at the level of the pubic symphysis with the flow on and the patient in a supine position. The entire process is visualized fluoroscopically on a screen where a digital pressure readout is instantaneously available. The bladder is filled, and the catheter is manually withdrawn through the proximal urethra until the urethral pressure–sensing aperture rests in the site of maximum urethral pressure or the external sphincter. The catheter is fixed in place in that position.

Compliance checking before determination of ALPP. It is essential when one is performing ALPP testing that the cystometrogram be normal, that is, that no significant increase in detrusor pressure during filling exists. If abnormal bladder compliance occurs during the cystometric part of the procedure, leak point pressure testing will grossly underestimate urethral sphincter efficiency. In other words, the condition of type III stress incontinence exists when intravesical and intraurethral pressures measured in the proximal 1.5 cm of urethra or the urethra superior to the external sphincter in the pelvic diaphragm are isobaric. If bladder compliance is abnormal and detrusor pressure rises with filling, pressures are directed at the internal meatus. At some point, the detrusor pressure rise will result in a situation where the bladder and proximal urethra are isobaric. When that happens, even though the detrusor pressure is the major expulsive force, type III stress incontinence exists solely by virtue of the abnormal change in detrusor pressure. If at this time an elevation in abdominal pressure occurs, a very low ALPP will be recorded. It is therefore important to be certain that the detrusor pressure component during filling is minimal.

When the bladder pressure in response to filling to 200 ml has been normal, the patient, in an upright position, is asked to perform a gradually more vigorous Valsalva maneuver until leakage occurs. The lowest total bladder pressure at which leakage occurs is the ALPP. If the Valsalva maneuver does not by itself generate sufficient abdominal pressure to induce leakage, the next step is to ask the patient to perform a series of coughs and again watch fluoroscopically for the lowest total bladder pressure at which leakage occurs in response to that abdominal pressure excursion. Urethral mobility can be assessed simultaneously. One final step is necessary if patients do not leak with either the Valsalva maneuver or repetitive coughing. The catheter must be removed and the abdominal pressure maneuvers repeated with use of fluoroscopic screening. Occasionally with a rigid urethra or one with a narrow outlet that does not function well as a continence organ, a urodynamic catheter of 10 Fr diameter may be sufficiently large to occlude the urethra and make ALPP testing artificially high.

Although this method utilizes expensive fluoroscopic urodynamic equipment, a much less expensive system could provide most of the same data. An ALPP and compliance testing can easily be performed with any urodynamic system, including a simple manometer.

Pitfalls in ALPP Testing

Genital prolapse. Genital prolapse interferes with the evaluation of urethral function because in cystoceles and other forms of genital prolapse abdominal pressure becomes dissipated in the production of the prolapse. The latter results in a falsely high ALPP, or, despite the best efforts of the examiner and patient, no leakage may occur with coughing or straining.[19] This is analogous to the effect that genital prolapse has on the symptom—stress incontinence—since most patients with very severe degrees of genitourinary prolapse do not complain of urinary stress incontinence, despite the fact that they have either urethral hypermobility or intrinsic sphincter deficiency, or both, in conjunction with the genital prolapse. In one study of 62 women with moderate and large cystoceles, 45 had symptomatic stress incontinence, but a further 13 did not, despite having very clear urodynamic evidence of intrinsic sphincter deficiency or urethral hypermobility. It is therefore important to reevaluate urethral function when the genital prolapse has been reduced.[20] If no leakage occurs with reduction of the genital prolapse, a situation that is not unusual, if the urethra is mobile or any leakage at all is produced through coughing or straining with prolapse, a tentative diagnosis of stress incontinence may be made. The ALPP may be remeasured after reduction of the genital prolapse with a vaginal pack or sponge stick.[20]

Conclusions

Bladder leak point pressure testing involves the determination of the amount of detrusor pressure required to induce leakage in the absence of maneuvers that increase abdominal pressure. That measurement reflects a relationship between bladder outlet resistance and detrusor factors. Although the mechanisms underlying this process are not completely understood, elevated outlet resistance in the face of detrusor expulsive activity seems to trigger the development of poor bladder compliance. In turn, poor compliance results in high storage pressures, which at pressures around 40 cm H_2O result in impaired ureteral delivery of urine into the bladder. This then is associated with the development of upper tract deterioration manifested by ureteral dilatation, vesicoureteral reflux, chronic pyelonephritis, renal scarring, or even end-stage renal failure. Either lowering the outlet resistance or decreasing the bladder pressure improves bladder storage function and upper tract function.

One should keep in mind that some patients may develop upper tract deterioration because of high bladder outlet resistance, elevated bladder outlet resistance, or fixed outlet resistance, though they have extremely severe incontinence related to poor function of the internal sphincter mechanism. Evaluation of incontinence in these patients does indicate that when the internal sphincter is nonfunctional, severe incontinence can result from maneuvers that raise abdominal pressure. Similarly the abdominal leak point pressure represents the ability of the urethra to oppose abdominal pressure as an expulsive force.

Both the abdominal leak point pressure and the bladder leak point pressure act as relatively simple tests for permitting measurement of total bladder pressure at the time of leakage. It is the way that pressure is generated in each instance that gives them their differential value.

References

1. Schafer W: Urodynamic concepts of physiological and pathological bladder outlet function during voiding, *Neurourol Urodyn* 4:161-201, 1985.
2. McGuire EJ, Woodside JR, Borden TA, Weiss RM: Prognostic value of urodynamic testing in myelodysplastic patients, *J Urol* 126:205-209, 1981.
3. Sidi AA, Dykstra DD, Gonzales R: The value of urodynamic testing in the management of neonates with myelodysplasia: a prospective study, *J Urol* 135:90, 1986.
4. Gerianiotis E, Koff SA, Enrile B: The prophylactic use of clean intermittent catheterization in the treatment of infants and young children with myelomeningocele and neurogenic bladder dysfunction, *J Urol* 139:85, 1988.
5. Wang SC, McGuire EJ, Bloom DA: A bladder pressure management system or myelodysplasia: clinical outcome, *J Urol* 140:1499-1502, 1988.
6. Ghoniem GM, Bloom DA, McGuire EJ, Stewart KL: Bladder compliance in meningomyelocele children, *J Urol* 141:1404, 1989.
7. Bloom DA, Knechtel JM, McGuire EJ: Urethral dilation improves bladder compliance in children with myelomeningocele and high leak point pressures, *J Urol* 144:430, 1990.
8. Flood HD, Ritchey ML, Bloom DA, et al: Outcome of reflux in children with myelodysplasia managed by bladder pressure monitoring, *J Urol* 152:1574, 1994.
9. Decter RM, Harster L: Pitfalls in determination of leak point pressure, *J Urol* 148:588-59, 1992.
10. Wan J, McGuire EJ, Bloom DA, Ritchey ML: Stress leak point pressure: a diagnostic tool for incontinent children, *J Urol* 150:700-702, 1993.
11. Woodside JR, McGuire EJ: Technique for detection of detrusor hypertonia in the presence of urethral sphincteric incompetence, *J Urol* 127:740, 1982.
12. Woodside JR, Borden TA: Determination of true intravesical filling pressure in patients with vesicoureteral reflux by Fogarty catheter occlusion of ureters, *J Urol* 127:1149, 1982.
13. McGuire EJ, Fitzpatrick CC, Wan J, et al: Clinical assessment of urethral sphincter function, *J Urol* 150:1452-1454, 1993.
14. McGuire EJ: Myelodysplasia: pathophysiology, applied neuroanatomy and urologic manifestations, *J Pediatr Neurosci* 1:4, 1985.
15. McGuire EJ: Combined radiographic and manometric assessment of urethral sphincter function, *J Urol* 118:632, 1977.
16. McGuire EJ, Lytton B, Kohorn EI, Pepe V: The value of urodynamic testing in stress urinary incontinence, *J Urol* 124:256, 1980.
17. Ghoniem GM, Walters F, Lewis V: The value of the vaginal pack test in large cystoceles, *J Urol* 152:931, 1994.
18. Gudziak MR: Assessment of urethral sphincter function after prostatectomy, *Adv Urol* 8:195, 1995.
19. Usui A, McGuire EJ, O'Connell HE, Aboseif SR: Abdominal leak point pressures in stress incontinence, *J Urol* 153:493A, 1957 (abstract).
20. Gardy M, Kozminski M, DeLancey JO, et al: Stress incontinence and cystoceles, *J Urol* 145:1211, 1991.

Chapter 14

Electromyography in Urodynamics

Mike B. Siroky, Robert J. Krane

The clinical status of the external urethral sphincter is reflected in the electromyographic activity of that sphincter and the perineal floor. The measurement of the electromyographic activity of the perineal floor provides immense clinical information for the physician about the function of the bladder and urethra. Because of the upright posture of humans, an important function of the perineal floor is to support the pelvic organs against the constant force of gravity. While performing this critical function, the muscles of the perineal floor must also act as specialized sphincters for the urinary, genital, and alimentary tracts. Thus the perineal floor muscles play a significant role in the elimination of body wastes, reproduction, and socialization. The role of these important muscle groups in the function of the bladder and urethra are studied by the techniques of electromyography (EMG).

Electrophysiologic Principles

The basic unit of motor function, the *motor unit,* includes the anterior horn cell, its axon, the neuromuscular junction, and the muscle fibers innervated by that neuron[1] (Fig. 14-1). Activation of a motor unit occurs through depolarization of the anterior horn cell resulting in propagation of a nerve action potential along the rapidly conducting myelinated motor axon. On reaching the neuromuscular junction, the action potential causes acetylcholine to be released and subsequent depolarization of the motor end plate in the muscle membrane. This in turn results in propagation of a depolarizing current along the muscle membrane—the motor unit potential.[1] It is this muscle current that is detected during electromyography.

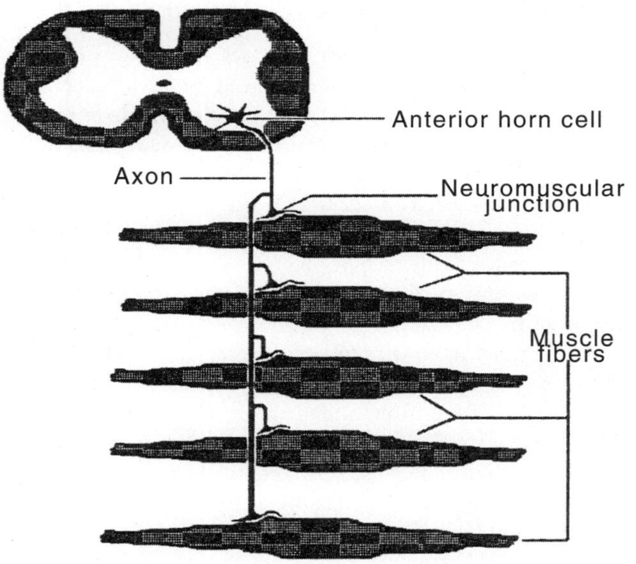

FIG. 14-1 *The motor unit consists of the anterior horn cell, its axon, the neuromuscular junction, and the muscle fibers innervated by that neuron.*

The number of muscle fibers within one motor unit varies according to the function of the muscle group. Muscles requiring fine motor control, such as hand muscles, typically have very few muscle fibers per motor unit. In contrast, muscle groups responsible for maintaining posture such as the back muscles have thousands of muscle fibers per motor unit. The perineal floor is also a sparsely innervated muscle group.

Electromyographic abnormalities may result from lesions in any part of the motor unit. For example, poliomyelitis is characterized by a loss of anterior horn motor cells resulting in wallerian degeneration of the axon and its branches. Similarly, amyotrophic lateral sclerosis affects anterior horn cells while sparing sensation and autonomic neurons. In contrast, Guillain-Barré syndrome is characterized by dysfunction of the nerve axon with temporary or permanent loss of conduction. Myasthenia gravis results from blockade at the neuromuscular junction, whereas a large variety of myopathies may cause muscle weakness or wasting.

Depolarization of muscle causes minute electrical potentials; electromyography is the acquisition, recording, and interpretation of these muscle potentials. Acquisition of these signals requires an electrical conductor (electrode) placed close to the origin of the signal. This may be accomplished either with intramuscular needle electrodes or surface electrodes placed on the skin or mucosa overlying the muscle of interest (Fig. 14-2). Although surface electrodes are easier to place and more comfortable for the patient, they cannot detect individual motor unit potentials. Also, using surface electrodes, one cannot very easily study a specific muscle.

Types of Electrodes

Surface Electrodes

Anal plug. The anal plug, as a type of electrode, records electrical activity from the circumanal striated muscles through the rectal mucosa. The anal plug may induce some artifact, increasing the baseline activity of the perineal floor as the patient attempts to hold the plug within the rectum.

Vaginal surface electrodes. The vaginal surface electrode records perineal floor activity through the vaginal mucosa and provides information similar to that derived from periurethral needle recordings.[2]

Catheter-mounted electrodes. The catheter-mounted electrode, consisting of two concentric rings mounted on a urethral catheter, is designed to detect perineal floor activity through the urethral mucosa. Although this type of electrode has the theoretical advan-

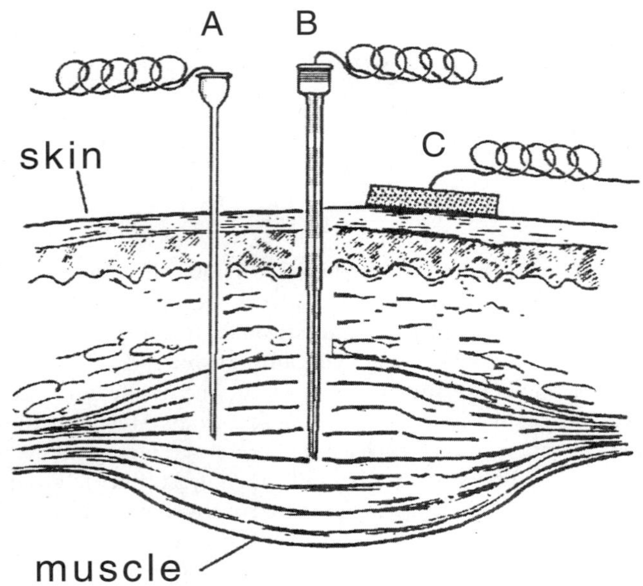

FIG. 14-2 *Diagram of some commonly used electromyograph electrodes.* ***A,*** *Monopolar electrode.* ***B,*** *Concentric needle electrode incorporating a single active electrode and a reference electrode.* ***C,*** *Surface electrode applied to the skin overlying a muscle.*

tage of recording activity from the urethral striated sphincter, in practice it is difficult to be certain which perineal floor muscle is contributing most of the recorded activity. The incidence of artifacts is high. Because of these factors and the fragility of these electrodes, they are little used in urodynamics today.

Skin-patch electrodes. Self-adhesive electrocardiographic (ECG) electrodes used as skin patches have been successfully adapted to urodynamic monitoring. These electrodes provide good surface recordings and have the added advantage of allowing the patient considerable mobility. In contrast to the anal-plug electrode, various muscles in the perineum may be sampled by use of ECG electrodes. These electrodes are very widely used in pediatric urodynamics.

Needle Electrodes

Needle electrodes are manufactured in various configurations. To obtain satisfactory recordings from single motor units, one should have the active tip of the electrode less than 1 mm^2 in area.[3] The duration and especially the amplitude of the recorded potential depend on the configuration and size of the electrode tip. The type of needle electrode selected is simply a matter of convenience and custom for the individual electromyographer, but the type of electrode used to obtain EMG recordings should be described when one is reporting the results of an EMG examination. Although needle electrodes provide excellent recording quality, their disadvantage is that patient mobility must be restricted to prevent their displacement during the examination. This problem is obviated by wire electrodes that can be placed into a muscle through a needle and then taped in place (see below). The problem of restricted patient mobility during electromyography is especially important in pediatric urodynamics and explains the popularity of wire and surface electrodes in children.

Wire electrodes. Wire electrodes are made of insulated, narrow-gauge stainless steel, platinum, or copper wire. The insulation is removed for several millimeters from the tip of the wire, which is then passed through a 25-gauge needle. The needle serves as a cannula to introduce the wire into the muscle and is removed after placement of the wire. The wire electrode is essentially a flexible monopolar electrode. The major advantage of wire electrodes is that they permit a great deal of patient mobility during the urodynamic examination. The major disadvantage is their fragility and the need for a separate reference grounding electrode.

Monopolar electrodes. Monopolar electrodes consist of a thin, solid conductive needle (approximately 30-gauge) coated with an insulating material (usually Teflon) except at its tip. The reference electrode most commonly used is a small metal disk placed on the skin near the muscle being examined. One may use another monopolar needle placed subcutaneously as the reference electrode. Since the active area of the monopolar electrode is extremely small, excellent recordings of muscle potentials are obtained.

Concentric electrodes. Concentric electrodes consist of a single wire cemented inside an outer cannula that serves as a reference ground. The outer cannula and the internal wire electrode are separated by insulating material. The concentric needle electrode has a larger outside diameter (about 22 gauge) than a monopolar electrode has. Concentric needle electrodes exclusively are more convenient than monopolar electrodes in that a separate reference electrode is not required. Also they are durable enough to easily penetrate the perineal skin, which can occasionally be quite tough. At the same time, the concentric electrode is small enough to permit recording from one to three motor units simultaneously.

Comparison of Surface and Needle Electrodes

Although the surface electrode provides an average or composite picture of muscle activity, the needle or wire electrode is influenced primarily by electrical activity within a radius of approximately 0.5 mm from the tip. This permits recording from a few or even a single motor unit. With appropriate electrodes, recordings can even be made from a single muscle fiber. In comparison to surface electrodes, the major advantage of needle or wire electrodes is their ability to record individual motor unit potentials, thus enabling one to assess the integrity of a single motor unit.

At the same time, wire or needle electrodes have several disadvantages, including the requirement of greater technical expertise, patient discomfort, and problems of muscle sampling. Although the small sampling area characteristic of needle electrodes is generally advantageous, sometimes it can be misleading. For example, the motor unit examined by the needle or wire electrode may not be representative of the many motor units making up the muscle. Theoretically this can be overcome by use of multiple needle electrodes distributed throughout the muscle with simultaneous recording. Multiple factors enter into the selection of the appropriate electrode, including the type of information desired (coordination versus innervation), the age and cooperativeness of the patient, and the type of study planned (cystometrogram, videourodynamics study, uroflow study).

TECHNIQUE OF ELECTRODE PLACEMENT

Surface Electrodes

Anal plug. The electrode is lubricated and placed into the anus until satisfactory EMG signals are recorded. The patient is instructed to maintain the electrode in place, but this may be difficult for patients with poor anal tone.

Vaginal electrodes. The vaginal electrode is placed under direct vision using a speculum against the anterior vaginal wall.

Intraurethral electrodes. The electrode-bearing catheter is inserted through the urethra in a manner similar to any urethral catheter. The retention balloon is inflated and pulled snugly against the bladder neck. The electrode rings are situated on the catheter in a way that places them close to the external urethral sphincter. However, because of the variations in anatomy, this proximity is often a problem and leads to poor recording quality.

Skin patch. The skin-patch electrodes are self-adhesive and are placed on the skin overlying the muscle to be studied.[4] They already contain conductive gel. The skin should be shaved and prepared with alcohol to reduce surface resistance.

Needle and Wire Electrodes

In most cases we use the bulbocavernosus muscle in men and the superficial anal sphincter in women as representatives of the perineal floor.[5] These muscles are easily accessible and have sufficient bulk to provide satisfactory EMG recordings. With experience, a single attempt should be sufficient to place the needle tip within the muscle.

The male patient is instructed to raise and abduct one or both legs while in the supine position. The examiner places two fingers over the bulb of the urethra and instructs the patient to "squeeze" or "hold urine." Except in the most obese patients, the contraction of the bulbocavernosus muscle is easily palpable. If one suspects unilateral neurologic lesions (for example, ruptured intervertebral disk or nerve trauma), each side of the bulbocavernosus muscle may be examined separately. This may be done either simultaneously using two needle electrodes or sequentially using one needle.

The needle electrode is passed through the overlying perineal skin and advanced into the bulbocavernosus muscle, aiming for the part of the muscle that surrounds the bulb (Fig. 14-3). In most cases this is minimally painful for the patient who rapidly becomes unaware of the needle's presence. Local anesthesia is not required. Proper needle placement is confirmed by audio and oscilloscopic monitoring. If the needle electrode is properly placed, one hears sharp pops or crackling sounds on the loudspeaker that vary in intensity with muscle contraction. A distant or muffled sound indicates that the needle is near the muscle but not in it and must be either withdrawn or advanced a few millimeters. If the needle is placed too far laterally, one is probably recording from the superficial transverse perineal muscle.

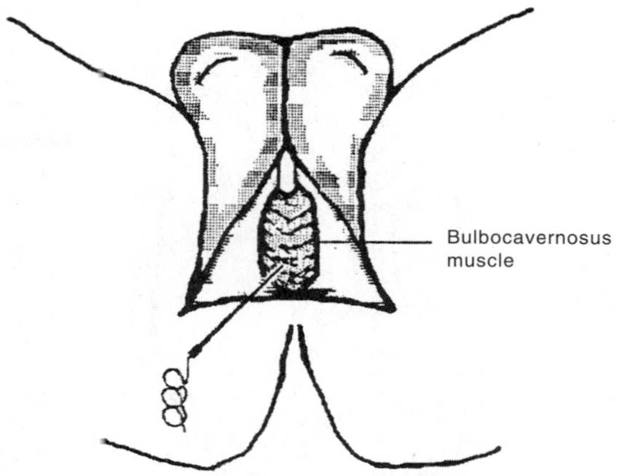

FIG. 14-3 *In men the needle electrode is most conveniently placed in the bulbocavernosus muscle.*

In cases in which it is deemed necessary or desirable to examine the external urethral sphincter in men, the following technique is used.[5,6] Usually the electromyographic needle must be at least 50 mm into this muscle. A finger is placed in the rectum to palpate the apex of the prostate. The needle is placed through the perineal skin just below the bulb of the urethra and advanced toward the apex of the prostate. Again, audio and oscilloscopic monitoring are used to detect the characteristic potentials of striated muscle. Even with the use of fluoroscopy, there is no way to be certain which striated muscle, anatomically speaking, has been entered, since the external urethral sphincter, the deep transverse perineal muscle, and the levator ani all lie close to the prostatic apex.

In women the position used is the same as in men. The superficial anal sphincter lies just below the surface of the circumanal skin, and a 25-mm electrode is adequate (Fig. 14-4). The examiner exposes the mucocutaneous junction and places the tip of the EMG electrode just below the skin surface at the 12 o'clock position. Lateralization is also possible using the superficial anal sphincter. Occasionally, this muscle is difficult to find because of loss of bulk, surgery, or obstetric injury. In such cases, the needle is advanced 1 or 2 cm until striated muscle potentials are observed. This most likely represents activity from levator ani muscle fibers anterior to the rectum.

Electromyography of the external urethral muscle in women is difficult, time consuming, and frequently uncomfortable for the patient. The needle is placed lateral to the urethral meatus (at a 3 or 9 o'clock position) and advanced parallel to the urethra a distance of about 1.5 cm (Fig. 14-4). The external urethral sphincter in women is thinnest at the 12 o'clock position. This is usually quite uncomfortable for the patient.

Recently a new technique has been described using transvaginal placement of the electrode that is much less uncomfortable for the patient and produces satisfactory EMG recordings[7] (Fig. 14-4). The patient is placed in the lateral decubitus position, and the anterior vaginal wall is exposed with a speculum. A needle electrode is placed through the vaginal mucosa lateral to the urethra.

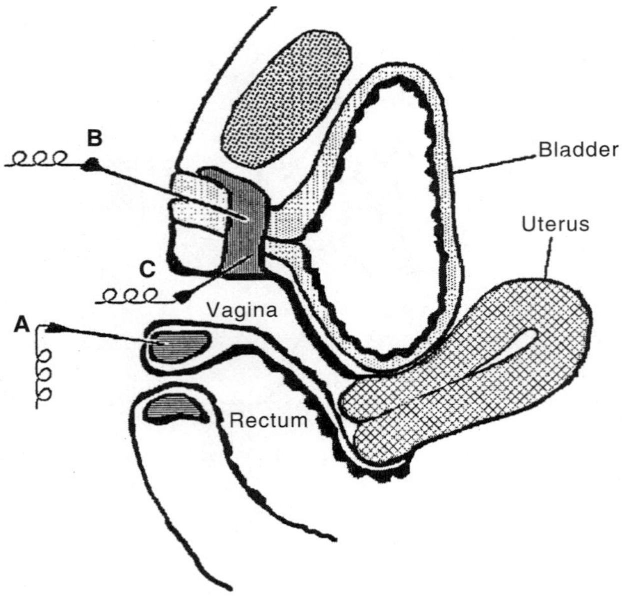

FIG. 14-4 *In women the needle electrode is most conveniently placed in the external anal sphincter,* ***A.*** *Placement in the external urethral is more difficult and time consuming,* ***B.*** *Transvaginal placement in the external urethral sphincter has recently been described,* ***C.***

Sources of Artifact

Elimination of artifacts is probably the greatest continuing problem for the electromyographer. Attention paid to this aspect of the examination will produce considerable dividends in the form of high-quality EMG recordings. An artifact is any recorded electrical potential that does not arise from depolarization of the striated muscle to be studied. In contrast to the electrocardiogram, EMG signals do not arise in a predictable sequence, and this irregularity makes it difficult to distinguish artifacts from true muscle potentials.

Probably the most common source of artifact is 60-cycle line voltage. This arises from electrical devices operating in the EMG room or sometimes from fluorescent lights, transformers, or light dimmers. Even devices that are turned off may be responsible and should be unplugged from the wall receptacle. Another extraneous source of interference is electrosurgical units used in operating rooms. These units cause short bursts of low-frequency interference and usually are picked up when there is a common line supplying both the EMG room and the operating room.

Improper grounding will usually cause a very poor or unreadable EMG recording. The ground plate as well as the skin should be thoroughly cleaned with alcohol before it is applied to the skin. Conductive paste should be used to reduce resistance. The best site for application of the ground plate is over the anterior portion of the iliac bone, since in this location there is little or no muscle immediately beneath the ground plate. If problems persist, a new ground plate and ground wire should be used, since the ground wire may be frayed or broken loose from the ground plate.

Defective insulation, especially in a concentric needle electrode, will cause bizarre artifacts. Problems may also arise from extraneous material, such as old blood, on the needle tip that causes a short circuit between the active electrode and the needle cannula. This problem can be reduced by proper cleaning of the needle electrode before sterilization and can be eliminated by the use of disposable needle electrodes. We now use disposable needle electrodes exclusively. Patient movement will cause a noticeable wandering of the baseline. This is usually not much of a problem in perineal electromyography but may be severe in patients in recording voluntary movement disorders such as Huntington's chorea.

Amplification and Recording

Most commercially available amplifiers are solid-state differential amplifiers with a high-input impedance, a wide-frequency response ranging from 30 to 10,000 hertz (Hz) and high common-mode rejection ratio. A high-frequency response is necessary to record potentials that are very brief (3 to 15 msec). In addition, the amplitude of EMG potentials varies from approximately 20 to 2000 microvolts (μV), a 100-fold range. The output from the amplifier is routed to one or more display devices such as a storage oscilloscope, loudspeaker, analog-to-digital converter, or physical recording device.

Auditory monitoring using a loudspeaker, though distinctly not "high-tech," remains one of the most useful methods of displaying and recognizing EMG activity. EMG potentials as well as many sources of artifact produce sounds that are distinctly recognizable and more useful than the visual display.

In urodynamic studies, the problem is to obtain a simultaneous recording of the EMG, a high-frequency signal, and the cystometrogram or flow rate, both very low-frequency signals, on the same recorder. A heat-writing recorder is the most commonly used method. However, a heat-writing pen usually has a frequency response of less than 60 Hz, which is insufficient to record faithfully single EMG potentials. Furthermore, it is difficult to quantify the degree of activation of the muscle (that is, the firing rate of the motor unit) using a heat-writing recorder.

We have approached this problem by using a memory-storage oscilloscope to record individual potentials permanently on paper. EMG activity may be quantitated by use of a frequency-to-voltage converter that produces an analog signal proportional to the number of potentials. Motor units in the perineum can fire at a rate of up to 40 per second. This maximum rate of firing is set to equal a full-scale deflection of the analog converter. Thus a semiquantitative record of the number of EMG potentials per second is achieved.

This problem has been obviated to a great degree in modern digital recording systems that allow recording of EMG and other signals in computer memory. These digitized signals can be displayed, permanently stored, or analyzed some time after they have been acquired.

Clinical Electromyography

Electromyography is a hybrid clinical tool that falls somewhere between the physical examination and a diagnostic test. For example, either a diagnostic test such as the electrocardiogram (ECG) will show depressed ST segments or it will not. Interpretation of the ECG does not require the examiner to obtain the ECG personally, does not require interaction with the patient, and does not depend on patient cooperation. All of these are required for EMG interpretation. Patient cooperation is extremely important to a successful electromyographic examination. The examiner should be present to ascertain that the patient's "voluntary maximal contraction" is in fact just that. Interaction with the patient is required to ascertain that instructions are fully understood and followed. For all these reasons, the EMG may be considered an extension of the neurologic examination rather than a pure diagnostic test in the usual sense of that word.

Indications for EMG studies in urodynamics include suspected or established peripheral neuropathies, spinal cord injury, lesions or disease, functional voiding disorders, medicolegal cases, and biofeedback therapy. A relative contraindication is coagulopathy or bleeding diatheses. Patients with cardiac valvular disease or prostheses should be considered for prophylactic antibiotics on an individual basis. The patient should be in a comfortable, relaxed position, that is, supine with legs extended. The room temperature should be somewhat warm to prevent involuntary shivering and movement. To reduce patient anxiety, the number of people in the examining room should be kept to a minimum, preferably no more than two.

The electromyographic examination begins immediately on insertion of the needle through the muscle membrane. In normal muscle, this produces an injury potential (insertional activity) that should cease immediately after needle placement (Fig. 14-5). Insertional activity is manifested as clusters of high-frequency discharges lasting several hundred milliseconds on the oscilloscope and as crisp static or pops on the loudspeaker. Persistence of insertional activity indicates membrane instability caused by denervation or myositis.[8] Miniature potentials, firing irregularly and lasting about 3 msec, may be observed if the needle is near the motor end plate (end-plate spikes) and requires moving the needle to another site. End-plate spikes may be difficult to differentiate from fibrillation potentials (see below).

The examiner then proceeds to observe the EMG activity with the muscle at rest. The normal striated muscle should be electrically silent at rest (Fig. 14-6). However, in contrast to skeletal muscles elsewhere in the body, it is difficult for many patients to relax their perineal muscles completely. Thus one typically observes a low level of activity even in relaxed perineal muscle. This low-level activity manifests as motor unit potentials (MUPs) of 100 to 500 μV at a firing rate of less than 10 per second.

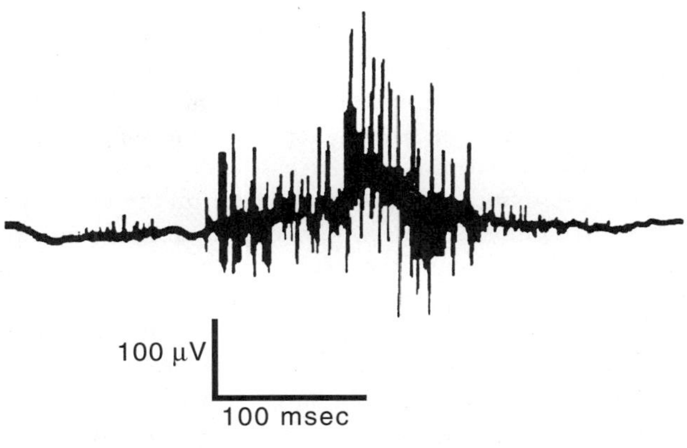

FIG. 14-5 *Burst of electromyographic activity associated with insertion of the needle electrode.*

Spontaneous potentials may be observed at rest, a state that indicates electrical instability of the muscle membrane (Figs. 14-6 and 14-7). *Fibrillation potentials* are small MUPs characterized by low amplitude (50 to 200 μV) and very short duration (1 to 5 msec). The fibrillation potential is probably the most consistent finding in cases of complete or nearly complete denervation. Most authors agree that the fibrillation potential represents spontaneous firing of single muscle fibers that becomes prominent after the loss of innervation, probably because of the denervation supersensitivity to circulating acetylcholine.[9] Although fibrillation potentials are usually present in cases of denervation, there are rare exceptions to this rule. Similarly, fibrillation potentials may be seen in myopathic processes as well as in atrophic muscle. Fibrillation potentials are small, short-duration potentials that fire in a regular pattern of approximately 15 impulses per second. Over the loudspeaker, they simulate a small outboard motor attempting to start.

In denervated muscle, *positive sharp waves* may also be observed (see Figs. 14-6 and 14-7). These are biphasic potentials with a major downward (positive) oscilloscopic deflection measuring 200 to 2000 μV followed by a longer-duration negative wave. Although the exact mechanism producing these potentials is unclear, it is known that they are closely associated with the appearance of fibrillation potentials and have the same significance. Both fibrillation potentials and positive sharp waves appear about 2 weeks following nerve injury.

Spontaneous firing of groups of muscle fibers may also be seen in denervated muscle and are termed *complex repetitive discharges*[10] (Fig. 14-8). These potentials are recognized by their abrupt onset and cessation. Over the loudspeaker they sound like a burst of machine gun fire. *Fasciculation potentials* also represent the firing of groups of muscle fibers in denervated muscle, but their activity is random rather than in bursts characteristic of complex repetitive discharges.

The patient is asked to contract the perineal muscles gradually to a maximum effort. As mentioned above, the maximum firing rate of a perineal muscle motor unit is up to 40 per second. On an oscilloscopic trace lasting 100 msec, therefore, one will observe a maximum of three or four potentials per screen from each motor unit. However, as other motor units in the area of the electrode are recruited, their potentials will overlap and "interfere" with the potentials of the earlier recruited motor units, producing the so-called *interference pattern* (Fig. 14-9). When a normal number of active motor units are present, the screen is filled with potentials, a situation described as a full interference pattern. In contrast, with dropout of motor units, the remaining motor units fire rapidly but are unable to produce a full interference pattern. Good patient cooperation is required for this assessment, since maximum voluntary effort is needed.

Abnormal potentials may be observed during muscle contraction. The normal muscle action potential is biphasic or triphasic with amplitude up to 3000 μV and duration up to 10 msec. One

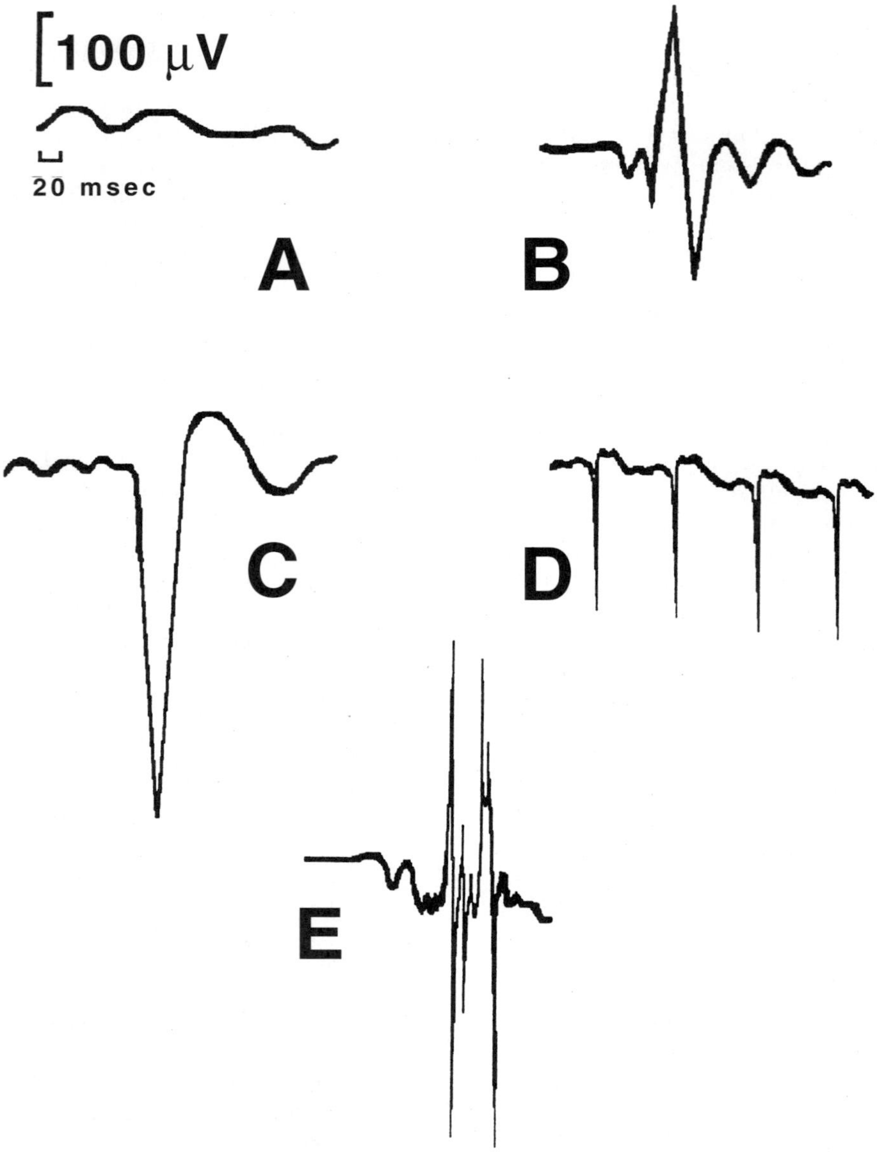

FIG. 14-6 *Representative electromyographic tracings redrawn from original records.* ***A,*** *Normal muscle at rest is nearly isoelectric.* ***B,*** *Normal motor unit potential.* ***C,*** *Positive sharp wave (by convention, a positive potential is displayed as a downward deflection).* ***D,*** *Fibrillation potentials.* ***E,*** *Polyphasic potential.*

may observe that interspersed with the normal potentials, there are larger, longer-duration potentials called *polyphasic potentials.* These potentials are believed to develop from the reinnervation process that occurs after nerve injury and are attributable to the larger number of muscle fibers innervated by the remaining motor units. Polyphasic potentials are defined as any potential with five or more phases. The polyphasic potential is of higher amplitude (up to 5000 μV) and longer duration (up to 25 msec) than the normal potential. The significance of polyphasic potentials is more difficult to assess than that of fibrillation potentials, since normal muscle may reveal polyphasia. It is generally agreed that up to 15% of potentials arising in the normal perineal muscle may be polyphasic. Therefore a significant proportion of potentials must be polyphasic before a diagnosis of neuropathy can be supported.

If the electromyogram thus far has been normal in every respect, the examiner may proceed to perform the rest of the urodynamic testing such as cystometroram, urethral pressure, and flow. However, if significant evidence of neuropathy or denervation is observed, an attempt should be made to assess its localization and distribution. This can be done in two ways. One method is to move the EMG electrode to other perineal muscles, especially the contralateral side. The finding of unilateral disease, for example, would be more consistent with a root lesion than with diabetic neuropathy.

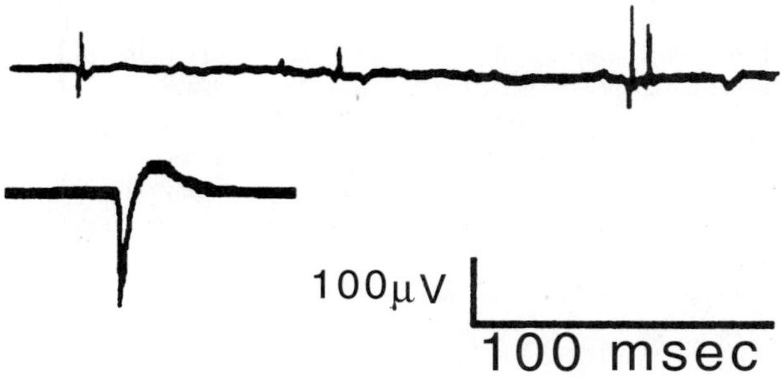

FIG. 14-7 *Spontaneous potentials seen in denervated muscle.* ***A,*** *Fibrillation potentials.* ***B,*** *Positive sharp wave.*

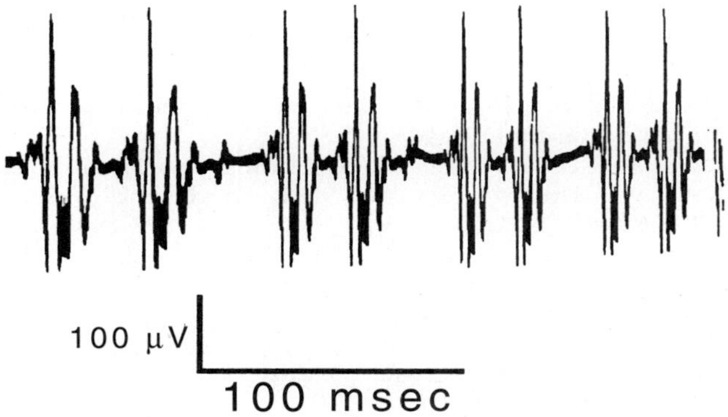

FIG. 14-8 *Complex repetitive discharges recorded in denervated muscle.*

Interpretation

Two kinds of information can be gained from electromyography of the perineal muscles. Sphincter coordination (or lack of it) with detrusor contraction may be considered a form of kinesiology study in which the presence or absence of electrical activity and its pattern are of prime importance. Thus surface, wire, or needle electrodes may be used interchangeably to obtain this kind of information. However, the needle electrode may have some disadvantages in this respect in that it samples only a small area of one muscle and may induce some artifactual contraction caused by discomfort. The second type of information, determination of the integrity of innervation, can be gained only by use of needle electrodes to detect characteristic signs of denervation and their distribution. However, electromyography can rarely provide a specific etiologic diagnosis, since no single finding or group of findings is pathognomonic of a specific disease.

Of all the components of the urodynamic examination, the electromyogram is a diagnostic technique that is most sensitive to operator technique and must be performed by the physician to arrive at a diagnosis. Needle electromyography should not be delegated to a technician, though he or she may be quite experienced or attentive to detail. The findings in electromyography are fleeting and evanescent and must be observed by the physician as they occur.

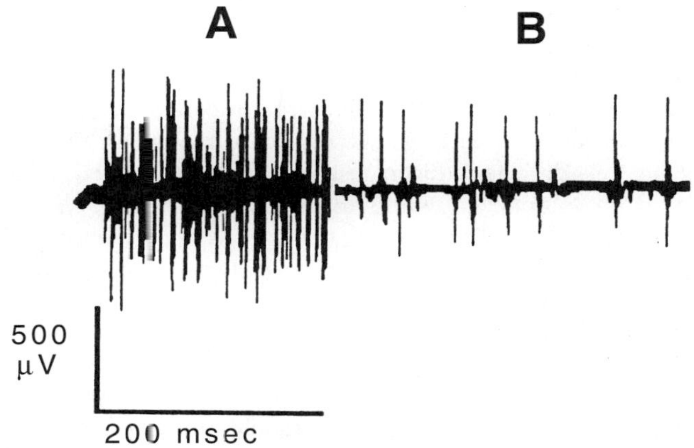

FIG. 14-9 ***A,*** *Full interference in normal muscle on maximum voluntary contraction.* ***B,*** *Interference pattern on maximum voluntary contraction in partially denervated muscle.*

Normal Perineal EMG

As mentioned above, the normal perineal muscle will usually demonstrate some activity even at rest. The normal perineal EMG should show normal biphasic or triphasic potentials without fibrillation potentials or positive sharp waves. With voluntary contraction, reflex activation, or bladder filling, EMG activity increases until a full interference pattern is seen. Some polyphasic potentials may be observed, but these should be distinctly rare. Cessation of EMG activity (electrical silence) should ensue just before the onset of a bladder contraction and should be maintained throughout most of micturition. With the bladder empty, EMG activity of the perineal floor will resume.

Sphincter Neuropathy

The EMG diagnosis of neuropathy relies heavily on signs of reinnervation after physically induced or other types of nerve injury. Thus EMG studies during the first 2 to 6 weeks after injury are likely to be inconclusive. After that time, if the injury or neuropathy is complete, fibrillation potentials and positive sharp waves will be observed in the resting muscle. If the neuropathy is incomplete, reinnervation from surviving neurons can take place, producing the characteristic polyphasic potential. During muscle activation, the interference pattern will be considerably less than full because of neuronal loss. EMG evidence of neuropathy is commonly seen in women because of vaginal childbirth. One recent report found electromyographic evidence of reinnervation of the perineal floor in 80% of women after their first delivery.[11] Those with longer labor and heavier babies showed more evidence of nerve damage. Others have reported abnormal EMG findings in women with stress incontinence.[12]

Lesions Above the Conus Medullaris

The most prominent feature is the presence of vesicosphincter dyssynergia (VSD), which is typically found in cases of complete spinal cord transection.[13-15] VSD is characterized by the presence or persistence of involuntary EMG activity during detrusor contraction (Fig. 14-10). Thus two conditions must be present to support the diagnosis of VSD; that is, a true detrusor contraction must occur, and the EMG activity must be involuntary. It is sometimes difficult to distinguish involuntary sphincteric activity from voluntary attempts to inhibit micturition, but it is essential to do so. The only way to do this is to encourage complete patient relaxation and observe whether the EMG activity can be suppressed. The second consideration is to differentiate true bladder contractions from abdominal straining. This is easily accomplished with intra-abdominal pressure recording to obtain detrusor pressure. In theory, the presence of a spinal cord lesion above the conus medullaris should not affect other features of the peripheral EMG. However, for reasons that are not understood, findings suggestive of peripheral neuropathy (such as polyphasic potentials) have been described in the peripheral EMG of patients with complete quadriplegia. In patients with suprapontine neurologic disease, the EMG is usually completely normal, though voluntary control of the perineum may be diminished. An example of this is the lack of voluntary sphincter control that occurs in parkinsonism.[16]

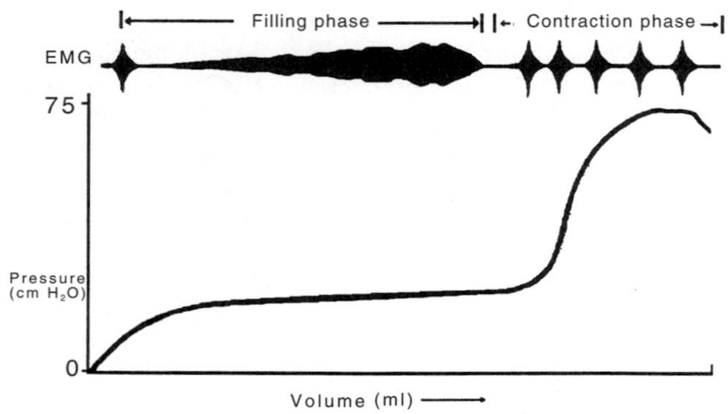

FIG. 14-10 *Diagram showing relationship between perineal floor electromyogram (EMG)* (top) *and cystometrogram* (bottom) *in a patient with vesicosphincter dyssynergia.*

REFERENCES

1. Buchthal F, Guld C, Rosenfalck P: The origin of the motor unit potential, *Acta Physiol Scand* 31(suppl. 114), 1954.
2. Lose G, Tanko A, Colstrup H, Andersen JT: Urethral sphincter electromyography with vaginal surface electrodes: a comparison with sphincter electromyography recorded via periurethral coaxial, anal sphincter needle and perianal surface electrodes, *J Urol* 133:815, 1985.
3. Goodgold S, Eberstein A: *Electrodiagnosis of neuromuscular disease,* ed 2, Baltimore, 1977, Williams & Wilkins.
4. Barrett DM: Disposable (infant) surface electrocardiogram electrodes in urodynamics: a simultaneous comparative study of electrodes, *J Urol* 124:663, 1980.
5. Siroky MB: Electromyography of the perineal striated muscles. In Krane RJ, Siroky MB, editors: *Clinical neuro-urology,* ed 2, Boston, 1990, Little, Brown.
6. Blaivas JG, Labib B, Bauer SB, Retik AB: A new approach to electromyography of the external urethral sphincter, *J Urol* 117:773, 1977.
7. Lowe, EM, Fowler CJ, Osborne JL, DeLancey JOL: Improved method for needle electromyography of the urethral sphincter in women, *Neurourol Urodyn* 13:29, 1994.
8. Weichers DO, Stow R, Johnson EW: Electromyographic insertional activity mechanically provoked in biceps brachii, *Arch Phys Med Rehab* 58:573, 1977.
9. Brumback RA, Bertorini TE, Engel WEK, et al: The effect of pharmacologic acetylcholine receptor on fibrillation and myotonia in rat skeletal muscle, *Arch Neurol* 35:8, 1978.
10. Dyro FM, Bauer SB, Hallet M, Koshbin S: Complex repetitive discharges in the external urethral sphincter in a pediatric population, *Neurourol Urodyn* 2:39, 1983.
11. Allen RE, Hosker GL, Smith AR, Warrel DW: Pelvic floor damage and childbirth: a neurophysiological study, *Br J Obstet Gynecol* 97:770, 1990.
12. Butler WJ: Pseudomyotonia of the periurethral striated muscle in women with stress urinary incontinence, *J Urol* 122:838, 1979.
13. Blaivas JG, Sinha HP, Zayed AAH, Labib KB: Detrusor-external sphincter dyssynergia: a detailed EMG study, *J Urol* 125:545, 1981.
14. DiBenedetto M, Yalla SV: Electrodiagnosis of striated urethral sphincter dysfunction, *J Urol* 122:361, 1979.
15. Siroky MB, Krane RJ: Neurologic aspects of detrusor-sphincter dyssynergia, with special reference to the guarding reflex, *J Urol* 127:953, 1982.
16. Staskin DS, Vardi Y, Siroky MB: Post-prostatectomy continence in the Parkinsonian patient: the significance of poor voluntary sphincter control, *J Urol* 140:117, 1988.

Chapter 15 Videourodynamics

Jerry G. Blaivas, Dianne M. Heritz

Videourodynamics refers to the simultaneous measurement and display of urodynamic parameters with radiographic visualization of the lower urinary tract during bladder filling, voiding, and provocative maneuvers to provoke incontinence. When coupled with a history, physical examination, micturition diary, and pad test, this is the most precise diagnostic tool available for evaluating incontinence. In these studies, radiographic contrast is used as the infusant for cystometry, and other urodynamic parameters such as abdominal pressure, urethral pressure, uroflow, and sphincter electromyography are recorded as well.[1] By simultaneously measuring multiple urodynamic variables, one gains a better insight into the underlying pathophysiology.

Moreover, since all variables are visualized simultaneously, one can better appreciate their interrelationships and identify artifacts with ease.

What are the indications for videourodynamics? The indications depend on the clinician's threshold for obtaining the most precise diagnostic information. More accurate information with less artifact can be derived from videourodynamics than by less sophisticated studies, but it is the role of clinical acumen to determine when this is necessary. In patients who complain of urge incontinence, one hardly needs videourodynamics (or even cystometry) to diagnose detrusor instability. But detrusor instability may be attributable to urethral obstruction, and only synchronous detrusor pressure and uroflow studies can diagnose obstruction with any degree of certainty.

In women who complain of stress incontinence and have obvious rotational descent of the urethra and leak urine during cough or a Valsalva maneuver, one hardly needs videourodynamics to diagnose incontinence caused by urethral hypermobility. But urethral hypermobility can and often does coexist with intrinsic sphincter deficiency; this can only be diagnosed with accuracy by measurement leak point pressure. Videourodynamics best evaluates detrusor function. If surgery is contemplated, the surgeon, armed with this information, can advise the patient with impaired or absent detrusor contractility that there is a higher risk for urinary retention, and the subtleties of surgical technique can be appropriately modified.

Men who have gravitational incontinence after radical prostatectomy hardly need videourodynamics to diagnose post-prostatectomy sphincteric incontinence, but many of these patients have a scarred, narrowed anastomotic site and paradoxically have concomitant outlet obstruction; others have concomitant detrusor instability. Only synchronous pressure and flow studies can make these distinctions.

We recommend videourodynamic studies for all these patients, but it makes little sense to do so unless the clinician bases his therapy on the results of the study. For the woman with stress incontinence, videourodynamics is only useful if intrinsic sphincter deficiency is treated differently from urethral hypermobility or if a woman with a strong detrusor is treated differently from a woman with a weak one.

General Guidelines for Videourodynamic Studies

The main purpose of urodynamic evaluation is to clearly document the underlying cause of the patient's complaints and to correlate symptoms with urodynamic findings. To this end, it is essential to understand the nature of the patient's complaints and to use the urodynamic evaluation as a provocative test to mimic those symptoms. The symptoms should be clearly documented before one begins the urodynamic evaluation on the basis of the history, the physical examination, the micturition diary, and, in the case of incontinence, the pad test.

The urodynamic study itself is an interactive process between examiner and patient. The examiner should clearly understand, at the time of the study, whether the patient's symptoms are reproduced, and, if they are, the underlying cause should be determined before completion of the study. The specific techniques for performing urodynamic studies differ according to the age and sex of the patient and the nature of the complaints, but for all patients, before starting the urodynamic study the following information should be known: (1) what symptoms are you trying to reproduce? (2) What is the functional bladder capacity (the usual voided volume based on the voiding diary)? (3) Does the patient usually empty his bladder (based on examinations and measurement of postvoid residual urine)? (4) Is the uroflow normal; that is, is there a likelihood of either urethral obstruction or impaired detrusor contractility? (5) Is urinary incontinence a complaint? If so, the nature of the incontinence and the severity should be determined from a diary, pad test, and exam with a full bladder. (6) Is there a neurologic lesion that could cause detrusor–external sphincter dyssynergia, detrusor hyperreflexia, or detrusor areflexia?

Technique

Videourodynamic studies are performed by infusion of radiopaque contrast into the bladder, usually at a medium fill rate of 50 to 100 ml/min with alterations in the rate based on patient response to filling. A double- or triple-lumen 8 to 10 French-gauge catheter is used to both fill and measure vesical and urethral pressures. Alternatively a two-catheter bi-stem (3 to 5 Fr for measuring pressure and 8 to 12 Fr for bladder filling) can be used. With this technique, the filling catheter is removed for the voiding phase. A rectal catheter is utilized to measure abdominal pressure. The external pressure transducers are zeroed at atmospheric pressure at the level of the pubic symphysis. Electronic subtraction of abdominal pressure from vesical pressure simultaneously displays detrusor pressure. Surface electrodes are applied to the perineum to record sphincter electromyography. Fluoroscopy is utilized to visualize the urinary tract during bladder filling, voiding, and provocative maneuvers such as coughing and straining. During the filling phase of the evaluation, one makes notation of the first sensation of bladder filling, first urge, and severe urge. The presence or absence of involuntary detrusor contractions is noted. At cystometric capacity, the patient is asked to do whatever ordinarily causes the incontinence. For most stress-incontinent patients, a strong cough or Valsalva effort will suffice. During the cough, it is noted either on direct examination or by x-ray whether there is descent of the vesical neck and proximal portion of the urethra associated with urinary leakage. If there is obvious descent, opening of the vesical neck, and urinary leakage, and the leakage ceases immediately after the cough is over, the patient has stress incontinence caused by urethral hypermobility. If during the cough there is opening of the urethra and urinary loss that occurs just during the cough without descent, the patient has intrinsic sphincter deficiency. Some patients have both intrinsic sphincter deficiency and urethral hypermobility; this can be diagnosed only by measurement of leak point pressure.

Stress hyperreflexia occurs when a cough, sneeze, or other straining maneuver induces an involuntary detrusor contraction. Clinically this is manifested either by incontinent flow that persists long after the cough is over or uncontrollable voiding that begins several seconds after the cough. With the urethral catheter in place, the involuntary detrusor contraction is usually obvious on the detrusor pressure channel. If continence is not demonstrated with the urethral catheter in place, it is removed, and the provocative maneuvers are repeated.

In women, the fluoroscopic portion of the videourodynamics is also used for evaluation of bladder contour, degree of cystocele and urethrocele at rest and with straining, the state of the bladder neck at rest and straining (closed, beaked, or open), the presence or absence of vesicoureteral reflux, bladder or urethral diverticula, or a fistula.

For patients with urge and mixed incontinence, it is noted whether the patient is aware of the involuntary detrusor contraction. If aware, can the patient abort it or does incontinence ensue? Not all patients who demonstrate detrusor instability during videourodynamics have symptoms consistent with this condition during their normal activities and, in addition, not all patients with a clinical history of detrusor instability will demonstrate them during urodynamic testing. If detrusor contractions do occur during bladder filling but the patient is unaware of them and there is not any associated incontinence, the diagnosis should be listed as asymptomatic detrusor instability. If the involuntary detrusor contraction is associated with an urge to void or there is urge incontinence and the patient does experience this symptom in his or her day-to-day life, it should be listed as detrusor instability. If the patient complains of urge incontinence but it is not demonstrated during the urodynamic evaluation, we consider that the test has simply failed to document the presence of detrusor instability.

In men with incontinence, the main purpose of videourodynamics is to evaluate the bladder and outlet to determine whether detrusor function is normal and whether there is concomitant urethral obstruction, which often coexists with incontinence.

When one is assessing a patient with a neurologic lesion, the purpose of the urodynamic evaluation is to provide objective documentation of the effect of the neurologic lesion on vesicourethral function, to assess the presence of urologic risk factors, and to document the cause of their symptoms. Urodynamic findings consistent with but not diagnostic of neurologic lesions include (1) absent electrical activity on EMG, (2) detrusor areflexia, (3) detrusor hyperreflexia, and (4) absent or diminished bladder-filling sensations. Findings diagnostic of a neurologic lesion include (1) detrusor–external sphincter dyssynergia and (2) an open vesical neck at rest (radiographic contrast within the urethra in the absence of a detrusor contraction or sudden increase in abdominal pressure) in a patient who has not previously undergone ure-

A

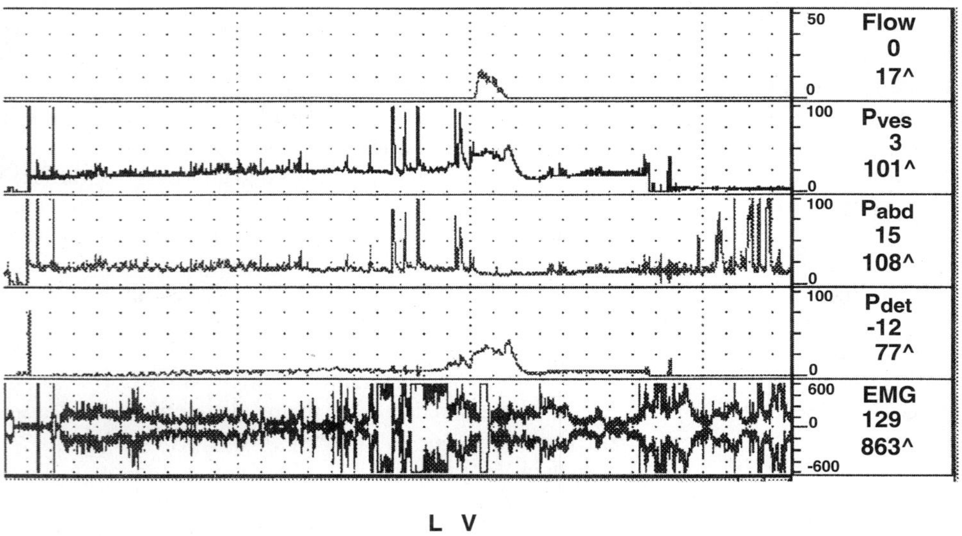

B

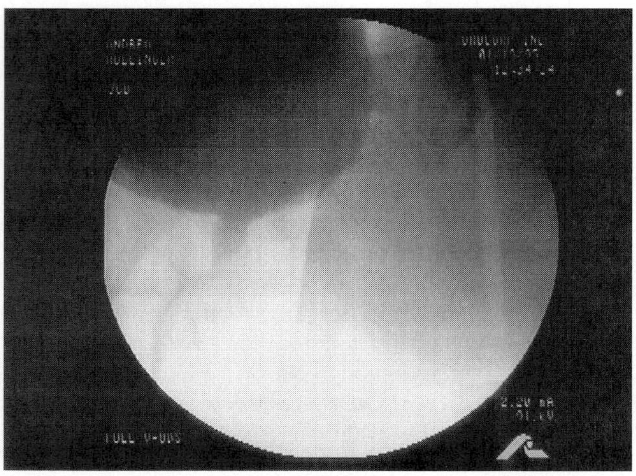

FIG. 15-1 *Videourodynamic study demonstrating stress incontinence caused by urethral hypermobility. The patient is a 41-year-old woman 2 years with no change in condition after repair of posthysterectomy vesicovaginal fistula who complains of stress incontinence.* ***A,*** *Urodynamic tracing. She has urinary leakage of a few drops at point L (she does not lose enough urine to activate the flowmeter). The leak point pressure is 100 cm H_2O. At point V, she voids with a detrusor contraction to 30 cm H_2O and a Q_{max} of 14 ml/sec.* ***B,*** *X-ray film obtained at L showing urethral hypermobility and stress incontinence.*

thral surgery. Urologic risk factors include (1) detrusor–external sphincter dyssynergia, (2) low bladder compliance, and (3) sustained high-magnitude detrusor contractions.

VIDEOURODYNAMIC EVALUATION OF URINARY INCONTINENCE IN WOMEN

Urinary incontinence in women may be caused by sphincteric abnormalities, detrusor instability, or extraurethral causes such as fistula or ectopic ureter. In most patients a clear differentiation can be made on a clinical basis between stress and urge incontinence. However, many patients have both types of incontinence. The purpose of the urodynamic study is to fill the bladder and provoke the incontinence either by bladder filling or by coughing and straining and so forth. If the nature of the patient's complaint is unclear, it is often possible to reproduce the incontinence during the urodynamic study and then simply ask the patient whether that is what happens to her during daily activities.

Stress incontinence has three major causes; urethral hypermobility, intrinsic sphincter deficiency, and stress hyperreflexia. Some patients have two or even all three causes. In urethral hypermobility there is rotational descent of the vesical neck and proximal part of the urethra, opening of the urethra, and occurrence of incontinence at a relatively high leak point pressure (Fig. 15-1). Patients with intrinsic sphincter deficiency usually have a low leak point pressure and often have an open vesical neck at rest (Fig. 15-2). Women with urethral hypermobility who have a low leak point pressure are considered to have both conditions. Stress hyper-

A

B

C

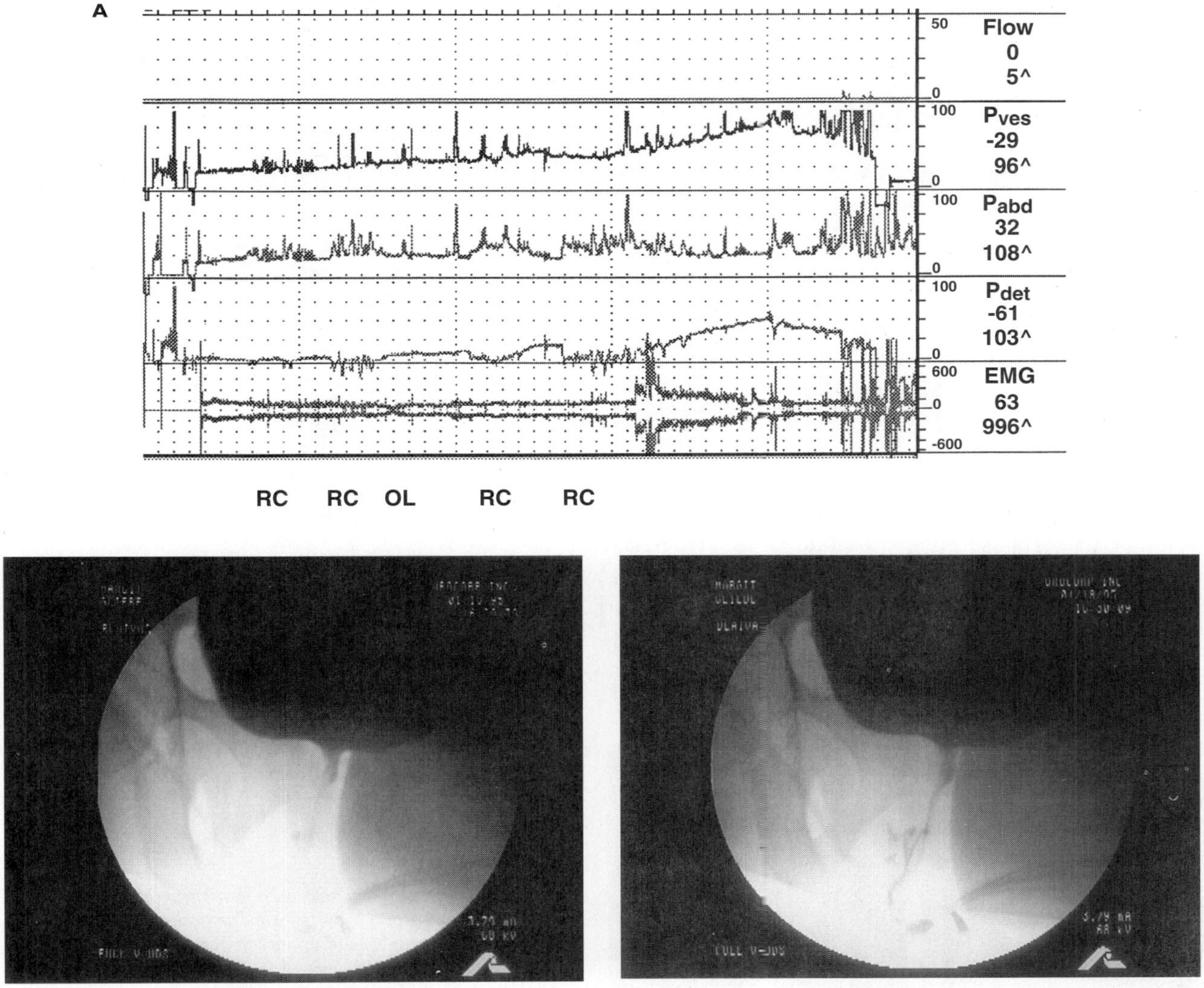

FIG. 15-2 *Videourodynamic view demonstrating intrinsic sphincter deficiency and low bladder compliance. The patient is a 50-year-old woman with no change in condition 2 years after radical hysterectomy and radiation therapy for carcinoma of the cervix.* ***A,*** *Low bladder compliance is evident on the cystometric tracing (P_{ves}) as a steep rise in pressure that reaches nearly 100 cm H_2O at a bladder capacity of 405 ml. Spontaneous rectal contractions (RC) cause an artifactual decrease in detrusor pressure (P_{det}). Intrinsic sphincter deficiency is diagnosed by the open bladder neck and proximal urethra at rest (point O) and the low Valsalva-strain leak point pressure (50 cm H_2O) at point L.* ***B,*** *X-ray view obtained at point O demonstrates an open vesicle neck at rest.* ***C,*** *X-ray view obtained at point L demonstrates sphincteric incontinence with a leak point pressure of 50 cm H_2O.*

reflexia is characterized by involuntary detrusor contractions precipitated by a sudden increase in abdominal pressure (Fig. 15-3).

Detrusor instability may be idiopathic or neurogenic or may be caused by bladder inflammation or urethral obstruction (Fig. 15-4). Once it has been determined that there are involuntary detrusor contractions, it is important to assess the degree of the patient's awareness, concern, and control. At the time of the first involuntary detrusor contraction, it should be determined whether the patient is aware of the contraction and whether she can contract the sphincter, interrupt the stream, and prevent incontinence by aborting the detrusor contraction.

Videourodynamic Evaluation of Incontinence in Men

Urinary incontinence in men may be caused by either involuntary detrusor contractions or intrinsic sphincter deficiency. Involuntary detrusor contractions may be idiopathic, caused by

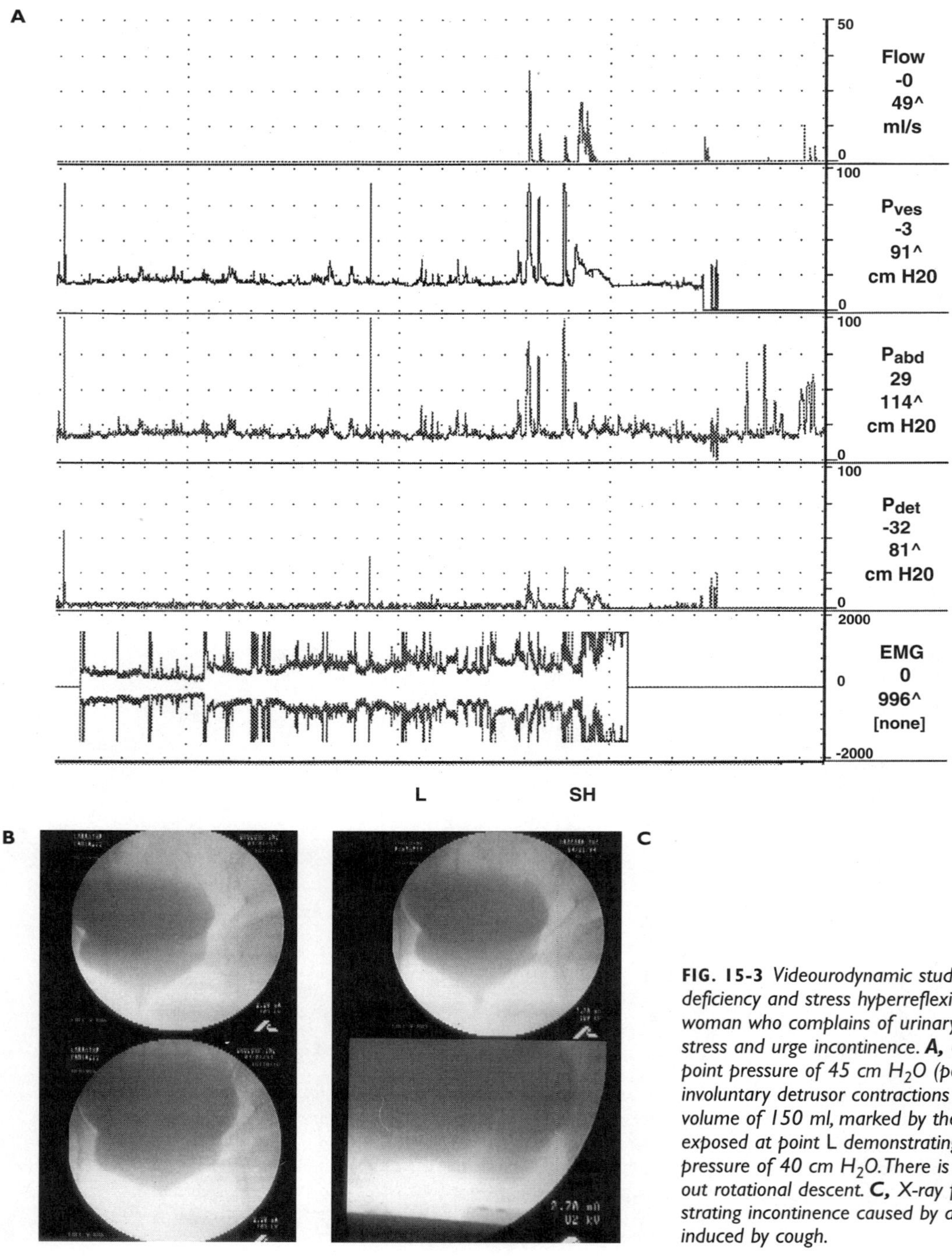

FIG. 15-3 *Videourodynamic study demonstrating intrinsic sphincter deficiency and stress hyperreflexia. The patient is a 70-year-old woman who complains of urinary frequency, urgency, and both stress and urge incontinence.* ***A,*** *Urodynamic tracing shows a leak point pressure of 45 cm H_2O (point L) and several stress-induced involuntary detrusor contractions (stress hyperreflexia) at a bladder volume of 150 ml, marked by the notation SH.* ***B,*** *X-ray film exposed at point L demonstrating urinary leakage at a leak point pressure of 40 cm H_2O. There is opening of the vesicle neck without rotational descent.* ***C,*** *X-ray film exposed at point SH demonstrating incontinence caused by an involuntary detrusor contraction induced by cough.*

A

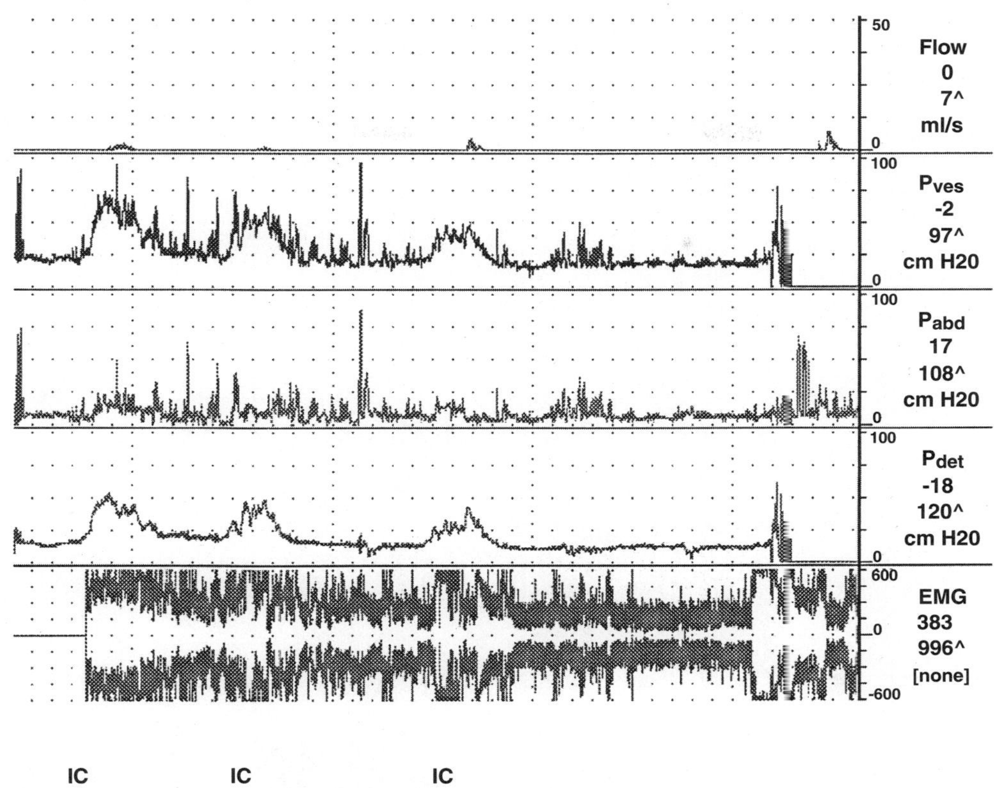

B

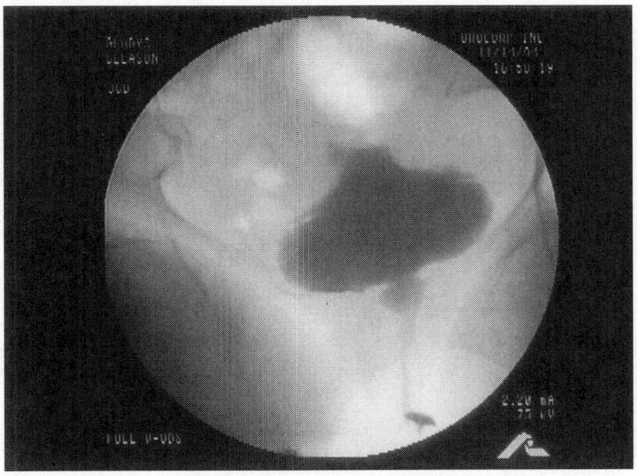

FIG. 15-4 *Videourodynamic study of a 74-year-old woman who complains of urinary frequency, urgency, and urge incontinence.* ***A,*** *Urodynamic tracing shows multiple involuntary detrusor contractions (IC). She contracts her sphincter in an attempt to abort them but is unsuccessful.* ***B,*** *X-ray film obtained during one of the involuntary detrusor contractions shows obstruction by the voluntary sphincter contraction.*

urethral obstruction or caused by neurologic conditions such as spinal cord injury, multiple sclerosis, and stroke. In addition, there may be low bladder compliance from long-standing benign prostatic hypertrophy (BPH) or neurologic conditions.

The most common cause of detrusor instability in men is BPH, but not all men with BPH have prostatic obstruction. Bladder outlet obstruction is defined by measurement of a detrusor contraction of adequate magnitude (pressure) and duration and a diminished uroflow.[2,3] Approximately two thirds of men with BPH have detrusor instability (Fig. 15-5), but detrusor instability may also occur without obstruction in men with BPH (see Fig. 15-7). Impaired detrusor contractility is characterized by a weak or poorly sustained detrusor contraction and a low flow (Fig. 15-6). Uroflow without synchronous measurement of detrusor pressure cannot allow one to distinguish between urethral obstruction, impaired detrusor contractility, and the normal state.[4]

Sphincteric incontinence is most commonly seen after radical prostatectomy (Fig. 15-7), but is occasionally encountered

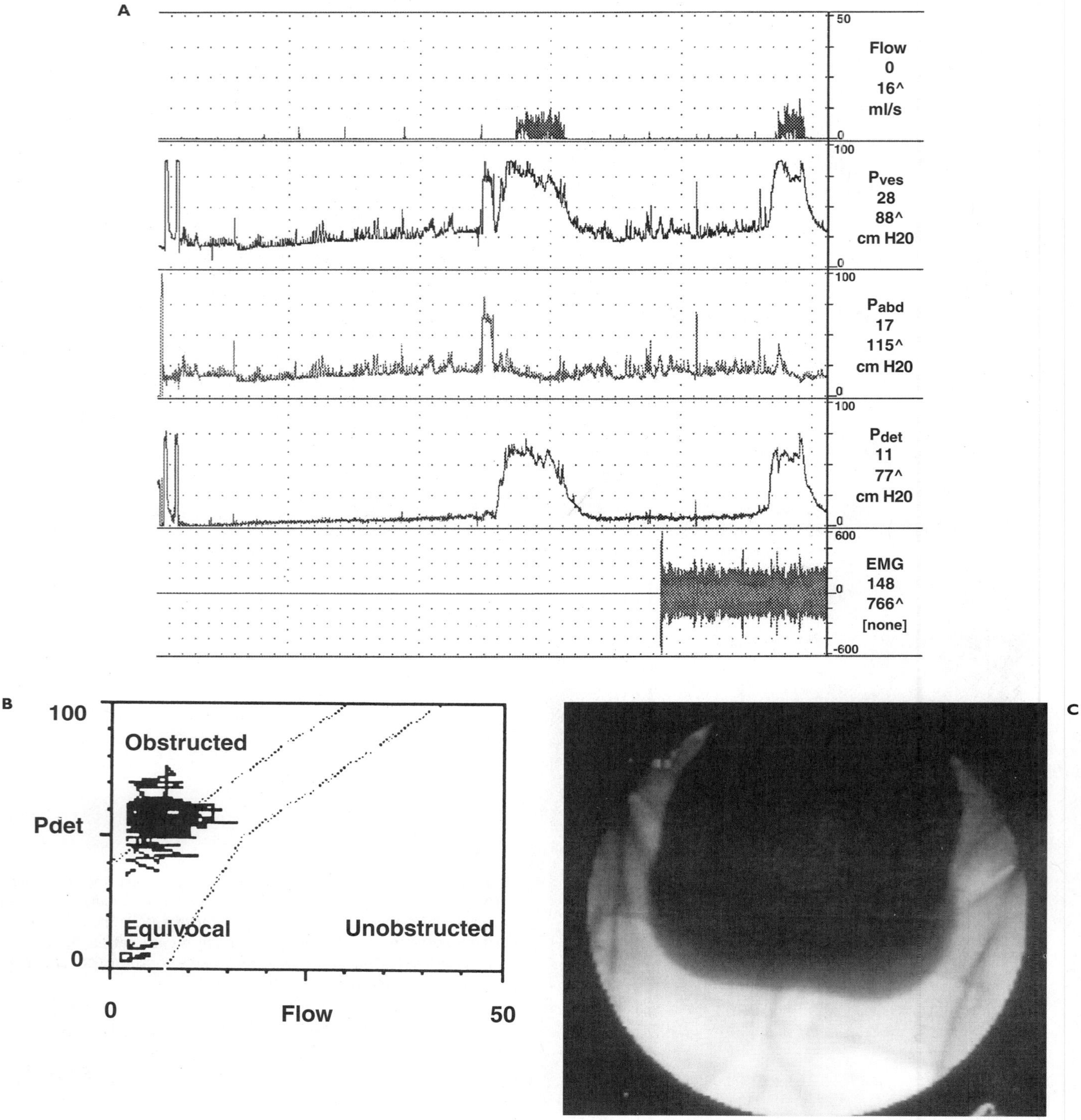

FIG. 15-5 *Videourodynamic study demonstrating urinary incontinence caused by detrusor instability in a 77-year-old white man with mild prostatic obstruction. He complains of urinary frequency, urgency, and urge incontinence. On examination, the prostate is 40 g in size and benign feeling.* ***A,*** *Urodynamic tracing demonstrates an involuntary detrusor contraction at a bladder volume of 300 ml to 60 cm H_2O (at the point marked IC). He voided about 230 ml with a Q_{max} = 10 ml/sec. He was refilled, and another involuntary detrusor contraction (IC) caused incontinence despite his attempts to inhibit micturition by contracting his sphincter (notice increased EMG activity).* ***B,*** *Pressure versus flow plot confirming urethral obstruction.* ***C,*** *X-ray film exposed at the first involuntary detrusor contraction showing a narrow prostatic urethra.*

after transurethral prostatectomy. Neurogenic causes include abdominoperineal resection of the rectum, myelodysplasia, anterior spinal artery syndrome, and Shy-Drager syndrome.

Videourodynamic Evaluation of Neurogenic Bladder

In patients with neurologic lesions the purpose of urodynamic evaluation is to (1) determine the cause of the symptoms, (2) provide objective documentation of the effect of the neurologic lesion on vesicourethral function, (3) confirm that the voiding dysfunction is caused by the neurologic lesion, and (4) assess for the presence of urodynamic risk factors. These risk factors include (1) detrusor–external sphincter dyssynergia (Fig. 15-8), low bladder compliance (see Figs. 15-2 and 15-3), and sustained high-magnitude detrusor contractions. Without effective therapy, patients with these risk factors have up to an 85% chance of developing hydronephrosis, vesicoureteral reflux, or urosepsis within 5 years.

A

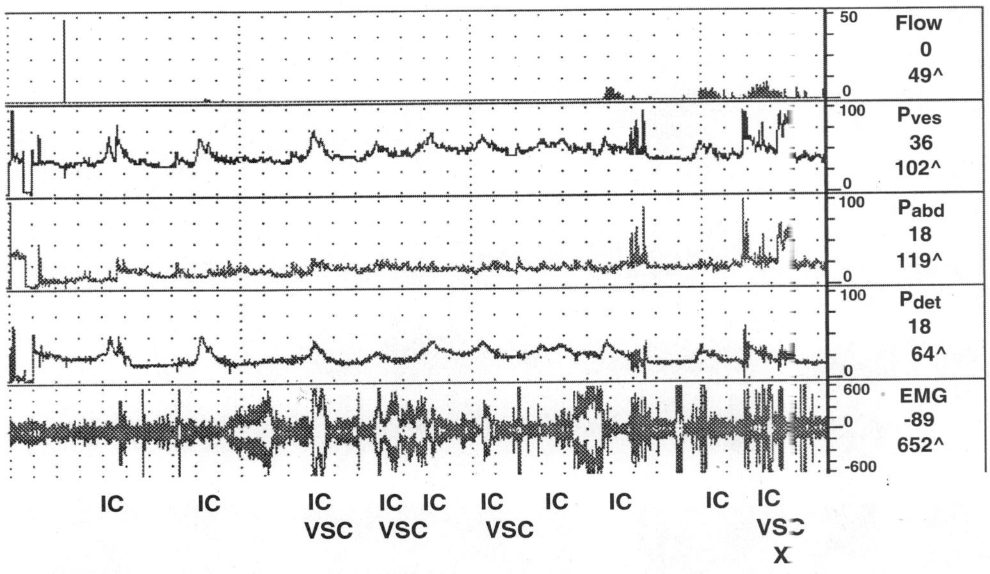

B

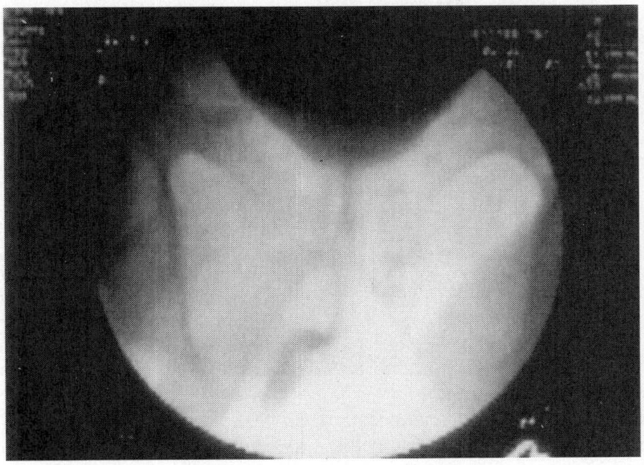

FIG. 15-6 *Videourodynamic study demonstrating detrusor instability and impaired detrusor contractility in a 51-year-old man with prostatism.* ***A,*** *Urodynamic tracing demonstrates multiple low-magnitude involuntary detrusor contractions (IC). Uroflow is low because of a combination of factors including weak, poorly sustained detrusor contractions, low voided volumes, and, on some occasions, voluntary sphincter contractions (VSC) in an attempt to inhibit micturition.* ***B,*** *X-ray film exposed at point marked X demonstrates a narrowed prostatic and membranous urethra.*

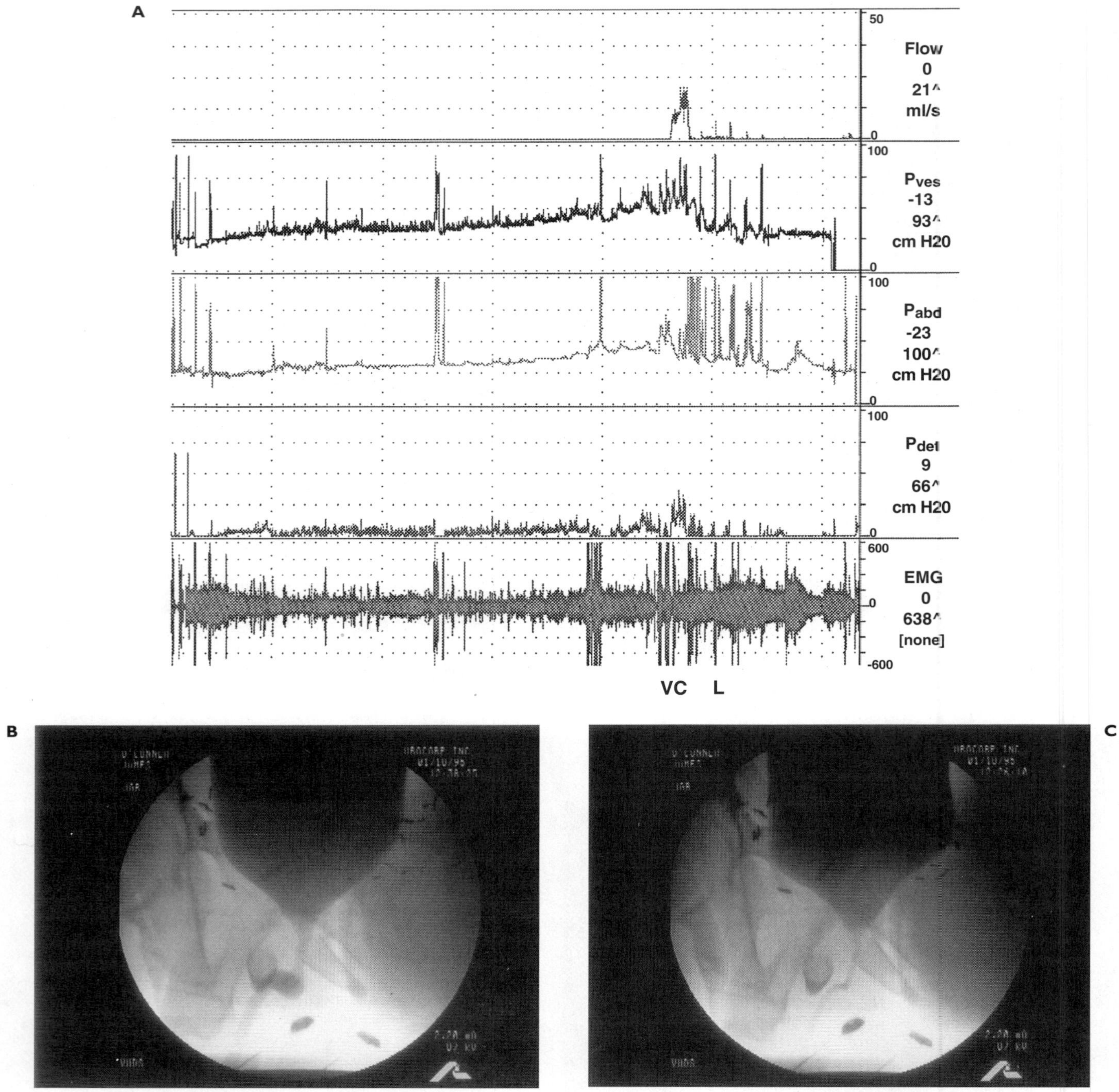

FIG. 15-7 *Videourodynamic study demonstrating postprostatectomy sphincteric incontinence in a 65-year-old man with no change in condition 3 years after radical prostatectomy. He describes a constant urinary leakage, and a 24-hour pad test showed 93 ml of urine loss.* ***A,*** *Urodynamic tracing showed that he voided with abdominal straining and a detrusor contraction of 25 ml and uroflow of 19 ml/sec at the point marked VC. The bladder was refilled to 200 and the leak point pressure was 26 ml at the points marked L.* ***B,*** *X-ray film exposed during the voluntary detrusor contraction showing unobstructed micturition at point VC.* ***C,*** *X-ray film exposed during incontinence at point L.*

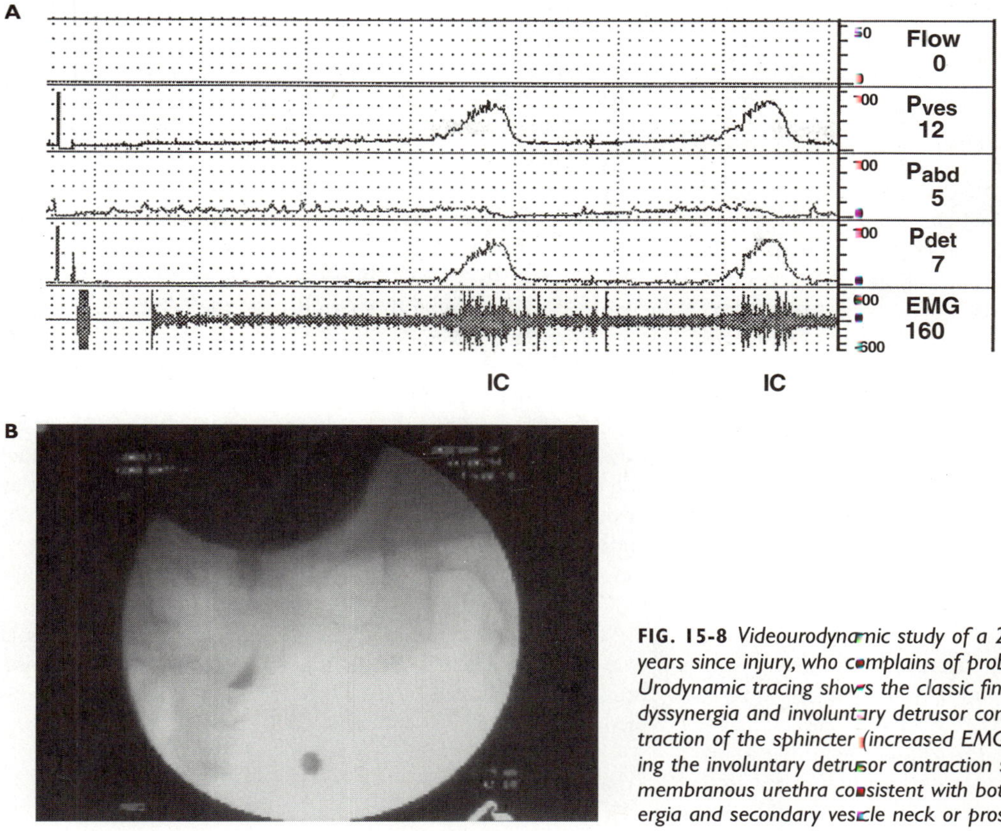

FIG. 15-8 *Videourodynamic study of a 25-year-old quadriplegic (C5-6) man, 5 years since injury, who complains of problematic autonomic dysreflexia.* ***A,*** *Urodynamic tracing shows the classic findings of detrusor–external sphincter dyssynergia and involuntary detrusor contractions (IC) accompanied by contraction of the sphincter (increased EMG activity).* ***B,*** *X-ray film obtained during the involuntary detrusor contraction showing a narrowed prostatic and membranous urethra consistent with both detrusor–external sphincter dyssynergia and secondary vesicle neck or prostatic obstruction.*

References

1. Blaivas JG: Urodynamic techniques. In Yalla S, McGuire EM, Elbadawi A, Blaivas JG, editors: *Principles and practice of urodynamics and neurourology*, New York, 1988, MacMillan.
2. Abrams PH, Griffiths DJ: The assessment of prostatic obstruction from urodynamic measurements and from residual urine, *Br J Urol* 51:129-34, 1979.
3. Blaivas JG. Multichannel urodynamic studies in men with benign prostatic hyperplasia: indications and interpretation, *Urol Clin North Am* 13:543-551, 1990.
4. Chancellor MB, Blaivas JG, Kaplan SA, Axelrod S: Bladder outlet obstruction versus impaired detrusor contractility: role of uroflow, *J Urol* 145:810, 1991.

Chapter 16 Endoscopic Evaluation

Richard F. Labasky

The endoscopic evaluation of the lower urinary tract is an office procedure that provides an immense amount of diagnostic information to the clinician that is not available by any other examination. Endoscopy of the bladder and urethra is minimally invasive, easy to perform, and safe for the patient. The diagnostic information derived from the endoscopic evaluation of the lower urinary tract is an essential part of the incontinence assessment by the clinician who is able to integrate the endoscopic observations with the clinical history, physical examination, radiographic evaluation, and urodynamic studies. The word *endoscopy* derives from the Greek roots for 'within' and 'examine.' Cystourethroscopy is the endoscopic procedure permitting visual examination of the lumen of the urinary bladder and urethra with a cystourethroscope. Panendoscopy is synonymous with rigid-instrument cystourethroscopy, meaning the total visualization of the urethra and bladder using multiple, angled lenses. Cystourethroscopy today is a minimally invasive, well-tolerated procedure that can be very useful in the evaluation of patients with urinary incontinence.

EQUIPMENT AND TECHNOLOGY

Despite the tremendous advances in endoscopic technology made since the development of the first endoscopes in the nineteenth century, the basic elements of a cystourethroscopic set remain the same: (1) a system to deliver light into the lumen of the urethra or bladder; (2) a system to transmit the image from the lumen to the examiner's eye, or a camera; (3) a fluid-delivery and flow-control system to facilitate visualization; and (4) a sheath system to enclose the light, image, and fluid transmission systems and to provide a channel through which manipulating instruments can be passed (Fig. 16-1). Since visualization quality is dependent on the quality and intensity of the light source, the optical qualities of the endoscope, and the clarity of the irrigating fluid, all technologic developments have been directed toward optimizing these characteristics. Variations in sheath configurations can alter the appearance of the lumen somewhat and patient comfort significantly.

The most significant advances in endoscopy have been improvements in the light delivery and lens systems. To replace the early candle and mirror light sources, electrically heated platinum wires and then incandescent bulbs within the lumen were used. Today, light-delivery systems are based on high-intensity, high-quality light sources (normally using xenon) that use fiberoptic (glass fiber) elements to dependably transmit the light from the source to the endoscope and then to the lumen of the urethra or bladder with little degradation.

Although endoscopy initially was performed under direct vision through a hollow tube, rigid lens systems today are built with alternating glass rods and air spaces along the long axis of the telescope; these varying configurations optimize the clarity of the object's magnified image as it is transmitted to the eyepiece. Different lens angles at the luminal end of the telescope permit several different fixed orientations of the centerline of the angle-of-view from the long axis of the rod, ranging from 0 to 120 degrees; these different lenses can be interchanged without removal of the endoscope from the lumen being examined. The arc of the angle of view varies with the fluid medium through which the object is viewed; it is about 70 degrees in air but somewhat less in the various liquids used to distend the bladder or urethra (Fig. 16-2). The illuminating light-carrying fibers of rigid-rod scopes are on the periphery of the telescopes with the visualizing lens system within the core. If desired, high-resolution cameras can be attached to the eyepiece of any cystourethroscope recording or monitor viewing.

A fluid (water or saline solution) or gas (CO_2) is infused through the cystourethroscope to distend the urethra and bladder and to help clear the visual field of any debris or blood that may be present. Gas provides a wider visual field than liquid, and some endoscopists believe that CO_2 permits a clearer visual image, though it can be irritating to the bladder wall. Urologists generally find the image with water or saline infused from a height of 2 to 3 feet above the bladder to be very adequate and consider a liquid essential to flush debris or blood from the urethra or bladder. Also, unlike gas, liquid can be left in the bladder to help detect stress incontinence when the endoscope is removed.

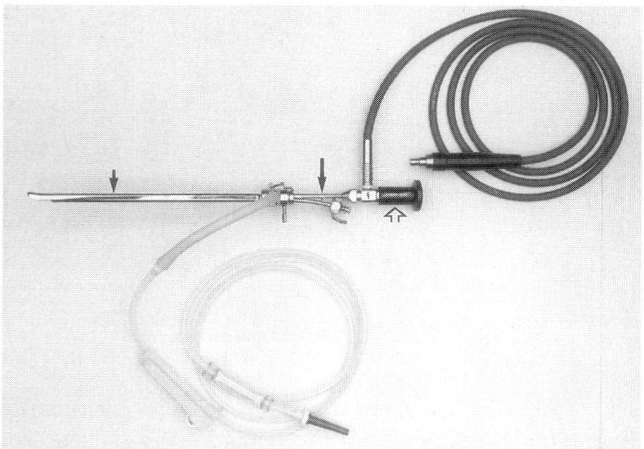

FIG. 16-1 *An assembled rigid cystourethroscopy set with a beak-tipped sheath* (short arrow) *attached to an operating bridge* (long arrow) *that connects the rod lens unit* (open arrow) *to the sheath element. Attached to the sheath is a water tubing with stopcock. Attached to the rod lens unit is a fiberoptic cable to transmit light from the light source to the lens unit.*

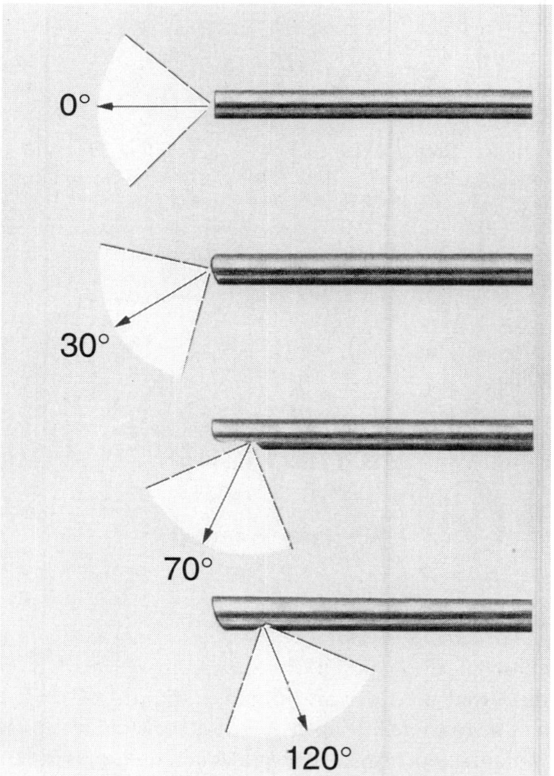

FIG. 16-2 *A diagram showing the center line of the angle of view and the arc of the angle of view for 0-, 30-, 70-, and 120-degree rigid rod lenses.* (Courtesy Karl Storz Endoscopy–America, Inc, Culver City, Calif.)

The rigid cystourethroscope sheath provides protection for the rod lenses and carries the infusion fluid and manipulating instruments for biopsies or foreign-body removal. Different shapes of the sheath tip facilitate different endoscopic procedures. A blunt-end sheath is better than the beaked sheath tip for female urethroscopy because the urethra can be distended immediately in front of the lens by the infusion fluid, and the urethral wall will not be distorted by the sheath during viewing (Fig. 16-3). A piece called a "bridge" connects the rod lenses to the sheath with a watertight connection and has valve adapters to allow attachment and control of the infusion fluid. An operating bridge has one or two other angled side ports, which permit passage of the manipulating instruments. Urologic endoscopes (and most urologic instrumentation and catheters) are sized by the French (Charriere) system. The French (Fr) size is the instrument's diameter times 3, that is, approximately the instrument's circumference. Rigid adult endoscope sheaths range in size from 17 to 25 Fr; rigid pediatric instruments are available in sizes down to 7 Fr.

Using fiberoptic elements to transmit both illuminating light and the image has led to the development of flexible sheath endoscopes. These endoscopes are about 16 Fr in size or smaller. They deflect passively along their length (Fig. 16-4). The lens within the endoscope tip is directed straight ahead (0 degrees), with an arc of the angle of view of about 110 degrees; the lens end can be actively deflected in one plane over a range of about 280 degrees. This easy tip and sheath deflectability and the ability to rotate the instrument 360 degrees allows complete visualization of the bladder and urethra. The object's image is transmitted through many individual glass fibers, and so the eyepiece image is composed of many tiny dots. Initially this image seems indistinct when compared with that of a rigid lens system, but with experience this apparent deficiency becomes insignificant. The flexible scopes contain channels through which manipulating instruments can be passed. Finally the flexibility and the caliber of the flexible scopes reduce patient discomfort versus the rigid cystourethroscopes. Thus these flexible cystourethroscopes blend technical and patient comfort qualities, which make them excellent instruments for urologic endoscopy, equal to rigid instruments.[1]

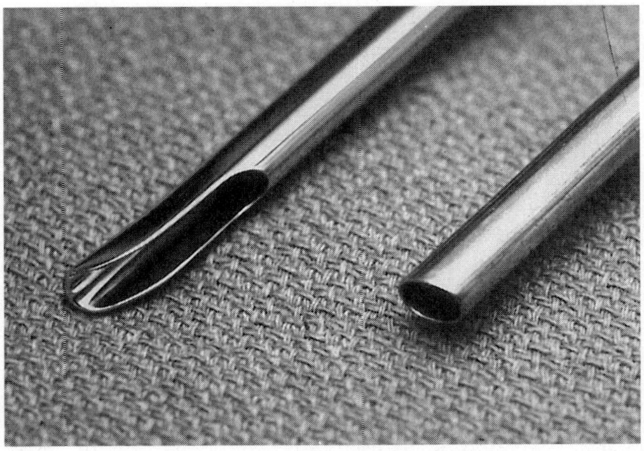

FIG. 16-3 *Blunt and beaked-end cystoscope sheath tips showing the difference in the configuration.*

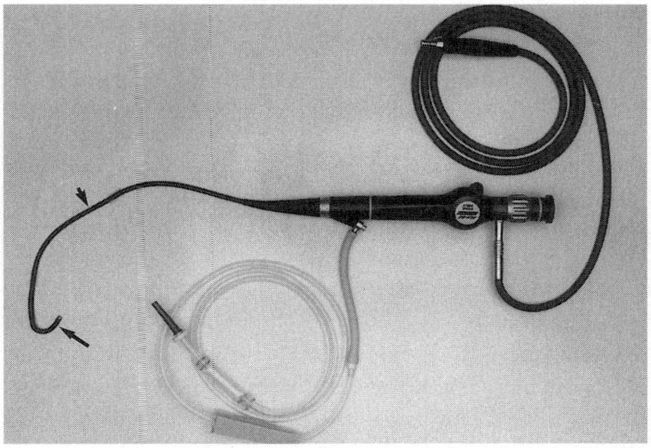

FIG. 16-4 *An assembled flexible cystourethroscopy set. The cystourethroscope is self-contained with a light cable and water tubing attached. Notice the flexible nature of the working portion of the endoscope* (short arrow) *and the lens tip* (long arrow).

Technique

Cystourethroscopy in the evaluation of urinary incontinence is a static and a dynamic assessment of urethral and bladder function. It is obviously static because we examine the lower urinary tract at rest. It is dynamic because we assess the active function of the urethra by asking the patient to voluntarily contract the urethral sphincter and to perform "stress" maneuvers such as coughing or Valsalva maneuvers. It is also dynamic because we assess tissue suppleness and changes from such processes as masses, filling defects, and involuntary contractions as we infuse the bladder and urethra. Successful cystourethroscopy for incontinent patients involves careful patient and physician preparation, thorough examination of the urethra and bladder, and thoughtful correlation of the endoscopic findings with the rest of the patient's evaluation.

Preparation

Cystourethroscopy in the adult is almost always performed with the patient fully awake, with no intravenous medications or anesthetic except, perhaps, intraurethral local anesthetic. Discomfort from an instrument passing through the urethra is most likely caused by tissue stretching. The discomfort is most notable in the periurethral striated sphincter muscles; it is increased by contraction or poor relaxation of these muscles. An anesthetic instilled into the urethral lumen can be absorbed into the urethra's subepithelial plexus and potentially reduce some of the discomfort from urethral tissue stretching. However, an intraurethral anesthetic will not likely block sensation of the striated sphincter muscles, and so the importance of allaying patient anxiety to facilitate pelvic and sphincteric muscle relaxation during cystourethroscopy is obvious.[2,3]

Studies evaluating the benefits of a topical intraurethral anesthetic instilled before cystourethroscopy have reached disparate conclusions because of the variety of types, volumes, and indwelling times of agents studied and the types and sizes of endoscopes used.[2-7] However, several findings are relatively consistent. Adding cocaine to a lidocaine gel lubricant offers no advantage to the lidocaine gel alone.[4] Discomfort levels with rigid endoscopy are higher in men than in women,[2,3] in younger than in older men,[2,4] in women with greater anxiety before the procedure than those with less,[3] and possibly higher in men without prior endoscopy experience than those with such experience.[3,4] Trends of patient and physician assessments of patient discomfort levels correlate,[2-5] but physicians tend to underestimate the levels stated by the patients.[3,5] With flexible endoscopes in men, younger age does not increase patients' discomfort levels. Finally and most importantly, with flexible or rigid endoscopy, double-blinded studies show that anesthetic gels offer no advantage to gel alone for women or for most men.[3,5,6]

Thus to minimize patient discomfort during an office or clinic cystoscopic procedure the following steps are useful:

1. Allay patient anxiety as much as possible before the procedure.
2. Use the smallest rigid endoscope sheath feasible or, preferably, a flexible instrument.
3. Use plain lubricating gel for flexible endoscopy and for rigid endoscopy in women and older men.[3,5,8]
4. Consider using a 2% lidocaine anesthetic gel intraurethrally 5 to 15 minutes before endoscopy for men younger than 55 years of age or for men or women with significant urethral or pelvic scarring or pain, in volumes of 20 ml in men and 11 ml in women.[2,3]
5. Use an anesthetic gel in spinal cord–injured patients at risk for autonomic dysreflexia.[9,10]

Considering that most patients who undergo endoscopy for incontinence are women or older men, one would suppose that flexible or rigid cystourethroscopy with lubricating gel alone would be adequate in the majority of circumstances. If necessary for women who find the endoscopy very painful despite an intraurethral anesthetic, lidocaine anesthetic solution can be injected transvaginally at the bladder base and periurethrally. Intravenous medications or general anesthetics can also be used, but the need for these techniques in the evaluation of incontinence would be extremely rare.

The primary risk of the use of intraurethral anesthetics is systemic absorption, but, although this occurs, systemic levels are far below toxic levels.[2] To minimize the amount of systemic anesthetic absorption, always instill it with low pressure and, if the urethral epithelium is injured, use smaller amounts of anesthetic. Some authors believe that injecting a lubricant with or without an anesthetic before insertion of the cystoscope will induce some inflammatory reaction within the urethra, which could be a misleading sign.[11]

Practice universal body fluid precautions during cystourethroscopy. Such precautions should include eye, mouth, and nose protection to prevent caregivers' contact with urine, blood, or semen, which may contain human immunodeficiency or hepatitis viruses. Obtain a urinalysis to rule out infection before endoscopy, and do not perform a cystourethroscopy in patients who have a significant, active genitourinary tract infection. About 2% of patients contract a urinary tract infection after a sterile cystourethroscopy; a short course of periendoscopic antibiotic therapy may reduce the infection risk.

Inform the patient of the purpose and nature of the cystourethroscopy and obtain consent to proceed. The patient should empty the bladder. If a rigid endoscope is used, place the patient in a dorsal lithotomy position. If a flexible endoscope is used, a male can be in the supine position and a female in a slight frog-leg position. Prep and drape the patient in a sterile fashion, and inject lubricating gel with or without anesthetic in a retrograde fashion into the urethra. Gently apply a clamp to the penis or insert a small cotton-tipped applicator into the female meatus to hold the gel in the urethra.

Examination and Correlation

Insert the cystourethroscope into the urethra as gently as possible. With a rigid lens system, use the smallest sheath possible and a forward-directed lens (one with a 0- to 30-degree viewing angle) to enter the urethra and the bladder. Ask the patient to relax the pelvic floor and sphincter muscles as much as possible to minimize discomfort. Turn the infusion fluid flow on to distend the urethra. Thoroughly examine the entire length of the male urethra and the bladder neck as you move toward the bladder, angling and rotating the scope as necessary. In the female you may find it easier to examine the urethra and bladder neck as you withdraw the instrument from the bladder, using a 0- or 5-degree lens, and the most blunt-tipped sheath available. The blunter sheath provides better water flow for urethral dilatation and does not distort the urethral shape as the beaked sheath tip can. You can facilitate the rarely difficult placement of a rigid scope into the urethra by streamlining the end of the sheath by placing an obturator within it. Calibrate the urethra if obstruction is present to the 17 Fr or smaller scopes.

Stop the fluid infusion, and the urethra should coapt at and distal to the bladder neck in females and the external sphincter in males. Failure of the urethra to coapt or evidence of scarred, pale, nonsupple epithelium may indicate neuromuscular damage, trauma, atrophy, hypoestrogenism, or radiation change. Patients with such changes may have sphincteric dysfunction and stress incontinence; those with notable radiation change, scarring in men, or a short bladder neck– to–external sphincter distance do not fare well with periurethral bulking substances such as collagen[12] (Figs. 16-5 and 16-6). Look for other abnormal urethral findings that only rarely contribute to incontinence such as urethritis, diverticula, foreign bodies; abnormal ducts, polyps, or fronds; and exudate or bleeding.

Turn the water flow on just enough to distend the urethra, and place the sheath tip just proximal to the midurethra area in women and just distal to the external sphincter in men to assess sphincteric closure capability and bladder neck mobility. Failed or sluggish coaptation of the urethra on command or with "stress" maneuvers may correlate with neuromuscular damage, which may be contributing to stress incontinence. In women, "stress"

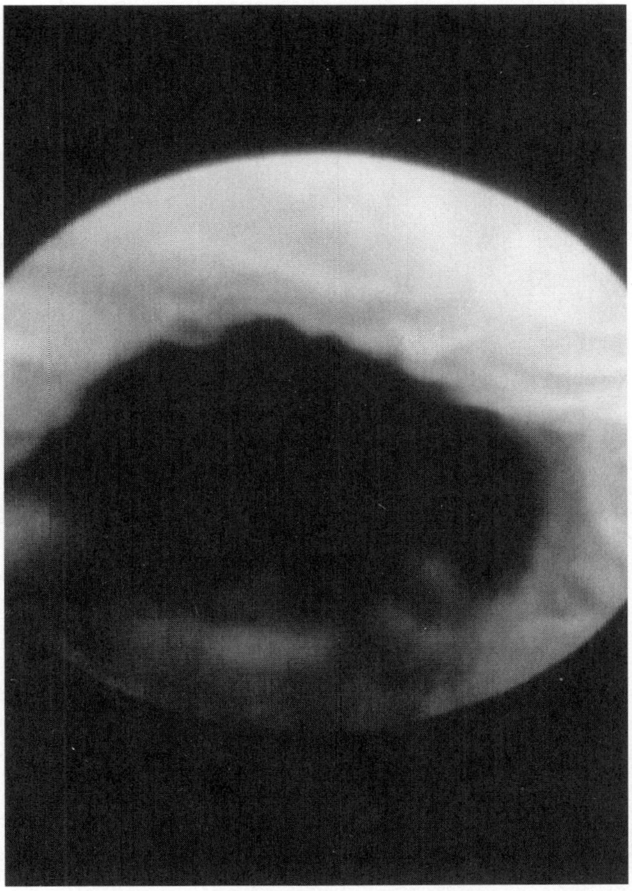

FIG. 16-5 *An open bladder neck at rest with water flow on very slowly. This is a totally nonfunctional sphincter consistent with severe intrinsic sphincteric deficiency. The tissue is relatively supple.*

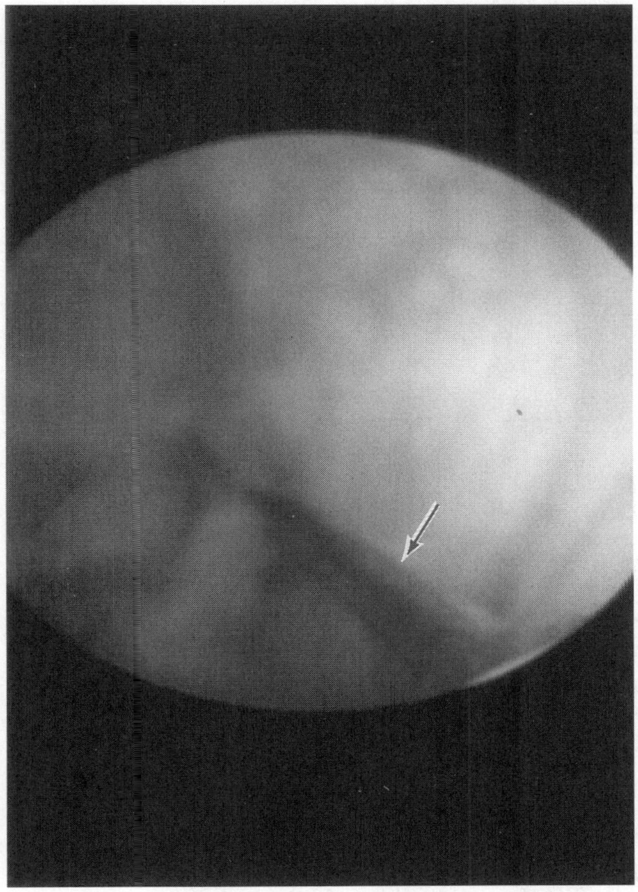

FIG. 16-6 *Same bladder neck and proximal urethra as that in Fig. 15-5. The periurethral tissue has been injected with collagen, which has coapted the epithelium completely.* Arrow, *the needle used in the injection.*

maneuvers that cause descent or opening of the bladder neck and proximal urethra add further but not unique support to the diagnosis of anatomic stress incontinence (Figs. 16-7 and 16-8).

An involuntary contraction may be observed as a funneling and opening of the bladder neck and proximal urethra with the patient at rest and not performing a "stress" maneuver; the patient may simultaneously report bladder fullness, urgency, pain, or voiding. These findings may correlate with urge incontinence from detrusor instability or hyperreflexia.

If a 17 Fr or smaller scope does not pass easily through the bladder neck or urethra, the patient has an anatomically significant bladder neck contracture or urethral stricture. Such fixed obstructions may cause incontinence by inducing detrusor instability or instead may be contributing to some of the patient's passive and stress continence. True urethral stenosis has been found in only 2% of women presenting with symptoms of urge or stress incontinence[13] and can be found during insertion of the endoscope; thus dilatation or routine sounding of the urethra for patients with an incontinence history is unnecessary. Some patients who have undergone surgery for stress incontinence may have an irregular course or high retropubic position to the bladder neck and urethra. These situations deserve careful urodynamic evaluation to rule out obstruction, since endoscopic assessment of obstruction from processes other than fixed stricture or contracture is poor.

After entering the bladder, examine it thoroughly and systematically with 25- or 30-, 70-, and 120-degree lenses, as needed. If the anterior bladder neck region cannot be seen clearly with the rigid rod lenses to rule out suture foreign bodies after prior surgeries and tumors, use a flexible cytourethroscope to perform the examination. Distend the bladder with enough fluid to smooth the bladder epithelium completely. Inspect the entire bladder epithelium, including the interior of any bladder diverticula, for evidence of pallor, squamous metaplasia (a normal finding on the female trigone), mass, tumor, bleeding, foreign body, hyperemia, erythema, edema, disruption, and inflammation. Assess the position of the ureteral orifices, and the urine efflux from the orifices. Notice the degree of bladder-wall trabeculation, usually indicative of detrusor hypertrophy. Although trabeculation does not uniquely correlate with a specific diagnosis, it is sometimes found in patients who have detrusor instability with hyperreflexia or have bladder outlet obstruction. Detrusor instability with hyperreflexia or low compliance might be suspected if the infusion stops because of fluid pressure

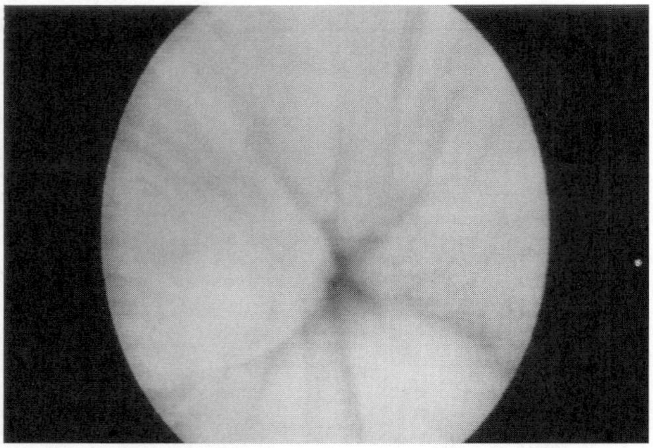

FIG. 16-7 *A normal bladder neck and proximal portion of the urethra in a female viewed from the midurethra with waterflow on enough to distend the urethra slightly. Notice the stellate appearance of the closed bladder neck at rest and the full and supple nature to the normal urethral epithelium.*

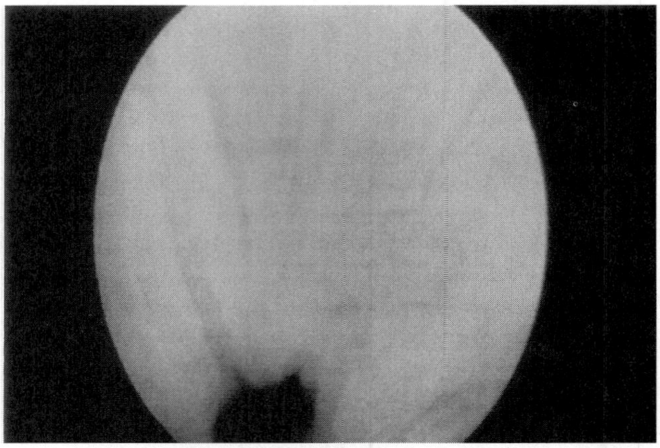

FIG. 16-8 *The same patient and lens position as that in Fig. 16-7 with the patient performing a Valsalva maneuver. Notice that the bladder neck, which had been in the middle of the lens in Fig. 16-7, has shifted to the lower portion of the lens, indicating bladder neck mobility. There is also opening of the bladder neck with straining.*

backup in the bladder; the same bladder problems or sphincteric incompetence might be suspected if the fluid leaks around the sheath at the external meatus. Notice the cystoscopic bladder capacity for comparison with the capacity found with a voiding diary or a cystometrogram. While removing the scope, examine the entire urethra with a forward-directed lens to ensure that no pathosis was missed during the entry urethroscopy, especially in a female. The endoscope can also be used to examine the vagina if ectopic ureters or fistulas are suspected.

The general techniqes of flexible cystourethroscopy are identical to those of the rigid scopes, though no lens changes occur during a single patient examination. Many of the nuances of flexible cystourethroscopy in evaluation of patients with spinal cord injuries is summarized by Rivas and Chancellor.[10] Whatever equipment is used, prevent autonomic dysreflexia in spinal cord–injured patients by preventing bladder overdistension. If dysreflexia occurs, drain the bladder immediately, and start to combat the hypertension with subinguinal nifedipine 10 mg every 5 minutes.[9,10]

At the end of the endoscopy, drain the bladder if a rigid scope sheath is in the bladder, or leave the bladder full if you wish to have the patient perform stress maneuvers before voiding. Voiding after endoscopy may cause some dysuria or hematuria for about 24 hours. If necessary, dysuria can be alleviated by mild analgesics such as phenazopyridine HCl.

Cystourethroscopy may be performed with pressure measurement to obtain simultaneous urodynamic information. This was first suggested by Robertson, who used a rigid urethroscope infusing with CO_2 for women,[14] and was extended to a flexible cystourethroscope with liquid infusate by Belville et al. in patients with neurogenic bladder.[15] The latter concluded that the synchronous technique produced accurate and reproducible pressure tracings with little artifact, combined with good speed, ease, and simplicity. Hadley et al. performed simultaneous flexible cystourethroscopy, cystometry, and retrograde perfusion sphincterometry in the evaluation of men with urinary incontinence.[16] They concluded that most men with findings of stress incontinence could be treated on the basis of information obtained from this simplified, synchronous technique.

Cystourethroscopy can be useful during surgical procedures on or near the bladder or urethra, such as bladder neck suspension, pubovaginal sling, or cystocele repair, to confirm the integrity of the bladder and urethra and patency of the ureters. This examination can be done transurethrally with a rigid or flexible endoscope for a patient thoroughly prepped in lithotomy position, or with a flexible instrument for a supine or a frog-legged patient. With an open abdominal incision, cystoscopy also can be performed when one makes a small cystotomy, inserting the instrument through that incision, and closing the incision once the cystoscopy is completed.

Usefulness and Indications for Endoscopy

With the discussion of cystourethroscopic equipment and technique complete it is now possible to address the question of which patients with urinary incontinence should undergo the procedure. On the basis of their extensive clinical experience some advisors in the general incontinence medical literature recommend that we routinely employ cystourethroscopy in the evaluation of patients with urinary incontinence. These advisors consider the technique useful, helpful, valuable and even essential, though they do not present specific data to support their recommendations.[14,17-22] Other advisors, also basing themselves only on their clinical experience, are less enthusiastic about the usefulness of cystourethroscopy, considering it clearly[23] or possibly[24] helpful only in selected situations. Many authors, including proponents of endoscopy, warn endoscopists that only anatomy and not function can be gleaned from cystourethroscopy[8,18,19,25,26] and that it is unnecessary and wasteful.[27] Many other authors report using endoscopy in their evaluation of incontinent patients but have not stated whether the technique was of value in those evaluations.

Fortunately, some authors have evaluated the usefulness of cystourethroscopy in the evaluation of patients with urinary incontinence more intensively. Aldridge et al. found that patients with complaints of stress incontinence had endoscopic abnormalities indicative of anatomic stress incontinence three times more often than patients with urge incontinence complaints. However, only 43% of patients with stress incontinence had the pertinent endoscopic abnormalities, raising the question of the specificity and sensitivity of endoscopy as a test in incontinent patients.[20] Fischer-Rasmussen et al. found that cystoscopy did not contribute to the classification of incontinence in any of 212 women with urinary incontinence. They concluded that cystoscopy should not be used in the routine evaluation of patients with incontinence, though it is not clear that they assessed the role of urethroscopy in these patients.[28] Horbach and Ostergard found that only 6 (2.3%) of the 263 women they evaluated had cystourethroscopic findings consistent with stress incontinence. These authors also concluded that endoscopy has little to no value in the evaluation of women with stress incontinence.[29]

In patients with urodynamic diagnoses of incontinence, Cardozo and Stanton found no cystoscopic abnormality in 100 patients with stress incontinence, and only 13 of 100 patients with detrusor instability had bladder wall abnormalities, all of which were benign.[30] Govier et al. found that cystoscopy cannot allow one to predict the functional integrity of the bladder neck and proximal urethra when compared with findings from videourodynamic studies generally.[31] Scotti et al. found urethral characteristics during urethroscopy consistent with stress incontinence in 53 of 99 patients with genuine stress incontinence by urodynamic testing, though none of the endoscopic findings were unique. They concluded that urethroscopic findings did not have enough sensitivity or specificity to be of value in the evaluation of most patients with stress incontinence.[32] In a geriatric female population, Ouslander et al. likewise concluded that cystoscopy is not adequately specific or sensitive enough as a test to confirm the type of incontinence present[33] and that the appropriate role of cystoscopy in the evaluation of incontinence remains to be defined.[34] Sand et al. compared the accuracy of urethroscopic supine cystometry with multichannel urethrocystometry (without urethroscopy) in 182 women with incontinence. Although they reported no specific, visual urethroscopic findings, their statistical analysis showed that the urethroscopic cystometry was a poor screening procedure for patients at risk for detrusor instability.[35] Even concurrent conditions such as urethral diverticula are always suspected on the basis of simpler examinations than cystoscopy, making the procedure merely a confirmatory rather than a diagnostic step.[36]

These studies of the usefulness of endoscopy indicate that it provides no unique value when compared with other routine, less invasive tests such as a history, physical examination, and urodynamic studies. There is no indication that endoscopy is necessary or useful for evaluation of simple stress or urge incontinence; before bladder neck suspension surgery; among the elderly; for assessment of an obstruction except in visualization of a suspected bladder neck contracture, stricture, or a surgically or traumatically altered urethral position or anatomy; or for routinely ruling out other remotely possible or benign and insignificant diagnoses not already suspected on the basis of other basic tests. Despite these conclusions, experience and common sense show that there are selected patients with urinary incontinence for whom cystourethroscopy is useful:

1. For women with urethral trauma or foreshortening to assess urethral anatomy.
2. For men after prostatectomy or other urethral or pelvic trauma to assess urethral anatomy and rule out bladder or urethral foreign body.
3. For any patient with continuous incontinence to rule out ectopic ureter, fistula, or complete sphincter deficiency.
4. For any patient with significant irritative symptoms (urgency, frequency, nocturia, dysuria, or hypersensitivity) unexplained by other basic tests, including urodynamics, and unresponsive to empiric therapy. This would be especially useful for women with these new symptoms after surgery near the bladder or urethra to rule out foreign bodies, especially sutures.
5. For patients with severe detrusor instability and hyperreflexia or low compliance with inadequate or sudden loss of response to aggressive, noninvasive therapy, unexplained by other tests, to rule out bladder pathosis.
6. For patients, especially those with histories of neurologic injury, who have used indwelling urethral catheters for lengthy periods, to rule out urethral damage, bladder pathosis, or foreign body.
7. In any patient with no evident cause for the incontinence on the basis of other tests, including history, examination, and urodynamic, laboratory, or radiologic studies.
8. To confirm the absence of other urethral or bladder conditions such as condyloma, neoplasms, foreign bodies, stones, or other types of urethral or bladder inflammations *only if these are strongly suspected on the basis of the history, examination, urodynamic, laboratory, or radiologic studies.*

CONCLUSION

Cystourethroscopy is a safe, well-tolerated procedure that can provide useful information for clinicians in their evaluation of patients with urinary incontinence. However, it should only be used in selected circumstances to allow its unique potential value to be demonstrated. Indeed, diagnosis of the cause of incontinence is more often a question of what functions abnormally rather than what looks abnormal. Knowledge of the dysfunction is always more important in guiding treatment than knowledge of the endoscopic abnormality.

REFERENCES

1. Clayman RV, Reddy P, Lange PH: Flexible fiberoptic and rigid-rod lens endoscopy of the lower urinary tract: a prospective controlled comparison, *J Urol* 131:715-716, 1984.
2. Brekkan E, Ehrnebo M, Malmström PU, et al: A controlled study of low and high volume anesthetic jelly as a lubricant and pain reliever during cystoscopy, *J Urol* 146:24-27, 1991.

3. Stein M, Lubetkin D, Taub HC, et al: The effects of intraurethral lidocaine anesthetic and patient anxiety on pain perception during cystoscopy, *J Urol* 151:1518-1521, 1994.
4. Pliskin MJ, Kreder KJ, Desmond PM, Dresner ML: Cocaine and lidocaine as topical urethral anesthetics, *J Urol* 141:1117-1119, 1989.
5. Birch BRP, Ratan P, Morley R, et al: Flexible cystoscopy in men: is topical anaesthesia with lignocaine gel worthwhile? *Br J Urol* 73:155-159, 1994.
6. Fisher HE: Dyclonine hydrochloride, *Missouri Medicine* 52:943-944, 1955.
7. Getzoff PL: A safe and effective topical anesthetic for office cystoscopy, *J Urol* 99:118-121, 1968.
8. Worth PHL: Cystourethroscopy. In Stanton SL, editor: *Clinical gynecologic urology,* St. Louis, 1984, Mosby.
9. Trop CS, Bennet CJ: Autonomic dysreflexia and its urological implications: a review, *J Urol* 146:1461-1469, 1991.
10. Rivas DA, Chancellor MB: Flexible cystoscopy in spinal cord injury: review article, *Paraplegia* 32:454-462, 1994.
11. Scotti RJ, Ostergard DR: Practical guide for triage of patients with lower urinary tract symptoms. In Ostegard DR, editor: *Gynecologic urology and urodynamics: theory and Practice,* ed 2, Baltimore, 1985, Williams & Wilkins.
12. Liu J, Flood HD: Selection of patients with intrinsic sphincter deficiency for treatment with collagen: can we do better? *J Urol* 153:277A, 1995.
13. Awad SA, Gajewski JB, Katz NO, Acker-Roy K: Final diagnosis and therapeutic implications of mixed symptoms of urinary incontinence in women, *Urology* 39:352-357, 1992.
14. Robertson JR: Urethroscopy: the neglected gynecologic procedure, *Clin Obstet Gynecol* 19:315-340, 1976.
15. Belville WD, Swierzewski SJ III, Wedemeyer G, et al: Synchronous cystoscopy and cystometry in the management of neurogenic bladder dysfunction, *J Urol* 150:431-433, 1993.
16. Hadley R, Ruckle H: Simplified urodynamic assessment of the incontinence male patient: perfusion sphincterometry, cystourethroscopy and cystometrics, *J Urol* 151:326A, 1994.
17. Wein AJ: Diagnostic evaluation of neuromuscular disorders of the bladder. In Seidman EJ, Hanno PM, editors: *Current urologic therapy* 3, Philadelphia, 1994, Saunders.
18. Stanton SL: Preoperative evaluation of the incontinent patient. In Ostergard DR, editor: *Gynecologic urology and urodynamics: theory and practice,* ed 2, Baltimore, 1985, Williams & Wilkins.
19. Stanton SL: Evaluation of female incontinence: definition and treatment. In Barret DM, Wein AJ, editors: *Controversies in neuro-urology,* New York, 1984, Churchill-Livingstone.
20. Aldridge CW Jr, Beaton JH, Nanzig RP: A review of office urethroscopy and cystometry, *Am J Obstet Gynecol* 131:432-437, 1978.
21. Bergman A: Office work-up of lower urinary tract dysfunctions and indications for referral for urodynamic testing, *Obstet Gynecol Clin North Am* 16:787-794, 1989.
22. Richardson DA: Investigative procedures in urogynecology, *Curr Opinion Obstet Gynecol* 3:513-519, 1991.
23. Raz S, Little NA, Juma S: Female urology. In Walsh PC, Gittes R, Perlmutter A, Stamey T, editors: *Campbell's urology,* ed 6, Philadelphia, 1992, Saunders.
24. Payne CK: Stress urinary incontinence in females. In Seidman EJ, Hanno PM, editors: *Current urologic therapy 3,* Philadelphia, 1994, Saunders.
25. Mundy AR: The unstable bladder, *Urol Clin North Am* 12:317-328, 1985.
26. Webster GD, Ramon J: Procedure selection in the management of stress urinary incontinence, *Prob Urol* 4:37-53, 1990.
27. Stamey TA: Urinary incontinence in the female: the Stamey endoscopic suspension of the vesical neck for stress urinary incontinence. In Walsh PC, Gittes R, Perlmutter A, Stamey T, editors: *Campbell's urology,* ed 6, Philadelphia, 1992, Saunders.
28. Fischer-Rasmussen W, Hansen RI, Stage P: Predictive values of diagnostic tests in the evaluation of female urinary stress incontinence, *Acta Obstet Gynecol Scand* 65:291-294, 1986.
29. Horbach NS, Ostergard DR: Predicting intrinsic urethral sphincter dysfunction in women with stress urinary incontinence, *Obstet Gynecol* 84:188-192, 1994.
30. Cardozo LD, Stanton SL: Genuine stress incontinence and detrusor instability: a review of 200 patients, *Br J Obstet Gynaecol* 87:184-190, 1980.
31. Govier FE, Pritchett TR, Kornman JD: Correlation of the cystoscopic appearance and functional integrity of the female urethral sphincteric mechanism, *Urology* 44:250-253, 1994.
32. Scotti RJ, Ostergar DR, Guillaume AA, Kohatsu KE: Predictive value of urethroscopy as compared to urodynamics in the diagnosis of genuine stress incontinence, *J Reprod Med* 35:772-776, 1990.
33. Ouslander J, Staskin D, Raz S, et al: Clinical versus urodynamic diagnosis in an incontinent geriatric female population, *J Urol* 137:68-71, 1987.
34. Ouslander JG, Leach GE, Staskin DR: Simplified tests of lower urinary tract function in the evaluation of geriatric urinary incontinence, *J Am Geriatr Soc* 37:706-714, 1989.
35. Sand PK, Hill RC, Ostergard DR: Supine urethroscopic and standing cystometry as screening methods for the detection of detrusor instability, *Obstet Gynecol* 70:55-60, 1987.
36. Ganabathi K, Leach GE, Zimmern PE, Dmochowski R: Experience with the management of urethral diverticulum in 63 women, *J Urol* 152:1445-1452, 1994.

Chapter 17 Radiographic Evaluation

Aaron Kirkemo

Many types of urinary incontinence can be effectively managed without the use of radiographic studies. For example, patients with urge incontinence or simple stress urinary incontinence may not need any imaging study in the course of the incontinence evaluation. Patients with suspected fistula or extravesical urine loss obligately require radiographic studies. The decision to obtain radiographic studies as part of an incontinence evaluation requires that the physician understand what type of anatomic or functional abnormalities can be expected based on the presenting history and physical examination of the incontinent patient. These studies may be obtained either to aid in the classification of the incontinence, to document any associated anatomic abnormalities preoperatively, or to evaluate some sequela of the dysfunctional voiding (such as vesical ureteral reflux).

Radiographic studies of women with stress incontinence have been a clinically valuable assessment of the anatomy of the urethra and bladder for decades. Historically these studies have provided physicians with essential information about incontinence that has been the basis for many clinical management decisions. Since urge or stress incontinence is a dynamic process, static x-ray films of the urethra and bladder do not provide the clinician with the same information that is available with videourodynamics. However, the traditional lateral resting and straining radiographic studies of the urethra provide the clinician with invaluable information about the anatomy of the urethra and bladder. This especially important clinical information if videourodynamic studies are not readily available. The selection of the appropriate imaging studies requires that the evaluating physician use some classification system of urinary incontinence to guide his or her choice of studies. The classification by Wein[1] describes urinary incontinence as a failure to store urine because of the bladder, the urethra (outlet), both, or other.

Failure to store because of the bladder may be attributable to detrusor overactivity, decreased compliance, or sensory urgency. Incontinence attributable to the outlet is either the result of anatomic abnormalities of the urethra and bladder neck (anatomic stress urinary incontinence) or the result of functional deficits of the bladder neck and proximal urethra (intrinsic sphincter deficiency). Clearly, more than one pathologic process can contribute to the incontinence. Frequently, both detrusor and bladder-outlet causes for the incontinence might coexist. Other causes such as fistula and diverticulum must be considered in certain patients (Fig. 17-1).

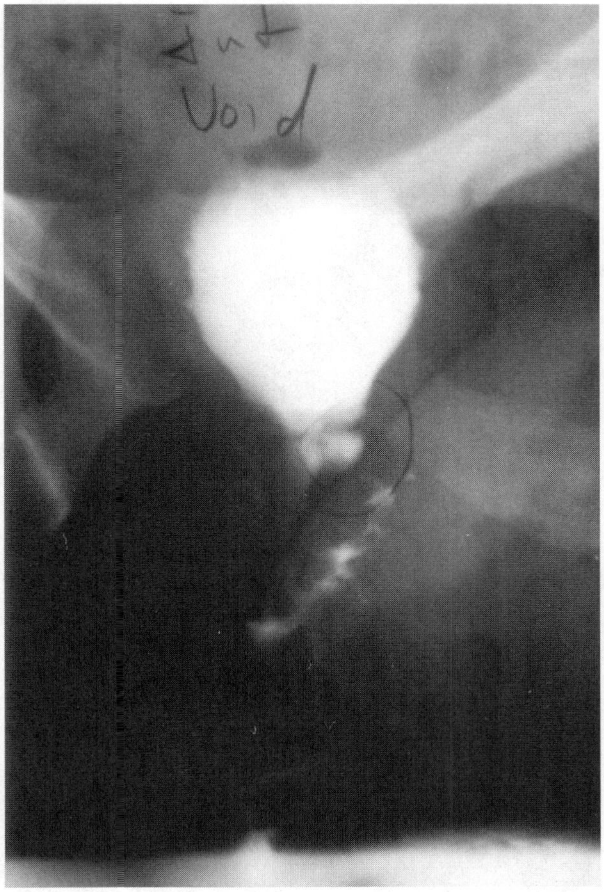

FIG. 17-1 *Patient presented with complaint of new onset of stress incontinence after a urethral diverticulectomy. A urethrovesical-vesicovaginal fistula was demonstrated with intrinsic sphincter dysfunction.*

If the cause of urine leakage is suspected to be bladder overactivity, the need for an imaging study is minimal. However, if the cause of the overactivity is suspected to be an anatomic abnormality such as urethral obstruction after a urethropexy, then a voiding cystourethrogram (VCUG) would be warranted. VCUGs would be warranted also for a patient with urge incontinence who is believed to have vesicoureteral reflux. Depending on the clinical history and the severity of reflux, an upper tract study may be reasonable (Fig. 17-5). Upper tract studies should be performed on patients with urodynamically proved high pressure or overactive bladders. Staskin has shown that patients with leak pressures over 40 cm H_2O and sustained motor overactivity with pressures over 40 cm H_20 in the presence of altered compliance run a high risk of upper tract deterioration even in the absence of reflux.[2]

Should the patient have symptoms compatible with stress urinary incontinence, a stress cystogram can help assess the severity of the anatomic support defect. It may also help evaluate the competency of the bladder neck. Additionally it will allow one to assess the severity and configuration of any coexistent cystocele.

If a urethral diverticulum is suspected as a cause for urine loss, the voiding portion of a stress cystogram, a double-balloon urethrogram, or urethral ultrasonography should be considered (Figs. 17-2 and 17-3). Urethral or vesicovaginal fistula can be evaluated with a stress cystogram. Extravesical causes of urine leakage such as ureterovaginal fistula are best evaluated with retrograde pyelography.

The boxed outline lists the studies that might be employed in the evaluation of a patient with urinary incontinence. The particular general diagnostic entities that can be gleaned from each study are listed. The primary radiographic study for evaluating patients with urinary incontinence is the stress VCUG. Since incontinence is a dynamic process, the VCUG ideally should be carried out under real-time fluoroscopic control. Incontinence is most easily provoked when patients are in an upright position. In patients with pelvic floor relaxation a supine study will fail to demonstrate many of the anatomic relationships that are seen only with the patient upright. For these reasons the study should be carried out with the patient either in a standing or a sitting position. It cannot be overemphasized that certain anatomic changes associated with normal voiding may mimic findings observed with anatomic stress urinary incontinence. Simultaneous recording of intra-abdominal and intravesical pressure can allow the observer to differentiate these events. If pressure recording cannot be carried out at the same time, extreme caution must be exercised when one is interpreting a stress VCUG.

A

B

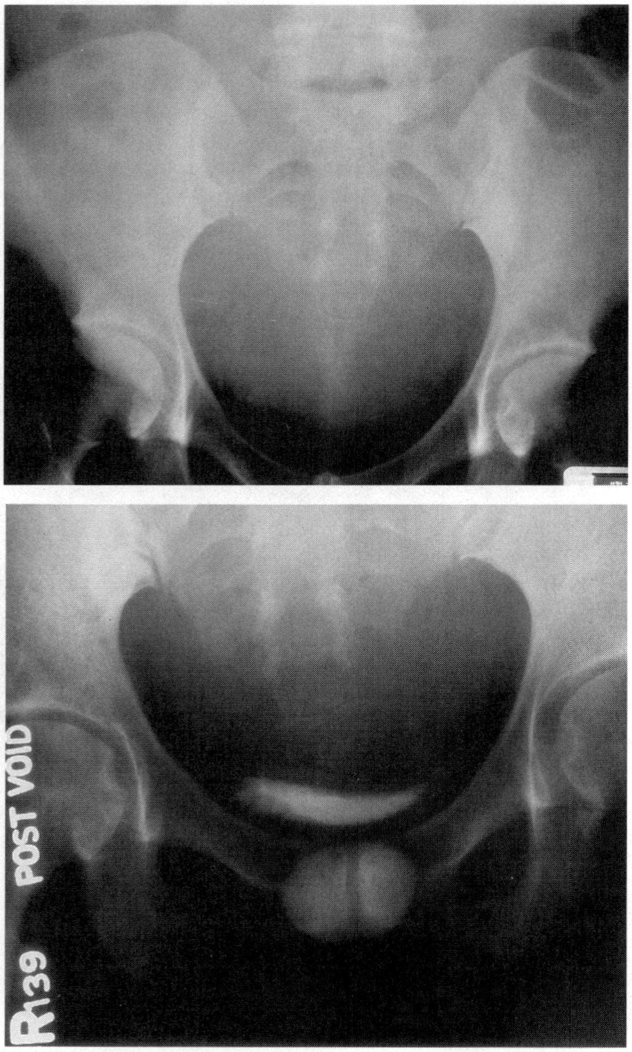

FIG. 17-2 ***A,*** *Notice the scout film, which shows a calcification overlying the pubic symphysis.* ***B,*** *The postvoid film reveals a massive diverticulum.*

List of Basic Radiographic Studies, the Urologic Structures that Can Be Evaluated by Them, and the Diagnostic and Structural Entities that Should Be Looked for

1. KUB (KIDNEYS, URETER, AND BLADDER)
- a. Assess potential upper tract abnormalities
  - (1) Stones caused by reflux or functional ureteral obstruction at the ureter
- b. Evaluate the spinal column
  - (1) Spinal bifida occulta
  - (2) Myelomeningocele
  - (3) Spinal cord injury
  - (4) Sacral agenesis
- c. Evaluate the pelvis
  - (1) Pelvic fracture
    - (a) Denervation of bladder or bladder neck
    - (b) Proximal urethral disruption
    - (c) Urethral or bladder fistula
  - (2) Diastasis of the pubic symphysis
    - (a) Exstrophy
    - (b) Epispadias
  - (3) Foreign bodies in bladder (such as bladder stones)
  - (4) Perivesical masses (such as uterine fibroids)
  - (5) Pelvic prolapse

2. UPPER TRACT IMAGING (RENAL ULTRASONOGRAM, INTRAVENOUS PYELOGRAM [IVP], NUCLEAR STUDIES, RETROGRADE PYELOGRAMS)
- a. Assess upper tract
  - (1) Hydronephrosis
  - (2) Stones
  - (3) Renal scarring
  - (4) Ureteral anatomy
  - (5) Dilatation
  - (6) Duplication anomaly
  - (7) Ectopic ureter
  - (8) Fistula

3. BLADDER IMAGING (CYSTOGRAM, VESICOURETEROGRAM [VCUG], STRESS VCUG)
- a. Bladder assessment
  - (1) Reflux
  - (2) Fistula
  - (3) Trabeculation
  - (4) Bladder configuration
  - (5) Christmas tree–shaped bladder
  - (6) Thickened bladder wall
- b. Bladder neck and urethra assessment (cystogram, VCUG, stress VCUG, ultrasonogram, balloon urethrogram)
  - (1) Degree of bladder neck and urethral support
  - (2) Bladder neck competency
  - (3) Fistula
  - (4) Diverticula
  - (5) Urethral obstruction

My choice for performing the study is similar to that described by Shapiro and Raz.[3] A noninvasive uroflow is performed and then followed by a postvoid residual check with use of a small-caliber (8 or 10 Fr) red rubber Robinson catheter. If a simultaneous electronic filling cystometrogram (CMG) is not carried out, the catheter is left in place and taped to the patient's leg. Otherwise a 7 Fr urodynamic catheter is inserted. A balloon catheter *should not be used!* The inflated balloon can occlude the bladder neck, making assessment of the continence and bladder neck function problematic.

The bladder is then filled at low pressure (15 to 20 cm H_2O pressure) with a contrast medium such as 30% Cystografin. A medium fill rate of 30 to 60 ml/min is used. If a urodynamic pressure transducer is not being used, a central venous pressure (CVP) manometer can be "Y'ed" into the system for an estimation of filling pressures. Ideally the study is carried out under fluoroscopy with simultaneous electronic measurement of intravesical, intra-abdominal, and subtracted pressure. The volumes and pressures at first sense of bladder filling, normal urge to void, and strong urge to void are recorded. At 200 ml of filling the patient is asked to perform a Valsalva strain and cough. Relaxed and straining anteroposterior and lateral films are obtained. The patient is placed obliquely at 30 degrees and

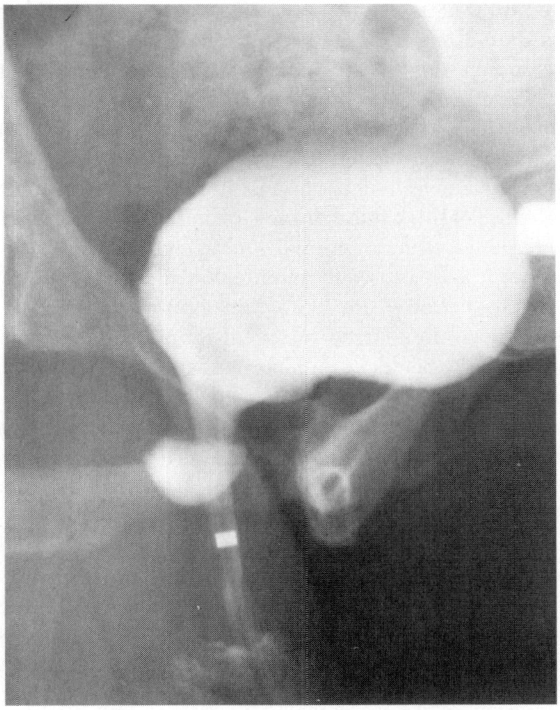

FIG. 17-3 *Voiding films will normally demonstrate urethral diverticula without the need for double-balloon urethrograms.*

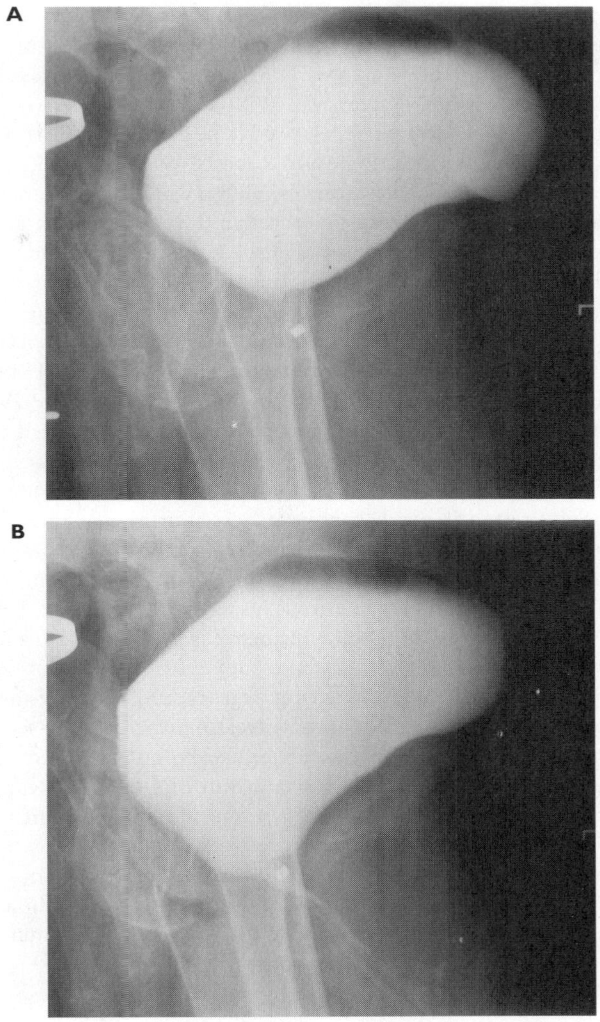

FIG. 17-4 ***A,*** *Patient straining without urine leakage.* ***B,*** *Same patient voiding. She was unable to stop her detrusor contraction and voided nearly to completion. Notice the descent and relation of the bladder neck and urethra as voiding occurs.*

asked to repeat the stress maneuvers. The oblique and lateral films are very important for assessment of the support of the urethra, bladder, and bladder neck. This positioning is mandatory in patients with cystoceles, since the superimposition of the bladder over the urethra and bladder neck precludes assessment of these structures. While the patient is still positioned obliquely, filling is continued until the patient reaches maximal cystometric capacity. Stress maneuvers are repeated and observed. If leakage occurs, it is important to document whether it happens coincidently with the stress maneuver or is delayed. This is particularly important to note if intravesical pressure monitoring is not done because delayed leakage may signal a detrusor contraction triggered by the stress maneuver rather than by stress incontinence. Once the stress films have been taken the patient is asked to void. A voiding and postvoid film is then taken.

As mentioned earlier, incontinence is a dynamic event. Evaluating static films of an incontinence event is very difficult unless the person interpreting the films either was present at the time point at which the films were obtained or has pressure data collected coincidentally with the captured event. A film of a patient voiding and one of a patient with stress urinary incontinence secondary to bladder neck hypermobility may look very similar (see Fig. 17-4). With this in mind one needs to evaluate the films for what they tell us about the static support of the bladder, urethra, and surrounding structures as well as the dynamic changes that occur with stress maneuvers and urine leakage.

Fluoroscopic Findings in Normal Bladder

Early fluoroscopic studies performed by Mueller[4] in 1949 reported that the base of the bladder sat at the upper border of the pubic symphysis in the continent prepartal female. With straining the bladder may descend some but still stays above the inferior border of the pubic symphysis. He noted that with normal voiding there was a loss of the posterior urethral vesical angle, as well as descent and funneling of the bladder neck preceding the detrusor contraction that initiated voiding. These same anatomic changes of the urethra and bladder neck were observed by him in women with stress urinary incontinence.

The static anteroposterior and lateral films help assess the level of bladder support. In the nulliparous female the base of the bladder should rest near the superior border of the pubic symphysis. Since the pubourethral ligaments and pubocervical fascia is intact, the urethra should be supported in a retropubic position behind the symphysis. Normally the urethral axis is 5 to 10 degrees off the vertical axis. With stress maneuvers it may open to 30 to 35 degrees. It is viewed to be pathologic if the angle exceeds 45 degrees. Jeffcoate and Roberts[5] popularized the concept of the posterior urethral vesical (PUV) angle. This angle is created when one draws a line through the urethra and another line tangent to the bladder wall at the level of the bladder neck. Their observations of both continent and incontinent women was that the normal PUV angle was 90 to 100 degrees. Any angle over 110 degrees was deemed pathologic and felt to be associated with a high incidence of incontinence. Hodgkinson[6] and others in the early 1950s measured the urethral axis and the PUV in patients preoperatively and postoperatively and noted that correction of these angle can ensure a high likelihood of restoration of urinary incontinence. The popularization of these concepts has give rise to an overly simplistic view of urinary incontinence leading some to believe that overcorrection of the urethral axis and posterior urethrovesical angle (PVA) can further improve the success rate of a bladder neck suspension.

One has to realize that incontinence is attributable to a host of factors that include anatomic support problems, intrinsic sphincter deficiencies of varying degrees, and detrusor-mediated factors. Blind selection of a treatment strategy based on anatomic findings alone is dangerous. Bergman et al.[7] compared stress cystograms from a group of continent women with a cohort of patients with genuine stress urinary incontinence. He found no difference between the two groups with respect to five cystographic criteria: posterior and anterior urethral angle, funneling of the proximal portion of the urethra on straining, the position of the urethrovesical junction, and flattening of the bladder base.

INTERPRETATION OF THE STRESS VCUG

The scout film is essential. A foreign body such as a stone in the bladder or urethra may be identified. Bony abnormalities of the pelvis may give clues to underlying patholosis for a person with incontinence. Diastasis of the symphysis pubis associated with a pelvic fracture can be suggestive of urethral and bladder neck trauma and incompetency. One should inspect the sacrum and lower spine to help predict whether any spinal dysraphism exists. Evidence of possible spinal cord injury should be looked for, including such things as disk-space narrowing, previous laminectomy, and residual myelogram contrast. The soft tissues in the pelvis should be evaluated also. Intramural bladder calcifications may be suggestive of a poorly compliant bladder resulting from chronic inflammation such as tuberculosis or schistosomiasis. Calcified and large noncalcified mass lesions in the colon, uterus, or ovaries may be seen.

The cystogram allows the physician to evaluate the certain structural characteristics of the urethra and bladder. It also contributes to the understanding of the functional status of the urethra-bladder unit. Again it cannot be overemphasized that a clear diagnosis of the functional status of the bladder and urethra requires simultaneous pressure measurements in conjunction with the radiographic functional assessment of the bladder and the urethra. If this is not possible, the person interpreting the films should be physically present when the films are taken in order to correlate the functional status of the patient with the film. For example, if a film shows a wide-open well-supported bladder neck and urine loss, it is virtually impossible to determine if the patient was voiding, was trying unsuccessfully to stop from voiding, or was leaking because of an incompetent sphincter. In the absence of this clinical or pressure information the film could be interpreted either as normal voiding, intrinsic sphincter deficiency, or leakage caused by an uninhibited detrusor contraction.

The evaluation of the cystogram should be carried out in a systematic fashion. First a comment should be made about the capacity of the bladder as well as its shape. The normal bladder should have a spherical appearance with a bladder wall that is thin. A small bladder with a thickened wall may be suggestive of bladder fibrosis with poor compliance, as might occur with radiation fibrosis. Bullous edema of the mucosa can be associated with poor bladder compliance. Urinary tract infections or allergic cystitis can create this finding. Trabeculation of the bladder is seen with either bladder outlet obstruction or motor overactivity. The presence of bladder diverticula except in the periureteral positions (Hutch diverticula) implies high detrusor pressures with voiding. Patients with a decentralized bladder may demonstrate a Christmas tree–shaped bladder (see Fig. 17-5). Extrinsic compression of the bladder by uterine fibroids or other pelvic structures may help identify an extravesical cause for the voiding dysfunction. Intravesical structures such as stones or tumors can be associated with incontinence and need to be looked for also.

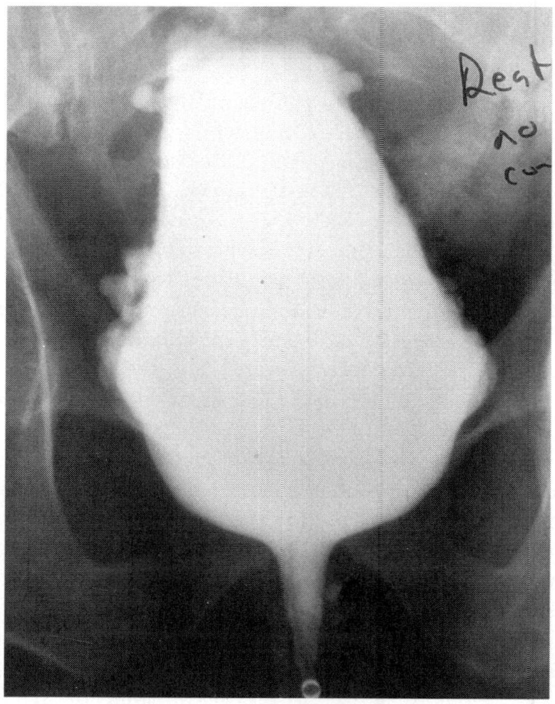

FIG. 17-5 *Christmas tree–shaped bladder in patient with stress incontinence. The patient had spinal bifida occulta and was found to have a poorly compliant atonic bladder.*

The position of the bladder and urethra in the pelvis both in the resting and the stress states is important both to evaluate from understanding the underlying voiding disorder and to guide the operative approach. Fischer et al. have shown that the pelvic exam underestimates the severity of bladder neck and urethral prolapse in approximately 40% of patients, especially if the patient has a history of prior anterior vaginal vault procedures.[8]

Cystoceles are graded on a I to III scale. A grade I cystocele drops just below the inferior border of the pubic symphysis (Fig. 17-6). Prolapse 2 to 5 cm below the pubic symphysis is classified as a grade II cystocele (Fig. 17-7). Grade III cystoceles are associated with gross protrusion beyond the vaginal introitus. In the absence of vault prolapse most cystoceles are the result of midline attenuation of the pubocervical fascia (Fig. 17-8). However, some cystoceles are the result of paravaginal defects. Variations in the configuration of the cystocele can help one determine where the defect in the pubocervical fascia is located. This knowledge is critical in planning the cystocele repair. The classic midline fascial defect results in a teardrop- or hourglass-shaped cystocele defect on a standard anteroposterior film. Paravaginal defects tend to produce an oblique configuration. Cystoceles associated with vaginal vault prolapse tend to produce a rounder symmetric bulge with only a minimal waist appearance at the level of the vaginal introitus. If the perineal body is torn, minimal indentation of the bladder may be seen.

The bladder neck and urethra are then evaluated. This evaluation is critical for distinguishing genuine stress urinary incontinence (GSUI, anatomic, or type II, incontinence) from intrinsic sphincter deficiency (type III incontinence). Observations that need to be noted include (1) a description of the bladder neck and urethral position both at rest and with straining, (2) the configuration of the bladder neck and the urethra, (3) the abdominal pressure and bladder volume at which leakage occurred, and (4) whether a bladder contraction was occurring.

With classic anatomic, or type II, stress urinary incontinence one should observe descent and posterior rotation of the bladder neck and urethra associated with loss of urine *in the absence of a detrusor contraction* (Fig. 17-9). The abdominal pressures required to produce the leakage associated with the demonstrated hypermobility should occur at "reasonable pressures." Classically this is defined as a Valsalva leak point pressure of greater than 100 cm H_2O pressure with 260 ml in the bladder.[9] This pressure definition has not been completely validated. The size of the urodynamics catheter, position of the patient, and volume of the bladder have all been shown to alter leak point

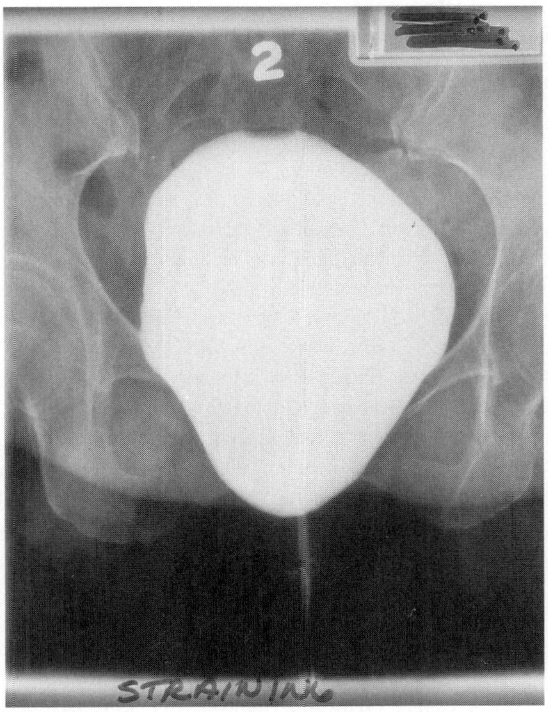

FIG. 17-6 *Patient with anatomic stress urinary incontinence and grade I cystocele.*

A, B

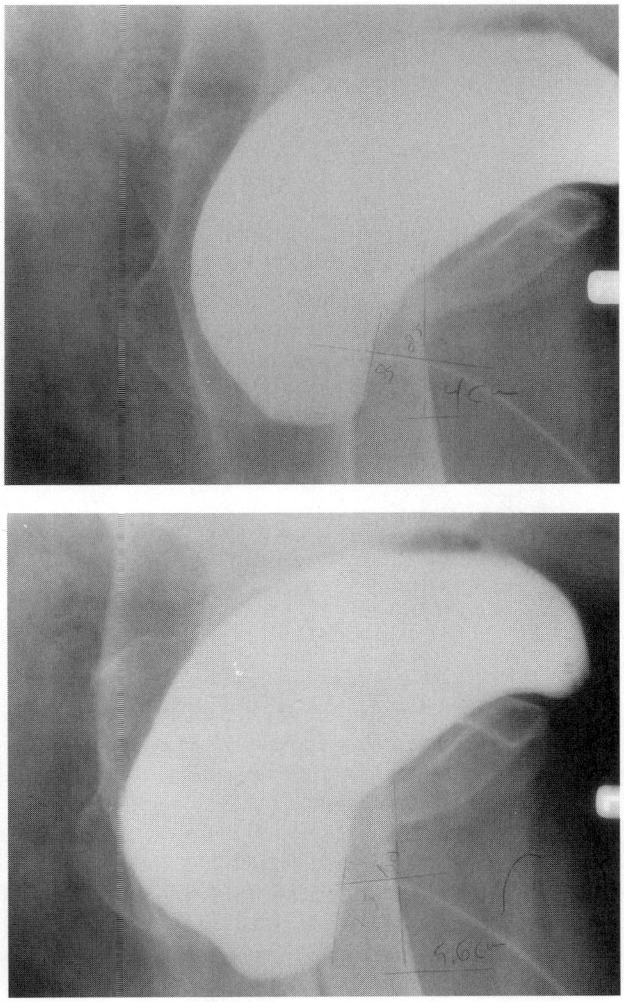

FIG. 17-7 *Grade II cystocele that prolapses from 4 cm below the pubic symphysis at rest to 5.6 cm with Valsalva effort. This patient had associated vaginal vault prolapse with both a rectocele and an enterocele. The rectal catheter encircled by a gas-density shadow is seen inferior and posterior to the ischial tuberosities.*

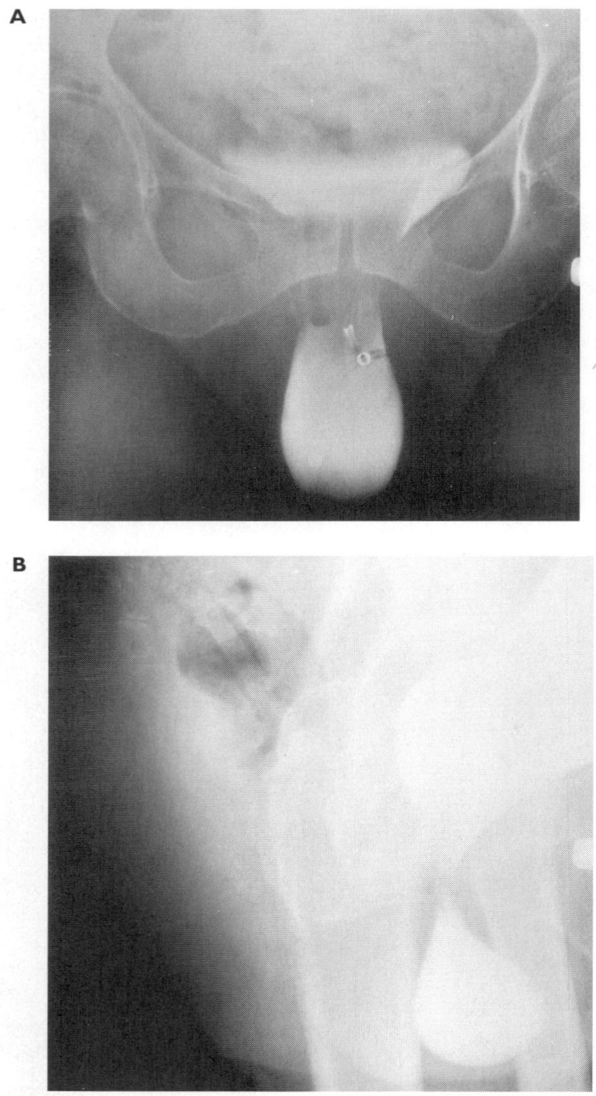

FIG. 17-8 *Grade III cystocele. This defect is the result of a midline fascial defect in the pubocervical fascia. A cavernous midline defect was seen on the floor of the bladder at the time of cystoscopy.*

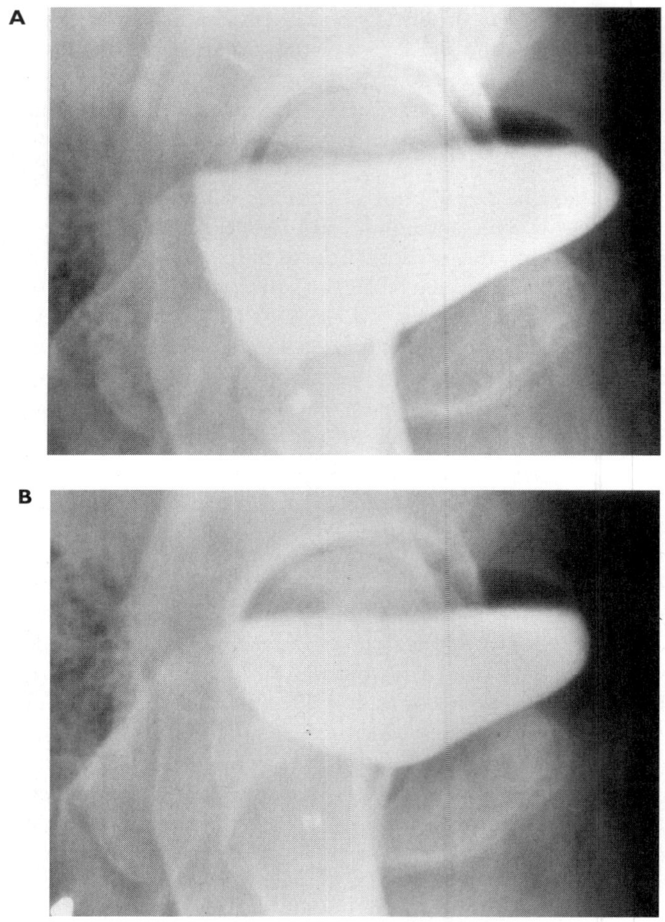

FIG. 17-9 *Patient developed stress incontinence after first delivery. Leaks with sneezing, laughing, and aerobics. Posterior descent of the urethra and bladder neck associated with straining produces discrete episodes of urinary leakage.*

pressures. Clinical correlation plays an integral role in making the diagnosis. If the patient reports discrete episodes of leakage with high-stress maneuvers, the diagnosis of GSUI can be made with a high degree of confidence.

The classic findings of intrinsic sphincter deficiency (ISD) are a fixed open bladder neck and a urethra that does not move with stress maneuvers and is associated with low Valsalva leak point pressure (<70 cm H_2O). An open bladder neck on a resting film does not automatically infer intrinsic sphincter deficiency. It should, however, heighten one's concern that ISD may exist. Most neurologically intact patients with ISD have had prior anti-incontinence surgery. The urethra and bladder neck are usually fixed against the pubic bone and do not move with stress maneuvers. Frequently the prior suspension sutures produce an elevation of the bladder base on either side of the bladder neck (Fig. 17-10). Valsalva leak point pressures are low, and most patients report significant urinary leakage with minimal stress maneuvers. ISD is unlikely in the patient who demonstrates a slight degree of bladder neck beaking and has demonstrable bladder neck and urethral hypermobility with leakage at high leak point pressures. This is especially true if the patient is neurologically normal, has not had prior surgery, and relates that she has small episodes of leakage with vigorous activity. The assessment of urethral competency is more problematic in the patient who demonstrates some degree of bladder neck beaking, has urethral and bladder neck hypermobility, and has low to indeterminate Valsalva leak point pressures. Further discussion of this group is reserved for Chapter 28 on urodynamic testing and evaluation and treatment of ISD.

Another issue that needs to be addressed is the evaluation of the bladder neck and urethra in patients with large cystoceles or enteroceles. The prolapse of these structures may serve as a pressure popoff that dampens the Valsalva pressure, precluding a meaning-

A

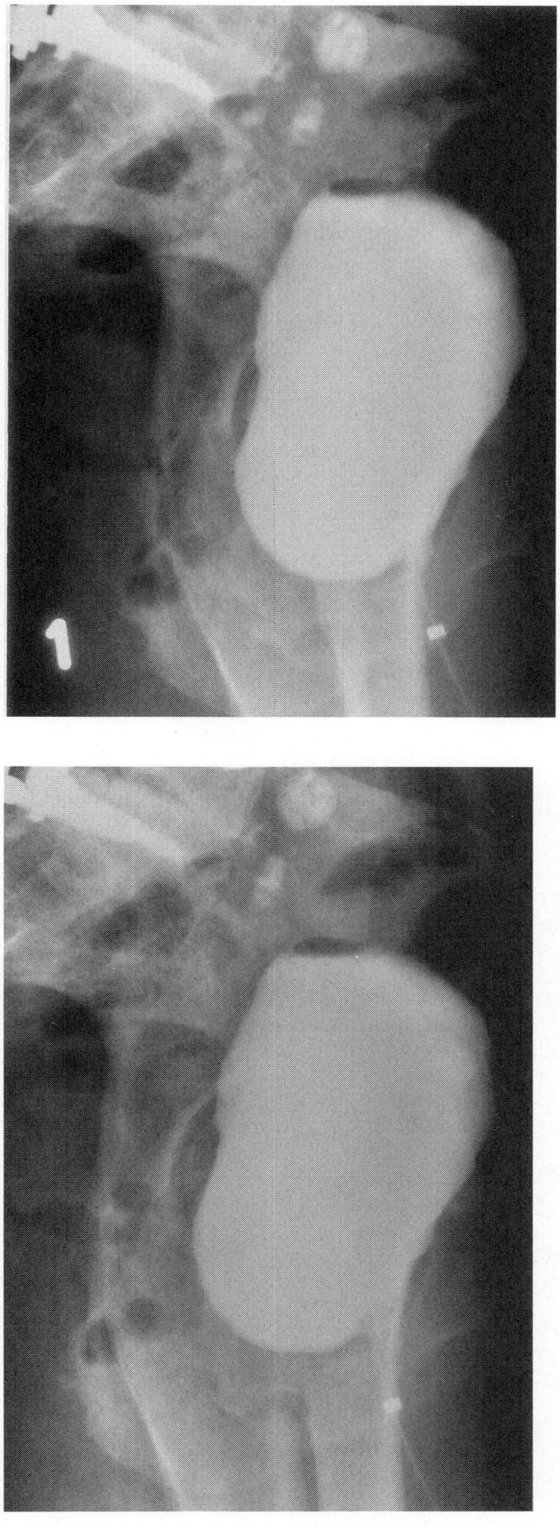

B

FIG. 17-10 *A,* *This patient continued to leak despite having had a previous MMK. Notice that the urethra and bladder neck are fixed to the pubic symphysis.* ***B,*** *At rest the bladder neck is open. A minimal Valsalva maneuver produces gross leakage despite the absence of any demonstrable hypermobility. These findings are the hallmark of intrinsic sphincter dysfunction.*

ful assessment of the force needed to overcome the urethra–bladder neck sphincter mechanism. Additionally the cystocele may partially obstruct the urethra or bladder neck and falsely elevate the Valsalva leak point pressure. For this reason, if there is any concern about the competency of the bladder outlet, a pessary or vaginal pack should be placed to reduce the prolapsed structures before one assesses the sphincter mechanism (Fig. 17-17). Usually, for patients with significant prolapse it is most convenient to place the pessary at the start of the procedure when the catheters are placed. Once the functional portion of the exam has been completed, the pessary is removed. Resting and straining films are obtained in both the anteroposterior and the lateral views.

Methodology for Creating a Videourodynamic Unit from a "Nonvideo" System

Modern videourodynamic equipment facilitates the collection of both the pressure and the anatomic information. These integrated machines tend to be very expensive, however. Many clinics have older computer-based urodynamic machines as well as access to fluoroscopic suites. Unfortunately, they are not integrated. It is possible, in many circumstances, to integrate the two systems without having to purchase a new videourodynamic suite. Many video converters are available to convert variable graphics array (VGA) signals to television video signals (NTSC and PAL).

The VGA-to-video converter is connected to the video output of the computer. This device splits off part of the signal and converts it to a standard video signal. The remainder of the signal goes to the computer's VGA monitor screen. As a result it is possible to simultaneously display information on both a computer screen and a TV video monitor. Most of these conversion devices will also permit a standard video input signal to be fed into it. Because of this feature, the video signal from the fluoroscopy unit can be fed into the composite video input port. Both signals are merged into a single output signal containing both the fluoroscopic image and the computer graphics image. This "overlay" image can be sent to a videotape machine for both taping the study and amplifying the signal. The output from the video is then sent to a conventional monitor for viewing (Fig. 17-11).

Many of these video converter systems can now be purchased for low cost. One can install them without inserting any boards into the computer and without having to install any computer software. A matrix film recorder such as those commonly used for capturing prostate ultrasound images can be connected to the television monitor. This allows for immediate capture of video and pressure images, which can be pasted into the patient chart.

Conclusion

Radiographic imaging studies can be useful for helping the clinician diagnose and plan the treatment of patients with urinary incontinence. Static images, however, constitute only "one piece of the puzzle." The images must be interpreted within the context of what was happening to the patient at the time the image was obtained. This is most easily accomplished with simultaneous pressure measuring.

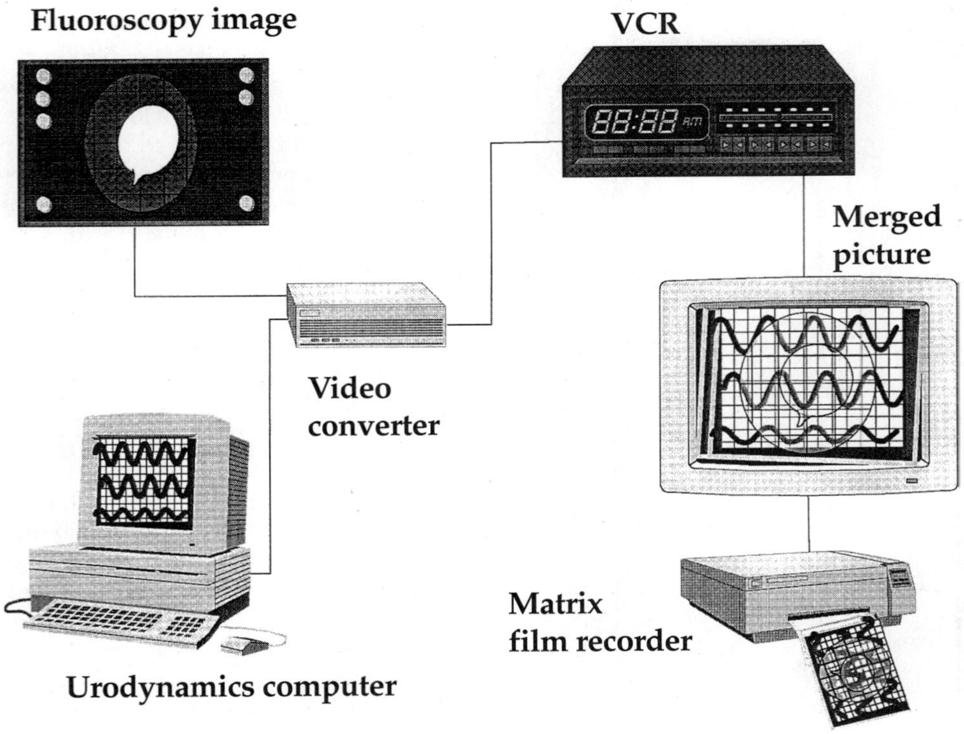

FIG. 17-11 *The availability of inexpensive converters of a variable graphics array (VGA) to a video image makes it possible to make a videourodynamic unit by integrating the image from a computer urodynamics machine with the fluoroscopy unit image output. See text for details.*

REFERENCES

1. Wein AJ: Classification of neurogenic voiding dysfunction, *J Urol* 125:605, 1981.
2. Shapiro RA, Raz S: Clinical applications of the radiologic evaluation of female incontinence. In Raz S, editor: *Female urology*, Philadelphia, 1983, Saunders.
3. Muellner SR, Fleischner FG: Normal and abnormal micturition: study of bladder behavior by means of the fluoroscope, *J Urol* 61:233, 1949.
4. Jeffcoate TNA, Roberts H: Observations on stress incontinence of urine, *Am J Obstet Gynecol* 64:721, 1952.
5. Hodgkinson CP: Relationships of the female urethra and bladder in urinary stress incontinence, *Am J Obstet Gynecol* 65:560, 1953.
6. Bergman A, McKenzie C, Ballard CA, Richmond J: Role of cystourethrography in the preoperative evaluation of stress urinary incontinence in women, *J Reprod Med* 33:372-6, 1988.
7. Fischer W, Schwenke A, Natho W: Usefulness of the Watup test in practice, *Zentralbl Gynskäl* 113:121-126, 1991.
8. McGuire EJ: Urodynamic evaluation of stress incontinence, *Urol Clin North Am* 22:551-555, 1995.

PART FOUR INCONTINENCE IN CHILDREN

Chapter 18

Clinical Management Decisions

Anthony J. Casale, Richard C. Rink

Children who have urinary incontinence usually present initially to the family physician or pediatrician. The question of urinary control in children and associated problems are a common concern of parents and physicians. The following is an outline of the normal development of urinary control and the many factors that affect control. We define which children have control problems and provide guidelines for their initial evaluation. Lastly, we suggest criteria that physicians can use to decide which children should be referred to specialists and which specialists are the most appropriate for various problems.

DEVELOPMENT OF BLADDER CONTROL

Infants are born with an autonomous bladder. They have no voluntary control of voiding and have little sensation of either filling or voiding. During the first year of life they begin to develop sensation as witnessed by levels of discomfort when the bladder is full and relief when they void. During the first year of life the number of voiding episodes per day decreases from approximately 20 to around 10 and the volume of each void increases accordingly. They remain in this state for about 2 years.[1]

Toddlers (2 to 4 years of age) usually begin to develop true bladder control and ultimately undergo "potty training." The first manifestation of this control is the ability to defer the desire to void, a skill that develops around 18 months of age. Since control of voiding requires both physical maturation of the nervous system and adequate emotional development to cooperate with their parents in toilet training, there is a considerable age range during which this step is achieved. Children are considered trained when they can sense a full bladder and can either empty appropriately or delay emptying as necessary. The last step in complete volitional bladder control is the ability to initiate voiding at any time on demand. This step may be delayed even into adulthood.[2] By 4 years of age all healthy children should have mastered the basics of daytime bladder control except for voiding on demand. While variable, the general order of development of urine and fecal continence is nighttime fecal control, followed by daytime fecal continence and then daytime urinary continence, with nighttime urinary control the last step to be achieved.

Preschoolers (4 to 6 years of age) should be completely trained during the day. Occasional daytime wetting accidents are not unusual and are often the result of poor decision making by the children. This is commonly attributable to the child's decision to delay voiding, even with a full bladder, until an involuntary bladder contraction leads to leaking of urine. This behavior tends to occur infrequently and usually improves spontaneously as the child matures. In some children it may escalate to the point where the parents seek help from a physician ("busy little girl syndrome").[3] Occasional (once every few weeks) wetting in this age range should be tolerated, but if the incontinence occurs once per week, a physician evaluation would be appropriate.

Normal school-age children should have uniform daytime continence with few exceptions. They should be able to conform to school schedules and void at the times appropriate with their peers. Recurrent daytime wetting in this age group is always abnormal and deserves medical attention.

DEVELOPMENTAL FACTORS AFFECTING CONTINENCE

Since control of the urinary tract involves decision making and judgment, children must reach a certain level of behavioral maturity to perform this successfully. Any delay in general development of the child may lead to a delay in development of urinary control. Behavioral parameters that are critical are attention span, the ability to concentrate on a single task, and the ability to follow instruction.

A simple but common problem occurs when the parent brings a very young child in for evaluation who is normal but who cannot be adequately toilet trained. Many of these parents start training too young in chronologic terms, and others have children who are simply immature for their age. It is helpful to ask about their developmental milestones and for the opinions of teachers and others besides the immediate family in deciding about the child's level of development. It is important to rule out other factors besides immaturity, which may cause the delay in learning toilet skills.

Other children fail in toilet training because of behavioral problems. These patients generally have incontinence as one manifestation of a multitude of problems. The family may be having problems in other areas of the child's life, especially school. These children may be receiving some form of counseling in behavioral modification, and the clinician who sees the patient for incontinence may combine treatment strategies with these counselors or decide that it is proper to wait until other behavioral problems are corrected before focusing on continence. It is rare to make significant progress in the isolated area of bladder control without making overall progress with the other behavioral problems. In certain children with severe dysfunctional voiding, psychologic problems may be secondary to recurrent wetting. The guilt associated with this wetting or the punishment by the parents for a problem the child has little control over results in significant loss of self-esteem. At times it can be difficult to know which is the primary and which is the secondary problem. We have at times seen a child's life dramatically improve in all areas of behavior after successful treatment of urinary incontinence.

True psychologic problems are even more uncommon, but these children often have continence problems as well. Again, as with those with less severe behavioral problems, the physician must focus on the entire situation in which the child is involved. Some treatment of psychologic disorders may interfere with continence, and the daily baseline level at which the child functions may make toilet training impractical at this time. In these children it is extremely important to consult with the psychiatrist or counselor working with the patient and to reach a common level of expected functionality. In some cases treatment of incontinence must be delayed until other more pressing problems are under control.

Finally, there is a wide range of physical impairments to development of bladder control. Most of these affect global development, and the most common are the various forms of mental retardation. These children usually develop functional bladder control that correlates with their age of function. Again, consultation with the other health care professionals can lead to a logical level of expected function for each patient. We want each child to maximize his or her potential but never want to demand more from any child than what each can reasonably achieve.

WHOM ARE YOU TREATING?

When a parent and child present with the complaint of voiding difficulties and incontinence, the physician must first judge the validity of the complaint. Many parents, especially young or first-time parents, will have unrealistic expectations. They may be motivated by the cost of diapers, the inability to place children in some day-care situations, pressure from friends or family, or just a poor understanding of the normal development in childhood. This most often leads to potty training at too young of an age. They may also expect perfect control and judgment when their children are not developmentally able to comply. The physician must therefore make a judgment of the child's level of function and whether the complaint is reasonable. Often the family just needs some advice and information to understand what their children are doing at a developmental level.

If you as a physician believe that there is a real problem, you must decide who is most bothered by this problem, the parent or the child. This will have a dramatic effect on the ability of the family to understand and to help solve the problem. Often the perception of the problem and its significance vary considerably between parent and child, and the treating physician must find some agreed starting point. To successfully treat incontinence in children, all involved must agree on the specific nature of the problem and the specific goals to be achieved in order of importance. For example, a 7-year-old may wet at school, when he takes naps in the afternoon, and also at night. The parents are concerned about nighttime wetting, and the child is more concerned about wetting at school in front of his friends. It is important to get all to recognize that day wetting is the highest priority problem and to focus on this aspect first with specific attainable goals to this end. Another difficult, but common problem arises in the case where the child apparently does not care about his or her incontinence. Parents and teachers bring the problem to light, and this situation occurs mostly with boys who are often having other behavioral problems. If the adults involved cannot entice the child to cooperate willingly or at least to take an interest, then treatment is fruitless. These are extremely frustrating cases for all involved, but the physician can do little without the child's cooperation.

GENERAL CLASSIFICATION OF INCONTINENCE

Enuresis, involuntary voiding beyond the anticipated age for control in children, may fall into several categories. Nocturnal enuresis, or bed-wetting, is defined as the inability to defer voiding while asleep. This is the last developmental step in learning bladder control and occurs in most children by 6 years of age. Most physicians recommend no treatment of children under 6 years of age because the condition is so common in younger children (15% to 20% of 5-year-olds).

There is a rapid period of resolution so that by 10 years of age only 5% of the population still suffer from nighttime wetting, and this number falls to only 1% at 15 years of age.[4,5] Many families who present with this complaint want only information and the reassurance that their child will eventually stop.

Daytime wetting is a completely different problem with different ramifications. It is never normal for school-age children to have daytime incontinence, and all such children deserve an evaluation. Causes occur in a wide range, from poor toilet habits to spinal cord tumors, and the work-up may need to be quite extensive, including neurosurgic consultation. Complete urinary incontinence, both day and night, carries the same weight as daytime incontinence and must be evaluated fully. Anatomic anomalies of the genitourinary tract such as epispadias or ectopic ureter and diseases of the nervous system are the most significant causes and must be ruled out.

A word must be said about the influence of stool incontinence and bowel dysfunction on bladder function. It is clear that constipation has a profound effect on bladder control and function in children.[6,7] The incidence of urinary incontinence, urgency, frequency, and urinary tract infection all are significantly increased in children with bowel dysfunction. If both bowel and bladder control problems exist, in our experience it has been very difficult to have any success treating urinary problems without treating the bowel problems simultaneously. In fact, in some cases the urinary incontinence will resolve completely when the bowel dysfunction improves. The combination of fecal and urinary incontinence always warrants further evaluation.

Initial Evaluation

General History

In this era of high technology, incontinence is one area where the clinical history remains the most important diagnostic tool. Time spent obtaining an accurate history can often allow detection of the exact cause of the incontinence without the need for further costly and often painful diagnostic studies. To understand the clinical significance and cause, one must know other factors. The duration and pattern of the symptoms is extremely important. For example, in children, a single episode of involuntary wetting is not cause for concern, nor is a short period of nocturnal enuresis in a child previously completely potty trained. In our experience, daytime wetting generally occurs in one of the following categories: sudden urge urinary leakage, vaginal voiding, or incontinence associated with anatomic or neurologic abnormalities. Every effort should be made by the history and physical examination to identify these various types of incontinence. The potty-training history is important and should include the age at which this occurred or was attempted, any difficulty associated with potty training, and notation of whether the child has been dry continuously since initial training. The timing of the wetting episode is also critical. Is the child wet continuously (regardless of when the parents check, the underwear is damp)? In girls this is very suggestive of an ectopic ureter, which warrants further x-ray evaluation. This is very different from the girl who is wet immediately after normal voiding. Postvoid dribbling is most often associated with vaginal voiding and requires no further evaluation. One of the more common types of incontinence in children is manifested by sudden involuntary wetting associated with a bladder contraction. These children with bladder instability or uninhibited contractions generally do not have a warning signal or a sensation that this will occur. The parents may notice the child posturing (dancing, leg crossing, squatting with a heel in the perineum), which is an effort to further compress the urethra to prevent urinary leakage. When the posturing is over, the child may have no desire to void as the bladder pressures have returned to a baseline condition. This sudden urge type of incontinence is generally a learned voiding dysfunction, but it may be secondary to bladder irritability associated with urinary tract infection, bladder inflammation, or even constipation. The severity, frequency, and duration of the incontinence should all be noted. Is the wetting significant enough to require the child to change clothes? Is this new-onset wetting or has it been ongoing throughout life?

The parents should be questioned regarding the child's urinary stream. Does the child start and stop the stream with dribbling, or is there a sudden forceful stream that stops abruptly? Both types of voiding are suggestive of detrusor-sphincter dyssynergia. Does the child strain to void? The parents should be questioned regarding the child's coordination, lower extremities, or fecal continence, all factors that may be suggestive of neurologic dysfunction. A good family history regarding similar problems as well as the family's approach and attitude regarding the incontinence is important. Has the child been punished? Does the wetting bother the child? Has there been prior treatment that has failed? If so, what type and how long ago was it tried? If medication was used, identify the dosage schedule. As a general rule, if the parents are seeking medical attention for the wetting, it is a significant problem for the family.

Physical Examination

When one is evaluating a child for incontinence, it is important not only to examine the child but also to observe the maturity of the child, as well as the child-parent interaction. The enuretic's gait should be observed. The abdomen should be palpated for any areas of tenderness and for any mass such as a distended bladder or stool in the sigmoid colon. Likewise, the genital exam is a critical portion of the overall evaluation. Any erythema or rash should be noted. In the male, the penis and urethra should be examined and the urethra palpated for tenderness. In the female, the labia should be spread to rule out labial fusion, and separate urethral and vaginal openings should be noted. A bifid clitoris is present in girls incontinent from epispadias. In a girl suspected of having an ectopic ureter, continual urinary dribbling may be found. Compression over the kidney and ureter may make this more evident. The child's back should be examined for vertebral abnormalities, in particular the lumbosacral area. Any area of pigmentation, hair patch, dimple, or sinus tract may represent underlying spinal dysraphism. The lower extremities in children with spinal dysraphism may be found to have muscle wasting, decreased sensation, and changes in the reflexes, and the feet are often noted to have high arches and clawed toes.

Laboratory Evaluation

In all children with incontinence, a urinalysis should be obtained to rule out urinary tract infection, proteinuria, and glucosuria, which may result in poor urinary control. If urinary concentrating ability is questioned, a first-morning-specimen specific gravity is helpful. Radiographic evaluation is always obtained if there are concomitant urinary tract infections (UTIs). In the remaining children, one should obtain x-ray studies based on the history and physical examination. For example, in those wet from vaginal voiding no studies are needed. However, in the girl with continual dampness suspected of an ectopic ureter, upper (intravenous pyelogram or renal ultrasonogram) and lower (voiding cystourethrogram) tract evaluation is indicated. These studies are also needed in children with epispadias. In a child believed to have neurogenic incontinence, a renal bladder ultrasonogram is warranted, as well as a magnetic resonance imaging study of the lumbosacral spine. Further radiographs are directed by the results of these initial studies.

It is more difficult to determine which children with voiding dysfunction require radiographic studies. It has been noted that up to 50% of children with significant uninhibited contractions will have vesicoureteral reflux. However, minimal degrees of wetting or posturing and no infection history is generally not further evaluated. Prevoid and postvoid bladder ultrasonography in these children can be very helpful to determine their ability to empty and to note bladder wall thickness, which may be quite impressive in those having detrusor-sphincter dyssynergia. It is also a painless in-office study that can be used for teaching the parents and children the importance of sphincter relaxation and voiding to completion. It can be easily used to demonstrate progress in emptying when the patients are working through their voiding abnormalities and is easily understood by the children. The child with pure nocturnal enuresis (no daytime incontinence, no history of UTI, and no suspected anatomic or neurologic abnormalities) does not require radiographic studies.

Urodynamic studies can be extremely useful in the evaluation of children with urinary incontinence.[8] When this study should be performed and what information it can provide are often confusing for the primary care physician. It can provide information regarding bladder compliance and contraction, sensation of bladder fullness, pressure levels at the time of sensation, voiding pressures, sphincteric function, and coordination of the bladder with the sphincter. Despite all the information obtainable, it is not necessary in most children with urinary incontinence. For example, most children with mild dysfunctional voiding can be treated successfully without urodynamics, and it has essentially no role in the evaluation of primary nocturnal enuresis or ectopic ureter. On the other hand, it is invaluable in the assessment of those with neurogenic dysfunction and in many with anatomic sphincteric problems or more severe dysfunctional voiding problems (Hinman's syndrome).[9]

WHEN TO REFER AND TO WHOM

The majority of patients with incontinence can be managed by the pediatrician or family physician if they have an interest in these problems. Children are often mismanaged by either ignoring the wetting ("it's normal; it will go away") or by overevaluating it. As noted previously, if the family seeks medical help, it is a problem in that home. That is not to say that every child needs treatment but that every child does warrant a thorough history and physical examination. Many times the family wants only reassurance that there is no significant disorder. If the primary care physician does not have an interest in voiding disorders or has not made progress with treatment, referral to a specialist is in order. Many general urologists are comfortable managing childhood incontinence, particularly in otherwise healthy children or those with incontinence of short duration. Incontinence therapy in children is time intensive, and only rarely are surgical procedures or cystoscopy warranted.

In those children with chronic or progressive incontinence who are unresponsive to therapy or in those with significant associated abnormalities, referral to a pediatric urologic center is appropriate. This holds true for those with significant anatomic problems such as epispadias or imperforate anus or in those with spinal dysraphism also. These centers generally have experience with severe voiding dysfunction and the personnel available for prolonged child and family therapy. Furthermore, there is urodynamic and surgical expertise for the more severe disorders.

SUMMARY

In summary, children who present with urinary incontinence represent a wide range of psychologic, anatomic, neurologic, and psychologic disorders. Therapy requires a keen interest on the part of the physician. Radiographic and laboratory evaluation is based on the underlying abnormality but is generally required in those with urinary tract infections and those suspected of having anatomic or neurologic incontinence. Incontinence therapy can be very time consuming with the accurate diagnosis relying heavily on history and physical findings. Successful therapy can also be quite rewarding. Incontinence can be a devastating social problem for developing school-age children, and successful treatment can dramatically change their lives in a positive fashion.

Few things are more pleasing than to improve a child's self-esteem. Certain warning signs must send up a red flag to the physician. Continual dampness day and night (ectopic ureter), bifid clitoris (epispadias), dermatologic changes over the lumbosacral spine, lower extremity changes or associated fecal incontinence (neurologic dysfunction), or recurrent urinary tract infections cannot be ignored and warrant further evaluation. Referral to a pediatric urologic center is in the child's best interest for these more severe problems, as well as for those children who fail to respond to initial management.

REFERENCES

1. Goellner MH, Ziegler EE, Fornan SJ: Urination during the first three years of life, *Nephron* 28:174, 1981.
2. Muellner SR: Development of urinary control in children, *JAMA* 172:1256, 1960.
3. Bauer SB, Retik AB, Colodny AH, et al: The unstable bladder of childhood, *Urol Clin North Am* 7:321, 1980.
4. DeJonge DA: Epidemiology of enuresis: a survey of the literature. In Kolvin I, MacKeith RC, Meadow SR, editors: *Bladder control and enuresis,* London, 1973, Heineman.
5. Crawford JD: Treatment of nocturnal enuresis: introductory comments, *J Ped* 114:687, 1989.
6. Gallo D, Presman D: Urinary retention due to fecal impaction in children, *Pediatrics* 45:292-294, 1970.
7. Shopfner CE: Urinary tract pathology associated with constipation, *Radiology* 90:865-877, 1968.
8. Bauer SB: Pediatric neuro-urology. In Krane RJ, Siroky MB, editors: *Clinical neuro-urology* 24:375-409, 1991.
9. Hinman F, Baumann FW: Vesical and ureteral damage from voiding dysfunction in boys without neurologic or obstructive disease, *J Urol* 109:727, 1973.

Chapter 19

Clinical Evaluation of Children

Helen E. O'Connell, Michael L. Ritchey, David A. Bloom

Urinary incontinence is a common phase between infantile and adult lower urinary tract function. The definition and evaluation of abnormal leakage is important to determining when a problem truly exists and what should be done about it. Parental concerns about toileting are common and often supersede the child's anxiety.[1] Many children are punished for wetting.[2] It is important therefore that health professionals dealing with children have a good working knowledge of normal patterns of the acquisition of day and night urinary control and significant departures from those normal patterns.

Definitions of Incontinence

Important terms that require definition include enuresis, primary nocturnal enuresis, secondary nocturnal enuresis, and incontinence.[3]

Enuresis has been defined as involuntary urine loss not related to any identifiable structural problem (central nervous system and genitourinary structures are normally formed), though when related to dysfunctional voiding the term "enuresis" may be applied.[3] This term clearly differs from the situation in adults where incontinence or involuntary leakage is defined as an objectively demonstrable social or hygienic problem that occurs regardless of a definable structural problem. The International Continence Society defines enuresis as any involuntary loss of urine, thereby not distinguishing this symptom from incontinence. Enuresis must be defined by whether it occurs during the day only (diurnal), night only (nocturnal), or both.

The American Psychiatric Association defines the condition *primary nocturnal enuresis* on the basis of the following diagnostic criteria: repeated voiding of urine into bed or clothes (whether involuntary or voluntary); the behavior is clinically significant as manifested by either a frequency of twice a week for at least 3 consecutive months or the presence of clinically significant distress or impairment in social, academic (occupational), or other important areas of functioning; chronologic age of at least 5 years (or developmental equivalent); and the behavior is not attributable exclusively to the direct physiologic effect of a substance (such as a diuretic) or a general medical condition (such as diabetes mellitus, spina bifida, a seizure disorder). However, we do not generally treat children under 7 years of age. Before this age there is a high spontaneous cure rate.

Secondary nocturnal enuresis occurs when day and night control have been present for at least 6 months and nocturnal enuresis develops.[3]

Prevalence of Nocturnal and Diurnal Enuresis

The prevalence of nocturnal enuresis is age dependent. In two large population studies the prevalence of 3-year-olds with regular bed-wetting was approximately 43%.[5,6] The rates of bed-wetting among 4- to 8-year-olds varies somewhat. In a study of children in southeast Michigan, Bloom et al. found that the incidence of nocturnal enuresis among 4-, 5-, 6-, 7-, and 8-year-olds was 24%, 23%, 28%, 20%, and 8% respectively.[5] This is compared with an incidence of 20%, 16%, 13%, 10%, and 7% respectively in a study of children in New Zealand by Fergusson et al.[6] The differences between the populations were difficult to explain, though cultural factors do play a role in toilet training, with some cultures commencing toilet training as early as 6 months of age. A difference between boys and girls at 7 years of age has been identified by Hellström et al.,[7] with bed-wetting rates of 7% and 12% respectively when defined as bed-wetting occurring at least once per month.

The incidence of diurnal enuresis is also age dependent. Diurnal enuresis occurred in 29% of 3-year-olds, 13% of 4-year-olds, or 5% to 10% of children 5 to 8 years old.[5] Hellström et al. found sex differences in the diurnal enuresis: 6% of girls at 7 years and 3.8% of boys.[7] Bloom et al. also noted that the prevalence of daytime accidents was higher for girls than for boys and higher among those with a history of urinary infection.[5] Interestingly, enuretic children voided more often than nonenuretic children, though the voiding frequency did not correlate with infection incidence. This pattern of incontinence with an increased urinary frequency is similar to patterns observed among incontinent elderly patients. Urodynamic studies of enuretic patients have shown that these symptoms are associated with sudden detrusor contractility that is provoked by filling. These patients have a poor warning system,[8] and the first bladder sensation coincides with detrusor instability rather than low-pressure filling. Although there is a common clinical impression that encopresis and bowel dysfunction parallel enuresis or nocturnal enuresis, no such correlation was observed.[5]

Clinical Evaluation and Decision Making

Incontinence can be the presenting symptom provoking the search for an underlying disorder. Alternatively the underlying disorder may be well established and incontinence a new manifestation of the disorder. The following box lists underlying conditions that may cause or contribute to incontinence. In later

Causes of Childhood Incontinence

Bladder outlet obstruction
Constipation
Detrusor instability
Diabetes mellitus
Diabetes insipidus
Ectopic ureter
Infection
Neurogenic bladder
Sleep disorders
Psychologic stress
Vaginitis

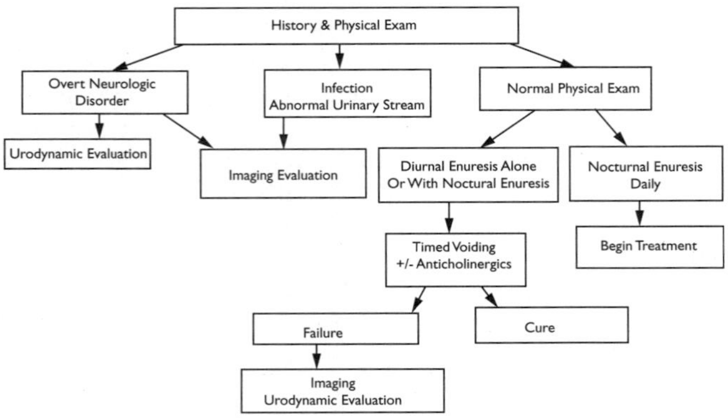

FIG. 19-1 *Algorithm for evaluation of incontinent child.*

childhood, 7 years of age or older, an underlying cause is rarely found. Once underlying disorders have been excluded, an enuretic child can be managed according to conventional algorithms (Fig. 19-1). The major questions to ask are as follows:

1. Is there neurologic disease?
2. Is there another underlying problem, structural or otherwise?
3. Is diurnal enuresis present (with or without nocturnal enuresis)?
4. Is this isolated nocturnal enuresis?

CLINICAL INFORMATION SOUGHT TO EXCLUDE OR IDENTIFY AN UNDERLYING NEUROLOGIC DISEASE

When an overt neurologic disorder such as myelodysplasia exists, the cause of incontinence is obvious. These patients have neurogenic vesical dysfunction with predictable patterns of bladder and urethral dysfunction. Early urodynamic evaluation and appropriate intervention should prevent upper tract deterioration[9] and facilitate continence. Neurologic disorders do not always lead to overt neurologic manifestations, and careful evaluation may be necessary to recognize a neurologic basis for childhood incontinence. History and physical examination will generally determine whether further neurourologic evaluation or imaging studies are needed before one formulates a treatment plan (see box below). Potential causes of a neurogenic bladder in childhood are listed in the next box.

History taking should include events that increase suspicion of a neurologic cause such as childbirth with anoxic injury, head or back trauma, or a seizure disorder. Developmental delays or delayed achievement of normal motor skills demand further evaluation.

Parents and child should be carefully questioned about the characteristics of the urinary stream. Does the child void by straining with a Valsalva maneuver, is the stream weak or interrupted, does leakage occur with crying, are there dry intervals between incontinent episodes, or does the child sense bladder fullness? Although structural problems can produce similar voiding abnormalities, these findings indicate the need for further imaging or neurourologic evaluation. Likewise prior episodes of urinary tract infection may be unrelated to neurologic disorders but mandate imaging of the urinary tract.

Parents should be questioned whether the enuresis is secondary or there is associated encopresis. Although the latter is a common problem in early childhood, the association of encopresis and enuresis raises the suspicion of a voiding neuropathy. The nature of the incontinent episodes is important. Stress incontinence can be related to structural as well as neurologic causes. Urge incontinence is a clinical diagnosis but is frequently associated with detrusor instability. In the presence of detrusor overactivity the child may adopt tricks to prevent leakage such as sitting on a heel (Vincent's curtsy), crossing his or her legs, or holding the perineum or penis. This reflects the child's attempt to suppress the bladder activity. The majority of children with urge incontinence do not require extensive investigation for neurologic disorders. This topic is discussed more extensively below.

It is often difficult to obtain an accurate record for the frequency of micturition or episodes of enuresis. Thus a micturition, incontinence, and fluid intake record is very helpful. This

Conditions Indicating Neurourologic Evaluation

Overt neurologic disease
Urosepsis
Hematuria
Urinary retention
Abnormal voiding positions
Dribbling
Painful urination
Secondary enuresis
Encopresis

Neurogenic Causes of Incontinence

CONGENITAL
Spinal dysraphism
Tethered cord syndrome
ACQUIRED
Spinal cord tumors
Pelvic surgery
Transverse myelitis
Spinal cord injury

allows objective quantification of the problem, correlation of incontinent episodes with voiding, and use as a monitor of the results of treatment. A version of the voiding chart that we find helpful is included in Appendix D.

Physical examination should include inspection of the abdomen, genitalia, and particularly the back, as well as a neurologic examination. Abdominal sensation is checked, and the lower abdomen is percussed to detect a distended bladder caused by poor bladder emptying. The genitalia are inspected, and the perineal sensation is assessed. A rectal examination with determination of anal sphincter tone and reflexes including the bulbocavernosus reflex is mandatory. The lower back is inspected for dimples, hairy patches, depressions, and lipomas, and the sacrum and coccyx are carefully palpated for evidence of spinal dysraphism or sacral agenesis. If there is any suspicion of an underlying neurologic disorder, further evaluation by a pediatric neurologist is indicated.

Clinical Information Sought to Exclude or Identify Other Underlying Disorders

Vaginal voiding, also referred to as urethrovaginal reflux,[3] refers to a dribbling type of leakage that occurs from the vagina after voiding as a result of pooling of urine in the vagina. In the presence of a normal perineum, the cause of this condition is the use of a toilet that is too big for a small girl, resulting in the child keeping her legs together to prevent herself from falling into the toilet, or in some obese older girls the problem may result from insufficient abduction of the thighs during voiding.

The important differentiating factor in this type of leakage is that it occurs a few moments after voiding. Vaginitis and even buttock pain[3] may occur. The child is instructed to separate the thighs widely during voiding. This may be facilitated by the removal of undergarments from one leg to allow the thighs to be widely separated. Alternatively the child can be instructed to sit on the commode facing backwards, that way mandating the corrective voiding position.

Labial fusion must be excluded as the cause of vaginal voiding. Topical estrogen cream or a minor surgical procedure usually solves the problem.

Ectopic ureters do not typically cause incontinence. However, if the ectopic ureter in girls inserts distally to the bladder neck, incontinence may occur. An ectopic ureter is associated with continuous dribbling incontinence, and the physical examination is normal except for constant leakage of urine. In boys, the ureter always inserts proximally to the external sphincter, and consequently leakage does not occur with ureteral ectopia.

Incontinence is a chronic problem in children born with *epispadias.* Usually the diagnosis is clinically obvious in the neonate. Occasionally a girl with epispadias presents with severe incontinence later in childhood. The history of incontinence may include day and night leakage, that is, total incontinence, though stress incontinence is more common. Physical examination reveals a bifid mons pubis, bifid clitoris, failure of fusion of the anterior labia, and a patulous open urethra. Urinary tract imaging and urodynamic testing before reconstruction is required.

If posterior urethral valves are not suspected antenatally, the diagnosis of *obstructive uropathy at the posterior urethral valves* may then be discovered early in the neonatal period. Children with posterior urethral valves can develop significant vesical dysfunction secondary due to decreased bladder compliance or detrusor hyperreflexia.[10] This leads to incontinence later in childhood despite previous successful surgical treatment of the posterior urethral valves. Bladder dysfunction can also lead to renal impairment. Less commonly, older boys will be diagnosed with posterior urethral valves (PUV). The presentation in older children may include incontinence, poor urinary stream, and infection.

Although the exact basis for the interaction between a full rectum and bladder dysfunction is unclear, an association is strong; *constipation* occurs in about 50% of enuretic children.[3]

Diabetes mellitus and diabetes insipidus may cause or exacerbate incontinence, though data indicating the prevalence of diabetes as an underlying cause of enuresis are limited. Polydipsia, polyuria, polyphagia, and weight loss may accompany the incontinence. To assess whether polyuria and polydipsia are contributing to incontinence, a knowledge of the 24-hour fluid intake and urine output is required. A fluid-balance chart completed by the parent will be more helpful than memory of such information.

Polyuria associated with fixed low-specific-gravity urine has also been associated with sickle cell disease.[11] Nocturnal polyuria may also relate to abnormal secretion of anitdiuretic hormone (ADH) in enuretic children with diminished nocturnal ADH compared to normal controls.[12] Although this abnormality may be a contributing factor in nocturnal enuresis, the presence of polyuria does not fully explain why some children wake and have nocturia and others remain asleep and wet the bed when the bladder is full. This may be an arousal failure.

Clinical Information Sought When Enuresis is Both Nocturnal and Diurnal

The *Hinman syndrome,* or nonneurogenic neuropathic bladder, is characterized by urodynamic and structural urinary tract changes suggestive of an underlying neurologic lesion in the absence of a neurologic lesion. This disorder of vesicourethral function was first described by Beer in 1915 and more fully appreciated and studied by others including Hinman,[13] who recognized that behavioral intervention, such as hypnosis, could effect resolution of the problem.

Characteristic urodynamic findings of high detrusor filling pressures followed by poor detrusor contractility during voiding and a tendency to upper tract deterioration with upper tract dilatation, vesicoureteral reflux, bladder trabeculation and associated encopresis increase the resemblance to a neuropathic bladder.[8] Electromyographic (EMG) activity in the external sphincter is normal, though maximum urethral pressures are sustained throughout a detrusor contraction associated with an open proximal urethra. Although this has been regarded as a form of detrusor sphincter discoordination, in fact the external sphincter activity begins as an attempt to control reflex detrusor activity and may be more of an exaggerated normal response to detrusor overactivity rather than true discoordination. In the later stages this may resemble simple dyssynergia. McGuire and Savastano observed a urodynamic sequence of poor appreciation of bladder filling, a decrease in EMG activity, and maximum urethral pressure, which herald the beginning of a reflex contraction.[8] The next step in the sequence was recognition that a contraction associated with an external sphincter contraction was occurring. Typically the external sphincter contraction does not control leakage, although in some patients it did. In a high proportion of patients, efforts directed at the detrusor, such as anticholinergic medication, were effective, and in this setting the drugs were not associated with retention. Nevertheless, anticholinergic medication alone may not be sufficient, particularly in the more severe cases. Attention to the secondary pelvic floor dysfunction and behavioral disorder is the principal therapeutic intervention.

The patient is typically a boy, with diurnal or nocturnal enuresis, urosepsis, high residual urine, and constipation and encopresis. The physical examination is usually normal, though the bladder is percussible or visible with a large residual volume and impacted stool may be found on rectal examination. Importantly, the neurologic examination is normal.

A variant of Hinman syndrome associated with a classic inverted smile to suppress laughing is called Ochoa syndrome.[14] This has an autosomal recessive genetic pattern. Presumably the facial expression is a means of reinforcing the closure of the external sphincter as would occur in the combination of laughing and straining.

There is *a continuum of effects of detrusor instability.* The major symptom in diurnal enuresis is urge incontinence, which is suggestive of detrusor instability. This usually results in storage symptoms, though normal children will adopt measures such as perineal pressure to help minimize leakage. Most children probably have some episodic instability, particularly at large bladder volumes, as they struggle to become socially continent. A continuum no doubt exists wherein most children with detrusor instability and enuresis eventually develop the neurologic maturity to prevent the uninhibited contractility before adverse sequelae develop. At the other end of the continuum one finds a small group of children with recurrent infections and vesicoureteral reflux.[15] In these children the associated symptoms are typically urgency, frequency, and urge incontinence often despite having just voided. The physical examination is normal, and residual urine volumes are unremarkable.

Because diurnal enuresis is such a common clinical problem in children, those under 5 years of age do not usually require evaluation. The majority of children with persistent diurnal enuresis after this age have both daytime and nocturnal wetting, but 10% to 20% have isolated daytime wetting. The proper evaluation of enuretic children includes history, physical examination, and urinalysis. Neuroanatomic cause for enuresis will usually be identified by these measures. Diurnal enuresis without neurologic or structural cause is initially managed by a timed voiding program and anticholinergic medication. For children with persistent wetting after medical management or those with obvious neurologic abnormalities on physical examination, imaging of the spine and urodynamic studies are warranted.

Spina bifida occulta in refractory diurnal enuresis. Recent reports have suggested that enuretic children with spina bifida occulta (SBO) may not do as well as other simple enuretics. Khoury et al. identified 31 diurnal enuretic children with SBO who failed to respond to conservative measures. After division of the filum terminale resolution of the incontinence was achieved in 70%.[16] The total number of enuretic children with and without SBO from which these patients were selected is not given. In a tertiary referral population of enuretic children, radiologic evidence of spina bifida occulta exists in nearly 10% (48 of 456), though not all children underwent radiologic examination.[17] Excluding all children with neurologic deficits, established tethered-cord syndrome, or lipomeningocele, the clinical course of children with SBO was compared with enuretic children with normal spines. The spina bifida occulta group actually had a higher rate of resolution of diurnal enuresis than the normal group had. Only 8% failed to improve with standard management, again a lower percentage than for those children with a normal spine x-ray film. In both groups prolonged follow-up study was required to the point of resolution of enuresis, that is, approximately 3 years in both those with and those without normal spine films. The retrospective nature of this study therefore limits the conclusions that could be drawn. Nevertheless, in the majority of enuretic patients with SBO the enuresis will resolve. Further radiologic imaging or urodynamic testing should be reserved for refractory cases provided that the neurologic examination is normal.

Infrequent voiding is a frequent cause of childhood incontinence. In a series of 636 children without neurologic disease or outflow obstruction, 7% had large-capacity hyporeflexic bladders.[18] In these children the threshold for initiating micturition is high, with voiding occurring only two or three times per day. Typically the child does not void on waking, and may not void until several hours later in the morning. Paradoxical urge incontinence may occur when the bladder reaches its large capacity. Associated problems include constipation and urinary infection. Apart from possible fecal impaction and percussible bladder, the physical findings are normal.

Another childhood urinary disorder that may cause parental concern is that of *extraordinary daytime urinary frequency.* Children with a normal urinary history develop severe urgency with voiding as often as every 15 minutes or less.[19] Other symptoms such as dysuria or incontinence are usually absent, and there is rarely any underlying condition. If nocturia is present, it is disproportionate to the diurnal pattern and rarely exceeds three or four times at night. An infectious or postinfectious cause has been proposed, but substantive data are lacking. The disorder is self-limiting, though the frequency can persist for many months or recur in cycles. Investigation should consist of a history, physical examination, and urinalysis.[19] Only occasionally is further study necessary.

Stress incontinence in children is unusual. Typically this is associated with a full bladder with activity and usually responds to bladder emptying before exertion. An underlying disorder such as epispadias, myelodysplasia, or trauma, such as pelvic fracture or bladder neck incision, should be sought in bona fide childhood stress urinary incontinence.

Giggle incontinence is an unusual condition involving leakage of urine with laughter and is not simply stress incontinence. This often occurs as an isolated symptom, and physical findings are normal. In some cases, detrusor instability is found on urodynamic study. Whether this is the cause or an associated finding is not clear.

Clinical Information Sought When Nocturnal Enuresis Alone Is the Problem

Whether the nocturnal enuresis is primary or secondary should be determined; that is, was the child ever continent at night and relapsed after primary attainment of toilet training? Secondary nocturnal enuresis is more commonly associated with psychologic factors and stressful life events than with primary nocturnal enuresis.[3] Although there is no particular value in attributing the problem of nocturnal enuresis to one parent, family history is a risk factor and is more likely associated with primary nocturnal enuresis without significant underlying neuroanatomic disorder.[3] When nocturnal enuresis alone is the only symptom, physical examination and urinalysis should be performed before treatment is initiated.

Urinary tract infection and vesicoureteral reflux in nocturnal enuresis. Most urologists do not recommend imaging of children with monosymptomatic nocturnal enuresis. However, one study found that, of children with nocturnal enuresis but no history of urinary tract infection, 16% have vesicoureteral reflux.[20] The presence of diurnal enuresis, urgency, frequency and secondary enuresis were not predictive for vesicoureteral reflux either as individual symptoms or collectively. In a nonenuretic population vesicoureteral reflux occurs in less than 1%. Prospective data are required to conclusively determine the value of imaging in nocturnal enuresis.

References

1. Howe AC, Walker CE: Behavioral management of toilet training, enuresis and encopresis, *Pediatr Clin North Am* 39:413-32, 1992.
2. Haque M, Ellerstein NS, Gundy JG, et al: Parental perceptions of enuresis: a collaborative study, *Am J Dis Child* 135:809-811, 1981.
3. Maizels M, Gandhi K, Keating B, Rosenbaum D: The wet child, *Curr Prob Pediatr* 23:402-450, 1993.
4. Abrams P, Blaivas JG, Stanton SL, Andersen JT: Standardization of terminology of lower urinary tract function, *Neurourol Urodyn* 7:403-427, 1988.
5. Bloom DA, Seeley WW, Ritchey ML, McGuire EJ: Toilet habits and continence in children: an opportunity sampling in search of normal parameters, *J Urol* 149:1087-1090, 1993.
6. Fergusson DM, Horwood LJ, Shannon FT: Factors related to the age of attainment of nocturnal bladder control: an 8 year longitudinal study, *Pediatrics* 78:884, 1986.
7. Hellström AL, Hanson E, Hansson S, et al: Micturition habits and incontinence in 7 year old Swedish school entrants, *Eur J Ped* 149:434, 1990.
8. McGuire EJ, Savastano JA: Urodynamic studies in enuresis and the non-neurogenic bladder, *J Urol* 132:299, 1984.
9. Wang SC, McGuire EJ, Bloom DA: A bladder pressure management system for myelodysplasia: clinical outcome, *J Urol* 140:1499, 1988.
10. Bauer SA, Dieppa RA, Retik AB, et al: The bladder in boys with posterior urethral valves: a urodynamic assessment, *J Urol* 121:769, 1979.
11. Readett DR, Morris J, Serjeant GR: Determinants of nocturnal enuresis in homozygous sickle cell disease, *Arch Dis Child* 65:615, 1990.
12. Norgaard JP, Pedersen EB, Djurhuus JC: Diurnal antidiuretic hormone levels in enuretics, *J Urol* 134:1029-1031, 1985.
13. Hinman F Jr: Non-neurogenic neurogenic bladder (the Hinman syndrome): 15 years later, *J Urol* 136:769, 1986.
14. Ochoa B: The urofacial (Ochoa) syndrome revisited, *J Urol* 148:580, 1992.
15. Koff SA, Murtagh DS: The uninhibited bladder in children: effect of treatment on recurrence of urinary infections and on vesicoureteral reflux resolution, *J Urol* 130:1138-1142, 1983.
16. Khoury AE, Hendrick EB, McLorie GA, et al: Occult spinal dysraphism: clinical and urodynamic outcome after division of the filum terminale, *J Urol* 144:426, 1990.
17. Ritchey ML, Sinha A, DiPietro MS, et al: Significance of spina bifida occulta in children with diurnal enuresis, *J Urol* 152:815-818, 1994.
18. Ruarte AC, Quesada EM: Urodynamic evaluation in children, *Int Perspect Urol* 14:114, 1987.
19. Zoubek J, Bloom DA, Sedman AB: Extraordinary urinary frequency, *Pediatrics* 85:1112-1114, 1990.
20. Sujka SK, Piedmonte MR, Greenfield SP: Enuresis and the voiding cystourethrogram: a re-evaluation, *Urology* 38:139-142, 1991.

Chapter 20 Urodynamics

Stuart B. Bauer

Urodynamic assessment has become an essential element in the evaluation of children with lower urinary tract dysfunction. During the last 15 years, development of small catheters, refinements in technique, dedication of trained personnel acutely aware of the needs of children, and ambulatory monitoring have advanced the procedure so that meaningful and reproducible data can be easily obtained.[1,2] These factors have permitted an evaluation of bladder and urethral sphincter function that has helped us to understand the pathophysiologic processes involved in the majority of voiding abnormalities occurring in children. With the improved reliability of data collection, the applicability of urodynamic testing has expanded to the point where those in many pediatric centers now believe that functional assessment of the lower urinary tract is as important as x-ray visualization in characterizing and managing these abnormal conditions.[3] In the course of this chapter the testing process, the diseases that warrant investigation and when and the expected findings are detailed so that one will grasp a better understanding of the specific problems encountered in children (see following box).

Urodynamic Testing

Before a urodynamic study is performed, a substantial amount of time and effort goes into its preparation.[4] It is important for

Aspects of the Urodynamic Examination

PREPARATION
Booklet explaining the test
Questionnaire on maternal, birth, and childhood history
URINARY FLOW RATE
Determine initial representative flow
Record peak and mean flow rate
Determine residual urine on subsequent catheterization
Calculate urine production per unit time
CYSTOMETROGRAM
Assess bladder filling pressures (compliance)
Denote uninhibited contractions and the ability to prevent voiding
Attempt to elicit uninhibited contractions by coughing or by Credé maneuver
Record pressure and sustainability of contraction while voiding
SPHINCTER ELECTROMYOGRAPHY
Characterize individual motor unit action potentials
Search for abnormal potentials or absence of sacral reflexes
Continuously monitor activity during bladder filling, looking for periodic relaxation or inappropriate responses to uninhibited contractions
Notice sphincter reaction to a voluntary or involuntary voiding contraction
URETHRAL PRESSURE PROFILE
Measure initially with the bladder empty
Position pressure-sensing point of catheter in midurethra area or another area of interest
Record measurement throughout bladder filling and voiding

the child and the family to have full knowledge of the procedure beforehand. Therefore an explanation of the test and a questionnaire are sent to each family before their appointment. A booklet is provided so that parents know what to expect and can explain the test to their child. If the boy or girl is old enough, he or she can read about it himself. Every attempt is made to reduce the anxiety level in those children who are able to understand what will happen by providing reasons for specific portions of the test and expounding exactly what the child will experience. The questionnaire tries to elicit information about the mother's pregnancy history, the child's birth and development, his or her current bladder and bowel habits, and any other information that might be pertinent to know at the time of the procedure.

In rare instances when children over 1 year of age are very anxious and cannot be consoled, meperidine, 1 mg/kg of body weight, is administered intramuscularly to reduce the individual's discomfort and anxiety level; this does not alter the child's cooperativeness or responsiveness.[5] If at all feasible, however, no medication is given, but the child is conscientiously attended to in order to minimize his or her fears. Parents are always allowed in the urodynamic suite to interact and comfort their child. Since 1993, EMLA cream, a topical anesthetic composed of lidocaine and prilocaine, has been applied to the perineum about 45 minutes before the electromyographic needle is inserted (if needed) to record urethral sphincter activity. If possible, the child is instructed to come to the urodynamic suite with a full bladder to obtain an initial representative urinary flow rate. The flowmeter computes out a flow-rate curve and calculates the peak and mean flow per second. The time of the child's previous urination is noted as well, to determine an average rate of urine production per unit of time. In addition, the nurse is able to record a reliable residual urine volume when the child is catheterized after voiding. The flowmeter is located in a private bathroom that contains a one-way mirror so that voiding can be viewed unobtrusively. This permits the investigator to see if the child employs a Credé method or Valsalva maneuver to help empty the bladder.

Next the nurse reviews the test and shows the child all the equipment in an attempt to assuage his or her fears and anxieties. The child is catheterized with either a 7 or 11 French-gauge triple-lumen urodynamic catheter (Cook Urological Inc., Spencer, Indiana) after a small amount of liquid lidocaine (1%) is injected into the urethra and prevented from leaking out for a moment or two. Then the residual urine is carefully measured. Sometimes it is necessary to aspirate the catheter to get an accurate volume of residual urine, especially if the bladder is hypotonic (that is, when the child is taking anticholinergic medication) or has been previously augmented with an intestinal segment because mucus from the segment may plug the catheter and impair drainage.

A small balloon catheter is passed into the rectum at this time to measure the intra-abdominal pressure during the cystometrogram to allow identification of artifacts of motion and monitoring of increases in abdominal pressure during filling and emptying of the bladder.[6] Uncontrolled detrusor (bladder muscle) contractions and straining to empty can be clearly differentiated by this maneuver (Fig. 20-1).

Before filling, a urethral pressure profile may be obtained by infusion of saline solution through the side-hole channel on the catheter at a rate of 2 ml/min as the catheter is withdrawn at a rate of 2 mm/sec.[7] Some urodynamicists advocate using a balloon or microtipped transducer catheter to measure urethral resistance.[8] When the maximum resistance is known, the catheter is positioned so that the urethral pressure port is located at that or any other point of interest. This area can be monitored throughout the urodynamic study. Urethral pressure profilometry (UPP) measures the passive resistance of a particular point

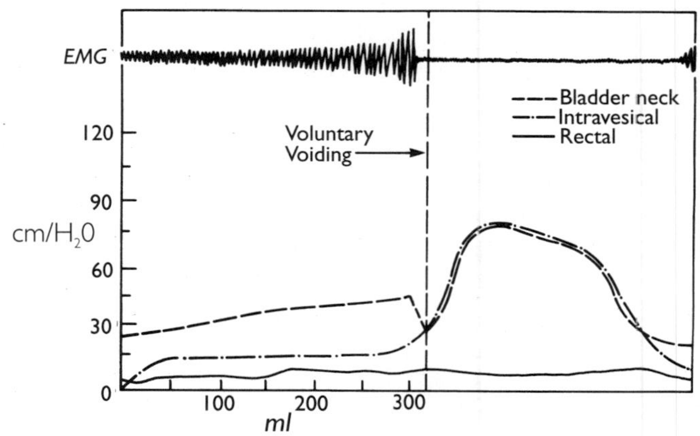

FIG. 20-1 *Normal lower urinary tract function. Interaction of intravesical, intraurethral, and rectal pressures and electromyographic activity (EMG) of the external sphincter during a micturition cycle.*

within the urethra to stretch.[9] Many factors contribute to this resistance including the elastic properties of the tissues surrounding the lumen and the tension generated by the smooth and skeletal muscles of the urethra, which are in a state of flux throughout the micturition cycle.[10,11] The static UPP is a measure of that resistance under one specific set of circumstances.[12] It may be fruitless and misleading to extrapolate data when one is obtaining a UPP while the bladder is empty and applying it to other conditions, that is, when (1) the bladder is full, (2) it responds to increases in abdominal pressure, or (3) emptying takes place.

External urethral sphincter electromyography (EMG) is recorded using a 24-gauge concentric needle electrode inserted perineally in males or paraurethrally in females and advanced into the skeletal muscle component of the sphincter until individual motor unit action potentials are seen or heard on a standard electromyographic recorder[13,14] (Fig. 20-2). EMLA cream applied 45 minutes before insertion of the electrode has greatly reduced the discomfort of this maneuver. Alternatively, perineal patch or wire electrodes placed the day before under anesthesia have been used to record the bioelectric activity in the sphincter. Needles are preferred over patch or wire[15,16] electrodes because of their greater accuracy for detecting denervation potentials and for recording dyssynergy (incoordination between the bladder and sphincter) during voiding in patients with a suspected neurologic condition. In addition, the intactness of sacral cord function is easily measured by observation of individual motor unit potentials when the patient is relaxed and the bladder is empty and by observation of responses to bulbocavernosus muscle and anal stimulation, Credé and Valsalva maneuvers, filling and emptying of the bladder, and voluntarily contraction and relaxation of the sphincter[17] (Fig. 20-3).

The rate of bladder filling per minute is set at 10% of the child's known or predicted capacity according to one of the following formulas: age [years] + 2 × 30 for children over 2 years,[18] or weight [kg] × 7 for those under the age of 2.[19] Ninety percent of children have bladder capacities that fall within these ranges. More rapid filling rates may yield falsely low levels of compliance and mask uninhibited contractions.[20,21] Other ways to achieve accurate measurements of compliance, hyperreflexia, and capacity include warming the saline to 37° C, employing even slower rates of filling,[22] asking the child to cough during filling, or diverting the child's attention by asking unrelated questions, reading a story, or showing a videotape cartoon.[23] We have found that uninhibited contractions are not suppressed when noxious stimuli are minimized.

The study is not considered complete unless the child urinates and voiding pressures are measured. The small size of the urodynamic catheter does not seem to adversely affect micturition pressures, even in the very young child. Normal voiding pressures in boys vary between 55 and 80 cm H_2O and in girls between 30 and 65 cm H_2O.[1,24,25] Occasionally it is difficult to get the child to void; patience, encouragement that it will not hurt, and a great deal of time are needed to accomplish this. Placing a bedpan under the buttocks in girls, having them assume a supine position or boys a standing position, or dripping tepid water on the genital area will often stimulate the child sufficiently to begin urination. Having the child listen to the audio channel of the EMG amplifier while he or she tightens and

A

B

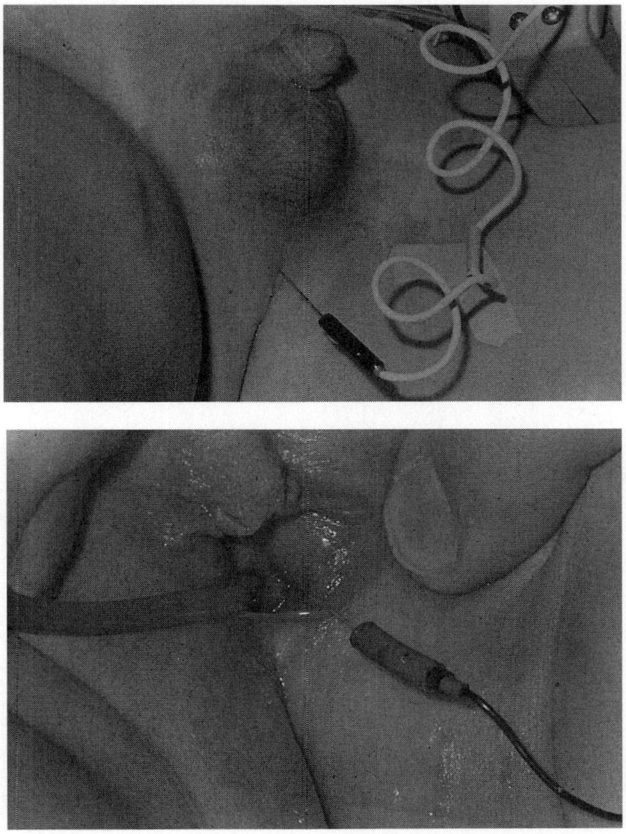

FIG. 20-2 *Placement of a concentric needle electrode to measure electromyographic activity of the external urethral sphincter is shown for* **A,** *males, and* **B,** *females.*

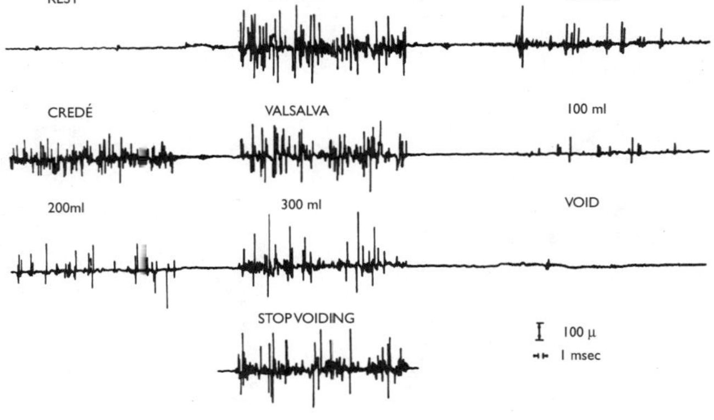

FIG. 20-3 *Normal external urethral sphincter electromyogram. Minimal activity is noted with the bladder empty. A complete interference pattern is seen with a bulbocavernosus (BC) reflex, cough, and Credé and Valsalva maneuvers. A gradual increase in electrical activity occurs with bladder filling. Voiding results in complete electrical silence. A command to stop voiding produces a complete interference pattern with cessation of the urine stream several seconds later.*

relaxes the sphincter provides a means of biofeedback training to get him or her to void. Once the child has voided, the following parameters are analyzed: the intensity and sustainability of the bladder contraction, the use of straining to facilitate emptying, the firing rate of the sphincter muscle, the appearance of after-contractions of the bladder, and the flow-rate characteristics.

Often it is appropriate to see the effects of drugs on the lower urinary tract, and so studies are repeated under similar circumstances several weeks to months later after medical therapy has been initiated. This is especially true when hypertonicity and hyperreflexia are being treated. To determine its maximal effect, the prescribed dose of the drug is taken 2 to 3 hours before the test is performed a second time. A list of commonly used drugs and their dosages is displayed in Table 20-1.

Conditions Appropriate for Urodynamic Studies

Neurospinal Dysraphisms

Myelomeningocele is the commonest cause of neurogenic bladder dysfunction in children. It stems from a failure of complete closure of the spinal canal by 35 days of gestation. The meningeal sac that protrudes from the surface of the back may or may not contain neural elements, thus producing a disease state that is highly variable in its extent of neurologic injury. Therefore urodynamic studies early in the neonatal period can provide information regarding the type of lower urinary tract function that is present, who is at risk for upper urinary tract decompensation over time if left untreated, and who is suffering from progressive neurologic deterioration when findings at this time are compared with subsequent studies[26-29] (see box). Studies are easy to perform in babies at this age because once the catheter and electrode are in place the child can be pacified with a bottle and often falls asleep.

It has been determined that certain patterns of dysfunction predispose the child to urinary tract deterioration[30] (Fig. 20-4). When bladder pressures rise steadily throughout the cystometrogram or reach levels above 40 cm H_2O later in filling, or the external urethral sphincter increases its activity later in filling and either remains very active or becomes even more active when the bladder contracts (at capacity), then reflux, hydronephrosis, and large residual urines leading to recurrent infection are likely to occur in more than 50% of affected indi-

Indications for Urodynamic Studies in Children with Myelodysplasia

NEWBORNS
Identifies who is at risk for urinary tract deterioration
Determines unequivocally who is showing signs of denervation on subsequent studies
REFLUX
Who needs clean intermittent catheterization
Who should be given anticholinergic medication
CONTINENCE
Helps select most suitable drug therapy
Assesses efficacy of drug therapy and alternatives if it is not
Determines necessity for augmentation cystoplasty
Small-capacity, poorly compliant bladder
Uncontrolled, uninhibited contractions
Directs the suitability of various bladder neck reconstructive procedures based on level of urethral resistance and sphincter innervation

Table 20-1 Drug Therapy in Neuropathic Bladder Dysfunction

Type	Minimum (mg/kg)	Maximum (mg/kg)
Cholinergic		
Bethanechol (Urecholine)	0.7 TID	0.8 QID
Anticholinergic		
Propantheline (Probanthine)	0.5 BID	0.5 QID
Oxybutynin (Ditropan)	0.2 BID	0.2 QID
Glycopyrrolate (Robinul)	0.01 BID	0.03 TID
Hyoscyamine (Levsin)	0.03 BID	0.1 QID
Sympathomimetic		
Phenylpropanolamine (alpha)	2.5 BID	2.5 TID
Ephedrine (alpha)	0.5 BID	1.0 TID
Pseudoephedrine (alpha)	0.4 BID	0.9 TID
Sympatholytic		
Prazosin (alpha)(Minipress)	0.05 BID	0.1 TID
Phenoxybenzamine (alpha)	0.3 BID	0.5 TID
Propanalol (beta)	0.25 BID	0.5 BID
Smooth muscle relaxant		
Flavoxate (Urispas)	3.0 BID	3.0 TID
Dicyclomine (Bentyl)	0.1 TID	0.3 TID
Other		
Imipramine (Tofranil)	0.7 BID	1.2 TID

alpha, Alpha-adrenergic receptor activity; *beta,* beta-adrenergic receptor activity.

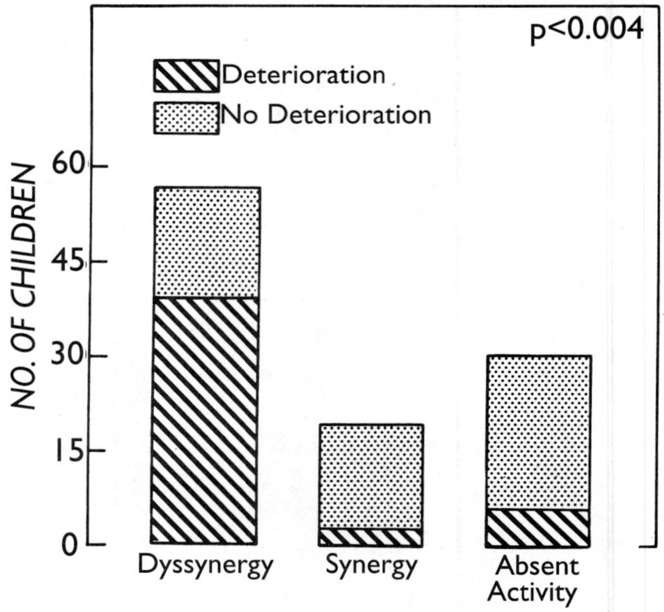

FIG. 20-4 *Urinary tract changes in relation to external urethral sphincter function in newborns with myelodysplasia. The incidence of deterioration in children with detrusor-sphincter dyssynergia is significantly higher than in those with synergy or absent activity (p <0.004).*

viduals.[26,28] This phenomenon has been labeled sphincter dyssynergy. Treating these children prophylactically with intermittent catheterization and anticholinergic medication, even in the newborn period when the urinary tract is normal radiologically, has prevented these changes from taking place. The incidence of deterioration has been reduced to a risk of less than 10%.[31]

It has been shown that a majority of newborns have bladder contractions and intact sacral reflex function, but in 15% there is progressive loss of function in the sphincter[32] (Fig. 20-5). This may take the form of an injury to peripheral nerve roots that innervate the sphincter with a lowering of urethral resistance and the development of incontinence, or interruption of communicating nerve pathways within the spinal cord to cause conversion of coordinated urethral sphincter activity to uncoordinated activity with a bladder contraction. The development of dyssynergy (uncoordinated sphincter activity) leads to the potential changes in urinary tract drainage alluded to above.

Children who have or develop vesicoureteral reflux should have urodynamic studies to determine the presence of hypertonic or hyperreflexic filling curves during cystometry and the necessity for anticholinergic therapy.[33] Fifty percent of children will resolve their reflux when treated with intermittent catheterization and anticholinergic medication.[34-36]

Continence is a paramount issue for these children and their parents as they grow and are mainstreamed in society. Although intermittent catheterization is the mainstay of initial treatment for incontinence, modulation of lower urinary tract function with appropriate drug therapy can be highly successful in achieving dryness. Therefore, before and sometimes after a specific drug is administered to achieve continence, a urodynamic study is performed to see its effect (Fig. 20-6). Specific drugs directed at reducing hypertonicity or hyperreflexia as well as medicines that increase bladder neck resistance by stimulating alpha-adrenergic receptor sites in this region are available. Failure to achieve continence necessitates surgical intervention, and the type of surgery (bladder enlargement or a bladder outlet procedure or both) is more easily dictated by the urodynamic findings than by any other test. As a result of these observations, a protocol has been devised for surveillance urodynamic studies in these children (Table 20-2).

Other causes of neurospinal dysraphism include all the "occult" types that are not associated with any specific syndromes: lipoma and lipomeningocele, diastematomyelia, dermal sinus, thickened filum terminale, or anterior meningocele. In 90% there is a lesion of the skin overlying the lower spinal column[37] (Fig. 20-7). Often urodynamic studies have shown that the lower extremities are totally unaffected while sacral cord function is impaired.[38,39] Magnetic resonance imaging invariably demon-

Table 20-2 Surveillance in Infants and Children with Myelodysplasia up to 5 Years of Age

SPHINCTER ACTIVITY	RECOMMENDED TESTS	FREQUENCY
Intact synergic	Postvoid residual	q 4 mo
	Intravenous pyelogram or renal ultrasonogram	q 12 mo
	Urodynamic study	q 12 mo
Intact dyssynergic*	Intravenous pyelogram or renal ultrasonogram	q 12 mo
	Urodynamic study	q 12 mo
	VCUG or RNC†	q 12 mo
Partial denervation	Postvoid residual	q 4 mo
	Intravenous pyelogram or renal ultrasonogram	q 12 mo
	Urodynamic study‡	q 12 mo
	VCUG or RNC†	q 12 mo
Complete denervation	Postvoid residual	q 6 mo
	Renal ultrasonogram	q 12 mo

*Patients receiving intermittent catheterization and anticholinergic agents.
†If detrusor hypertonicity or reflux already present.
‡Depending on degree of denervation.
RNC, Radionuclide cystogram; *UDS*, urodynamic study; *VCUG*, voiding cystourethrogram.

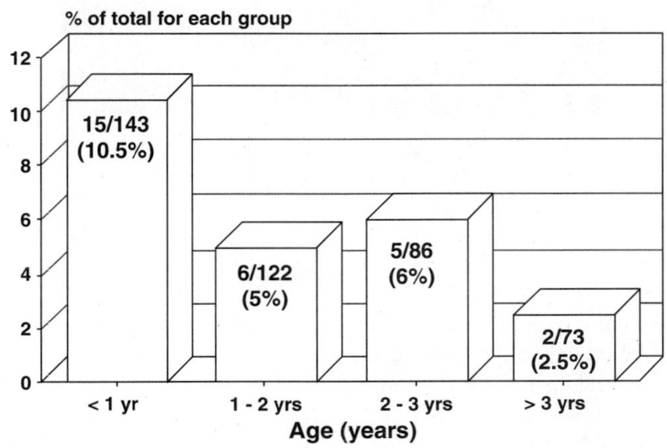

FIG. 20-5 *The incidence of deterioration in external urethral sphincter function in children with myelodysplasia in relation to increasing age.*

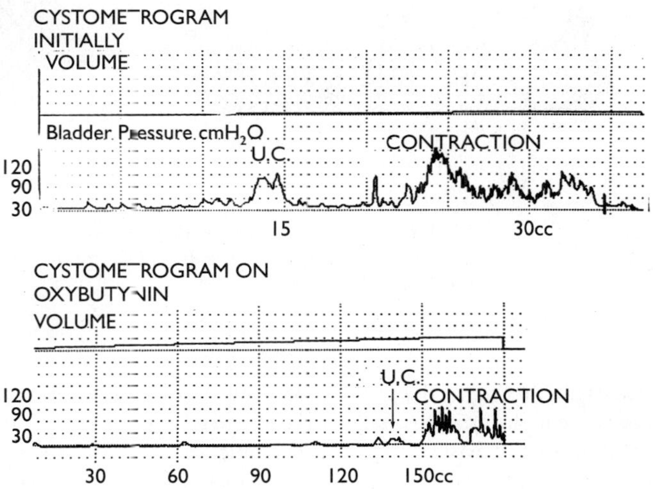

FIG. 20-6 *Oxybutynin HCl is very effective in abolishing uninhibited contractions (UC) and increasing bladder capacity in children with myelodysplasia who have this urodynamic picture.*

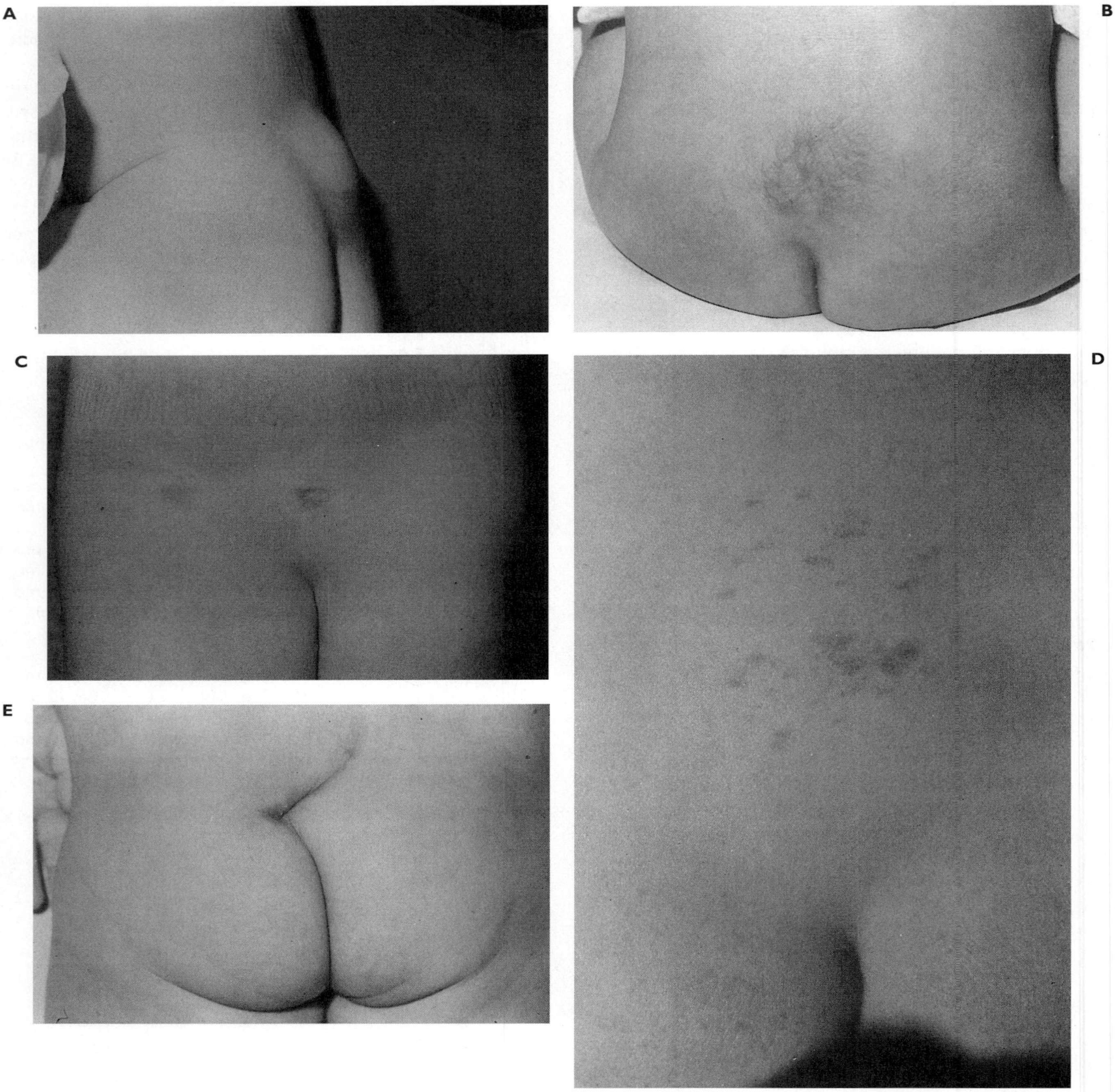

FIG. 20-7 *Common cutaneous manifestations of an occult spinal dysraphism that are present in over 90% of cases.* ***A,*** *Subcutaneous lipoma;* ***B,*** *hair patch;* ***C,*** *midline lumbosacral dimple;* ***D,*** *dermal vascular malformation;* ***E,*** *asymmetric gluteal cleft.*

strates a tethering of the spinal cord,[40] but functional studies of the nerve pathways potentially at risk are needed to determine if an abnormality exists. Thus a urodynamic investigation is warranted to delineate the extent of any dysfunction either initially or over time and to measure the response to treatment if the child undergoes an untethering procedure.[41] Studies are usually performed when the diagnosis is made, if the child does not toilet train at a reasonable age or has incontinence recur after a period of being dry or develops recurrent urinary infection.[42]

Sacral agenesis is a condition associated with the absence of one or more sacral vertebrae (Fig. 20-8). Motor and sensory function to the lower extremities is intact but motor function to the sacral cord is affected in 75%.[43] This pattern of denervation makes it difficult to diagnose in early infancy unless the clinician

A

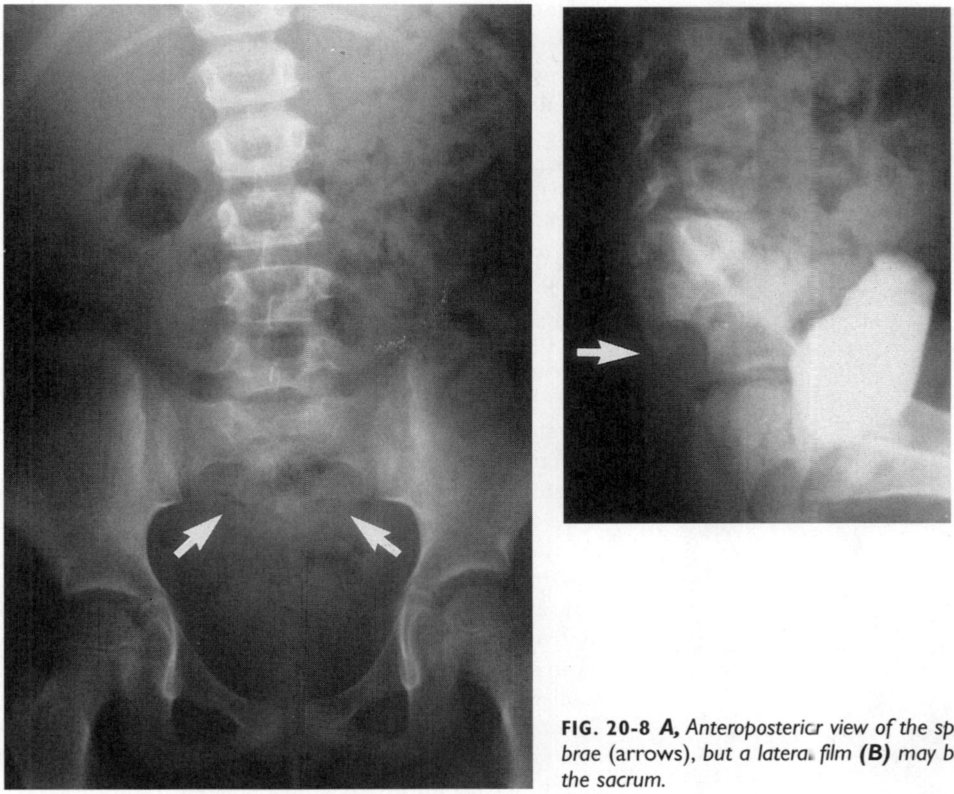

B

FIG. 20-8 ***A,*** *Anteroposterior view of the spine may show absence of sacral vertebrae* (arrows), *but a lateral film* ***(B)*** *may be more revealing if bowel gas obscures the sacrum.*

is sensitive to its cause. Insulin-dependent diabetic mothers have a 1% chance of having an affected child. One reliable pathognomonic sign is a low short gluteal cleft and flattened buttocks (Fig. 20-9). The type of lower urinary tract function varies between bladder hyperreflexia or areflexia and intact but dyssynergic versus complete denervation in the external sphincter.[44] The type of neurourologic picture present is independent of the number of affected vertebrae. This condition is not progressive over time.[45] Characterization of the lesion with urodynamic studies is mandatory to efficiently treat these affected children.

An occult spinal dysraphism may be associated with other abnormal conditions. Only recently has this come to light with the expanded use of magnetic resonance imaging.[46] Approximately 30% of children with imperforate anus[47,48] and 15% of babies with a sacrococcygeal teratoma[49] have a tethered cord. The development of incontinence in these children is more likely caused by this heretofore unrecognized condition than to any surgical procedure that was used to remove the tumor initially. The findings of an abnormality need to be confirmed, however, for accurate diagnosis and treatment of symptoms.

Central Nervous System Abnormalities

Cerebral palsy. Cerebral palsy is a condition that occurs as a result of a prenatal, natal, or early postnatal injury to the cerebral cortex from an anoxic episode such as apnea, infection, or seizure.[50-52] The resulting neuromuscular disorder is self-limited and may not become manifest until later in the child's development. Most children become continent, albeit at a later than usual age, but some never achieve dryness.[53] Urodynamic studies are indicated when children do not train at a reasonable age or have recurrent urinary infection. This is caused by bladder hyperreflexia that may need treatment with anticholinergic medication[54,55] (Table 20-3). The urethral sphincter is rarely denervated and usually reacts appropriately, being synergic (or coordinated) with a bladder contraction.[56]

Spinal cord injuries. Spinal cord injuries rarely occur in children, but when they do, they are usually the result of a sports injury or motor vehicle accident.[57,58] Some newborns suffer from cervical cord trauma when a forceps delivery produces a hyperextension injury.[59] Infants are prone to a hyperextension injury as well because the cervical spine acts as a fulcrum between the heavy cranium and the spine.[60]

In the early postinsult period the child needs to be treated with intermittent catheterization to empty the bladder on a regular basis.[61] However, once the neurologic condition stabilizes, urodynamic studies are a useful adjunct to determine if the child has coordinated bladder and urethral sphincter function during a detrusor contraction.[62,63] Residual urine volume after voiding is not a sufficient measure of function because the child may empty his or her bladder at high voiding pressures from bladder sphincter incoordination.[60] If there is coordinated or synergistic sphincter activity and normal voiding pressure, the child should be allowed to void on his or her own. However, if the pressure is high because of dyssynergy, then intermittent catheterization and anticholinergic medication or sometimes urethral sphinc-

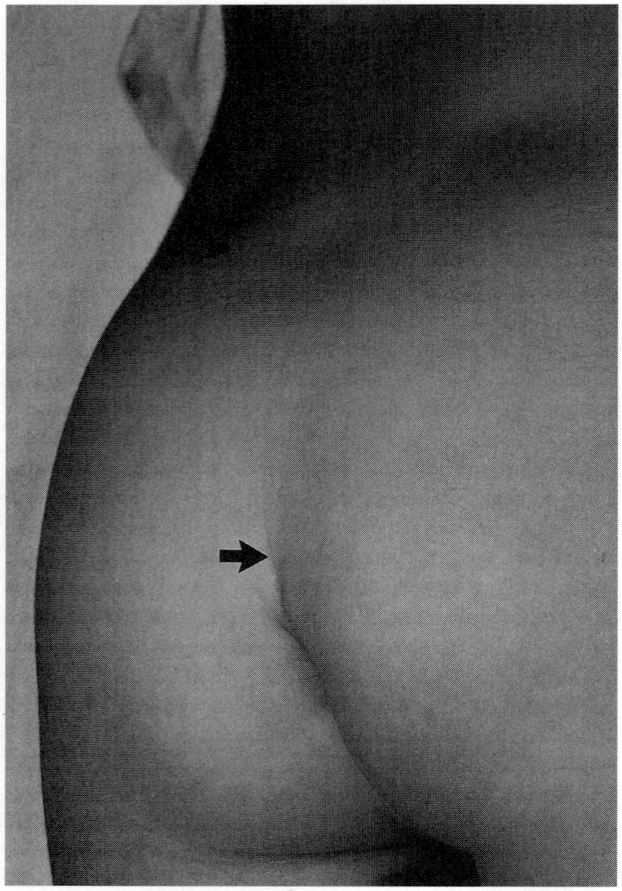

FIG. 20-9 *Pathognomonic sign of sacral agenesis is flattening of the buttocks with a low-lying or absent gluteal cleft* (arrow).

Table 20-3 Urodynamic Findings in Cerebral Palsy

UPPER MOTOR NEURON	
Uninhibited contractions	35
Detrusor sphincter dyssynergy	7
Hyperactive sacral reflexes	6
No voluntary control	3
Small capacity bladder	2
Hypertonia	2
LOWER MOTOR NEURON	
Excessive polyphasia	5
↑Amplitude + ↑duration potentials	4
Some had more than one finding	

terotomy should be undertaken.[61,64] Generally, it takes time for lower urinary tract function to stabilize after a spinal cord injury, and so waiting a period of 6 to 12 weeks after the insult may be needed before urodynamic studies can be performed. Periodic assessment of lower urinary tract function when dyssynergy is present is warranted to determine if continued catheterization and anticholinergic medication are necessary.[65]

Anatomic Abnormalities

Posterior urethral valves. Posterior urethral valves (PUV) are mucosal leaflets that arise from the verumontanum and extend distally toward the external sphincter. They billow and obstruct the flow of urine causing the bladder muscle to increase its contractile force in an attempt to empty (Fig. 20-10, *A*). Today, PUV are increasingly being diagnosed when prenatal ultrasonic screening demonstrates bilateral hydroureteronephrosis and postnatal imaging reveals the lesion.[66] Unless the kidneys are dilated and the bladder wall is thickened (Fig. 20-10, *B*), the diagnosis may not be evident at this time. The abnormality can remain undetected until urinary tract infection occurs or the boy has persistent day and night incontinence at an age when he should be dry, signs and symptoms that lead to a radiologic evaluation of the lower urinary tract.[67] In addition, boys with daytime incontinence over 5 years of age should undergo voiding cystography to determine the presence of PUV. On rare occasions, urinary retention may be the presenting sign.

Once a diagnosis of posterior urethral valves is made, transurethral resection of the valve leaflets is curative of the obstruction, but the bladder dysfunction that often accompanies it can persist for several months to years afterwards. Urodynamic studies are indicated when the voiding dysfunction that led to the diagnosis does not abate after a reasonable time after valve ablation, regardless of whether anticholinergic drugs have been administered, or hydroureteronephrosis that sometimes is noted with the valvular obstruction does not diminish.[68]

Urodynamic studies performed after valvular resection have revealed three patterns of bladder dysfunction: hyperreflexic, hypertonic, or myogenic failure[69,70] (Fig. 20-11). Hyperreflexia is a term that is used in this discussion of children that describes uninhibited detrusor contractions occurring before capacity is reached and a voiding contraction takes place. This term will be used to describe some patients who do not have overt neurologic disease as recommended by the International Continence Society. A hypertonic bladder is one in which the pressure within the bladder rises inexorably with the start of the cystometrogram or soon thereafter. Myogenic failure is the absence of a sustained bladder contraction at capacity so that the bladder fails to empty each time attempts are made to do so. This delineation of function may not be practical because it might be difficult to fit the bladder findings into a single discrete entity. Rather, the bladder dynamics may show a combination of patterns but with one type predominating. The boys with hyperreflexia or myogenic failure are likely to have incontinence as a predominant feature, whereas a hypertonic detrusor is most likely responsible for a dilated upper urinary tract.[69]

Treatment of the bladder dysfunction with anticholinergic medications is the first choice for patients with hyperreflexia or hypertonia, or both, whereas intermittent catheterization is necessary for those boys with myogenic failure. The use of anticholinergic drugs for the latter condition would only aggravate the ability to empty the bladder. Even after the administration of anticholinergic medication, urinary continence or hydronephrosis may not improve, and so urodynamic studies might be needed to determine the effect of this medication on detrusor function.[70,71]

A

B

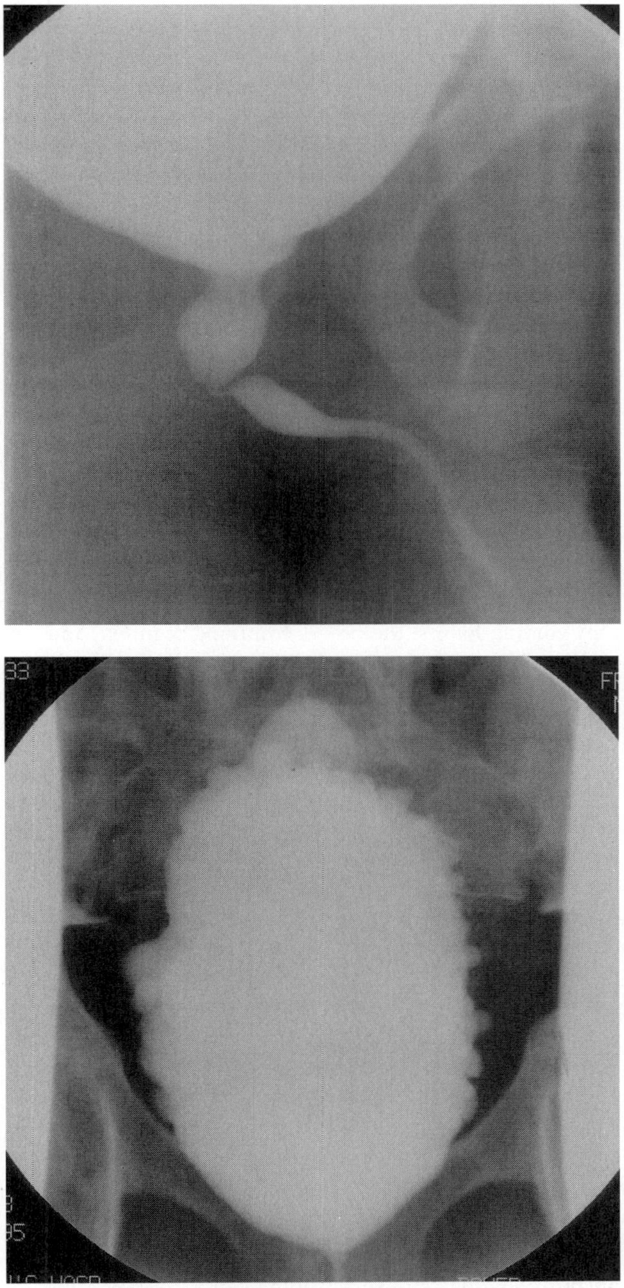

FIG. 20-10 *Posterior urethral valves are mucosal leaflets that emanate from the verumontanum and extend distally as they course anteriorly. Their obstructive effect leads to dilatation of the posterior urethra on the voiding phase of a cystogram,* ***A,*** *and possibly to profound trabeculation or hypertrophy of the bladder muscle as it attempts to overcome the increased resistance to flow in the urethra,* ***B.***

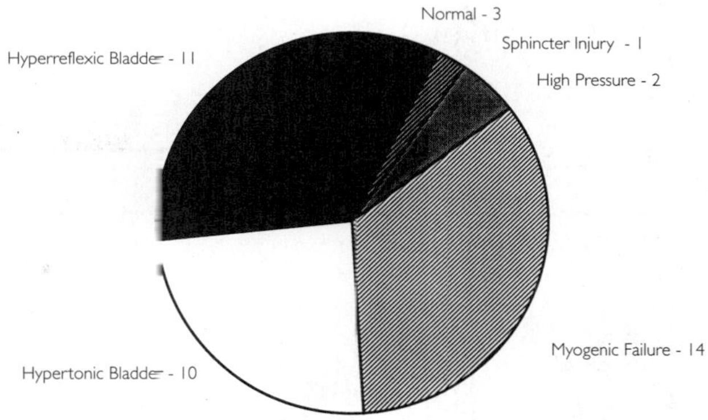

FIG. 20-11 *Profound changes in bladder muscle function can occur when posterior urethral valves are present.*

Functional Disorders

Recurrent Urinary Tract Infection

The urinary tract is the most common site for bacterial infection in childhood after the respiratory system. Five percent of all school-age girls are likely to get an infection before their teenage years. Most infections are easily treated, and the children usually become symptom free within a day or two. Some children with normal x-ray studies develop recurrent infection despite continuous antibiotics, or whenever they come off medication. A small number of children suffer from urgency, frequency, or incontinence even though their urine cultures become negative after a bout with infection. To determine if these children have a voiding-pattern abnormality as a cause for their recurrent urinary infection or persistent voiding symptoms, urodynamic studies may be needed.

Most children void four or five times a day and have bowel movements either daily or every other day.[72,73] When they void, there should be a steady stream of urine. However, some girls with recurrent infection may have an intermittent or staccato flow pattern[74] (Fig. 20-12). The interrupted flow is the result of either a tightening of the external sphincter or unsustained contractions of the bladder. This produces nonlaminar flow, and the eddy currents set up by this pattern of voiding leads to the ascension of bacteria at the meatus opening into the bladder[75,76] (Fig. 20-13). Failure to empty the bladder allows this inoculation of bacteria into the bladder to multiply and cause urinary tract infection.[77] Infrequent or incomplete emptying of the bladder may also lead to urinary infection even with a normal flow rate. In addition, recurrent urinary infection can affect how the detrusor muscle functions. Hyperreflexia is not an uncommon aftermath of infection because of irritability of the mucosa or submucosa from the inflammation.[76] Repeated infection with its attendant inflammatory process may produce a transmural inflammatory process that reduces the elasticity of the bladder wall and produces hypertonicity over time.[78]

Thus abnormal voiding patterns can either cause or develop from recurrent urinary infection. Despite careful questioning of a child about his or her bladder or bowel habits, it may be difficult to discern a pattern of voiding dysfunction unless urodynamic studies are performed.[75] Measuring the flow rate and its characteristics, determining the residual urine volume on catheterization of the bladder immediately afterwards, filling the bladder and observing the pressure responses of the detrusor to this maneuver, and denoting voluntary attempts at emptying provide a wealth of information regarding the causes of recurrent urinary infection in children.

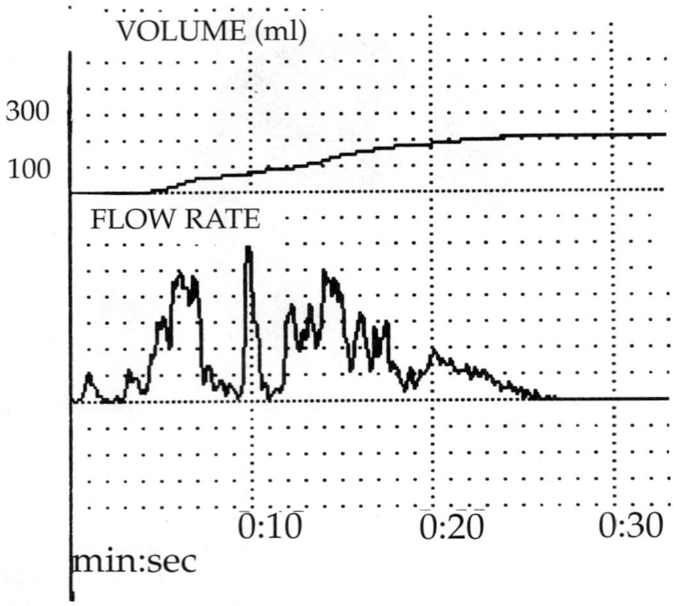

FIG. 20-12 *An intermittent or interrupted urinary flow rate can lead to recurrent urinary infection.*

Treatment is aimed at the specific pattern of dysfunction encountered. Infrequent or intermittent voiding is dealt with by encouragement of a regular schedule of emptying and relaxing the sphincter during urination.[79] Behavioral therapy and in some cases biofeedback training are necessary to achieve a normal voiding pattern.[76] Incomplete emptying can be managed after one asks the child to take sufficient time to empty and not rush from the toilet until he or she has completely emptied the bladder. Double and triple voiding may be used as well. Consistently high urine residuals might dictate the need to start clean intermittent catheterization to ensure complete emptying of the bladder. Even though it is done cleanly but not sterilely, urinary tract infection is not a common sequela because the bladder is emptied regularly. Once the child demonstrates the ability to empty with low residuals at the end of a voluntary void, the catheterization program may be discontinued with no long-term effects. Periodic reinforcement of appropriate toiletting habits may be necessary to ensure no further infection.

Urinary Incontinence

Most children show some if not a complete ability to control urination by 2½ to 3 years of age.[80] It is not unusual, however, to find that a substantial number of children are still wet at night beyond that age. For each year after that about 10% to 15% become totally trained at night so that less than 5% are still enuretic by the time they reach puberty.[81,82] Even this delay in achieving total control may not be pathologic, especially in children with a family history of enuresis that persisted until later childhood.[83] On the other hand, daytime incontinence beyond the start of school may be a sign of either abnormal function of the lower urinary tract or an anatomic abnormality. Voiding cystourethrography should be performed to exclude the latter, whereas urodynamic studies are needed to diagnose the former. As part of the urodynamic evaluation, a complete assessment of the child's past history needs delineation. This should include the mother's pregnancy, the events surrounding the child's birth and early postnatal period, his or her developmental milestones, the ease or difficulty in becoming toilet trained, the child's current voiding habits, the bowel-emptying regimen, and school and intellectual performance. A history of delayed training or enuresis in other family members should be sought. A careful neurologic examination including sensation, strength, tone and reflexes in the lower and upper extremities, perianal and perineal sensation, assessment of gait and fine motor coordination, and inspection of the lower spine are important components of the physical examination and must not be overlooked.

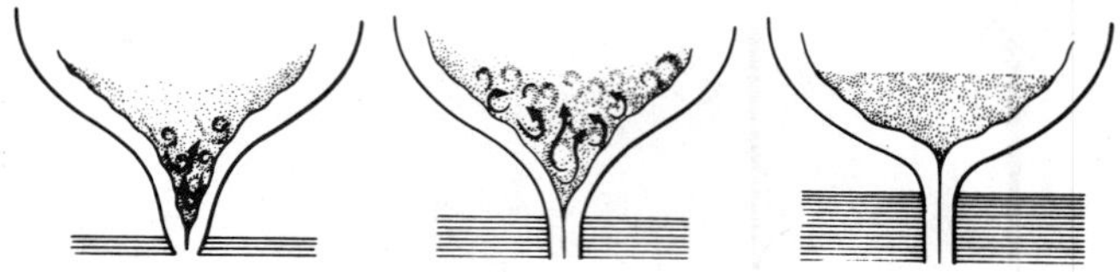

FIG. 20-13 *Eddy currents set up when the sphincter contracts (however evanescently), preventing the normal laminar flow of urine and allowing bacteria from the introitus to ascend into the bladder. If the child fails to empty his or her bladder, the residual urine acts as fertile ground for an infection to develop.*

Urodynamic studies in neurologically normal children who are incontinent has delineated four distinct patterns of dysfunction.[79] They have been labeled as follows: small-capacity hypertonic; hyperreflexic; hypotonic (lazy bladder syndrome); and nonneurogenic versus eurogenic (Hinman-Allen syndrome).

The small-capacity, hypertonic bladder is as its name implies. Although most commonly associated with recurrent infection, it may occur in children with an intense uncontrolled contraction relatively early in filling that leads to urinating despite the child's best efforts to prevent it by tightening the external urethral sphincter.[79] Over time, the detrusor muscle hypertrophies in response to the high outlet obstruction caused by the closed sphincter at the start of voiding.[78] The urodynamic study will show a small capacity, somewhat hypertonic filling curve, an uncontrolled high-pressure voiding contraction at a low filling volume, and a sphincter that does not relax but actually contracts during the early phase of micturition (Fig. 20-14).[75,76] Treatment with anticholinergic medication may resolve the condition if it is diagnosed before irreversible changes take place in the detrusor muscle. Biofeedback training to teach the child to relax his or her sphincter has also been helpful.

A hyperreflexic bladder is one that exhibits multiple small contractions during filling that the child may or may not be aware of. If the child does not recognize the occurrence of these contractions, there is relaxation of the sphincter muscle and leakage of urine until the child realizes he or she is wetting. Then the child stops the contraction by tightening the sphincter. If the child senses the contraction early enough (urgency), he or she tightens the sphincter in an attempt to stop it before they wet.

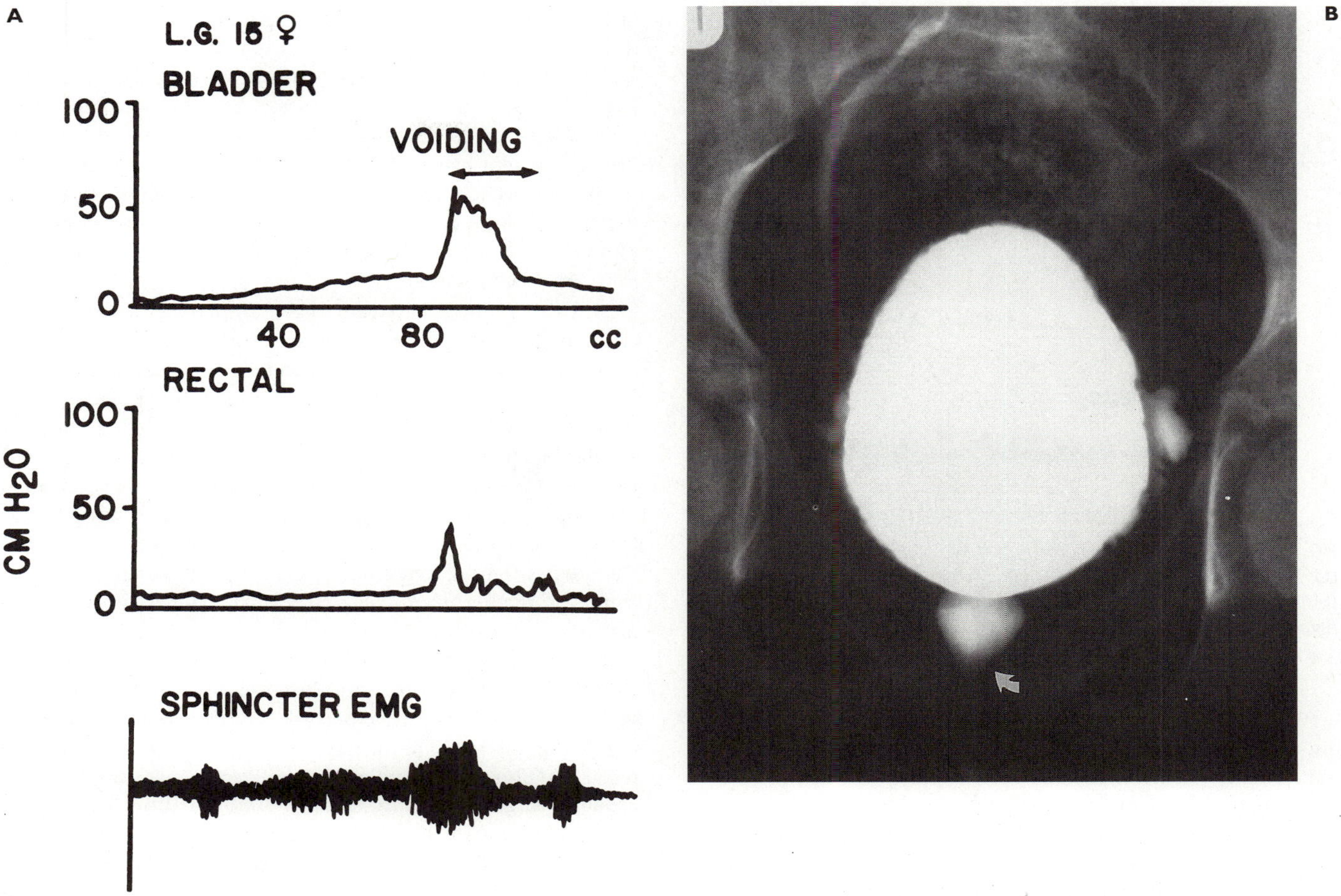

FIG. 20-14 *Fifteen-year-old girl with recurrent urinary infection had this urodynamic pattern of poor compliance (high filling pressure), small bladder capacity, and a highly active sphincter that failed to completely relax during voiding,* **A.** *Her voiding cystogram,* **B,** *revealed bladder trabeculation, multiple small diverticula, right reflux, and a functional narrowing of the urethra* (arrow) *secondary to increased electrical activity in the sphincter.*

When capacity is reached, these children void normally. They may experience urgency, frequency, or wetting despite normal micturition. It is not unusual for them to exhibit a characteristic squatting behavior, placing a heel in the perineum in an attempt to prevent wetting.[84] Once the sensation passes the child resumes his or her activities and eventually voluntarily voids when the bladder is full. This condition may be associated with recurrent urinary infection, which irritates the bladder and causes the instability, but most commonly it is seen in children who have a family history of enuresis.[85] It may also be seen in children who have suffered a perinatal insult that partially removes the central nervous system modulation of bladder function.

Urodynamic studies demonstrate low detrusor pressure but multiple small contractions of the bladder, especially during the early phase of filling.[79] At capacity there is a normal voiding contraction with normal pressure and complete emptying. If the sphincter muscle has been monitored during the study, there may be either a total relaxation or an increase in activity with the uninhibited contraction (depending on whether the child senses it) but complete silencing with voluntary voiding (Fig. 20-15).

Treatment is based on controlling the uninhibited contractions. Anticholinergic drugs are effective regardless of the cause. If urinary infection has occurred, antibiotics may need to be administered as well.

The hypotonic, or lazy, bladder syndrome is seen in children who make a conscious effort not to use the toilet. There are numerous reasons for this—parental mimicking, aversion to dirty places like bathrooms, or an adverse experience during toilet training that led to a fear with regard to using the toilet.[79] The behavior becomes a habit, and the bladder enlarges because of progressive loss of the sense of the need to void.[77] The children learn to relieve themselves only two or, at most, three times a day.[86] Their bowel-emptying regimen is similarly affected, and they become chronically constipated with bowel movements occurring about once or twice a week. This condition usually affects girls much more frequently than boys. It does not manifest itself before the onset of toilet training, and for this reason it is considered a learned or an acquired abnormality.

Urodynamic studies reveal several interesting findings.[79] The initial flow rate is often greatly interrupted with long periods

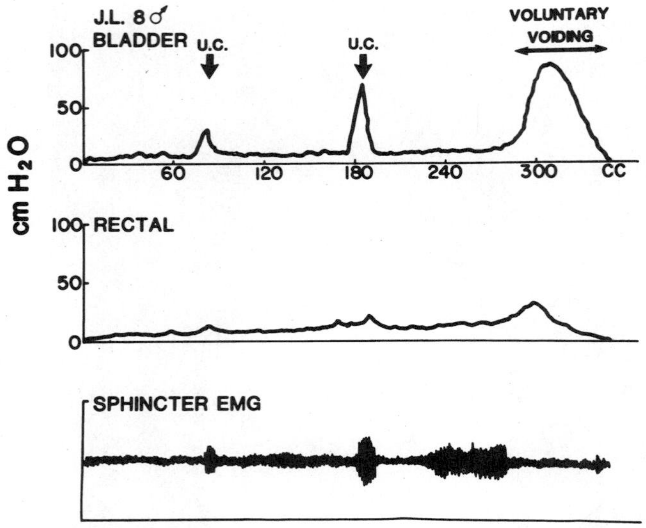

FIG. 20-15 *Hyperreflexia is characterized by uninhibited contractions (UC) of the bladder accompanied by a rise in electromyographic (EMG) activity of the external sphincter during filling but with a coordinated vesicourethral unit during voluntary voiding.*

between spurts of urine. The children will say they are finished, but when cajoled to void some more they are capable of urinating again. If one watches unobtrusively how the child urinates, straining or a Credé maneuver may be used to facilitate emptying. After the child has numerous encouragements to empty, the bladder will contain a sizable residual when catheterized. As the bladder is being filled, the child will not experience a desire to urinate until considerably more than the predicted volume of fluid has been instilled. Then the child might feel full and say he or she has to void. When voiding takes place, there may be either no contraction or an unsustained contraction of the bladder.[87] Detrusor pressures may seem normal or possibly high unless a rectal probe monitors intra-abdominal pressure as well, in order to obtain a subtracted or true intravesical pressure because voiding is usually enhanced by straining or even a Credé maneuver. The urethral sphincter muscle will remain quiet during voiding.

Studies in these children reveal normal kidneys and ureters by radiography or by ultrasonography, and a larger-than-normal capacity, smooth-walled bladder without reflux, but a large postvoid residual on voiding cystourethrography.[77]

Treatment is aimed at increasing the frequency of emptying both the bladder and the rectum. Setting up a schedule of regular emptying even though the child does not feel the urge to void and having a system of rewards for adhering to the program is a useful way to modify the child's behavior pattern.[88] Adjunctive therapy with cholinergic drugs may help to restore adequate bladder contractility to empty effectively. Occasionally, intermittent catheterization is needed to reduce very high residual urines and minimize recurrent infection. At the same time a program for emptying the bowels should be instituted because this improves the efficacy of treating each system alone.

The nonneurogenic, neurogenic bladder, or Hinman-Allen syndrome, is the most serious functional derangement of the lower urinary tract.[89,90] It is caused by a conscious contraction of the external urethral sphincter every time the child attempts to urinate.[91] This incoordination between the bladder and sphincter during voiding leads to very high voiding pressure, hypertrophy of the detrusor muscle, hydroureteronephrosis, high-pressure vesicoureteral reflux, large postvoid residual urine, recurrent urinary infection, and eventual renal failure. In the past it was believed that the cause was neurologic because of the characteristic appearance of the bladder on voiding cystography, but now it is believed to be a learned response to environmental factors.[79,92]

Affected children have remarkable similarities in the pattern of family dynamics.[92] The parents, especially the father, tend to be domineering, exacting, and intolerant of weakness or failure. Divorce and alcoholism are common threads that exacerbate the situation. Wetting is perceived as an immature, defiant, or purposeful behavior that the parents believe must be counteracted with stern reprimands manifesting as mental or physical punishments. The children often withdraw for fear of wetting and try to withhold urination and defecation by keeping the sphincter muscles tight.[79] Retention of urine and feces aggravates the condition further until severe structural changes appear in the urinary and gastrointestinal tracts.[93]

Urodynamic studies demonstrate a large-capacity poorly compliant bladder with uninhibited contractions and either high pressure or ineffective detrusor contractions during voiding[92] (Fig. 20-16). The urinary flow rate is intermittent as a result of failure of the external sphincter to relax, and there is usually a large postvoid residual. X-ray evaluation reveals profound changes in the urinary tract[79] (Fig. 20-17). Hydroureteronephrosis with pyelonephritic scarring from recurring infection is seen in two thirds of the children. Fifty percent have reflux. Nearly every one has a grossly trabeculated, large-capacity bladder. Voiding films show either persistent or intermittent narrowing in the region of the external urethral sphincter with a weak, thin stream beyond that point and a substantial postvoid residual at the end of voiding. A scout film before either the

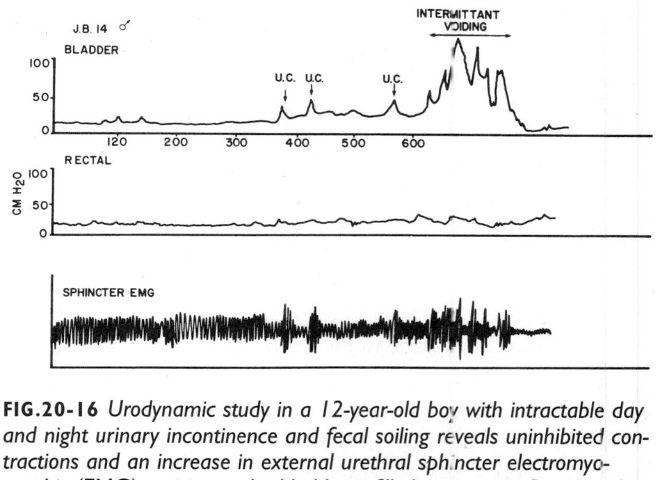

FIG.20-16 *Urodynamic study in a 12-year-old boy with intractable day and night urinary incontinence and fecal soiling reveals uninhibited contractions and an increase in external urethral sphincter electromyographic (EMG) activity as the bladder is filled to capacity. During voluntary voiding, high detrusor pressures (>100 cm H_2O) are generated from the increased EMG activity and only intermittent relaxation of the external sphincter.*

A

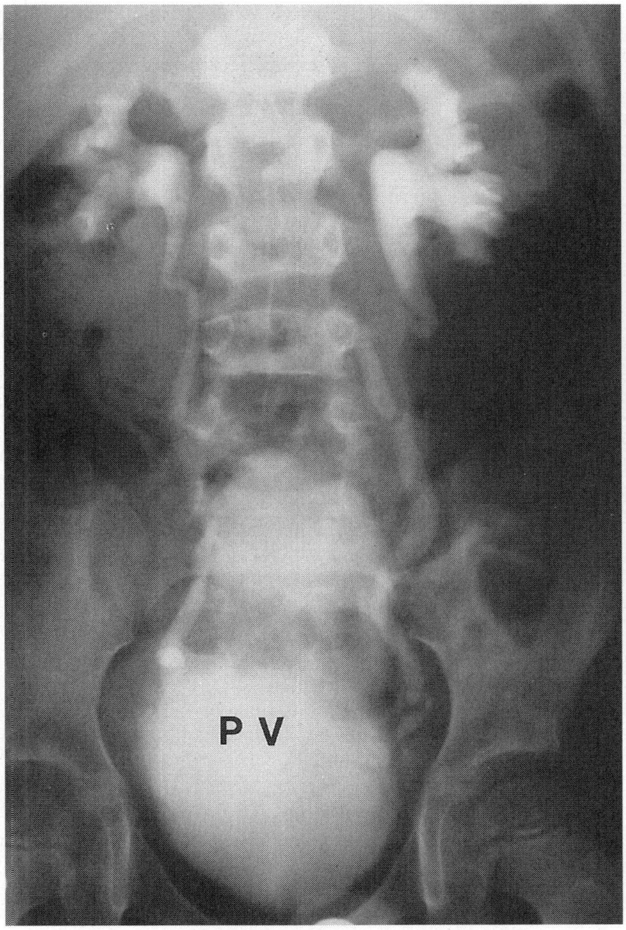

B

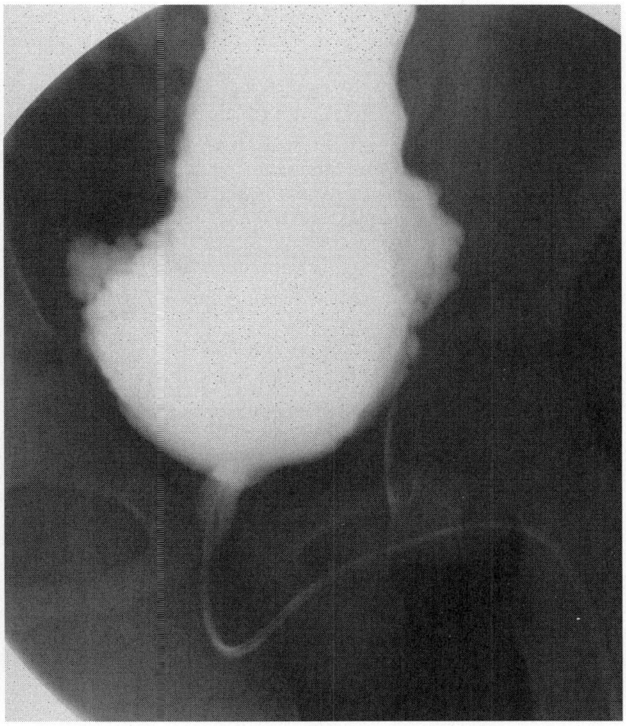

FIG. 20-17 *As a result, the child had substantial hydronephrosis and a large residual urine on excretory urography,* ***A.*** *PV, His voiding cystogram demonstrates narrowing in the region of the external sphincter and extensive trabeculation throughout the fundus of the bladder,* ***B.***

voiding cystogram or excretory urogram displays considerable fecal material in the colon consistent with chronic constipation.

Before the pathophysiologic characteristics of this "syndrome" were recognized, many children underwent multiple operations to improve emptying and correct reflux only to have these procedures fail. Consequently, urinary diversion was not an uncommon avenue for them to follow. Today, treatment is focused on alleviating the psychosocial pressures that contributed to the voiding dysfunction coupled with improving the child's ability to empty.[88] Psychotherapy is initiated to reeducate the child and his parents to tolerate the wetting (to an extent) and to eliminate punishments as a means of managing the problem. Biofeedback techniques to relax the sphincter during voiding along with a scheduled program of bladder emptying are instituted initially. Drug therapy may be added to either help control uninhibited contractions or increase contractility of the detrusor muscle. Intermittent catheterization may be needed in children who fail to respond or have renal failure that requires immediate decompression of their upper urinary tract.

References

1. Blaivas JG, Labib KB, Bauer SB, Retik AB: Changing concepts in the urodynamic evaluation of children, *J Urol* 117:777, 1977.
2. Blaivas JG: A critical appraisal of specific diagnostic techniques. In Krane RJ, Siroky MB, editors: *Clinical neurourology,* Boston, 1979, Little, Brown.
3. Bauer SB: Pediatric neurourology. In Krane RJ, Siroky MB, editors: *Clinical neurourology,* Boston, 1979, Little, Brown.
4. Bauer SB: Urodynamics in children: indications and methods. In Barrett DM, Wein AJ, editors: *Controversies in neuro-urology,* New York, 1983, Churchill Livingstone.
5. Ericsson ND, Hellström B, Negardth A, Rudhe U: Micturition urethrocystography in children with myelomeningocele, *Acta Radiol Diagn* 11:321, 1971.
6. Bates CP, Whiteside CG, Turner-Warwick RT: Synchronous cine/pressure/flow/cysto-urethrography with special reference to stress and urge incontinence, *Br J Urol* 42:714, 1970.
7. Yalla SV, Rossier AB, Fam B: Vesico-urethral pressure recordings in the assessment of neurogenic bladder functions in spinal cord injury patients, *Urol Int* 32:161, 1979.
8. Tanagho EA: Membrane and microtransducer catheters: their effectiveness for profilometry of the lower urinary tract, *Urol Clin North Am* 6:110, 1979.
9. Gleason DM, Reilly RJ, Bottacini MR, Pierce MJ: The urethral continence zone and its relation to stress incontinence, *J Urol* 112:81, 1974.
10. Abrams PH: Perfusion urethral profilometry, *Urol Clin North Am* 6:103, 1979.
11. Evans AT, Felker JR, Shank RA, Sugarman SR: Pitfalls of urodynamics, *J Urol* 122:220, 1979.

12. Yalla SV, Sharma GURK, Barsamian EM: Micturitional static urethral pressure profile method of recording urethral pressure profiles during voiding and implications, *J Urol* 124:649, 1980.
13. Diokno AC, Koff SA, Bender LF: Periurethral striated muscle activity in neurogenic bladder dysfunction, *J Urol* 112:743, 1974.
14. Blaivas JG, Labib KB, Bauer SB, Retik AB: A new approach to electromyography of the external urethral sphincter, *J Urol* 117:773, 1977.
15. Maizels M, Firlit CF: Pediatric urodynamics: clinical comparison of surface vs. needle pelvic floor/external sphincter electromyography, *J Urol* 122:518, 1979.
16. Koff SA, Kass EJ: Abdominal wall electromyography: a noninvasive technique to improve pediatric urodynamic accuracy, *J Urol* 127:736, 1982.
17. Blaivas JG: EMG: other uses. In Barrett DM, Wein AJ, editors: *Controversies in neuro-urology,* New York, 1979, Churchill Livingstone.
18. Koff SA: Estimating bladder capacity in children, *Urology* 21:248, 1983.
19. Fairhurst JJ, Rubin CME, Hyde I, et al: Bladder capacity in infants, *J Pediatr Surg* 26:55, 1991.
20. Scott FB, Quesada EM, Cardus D: Studies on the dynamics of micturition, *J Urol* 92:455, 1964.
21. Joseph DB: The effect of medium-fill and slow-fill cystometry on bladder pressure in infants and children with myelodysplasia, *J Urol* 147:444, 1992.
22. Kerr LA, Bauer SB, Staskin DR: Abnormal detrusor function precipitating hydronephrosis identified by extended voiding cystometry, *J Urol* 152:89, 1994.
23. Scott FB, Quesada EM, Cardus D: Studies on the dynamics of micturition, *J Urol* 92:455, 1964.
24. Gierup J, Ericsson NO, Okmain L: Micturition studies in infants and children, *Scand J Urol Nephrol* 3:1, 1969.
25. Blaivas JG: A critical appraisal of specific diagnostic techniques. In Krane RJ, Siroky MB, editors, *Clinical neurourology,* Boston, 1979, Little, Brown.
26. Bauer SB, Hallet M, Khoshbin S, et al: The predictive value of urodynamic evaluation in the newborn with myelodysplasia, *JAMA* 152:650, 1984.
27. McGuire EJ, Woodside JR, Borden TA, Weiss RM: The prognostic value of urodynamic testing in myelodysplastic patients, *J Urol* 126:205, 1981.
28. Sidi AA, Dykstra DD, Gonzalez R: The value of urodynamic testing in the management of neonates with myelodysplasia: a prospective study, *J Urol* 135:90, 1986.
29. Kaufman AM, Roberts AC, Rudy DC, et al: Decreased bladder compliance in myelomeningocele patients managed by radiologic observation, Presented at annual meeting of American Urological Association, Las Vegas, April 24, 1995, abstract 199.
30. Perez LM, Khoury J, Webster GD: The value of urodynamic studies in infants less than one year old with congenital spinal dysraphism, *J Urol* 148:584, 1992.
31. Edelstein RA, Bauer SB, Kelly MD, et al: The long-term urologic response of neonates with myelodysplasia treated proactively with intermittent catheterization and anticholinergic therapy, *J Urol* 154:1500-1504, 1995.
32. Lais A, Kasabian NG, Dyro FM, et al: Neurosurgical implications of continuous neuro-urological surveillance of children with myelodysplasia, *J Urol* 150:1879-1883, 1993.
33. Flood HD, Ritchey ML, Bloom DA, et al: Outcome of reflux in children with myelodysplasia managed by bladder pressure monitoring, *J Urol* 152:1574, 1994.
34. Kass EJ, Koff SA, Lapides J: Fate of vesico-ureteral reflux in children with neuropathic bladders managed by intermittent catheterization, *J Urol* 125:63, 1981.
35. Bauer SB: Myelodysplasia: newborn evaluation and management. In McLaurin RL, editor: *Spina bifida: a multidisciplinary approach,* New York, 1984, Praeger.
36. Joseph DB, Bauer SB, Colodny AH, et al: Clean intermittent catheterization in infants with neurogenic bladder, *Pediatrics* 84:78, 1989.
37. Anderson FM: Occult spinal dysraphism: a series of 73 cases, *Pediatrics* 55:826, 1975.
38. Keating MA, Rink RC, Bauer SB, et al: Neuro-urologic implications of changing approach in managment of occult spinal lesions, *J Urol* 140:1299, 1988.
39. Foster LS, Kogan BA, Cogan PH, Edwards MSB: Bladder function in patients with lipomyelomeningocele, *J Urol* 143:984, 1990.
40. Tracey PT, Hanigan WC: Spinal dysraphism: use of magnetic resonance imaging in evaluation, *Clin Pediatr* 29:228, 1990.
41. Satar N, Bauer SB, Shefner J, et al: The effects of delayed diagnosis and treatment in patients with an occult spinal dysraphism, *J Urol* 154(2pt2):754-758, 1995.
42. Mandell J, Bauer SB, Hallett M, et al: Occult spinal dysraphism: a rare but detectable cause of voiding dysfunction, *Urol Clin North Am* 7:349, 1980.
43. Schlussel RN, Bauer SB, Kelly MD, et al: The clinical and urodynamic findings in 35 patients with sacral agenesis, Presented at annual meeting of American Urological Association, San Francisco, May 16, 1994, abstract 412.
44. Guzman L, Bauer SB, Hallett M, et al: The evaluation and management of children with sacral agenesis, *Urology* 23:506, 1983.
45. Boemers TM, van Gool JD, de Jong TPVM, Bax KMA: Urodynamic evaluation of children with caudal regression syndrome (caudal dysplasia sequence), *J Urol* 151:1038-1041, 1994.
46. Rivosecchi M, Lucchetti MC, Zaccara A, et al: Spinal dysraphism detected by magnetic resonance imaging in patients with anorectal anomalies: incidence and clinical significance, *J Pediatr Surg* 30:488-490, 1995.
47. Greenfield SP, Fera M: Urodynamic evaluation of the patient with imperforate anus: a prospective study, *J Urol* 146:539, 1991.
48. Kakizaki H, Nonomura K, Asano Y, et al: Preexisting neurogenic voiding dysfunction in children with imperforate anus: problems in management, *J Urol* 151:1041-1044, 1994.
49. Boemers TM, van Gool JD, de Jong TPVM, Bax KMA: Lower urinary tract dysfunction in children with benign sacrococcygeal teratoma, *J Urol* 151:174, 1994.
50. Kuban KCK, Levitton A: Cerebral palsy, *N Engl J Med* 330:188-195, 1994.
51. Nelson KB, Ellenberg JH: Antecedents of cerebral palsy, *N Engl J Med* 315:81, 1986.
52. Naeye RL, Peters EC, Bartholomew M, Landis R: Origins of cerebral palsy, *Am J Dis Child* 143:1154, 1989.
53. McNeal DM, Hawtrey CE, Wolraich ML, Mapel JR: Symptomatic neurogenic bladder in a cerebral-palsied population, *Dev Med Child Neurol* 25:612, 1983.
54. Mayo ME: Lower urinary tract dysfunction in cerebral palsy, *J Urol* 147:419-420, 1992.
55. Reid CJD, Borzyskowski M: Lower urinary tract dysfunction in cerebral palsy, *Arch Dis Child* 68:739-742, 1993.
56. Decter RM, Bauer SB, Khoshbin S, et al: Urodynamic assessment of children with cerebral palsy, *J Urol* 138:1110, 1987.
57. Cass AS, Luxenberg M, Johnson CF, Gleich P: Management of the neurogenic bladder in 413 children, *J Urol* 132:521, 1984.
58. Hadley MN, Zabramski JM, Browner CM, et al: Pediatric spinal trauma: review of 122 cases of spinal cord and vertebral column injuries, *J Neurosurg* 68:18-24, 1988.
59. Lanska MJ, Roessmann U, Wiznitzer M: Magnetic resonance imaging in cervical cord birth injury, *Pediatrics* 85:760, 1990.
60. Decter RM, Bauer SB: Urologic management of spinal cord injury in children, *Urol Clin North Am* 20:475-483, 1993.
61. Barkin M, Dolfin D, Herschorn S, et al: The urologic care of the spinal cord injury patient, *J Urol* 129:335, 1983.
62. Iwatsubo E, Iwakawa A, Koga H, et al: Functional recovery of the bladder in patients with spinal cord injury: prognosticating programs of an aseptic intermittent catheterization, *Acta Urol Japonica* 31:775, 1985.

63. Fanciullacci F, Zanollo A, Sandri S, Catanzaro F: The neuropathic bladder in children with spinal cord injury, *Paraplegia* 26:83, 1988.
64. Donnelly J, Hackler RH, Bunts RC: Present urologic status of the World War II paraplegic: 25-year follow-up comparison with status of the 20-year Korean War paraplegic and 5-year Vietnam paraplegic, *J Urol* 108:558, 1972.
65. Ogawa T, Yoshida T, Fujinaga T: Bladder deformity in traumatic spinal cord injury patients, *Acta Urol Japonica* 34:1173, 1988.
66. Scott JE: Management of congenital posterior urethral valves, *Br J Urol* 57:71, 1985.
67. Gonzales ET: Posterior urethral valves and other urethral anomalies. In Walsh PC, Gittes R, Perlmutter A, Stamey T, editors: *Campbell's urology,* Philadelphia, 1992, Saunders.
68. Kaefer M, Keating MA, Adams MC, Rink RC: Posterior urethral valves, pressure pop-offs and bladder function, *J Urol* 154:708-711, 1995.
69. Peters CA, Bolkier M, Bauer SB, et al: The urodynamic consequences of posterior urethral valves, *J Urol* 144:122, 1990.
70. Holmdall G, Sillen U, Bachelard M, et al: The changing urodynamic pattern in valve bladders during infancy, *J Urol* 153:463-67, 1995.
71. Glassberg K: Persistent ureteral dilatation following valve resection, *Dialogues in Pediatr Urol* 5:4, 1982.
72. Weaver LT, Steiner H: The bowel habits of young children, *Arch Dis Child* 59:649, 1984.
73. Bloom DA, Seeley WW, Ritchey ML, McGuire EJ: Toilet habits and continence in children: an opportunity sampling in search of normal parameters, *J Urol* 149:1087-1090, 1993.
74. Tanagho EA, Miller EA, Lyon RP: Spastic striated external sphincter and urinary tract infection in girls, *Br J Urol* 43:69, 1971.
75. van Gool JD, Tanagho EA: External sphincter activity and recurrent urinary tract infection in girls, *Urology* 10:348, 1977.
76. Hansson S, Hjälmas K, Jodal U, Sixt R: Lower urinary tract dysfunction in girls with untreated asymptomatic or covert bacteriuria, *J Urol* 143:333, 1990.
77. Webster GD, Koefoot RB, Sihelnik S: Urodynamic abnormalities in neurologically normal children with micturition dysfunction, *J Urol* 132:74, 1984.
78. Mayo ME, Burns MW: Urodynamic studies in children who wet, *Br J Urol* 65:641, 1990.
79. Bauer SB, Retik AB, Colodny AH, et al: The unstable bladder of childhood, *Urol Clin North Am* 7:321, 1980.
80. Yeats WK: Bladder function in normal micturition. In Kolvin I, MacKeith RC, Meadow SR, editors: *Bladder control and enuresis,* Philadelphia, 1973, Lippincott.
81. Bellman N: Encopresis, *Acta Paediatr Scand* 70(suppl 1):1, 1966.
82. Fergusson DM, Hons BA, Horwood LJ, Shannon FT: Factors related to the age of attainment of nocturnal bladder control: an eight year longitudinal study, *Pediatrics* 78:884, 1986.
83. MacKeith RL, Meadow SR, Turner RK: How children become dry. In Kolvin I, MacKeith RL, Meadow SR, editors: *Bladder control and enuresis,* Philadelphia, 1973, Lippincott.
84. Kondo A, Kobayashi M, Otani T, et al: Children with unstable bladder: clinical and urodynamic observation, *J Urol* 129:88, 1983.
85. Torrens MJ, Collins CD: The urodynamic assessment of adult enuresis, *Br J Urol* 47:433, 1975.
86. DeLuca FG, Swenson O, Fisher JH, Loutfi AH: The dysfunctional "lazy" bladder syndrome in children, *Arch Dis Child* 37:117, 1962.
87. Koefoot RB, Webster GD, Anderson EE, Glenn JF: The primary megacystis syndrome, *J Urol* 125:232, 1981.
88. Masek BJ: Behavioral management of voiding dysfunction in neurologically normal children, *Dialogues in Pediatr Urol* 8:7, 1985.
89. Hinman F: Urinary tract damage in children who wet, *Pediatrics* 54:142, 1974.
90. Hinman F: Non-neurogenic bladder (the Hinman Syndrome) fifteen years later, *J Urol* 136:769, 1986.
91. Allen TD: The non-neurogenic bladder, *J Urol* 117:232, 1977.
92. Allen TD, Bright TC: Urodynamic patterns in children with dysfunctional voiding problems, *J Urol* 119:247, 1978.
93. Williams DI, Hirst G, Doyle D: The occult neuropathic bladder, *J Pediatr Surg* 9:35, 1975.

Chapter 21

Enuresis

Curtis A. Sheldon, Jeffrey Wacksman

I knew that bedwetting was a) wicked and b) outside of my control. . . . It was therefore possible to sin without knowing you committed it, without wanting to commit it, and without being able to avoid it. . . . The double beating was a turning point for it brought home to me for the first time the harshness of the environment into which I had been flung. . . had a conviction of sin and folly and weakness such as I don't remember to have had before.

George Orwell in Moffatt[1]

Enuresis is a nonspecific term referring to the involuntary passage of urine. Diurnal enuresis refers to incontinence during the day. By contrast, nocturnal enuresis involves wetting at night, or bedwetting. Generally, however, this term denotes incontinence occurring during sleep. It is important for the caregiver to realize that children with nocturnal enuresis often wet in the daytime during naps and should not be labeled as having diurnal enuresis on this basis alone. Children with primary enuresis have never developed urinary control. There has been no significant interval of consistent continence. In contrast, children with secondary enuresis have had a significant, consistent dry interval, usually at least 6 months in duration. Nocturnal enuresis is generally defined as sleepwetting occurring more than twice monthly in a child over 5 years of age.

Enuresis is a symptom and is not itself a disease. Multiple causes may be identified (Fig. 21-1). More than one cause is

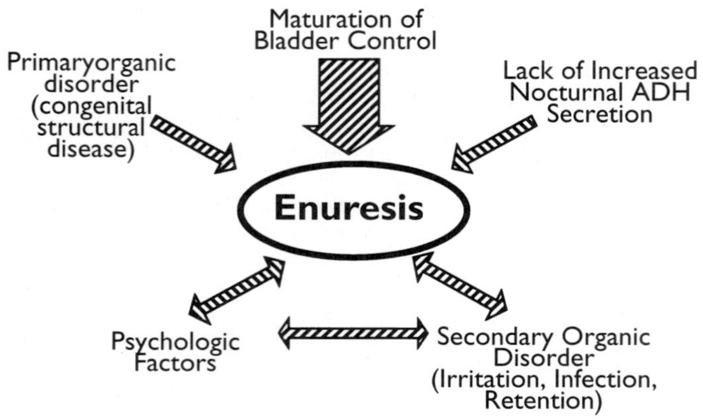

FIG. 21-1 *Multiple etiologies may interact and contribute to the genesis enuresis.*

often operative in any given patient. Further, there may be multiple conditions or factors that facilitate the pathogenesis of this symptom complex. Despite the frequency of this diagnosis, the cause and pathophysiologic characteristics remains incompletely understood. Review of available data raises several unanswered questions. Given the refractory nature of some cases and the high incidence of relapse after successful medical control, why is the spontaneous resolution rate so high? Why do some controlled therapeutic trials reveal such a high placebo response rate? Why do studies reveal such dramatically divergent success rates for virtually all commonly employed therapeutic modalities? Why is there such a high relapse rate associated with such modalities as pharmacologic agents and alarm conditioning despite often rather prompt and complete initial symptomatic control? It is important to be cognizant of these observations because they relate strongly to many of the misconceptions that envelope this entity.

SOCIAL SIGNIFICANCE

Enuresis is often given a very low priority by health care professionals. The importance of bedwetting to the family, however, is indicated by the fact that only 5.2% of parents surveyed by Haque did not seek some form of intervention.[2] Additionally, it is imperative for the caregiver to be aware that there is often a significant difference in attitude regarding the significance of enuresis between the child, the child's parents, and the child's physicians.[2] Parents tend to believe that their children should become dry at an earlier age than physicians regard as normal. In contrast, only 63% of parents believe that medical therapy is appropriate for enuresis, whereas over 90% of physicians believe that medical therapy is appropriate. Further, in contrast to physicians, over a third of parents believe that enuresis is an emotional problem rather than one having a physical or physiologic basis.

Although enuresis is often considered a nuisance by the medical community or at least produces a diagnosis that warrants a low degree of medical concern, the effect on the family and the life of the child can be intense, even precipitating abusive relationships. The anxiety associated with enuresis is underscored by a rather morbid history of management that has embraced painful punishment, public humiliation, and even urethral occlusion.

The history of enuresis has been reviewed by Glicklich.[3] Its treatment was addressed in medical texts dated as early as 1550 B.C. One of the earliest texts devoted to pediatrics in the English literature was published in 1544 by Thomas Phaer, entitled *Boke of Children*; contained therein was a section labeled "Of pyssying in the bedde."

In addition to public humiliation and beating, primitive concoctions involving not only a variety of plants but even such extreme substances as the comb of a cock, the testicle of a hare, the lung of a kid, the bladder of a sow, and the cerebrum of a hare testify to the influence of this symptom complex throughout history. The application of painful "blisters" to the sacrum or genitalia was employed, as were urethral occlusion techniques. Cauterization of the urethral orifice with silver nitrate and chromic acid was also employed. Further, urethral dilatation and circumcision were prescribed for the treatment of enuresis.

Urethral occlusion techniques included the inflation of a "rubber bag" within the vagina of a little girl and the application of collodion to the meatus or penile constriction in little boys. At least two instances of penile amputation complicating the latter technique have been documented. Some attempted to prevent the child from sleeping in a supine position by applying "blisters" to the sacrum or by the attachment of instruments that applied pain (as by steel spikes) when the child laid supine.

The more modern era of therapy was ushered in by the availability of various medications, such as belladonna and a chlorhydrate, and early alarm devices. Such alarm devices employed a soluble substance to detect an enuretic episode by dissolving and triggering a blast of cold water or air or the unwinding of a twisted strip of rubber as the awakening stimulus. With the development of electricity, urine as an electrical conductor to complete a circuit became the detector and a bell became the stimulus. Unfortunately, so also did an electrical shock.

The incidence of both diurnal and nocturnal enuresis varies dramatically with age.[4-9] Fig. 21-2 demonstrates the prevalence of both daytime and nighttime wetting as a function of age.[5] The prevalence of diurnal enuresis declines most rapidly. Of note is the observation that beyond the age of maturation (4 years) a high spontaneous cure rate for nocturnal enuresis is evident. Forsythe documented this rate at 14% to 16% per year.[9] A slight prolongation to the attainment of dryness has been documented in the male, the white, and the low-birth weight child.[5]

The actual development of urinary control remains incompletely understood. The newborn bladder functions by reflex voiding, emptying approximately 20 times daily.[10] Several stages have been identified through which most children proceed during the first 3 years of life.[11,12] With age, a progressive increase in bladder capacity is demonstrated[13] (Fig. 21-3). With time, the child develops a conscious sensation of bladder filling. Subsequently volitional control of periurethral striated muscle is attained, and, finally, volitional control over the spinal micturition reflex itself is achieved so that bladder contraction can be inhibited. Generally, children have developed the necessary components for an adult pattern of control by 4 years of age.[14]

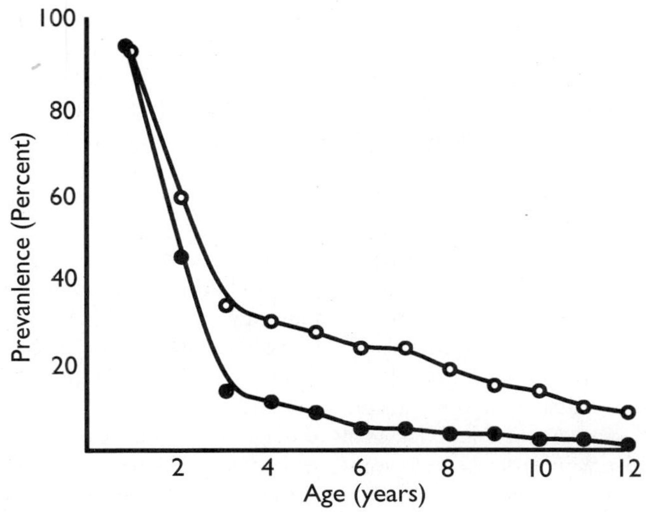

FIG. 21-2 *Prevalence of daytime and nighttime wetting as a function of age.* (From Oppel WC, Harper PA, Rider RV: *Pediatrics* 42:614-626, 1968.)

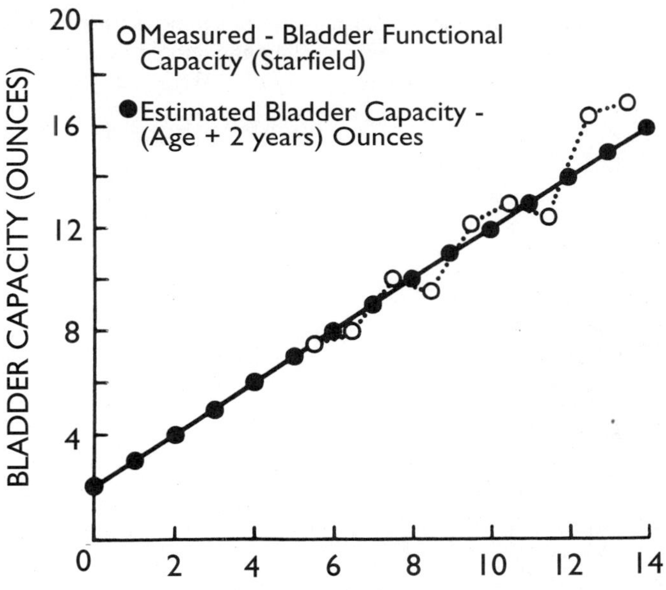

FIG. 21-3 *Age-related increment in bladder capacity.*

Whereas control of bowel continence is achieved by the age range of 18 to 24 months, bladder control during the day is reached at a median age of 4 years, and bladder control during the night is achieved at a median age of 4.5 years.

ETIOLOGY

The major causes proposed for enuresis are listed in the box at right. That delayed maturation of bladder control is important in the pathogenesis of enuresis is suggested by the high incidence of spontaneous resolution of this symptom. This cause has numerous advocates.[15-19] Further, the sequence of resolution is the same in the enuretic child as in the normal child. Most commonly, daytime control is followed by the subsequent attainment of nighttime control. Further, a reduced functional (not structural) bladder capacity has been documented in enuretics. Urodynamically documented bladder instability may be seen but is more frequent if there is a significant component of daytime symptoms.

Without question, developmental delay can play a role in some children.[20-22] This is suggested by the strong correlation between the general developmental level of such children and their age of attainment of control of urine. Additionally, environmental stress and socioeconomic level have epidemiologically been correlated with the risk of enuresis and are believed to be contributory to developmental delay in some children.

Lack of normal nocturnal excretion of antidiuretic hormone (ADH) has been documented in some enuretics compared to controls.[23-25] This loss of normal circadian variation in ADH excretion has been associated with a higher mean nocturnal urinary volume and a lower mean nocturnal urine osmolality. Although some have attributed enuresis to a sleep disorder, enuretic episodes appear to be independent of electroencephalographically identifiable sleep stages. Further, the sleep patterns in enuretics are not significantly different from those identified in normal controls.[26] Similarly, psychologic factors have been implicated and are certainly contributory in some instances. There is, however, no consistent evidence to support an increased incidence of significant psychopathologic states in children with enuresis or in adults who had childhood enuresis.[27,28] In addition, nocturnal enuresis is a significant stressor to children, and its resolution is demonstrated to be associated with a considerable increase in self-esteem. Consequently, it is not surprising that it may be associated with various behavioral abnormalities. Evidence for true psychologic disturbance is restricted to the occasional patient.[1]

As demonstrated in Fig. 21-4, there is an extremely strong genetic input into the pathogenesis of enuresis.[30] In this study, children where neither parent was enuretic had only a 15% risk of enuresis. If one parent was enuretic, this risk rose to 44%. If both parents were enuretic, this risk rose further to 77%. Additional evidence for a strong genetic influence is suggested by twin studies in which dizygotic twins of enuretic children have a 36% rate of enuresis as contrasted to monozygotic twins in which the incidence is 68%.

Proposed Pathophysiologic Characteristics of and Contributing Factors for Enuresis

- Delayed maturation of bladder control
- Developmental delay
- Abnormal nocturnal secretion of antidiuretic hormone
- Sleep disorder
- Psychologic disorder
- Genetic influence
- Irritation, infection, retention
- Anatomic abnormalities
- Polyuria

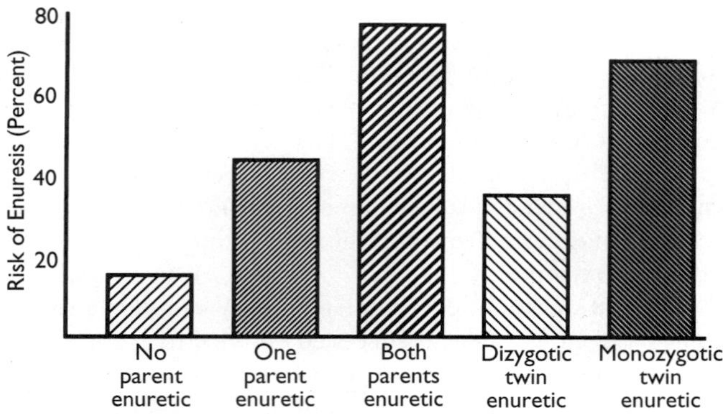

FIG. 21-4 *Familial risk of enuresis.*

EVALUATION

Urinary tract infection and irritative and retentive disorders may also contribute to the symptom of enuresis.[31-35] Perineal inflammation caused by irritants such as harsh soaps or pinworms may contribute to enuresis, and elimination of these inflammatory processes may considerably facilitate therapy. Some authors have demonstrated a correlation with food intolerances, constipation, encopresis, infrequent voiding, and hypercalciuria. An increased incidence of hayfever, urticaria, and food and drug allergies has been demonstrated,[33] as has an increased incidence of bacteriuria, primarily in little girls.[31]

It is of critical importance that the caregiver be aware that urethral obstruction (such as posterior urethral valves or stricture), occult neurogenic bladder dysfunction, and ectopic ureteral insertion may present as enuresis. Although generally such entities present with symptoms suggestive of anatomic abnormalities, such as diminished stream or continuous dribbling, these symptoms may be absent or unnoticed. In general, the risk of anatomic abnormalities in children with nocturnal enuresis alone is low. This risk is increased when diurnal symptoms are present, especially if they predominate. One must additionally be cognizant of the fact that polyuria caused by primary renal disease, diabetes insipidus, or diabetes mellitis may contribute to enuresis.[37] The goals of diagnostic evaluation of children with enuresis are to avoid a missed diagnosis of organic disease, to prevent the progression of functional to organic disease, and to avoid frightening and painful procedures whenever possible while promoting time and cost effectiveness.

Fig. 21-5 presents a clinical pathway that is responsive to these considerations. Children presenting with enuresis begin with a first stage of evaluation that includes a careful history and physical examination, urinalysis and urine culture, and estimation of the functional bladder capacity. A history should define the type of enuresis with which one is dealing and should also look for such urinary symptoms as frequency, infrequency, urgency,

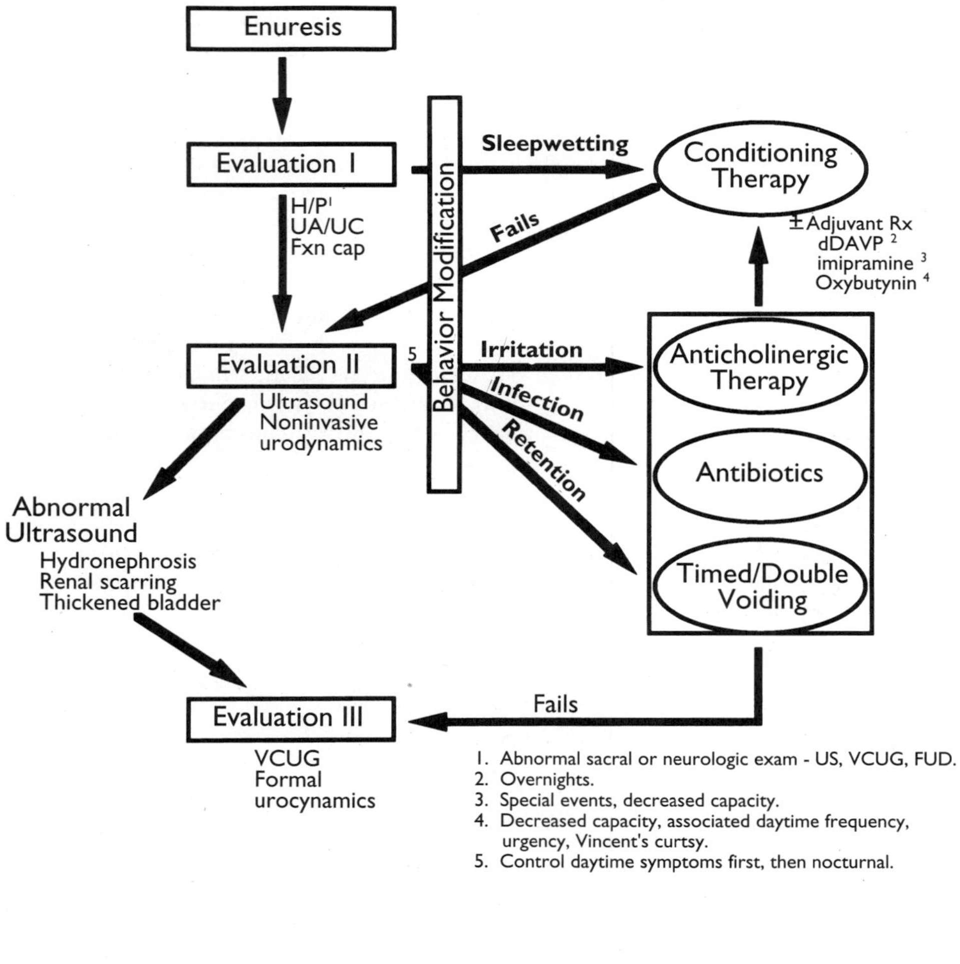

FIG. 21-5 *Clinical pathway for the diagnostic evaluation and treatment of enuresis.* dDAVP, *l-Deamino-8-D-arginine vasopressin;* FUD, *fluorodeoxyuridine;* Fxn cap, *functional capacity;* H/P, *history and physical examination;* UA/UC, *urinalysis/urea clearance;* US, *ultrasonography;* VCUG, *voiding cystourethrogram.*

urgency incontinence, constant dribbling, and Vincent's curtsy (Fig. 21-6). One should search for pertinent bowel symptoms such as constipation and encopresis, as well as the use of tub baths, especially those involving the use of bubble baths and harsh soaps such as shampoos. Physical examination should include a careful evaluation of the abdomen and genitalia. One should carefully examine the sacrum, looking for tufts of hair, lipomas, abnormal dimpling, and abnormal cutaneous pigmentation, all of which may be associated with underlying spinal abnormalities causing a neurogenic bladder. A neurologic examination is tailored to the needs of the individual patient and generally includes an examination of lower-extremity strength and reflexes and observation of gait. Some children require estimation of anal tone and the integrity of the bulbocavernosus reflex.

It is important to document the frequency of accidents and their distribution throughout the day, because it is quite common for these to be poorly represented by the parents on initial questioning. Additionally it is important to obtain a diary of voided volumes to estimate the frequency of urination as well as the functional voiding capacity.

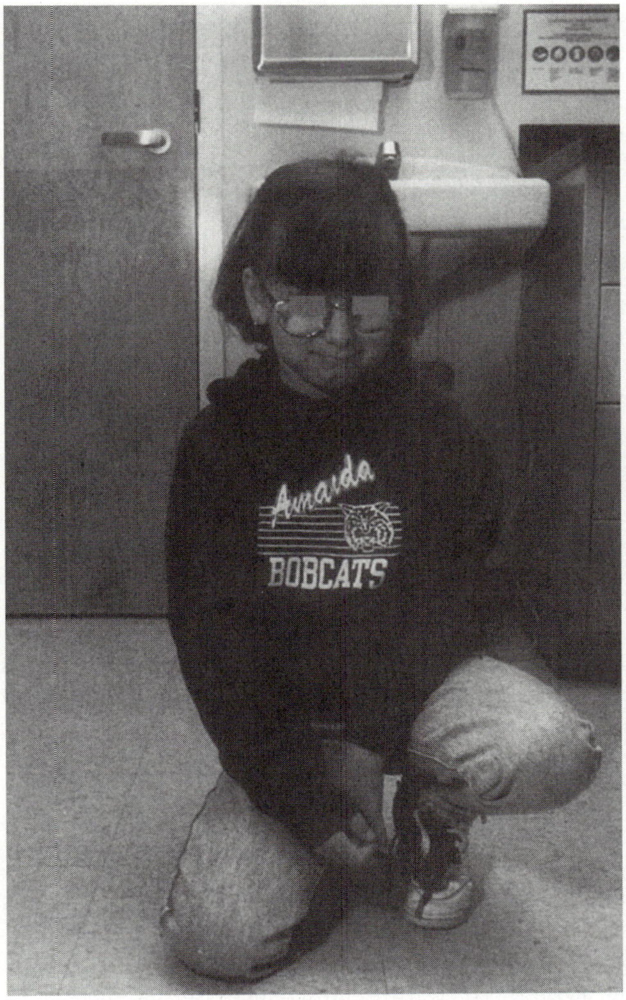

FIG. 21-6 *Vincent's curtsy is commonly manifested by squatting or sitting on the heel of the foot to minimize incontinence episodes.* (From Sheldon CA, Bukowski T: Bladder function. In Rowe MI, O'Neill JA Jr, Grosfeld JL, et al: *Essentials of pediatric surgery,* St. Louis, 1995, Mosby.)

Children with abnormal findings from a sacral or neurologic examination proceed directly to a renal ultrasonogram, a contrast voiding cystourethrogram, and a formal urodynamics investigation. Selected children require spinal imaging generally by magnetic resonance imaging. Those with evidence of urinary tract infection or daytime symptoms, as well as those with apparently uncomplicated nocturnal enuresis who fail initial therapy, undergo a secondary evaluation. This includes ultrasonography and noninvasive urodynamics to include uroflowmetry, electromyography, and measurement of postvoid residual by ultrasound technique. Children with an abnormal renal ultrasonogram or who fail aggressive medical therapy for enuresis undergo a tertiary evaluation that includes a voiding cystourethrogram and formal urodynamic investigation.

Management

Tremendous variation exists in the treatment of enuresis. It is crucial that the caregiver remember that the child is the consumer of this care. Consequently treatment should not be morbid. It is important to avoid instilling a sensation of punishment in a child by introducing either painful or fearful diagnostic or therapeutic interventions whenever possible. Side effects or excessive cost of therapy is intolerable if the child himself or herself does not desire symptomatic resolution of nocturnal enuresis. In this instance treatment efficacy is dramatically lowered. Parents should be counseled to await the child's pursuit of nocturnal dryness that is, when the child wishes to be dry at night and is capable of being an active participant in therapy. In contrast, daytime dryness in the school-aged child is important to allow the child to participate maximally and effectively in scholastic endeavors. Consequently treatment of daytime incontinence should be strongly encouraged. When treatment is undertaken, one should attempt to attain prompt symptomatic relief and sufficient symptomatic relief to allow the child to integrate socially. This endeavor will prevent discouragement and encourage active participation. Cost-effective and understandable therapy must be employed to facilitate compliance on the part of both the parents and the child. Additionally treatment should be conceptually simple and cost effective to allow long-term application, if necessary, to minimize or treat relapse.

The methodology of studying enuresis therapy has been extensively reviewed by Blackwell and Currah. It is clear that randomized, prospective, crossover, large-volume studies employing a double-blind approach are optimal to achieve adequate results and are often not achieved in clinical trials.[37] It is important to obtain accurate baseline information with which to compare therapeutic efficacy because parents often overestimate their child's incontinence by history, and this can cause an overestimation of the therapeutic effect of an intervention. This also probably explains a significant component of the observed "placebo effect" As previously noted, studies evaluating the same therapeutic agent may give drastically different results. One must remember that enuresis is multifactorial in its pathogenesis, and there may be significant population variance between studies. In addition, the degree to which other therapeutic interventions, such as behavior modification and bladder training, are applied may vary as well. For example, a child's nocturnal urinary output may be so high and his functional bladder capacity so small that the child is refractory to conditioning therapy. The use of a regulated fluid-intake regimen, bladder exercises, and even the use of anticholinergic agents may considerably facilitate the response to conditioning therapy. Further, if conditioning therapy is not continued beyond the point where nocturnal fluid intake is liberalized and anticholinergic agents are withdrawn, a high rate of relapse would be expected.

Fig. 21-5 illustrates the multimodal approach to therapy, which we have found most effective. Patients with simple bedwetting are begun with a behavior-modification program and conditioning therapy that is detailed later in this chapter. Those who fail this regimen or those who have associated daytime symptoms or evidence of a significantly diminished functional bladder capacity undergo renal and bladder ultrasonography and noninvasive urodynamics testing. Patients with retentive pathophysiologic features (elevated postvoid residual or infrequent voiding) are begun on a timed and, if indicated, double-voiding regimen. An occasional patient will require alpha-adrenergic blockade or biofeedback for failure to empty. Patients with evidence of chronic infection are cleared of infection and and placed on prophylaxis. Those who have irritative voiding symptoms such as frequency, urgency, urgency incontinence, and Vincent's curtsy in the absence of infection are excellent candidates for anticholinergic therapy. Once daytime symptoms are controlled by these measures, nocturnal wetting is addressed. Patients who fail to achieve control by this regimen proceed to voiding cystourethrography (VCUG) and formal urodynamics testing.

The box outlines the most commonly employed modalities available to the practitioner. Motivational therapy for some children may result in symptomatic improvement with a response and relapse rate comparing favorably to other types of therapeutic modalities.[38] There is a diminished hope for resolution of nocturnal enuresis if a child does not himself or herself desire to be dry. Children who become active participants in therapy have a greater response rate and a lower relapse risk compared to those children with more passive involvement.[38]

With motivational therapy, wet and dry nights are recorded, and the child is rewarded not only for dry nights but also for overall progress as assessed at regular intervals. The child is made responsible for his or her hygiene. The morning after each wet night the child is required to shower, pull off the bed clothing, and place this clothing in the washing machine. Additional

Proposed Therapeutic Modalities for Enuresis

1. Motivational or responsibility training
2. Bladder training
3. Conditioning therapy
4. Tricyclic antidepressants
5. Anticholinergics
6. Desmopressin acetate
7. Psychotherapy
8. Hypnotherapy

behavior modification may include evening fluid restriction, voiding immediately before going to bed, encouraging vigorous hydration during the day, avoidance of bladder irritants in the diet, and the avoidance of tub baths associated with harsh soaps. We routinely request that our patients greatly lower the intake of carbonated beverages, caffeine, citrus products, and chocolate.

Bladder training routinely plays a role in management. Resolution of enuresis, irrespective of the therapy employed, is generally associated with a decrease in diurnal frequency and an increase in bladder capacity.[39] Bladder-retention exercises alone in some series have demonstrated response rates as high as 66% and cure rates as high as 30%.[40] Those children who respond to such regimens demonstrate an increase in bladder capacity compared to those who do not. Such therapy has been found to be a good adjunct to conditioning therapy allowing symptomatic resolution in over 90% of patients in some series.[41,42]

With bladder-training exercises, the child practices inhibiting micturition and attempts to increase the interval between voiding. Additionally the child measures and records voided volume and aims for ultimately achieving a bladder capacity that is expected for his or her age. We employ the formula:[2]

$$\text{Capacity (oz)} = \text{Age (years)} + 2$$

Forced daytime hydration is employed to facilitate the response to this therapy.[42] Progress is rewarded. Because therapies directed solely at attaining greater bladder capacity have not proved effective for most children with nocturnal enuresis, this intervention is employed as an adjuvant form of therapy only.[43,44]

Several controlled trials have demonstrated a greater effectiveness with conditioning therapy than with either pharmacologic or psychotherapy.[45,49] It is important to realize, however, that there may be a significant relapse rate, as high as 20% to 30%.[50,51] Conditioning therapy, for the most part, employs a urine-sensing auditory alarm. Although the mechanics for this therapy are incompletely understood, it is believed that repeated episodes where bladder distension, by stimulating reflex micturition, results in the activation of an alarm that awakens the child, forcing inhibition of micturition. This is immediately followed by normal voiding. Over time, bladder distension itself is felt to elicit the inhibition response without the intermediary alarm stimulus.[43]

The most common cause for a therapeutic failure is a lack of understanding of the use of the alarm by either the child or the parent. It is critical that the child be allowed to awaken from the alarm and that he or she get up to void immediately after awakening. Before going to sleep, the patient rehearses what to do when the alarm sounds. The urine stream is interrupted, the sensor is disconnected, and the child goes to the toilet to finish voiding. Patients fearful of the dark may benefit from a flashlight or nightlight. The child changes his or her bedclothes, reconnects the sensor, and rehearses what to do if the alarm sounds again.

Overlearning helps to minimize the risk of relapse to rates below 10%.[50-52] Here, one intensifies the therapeutic effect of the alarm by tapering off any adjunctive medications such as imipramine, oxybutinin, or antidiuretic hormone analog (dDAVP, 1-deamino-8-D-arginine vasopressin). Subsequently, evening fluid restrictions are released, and ultimately fluids are encouraged before bedtime to achieve diuresis and maximize the child's ability to practice the inhibition response. It is important to realize that should relapse recur excellent response to retreatment is generally experienced.[50,51]

Anticholinergic agents commonly employed for enuresis include oxybutinin chloride and propantheline bromide. Because therapies directed solely at attaining greater bladder capacity are not effective for children with pure nocturnal enuresis, anticholinergic therapy in this setting has generally proved to be refractory.[51-53] In fact, anticholinergic therapy when applied as monotherapy has demonstrated little benefit over placebo.[54-56] Unfortunately, many of these studies incorporated a relatively small numbers of patients. Anticholinergic therapy has clearly been demonstrated to result in an increased bladder capacity in enuretic children[53,57] and therefore would be expected to be good adjunctive therapy in those children whose functional bladder capacity is small. Anticholinergic therapy has proved to be highly effective in correcting nocturnal enuresis in patients with daytime frequency and urgency or those who have concomitant diurnal enuresis.[57,58] Children, particularly female, with a strong history of urinary tract infection have also been demonstrated to respond to this therapy.[58] Significant complications may be associated with anticholinergic therapy and must be carefully monitored. Hyperpyrexia is not uncommon. Children should be warned to avoid excessively strenuous activity in hot environments. Cutaneous flushing (particularly the cheeks) and dry mucous membranes are routinely encountered. Some children will develop elevated residual urines, which may potentiate infection, whereas some children will experience personality changes, vision changes, hallucination, and nightmares. This therapy is begun at a relatively low dosage and is administered twice daily. Oxybutynin may be administered as a tablet (5 mg) or as a syrup (5 mg/5 ml). Children over 5 years of age may begin with a dosage of 2.5 mg PO bid. The dosage is titrated to control symptoms, but the postvoid residual is monitored noninvasively. If symptoms cannot be controlled without avoidance of an elevated postvoid residual, urosuppression may be required.

The tricyclic antidepressant series has proved to have a very significant antienuretic effect. The most commonly employed drug is imipramine; however, other tricyclic agents have a similar effect. An extensive literature review by Blackwell demonstrates an initial control rate exceeding 50%, with a further 15% to 25% showing improvement in enuresis symptoms.[59] This review also documents a very large variation in effectiveness, and a high risk of relapse, reaching a rate of 60% in some series. The mechanism of action of imipramine is incompletely understood. Several mechanisms have, however, been proposed. As reviewed by Stephenson, probably the most important mechanism is an increase in bladder capacity.[60] That this is important is suggested by the fact that an increased capacity is demonstrated in most responders as compared to nonresponders who show a very blunted effect on bladder capacity. The increase in bladder capacity may in part be related to anticholinergic effects.[61] These anticholinergics effects are, however, very weak and at the usual dose range employed are not capable of consistently abolishing uninhibited detrusor contraction. A direct antispasmodic effect on bladder smooth muscle has also been identified and is also quite weak.[62] Further, there is some suggestion of enhancement in beta-adrenergic receptor stimulation.

Another postulated mechanism of action is that of antidepressant activity itself. The antienuretic effect, however, occurs much more rapidly and at much too low a dose to be explained by this mechanism.[63] Additionally, some authors have documented an alteration in sleep pattern with imipramine. The ratio of REM (rapid eye movement) to non-REM sleep is decreased with imipramine. Of note, however, is the fact that the effect on sleep stage appears to be independent of its effect on enuresis.[26,64] Another proposed mechanism has been an alteration in the excretion pattern of ADH.[65]

Imipramine is generally reserved for children over 6 years of age. It is generally administered once daily shortly before bedtime. Those patients whose enuresis occurs before 1 o'clock AM may benefit from having the dosage given in the afternoon at 3 to 4 PM or split between afternoon and bedtime.[66] There is a poor correlation between clinical effect and plasma level, and dosages are generally begun in a low range and titrated according to symptomatic effect. Imipramine is administered as a tablet (10, 25, or 50 mg). Children over 6 years of age begin with 25 mg daily. The dosage may be increased to 50 mg daily or, if the child is over 12 years of age, 75 mg. Dosage should not exceed 2.5 mg/kg/day. The potential for cardiac toxicity has prompted some clinicians to obtain a baseline electrocardiogram and to avoid imipramine when a family history of sudden death, a prolonged P-R interval, or any abnormality in intraventricular conduction is encountered.

Side effects of imipramine administration are similar to those of anticholinergics and include personality changes, sleep disturbance, alteration in appetite, nervousness, anxiety, nausea, and dry mucous membranes. Probably the greatest impediment to the use of imipramine is the risk of fatal overdosage. Overdosages are associated with cardiac conduction abnormalities, hypotension, respiratory insufficiency, and seizure activity.[67,68] Treatment of overdosage always involves cardiac monitoring. If children present early, gastric lavage and the administration of activated charcoal may be beneficial. Seizures may be managed with diazepam or phenobarbital, whereas arrhythmias, hypotension, and respiratory insufficiency may respond to serum alkalinization with bicarbonate.[69,70] Phisostigmine may be used but can result in prescription collapse.[70]

Desmopressin acetate (dDAVP), an ADH analog, is a relatively new option of management.[71] The mechanism of action is the reduction of nighttime urinary output below the functional bladder capacity. Maximal plasma concentration is achieved 40 to 55 minutes after intranasal administration. The duration of action ranges between 6 and 24 hours. dDAVP is supplied at a concentration that delivers 10 μg per nasal spray. The initial dosage is usually 20 μg (one spray in each nostril) administered at bedtime. Dosages are titrated, generally not to exceed 40 μg. Side effects include rhinorrhea, nasal stuffiness, and epistaxis. Of note is the fact that water intoxication with severe hyponatremia, seizure, and coma have been reported even after relatively short-term usage.[72,73] Desmopressin acetate can be used on a daily basis; however, we reserve its use for special events such when children spend the night with their friends. One must be cognizant of the relative expense of these agents (Fig. 21-7).

Fig. 21-8 presents a conceptual approach to the management of nocturnal enuresis. A review of the fluid intake of many children with enuresis will reveal a very low fluid intake during the

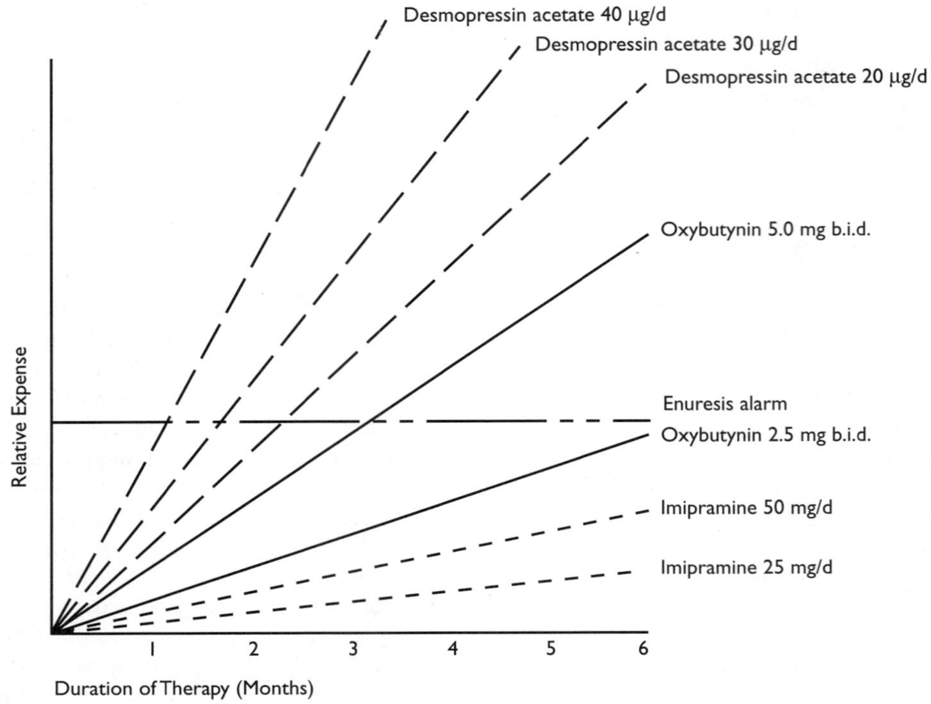

FIG. 21-7 *Relative expense of commonly employed therapeutic modalities for enuresis.*

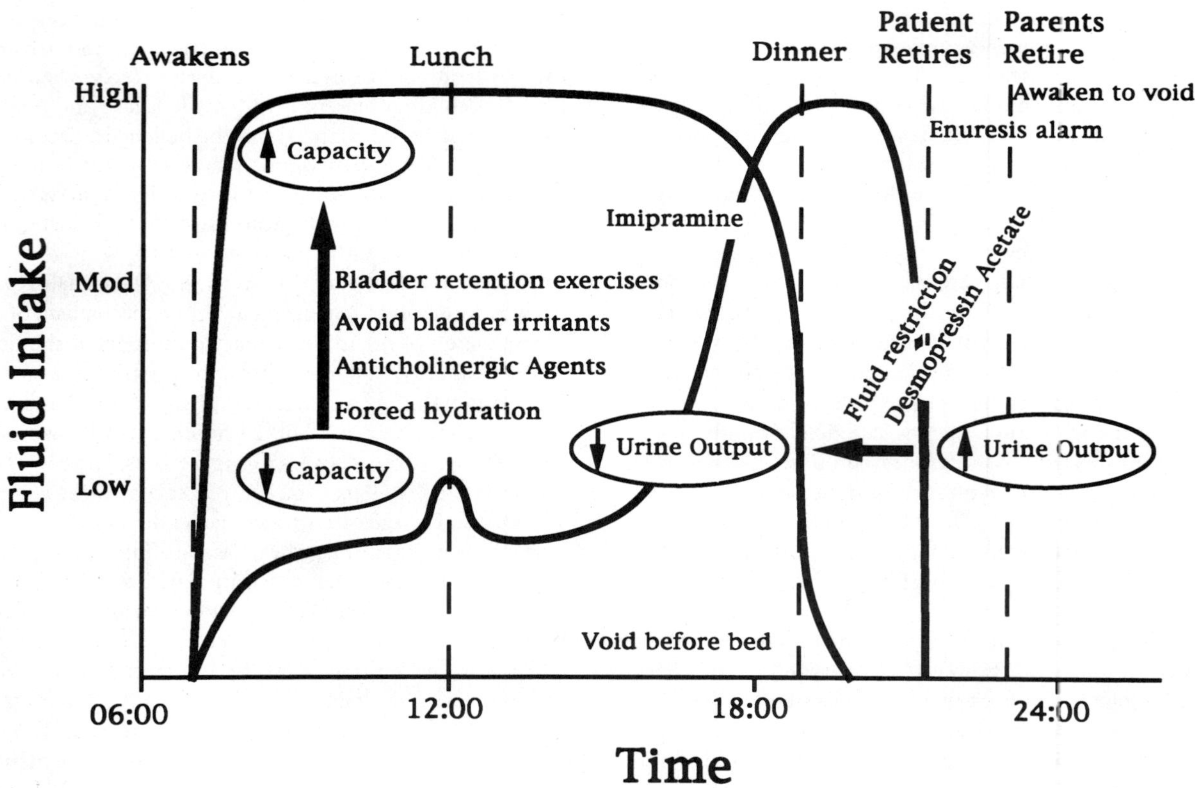

FIG. 21-8 *A conceptual approach to the management of nocturnal enuresis.*

early part of the day followed by a very high fluid intake in the afternoon and evening. Because these children often have a very low bladder capacity, the resultant high urine output at night fills this small bladder relatively quickly. Because children sleep very soundly at night, this stimulus may not result in the child awakening to a sufficient degree to allow normal voiding. Treatment is begun with the encouragement of daytime hydration, bladder-retention exercises, avoidance of bladder irritants in the diet, and if necessary for a significantly low-functional bladder capacity, an anticholinergic may be added.

In the evening, fluid intake is restricted to decrease nighttime urine output. The child voids before going to bed. By beginning the night with an empty bladder, an increased bladder capacity, and a diminished nighttime urine output, the child's potential for staying dry is greatly facilitated. Occasionally a patient will benefit from having the parents awaken the child to void before their retiring to bed. Nighttime urine output can also be diminished by desmopressin acetate.

Conditioning therapy with the enuresis alarm remains the mainstay for uncomplicated enuresis in those children who fail to respond to motivational therapy and behavior modification alone and for those children whose daytime symptoms or diminished capacity have been controlled (as by anticholinergics) but whose nocturnal enuresis remains. This therapy is cost effective, safe, and successful when employed in children who are motivated and capable of comprehending their therapy. Once continence has been achieved, anticholinergic agents are tapered and eliminated while the evening fluid intake is initially liberalized and ultimately encouraged to facilitate "over-learning" by conditioning therapy.

Desmopressin acetate is extremely effective as an adjunct to therapy and is particularly valuable for special events such as sleep-overs or slumber parties, providing the child with the immediate reward of socialization without embarrassment. Because it does not address what we interpret the underlying pathophysiologic problem to be, because it is costly, and because it may interfere with optimal conditioning therapy, we do not employ desmopressin on a daily basis.

Imipramine is a potentially valuable therapeutic modality, particularly in the patient whose bedwetting is not associated with daytime symptoms but where a mild diminished functional capacity is observed. It is particularly valuable for vacations and prolonged stays with relatives where conditioning therapy may be inapplicable. Once control has been attained, imipramine is tapered slowly, and relapse is not infrequent. Conditioning therapy is appropriate in this setting and may be used as an adjunct to the reintroduction and subsequent retapering of imipramine.

With a balanced and individualized approach to therapy, it is rare to have a child fail to achieve continence in the absence of true developmental delay.

References

1. Moffatt MEK: Nocturnal enuresis: psychologic implications of treatment and nontreatment, *J Pediatr* 114:697-704, 1989.
2. Haque M, Ellerstein NS, Gundy JH, et al: Parental perceptions of enuresis, *Am J Dis Child* 135:809-811, 1981.
3. Glicklich LB: An historical account of enuresis. In Stokes J Jr, editor: Special reviews, *Pediatrics* 8:859-876, 1951.
4. Fergusson DM, Hons BA, Shannon FT: Factors related to the age of attainment of nocturnal bladder control: an 8-year longitudinal study, *Pediatrics* 78(5):884-890, 1986.
5. Oppel WC, Harper PA, Rider RV: The age of attaining bladder control, *Pediatrics* 42(4):614-626, 1968.
6. Verhulst FC, van der Lee JH, Akkerhuis GW, et al: The prevalence of nocturnal enuresis: do DSM III criteria need to be changed? A brief research report, *J Child Psychol Psychiatry* 26(6):989-993, 1985.
7. Blomfield JM, Douglas JW: Bedwetting: prevalence among children aged 4-7 years, *Lancet* June:850-852, 1956.
8. Hallgren B: Enuresis, *Acta Psychiatr Neurol Scand* 31(4):379-401, 1956.
9. Forsythe WI, Redmond A: Enuresis and spontaneous cure rate, *Arch Dis Child* 49:259-264, 1974.
10. Goellner MH, Ziegler EE, Foman SJ: Urination during the first three years of life, *Nephron* 28:174, 1981.
11. Yeates WK: Bladder function in normal micturition. In Kolvin I, MacKeith RC, Meadow SR, editors: *Bladder control and enuresis,* London, 1973, Heinemann.
12. Nash DFE: The development of micturition control with special reference to enuresis, *Ann R Coll Surg Engl* 5:318, 1949.
13. Koff SA: Estimating bladder capacity in children, *Urology* 21(3):248, 1988.
14. Stein Z, Susser M: Social factors in the development of sphincter control, *Develop Med Child Neurol* 9:692-706, 1967.
15. Mahoney DT, Laferte RO, Blais DJ: Integral storage of voiding reflexes, *Urology* 9(1):95-107, 1977.
16. McGuire EJ, Savastano JA: Urodynamics studies in enuresis and the nonneurogenic neurogenic bladder, *J Urol* 132:299-302, 1984.
17. Pompeius, R: Cystometry in paediatric enuresis, *Scand J Urol Nephrol* 5:222-228, 1971.
18. Troup CW, Hodgson NB: Nocturnal functional bladder capacity in enuretic children, *J Urol* 105:129-132, 1971.
19. Webster GD, Koefoot RB, Sihelnik S: Urodynamic abnormalities in neurologically normal children with micturition dysfunction, *J Urol* 132:74-77, 1984.
20. Essen J, Peckham C: Nocturnal enuresis in childhood, *Develop Med Child Neurol* 18:577-589, 1976.
21. MacKeith RC: Is maturation delay a frequent factor in the origins of primary nocturnal enuresis? *Develop Med Child Neurol* 14:217-223, 1972.
22. McKendry JBJ, Williams HAL, Broughton C: Enuresis: a study of untreated patients, *Appl Therapeutics* 10(12):815-817, 1968.
23. Norgaard JP, Pedersen EB, Djurhuus JC: Diurnal anti-diuretic hormone levels in enuretics, *J Urol* 134:1029-1031, 1985.
24. Puri VN: Urinary levels of anti-diuretic hormone in nocturnal enuresis, *Indian Pediatr* 17:675-676, 1980.
25. Rittig S, Knudsen UB, Norgaard JP, et al: Abnormal diurnal rhythm of plasma vasopressin and urinary output in patients with enuresis, *Am J Physiol* 256:664-671, 1989.
26. Kales A, Kales JD, Jacobson A: Effects of imipramine on enuretic frequency and sleep stages, *Pediatrics* 60(4):431-36, 1977.
27. Bindelglas PM, Dee GH, Enos FA: Medical and psychosocial factor in enuretic children treated with imipramine hydrochloride, *Am J Psychiatry* 124:1107-1112, 1968.
28. Moffatt MEK, Kato C, Pless IB: Improvements in self-concept after treatment of nocturnal enuresis: randomized controlled trial, *J Pediatr* 110:647-652, 1987.
29. Shaffer D: The association between enuresis and emotional disorder: a review of the literature. In Kolvin IM, MacKeith RC, Meadow SR, editors: *Bladder control and enuresis,* London, 1973, Heinemann.
30. Bakwin H: The genetics of enuresis. In Kolvin IM, MacKeith RC, Meadow SR, editors: *Bladder control and enuresis,* London, 1973, Heinemann.
31. Dodge WF, West EF, Bridgforth EB, et al: Nocturnal enuresis in 6- to 10-year old children, *Am J Dis Child* 120:32-35, 1970.

32. Sachdev YV, Howards SS: *Enterobius vermicularis* infestation and secondary enuresis, *J Urol* 113:143-144, 1975.
33. Zaleski A, Shokeir MK, Gerrard JW: Enuresis: familial incidence and relationship to allergic disorders, *Can Med Assoc J* 106:30-31, 1972.
34. O'Regan S, Yazbeck S, Schick E: Constipation, bladder instability, urinary tract infection syndrome, *Clin Nephrol* 23(3):152-154, 1985.
35. Vachvanichsanong P, Malagon M, Moore ES: Urinary incontinence due to idiopathic hypercalciuria in children, *J Urol* 152:1226-1228, 1994.
36. Novello AC, Novello JR: Enuresis, *Pediatr Clin North Am* 34(3):719-733, 1987.
37. Blackwell B, Currah J: The psychopharmacology of nocturnal enuresis. In Kolvin I, MacKeith RC, Meadow SR, editors: *Bladder control and enuresis,* London, 1973, Heinemann.
38. Marshall S, Marshall HH, Lyon RP: Enuresis: an analysis of various therapeutic approaches, *Pediatrics* 52(6):813-817, 1973.
39. Zaleski A, Gerrard JW, Shokeir MHK: Nocturnal enuresis: the importance of a small bladder capacity. In Kolvin IM, MacKeith RC, Meadow SR, editors: *Bladder control and enuresis,* London, 1973, Heinemann.
40. Starfield B, Mellits ED: Increase in functional bladder capacity and improvements in enuresis, *J Pediatr* 72(4):483-487, 1968.
41. Geffken G, Johnson SB, Walker D: Behavioral interventions for childhood nocturnal enuresis: the differential effect of bladder capacity on treatment progress and outcome, *Health Psychol* 5(3):261-272, 1986.
42. Hagglund TB: Enuretic children treated with fluid restriction or forced drinking, *Ann Paediat Fenn* 11:84-90, 1965.
43. Doleys DM: Behavioral treatments for nocturnal enuresis in children: a review of the recent literature, *Psychol Bull* 84(1):30-54, 1977.
44. Harris LS, Purohit AP: Bladder training and enuresis: a controlled trial, *Behav Res Ther* 15:485-490, 1977.
45. DeLeon G, Mandell W: A comparison of conditioning and psychotherapy in the treatment of functional enuresis, *J Clin Psychol* 22:326, 1966.
46. Moffatt MEK, Kato C, Pless IB: Improvements in self-concept after treatment of nocturnal enuresis: a randomized clinical trial, *J Pediatr* 110:647, 1987.
47. Turner RK: Conditioning treatment of nocturnal enuresis: present status. In Kolvin IM, MacKeith RC, Meadows SR, editors: *Bladder control and enuresis,* London, 1973, Heinemann.
48. Wagner W, Johnson SB, Walker D, et al: A controlled comparison of two treatments of nocturnal enuresis, *J Pediatr* 101:302, 1982.
49. Wille S: Comparison of desmopressin and enuresis alarm for nocturnal enuresis, *Arch Dis Child* 61:30, 1986.
50. Morgan RTT: Relapse and therapeutic response in the conditioning treatment of enuresis: a review of recent findings on intermittent reinforcement, overlearning, and stimulus intensity, *Behav Res Ther* 16:273-279, 1978.
51. Young GC, Morgan RTT: Overlearning in the conditioning treatment of enuresis, *Behav Res Ther* 10:147-151, 1972.
52. Brooksbank DJ: The conditioning treatment of bedwetting in secondary school aged children, *J Adolescence* 2:239-244, 1979.
53. Johnstone JMS: Cystometry and evaluation of anticholinergic drugs in enuretic children, *J Ped Surg* 7(1):18-20, 1972.
54. Harrison JS: An investigation into the effects of imipramine hydrochloride on the incidence of enuresis in institutionalized children, S Afr Med J 44:253-255, 1970.
55. Leys D: Value of propantheline bromide in treatment of enuresis, *Br Med J* 10:549-552, 1956.
56. Lovering JS, Tallett SE, McKendry JBJ: Oxybutynin efficacy in the treatment of primary enuresis, *Pediatrics* 82(1):104-106, 1988.
57. Thompson IM, Lauvetz R: Oxybutinin in bladder spasm, neurogenic bladder, and enuresis, *Urology* 8(5):452-454, 1976.
58. Kass EJ, Diokno AC, Montealegre A: Enuresis: principles of management and result of treatment, *J Urol* 121:794-796, 1979.
59. Blackwell B, Currah J: The psychopharmacology of nocturnal enuresis. In Kolvin IM, MacKeith RC, Meadow SR, editors: *Bladder control and enuresis,* London, 1973, Heinemann.
60. Stephenson JD: Physiologic and pharmacologic basis for the chemotherapy of enuresis, *Psychol Med* 9:249-263, 1979.
61. Diokno AC, Hyndman CW, Hardy DA, et al: Comparison of action of imipramine (Tofranil) and propantheline (Probanthine) on detrusor contraction, *J Urol* 107:42, 1972.
62. Labay P, Boyarsky S: The action of imipramine on the bladder musculature, *J Urol* 109:385-387, 1973.
63. Sigg EB: Pharmacological studies with Tofranil, *Can Psychiatr Assoc J* 4:S75-S83, 1959.
64. Rapoport JL, Mikkelsen EJ, Zavadil A, et al: Childhood enuresis, *Arch Gen Psychiatry* 37:1146-1152, 1980.
65. Puri VN: Increased urinary antidiuretic hormone excretion by imipramine, *Exp Clin Endocrinol* 88(1):112-114, 1986.
66. Alderton HR: Imipramine in childhood enuresis: further studies on the relationship of time of administration to effect, *Can Med Assoc J* 102:1179-1180, 1970.
67. Fouron J-C, Chicoine R: ECG changes in fatal imipramine (Tofranil) intoxification, *Pediatrics* 48(5):777-781, 1971.
68. Rohner TJ, Sanford EJ: Imipramine toxicity, *J Urol* 114:402-403, 1975.
69. Greene AS, Cromie WJ: Treatment of imipramine overdose in children, *Urology* 18(3):314, 1981.
70. Sidford C: Cyclic antidepressants. In McGuigan MA, Gaudreault P, Woolf A, editors: *Clinical toxicology review,* 13(9):1-4, 1991.
71. Richardson DW, Robinson AG: Desmopressin, *Ann Intern Med* 103:228-239, 1985.
72. Simmonds EJ, Mahoney MJ, Littlewood JM: Convulsion and coma after intranasal desmopressin in cystic fibrosis, *Br Med J* 297:1614, 1988.
73. Bamford MFM, Cruickshank G: Dangers of intranasal desmopressin for nocturnal enuresis, *J R Coll Gen Pract* 39(325):345-346, 1989.

Chapter 22

Anatomic Incontinence

Michael C. Carr, Michael E. Mitchell

Incontinence in children can have many causes. Parents are most anxious to rule out a "physical cause" for incontinence particularly if the incontinence occurs both during the day and at night. The majority of the time there is no anatomic abnormality because the wetting relates to a functional or behavioral mechanism. This is often evident after a careful voiding history is obtained.[1-3] Voiding dysfunction has been used to describe a clustering of symptoms that include infrequent or ineffective bladder emptying, inconsistent bladder emptying, and detrusor-sphincter discoordination. With this problem we observe two distinct patterns: the nonneurogenic neurogenic bladder (Hinman's syndrome) and bladder instability (uninhibited bladder). See Chapter 20. Although boys may be affected, the majority of these children are girls, and boys who present with both daytime and nighttime urinary incontinence may have true mechanical obstruction, that is, posterior urethral valves. A small segment of incontinent children may have an underlying neurovesical abnormality. This can include patients born with other problems such as imperforate anus, sacrococcygeal teratoma, or spinal dysraphism.[4,5] The latter may be manifested by cutaneous abnormalities of the back such as presacral lipoma, hair patch, dermal vascular malformation, hemangioma, sacral dimple, or aberrant gluteal cleft. The dysraphic state refers to structural anomalies of the caudal end of the spinal cord and the vertebral column. It includes lipomas, lipomeningocele, diastematomyelia, dermoid cyst or sinus, aberrant roots, and tight filum terminale.[6] Sacral agenesis, an absence of part or all of one or more sacral vertebrae, can also result in a neurogenic cause of urinary incontinence. Finally, clinically overt neurogenic causes such as myelodysplasia or spinal cord injuries can contribute to urinary incontinence. These conditions are dealt with in the next chapter.

This chapter specifically addresses those children who are born with a nonneuronal anatomic abnormality that contributes to urinary incontinence. Specifically the bladder neck is maldeveloped or damaged. These causes are better understood by definition of the anatomic and underlying embryologic features. Malformations causing incontinence can be divided into anterior (ventral) or posterior (caudal) defects. The anterior conditions include exstrophy and epispadias, whereas the posterior conditions include urogenital sinus, persistent cloaca, ectopic ureter or ureters, and cecoureteroceles.

Anterior Malformations

Bladder exstrophy and epispadias represent unique abnormalities in the development of the genitourinary tract. Whether resulting from failure of the infraumbilical membrane to be resorbed and reinforced by mesodermal ingrowth or a primary herniation that prevents the medial migration of mesenchymal tissue in the lower abdominal wall has not been resolved. The result is symphyseal diastasis, flattening of the pelvis, and anterior displacement of the bladder, bladder neck, and urethra with or without failure of closure of these structures. The timing of the original event is crucial because earlier herniation at the cloacal phase results in exstrophy of the cloaca; later herniation leads to bladder exstrophy. An even later event leads to epispadias in which the bladder is formed but the urethra remains only as a plate rather than as a tube.[7] Pubic diastasis and altered pelvic anatomy represent a significant part of the anterior displacement process and contribute to incontinence. The total repair of bladder exstrophy usually requires several staged procedures. The first procedure is that of reduction of the anterior abdominal hernia and closure of the bladder in the neonatal period. Exstrophy of the bladder has a window of about 48 hours after birth in which the bladder can be closed and the symphysis approximated without need for pelvic osteotomy. Circulating maternal relaxins facilitate pelvic closure in this period. The most important operation of the exstrophy patient is this primary early closure. If done well, subsequent procedures are much easier. In the female patient, this may be the only surgery that is necessary, because it is possible to secure good bladder and urethral function with the primary closure in some patients.

The most important components of primary bladder closure include (1) aggressive dissection and mobilization of the bladder and bladder neck to permit relocation deep in the pelvis and proper closure of the bladder neck behind the approximated symphysis, (2) meticulous bladder closure, (3) symphyseal approximation, (4) abdominal wall closure, and (5) patient immobilization. The importance of the primary closure cannot be overemphasized because future success for continence and genital reconstruction is predicated on the initial surgery. Repeated operations can lead to scarring and ultimately reduce the potential for spontaneous voiding. Furthermore, it is possible that some bladder outlet resistance is essential to appropriate bladder growth and development in the first year of life.

The techniques for exstrophy closure and bladder neck reconstruction have evolved in the past 50 years. Hugh H. Young reported in 1942 on the first successful reconstruction of a 6-year-old girl born with bladder exstrophy.[8] She was continent and able to void volitionally. In those days the initial bladder closure was not done until the patients were older. This particular patient had her bladder closure done at 5 years of age. John E. Dees reported on his series of six patients with congenital epispadias and incontinence in 1949.[9] He was able to correct their incontinence with a bladder neck reconstruction that involved an extension of Young's technique. The basic concept was to expose the bladder, dissect the prostatic urethra in males or proximal urethra in females free from the dorsal surface of the intersymphyseal band, and then open the bladder in the midline from its dome to the level of the external sphincter. Triangular wedges of tissue were then excised from the roof and the lateral wall of the posterior urethra and adjacent bladder wall (Fig. 22-1). Subsequent closure resulted in a snug internal and external sphincter and a tubular rather than conical urethra. The bladder wall adjacent to the neourethra is denuded of its mucosa. This tissue is then used as a second layer of closure over the neourethra. (Fig. 22-2) Dees was successful in obtaining continence in all six of the patients who were reported on.

These early successes in patients with exstrophy or epispadias led some surgeons to abandon the earlier procedures of urinary diversion. In 1964 Leadbetter reviewed the various surgical techniques for bladder neck reconstruction.[10] Previous work had been performed with plication of the urethra and vesical neck as previously described, the use of slings around the bladder neck, creation of a sphincter with muscle grafts, and formation of a new urethra with bladder muscle, vaginal flaps, or denervated ileum. He recommended opening the bladder in the midline and extending an incision through the urethra down to the triangular ligament. After reimplantation of the ureters the bladder neck is tubularized over an 8 or 10 French catheter with a two-layer closure. Bladder muscle is then used to imbricate the proximal urethra. He believed that continence is achieved principally because the tube formed from muscle of the bladder floor, particularly the trigone, is long enough, has an undisturbed blood supply, and thereby has sufficient tone to produce sphincteric action.

Williams reviewed the experience of The Hospital for Sick Children in London with the complete form of exstrophy of the bladder from 1946 to 1963.[11] In male infants the initial surgery involved correction of chordee 6 months before actual closure of the bladder. The next stage included bilateral pelvic osteotomy and actual bladder and urethral closure. The fibromuscular tissue that had been freed from the pelvis was wrapped around the front of the bladder neck area if possible. The rectus sheath was then closed over the bladder in the midline. He was able to demonstrate acceptable continence in 10% of his patients who underwent primary bladder closure. The second series of patients treated between 1963 and 1969 faired somewhat better, with acceptable continence in 30% of patients. He believed that the best results were obtained when muscle tissue in the region of the bladder neck is well formed and no attempt at extreme urethral narrowing is made. The improvement in the continence and decreasing complication

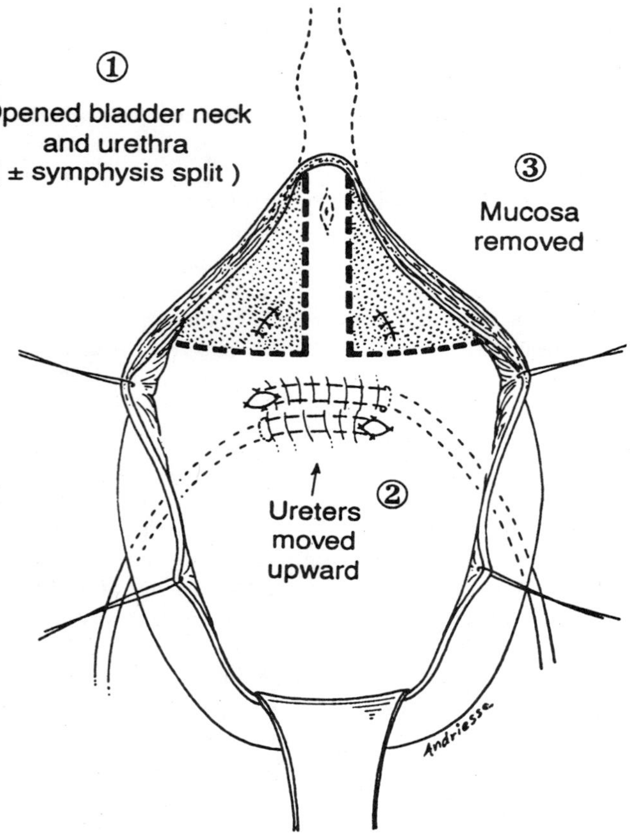

FIG. 22-1 *The bladder neck and urethra are opened, often after the symphysis is split. The ureters are reimplanted by the cross trigone method. Triangular areas are demucosated to allow for tubularization of the urethra.*

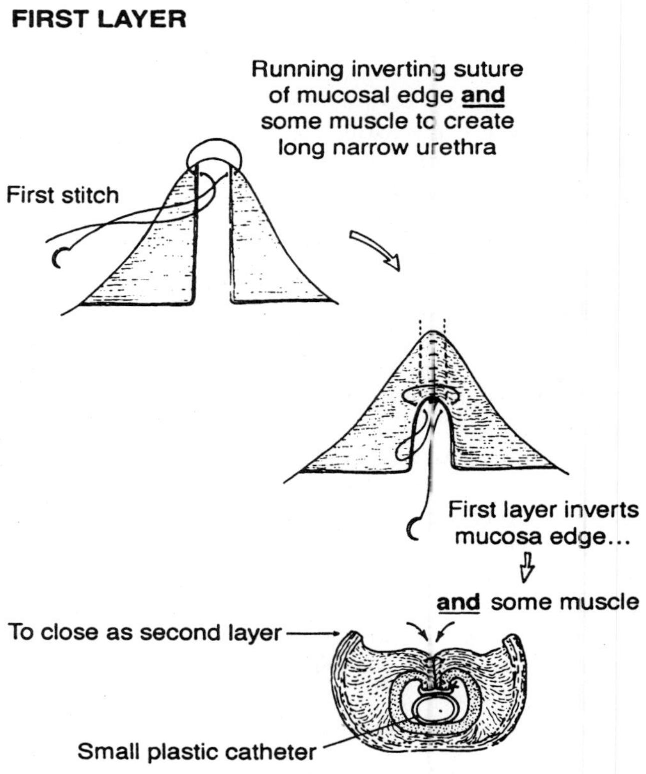

FIG. 22-2 *Closure of the bladder neck and proximal urethra is accomplished in two layers. The first layer incorporates the mucosal edge and some muscle. The second layer is closure of the detrusor muscle over the bladder neck and neourethra. A catheter is left in place during the closure.* (From Hendren WH, Hendren RB: *AUA Today* 8, 12, 1995, American Urological Association, Baltimore, Md.)

rate provided a further impetus to attempt bladder closure rather than urinary diversion, which was the preferred mode of treatment for the exstrophy patient at that time.

Mollard in 1980 described a modification of the Young-Dees-Leadbetter bladder neck reconstruction.[12] This reconstruction was usually done when the child was 4 or 5 years of age. Tubularization of the urethra was performed along with the creation of a muscular triangle that was wrapped upward in front of the new bladder neck and the lowest part of the detrusor. This reconstitutes a muscular loop in front of the new bladder neck and creates a clear urethrovesical angle. A more recent review of 49 cases using his technique confirmed his preliminary results with normal continence and transurethral voiding in 77% of female patients and 63% of male patients. All these children were dry during the day under all circumstances including sports and had transurethral voiding every 3 hours. Nocturnal continence was always delayed, but all patients over 15 years of age were dry at night. Some of these patients did require a secondary endourethral procedure including a periurethral sling, further bladder neck reconstruction, or bladder neck reconstruction combined with bladder augmentation. He believed that continence results could not adequately be assessed until 18 months after the bladder neck reconstruction. Beyond this point improvement was rare. A repeat bladder neck reconstruction remained his preferred procedure in cases of persistent urinary incontinence. Creation of a very narrow bladder neck combined with the so-called Mitrofanoff procedure is recommended. This procedure involves the creation of a catheterizable channel using either an appendix, a ureter, or a tubularized segment of small bowel that is tunneled into the bladder and brought out to the skin. He stressed that the reconstruction does not create a normal bladder neck or active sphincter but simply aims to enhance the outlet resistance. This resistance should be high enough to retain a sufficient volume of urine without leakage and yet low enough to allow complete micturition without inducing too high of an intravesical pressure. In his series of exstrophy patients, he found that micturition was generally abnormal and involved relaxation of the perineal muscles along with abdominal straining. Only two thirds of exstrophic detrusors urodynamically assessed were contractile. A modification of his technique has been used to create a regular muscular and mucosal tube that is then suspended from the abdominal wall. Early results are encouraging, but the follow-up study has been too short to draw definitive conclusions.[13]

Hendren provided a description of female epispadias repair in which he used a combined perineal and transvesical approach. This procedure included narrowing of the abnormally wide urethra by making parallel incisions along the urethra up into the bladder neck and using the fat from the mons in order to cover the neourethra and obliterate the space behind the pubic symphysis. Hendren underscored the need to deal with the underlying disorder: a lack of urethral resistance in such patients. What had previously been performed in several stages was now able to be performed in a single stage combining the perineal and transvesical approaches.[14]

Jeffs defined the factors necessary to complete a successful exstrophy closure.[15] This early series underscored the staged approach to functional closure of classical bladder exstrophy. After bladder closure at an early age, bladder neck reconstruction and an antireflux procedure were performed in patients at approximately 3 years of age. This was followed by an epispadias repair at 4 to 5 years of age. This earlier review noted that the successes were greater in girls than in boys. Daytime and nighttime continence along with normal upper tracts was achieved in 60% of the patients who completed these staged closures. He stressed that those patients with small bladders, diverted and severely scarred bladders, or those with extensive ectopic bowel mucosa tended to do more poorly with respect to continence. The use of osteotomies was helpful to allow for placement of the urethra within the pelvic ring and to prevent an excessively acute urethrovesical angle. The use of urethral suspension after the bladder neck plasty makes use of the levator ani action to aid in voluntary control. He preferred the Young-Dees-Leadbetter bladder neck reconstruction along with the cross trigonal ureteral reimplantation. He stressed the importance of a urethral length of 2.5 cm along with a urethral closure pressure of 60 to 80 cm H_2O.

A subsequent review from the Johns Hopkins group addressed the issue of management of the failed exstrophy closure.[16] Either posterior iliac osteotomy or anterior innominate osteotomy was performed at the time of reclosure. This was often coupled with epispadias repair. Eight patients subsequently underwent bladder reconstruction, seven of whom were dry for 4 hours. The most common factor in all the patients who had a failed exstrophy closure was the lack of any osteotomy being performed at the time of the initial closure. It was concluded that even though closure of the pelvis in the first 48 hours of life is possible, osteotomies should be considered if the pelvis is not malleable or the pubic bones are widespread. The option to perform an epispadias repair at the time of the bladder reclosure can be very helpful.

Recent work from the Hopkins group has detailed their approach to genitourinary reconstruction and female epispadias patients.[17] The approach has been to perform the urethral and genital reconstruction at 18 months of age followed by a Young-Dees-Leadbetter (Y-D-L) bladder neck reconstruction at approximately 4 to 5 years of age. The average bladder capacity in those patients who underwent bladder neck reconstruction after prior urethral and genital reconstruction was 121 ml. Thus the bladder was suitable for a bladder neck reconstruction without the use of augmentation cystoplasty and the need for intermittent catheterization. The interval to achieve continence ranged from a mean of 18 months for those who had reconstruction at one time to 23 months in patients who underwent a staged repair. This may represent an ongoing development of the pelvic musculature as it occurs over time. Their results strongly support the use of urethroplasty and genital reconstruction before the bladder neck reconstruction. The increased bladder capacity facilitates the ultimate bladder neck reconstruction.

A modification of the Y-D-L bladder neck reconstruction has recently been described.[18] This technique has been applied to a broad range of patients including those with exstrophy/epispadias, myelomeningocele, and cecoureteroceles. The modified Y-D-L repair was compared to several different types of bladder neck reconstruction. The greatest success was seen in those patients who underwent a modification of the Y-D-L bladder neck reconstruction. Incontinence was seen in only one of 11 patients, whereas reoperation was needed in three out of 11 patients. The modified Y-D-L procedure involves performing a transverse incision through the anterior half of the distal pelvic urethra (Fig. 22-3, *A*). The incision is extended cephalad along the posterolateral proximal area of the urethra and then cephalad along the posterior bladder wall to the ureteric orifices bilaterally. With gentle traction the incision is then elongated (Fig. 22-3, *B*). Reimplantation of the ureters is accomplished by either the cross trigonal or standard Politano-Leadbetter technique. The urethra is then tubularized in two layers using a 6-0 polydimethylsiloxane (PDS) in the mucosa and a running 4-0 PDS in the muscularis (Fig. 22-3, *C*). The neourethra is constructed over an 8 or 10 Fr catheter depending on the size of the patient (Fig. 22-3, *D*). A 5 Fr feeding tube is left indwelling in the immediate postoperative period. This technique can be combined with a urethral sling or suspension procedure, but this is usually not necessary. The bladder is then closed vertically in the midline (Fig. 22-3, *E*). With this technique little volume is lost from the bladder capacity. The success of this technique was greatest as a primary procedure (?%), with only a 50% success rate being seen when used as a secondary procedure. Certainly the effectiveness of this modification is offset by scarring and fibrosis that can occur at the bladder neck after an initial reconstructive procedure. It has been postulated that postoperative scarring can result in fixation and ultimate loss of the contractility of the circular and obliquely oriented muscular fibers that traverse the bladder neck and ultimately produce mucosal coaptation.

Another approach in treating anatomic urinary incontinence has been the use of an artificial urinary sphincter. With the successes in adult patients the procedure has been applied to incontinent children and young adults.[19] The greatest numbers have been used in those with myelodysplasia. It has also been successfully applied to patients with epispadias/exstrophy complex, spinal cord injury, those with posterior urethral valves, and even a patient with Ewing's sarcoma of the sacrum. The criteria for patient selection included motivated, cooperative family and patient, a minimum age of 6 years, and the ability to empty the bladder with minimal residual urine (which can include intermittent self-catheterization). Other important criteria include a reasonable detrusor compliance and contractility, no significant vesicoureteral reflux or urinary infection, and acceptance of the mechanical limitation and potential need for eventual revision of the device. Finally the family must accept responsibility for lifelong follow-up study. The overall continence rate was good in 80% of the patients. Continence was defined as day and night continence with one pad or none and no physical restrictions. Fair continence, those who used up to three pads a day with occasional

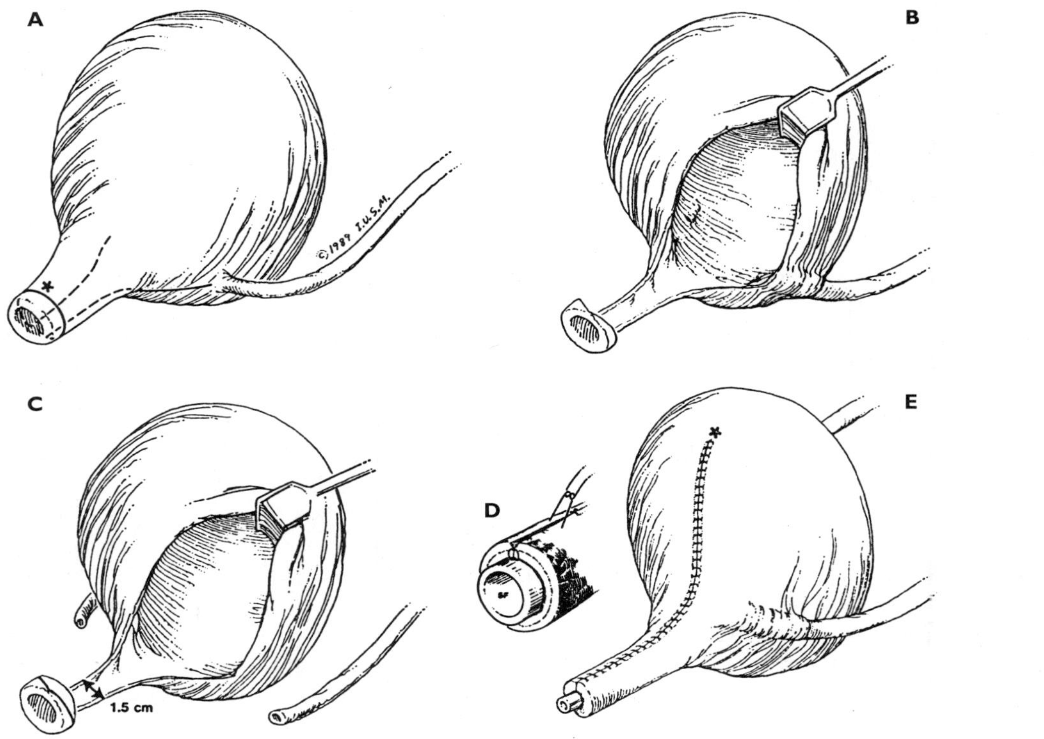

FIG. 22-3 ***A,*** *Transverse incision is made distal to the original bladder neck area. Notice the location of the asterisk relative to the incision.* ***B,*** *The incision is extended laterally, posteriorly, and then cephalad toward the ipsilateral ureteric orifice on each side.* ***C,*** *The ureters are dissected free from the bladder and reimplanted cephalad in the posterior bladder wall.* ***D,*** *The resultant posterior strip of bladder is tubularized in two layers.* ***E,*** *The bladder is closed longitudinally as an extension of the bladder neck closure. The site of the original bladder neck,* asterisk, *is now located near the dome.* (From Jones JA, Mitchell ME, Rink RC: *Br J Urol* 71:555, 1993.)

leakage at night, was seen in 14% of the patients. The remaining (6%) had failure of the sphincter and required removal of the device. Secondary procedures were required in nearly 50% of the patients. All male patients who were sexually active before the implantation of the sphincter remained so after surgery.

A major issue concerning the artificial urinary sphincter is that prolonged ischemia caused by cuff compression around the bladder neck may lead to tissue atrophy. This can ultimately manifest as a return of incontinence or even bladder neck erosion. A newer narrow-backed cuff design has recently been developed and should help this problem.[20] The design of the cuff allows for more uniform compression of urethral tissue, a feature that may be particularly important when the cuff is applied to tissue with underlying atrophy. Other important technical points include using a lower pressure balloon, generally 61 to 70 cm H_2O. Finally, nocturnal deactivation of the device in which the patient manually deactivates the sphincter has contributed to a decreased reoperation rate.

A novel approach for those patients who remain incontinent after implantation of an artificial urinary sphincter is to add a second sphincter cuff around the bulbous urethra.[21] This technique has been used most often in men with incontinence after radical prostatectomy but has also been used in patients with myelodysplasia and sacral agenesis. A three-way connector is used to connect the tandem cuffs to a single control pump tubing. Thus the cuffs can be activated simultaneously. The use of two cuffs leads to doubling the area of compression of the urethra and thus increasing the resistance to urine leakage without ultimately decreasing tissue perfusion. Eighty percent of the patients who underwent this procedure were either totally dry or required only the use of one to three pads per day. Thus the overall success rate for the artificial urinary sphincter in all patients is 95%.

A final approach to gaining urinary continence in patients with anterior anatomic defects is the use of biomaterials injected into the submucosal periurethral space. Investigators in the early 1960s attempted to use sclerosing agents and then agents to add bulk and narrow the region of the urethral sphincter. Polytetrafluoroethylene (Teflon) paste was injected in the urinary sphincter in male and female patients to improve incontinence. Subsequent studies have shown that this inert paste migrates from the site of injection. Distant polytetrafluoroethylene granulomas and emboli have been found in the liver, lung, and spleen. A newer biomaterial, glutaraldehyde, cross-linked collagen, has gained increasing acceptance in the treatment of urinary incontinence.[22] The collagen has been injected after bladder neck reconstruction that only provided partial continence to the exstrophy and epispadias population.[23] Improvement was seen in all cases for those injected after their bladder neck reconstruction. The need for intermittent catheterization to ensure bladder emptying should be anticipated. Collagen also has been used before formal bladder neck reconstruction to increase the urethral resistance and ultimately increase the bladder capacity. Repeated injections are often necessary to maintain a good degree of continence. There have been no significant complications with this approach. Thus it seems to be both a simple and safe approach with a reasonable success rate that can be used as an adjunct to improving continence in patients with the exstrophy-epispadias complex who have failed to gain complete control after reconstructive surgery. Continued follow-up study of these patients will be necessary because the collagen may be degraded over time. The durability of the collagen and the ability to reinject in the bladder neck region will be important issues to address over the long term.

A review from St. Peter's Hospital and The Hospital for Sick Children in London underscored the importance of urodynamic investigation to evaluate the causes of incontinence after bladder neck reconstruction in exstrophy and epispadias patients.[24] The bladder neck reconstruction often is performed independently of other procedures on the bladder. Yet the bladder neck does not function as a separate entity but rather as part of an integrated unit. The importance of urodynamic evaluation underscores the need to determine how the properties of the bladder as well as the bladder neck and urethra interact to achieve continence. Thus the bladder stability, compliance (measure of bladder pressure versus capacity), capacity, and the maximum urethral closure pressure all become important variables. This study demonstrated that detrusor behavior was not normal in most of the children studied during both the filling and the voiding phases. The authors attempted to classify the function of the bladder and bladder neck with the assumption that an adequate capacity was 250 ml. Four different types of lower tract behavior were defined to classify the underlying problem based upon the urodynamic findings. It is only with detailed urodynamic investigation that the function of the bladder and the bladder neck as well can be understood, particularly when further reconstructive surgery is contemplated.

Posterior Malformations

The second broad group of anatomic abnormalities relate to the posterior bladder wall and bladder neck. Within this broad group is included ureteral ectopia. The hallmark sign of ectopic ureteral orifices in girls is continuous urinary incontinence with an otherwise normal voiding pattern after toilet training. The ectopic ureter is often associated with renal duplication and an upper pole moiety but is dependent on an abnormal cephalad position of the ureteric bud on the mesonephric duct. An ectopic ureter can completely fail to become incorporated into the lower urinary tract. Thus it can end in a seminal vesical or vas deferens in the male or in Gartner's duct, upper vagina, cervix, uterus, or fallopian tubes in females. *Females* will present with urinary incontinence, whereas *males* may develop a urinary tract infection but *not incontinence* (Fig. 22-4). The incontinence in young girls can be continuous, occur when the child is upright, or diurnally when the renal moiety is poorly functioning. Other clinical manifestations include "stress" incontinence, a persistent vaginal discharge, or episodes of recurrent urinary tract infections, or even failure to thrive and chronic infections.[25]

Diagnosis of ectopic ureters can sometimes be made by ultrasonography. A duplex kidney with upper-pole hydronephrosis in a normal bladder is suggestive of an obstructed upper-pole ectopic ureter. The dilated ureter is clearly extravesical, with a thick bladder wall between ureteral lumen and bladder lumen. The renal parenchyma of the upper pole is often thinned because of the hydronephrosis. This can be confirmed by excretory urography or renal scan. The nonvisualizing or poorly visu-

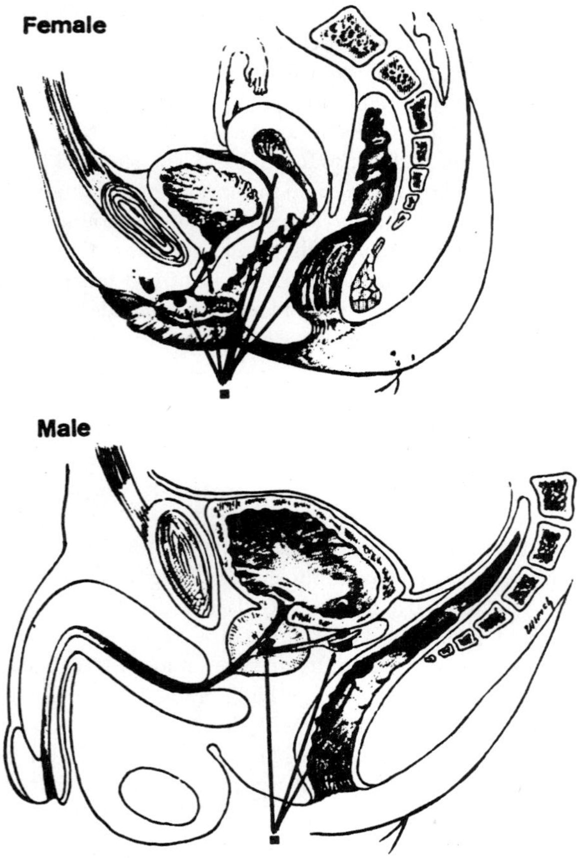

FIG. 22-4 *Ectopic ureteral orifices are found in the bladder neck, proximal or distal parts of the urethra, and vestibule. The ureter may empty into the vagina, uterus, or cervix in females. In the male, ectopic ureters usually drain into the prostate, urethra, prostatic utricle, seminal vesicle, vas deferens, or ejaculatory duct.* (From Retik AB, Peters CA: Ectopic ureter and ureterocele. In Walsh PC, Gittes R, Perlmutter A, Stamey T, editors: *Campbell's urology,* ed 6, Philadelphia, 1992, Saunders.

alizing upper pole of a duplex system that is massively dilated can be seen. This upper pole displaces the lower pole downward and outward. On the other hand, an ectopic ureter can drain a nonvisualizing, diminutive, dysplastic upper pole segment. The typical radiographic criteria may no longer be seen. The contralateral kidney may demonstrate ureteral ectopia as well, with an incidence of 5% to 15% of cases.

Voiding cystourethrography can demonstrate vesicoureteral reflux into the lower pole moiety in up to 50% of the cases. Reflux can intermittently also be seen in the upper pole, depending on the location of the ectopic ureteral orifice. If reflux occurs before voiding, the orifice is proximal to the bladder neck (that is, no incontinence); reflux during voiding may be suggestive of an orifice in the urethra. Sphincteric orifices may not undergo reflux at all. Finally, large ectopic ureters may impinge against the bladder and create an indentation much like that of a ureterocele (pseudoureterocele).[26]

Treatment of an ectopic ureter is dependent on the function of the upper-pole moiety. A poorly functioning upper-pole segment will be excised. If the upper-pole moiety functions well enough to warrant salvage, the upper-pole ureter can be anastomosed to the lower-pole pelvis or to the proximal lower-pole ureter of adequate caliber. Finally, a common sheath ureteral reimplantation, which involves tunneling both ureters into the bladder, can be performed. This is most beneficial in instances when the lower-pole ureter undergoes reflux and the upper-pole ureter is not severely dilated and drains an upper-pole segment with adequate function.

Bilateral single-system ectopic ureters are a rare anomaly. The ureters end in the prostatic urethra in males or into the distal urethra in females. In females there is failure to develop a competent bladder neck as well as trigone and base plate. The kidneys may be dysplastic or hydronephrotic. The ureters are usually dilated, and reflux may be present. The bladder is small, and the bladder neck is patulous; therefore a child dribbles urine continuously. The male may have some continence because of the external sphincter function. This condition is similar to epispadias in that there is a short urethra and incompetent bladder neck. In contrast to epispadias, though, there is a high incidence of renal and ureteral abnormalities. Surgical treatment involves reimplanting the ureters into the bladder along with bladder neck reconstruction as previously described. The response of the bladder to increased urethral resistance and bladder cycling is crucial, with increases in bladder capacity often leading to satisfactory control. A bladder augmentation, using a segment of gastrointestinal tract, may be necessary to optimize the outcome.

Renal duplication can also be associated with a ureterocele, which is a cystic dilatation of the terminal ureter. In the pediatric population ureteroceles associated with duplex systems are the most common and can be the most problematic. Increasingly these ureteroceles can be recognized at the time of prenatal ultrasonography or in the work-up of a child who presents with a urinary tract infection. Various names are used to described the different types of ureteroceles. The rarest among these is the cecoureterocele, so named because the actual lumen extends through the bladder neck as a long tongue, or "cecum" ('blind gut') beneath the urethral submucosa (Fig. 22-5). Williams et al. noted the defective muscle backing of ureteroceles in the trigone and bladder neck.[27] This is exacerbated with cecoureteroceles because the muscles around the posterior half of the expanded urethra and bladder neck are further attenuated. Surgical excision of the cecoureterocele, in fact, rendered several patients incontinent. Stevens's careful analysis of a necropsy specimen of a cecoureterocele led to the following observations: (1) a muscle deficit of the bladder neck and urethra may predispose to incontinence; (2) after excision of the vesical and bladder neck parts of the ureterocele, surgery to the distal tongue should be limited initially to division of the coapting epithelial layers of the urethra and cecoureterocele; and (3) the hypomuscularity of the trigone, internal sphincter, and adjoining urethra that backed the ureterocele should be repaired by coaptation of the thicker muscle repairing the weakened area.[28]

The final broad category of posterior abnormalities relate to cloacal malformations in which the urinary, genital, and intestinal tracts converge into a common outflow structure, the cloaca (Latin for 'sewer'). A less severe condition involves a urogenital sinus, in which the intestinal tract is not involved but the urinary and genital systems communicate. These conditions are seen exclusively in

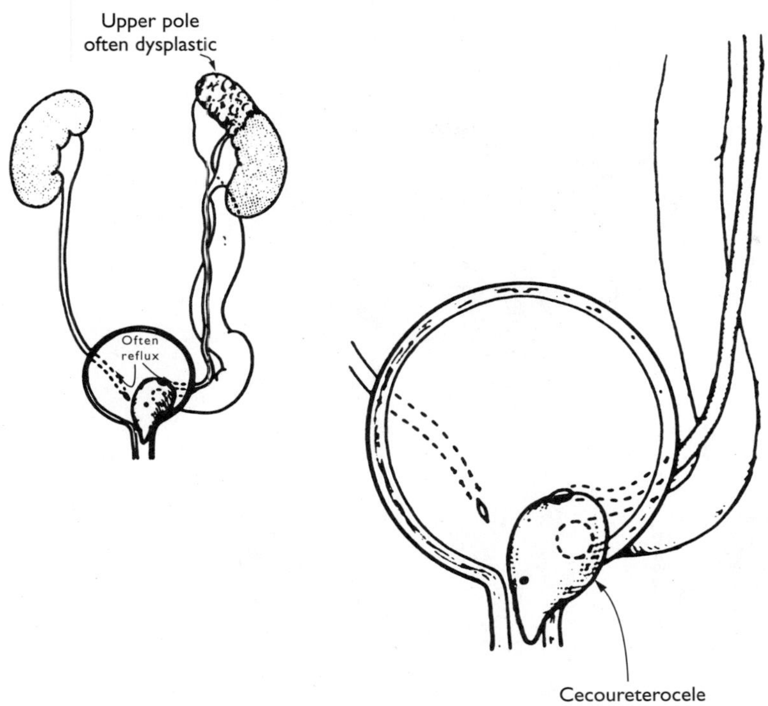

FIG. 22-5 *The cecoureterocele, associated with a poorly functioning upper-pole moiety, extends through the bladder neck. The lower-pole moiety often will be associated with vesicoureteral reflux.*

phenotypic females, where there is a single perineal opening for passage of urine, genital secretions, and feces or meconium (cloacal malformation) or a perineal opening and anus as seen in urogenital sinus. Both of these defects relate to failure of the urogenital sinus or urorectal septum (cloaca) to completely form.

The prognosis of infants with the cloacal malformation has dramatically improved in recent years. The imperative is to preserve renal function, which is the most significant potential cause for morbidity in these patients. Thus imaging studies and cystoscopy become very important in defining the anatomic characteristics and documenting whether obstruction or vesicoureteral reflux is present. Early diversion of the fecal stream by colostomy is necessary in the patient with a cloaca. In addition, further radiographic evaluation of the genitourinary tract, intestine, lower spinal cord, and pelvic wall is necessary because of the high potential for spinal malformation.[29]

A helpful way to categorize the cloacal malformation is by defining the level of confluence of the vagina, rectum, and urinary tract.[30] The cloacal configuration has been categorized as either urethral or vaginal (Fig. 22-6, *A*). The former involves a narrow, long, and curved cloaca (continuation of urethra), whereas the latter is a wide, straight continuation of the vagina. The urinary-cloacal communication is categorized as urethrocloacal when a well-formed urethra joins the bladder or vesicocloacal when the urethra is absent or diminutive (Fig. 22-6, *B*). It is unlikely that the vesicocloacal configuration would have a continent bladder neck. In addition, a good number of these patients can have spinal anomalies including dysraphism, segmentation anomalies, and spinal stenosis. Spinal cord tethering has been increasingly recognized, since magnetic resonance imaging has been used to assess the spinal cord.

The repair of cloacal anomalies mandates that the anatomy is very well defined both radiographically and endoscopically. The approach now favored is a posterior sagittal incision that allows correction of the anorectal, vaginal, and urogenital anatomic anomalies. A diverting colostomy is performed on the first day of life once the anomalies have been recognized. The subsequent surgery involves dividing the common cloaca into its component parts. Thus, with the posterior sagittal approach, the first structure to be identified is the rectum. In the case of a cloaca the rectum is mobilized and can be brought down into the correct position. The vagina is then separated from the urethra, with the plane of dissection being the anterior vaginal wall and the posterior urethral wall. The vagina can then be mobilized and the urethra lengthened the necessary amount so that each structure is brought out to the perineum. The key to this entire surgery is maintaining a midline dissection, which is aided by the use of an electrical stimulator. If a posterior sagittal approach is used for the urogenital sinus, a diverting colostomy is necessary to protect the repair. The rectum is actually divided in the midline so that access can be gained to the urogenital sinus. As in the case of a cloacal repair, the vagina and urethra are separated, and each structure is brought out to the perineum. In situations in which the vagina is connected to the urethra very low and close to the external opening of the sinus, a perineal approach can be used. The vaginal opening is enlarged often by use of skin flaps.

CONCLUSION

Anatomic urinary incontinence in the pediatric patient can be attributable to such obvious causes as epispadias or exstrophy. On the other hand, the explanation may be very subtle as in uni-

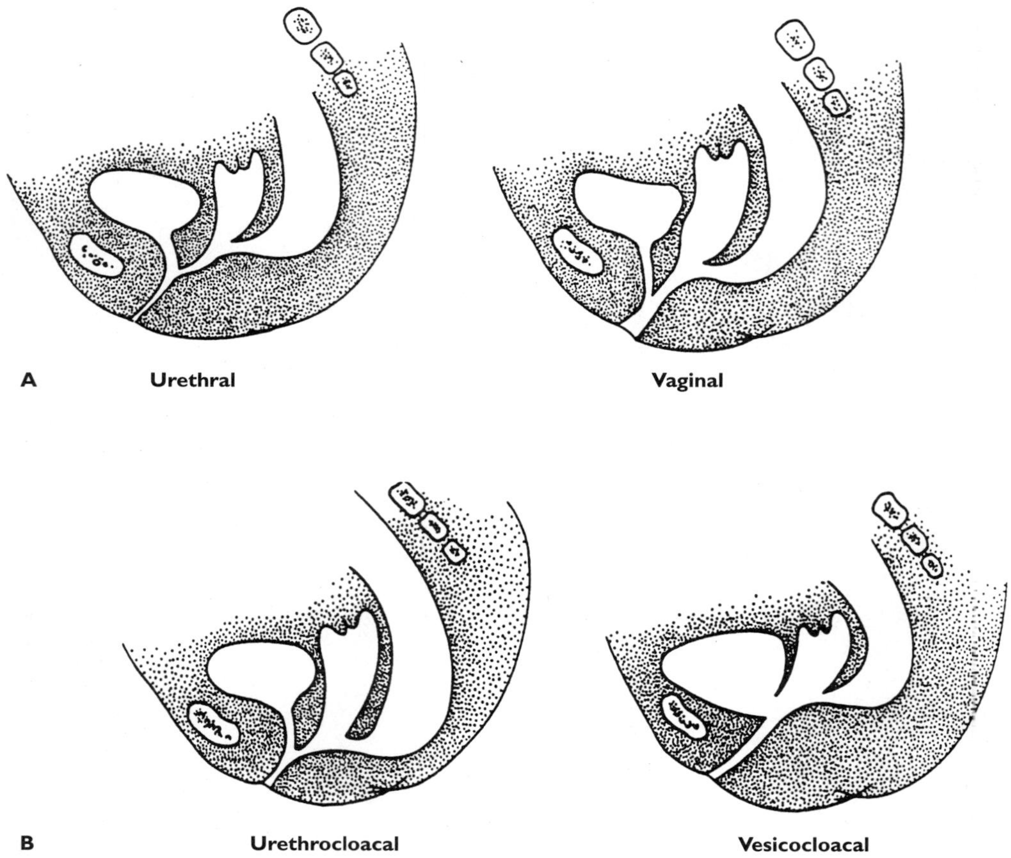

FIG. 22-6 *The cloacal malformation can be categorized as either urethral, with a narrow configuration, or vaginal with a wide configuration.* ***A,*** *The urinary-cloacal communication is called urethrocloacal when a well-formed urethra joins the bladder to the cloaca or vesicocloacal when the urethra is absent or rudimentary.* ***B,*** *A competent urinary sphincter would not be expected with these anatomic features.* (From Jaramillo D, Lebowitz RL, Hendren WH: *Radiology* 177:441, 1990.)

lateral or bilateral ureteral ectopia associated with duplicated collecting systems. The key is understanding the anatomy and ultimately the embryology. Treatment must be individualized to the patient. The most important surgical procedure is the initial procedure. Repeated operations generally lead to scarring and ultimately reduce the potential for ultimate success. Yet a lack of success does not mean that further attempts should be abandoned. Persistence is necessary particularly with the complicated cases. Careful urodynamic evaluation can lead to a better understanding of the bladder, bladder neck, and urethral functions. This information will prove of utmost importance before further attempts at reconstructive efforts are undertaken.

REFERENCES

1. Hinman F, Baumann FW: Vesical and ureteral damage from voiding dysfunction in boys without neurologic or obstructive disease, *J Urol* 109:727, 1973.
2. Allen TD: The non-neurogenic neurogenic bladder, *J Urol* 117:232, 1977.
3. van Gool JD, Hjälmås K, Tamminen-Möbius T, Olbing H: Historical clues to the complex of dysfunctional voiding, urinary tract infection and vesicoureteral reflux, *J Urol* 148:1699, 1992.
4. Greenfield SP, Fera M.: Urodynamic evaluation of the patient with an imperforate anus: a prospective study, *J Urol* 146:539, 1991.
5. Boemers TML, van Gool JD, de Jong TP, Bax KM: Lower urinary tract dysfunction in children with benign sacrococcygeal teratoma, *J Urol* 151:174, 1994.
6. Mandell J, Bauer SB, Hallett M, et al: Occult spinal dysraphism: a rare but detectable cause of voiding dysfunction, *Urol Clin North Am* 7:349, 1980.
7. Ambrose SS, O'Brien DP: Surgical embryology of the exstrophy/epispadias complex, *Surg Clin North Am* 54:1379, 1974.
8. Young HH: Exstrophy of the bladder: the first case in which a normal bladder and urinary control have been obtained by plastic operations, *Surg Gynecol Obstet* 74:729, 1942.
9. Dees JE: Congenital epispadias with incontinence, *J Urol* 62:513, 1949.
10. Leadbetter GW: Surgical correction of total urinary incontinence, *J Urol* 91:261, 1964.
11. Williams DI, Keeton JE: Further progress with reconstruction of the exstrophied bladder, *Br J Surg* 60:203, 1973.
12. Mollard P: Bladder reconstruction in exstrophy, *J Urol* 124:525, 1980.
13. Mollard P, Mouriquand PDE, Butten X: Urinary continence after reconstruction of classical bladder exstrophy (73 cases), *Br J Urol* 73:298, 1994.
14. Hendren WH: Congenital female epispadias with incontinence, *J Urol* 125:558, 1981.

15. Jeffs RD, Guice SL, Oesch I.: The factors in successful exstrophy closure, *J Urol* 127:974, 1982.
16. Gearhart JP, Jeffs RD: Management of the failed exstrophy closure, *J Urol* 146:610, 1991.
17. Gearhart JP, Peppas DS, Jeffs RD: Complete genitourinary reconstruction in female epispadias, *J Urol* 149:110, 1993.
18. Jones JA, Mitchell ME, Rink RC: Improved results using a modification of the Young-Dees-Leadbetter bladder neck repair, *Br J Urol* 71:555, 1993.
19. Barrett DM, Parulkar BG, Kramer SA: Experience with AS800 artificial sphincter in pediatric and young adult patients, *Urology* 42:431, 1993.
20. Leo ME, Barrett DM: Success of the narrow-backed cuff design of the AMS800 artificial urinary sphincter: analysis of 144 patients, *J Urol* 150:1412, 1993.
21. Brito CG, Mulcahy JJ, Mitchell ME, Adams MC: Use of a double cuff AMS800 urinary sphincter for severe stress incontinence, *J Urol* 149:283, 1993.
22. Shortliffe LMD, Freiha FS, Kessler R, et al: Treatment of urinary incontinence by the periurethral implantation of glutaraldehyde cross-linked collagen, *J Urol* 141:539, 1989.
23. Caione P, Capozza N, Lais A, et al: Female genito-urethroplasty and submucosal periurethral collagen injection as adjunctive procedures for continence in the exstrophy-epispadias complex, *Br J Urol* 71:350, 1993.
24. Hollowell JG, Hill PD, Duffy PG, Ransley PG: Evaluation and treatment of incontinence after bladder neck reconstruction in exstrophy and epispadias, *Br J Urol* 71:743, 1993.
25. Retik AB, Peters CA: Ectopic ureter and ureterocele. In Walsh PC, Gittes R, Perlmutter A, Stamey T, editors: *Campbell's urology*, ed 6, Philadelphia, 1992, Saunders.
26. Daird F, Chateil JF, Bondonny JM, et al: "Pseudo-ureterocele": buckling of an ectopic megaureter imprinting the urinary bladder, *J Radiol* 68:177-184, 1987.
27. Williams DI, Fay R, Lillie JG: The functional radiology of ectopic ureterocele, *Br J Urol* 44:417, 1972.
28. Gomez F, Stephens FD: Cecoureterocele: morphology and clinical correlations, *J Urol* 129:1017, 1988.
29. Jaramillo D, Lebowitz RL, Hendren WH: The cloacal malformation: radiologic findings and imaging recommendations, *Radiology* 177:441, 1994.
30. Hendren WH: Cloacal malformations: experience with 105 cases, *J Pediatr Surg* 27:890, 1992.
31. Pena A, deVries PA: Posterior sagittal anorectoplasty: important technical considerations and new applications, *J Pediatr Surg* 17:796, 1982.

Chapter 23

Spina Bifida and Other Spinal Disorders

Julian Wan, Saul P. Greenfield

Incontinence is a common urologic symptom of pediatric spinal cord abnormalities. This chapter is a discussion of the evaluation and treatment of incontinence in prevalent pediatric spinal cord disorders. Much progress has been made in the care of patients with spinal disorders over the past 50 years. They are living longer, staying healthier, and having better prospects of functioning effectively in society. Many of these advances are attributable to the successful recognition and management of their urologic concerns. The first part of this chapter deals with the most common of pediatric spinal disorders: spina bifida. The second part covers other important spinal conditions, which include occult spina dysraphism, caudal regression syndrome, sacral agenesis, imperforate anus, the VACTERL* syndrome, transverse myelitis, and physically induced injury.

Spina Bifida

Classification and Epidemiology

In patients with spina bifida, there is an abnormal innervation of the bladder that leads to neurogenic bladder dysfunction. This in turn has consequences for urinary continence and renal development and growth. The abnormality occurs as a result of a failure of fusion of the posterior aspects of one or more vertebrae.[1] This happens early in pregnancy, during the first trimester, and can cause maldevelopment not only of the bony vertebral bodies, but also of the underlying spinal cord and overlying skin. Disruption of the spinal cord is variable, and therefore the spinal level of the defect cannot be predictive of the neurologic deficit. Furthermore, there can be associated intracranial abnormalities, such as hydrocephalus and Arnold-Chiari malformation, which may also compound the neurologic difficulties.[2] Each child must be considered individually, since the urologic dysfunction will be unique and not easily categorized by the level of bony abnormality. The majority of these occur in the lower thoracic, lumbar, or sacral vertebrae.

Spina bifida is further classified into three subtypes: myeloschisis, myelomeningocele, and meningocele. Myeloschisis is the most severe. There is a flat, exposed neural plate, without any covering of skin, dura, or meningeal tissue and open spinal fluid leakage. Myelomeningocele is the most common, around 50%, and there is a meningeal covering over the neural plate. Meningoceles are herniations of dura through the vertebral defect, often without any neural elements. This subtype therefore has the mildest of neurologic or urologic deficits. All forms of spina bifida are usually surgically closed within the first 48 hours of life.[1]

The incidence of spina bifida has declined by half over the last decade from six to three per 10,000 live births.[3] Improvement in

*VACTERL is an association of vertebral abnormalities, anal atresia, cardiac abnormalities, tracheoesophageal fistula or esophageal atresia, renal agenesis and dysplasia, and limb defects.

maternal prenatal nutrition and early diagnosis are believed to be responsible. Maternal folic acid deficiencies have been implicated, and oral folic acid supplementation has reduced but not eliminated the incidence of spina bifida.[4] Prenatal alpha-fetoprotein testing and early termination of pregnancy have also contributed to the decline.[5] The incidence is higher in England, Ireland, and Wales and, in general, lower among Africans and Asians than in whites.[6,7] Girls are more commonly affected than boys.[8] Some families with multiple children with spina bifida exhibit a genetic predisposition.[9] If there is already one affected child, the risk of having a subsequent affected sibling increases to 5%, and if there are two affected siblings, the risk of having a third rises to 15%.

With improvement in neurosurgical care, over 90% of newborns survive.[10] Eighty percent or more will have normal intelligence, especially those without hydrocephalus, cerebral hemorrhage, or meningitis. The majority complete secondary school, and about one third receive additional education. Nearly 85% are capable of functional ambulation with bracing, canes, or walkers.[10,11]

Urologic Aims and Principles

Although incontinence is a visible and often distressing symptom to the child and parents, it must be remembered that *it is only a single symptom of a complex urologic problem.* This fact cannot be overemphasized, especially when discussing care with parents whose child's other symptoms may be minimal. A "dry" child is not necessarily urologically well, nor is a "wet" child necessarily a urologic cripple. The treatment of incontinence in spina bifida patients therefore should be part of an overall urologic management plan. Such a plan seeks two distinct but related goals: preservation of renal function and attainment of complete urinary continence.

The aberrant innervation of the bladder detrusor muscle and the sphincter causes various combinations of dysfunction. Incontinence in a diaper is expected in infancy, and so this is not addressed at first. Some of the infants, however, have bladder and sphincter dysfunction leading to abnormally high bladder pressures. These pressures can result in vesicoureteral reflux, hydronephrosis, recurrent urinary tract infection with pyelonephritis, and subsequent renal damage.[12-15] Abnormally high bladder pressures with chronic infection can also result in the bladder wall changes of muscular hypertrophy and fibrosis. This in turn causes a less compliant bladder wall and decreased bladder capacity.[16] These children will have greater difficulty with continence when older, since the ability of the bladder to act as an adequate, low-pressure reservoir will be compromised.[17] The earliest urologic effort in infancy therefore is to categorize the neurovesical dysfunction and identify those who require early intervention to prevent both the bladder and the upper urinary tract changes. Therefore, even though the child's continence is not a critical concern at this time, the process of monitoring and treating any bladder dysfunction has a direct effect on future potential continence.

At around school age of the child families start to worry more about continence, and the exact age for addressing the problem will differ from family to family. Normal toilet training is relatively uncommon in these children, but many families would like to try before moving on to other modalities. Depending on the type of neurovesical dysfunction, getting out of diapers will require management with drugs, self-catheterization, or surgery. Monitoring of dysfunction must continue beyond the early school years and well into adolescence, since the neurologic lesion may change with time.[18,19] The cord may become tethered as the child grows and the spine elongates, thus causing changes in bladder and sphincter function.[20]

Urologic Evaluation in Infancy

The urologist usually sees the newborn with spina bifida after the back is closed. Some infants may have a distended bladder and urinary retention secondary to spinal shock after back closure, which can be transient.[21] Intermittent catheterization should be started until urodynamics are obtained. Undescended testes are more common in these children, and so examination of the inguinal canal is important in boys. Circumcision is often deferred until later. A urinalysis and culture should also be obtained initially.

A renal and bladder ultrasound along with a contrast voiding cystourethrogram (VCUG) are performed as soon as the baby can be placed supine after back surgery and at intervals over the ensuing years. If videourodynamic facilities are available, the VCUG can be combined with the urodynamic study initially. The early radiographic studies will reveal other congenital urologic anomalies, which might be coincident with spina bifida, but most important, serve as a baseline reference. The renal ultrasound can detect the development of hydronephrosis over time (Fig. 23-1). The VCUG is inspected for bladder shape, bladder wall outline and vesicoureteral reflux (Fig. 23-2). Vesicoureteral reflux, if present at birth, may be caused by congenital deficiency of the antireflux valve mechanism at the ureterovesical junction, as in most children, or a manifestation of neurovesical dysfunction and high bladder pressures, which can begin in utero.[22,23] Management of the reflux, therefore, might require more than antibiotic prophylaxis or antireflux surgery, but it might also entail reduction of bladder pressures.[24]

Urodynamics is the cornerstone of urologic management and along with the radiographic findings guide therapy.[10,15] Videourodynamics, which combine the pressure tracings with a simultaneous VCUG under fluoroscopy, are ideal. A standard cystometrogram (CMG), however, will suffice to diagnose worrisome neurogenic bladder behavior. Sphincter electromyograms (EMG) using needle or patch electrodes also help to characterize external sphincter function. The bladder pressure observed when urethral leakage occurs, called "leak point pressure" (LPP), should remain below 40 centimeters of water (cm H_2O) to avoid deleterious effects on the bladder wall and upper urinary tracts (Fig. 23-3).[13] Early bladder contractions with high pressures are also of concern. Inappropriate neural stimulation and muscular contraction of the detrusor are responsible for these elevated bladder pressures. The sphincter EMG is watched for detrusor-sphincter dyssynergia (DSD), that is, an inappropriate increase in electrical activity during bladder contraction.[25,26] Failure of the external sphincter to relax during bladder contraction is also often found with high leak point pressures.

A

B

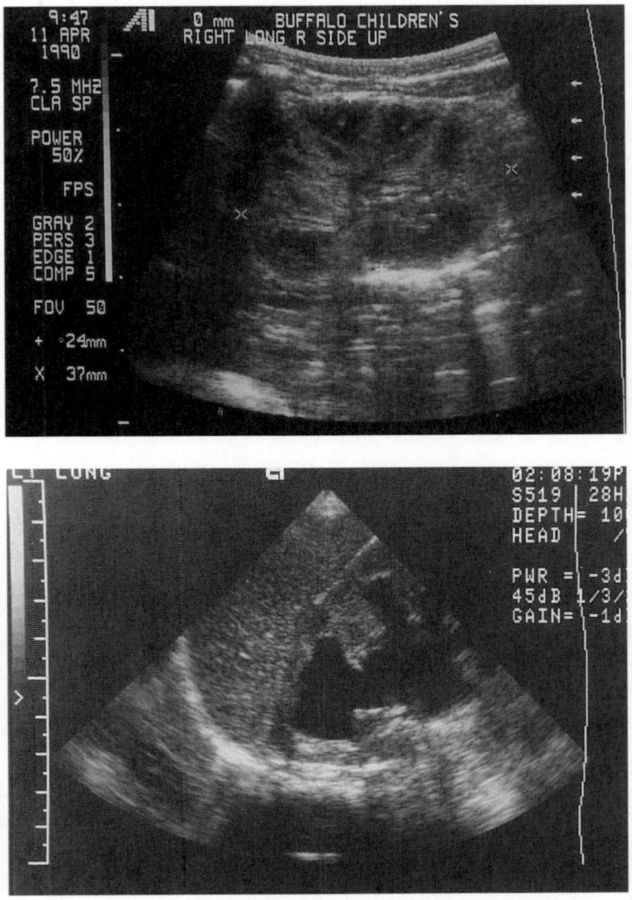

FIG. 23-1 ***A,*** *Normal renal ultrasonogram without hydronephrosis in an infant with spina bifida and a high leak point pressure who was observed without therapy.* ***B,*** *Renal ultrasonogram in the same infant 22 months later demonstrating new hydronephrosis.*

A

B

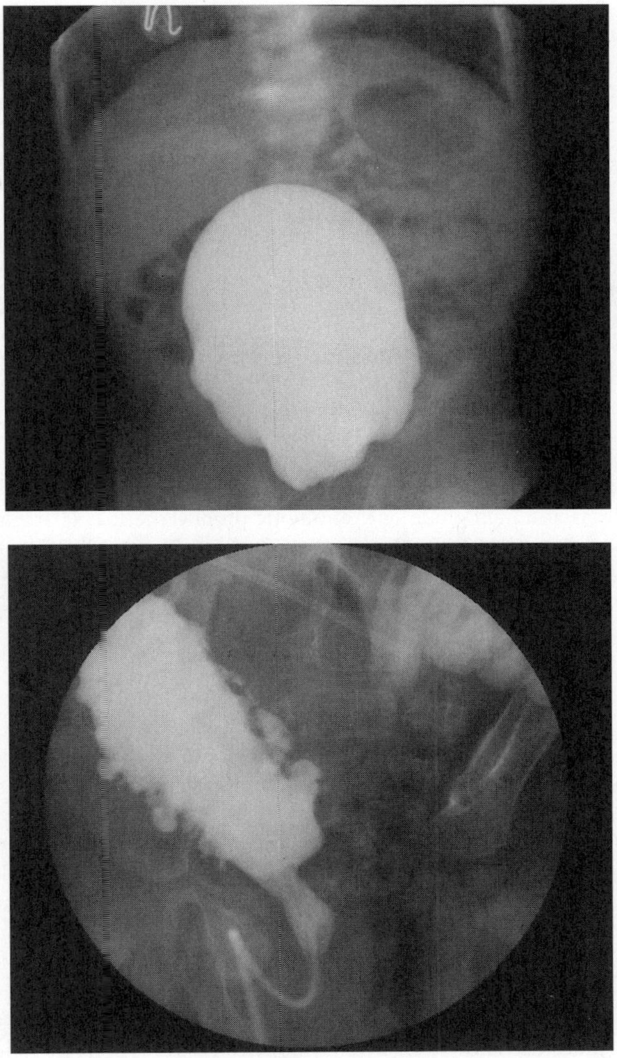

FIG. 23-2 ***A,*** *Normal voiding cystourethrogram (VCUG) in an infant with spina bifida and a high leak point pressure who was observed without therapy. Notice that the bladder wall outline is round and smooth.* ***B,*** *Follow-up VCUG in the same infant 8 months later showing the development of bladder wall trabeculation, cellules, and elongation.*

An LPP greater than 40 cm H_2O mandates early intervention with intermittent catheterization and oral anticholinergics.[13] Catheterization alone may be recommended for those bladders that are at low pressure and atonic but do not empty at all. A temporary cutaneous vesicostomy, which can be reversed when the child is older, may be required in infants in whom either medication fails or there is inability to comply with a catheterization and medication schedule.[27,28] Plastic 8 French gauge feeding tubes are used in the smallest infants, and latex products are avoided, because of the high incidence of latex allergies in these children.[29,30] Since efforts to gain continence often require catheterization when older, early familiarity with catheterization techniques results in greater acceptance in the future.[31,32] A regimen of catheterizing 4 to 6 times per day and allowing the child to sleep overnight is usually well tolerated by families. Oxybutynin or hyoscyamine are commonly used anticholinergic medications that inhibit detrusor contractions and cause smooth muscle relaxation. If oral medication is ineffective or anticholinergic side effects are debilitating (dry mouth, heat intolerance, constipation), intravesical oxybutynin can be used. Crushed oxybutynin tablets are dissolved in water and then instilled at the end of a catheterization.[33] Delivered in this manner, there are fewer side effects and a greater drug effect on the bladder muscle.

No urologic intervention is instituted for those infants who have leak points below 40 cm H_2O. These infants are allowed to be incontinent in their diapers. The Credé maneuver, which is the manual application of force to expel urine from the bladder, is not recommended, since very high pressures are generated.[34] Urodynamics are repeated at 6 months and one year of age and at intervals thereafter. The VCUG and renal ultrasonogram are also repeated at intervals along with urine cultures. A change in the urodynamic or radiographic parameters may mandate a shift from observation to intervention. In addition, cord tethering may be signified by a change in urodynamic findings. Those with high-pressure bladders are reevaluated more frequently to judge the success of therapy. Vesicoureteral reflux might require surgical correction if

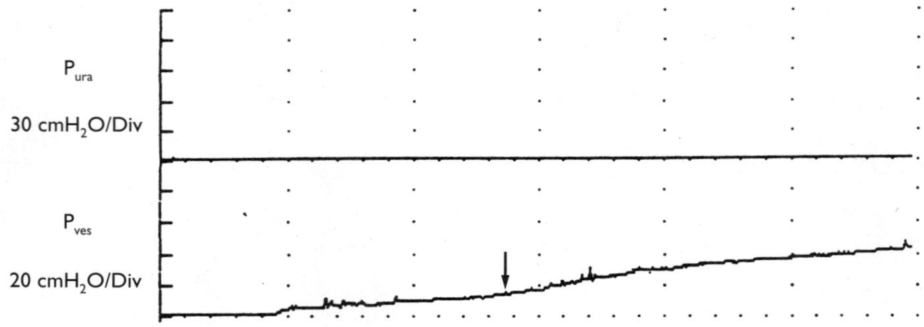

FIG. 23-3 *Pressure tracing seen during a cystometrogram performed on a child with spina bifida reveals a low bladder pressure (<40 cm H_2O). The arrow indicates when leakage from the urethra was observed, thereby marking this point as the leak point pressure.* (From Wan J, Greenfield SP: Pediatric urodynamics. In Chancellor M, Blaivas J, editors: *Atlas of urodynamics,* Baltimore, 1995, Williams & Wilkins.)

it is at a high grade or if antibiotic prophylaxis fails to maintain sterile urines. Maintenance of sterile urines can be difficult along with intermittent catheterization, since the majority of those children will have bacteriuria.[35] The success of reimplantation surgery may also be compromised if bladder pressures remain high.

Continence in the Older Child

As mentioned earlier, the age at which both family and child wish to pursue continence is variable. An understanding of the nature of both the bladder and the urethral sphincter dysfunction is the key to devising a program of continence. For most children who cannot voluntarily void, continence depends on having both a low-pressure, compliant bladder that stores adequate volumes of urine and a competent proximal urethral sphincter. The bladder is then artificially emptied with intermittent catheterization. Both families and physicians must be realistic about the level of continence that can be attained. The wearing of one or two pads a day with regular underwear allows for a normal lifestyle in the eyes of many patients and families.[36] For many, even after aggressive surgical procedures, this is the result. Bowel habits and fecal continence also become important at this time. Failure to eliminate fecal soiling will leave the child in diapers, despite good urinary control. For this reason it is important to establish a bowel program that ensures predictable periodic emptying of the rectum. Once continence is established, new onset wetting may signify cord tethering, which is occurring along with somatic growth of the child. Prompt neurosurgical intervention will often restore continence.

Clean intermittent catheterization (CIC) performed at first by family members and then by the patient is the basis for continence in most of these children. Strict technique using sterile gloves and fields is not necessary.[35] Bacteriuria is present in the majority but is most often asymptomatic and is not treated. Attempts to prevent this bacteriuria with antibiotic prophylaxis are frustrating and lead to resistant organisms. This is only an issue in those children who have vesicoureteral reflux and the relatively rare patient with a symptomatic infection. Children and families who are unprepared for CIC or rebellious adolescents who refuse to comply remain a challenge to the clinician. Often the problem lies in a misunderstanding or incomplete comprehension of the reasons why CIC needs to be done. Occasionally it is a very simple matter that the wrong-sized catheter is being used. This sometimes can be seen in children who have been followed from birth. As the child grows, it is forgotten that the urethra also expands and can accommodate a larger size of catheter. We have discovered teenage patients still using 8 and 10 Fr tubes. These smaller tubes worked well when the child was younger but now prolong the drainage process, making CIC a very tedious process. When a larger, appropriately sized catheter was substituted, drainage times became more reasonable, and patient compliance with CIC improved.

Assuming adequate urethral sphincter resistance, to remain dry a child must have a low-pressure, compliant bladder. Clean catheterization alone or with either oral or intravesical anticholinergics may then be all that is required. Early urologic management from infancy onward ensures that most children will not reach the age of continence with permanently altered bladder walls or upper urinary tracts. A small number will require surgical bladder augmentation (see Chapter 55). This is most often accomplished by use of detubularized segments of the gastrointestinal tract—stomach, ileum, or colon.[37,38] Compliance and commitment are more important in these individuals, since failure to catheterize an augmented bladder may lead to intraperitoneal rupture and death.[39] A newer technique, termed "autoaugmentation," refers to increasing bladder capacity by removal of only the detrusor muscle from the bladder dome so as to allow the bladder epithelium to expand.[40,41] This has met with mixed success but is a simpler and less morbid procedure. In general, among properly selected and motivated patients, bladder augmentation is highly successful and gratifying.

A dysfunctional urethral sphincter remains the greatest challenge to continence. Pharmacologic manipulation is rarely successful. Alpha-adrenergic medications, such as ephedrine or imipramine, can be tried, but most often fail. Very low LPPs are suggestive of a poorly functioning urethra.[42] This can be confirmed radiographically by observation of leakage through a patulous bladder neck. Another related parameter is known as the stress leak point pressure (SLPP, also known as the Valsalva leak point pressure, or VLPP), which is the measurement by which dysfunctional urethras can be reproducibly and reliably identified.[43] It is the pressure at which a patient leaks with a full bladder, after abdominal pressure is applied by a Valsalva maneuver or external compression. A SLPP of less then 90 cm H_2O suggests that a urethral procedure will be necessary (Fig. 23-4).

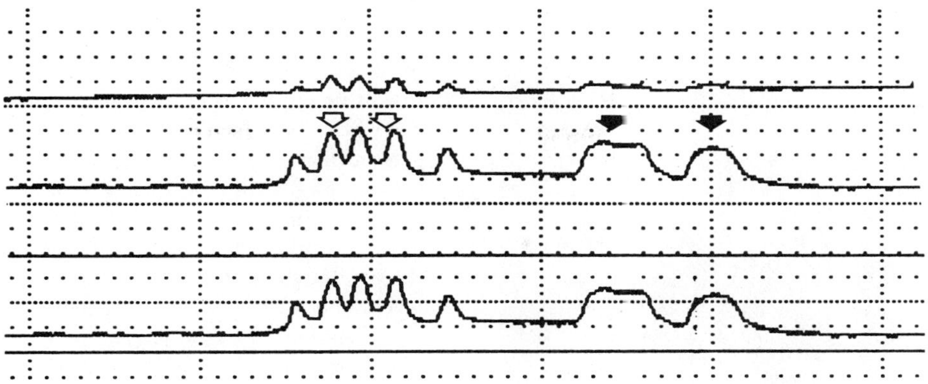

FIG. 23-4 *A stress leak point pressure (SLPP), also known as a Valsalva leak point pressure (VLPP), is shown on this tracing from a patient with spina bifida. Leakage is observed with the rise in bladder pressure during both coughing* (open arrows) *and Valsalva maneuvers* (closed arrows). (From Wan J, Greenfield SP: Pediatric urodynamics. In Chancellor M, Blaivas J, editors: *Atlas of urodynamics,* Baltimore, 1995, Williams & Wilkins.)

There are several approaches to correcting an incompetent urethra, and no one ideal method exists for all patients. Current options include periurethral collagen injection, periurethral fascial sling, bladder neck reconfiguration, and the artificial urinary sphincter.[44-48] Of these, periurethral collagen injection is the simplest, since it is an outpatient procedure that can be repeated and does not preclude performance of other procedures. In some spina bifida patients it can be accomplished with little or no anesthesia.

A small number of patients, for reasons of posture or a lack of motor coordination, cannot catheterize the urethra in its orthotopic location. Catheterizable and continent abdominal stomas, using appendix, native ureter, or tubularized bladder wall have been devised.[49-51] These can also be employed when surgical approaches to the sphincter fail. In that circumstance, the bladder neck is divided, closing off urinary egress via the urethra. The patient can then catheterize through an abdominal stoma.

Older treatment concepts for incontinence should be avoided. Long-term indwelling Foley catheters or suprapubic tubes are to be condemned. They result in urethral stricture and fistula, bladder stones, chronic bladder inflammation and contraction, bladder malignancies, and upper urinary tract damage.[52] Standard ileal loop diversion is unsuitable for children or young adults with many years ahead of them, since upper urinary tract damage will ensue over time.[53] Diversion to an abdominal stoma with a collection bag also implies that the bladder cannot be rehabilitated or modified, a rare circumstance with contemporary management techniques.[54]

Occult Spinal Dysraphism

Unlike the defects seen in spina bifida, the spinal abnormalities associated with occult spinal dysraphism (OSD) occur beneath an intact skin covering. There is still a posterior bony defect, but because the overlying dermis and epidermis are intact, it is often undetected until it manifests itself neurologically. The term "occult spinal dysraphism" should not be confused with "spina bifida occulta," which refers to the radiologic finding of a small gap between the bony posterior elements of the vertebral bodies. These patients only rarely have spinal cord abnormalities with neurologic or urologic sequelae.[55]

It is theorized that the abnormality of OSD occurs because of an abnormality during the separation or disjunction of the ectoderm and the underlying neural tube. An important consequence of this failure in disjunction is that the ectoderm as it differentiates can give rise to a cutaneous marker that acts as a clue to the presence of OSD. Cutaneous abnormalities of the lumbosacral back are not always present but have been found in up to 80% of patients with OSD.[56-59] These include classic findings such as a dermal sinus tract, hairy tufts, deep skin pimples, and hemangiomas (Fig. 23-5).

Neurologically the failure in disjunction can lead to abnormal attachments of the spinal cord. These attachments prevent the cord from floating freely within the spinal canal. With activity and growth they act as points of fixation, hence the term "tethered spinal cord." The most common point of tethering occurs in the lumbosacral region at the end of the spinal cord. When the cord is tethered, it experiences traction and tension. Repetitive stretching causes venous congestion, arteriolar and capillary spasm, which can lead to ischemia and hypoxia of the cord and nerve roots. Because this occurs most commonly at the end, or conus, of the cord, the manifestations of tethering are usually first seen in the lower limbs, bowels, and bladder. Leg pain, paresthesia, bowel incontinence and severe constipation, bladder areflexia, dyssynergia, and hyperreflexia are all possible symptoms.[60]

The evaluation of suspected OSD should include imaging of the spine, upper urinary tract (by ultrasonogram or intravenous pyelogram) and urodynamics. In infants up to 6 months of age, spinal ultrasonography is a useful modality to determine the appearance of the cord (Fig. 23-6).[61] After 6 months of age, spinal ossification precludes the use of this study. Because many children present when older, often after failing to acquire toilet control, an MRI scan of the spine is the preferred diagnostic modality. It can clearly determine the level of the conus, particularly on a sagittal view. The conus should be at or above the L2 vertebral body regardless of age. Upper urinary tract findings are dependent on the severity of the bladder dysfunction. Although

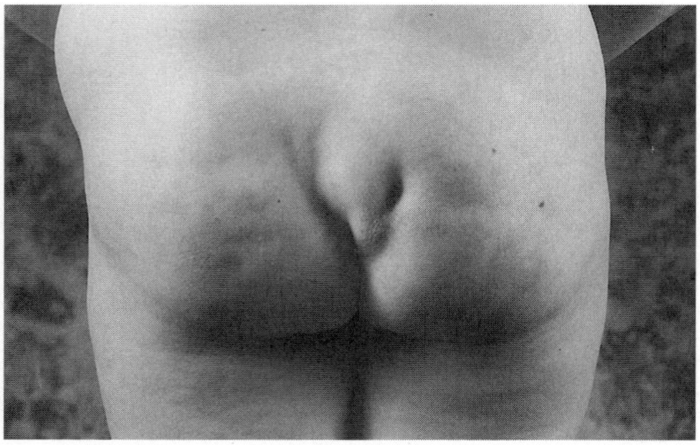

FIG. 23-5 *Teenage girl who presented with day and night wetting. On physical examination, there was found an abnormal gluteal skin fold and a hair tuft arising from this cleft. This patient was found to have occult spinal dysraphism.* (From Wan J, Greenfield SP: Pediatric urodynamics. In Chancellor M, Blaivas J, editors: *Atlas of urodynamics,* Baltimore, 1995, Williams & Wilkins.)

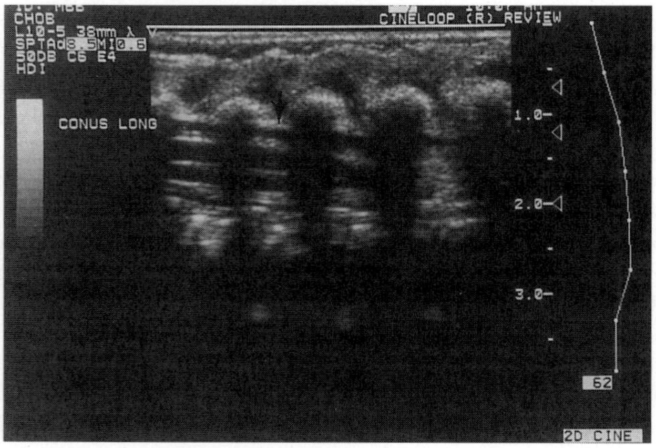

FIG. 23-6 *A spinal ultrasonogram from a newborn child being evaluated for possible occult spinal dysraphism. The conus can be seen between the gaps of the not yet ossified vertebral bodies* (arrow). *This child was normal.*

the whole gamut of urodynamic findings can occur (normal to hyperreflexic to flaccid), the usual finding is of a poorly compliant bladder with incomplete emptying.

The treatment of OSD is aimed at relieving the spinal cord tethering. When the onset of symptoms is acute, there can be reversal with recovery, but often when detection has been delayed, there can only be the hope for prevention of further damage and deterioration. In such cases where normal voiding and continence does not return, management with self-catheterization and anticholinergics may be required life long.

Caudal Regression Syndrome, Sacral Agenesis, Imperforate Anus, VACTERL Syndrome

The caudal regression syndrome is an umbrella term given to a range of associated anomalies that have vertebral and spinal cord abnormalities that in turn can give rise to abnormal bladder innervation and function. First noted by Duhamel in 1961, in its most severe form it includes sacral agenesis, imperforate anus, fusion of the lower extremities (a process giving rise to the descriptive "mermaid syndrome"), and complete absence of the genitourinary tract except for the gonads.[62] The disorder occurs during the fourth to fifth weeks of gestation when the lumbosacral spine and nephrogenic blastema are forming. It is also during this time that the cloacal septum is advancing to divide the genitourinary sinus from the rectum. Although the most severe "mermaid" form is fortunately rare, the other less extreme manifestations, notably sacral agenesis and imperforate anus, are more common. The VACTERL syndrome includes imperforate anus as one of its salient features, as well as other anomalies unrelated to caudal regression.

Sacral Agenesis

Sacral agenesis is characterized by the absence of part or all of the lowermost vertebral bodies.[63] The exact cause remains undefined, but vascular compromise or teratogenic factors have been implicated by the observation that insulin-dependent diabetic mothers have a 1% chance of bearing a child with sacral agenesis. Conversely, about 15% to 20% of children with sacral agenesis have a diabetic mother. This diabetes need only be of the gestational insulin-dependent type.[64,65] There can be spinal cord and root abnormalities, intradural lipomas, dermoid cysts, and cord tethering. The neurourologic manifestations of sacral agenesis can develop because of these intrinsic abnormalities or from the subsequent effects of the cord tethering. Sacral agenesis can present later in life when the child fails to be toilet trained. Since there is usually normal lower limb function and sensation, up to 20% of patients with sacral agenesis are found only after their third or fourth birthdays.[66] A physical examination commonly reveals flattened buttocks with a short gluteal cleft and no palpable coccyx.[65] A plain radiograph would show an absent sacrum (Fig. 23-7). Urodynamically about 25% have normal functioning bladders; another 33% have areflexic bladders, which can overfill and thereby cause wetting; and the remainder exhibit bladder hyperreflexia with and without dyssynergia. The severity of the urodynamic findings do not correlate with the severity of the bony defect. Thus patients with a complete sacral absence can still have normal bladder function, and those missing just one vertebral body can have very severe bladder dysfunction.[65]

Imperforate Anus

Imperforate anus occurs approximately once in every 4000 to 5000 newborns with a male predominance.[67] This anomaly is described and classified according to the level of the imperforation. The higher the lesion, the more likely there will be other associated vertebral and genitourinary abnormalities. Spinal column malformations occur in up to 40% of patients with anorectal defects and usually present as partial or complete sacral agenesis.[68] High rectal pouches that end well above the pelvic floor musculature characteristically have a fistula linking the pouch with the prostatic urethra in boys and the vagina or uterus in girls. Lower lesions

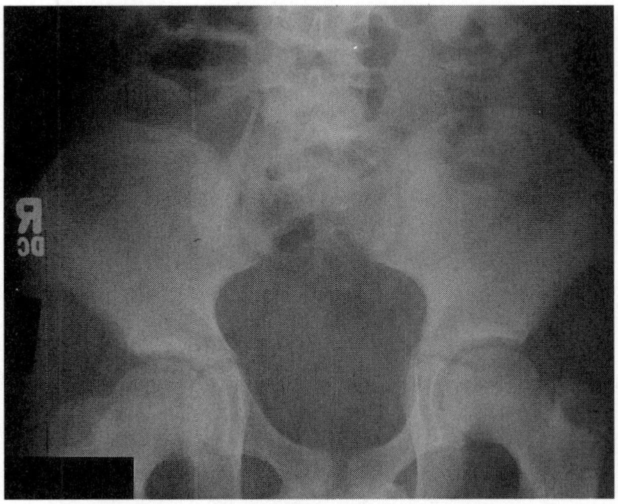

FIG. 23-7 *This child was evaluated for failure of toilet training. On physical exam flat buttocks and no palpable coccyx were noted. The subsequent radiograph shows no sacral bony elements consistent with sacral agenesis.*

(below the pelvic floor musculature) may manifest only as a stenotic anus or a fistula to the perineum or distal area of the vagina. Other urologic problems that can be found in the presence of imperforate anus include concomitant vesicoureteral reflux, unilateral renal agenesis or dysplasia, and neurogenic bladder. For these reasons, patients with an imperforate anus should undergo a thorough urologic evaluation of the upper and lower urinary tracts: VCUG, ultrasonogram, or intravenous pyelogram. This work-up should include urodynamics because around 10% to 20% of the patients studied will have a dysfunctional neurogenic bladder, and some of these children will have no bony abnormalities.[69] Regular periodic testing should begin shortly after birth and is particularly important before and after any anorectal repair. Reconstructive surgery can affect bladder innervation and thereby alter bladder behavior. A cooperative effort therefore should be made by the pediatric surgeons and the pediatric urologists.[67]

VACTERL Syndrome

The VACTERL syndrome is a non-random association of multiple congenital anomalies first noted in 1968.[70] The acronym denotes the site of the various abnormalities: V, *v*ertebral (usually a hemivertebra); A, *a*norectal malformation, imperforate anus; C, *c*ardiac (ventricular or atrial septal defect); TE, *t*racheo*e*sophageal fistula; R, *r*enal agenesis/dysplasia and *r*adial absence; L, *l*imb lesions. Patients with any two of these findings should be suspected of having the syndrome, and a full search should be conducted in the remaining categories. The degree of lower limb function can be totally normal; hence it is a misleading sign and should not be used to gauge the severity of the syndrome. As with the anomalies mentioned earlier, the emphasis should be on the recognition that a neurourologic abnormality can exist and should be actively identified. A thorough urologic evaluation with upper tract studies and urodynamics is therefore warranted (Fig. 23-8).[71-73]

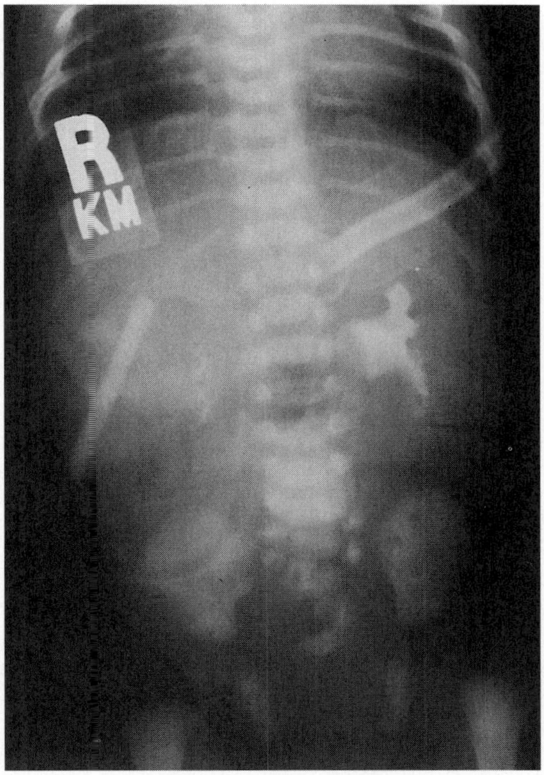

FIG. 23-8 *An infant with VACTERL syndrome underwent an intravenous pyelogram. This child has unilateral renal agenesis, and no kidney is visualized on the right side. There is a normal left kidney, and the distorted sacrum is clearly visible.*

Transverse Myelitis

The term "transverse myelitis" is applied to those conditions that cause partial or total motor paralysis, paresthesia, and bowel or bladder dysfunction.[74] There are many different known causes, chiefly inflammatory and infectious, and it can also occur idiopathically.[75-80] The causes are listed in the box on p. 178.

Symptoms develop at or below the level of the lesion. It is characterized by patchy spinal cord inflammation and will occasionally result in demyelination and focal destruction. The symptoms may evolve over several days to weeks and months. Resolution is equally languorous. Classically there is a loss of bladder function with an inability to empty. Wetting usually occurs as a form of overflow incontinence. Supportive care is normally all that is required while the underlying cause is sought and treated. Where possible, clean intermittent catheterization (CIC) should be used. Serial urodynamic studies should be done to track the course of the disease and during recovery (Fig. 23-9). The mere fact that the patient is "voiding" or wetting the diaper should not be taken as evidence of good bladder function. The patient may not be voiding normally, and urodynamic testing should be performed to confirm normal behavior. Essentially the goal is to protect the bladder and upper urinary tract until the cause is identified and treated and normal function can resume.

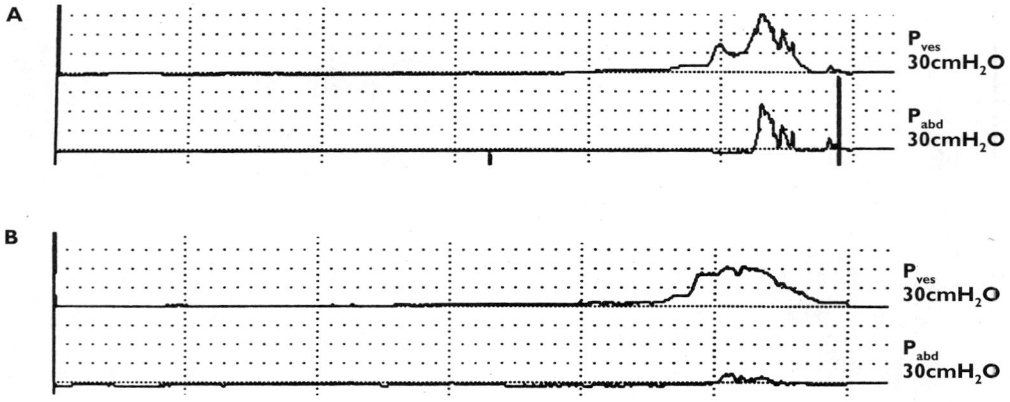

FIG. 23-9 ***A,*** *Twelve-year-old girl who had developed transverse myelitis. At the onset of the condition her voiding appeared strained. The tracing shows two pressure measurements. The upper line shows bladder pressure (P_{ves}), and the lower line shows intra-abdominal pressure (P_{abd}). Because her bladder was affected by her condition, she was unable to void except by abdominal straining. This is seen by the simultaneous rise in abdominal pressure with the bladder pressure.* ***B,*** *After several months this same patient shows improvement with a bladder contraction without a simultaneous rise in abdominal pressure. This confirms that her voiding is no longer caused by abdominal straining.* (From Wan J, Greenfield SP: Pediatric urodynamics. In Chancellor M, Blaivas J, editors: *Atlas of urodynamics,* Baltimore, 1995, Williams & Wilkins.)

Causes of Transverse Myelitis

VIRAL
Poliomyelitis
Coxsackie
Herpes zoster
Rabies
Epstein-Barr
Mumps
BACTERIAL
Syphilis
Tuberculosis
Bacterial meningitis sequelae
PARASITIC AND FUNGAL
VASCULAR AND INFLAMMATORY
Arteritis—systemic lupus erythematosus, polyarteritis nodosa
Arterial insufficiency—aneurysmal occlusion, malformations
NUTRITIONAL
Vitamin B_{12} deficiency
Vitamin B_6 deficiency
IDIOPATHIC

TRAUMA

The management of spinal cord trauma in pediatric patients is similar to that of adults[81,82] (see Chapter 50). Once the initial phase of spinal shock has worn off, regular urodynamic testing should be done to follow the bladder. As with the patients with spina bifida, CIC plays an important role in the management of spinal cord–injured patients. Long-term indwelling catheters, suprapubic tubes, and Credé methods of emptying should be avoided. A short duration of Foley drainage is acceptable if monitoring of fluid output is needed or if temporary diversion is required because of associated perineal or abdominal injuries.

As a rule-of-thumb, injuries to the pelvic nerves result in a flaccid areflexic bladder prone to overflow incontinence if unrecognized. Lesions within the spinal cord but below the level of the level of the pons usually result in bladder hyperreflexia and a discoordinated external sphincter. Lesions at or above the level of the pons usually manifest as bladder hyperreflexia with coordination. Finally, injuries above the T6 vertebral level can result in the loss of feedback inhibition to the sympathetic chain, which can result in an uncontrolled sympathetic discharge when the patient experiences any noxious stimulus. This is known as autonomic dysreflexia and results in a grouping of symptoms, most notably bradycardia, severe hypertension, sweating, and nausea. An undrained bladder or impacted rectum are classic stimuli and should be considered when one is faced with a patient having such symptoms.

REFERENCES

1. Reigel DH, Rotenstein D: Spina bifida. In Cheek WR, Marlin AE, McLone DG, et al, editors: *Pediatric neurosurgery,* ed 3, Philadelphia, 1994, Saunders.
2. Swaiman KF: *Pediatric neurology: priniciples and practice,* St. Louis, 1994, Mosby.
3. Centers for Disease Control: Spina bifida incidence at birth—United States, *MMWR* 41:497, 1992.
4. Laurence KM: In prevention of neural tube defects by improvement in maternal diet and preconceptional folic acid, supplementation in prevention of physical and mental congenital defects, Part B: Epidemiology, early detection and therapy and environmental factors, *Prog Clin Biol Res* 168:383, 1985.
5. Milunsky A, Alpert E, Neff RK, et al: Prenatal diagnosis of neural tube defects. IV. Maternal serum alpha-fetoprotein screening, *Obstet Gynecol* 55:60, 1980.
6. Elwood JH: Major central nervous system malformations notified in Northern Ireland, 1964-1968, *Dev Med Child Neurol* 14:731,1972.
7. Elwood JM, Elwood JH: *Epidemiology of anencephalus and spina bifida,* New York, 1980, Oxford University Press.
8. Sever LE, Saunders M, Monsen R: An epidemiologic study of neural tube defects in Los Angeles County. I. Prevalence at birth based on multiple sources of case ascertainment, *Teratology* 25:315, 1982.

9. Fraser F: Genetic counseling in some common paediatric diseases, *Am J Hum Genetics* 26:636, 1974.
10. Mclone DG: Continuing concepts in the management spina bifida, *Pediatr Neurosurg* 18:254, 1992.
11. Woodhouse CRJ: Neuropathic bladder. In Woodhouse CRJ, editor: *Long-term paediatric urology,* London, 1991, Blackwell Scientific Press.
12. Bauer SB, Hallet M, Khoshbin S, et al: The predictive value of urodynamic evaluation in the newborn with myelodysplasia, *JAMA* 152:650, 1984.
13. McGuire EJ, Woodside JR, Borden TA, et al: The prognostic value of urodynamic testing in myelodysplastic patients, *J Urol* 126:205, 1981.
14. McLorie GA, Perez-Morero R, Csima AL, et al: Determinants of hydronephrosis and renal injury in patients with myelomeningocele, *J Urol* 140:1289, 1986.
15. Sidi AA, Dyktra DD, Gonzalez R.: The value of urodynamic testing in the management of neonates with myelodysplasia: a prospective study, *J Urol* 135:90, 1986.
16. Kaufman AM, Roberts AC, Rudy DC, et al: Decreased bladder compliance in myelomeningocele patients managed by radiologic observation, Presented at American Urologic Association, 19th annual meeting, Las Vegas, Nevada, April 1995.
17. Bauer SB: Neuropathology of the lower urinary tract. In Kelalis PP, King LR, Belman AB, editors: *Clinical pediatric urology,* ed 2, Philadelphia, 1992, Saunders.
18. Spindel MR, Bauer SB, Dyro FM, et al: The changing neuro-urologic lesion in myelodysplasia, *JAMA* 258:1630, 1987.
19. Begger JH, Meihuizen de Regt MJ, Hogen Esch I, et al: Progressive neurologic deficit in children with spina bifida aperta, *Z Kinderchir* 41(suppl 1):13, 1986.
20. Reigel DH, McLone DG: Tethered spinal cord. In Cheek WR, Marlin AE, McLone DG, et al, editors: *Pediatric neurosurgery,* ed 3, Philadelphia, 1994, Saunders.
21. Kroovand RL, Bell W, Hart LJ, et al: The effect of back closure on detrusor function in neonates with myelodysplasia, *J Urol* 144:423, 1990.
22. Bauer SB: Vesico-ureteral reflux in children with neurogenic bladder dysfunction. In Johnston JH, editor: *International perspectives in urology,* vol 10, Baltimore, 1984, Williams & Wilkins.
23. Kopp C, Greenfield SP: Effects of neurogenic bladder dysfunction in utero seen in neonates with myelodysplasia, *Br J Urol* 71:739, 1993
24. Flood HD, Ritchey ML, Bloom DA, et al: Outcome of reflux in children with myelodysplasia managed by bladder pressure monitoring, *J Urol* 152:1574, 1994.
25. Blaivis JG, Sinka HP, Zayed AH, et al: Detrusor-sphincter dyssynergia: a detailed electromyographic study, *J Urol* 125:545 1986.
26. van Gool JD, Kuijten RH, Dockenwolcke R, et al: Detrusor-sphincter dyssynergia in children with myeolmeningocele: a prospective study, *Z Kinderchirg* 37:148, 1982.
27. Mandell J, Bauer SB, Colodny AH, et al: Cutaneous vesicostomy in infancy, *J Urol* 126:92, 1981
28. Duckett JW: Cutaneous vesicostomy in childhood, *Urol Clin North Am* 1:485, 1974.
29. Shapiro E: Complications of latex allergy, *Dialogues of Pediatric Urology* 15(3):1-8, 1992.
30. Slater JE: Allergic reactions to natural rubber, *Ann Allergy* 68:203, 1992.
31. Geraniotis E, Koff SA, Enrile B: Prophylactic use of clean intermittent catheterization in treatment of infants and children with myelomeningocele and neurogenic bladder dysfunction, *J Urol* 139:85, 1988.
32. Joseph DB, Bauer SB, Colodny AH, et al: Clean intermittent catheterization in infants with neurogenic bladder, *Pediatrics* 84:78, 1989.
33. Greenfield SP, Fera M: The use of intravesical oxybutynin chloride in children with neurogenic bladder, *J Urol* 146:532, 1991.
34. Barbalias GA, Klauber GT, Blaivis JG: Critical evaluation of the Credé maneuver: a urodynamic study of 207 patients, *J Urol* 130:720, 1983.
35. Lapides J, Diokno AC, Silber SJ, et al: Clean intermittent self-catheterization in the treatment of urinary tract disease, *J Urol* 107:458, 1972.
36. Hernandez RD, Hurwitz RS, Foote JE, et al: Nonsurgical management of threatened upper urinary tracts and incontinence in children with myelomeningocele, *J Urol* 152:1582, 1994.
37. Mitchell ME, Piser JA: Intestinocystoplasty and total bladder replacement in children and young adults: follow-up of 129 cases, *J Urol* 138:1140, 1987.
38. Adams MC, Mitchell ME, Rink RC: Gastrocystoplasty: an alternative solution to the problem of urological reconstruction in the severely compromised patient, *J Urol* 140:1152, 1988.
39. Elder JS, Snyder HM, Hulbert WC, et al: Perforation of the augmented bladder in patients undergoing clean intermittent catheterization, *J Urol* 140:1159, 1988.
40. Cartwright PC, Snow BW: Bladder autoaugmentation: early clinical experience, *J Urol* 142:505, 1989a.
41. Cartwright PC, Snow BW: Bladder autoaugmentation: partial detrusor excision to augment bladder without use of bowel, *J Urol* 142:1050, 1989b.
42. McGuire EJ, Fitzpatrick CC, Wan J, et al: Clinical assessment of urethral sphincter function. *J Urol* 150:1452, 1993.
43. Wan J, McGuire EJ, Bloom DA, Ritchey ML: Stress leak point pressure: a diagnostic tool for incontinent children, *J Urol* 150:700, 1993.
44. Barrett DM, Furlow WL: The management of severe urinary incontinence in patients with myelodysplasia by implantation of the AS791/792 urinary sphincter device, *J Urol* 128:44, 1982.
45. Raz S, Ehrlich RM, Zeidman EJ, et al: Surgical treatment of the incontinent female patient with myelomengocele, *J Urol* 139:524, 1988.
46. McGuire EJ, Wang CC, Usitalo H, et al: Modified pubovaginal sling in girls with myelodysplasia, *J Urol* 135:94, 1986.
47. Kropp KA, Angwafo FF: Urethral lengthening and reimplantation for neurogenic incontinence in children, *J Urol* 135:533, 1986.
48. Wan J, McGuire EJ, Bloom DA, et al: The treatment of urinary incontinence in children using glutaraldehyde cross-linked collagen, *J Urol* 148:127, 1992.
49. Sumfest JM, Burns MW, Mitchell ME: The Mitrofanoff principle in urinary reconstruction, *J Urol* 150:1875, 1993.
50. Mitrofanoff P: Cystometrie continente trans-appendiculaire dans le traitement des vessies neurologiques, *Chir Pediatr* 21:297, 1980.
51. Duckett JW, Snyder HM III: Continent urinary diversion: variations of the Mitrofanoff principle, *J Urol* 136:58, 1986.
52. Wan J, McGuire EJ, Fleenor S, et al: Urinary tract status of patients with neurogenic dysfunction presenting with upper tract stone disease, *J Urol* 148:1126, 1992.
53. Shapiro SR, Lebowitz RL, Colodny AH: Fate of 90 children with ileal conduit urinary diversion a decade later: analysis of complications, pyeloplasty, renal function and bacteriology, *J Urol* 114:289, 1975.
54. Hendren WH: Urinary diversion and undiversion in children, *Surg Clin North Am* 56:425, 1976.
55. Boone D, Parsons D, Lochman SM, et al: Spina bifida occulta: lesion or anomaly? *Clin Radiol* 36:159, 1985.
56. McAtee SJ, Hebert AA, Rapini RP, et al: Skin lesions of the spinal axis and spinal dysraphism: fifteen cases and review of the literature, *Arch Pediatr Adolesc Med* 148:740, 1994.
57. Hendrick EB, Hoffman JH, Humphreys RP: The tethered spinal cord, *Clin Neurosurg* 30:457, 1983.
58. Davis DA, Cohen PR, George RE: Cutaneous stigmata of occult spinal dysraphism, *J Am Acad Dermatol* 31(part 2):892, 1994.
59. Schmidt DM, Robinson B, Jones DA: The tethered spinal cord: etiology and clinical manifestations, *Orthoped Rev* 29:870, 1990.
60. Thompson WF, McKay M: Occult spina dysraphism: case report and review of the literature, *Orthopedics* 9:403, 1986.

61. Korsvik HE: Ultrasound assessment of congenital spinal anomalies presenting in infancy, *Semin Ultrasound CT MR* 15:264, 1994.
62. Duhamel B: From the mermaid to anal impeforation: the syndrome of caudal regression, *Arch Dis Child* 36:152-155, 1961.
63. O'Neill OR, Piatt JH Jr, Mitchell P, Roman-Goldstein S: Agenesis and dysgenesis of the sacrum: neurosurgical implications, *Pediatr Neurosurg* 22:20, 1995.
64. Passarge E, Lenz K: Syndrome of caudal regression in infants of diabetic mothers: observations of further cases, *Pediatrics* 37:672, 1966.
65. Guzman L, Bauer SB, Hallett M, et al: The evaluation and management of children with sacral agenesis, *Urology* 23:506, 1983.
66. Koff SA, DeRidder PA: Patterns of neurogenic bladder dysfunction in sacral agenesis, *J Urol* 118:87, 1977.
67. Brock WA, Pena A: Cloacal abnormalities and imperforate anus. In Kelalis PP, King LR, Belman AB, editors: *Clinical pediatric urology*, ed 2, Philadelphia, 1992, Saunders.
68. Greenfield SP, Fera M: Urodynamic evaluation of the patient with an imperforate anus: a prospective study, *J Urol* 146:539, 1991.
69. Sheldon C, Cormier M, Crone K, et al: Occult neurovesical dysfunction in children with imperforate anus and its variants, *J Pediatr Surg* 26:49, 1991.
70. Say P, Geral PS: A new polydactyly/imperforate anus/vertebral anomalies syndrome? *Lancet* 2:688, 1968.
71. Temtamy SA, Miller JD: Extending the scope of the VATER association: definition of the VATER syndrome, *J Pediatr* 85:345, 1974.
72. Uehling DT, Gilbert E, Chesney R: Urologic implications of the VATER association, *J Urol* 129:352, 1983.
73. Weaver DD, Mapstone CL: The VATER association: analysis of 46 patients, *Am J Dis Child* 140:225, 1986.
74. Altrocchi PH: Acute transverse myelopathy, *Arch Neurol* 9:112, 1963.
75. Carriere JP: Acute transverse myelitis and coxsackie A9 virus infection, *Pediatr Infect Dis J* 13:77, 1994.
76. Nussinovitch M, Brand N, Frydman M, et al: Transverse myelitis following mumps in children, *Acta Paediatr* 81:183, 1992.
77. Mills RW, Schoolfield L: Acute transverse myelitis associated with *Mycoplasma pneumoniae* infection: a case report and review of the literature, *Pediatr Infect Dis J* 11:228, 1992.
78. Heller L, Keren O, Mendelson L, et al: Transverse myelitis associated with *Mycoplasma pneumoniae*: case report, *Paraplegia* 28:522, 1990.
79. Boyce TG: Acute transverse myelitis in a 6-year-old girl with schistosomiasis, *Pediatr Infect Dis J* 9:279, 1990.
80. Propper DJ, Bucknall RC: Acute transverse myelopath complicating systemic lupus erythematosus, *Ann Rheum Dis* 48:512, 1989.
81. McGuire EJ: Spinal cord injury. In *Clinical evaluation and treatment of neurogenic vesical dysfunction*, Baltimore, 1984, Williams & Wilkins.
82. Fanciullacci F, Zanollo A, Sandri S, et al: The neuropathic bladder in children with spinal cord injury, *Paraplegia* 26:83, 1988.

PART FIVE INCONTINENCE IN ADULTS

Chapter 24 Practical Urodynamics

Jack Christian Winters, Rodney A. Appell

In present-day practice, urodynamic testing varies from simple uroflowmetry without instrumentation to complex multichannel urodynamic testing and plays a significant role in the evaluation of symptoms or complications associated with lower urinary tract dysfunction. A large number of tests and devices to perform individual urodynamic studies exist, and it is the responsibility of the clinician to perform the most accurate, least invasive, and least expensive study to assist in making the proper diagnosis by evaluating a reproduction of the patient's symptoms. Therefore a thorough neurourologic history and physical examination is essential before a urodynamic study is performed. The clinician should formulate a working diagnosis before the urodynamic evaluation, which will assist in the selection of the most precise study.

When one is considering urodynamic tests, it is important to think of voiding in two phases, filling and storage.[1] Also it is essential to identify activity in the bladder and bladder outlet (bladder neck and proximal urethra) during both the filling and the storage phases. Bladder filling and urine storage requires accommodation of increasing volumes of urine at low pressures with appropriate sensation, a closed bladder outlet at rest that remains closed during increases in intra-abdominal pressure, and the absence of involuntary bladder contractions. Bladder emptying requires a coordinated detrusor contraction of adequate magnitude and duration, concomitant lowering of resistance at the level of the smooth and striated sphincter, and the absence of anatomic obstruction. During the patient interview and physical examination, factors that may affect one or more of these parameters should be identified, with allowance for selection of the most appropriate urodynamic test.

It is important that urodynamics should reflect or reproduce the clinical symptoms of the patient. If the particular symptom of which the patient complains is not duplicated during the study, the study is not helpful in obtaining a diagnosis. For example, if the problem described by the patient is nocturnal enuresis, what would be the utility of performing awake urodynamics? As another example, if a patient states that she loses urine only in an upright position, nothing is to be gained by a supine cystometrogram. The urodynamic tests should confirm a specific diagnosis, allowing one to recommend the most appropriate therapy and aid in the determination of the patient's prognosis. If the test reveals information not expected by the clinician, he or she must repeat the history and physical exam to fully understand the cause or causes of the patient's urinary incontinence.

URODYNAMIC TESTING

It is important that urodynamics be performed without anesthesia in a setting as comfortable to the patient as possible. The tests may be tailored to performing a uroflow investigation with the patient voiding alone or a complex videourodynamic procedure involving several technicians and devices. Obviously the reduction in the equipment and people utilized for the study will make the patient more comfortable and allow the performance of a more physiologic study. However, the information gained from the study should not be compromised.

Uroflowmetry

Uroflowmetry is a basic urodynamic test recording the urinary flow rate throughout the course of voiding. The urinary flow rate is the volume of urine expelled through the urethra per unit time and is expressed in milliliters per second.[2] The uroflow is a simple test to assess the emptying phase of the voiding cycle. The uroflow may be affected by abnormalities in the bladder (decreased contractility) or bladder outlet (obstruction). Patients do not resist the idea of uroflowmetry because it is noninvasive; however, an important aspect of the test is to evaluate the residual urine (postvoiding residual, PVR) remaining in the bladder, which may require catheterization, especially if one is planning more invasive testing such as cystometry, or if one does not have ultrasound equipment readily available.

Of course, the simplest uroflowmetry is observation of the patient's stream and recording the time over which the patient's urinary volume in milliliters per second is voided. This, however, records only the average flow rate (Q_{avg}) and peak flow (Q_{max}), which has been accepted as the more accurate parameter of voiding efficiency, but even this is dependent on age, sex, voided volume, and position during voiding.[3]

The uroflow is more accurately measured by several varying techniques: rotating disk,[4] electronic dipstick method,[5] or the most common gravimetric method,[6] and the data are generated as a flow pattern (curve) with quantitative measurements of specific parameters of the voiding flow cycle. In addition to Q_{avg} and Q_{max}, the other individual variables recorded are volume voided (ml), voiding time (sec), and time to maximum flow (sec). These parameters are accompanied by a flow pattern that is extremely important in the adequate interpretation of uroflow data (Fig. 24-1). Certainly the quantitative measurements should not be interpreted in isolation without the flow pattern because abnormalities in the flow pattern may be suggestive of the cause of abnormal flow variables.

Abnormal flow patterns present in several types. An abnormally long, flat plateau with a low mean and peak rate of flow generally indicates outlet obstruction or decreased detrusor contractility. Intermittent flow is generally secondary to abdominal straining or sphincter dyssynergia. In rare instances, it may be attributable to undulating low-amplitude detrusor contractions[7] (Figs. 24-2, 24-3, and 24-4). Caution should be employed when one is interpreting a flow rate with a voided volume of less than 150 ml. In this way, Q_{max} should be more than 15 ml/sec. Low flow rates may reflect outlet resistance or impaired detrusor contractility, whereas high flow rates may be indicative of decreased outflow resistance.

A variety of nomograms exist to determine "acceptable flow rates" for a given age group. The Siroky[8] flow rate nomogram relates peak and average flow rate to intravesical volume. A particularly useful nomogram is the Drach[9] nomogram relating a maximum flow rate to voided volume. In males, these nomograms are useful in identifying flow rates worrisome for obstruction in a particular age group.

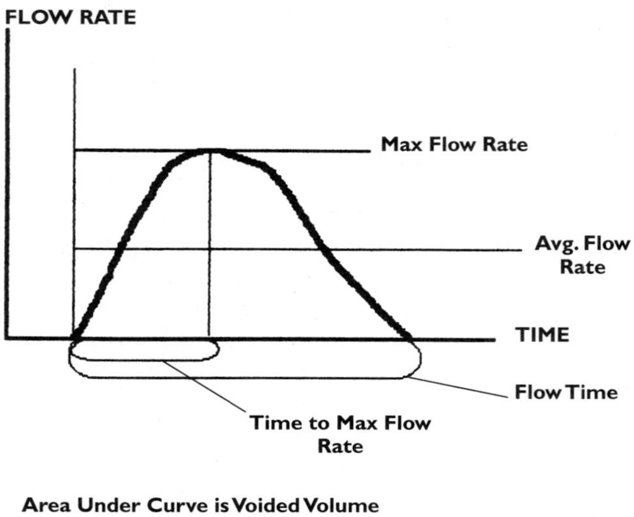

FIG. 24-1 *Normal uroflow curve depicting individual parameters of the flow cycle.*

Cystometry

Cystometry is the recording of intravesical pressure and is performed in two phases: filling cystometry and voiding cystometry. Filling cystometry is the measure of bladder pressure during the collecting or reservoir phase, whereas voiding cystome-

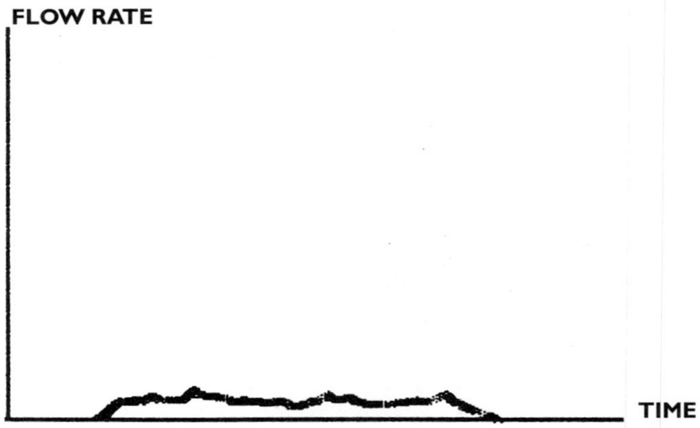

FIG. 24-2 *Prolonged, flat voiding curve seen in obstruction or impaired contractility.*

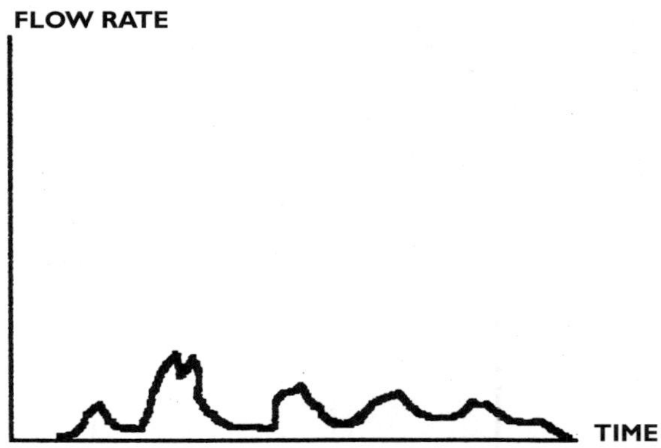

FIG. 24-3 *Intermittent flow curve with saw-toothed shape, commonly seen in abdominal straining or detrusor sphincter dyssynergia.*

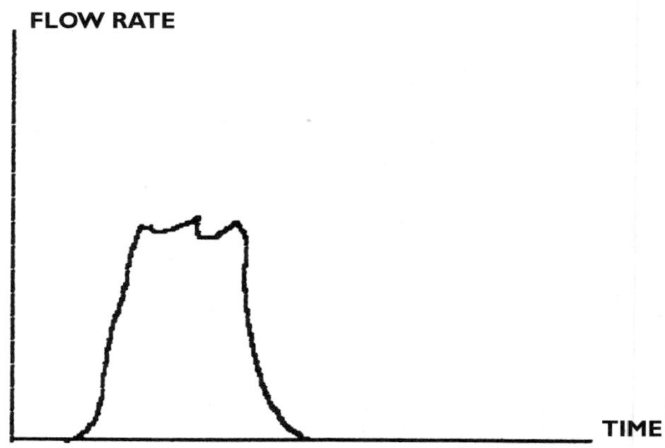

FIG. 24-4 *High rapid flow rate consistent with decreased urethral resistance, manifest in "supervoiders."*

try is the measurement of pressure during expulsion of urine. The media used for cystometry are water[10] or carbon dioxide gas.[11] Carbon dioxide (CO_2) has been noted to represent a rapid and simple method to measure changes in bladder pressure during filling, particularly detrusor instability.[12] However, CO_2 may act as vesical irritant, and leakage of it around the catheter, which is unnoticeable, may alter the result.[13] Additionally, gas expands in all directions at once, whereas water fills the bladder more physiologically from bottom to top. Also the use of water allows a uroflow study and voiding cystometry to be performed following the filling cystometrogram,[14] and contrast may be mixed with the water to allow radiographic anatomic studies when indicated.

Filling cystometry may be performed after the insertion of one small (7 to 10 Fr) multilumen bladder catheter. This catheter allows simultaneous instillation of water or gas and bladder pressure measurement during filling. A single-lumen catheter is not recommended because pressure changes would take place depending on the rate of filling (Bernoulli's principle). In other words, as the inflow of fluid through the catheter would be increased, the measurement of pressure within the bladder would also be increased. In a multilumen catheter any increase in inflow of fluid would not affect the measured pressure in the bladder. Since this is performed using one catheter within the bladder, it is known as a single-channel pressure measurement and measures total bladder (intravesical) pressure (P_{ves}): the sum of intrinsic detrusor muscle pressure (P_{det}) and intra-abdominal pressure (P_{abd}). Therefore any maneuver that increases intra-abdominal pressure will be reflected by an increase in total bladder pressure, which may be mistaken for a detrusor contraction; clinical observation by the physician during the study will betray obvious abdominal straining, but more subtle increases in intra-abdominal pressure may be overlooked. However, this can be obviated by use of a multichannel device by monitoring P_{abd} by means of a rectal balloon catheter. This P_{abd} value can be subtracted from the total bladder pressure to determine the true P_{det}. A simultaneous recording of intrarectal pressure is required to determine true detrusor pressure. The patient should be asked to cough at the beginning of the study, and the relationship between the intrarectal and intravesical pressure can be assessed and used throughout the cystometrogram to determine detrusor pressure. This is known as multichannel pressure recording and is useful for micturition (voiding) studies or in neurogenic and obstructive bladder conditions where abdominal straining is suspected. We prefer subtracted pressures, because they are easy to do and allow for a much more precise interpretation of the urodynamic study.

The rate of filling affects the pressure level at which the voiding reflex is activated and the presence of unstable bladder contractions.[15] Any nonvolitional rise in P_{det}, especially when associated with a sensation of the urge to void, is an unstable or uninhibited bladder contraction. The higher the rate of filling, the less physiologic it becomes, and the subject voids at lower volumes. Also, there are more unstable detrusor contractions elicited with a faster filling rate. Generally we use medium fill rates of 60 to 90 ml/min during our urodynamic studies. Maximum cystometric capacity is the filled volume at which the patient can no longer delay voiding and usually ranges from 350 to 500 ml. If the patient has this symptom complex but no involuntary contractions are noted, especially at a low filling volume, then the patient's condition is defined as *sensory with urge.*

During normal cystometry, an initial rise in bladder pressure occurs at a volume of less than 100 ml with an eventual flattening of the curve to a volume between 250 to 500 ml. This cycle of filling represents the time when compliance in the bladder is high, that is, the ability of the bladder muscle to accept an increase in volume without a concomitant rise in pressure. After this, a steep rise in bladder pressure is seen with increasing volume because the elastic properties of the bladder wall have reached their limit. This is followed by a uniform, coordinated bladder contraction seen as a sudden but smooth increase in pressure that then subsides after several seconds (Fig. 24-5).

In many patients, the initial rise in pressure at less than a 100 ml volume is commonly absent. No clinical significance is given to its absence During the phase of high bladder compliance, there should be a minimal rise of bladder pressure during filling, and bladder pressure should not exceed 6 cm H_2O during normal filling.[16] This period of high compliance lasts to a volume of approximately 250 to 500 ml in normal subjects. Abnormalities of pressure changes during this filling generally manifest as involuntary rises in detrusor pressure, known as detrusor instability.

Detrusor instability is seen in two forms: (1) A disorder of compliance, which is an abnormal rise in bladder pressure with increasing volume, is known as *tonic instability* (Fig. 24-6). These poorly compliant bladders generally result from neurologic injury or from inflammatory or infectious conditions or in patients with chronic indwelling catheters. Patients exhibiting no rise in bladder pressure despite an abnormally large bladder volume have bladders of increased compliance, which is characteristic of an individual with decreased sensation and bladder decompensation (Fig. 24-7). (2) Involuntary bladder contractions during filling with a return to baseline detrusor pressure is known as *phasic instability* (Fig 24-8). *Detrusor hyperreflexia*

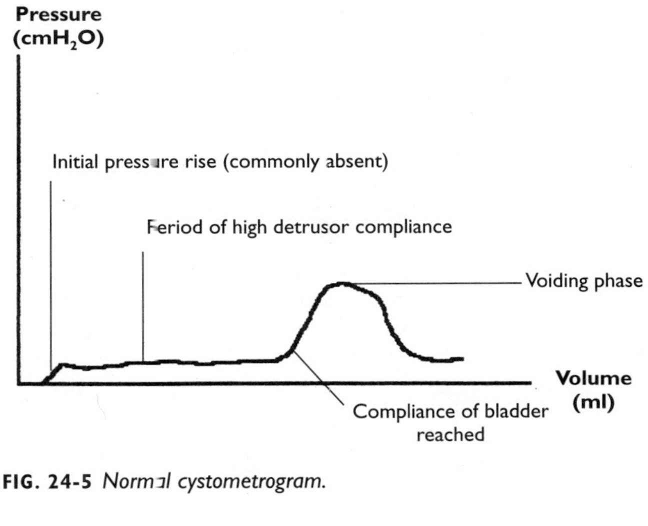

FIG. 24-5 *Normal cystometrogram.*

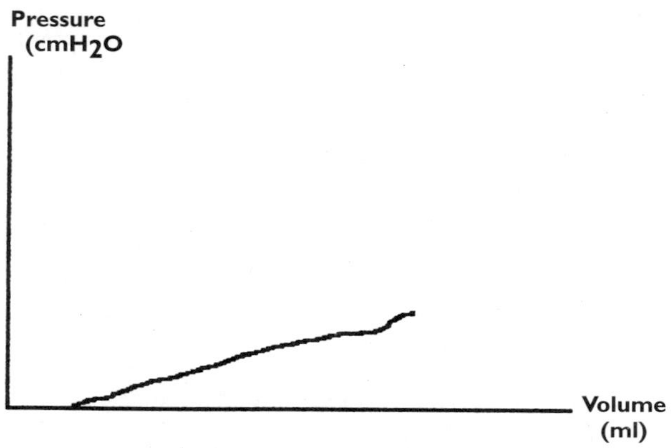

FIG. 24-6 *Detrusor instability. Low detrusor compliance known as "tonic instability."*

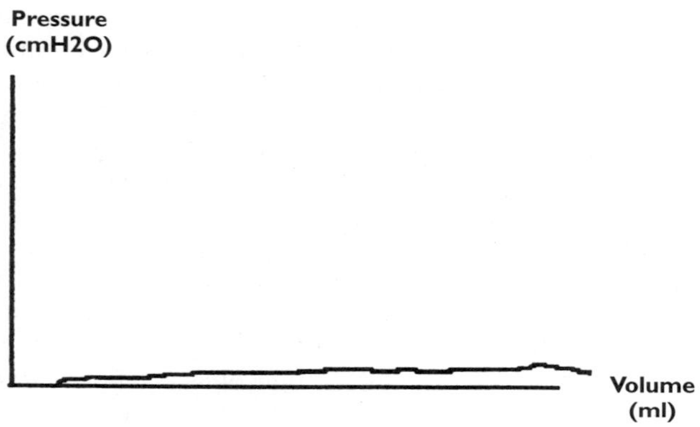

FIG. 24-7 *Abnormally high detrusor compliance. Patient with impaired sensitivity and contractility.*

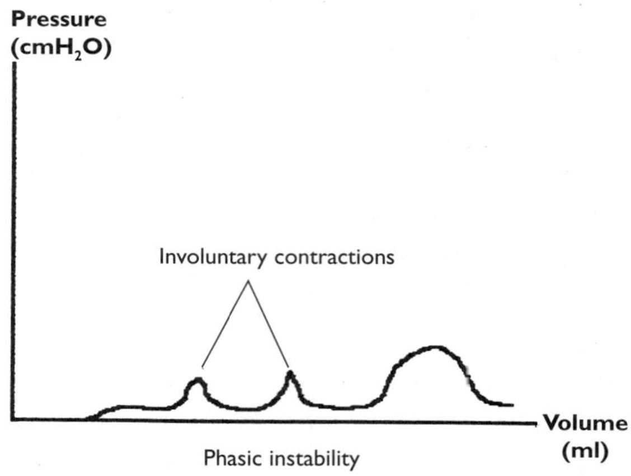

FIG. 24-8 *Detrusor instability, or detrusor hyperreflexia. Involuntary bladder contractions that return to baseline reference value, otherwise known as "phasic instability."*

refers to phasic involuntary bladder contractions in the presence of a known neurologic lesion such as multiple sclerosis, whereas *detrusor instability* is the presence of phasic involuntary bladder contractions in the absence of neurologic disease. It has been reported by the International Incontinence Society that phasic contractions of greater than 15 cm H_2O are required to obtain the diagnosis of detrusor instability.[17] However, it has been demonstrated that phasic contractions of less amplitude may certainly correlate with symptomatic detrusor instability evidenced by urgency to void, frequency of urination, and even urge incontinence.[18]

During the voiding phase, voiding cystometry or measurement of the voiding pressures simultaneously with uroflowmetry (pressure-flow study) allows determination of detrusor contractility. Detrusor contractility varies with patient age and sex. In men, voiding pressures of 45 to 60 cm H_2O are normal. Pressures higher than this one are suggestive of obstructive states, and pressures lower than this are suggestive of detrusor hypocontractility. In females, voiding pressures are certainly less, and it is not uncommon for females to void with detrusor pressures of 15 to 20 cm H_2O.

Electromyography

Electromyography (EMG) permits evaluation of the striated urinary sphincter during voiding. EMG recordings may be obtained by use of surface electrodes (skin patches), anal plugs, intraurethral electrodes, or needle and wire electrodes. Needle electrodes permit more accurate placement and recording, but in many patients surface electrodes provide a most useful signal that is clinically relevant.[19] In fact, in children, surface electrodes may be preferable because placement of the needle usually makes the child uncooperative for further study.

Normally, as the bladder fills with urine, there is a gradual and sustained increase in EMG activity recruited from the pelvic floor muscles. This reaches a maximum just before the voiding phase and is known as the "guarding reflex." Commonly, the first sign of voluntary voiding is complete electrical silence, signifying relaxation of the striated sphincter. This has been followed by a rise in detrusor pressure and coordinated voiding. During the study, abdominal straining (cough and Valsalva maneuvers) and other stimuli generally increase the EMG activity. Also, during the filling phase, an involuntary bladder contraction also produces an increase in EMG activity, a learned behavior from the patient to prevent urinary leakage. This may be commonly misinterpreted as detrusor-sphincter dyssynergia.

Detrusor-sphincter dyssynergia is obstruction to the outflow of urine during a bladder contraction caused by the involuntary contraction of the striated musculature surrounding the urethra. This is almost universally seen in patients with discrete neurologic disease such as multiple sclerosis or suprasacral spinal cord injury. This diagnosis must be made by means of a *voiding cystometrogram* only. During the voiding phase, the rise in bladder pressure during the bladder contraction is accompanied by a pronounced increase in activity from the striated musculature sphincter, which obstructs the flow of urine (Fig. 24-9). This is the hallmark of detrusor-sphincter dyssynergia and is almost universally seen in patients with an identifiable neurologic disease.[20] The diagnosis should be made with reservation in a patient with no neurologic history or other abnormal neurologic findings.

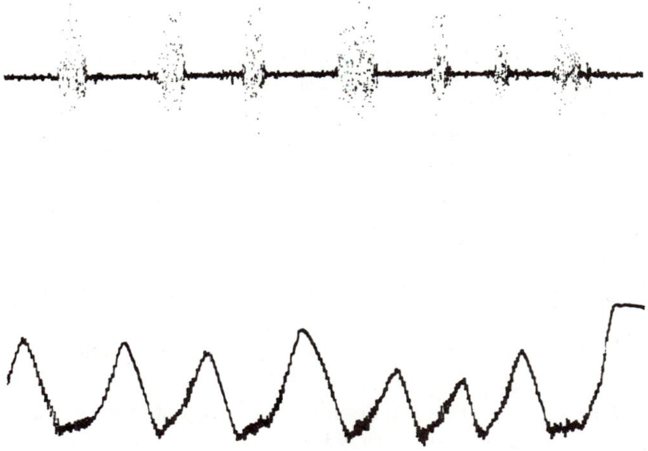

FIG. 24-9 *Detrusor sphincter dyssynergia.*

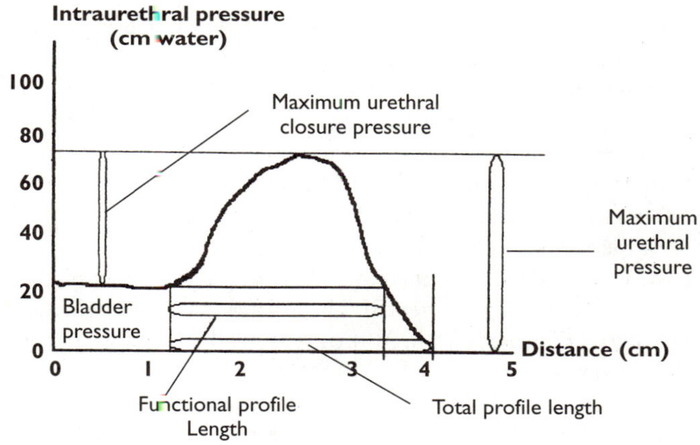

FIG. 24-10 *Urethral pressure profile curve depicting individual parameters of urethral profilometry.*

Urethral Pressure Profile

A static urethral pressure profile is a slow withdrawal of the catheter through the urethra with the patient at rest with the simultaneous recording of intraurethral pressure. The most widely used technique for urethral pressure profilometry is that described by Brown and Wickham in 1969.[21] The technique uses an 8 Fr single-lumen catheter with side holes placed about 2 to 3 cm from the tip. A motorized syringe pump is used to produce a constant flow through the catheter of 2 ml/min. The resistance to flow of infused fluid through the catheter side holes produced by the intraurethral pressure is recorded on a recorder from an externally mounted transducer. A catheter-withdrawal machine will allow constant catheter-withdrawal rates and may be synchronized to the selected paper chart speed. This will enable the extrapolation of the data to provide an accurate measurement of functional urethral length. Hand-pull techniques, not employing withdrawal equipment, may suffice; however, this technique will reduce the accuracy of urethral length measurements.[22]

The medium is infused through the catheter, and the catheter is withdrawn at a constant rate. The pressure required to push the medium through the side holes is recorded from inside the bladder out to a distance where the pressure becomes essentially equal with the bladder pressure. This generates an infusion profile curve representative of the urethral pressure profile (Fig. 24-10). Several parameters are obtained from the urethral pressure profile, and the International Continence Society recommended that a common terminology apply to the interpretation of urethral pressure measurements.[23] The parameters obtained from the urethral pressure profile are: intravesical pressure (P_{ves}), which is the pressure measurement within the bladder; maximum urethral pressure (P_{ura}), which is the highest pressure obtained during withdrawal of the catheter; maximum urethral closure pressure (UCP_{max}), which is the difference in pressure obtained when the P_{ves} is subtracted from the P_{ura} (which is the pressure gradient from the urethra to the intravesical pressure); the functional urethral length is the urethral length where the intraurethral pressure exceeds the bladder pressure; and the total profile length is the length of the urethra as measured using the withdrawal technique (Fig. 24-10).

A "stress urethral pressure profile" is performed with a catheter containing pressure sensors in the bladder and proximal area of the urethra. With coughing or straining, the change in pressure in the bladder and that in the urethra is recorded simultaneously. In normal subjects, the change in urethral pressure should always be equal or greater to the change in bladder pressure. However, in patients with stress incontinence, the change in urethral pressure will generally be less than the change in bladder pressure. This study has been advocated as a way to differentiate between normal urethral function and stress incontinence.[24]

Dynamic infusion profilometry also uses a catheter with sensors in the bladder and proximal urethra. Pressures are recorded during bladder filling and bladder emptying, and the interaction between bladder pressure and the pressure in the urethra at the level of the sphincter is recorded. These techniques have been advocated to assist in diagnosing stress urinary incontinence. However, it has been suggested that a significantly high false-positive and false-negative rate might make this technique difficult to interpret. Much overlap of pressure values exists with normal patients, and these measurements cannot be used as reliable indicators.[25-27]

It has been suggested that the urethral pressure profile is useful in evaluating patients with stress incontinence, detrusor sphincter dyssynergia, and obstruction. However, because of the reasons discussed above, this study has not gained universal acceptance for these applications. The urethral pressure profile can be an excellent means to evaluate function of an artificial urinary sphincter and to evaluate a neuropathic nonfunctioning bladder neck or proximal urethral segment with fluoroscopic assistance.[28] However, the shape and magnitude of the urethral pressure profile varies so much with individual techniques that it is currently impossible to define normal values.

Leak Point Pressure Determination

The most commonly performed leak point pressure up to now is known as the Valsalva leak point pressure.[29] This is a direct measurement of the abdominal pressure required to overcome urethral resistance, otherwise known as the urethral opening pressure. This Valsalva or abdominal leak point determination may be considered an indirect method of measuring the closure forces of the urethra during straining maneuvers. It is used primarily in females with stress urinary incontinence to differentiate between anatomic displacement of a normal functioning urethra (stress urinary incontinence) from poor urethral function otherwise known as intrinsic sphincteric dysfunction (ISD). The test is done with the patient's bladder half full. At 150, 200, and 250 ml, the patient is asked to strain, increasing the intra-abdominal pressure, and any leakage is documented. The leakage may be documented visually or fluoroscopically. At the point in which leakage occurs, the abdominal pressure (P_{abd}) is recorded and is known as the abdominal, or Valsalva, leak point pressure (LPP_{abd}). Patients with intrinsic sphincteric dysfunction demonstrate minimal urethral resistance to straining; therefore the urethral opening pressure is very low; whereas patients with an anatomic displacement of a normally functioning urethra have high urethral opening pressures; therefore, the LPP_{abd} will be higher. It is generally well accepted that LPP_{abd} of less than 65 cm H_2O constitute ISD, and these patients will do poorly with standard bladder neck suspension procedures. Patients with LPP_{abd} greater than 90 cm H_2O demonstrate normal urethral function and may be recommended for standard bladder suspension procedures. A "gray" zone exists at LPP_{abd} between 60 and 90. In a comparative study, patients were evaluated by both urethral pressure profilometry and the LPP_{abd}, and it was demonstrated that measurement of the LPP_{abd} was more reproducible and easier to perform, and that LPP_{abd} of less than 60 cm H_2O correlated with urethral closing pressures of less than 20 cm H_2O, which is indicative of ISD.[30]

Detrusor (subtracted) leak point pressures (LPP_{det}) are most commonly used in patients with neurogenic lower urinary tract dysfunction or outlet obstruction to identify patients who may be at risk for adverse upper urinary tract changes and must be distinguished from VLPP. Patients with incontinence and poorly compliant bladders are excellent candidates for the determination of the LPP_{det}. This is a passive measurement, and it is the detrusor pressure at which time leakage occurs. It is important to note that the detrusor pressure (P_{det}) is the pressure recorded. It appears that if leakage occurs at a P_{det} less than 40 cm H_2O, then upper tract decompensation will not occur in the absence of other complicating factors.[31] Therefore patients with neurogenic lower urinary tract dysfunction who exhibit poor compliance during the filling cystometrogram should be evaluated for an LPP_{det} to determine if they are at risk for upper tract deterioration.

In summary, when evaluating leak point pressures, it is important to make the distinction between the true LPP_{det} and the LPP_{abd}. To perform both tests, it is preferable to have multichannel measurements with subtracted intrarectal pressures to distinguish between the true P_{det} and the P_{abd}. It is difficult to interpret leak point pressures with a single channel filling cystometrogram. The true LPP_{det} is most commonly used in patients with incontinence and poor compliance and is a passive leak point pressure obtained at the time urine leaks around the catheter. The LPP_{abd} is an active process with the patient straining and the P_{abd} at which urine leaks per urethra is recorded. This is most commonly performed in patients with stress urinary incontinence.

Voiding dysfunction is a quality-of-life issue, and problems such as obstructive uropathy and incontinence are a major health issue. Urinary incontinence, for example, occurs in all patient types, ranging from children to the elderly, in both sexes, and in patients with a variety of neurologic disorders. There is a wide variety of causes of urinary incontinence in these patients; therefore the evaluation of these patients must be individualized, and a "cookbook" approach to the evaluation and urodynamic investigation cannot be utilized. A wide variety of urodynamic studies exist, and the urodynamic evaluation represents only a part of the neurourologic history and physical examination.

In the next section we address several areas of common voiding dysfunction problems and discuss the application of urodynamics in these areas. An attempt is made to identify the most appropriate urodynamic study in each situation and how it may be utilized clinically.

Female Stress Incontinence

When one is evaluating female patients with a history of stress urinary incontinence, the diagnosis cannot be established by history alone. Based on the history alone, the physician can expect to be wrong at least 20% of the time about the cause of the incontinence.[32] The physical examination is performed to determine if any associated prolapse is present. A postvoid residual urine is recommended in every patient as an indication of emptying function. An elevated postvoid residual urine may be the result of a poorly contractile bladder or outlet obstruction. This is not present in cases of pure stress urinary incontinence, and an elevated residual urine warrants further search for another cause of the urinary incontinence.

In patients with symptoms suggestive of stress urinary incontinence alone, documented urethral hypermobility, no significant associated prolapse, and minimal postvoid residual urine, a filling cystometrogram is all that is required to confirm a stable, compliant reservoir. This may be performed by use of a gas cystometrogram to assess bladder sensation, capacity, and compliance and also to document the presence or absence of uninhibited bladder contractions. Provocative maneuvers to elicit uninhibited contractions are performed.[33]

In patients with a suspected or established neurologic lesion, a history of prior surgery, or symptoms of mixed (urge) incontinence, a more complex urodynamic investigation is indicated before selection of a surgical procedure. In these patients, multichannel filling and voiding cystometry should be performed. During the filling phase, provocative maneuvers should be performed to elicit unstable bladder contractions, and the capacity and compliance of the bladder should be assessed. Also during the filling phase, the LPP_{abd} should be calculated as described above. After this, a voiding cystometrogram is obtained when bladder capacity is reached to obtain information regarding bladder contractility and the possibility of concomitant obstruction. In patients with a known neurologic lesion, an EMG tracing should be performed in addition to the multichannel cystometry to evaluate striated sphincter function during the voiding phase. In patients with associated urogenital prolapse, videourodynamic testing, the integration of multichannel urodynamics with fluoroscopic evaluation, is employed. The use of fluoroscopy allows one to stage the associated urogenital prolapse and also to obtain a leak point pressure. In cases of ISD, the bladder neck is open at rest in the absence of a detrusor contraction, and urine can be seen leaving through the urethra at an LPP_{abd} of less than 65 cm H_2O.

In our practice, we perform multichannel filling and voiding cystometry on all patients. During the filling phase, we obtain an LPP_{abd} using direct visualization. This is quite simply performed when one places a small piece of aluminum foil in the bottom of the beaker collecting urine from the commode chair used during a pressure-flow study (filling and voiding cystometrics). Voiding cystometry is obtained to assess detrusor contractility. Patients with impaired contractility may be at increased risk for developing retention problems postoperatively. We reserve videourodynamic testing for patients with a known neurologic lesion, in patients with significant associated urogenital prolapse, or in patients who had failed previous bladder neck suspension surgery.

Urethral pressure profilometry (UPP) may be performed to evaluate urethral function before proposed bladder suspension surgery. However, because of reasons previously described in this chapter, UPP is not routinely performed. We do find the performance of static UPP useful in patients who demonstrate detrusor instability on the filling cystometrogram. Commonly these patients exhibit detrusor instability during the Valsalva maneuver. It is impossible to determine an accurate LPP_{abd} during an involuntary contraction because the bladder must remain at rest so that one can obtain an accurate measurement. Therefore in these patients we perform static UPP to evaluate urethral function. Otherwise, we do not find the urethral pressure profile to be useful in the evaluation of stress urinary incontinence.

Benign Prostatic Hyperplasia with Outflow Obstruction

Prostatism is the symptom complex of irritative and obstructive symptoms believed to be caused by prostatic urethral obstruction. During the initial evaluation a formal quantitation of the patient's symptoms may be obtained with the American Urologic Association (AUA) prostate symptoms severity score (see Appendix E). The AUA symptom score is a self-administered test separating diseased from younger, normal controls and improves significantly after treatment for benign prostatic hyperplasia (BPH).[34] The AUA symptom score, however, correlates poorly at baseline reference with uroflowmetry, postvoid residual, prostate size, and degree of bladder trabeculation. After treatment there is a modest correlation between improvements in the score and the uroflow.[35] Also, it is noted that the severity of the AUA symptoms score does not correlate with future pressure-flow studies.[36]

The measurement of uroflow is a screening test of possible outflow obstruction because most men with obstruction have a decreased flow rate.[37] However, as mentioned previously, a poor flow can be from either obstruction or an impaired detrusor contractility.

In the patient care guidelines for BPH established by the AUA, the AUA symptom score is considered a standard in evaluation and treatment of BPH. Further urodynamic testing is considered optional and is based on the physician and patient preference.[38] The panel describes the use of uroflow as "useful" in evaluating patients with symptoms of prostatism. With regard to pressure-flow studies, the panel found that in patients with an unusual history, physical findings, or other objective parameters where the diagnosis is unclear, a pressure-flow study may clarify the situation. Therefore it was recommended as an option for management of prostatism.[38] It has been demonstrated, however, that there is a lack of correlation of the subjective information from the AUA symptoms score with objective data for assessment of bladder outlet obstruction. The AUA symptom index has been objectively demonstrated not to predict the presence or severity of bladder outlet obstruction.[39] Incorporating these data with the patient care guidelines for BPH, we also include a urodynamic evaluation of symptomatic BPH in our practice in this manner: patients with symptoms of prostatism and no complicating factor (diabetes, neurogenic component, previous surgery) are offered medical therapy if the symptom score and uroflow are reflective of obstruction. Before surgical intervention in any patient, we perform pressure-flow studies to confirm the diagnosis of outlet obstruction. In all patients with symptomatic prostatism and other associated factors (diabetes, neurogenic component, previous surgery) we embark on pressure-flow studies before administering therapy.

The pressure-flow studies are performed using multichannel filling and voiding cystometry. Videourodynamics is not necessary in this patient population. The use of multichannel filling and voiding cystometry allows one to confirm the diagnosis of outlet obstruction. In addition, during the filling cystometrogram, the presence of bladder instability, decreased compliance, and appropriate sensation can be ascertained. Increased bladder contractility in combination with a low flow rate is diagnostic for the presence of bladder outlet obstruction. During the voiding phase, the presence of impaired contractility with a low flow rate signifies impaired detrusor contractility as the major source of the patient's symptoms, and this patient will not likely benefit from prostatectomy.

In a small population of younger men between 30 and 50 years of age complaining of long-standing obstructive voiding symptoms, the level of obstruction may be at the bladder neck. This is known as primary bladder neck obstruction, or bladder neck dyssynergia.[40] In these patients, videourodynamics is useful to localize the level of obstruction.[41] The cystometric parameters are consistent with obstruction, and the fluoroscopic images localize this obstruction to the bladder neck level. However, this is most commonly seen in younger men with a long-standing history of obstructive symptoms. For the majority of the patients with symptomatic BPH, a multichannel pressure-flow study without fluoroscopic assistance is sufficient to establish an accurate diagnosis.

Postprostatectomy Incontinence

The incidence of urinary incontinence after transurethral resection of the prostate for BPH is 0.2% to 1.4%,[42] and the incidence reported after radical prostatectomy ranges from 2.5% to 87%.[43,44] During the evaluation of these patients, cystourethroscopy may demonstrate residual adenoma, stricture, or bladder neck contracture. However, it should be noted that urethroscopy is not an accurate method of assessing residual prostatic obstruction. Radiologic studies such as a voiding cystourethrogram are essential to delineate anatomic obstruction and the appearance of the bladder neck and sphincteric areas during straining maneuvers and the voiding phase. The presence of associated detrusor instability after prostatectomy has been noted as high as 50%.[45]

Because of the multiple factors involved in the cause of postprostatectomy incontinence, mainly sphincteric damage secondary to the prostatectomy, we commonly employ videourodynamic investigation in these patients. Videourodynamics allows combined radiographic evaluation of the bladder, bladder neck, and proximal portion of the urethra along with multichannel filling and voiding cystometry. During the filling phase, the presence of involuntary bladder contractions or poor bladder compliance may be identified. Also during filling, the appearance of the bladder neck and proximal urethra under fluoroscopic guidance is obtained. Initial images are obtained with the bladder at rest. After this, the patient is asked to perform various straining maneuvers, and the appearance of the bladder neck and proximal portion of the urethra is identified fluoroscopically. A leak point pressure is obtained as urine traverses through the bladder neck and proximal urethra. During voiding cystometry, bladder contractility is assessed for possible residual obstruction or decreased contractility.

In our experience, we find that the appearance of the bladder neck and proximal portion of the urethra fluoroscopically is important in directing future management. In patients with a severely deformed bladder neck and proximal portion of the urethra that remain opened during the resting phase, treatment with injectables (see Chapter 37) has not been universally successful. In the patients with a closed bladder neck at rest and incontinence associated with mild to moderate funneling of the bladder neck and proximal portion of the urethra during straining maneuvers, we have considered these patients acceptable candidates for injectable treatment.[46] Therefore we have found it very useful to perform videourodynamic investigation in males with postprostatectomy incontinence. EMG tracings are generally not useful unless, again, a known neurologic lesion is present.

NEUROGENIC BLADDER

After neurologic injury, the bladder and urethra respond to the neurologic disease in several different ways. The identification of bladder and urethral function after neurologic injury is essential to determine the cause of the urinary incontinence and most importantly to determine the risk of upper tract decompensation.

In patients with suprasacral spinal cord lesions (physically induced spinal cord injury, multiple sclerosis, and transverse myelitis) detrusor hyperreflexia and detrusor–external sphincter dyssynergia are prone to develop.[47] Patients with both sacral lesions (such as myelodysplasia and cauda equina injuries) are more likely to develop detrusor areflexia and low bladder compliance. In patients with neurologic lesions above the spinal cord, such as those occurring in stroke and Parkinson's disease, there is little risk of urologic complication unless there is a concomitant urologic condition such as BPH.[47]

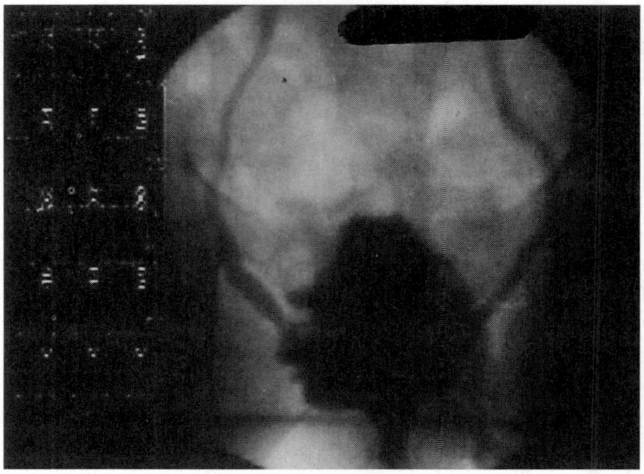

FIG. 24-11 *Fluoroscopic imaging of patient with suprasacral spinal cord injury demonstrating greatly trabeculated bladder, leakage across sphincteric mechanism, and bilateral vesicourethral reflux.*

The goal of urodynamic evaluation of the incontinent patient with a known neurologic disorder is to identify the abnormalities of vesicourethral dysfunction precisely and therefore to direct specific therapy. In addition to correcting the cause of the urinary incontinence, the urodynamic tests should allow assessment of the risk of upper tract deterioration and the associated presence of vesicoureteral reflux in this patient population. Significant derangements of vesicourethral function frequently coexist in these patients, and urodynamic testing should allow identification of these factors. Therefore we believe that the initial choice with thorough urodynamic evaluation in patients with a known neurologic disorder is multichannel videourodynamics with EMG tracings (Fig. 24-11). A voiding cystourethrogram may be done in the absence of simultaneous urodynamic studies; however, one cannot be certain of the existing circumstances where the bladder neck or sphincter opening closure is located.[48] After treatment, subsequent urodynamic investigation may be more selective in these patients for routine surveillance and to follow the results of treatment.[49]

CONCLUSION

It has been stated that the urodynamic study is the "reflex hammer" of the urologist. It is important for the treating physician to notice, however, that the urodynamic study represents one phase of the evaluation of these patients. Before ordering a urodynamic investigation, the physician should formulate a working diagnosis to allow him or her to order the most accurate study in the most cost-effective fashion, that is, a target-oriented investigation. A properly performed urodynamic study should reproduce the patient's symptoms and signs of an underlying disorder and therefore assist the physician in establishing the diagnosis. These studies are designed to confirm the clinician's diagnosis or to modify that diagnosis because of variables ascertained during the investigation, which may change thoughts on treatment and prognosis for the indiviual patient. Urodynamic studies have allowed physicians to select therapy that addresses the underlying pathophysiologic characteristics in patients with urinary incontinence and other voiding dysfunctions and therefore achieve successful outcomes of treatment while preventing upper urinary tract deterioration.

REFERENCES

1. Wein A, Barrett D: Practical urodynamics. In AUA Update Series: Lesson 39, 12:306-311, Baltimore, 1993, American Urological Association.
2. Bates P, et al: The standardization of terminology of lower urinary tract function, 1984. International Continence Society Committee.
3. Blaivas JG: A critical appraisal of specific diagnostic techniques. In Krane RJ, Siroky MG, editors: *Clinical neurourology,* Boston, 1979, Little, Brown.
4. Tammen H: Miktiography 7005, *Acta Medicotech* 19:10, 1971.
5. James E: Urodynamic equipment: technical aspects, *Proc Int Continence Soc Working Party,* 1985.
6. Drake W: The uroflometer: an aid to the study of the lower urinary tract, *J Urol* 59:650, 1948.
7. Wein A, English W, Whitmore K: Office urodynamics, *Urol Clin North Am* 15:609-623, 1988.
8. Siroky M, Olsson C, Krane R: The flow rate nomogram. II. Clinical corelations, *J Urol* 123:208, 1980.
9. Drach G, Laylon T, Bottaccini M: A method of adjustment of male peak urinary flow for varying age and volume voided, *J Urol* 128:960, 1982.
10. Gleason D, Bottaccini R, Reilly R: Comparisons of cystometrograms and urethral profile with gas and water media, *Urology* 9:155, 1977.
11. Merrill D, Bradley W, Markland C. Air cystometry. II. A clinical evaluation of normal adults, *J Urol* 108:85, 1972.
12. Bradley W, Clarren S, Shapiro R, et al: Air cystometry, *J Urol* 100:45, 1968.
13. Wein A, Hanno PM, Dixon DO, et al: The reproducibility and interpretation of carbon dioxide cystometry, *J Urol* 120:205, 1978.
14. Susset J: Cystometry. In Krane R, Siroky M, editors: *Clinical neurourology,* ed 2, Boston, 1991, Little, Brown.
15. Klevmark B: Motility of the urinary bladder in cats during filling at physiologic rates. I. Intravesical pressure pattern studied by a new method of cystometry, *Acta Physiol Scand* 90:565, 1974.
16. McGuire E: Neuromuscular dysfunction of the lower urinary tract. In Walsh P, Gittes R, Perlmutter A, Stamey T, editors: *Campbell's urology,* ed 5, Philadelphia, 1986, Saunders.
17. Abrams P, Blaivas J, Stanton J, Anderson J: Standardization of lower urinary tract function, *Neurourol Urodyn* 7:403, 1988.
18. Stone A: Detrusor instability management. In Webster B, Stone A, editors: *Urinary incontinence: problems in urology,* Philadelphia, 1990, Lippincott.
19. O'Donnell P: Pitfalls of urodynamic testing, *Urol Clin North Am* 18:257-268, 1991.
20. Yalla SO, Blunt K, Fam B, et al: Detrusor–urethral sphincter dyssynergia, *J Urol* 118:1026, 1977.
21. Brown M, Wickham J: The urethral pressure profile, *Br J Urol* 41:211, 1969.
22. Shaw J: Urethral pressure profile. In Krane R, Siroky M, editors: *Clinical neurourology,* ed 2, Boston, 1991, Little, Brown.
23. International Continence Society: First report on the standardization of terminology of lower urinary tract function, *Br J Urol* 48:39, 1976.
24. Richardson D: Value of the cough pressure profile in the evaluation of patients with stress incontinence, *Am J Obstet Gynecol* 155:808, 1986.
25. Laval K: Urethral stress profilometry: a reliable diagnostic procedure for stress incontinence? *Proc eleventh annual meeting of the International Continence Society,* pp 127-128, 1981.
26. Massey A, Abrams P: Urodynamics of the female lower urinary tract, *Urol Clin North Am* 12:236, 1985.
27. Constantinou C, Govan D: Special distribution and timing of transmitted and reflex generated urethral pressures in healthy women, *J Urol* 127:964, 1982.
28. Scott F: The artificial urinary sphincter: experience in adults, *Urol Clin North Am* 16:105-117, 1989.
29. Wan J, McGuire E, Bloom D, Ritchey M: Stress leak point pressure: a diagnostic tool for incontinent children, *J Urol* 150:700, 1993.
30. Appell R: Valsalva leak point pressure (LPP) versus urethral pressure profile (UPP) in the evaluation of intrinsic sphincteric deficiency (ISD), Abstract presented at the American Urogynecology Society annual meeting, Toronto, Canada, 1994.
31. McGuire E, Woodside J, Borden T: Upper tract deterioration in patients with myelodysplasia and detrusor hypertonia: a follow-up study, *J Urol* 129:823, 1983.
32. Shortcliffe L, Stamey T: Urinary incontinence in the female. In Walsh P, Perlmutter A, Gittes R, Stamey T, editors: *Campbell's urology,* ed 5, Philadelphia, 1986, Saunders.
33. Staskin D, Zimmern P, Hadley R, Raz J: The pathophysiology of stress incontinence, *Urol Clin North Am* 12:271-278, 1985.
34. Barry M, Fowler F, O'Leary M, et al: The AUA symptom index for BPH, *J Urol* 148:1549, 1992.
35. Barry M, Cockett A, Holtgrewe H, et al: Relationship of symptoms of prostatism to commonly use physiological and anatomical measures of the severity of BPH, *J Urol* 150:351, 1993.
36. Beek C, Rollema H, Boender H, et al: Relationship between AUA symptoms score and objective pressure flow parameters, *Neurourol Urodyn* 12:36•, 1993.
37. Blaivas J: Multichannel urodynamic studies in men with BPH: indications and interpretation, *Urol Clin North Am* 17:543, 1990.
38. Mebust W: BPH patient care policies/guidelines. In AUA Update Series: lesson 29, 12:226-231, Baltimore, 1993, American Urological Association.
39. Sirls L, Kirkemo A, Jay J: Lack of correlation of the American Urologic Symptom 7 Index with urodynamic bladder outlet obstruction, Abstract presented at the Urodynamic Society 17th annual meeting, Las Vegas, Nevada, 1995.
40. Marion G: Surgery of the neck of the bladder, *Br J Urol* 5:351, 1933.
41. Turner-Warwick R: Bladder outflow obstruction in the male. In Mundy A, Stephenson T, Wein A, editors: *Urodynamics: principles and applications,* Edinburgh, 1984, Churchill-Livingstone.
42. Wein A, Barrett D: Other voiding dysfunctions and related topics. In *Voiding function and dysfunction,* St Louis, 1988, Mosby.
43. Walsh P, Jewett A: Radical surgery for prostatic cancer, *Cancer* 45:1906, 1980.
44. Rudy D, Woodside J, Jeffrey R, et al: Urodynamic evaluation of incontinence in patients undergoing modified Campbell radical retropubic prostatectomy: a prospective study, *J Urol* 132:708, 1984.
45. Leach G, Yip C, Donovan B: Postprostatectomy incontinence: the influence of bladder dysfunction, *J Urol* 138:574, 1987.
46. Appell R: Personal communication, 1995.
47. Chancellor M, Blaivas J: Diagnostic evaluation in neurourology and its role in urologic disease: I. In Paulson D, editor: *Problems in urology,* Philadelphia, 1992, Lippincott.
48. Blaivas J, Fisher D: Combined radiographic and urodynamic monitoring: advances in techniques, *J Urol* 125:693, 1981.
49. Rudy D, Woodside J: The incontinent myelodysplastic patient, *Urol Clin North Am* 18:295, 1991.

Chapter 25

Stress Urinary Incontinence

D. Duane Baldwin, Roger Hadley

The involuntary leakage of urine resulting from increased abdominal pressure (stress) is clinically referred to as stress urinary incontinence. *Genuine stress incontinence* (GSI) is a term used to describe the involuntary loss of urine occurring when, in the *absence* of a bladder muscle contraction, the pressure inside the bladder is greater than the pressure generated by the urethra and sphincter. This pressure differential results in the leakage of urine. Patients with stress incontinence who present to their primary care physician will often describe their symptoms as leakage of urine with coughing or sneezing. *Urge incontinence* (UI) is a different condition where the loss of urine results from increased intravesical pressure attributable to an uninhibited bladder contraction. This distinction is important, since GSI may be effectively treated with surgical procedures designed to restore usual anatomic relationships, whereas urge incontinence is more effectively managed with medical and behavioral therapy designed to inhibit the spontaneous contractions of the bladder. The diagnosis and treatment of incontinence is complicated by the fact that both conditions may exist in the same patient.

Although stress incontinence affects millions of women, it rarely affects men in the absence of prior pelvic or prostatic surgery. Stress incontinence affects between 15% and 60% of women.[1,2] Although stress incontinence is often thought of as a disorder of the elderly, Wolin, who studied a large group of young nulliparous nursing students, found over half reported stress incontinence. One sixth of these nurses reported daily incontinence.[3] Although incontinence may be more common in those who are overweight,[2] Nygaard et al. found that over one fourth of nulliparous elite college varsity athletes reported stress incontinence while participating in their sports.[4] This very high incidence of incontinence even in young, nulliparous women should be kept in mind when one is interpreting the results of surgical therapy for incontinence.

Although stress urinary incontinence is a benign condition, its effect on the quality of life may be tremendous. Patients are often sensitive about losing control of this very important body function. Out of embarrassment they may delay seeking treatment. These patients need to learn that they are not alone and that many different treatment options do offer hope for improvement. Information about the disease, the options for treatment, and the potential outcomes of these treatments will allow the patient to select the treatment that is best for her.

Etiology

The cause of stress urinary incontinence is complex. Many different factors may contribute, including age, parity, and previous gynecologic surgery.[5-9] Other factors that may increase the risk of developing incontinence include an increased body mass index,[2] a positive family history,[6] straining at stool as a young adult,[10] and smoking.[11,12] The complex relationship that exists between each of these factors makes it difficult to predict who will become incontinent. The patient should be reassured that the condition is not her fault and that there probably was little she could have done to prevent it from occurring.

Mechanisms of Continence

We have already mentioned that GSI results from an increase in intra-abdominal pressure that is transmitted to the bladder in the absence of a bladder contraction. This increase in intravesical pressure is greater than the pressure generated by the bladder neck and sphincter resulting in the loss of urine. The reason for these inadequate urethral closing pressures may be multifactorial including deficiencies in the active mechanism of continence, the anatomic mechanism of continence, and the mucosal seal mechanism.

The active mechanism of continence is supplied by the active contraction of muscles in the urethra, sphincter, and bladder neck. The active contraction of these muscles provides a force that closes the bladder outlet. This contraction is separate and in addition to the force transmitted to the proximal urethra, which is discussed in the next paragraph. An active contraction has been noted to occur 250 msec before increases in intra-abdominal pressure, such as would be seen with sneezing or coughing. This contraction actively closes the bladder outlet countering the abdominal pressure, which can act to expel urine. Women with genuine stress incontinence have been noted to have lower peak contractions and decreased length of maximal contractions.[13,14] Traumatic deliveries or other precipitators of incontinence may damage the nerves to the muscles or the muscles themselves by replacement with scar tissue. This results in the qualitative and quantitative changes in the pelvic floor and sphincter muscles that lead to stress incontinence.[15-17] The second mechanism that participates in the maintenance of continence is the anatomic mechanism. Most surgical treatments for incontinence attempt to restore this mechanism. In an anatomically well supported bladder neck, increases in intra-abdominal pressure that are transmitted to the superior surface of the bladder are also transmitted to the proximal, intra-abdominal portion of the urethra. The rigidity of the ligaments and fascia supporting the urethra and bladder neck provide a counterforce to the abdominal force that is transmitted to the proximal portion of the urethra, thereby closing the bladder outlet[18] (Fig. 25-1). In a continent woman this transmitted compressive force begins just after and acts simultaneously with the active contractile force discussed in the previous paragraph.[13] In contrast, the woman with stress incontinence has ligaments that are lax and stretched, allowing

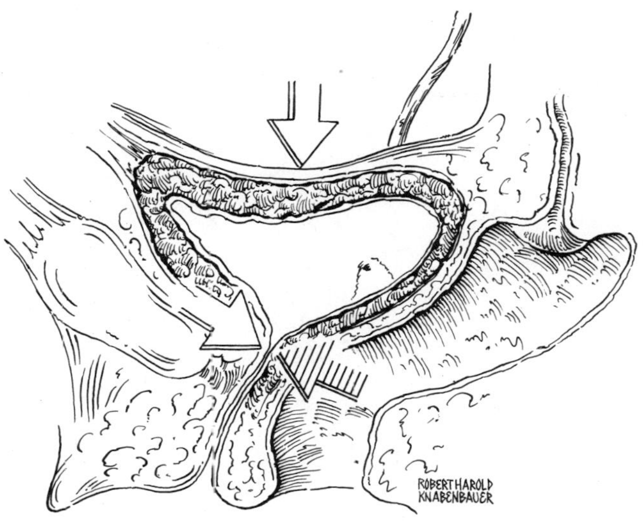

FIG. 25-1 *Anatomic support of a continent woman. In a continent woman with good anatomic support, increases in intra-abdominal pressure that act on the bladder also act on the proximal portion of the urethra* (open arrows). *This abdominal force acting upon the proximal portion of the urethra meets the support provided by strong ligaments* (shaded arrow), *resulting in compression of the urethra and continence.*

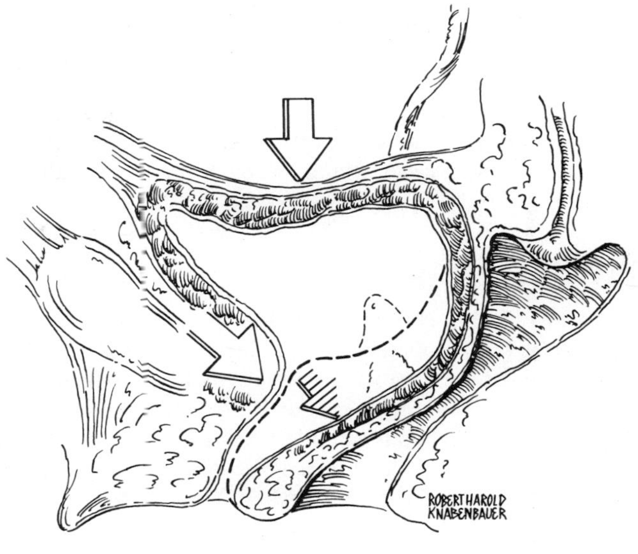

FIG. 25-2 *Loss of anatomic support in an incontinent woman. In the woman with poor anatomic support, increases in intra-abdominal pressure meet no resistive force. The weakened anatomic support* (shaded arrow) *allows the bladder neck and urethra to rotate down and posteriorly. The urethra is not compressed, and incontinence results.*

the bladder neck to descend into a location where increases in intra-abdominal pressure are not transmitted to the proximal urethra and bladder neck (Fig. 25-2). Hence, increases in intra-abdominal pressure during coughing or sneezing act only on the bladder but not on the bladder neck and proximal urethra. This produces a significant force for expelling urine.

Finally, the third mechanism that participates in maintenance of continence is the leakproof mucosal seal provided by the supple urothelium and the vascularity of the submucosal vessels of the urethra and bladder neck. A urethra that has lost its suppleness and whose submucosal blood supply has been compromised by prior surgery, radiation, or loss of estrogenization may require significantly more force from the active sphincteric mechanism to obtain a urine-tight closure.[19,20]

All three of the above mechanisms simultaneously interact to maintain continence. This may explain why a young female with multiple complicated deliveries and ligamentous weakening (loss of the anatomic mechanism of continence) does not develop stress incontinence until after menopause when she also loses estrogenization (mucosal seal mechanism). This may also explain why not all women who demonstrate hypermobility develop incontinence, since the increased efforts of the active mechanism and the intact mucosal seal mechanisms may be able to compensate for the lost anatomic mechanism. Finally, an understanding of the interplay between the three mechanisms of continence may explain why some women fail standard bladder neck suspension surgery. Despite a high retropubic fixation of the bladder neck (restored anatomic mechanism), they have damage to the mucosal seal and active mechanisms (intrinsic sphincter deficiency) and hence remain incontinent.

Classification of Incontinence

Determining which of these mechanisms are functional and which are not in a given patient is often quite difficult. In an attempt to describe the anatomic and physiologic changes that are responsible for stress incontinence, several classification schemes have been developed. The ultimate significance of these classification systems lies in their ability to predict later surgical success rates utilizing a given surgical repair. Historically, Green noted that in continent women a lateral view of the urethra showed the position of the upper urethra to have an angle of inclination of no more than 30 degrees from vertical. Normal continent women also had a posterior urethrovesical angle of 90 to 100 degrees. Green developed a categorization scheme with two parts. Incontinent women who retained a normal urethral axis but had lost the posterior urethrovesical angle were classified as type I. Those patients who had an increase in the urethral angle of inclination caused by rotational descent of the urethra during straining were classified as type II. These original classifications were believed to be significant because the standard anterior vaginal wall repair was much more successful with type I than with type II stress incontinence.[21]

Later, the concept of stress incontinence evolved to include both urethral anatomy and function. McGuire combined radiologic diagnostic techniques with manometric techniques to look simultaneously at urethral anatomy and function. He identified an additional category of incontinence that was attributable to intrinsic weakness of the sphincter, or type III, incontinence. This additional classification was significant because patients who had intrinsic sphincter deficiency were more likely to fail if treated with a standard bladder neck suspension than if treated with a urethral sling.[22,23] This concept of intrinsic sphincter deficiency (type III incontinence) has been one of the major advancements in the understanding and treatment of stress incontinence. Many surgeons currently recommend a urethral suspension procedure for both type I and type II incontinence (making distinction between the two less important), whereas they recommend a urethral sling operation for those with type III incontinence.[24,25]

CLINICAL EVALUATION

When a patient presents with symptoms of stress urinary incontinence, the history obtained by the physician is usually focused initially on determining whether the symptoms are consistent with simple stress incontinence or if urgency is also involved. This distinction between genuine stress incontinence and the more complicated urge, or mixed, incontinence is important because the appropriate evaluation and treatment will be determined by this classification. Stress incontinence is leakage of usually small amounts of urine at the time of significant increases in intra-abdominal pressure such as coughing, sneezing, or lifting. Urgency incontinence usually presents with an irresistible urge to urinate accompanied by a large volume of urine leakage, often the entire contents of the bladder. This irrepressible urge may occur when running water is heard, while watching TV, or upon placing the keys in the door lock while arriving home from a trip, or it may be precipitated by a cough or sneeze. Patients who are more likely to have complicated stress incontinence include those who have a history of previous bladder neck or pelvic surgery, other medical or neurologic conditions, obesity, and advancing age.[20]

Once the type of incontinence has been determined, the severity of symptoms and the effect that these symptoms have upon the patient's quality of life should be determined. An 80-year-old woman who soaks her underwear every time she participates in strenuous activity but participates in strenuous activities only twice a year must be considered differently from a 45-year-old gymnastics coach who participates in strenuous activity many times a day. Medical history, including the number of vaginal deliveries, previous gynecologic surgeries, hormonal status, neurologic history, childhood voiding dysfunction, medications (particularly alpha-adrenergic receptor blockers), and the previous attempts at therapy with the responses obtained using that therapy, must be elicited. A voiding diary quantifying frequency, quantity, and activity engaged in when incontinence occurs will greatly help the physician understand how the incontinence is affecting the patient.

A standard physical examination should be performed with special emphasis on the neurologic evaluation. The urethra should be palpated, and while the patient is straining, the anatomic support of the bladder neck should be determined. The presence of descent of the urethra and bladder neck (hypermobility) with straining is an important finding to document. The classic Q-Tip test may also be performed. An upward deflection of the tip by 2 to 3 cm is evidence of bladder neck hypermobility (Fig. 25-3). Obviously, it is also important to document incontinence by having the patient cough and strain both in the supine and standing position. The presence of additional abnormalities such as cystocele, rectocele, enterocele, and uterine support should also be made at this time.

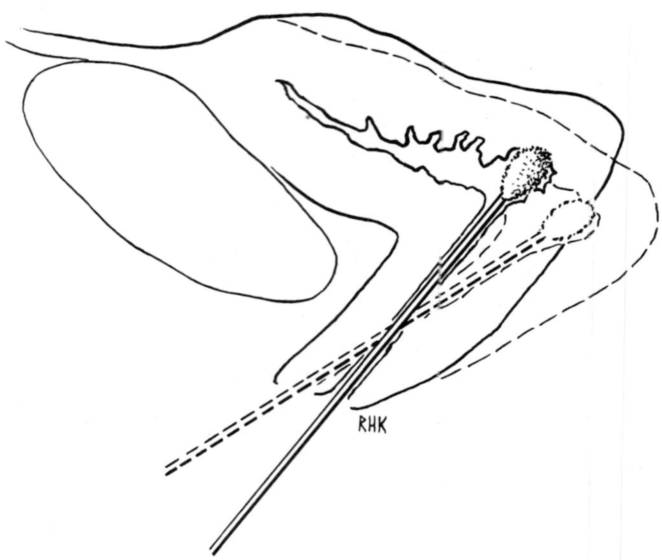

FIG. 25-3 *Q-tip test. An upward deflection of 2 to 3 cm is evidence of urethral hypermobility.*

Once the history and physical have been completed it is important to determine which treatment for stress incontinence will provide the patient with the best long-term results. The origin of a poor treatment outcome may be incomplete information resulting in a treatment that is not the best for the patient. Several additional studies are available to help confirm the factors responsible for stress incontinence. These additional studies include plain radiographs of the contrast-filled bladder, urodynamics, videourodynamics, and endoscopy.

Traditionally an important portion of the evaluation has included some form of objective documentation of anatomic relationships. Lateral standing radiographs of the bladder at rest and during straining represent one method of anatomic evaluation of incontinence. These radiographs may also provide evidence of intrinsic sphincter deficiency by showing an open bladder neck on the resting films (Fig. 25-4). An open bladder neck, however, may also be seen in continent women, and the significance of this finding in those who are continent is unclear.[26,27]

The extent of urodynamic evaluation required to adequately assess the patient with stress incontinence is controversial. Some physicians believe that uncomplicated stress incontinence requires little if any urodynamic testing.[23] Although most physicians believe that patients with mixed symptoms should undergo urodynamic testing,[29,30] others believe that the utility and necessity of determining preoperative detrusor instability is questionable, since the majority of those who do demonstrate preoperative bladder instability will have no difficulty with the syndrome postoperatively.[23,31]

Videourodynamic studies combine simultaneous radiographic and urodynamic studies. An important component of videourodynamics is the determination of the Valsalva leak point pressures (VLPP) of women with stress incontinence to

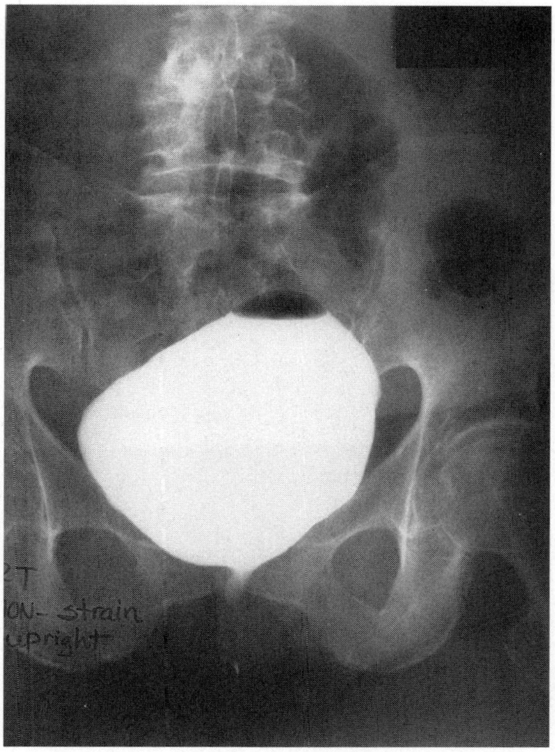

FIG. 25-4 *Open bladder neck. An upright radiograph of the bladder demonstrates an open bladder neck at rest.*

assess the presence or absence of intrinsic sphincter deficiency. Those with low Valsalva leak point pressures probably have intrinsic sphincter deficiency and should be considered for a sling procedure.[32]

Endoscopic evaluation in a patient with stress incontinence is helpful to confirm findings determined by radiologic and urodynamic testing and to rule out carcinoma in situ and other pathologic states.[33]

Treatment of Stress Incontinence

Once the type and severity of incontinence have been determined, along with the effect that these have upon the patient's quality of life, the attention is next directed toward selecting the appropriate treatment. The following is a summary of the nonoperative and operative techniques that have been developed and applied in the treatment of stress urinary incontinence.

Nonsurgical Treatment

As one might expect, surveys have shown that when given a choice, most patients will choose to undergo behavioral and medical therapy before surgical intervention.[34] Nonsurgical therapies include behavior modification, physiotherapy, biofeedback, electromyostimulation, and medical therapy. Those patients most likely to be benefited by nonsurgical therapy include young, highly motivated patients with milder forms of incontinence.[35,36] Since stress incontinence is not a life-threatening condition, nonsurgical therapy can be used without long-term risks or complications. Nonoperative therapy provides a time period for the patient to fully comprehend the effect of incontinence on her lifestyle. Nonsurgical therapies when used alone or in combination may provide some degree of effective cure, though the cure rates are quite modest.[37,38] Even if incontinence is not cured, the severity may be lessened to a degree where incontinence no longer has a significant impact upon the patient's lifestyle.

Surgical Treatment

Since the early years of the twentieth century, dozens of operative procedures have been described for the treatment of stress urinary incontinence in women. Many have been modifications of original procedures in an effort to improve results or make the operative procedure easier to perform or less invasive for the patient. Reports on the results of incontinence surgery vary widely, even when comparing similar surgical techniques.[39,40] The reasons for these differences are probably multifactorial. Certainly patient selection and the technical ability of the surgeon will vary. Additionally the definition of success and particularly the method used for follow-up study may have a tremendous effect on the reported outcomes of surgery. Questionnaire-based follow-up study gives profoundly lower (more accurate) cure rates than cure rates determined only by chart review.[41]

Although many issues of surgical decision making remain unreconciled, there are some general trends in the treatment of stress incontinence. The patient who has a poorly supported bladder neck and urethra with no suspicion of intrinsic sphincter deficiency is most commonly treated with one of the standard bladder neck suspension operations. Patients who have both poor anatomic support and a suspicion for intrinsic sphincter deficiency may be best treated by a urethral sling operation. Patients who already have a well-supported bladder neck but still have stress incontinence may be best served with periurethral collagen injection or a urethral sling.[24,25,42,43]

The surgical alternatives for the treatment of incontinence can be divided into categories based on the mechanism of continence that they attempt to restore. These categories include a surgical procedure designed to restore the active mechanism of continence (artificial urinary sphincter), procedures that restore the anatomic mechanism of continence either by indirect (bladder neck suspension) or direct (urethral sling) means, and finally a procedure that attempts to restore the mucosal seal mechanism of continence (periurethral collagen).

The only surgical technique for incontinence that is an attempt to mimic the active mechanism of continence is the artificial urinary sphincter (Fig. 25-5). The artificial sphincter uses a saline-filled cuff to actively close the proximal portion of the urethra in a manner designed to mimic the active contraction of the muscles of the urethra and pelvic floor (Fig. 25-5). Because they are an attempt to mimic the intrinsic contraction of the natural sphincter, the artificial sphincter may be most effective in women with type III incontinence. Relative contraindications to sphincter placement may include those with prior radiation and those with poor manual dexterity.[44,45] A drawback of the artifi-

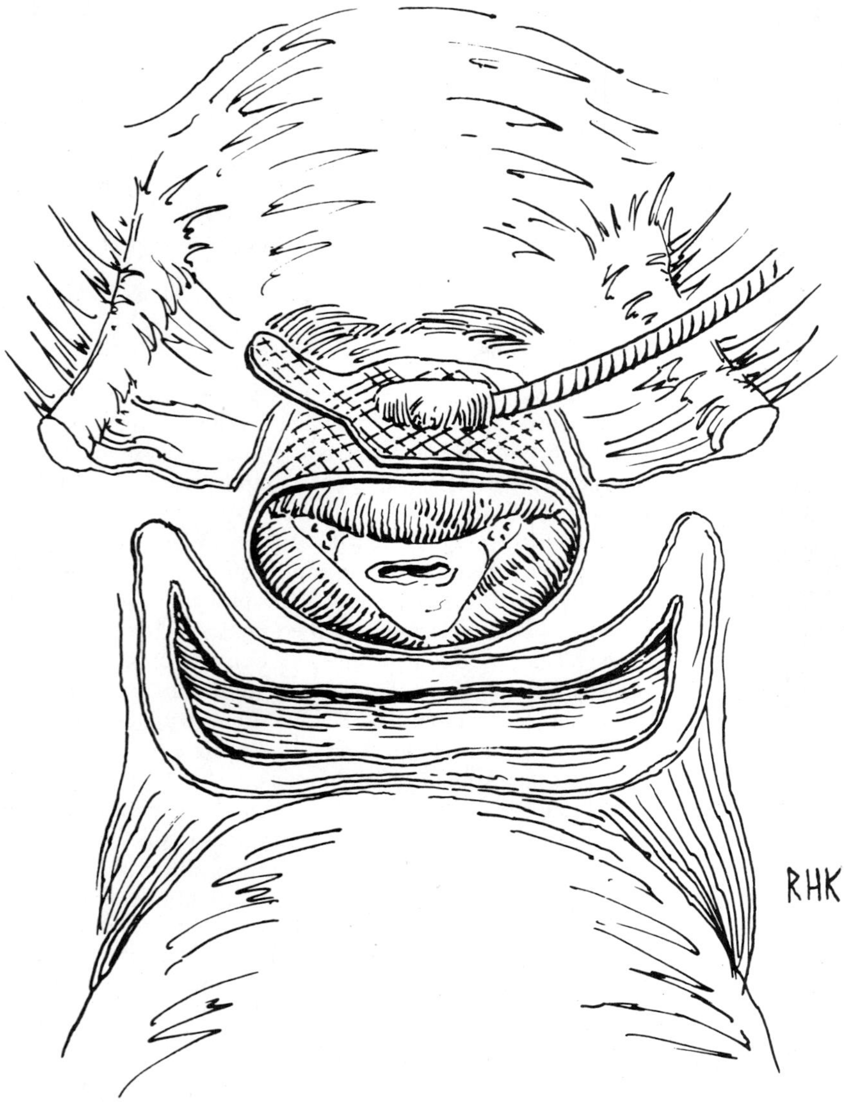

FIG. 25-5 *Artificial urinary sphincter. The artificial sphincter mimics the active compression of the native urethra and pelvic floor.*

cial urinary sphincter is the potential for infection, erosion, and equipment malfunction,[46] but these may be minimized in the hands of experienced surgeons.[47]

The most frequently utilized operative techniques to cure stress incontinence are those that are designed to restore the anatomic mechanism of continence. The goal of each of these procedures is to provide strong support for the bladder neck and urethra so that increases in intra-abdominal pressure will also be transmitted to the proximal urethra. These transmitted pressures act against the anatomic support supplied by the surgical repair to produce effective closure of the bladder neck. These surgical procedures may be considered in separate categories based on whether they support the urethra and bladder neck indirectly or directly.

The procedures that indirectly support the bladder neck and urethra include approaches that are abdominal (Burch), endoscopic (Stamey), and vaginal (Kelly, Pereyra, Raz). Because a common cause of failure is sutures pulling through the suspended tissue, it is important to obtain a solid anchoring of the appropriate periurethral structure in each of these indirect (suspension) type of operations.[42] One concern with all these procedures is the potential for damage to the periurethral vascular and nerve supply and also for urethral obstruction in the techniques with blind passage of suture. This may convert type I or II incontinence into type III. The Raz technique stays lateral to the bladder neck and periurethral plexus and suspends using the urethropelvic ligament in an attempt to minimize these factors[48] (Fig. 25-6). Direct comparison between operative repairs that indirectly support the bladder neck is very difficult and complicated by variations in technique, type of follow-up study, length of follow-up study, definition of terms, and patient selection. In general, the suprapubic approaches may trade a longer hospital stay and recovery for a slightly better cure rate.[49,50] Although still used by some gynecologists, the Kelly anterior repair, which merely reinforces anterior vaginal wall tissues, has been found to have a much higher recurrence rate than other procedures. For

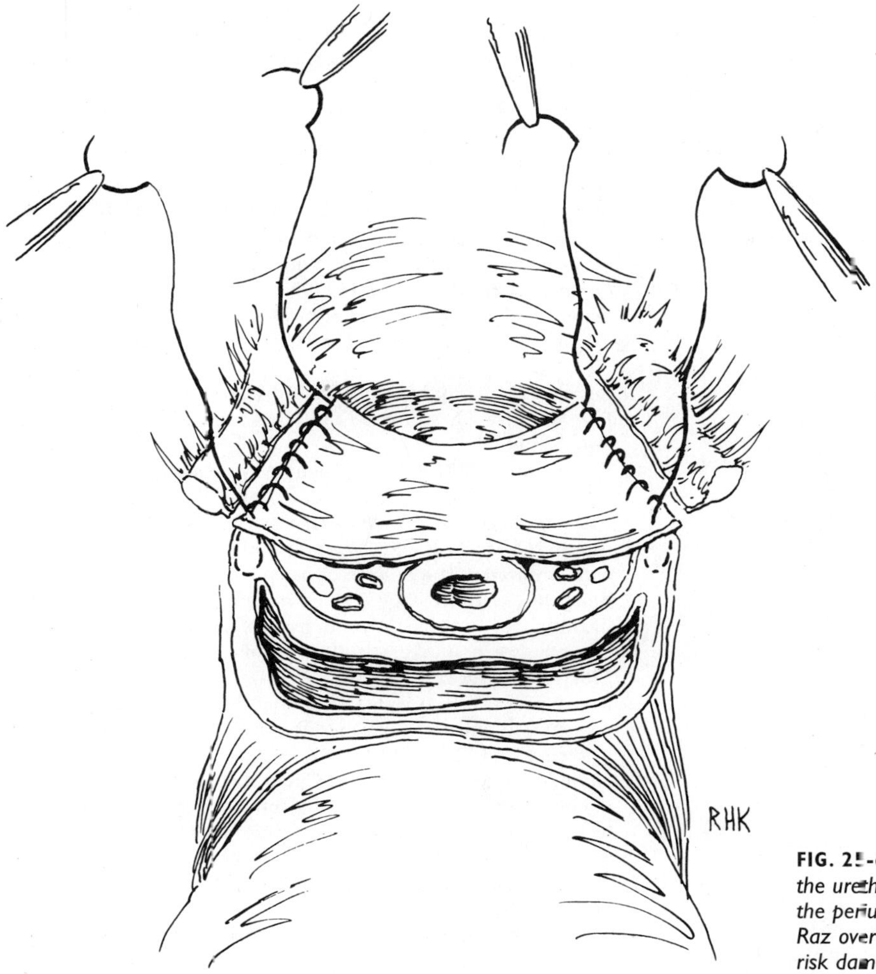

FIG. 25-6 *Raz bladder neck suspension. Sutures placed in the urethropelvic ligaments lateral to the bladder neck avoid the periurethral plexus. This is a potential advantage of the Raz over some other bladder neck suspensions, which may risk damage to the periurethral vascular and nerve supply.*

this reason it is not routinely used today in the treatment of stress incontinence.[51]

A second category of surgical procedures designed to restore the anatomic mechanism of continence is the group of procedures that are an attempt to create a direct suspension of the urethra and bladder neck. The difference between indirect and direct suspension may be illustrated by the playground swing. A small child wearing trousers desires to be swung back and forth. An indirect method of swinging him would be to suspend cables from an overhead bar and attach these to his belt loops. The child could probably swing, but his success would depend on the strength of the belt loops. Alternatively he could be directly supported by a large slab of rubber (seat of the swing) placed underneath him and attached to the overhead bar. This same principle may be applied to incontinence surgery. Standard bladder neck suspension operations are dependent on good strength of the periurethral tissues on either side of the urethra. These tissues have already demonstrated some anatomic weakness or the patient would not have developed incontinence in the first place. In contrast, the sling provides a good distribution of force to the entire undersurface of the urethra and is not dependent on strength of periurethral tissues.

Two direct procedures include the classic Marshall-Marchetti-Krantz (MMK) procedure and the urethral sling. The classic MMK used sutures into the urethra itself to create a direct suspension[52] (Fig. 25-7). These sutures placed directly into the urethra increased the possibility of urinary retention and damage to the delicate urethra.[53] Later descriptions of the technique do not include bites directly into the urethra and are hence actually indirect procedures.[54]

The remaining direct procedure is the urethral sling. Common to all urethral slings is a band of material placed directly beneath the urethra. Urethral slings avoid the placement of sutures directly into the urethra or the periurethral tissues, which might result in sphincter damage. One of the criticisms of slings has been the possible increased incidence in detrusor instability and potential for prolonged urinary retention. Modifications of the sling procedures have been developed to counter these disadvantages. Tying the slings loosely, however, may lower the incidence of these complications. Excellent cure rates along with low complication rates have led some, including us (D.D.B. and R.H.), to apply the urethral sling procedures to most types of incontinence.[55]

The bulking agents (that is, collagen) are designed to thicken the submucosal tissues at the level of the sphincter, thereby

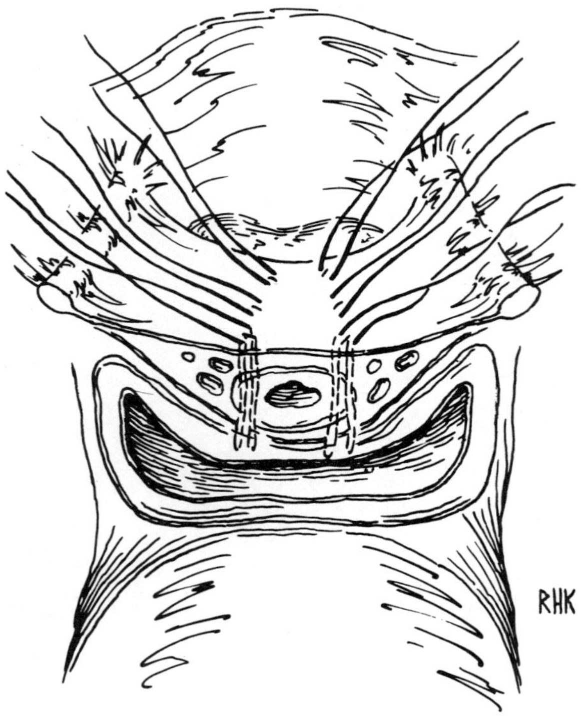

FIG. 25-7 *The classic Marshall-Marchetti-Krantz (MMK) procedure. The original description of the MMK procedure involved placement of sutures directly into the urethra to provide direct anatomic support. Later modifications, however, avoid placement of sutures directly into the urethra.*

improving urethral coaptation and restoring the mucosal seal mechanism of continence. Many materials have been used historically but currently the principal material used for injection therapy is glutaraldehyde cross-linked collagen. Since the bulk provided by collagen restores coaptation of the urethra, it is intuitive that its best indication for treatment may be in women who are incontinent despite a well-supported bladder neck (intrinsic sphincter deficiency, or type III). Short-term cure rates of 40% to 60% may be achieved in well-selected patients.[43,56]

In summary, many different treatment options are available to women with stress urinary incontinence. Nonsurgical therapy may benefit many patients, whereas others will choose an operative procedure. Increased consensus of terminology, long-term continence rates, objective self-administered questionnaire follow-up exam, and prospective, randomized, standardized studies are needed to make possible meaningful comparison of techniques. Ultimately individual decisions for treatment will be determined by the surgeon's expertise and preference in conjunction with the educated wishes of the patient.

REFERENCES

1. Foldspang A, Mommsen S: Adult female urinary incontinence and childhood bedwetting, *J Urol* 152:85-88, 1994.
2. Burgio KL, Matthews KA, Engel BT: Prevalence, incidence and correlates of urinary incontinence in healthy, middle-aged women, *J Urol* 146:1255-1259, 1991.
3. Wolin LH: Stress incontinence in young, healthy nulliparous female subjects, *J Urol* 101:545-549, 1969.
4. Nygaard IE, Thompson FL, Svengalis SL, Albright JP: Urinary incontinence in elite nulliparous athletes, *Obstet Gynecol* 84:183-7, 1994.
5. Mommsen S, Foldspang A, Elving L, Lam GW: Association between urinary incontinence in women and a previous history of surgery, *Br J Urol* 72:30-37, 1993.
6. Skoner MM, Thompson WD, Caron VA: Factors associated with risk of stress urinary incontinence in women, *Nurs Res* 43:301-306, 1994.
7. Foldspang A, Mommsen S, Lam GW, Elving L: Parity as a correlate of adult female urinary incontinence prevalence, *J Epidemiol Community Health* 46:595-600, 1992.
8. Dimpfl T, Hesse U, Schussler B: Incidence and cause of postpartum urinary stress incontinence, *Eur J Obstet Gynecol Reprod Biol* 43:29-33, 1992.
9. Resnick NM: Urinary incontinence in the elder woman. In Kursh ED, Mcguire EJ, editors: *Female urology*, Philadelphia, 1994, Lippincott.
10. Spence-Jones C, Kamm MA, Henry MM, Hudson CN: Bowel dysfunction: a pathogenic factor in uterovaginal prolapse and urinary stress incontinence, *Br J Obstet Gynaecol* 101:147-152, 1994.
11. Bump RC, McClish DK: Cigarette smoking and urinary incontinence in women, *Am J Obstet Gynecol* 167:1213-1218, 1992.
12. Bump RC, McClish DM: Cigarette smoking and pure genuine stress incontinence of urine: a comparison of risk factors and determinants between smokers and nonsmokers, *Am J Obstet Gynecol* 170:579-582, 1994.
13. Constantinou CE, Govan DE: Spatial distribution and timing of transmitted and reflexly generated urethral pressures in healthy women, *J Urol* 127:964-969, 1982.
14. Gunnarsson M, Mattiasson A: Circumvaginal surface electromyography in women with urinary incontinence and in healthy volunteers, *Scand J Urol Nephrol* 157(suppl):89-95, 1994.
15. Snooks SJ, Swash M: Abnormalities of the innervation of the urethral striated sphincter musculature in incontinence, *Br J Urol* 56:401-405, 1984.
16. Meyer S, de Grandi P, Kuntzer T, et al: Birth trauma: its effect on the urine continence mechanisms, *Gynäkol Geburtshilfliche Rundsch* 33:236-242, 1993.
17. Deindl FM, Vodusek DB, Hesse U, Schüssler B: Pelvic floor activity patterns: comparison of nulliparous continent and parous urinary stress incontinent women: a kinesiological EMG study, *Br J Urol* 73:413-417, 1994.
18. DeLancey JOL: Structural support of the urethra as it relates to stress urinary incontinence: the hammock hypothesis, *Am J Obstet Gynecol* 170:1713-1723, 1994.
19. Zinner NR, Sterling AM, Ritter RC: Role of inner urethral softness in urinary continence, *Urology* 16:115-117, 1980.
20. Romanzi LJ, Heritz DM, Blaivas JG: Preliminary assessment of the incontinent woman, *Urol Clin North Am* 22:513-520, 1995.
21. Green TH Jr: Development of a plan for the diagnosis and treatment of urinary stress incontinence, *Am J Obstet Gynecol* 83:632-648, 1962.
22. McGuire EJ, Lytton B, Pepe V, Kohorn EI: Stress urinary incontinence, *Obstet Gynecol* 47:255-264, 1976.
23. McGuire EJ, Lytton B, Kohorn EI, Pepe V: The value of urodynamic testing in stress urinary incontinence, *J Urol* 124:256-258, 1980.
24. Blaivas JG: Sphincteric incontinence in the female: pathophysiology, classification and choice of corrective surgical procedure, AUA Update Series, vol 6, lesson 25, Baltimore, 1987, American Urological Association.
25. McGuire EJ, Bennett CJ, Konnak JA, et al: Experience with pubovaginal slings for urinary incontinence at the University of Michigan, *J Urol* 138:525-526, 1987.
26. Chapple CR, Helm CW, Blease S, et al: Asymptomatic bladder neck incompetence in nulliparous females, *Br J Urol* 64:357-359, 1989.

27. Versi E: The significance of an open bladder neck in women, *Br J Urol* 68:42-43, 1991.
28. Lagro-Janssen ALM, Debruyne FMJ, VanWeel C: Value of the patient's case history in diagnosing urinary incontinence in general practice, *Br J Urol* 67:569-572, 1991.
29. Versi E, Cardozo L, Anand D, Cooper D: Symptoms analysis for the diagnosis of genuine stress incontinence, *Br J Obstet Gynaecol* 98:815-819, 1991.
30. Jensen JK, Nielsen FR Jr, Ostergard DR: The role of patient history in the diagnosis of urinary incontinence, *Obstet Gynecol* 83:904-910, 1994.
31. McGuire EJ, Lytton B: Pubgovaginal sling procedure for stress incontinence, *J Urol* 119:82-84, 1978.
32. McGuire EJ, Fitzpatrick CC, Wan J, et al: Clinical assessment of urethral sphincter function, *J Urol* 150:1452-1454, 1993.
33. Couillard DR, Webster GD: Detrusor instability, *Urol Clin North Am* 22:593-612, 1995.
34. Diokno A, Yuhico M Jr: Preference, compliance and initial outcome of therapeutic options chosen by female patients with urinary incontinence, *J Urol* 154:1727-1730, 1995.
35. Mouritsen L, Frimodt-Moller C, Moller M: Long-term effect of pelvic floor exercises on female urinary incontinence, *Br J Urol* 68:32-37, 1991.
36. Elia G, Bergman A: Pelvic muscle exercises: when do they work? *Obstet Gynecol* 81:283-286, 1993.
37. Hahn I, Milsom I, Fall M, Ekelund P: Long-term results of pelvic floor training in female stress urinary incontinence, *Br J Urol* 72:421-427, 1993.
38. McIntosh LJ, Frahm JD, Mallett VT, Richardson DA: Pelvic floor rehabilitation in the treatment of incontinence, *J Reprod Med* 38:662-666, 1993.
39. Stamey TA: Endoscopic suspension of the vesical neck for urinary incontinence in females: report on 203 consecutive patients, *Ann Surg* 192:465-471, 1980.
40. Spencer JR, O'Conor VJ, Schaeffer AJ: A comparison of endoscopic suspension of the vesical neck with suprapubic vesicourethropexy for treatment of stress urinary incontinence, *J Urol* 137:411-415, 1987.
41. Sirls LT, Keoleian CM, Korman HJ, Kirkemo A: The effect of study methodology on reported success rates of the modified pereyra bladder neck suspension, *J Urol* 154:1732-1735, 1995.
42. Leach GE, Zimmern PE: Vaginal suspension procedures, AUA Update Series, vol 9, lesson 40, Baltimore, 1990, American Urological Association
43. Eckford SD, Abrams P: Para-urethral collagen implantation for female stress incontinence, *Br J Urol* 68:586-589, 1991.
44. Duncan HJ Nurse DE, Mundy AR: Role of the artificial urinary sphincter in the treatment of stress incontinence in women, *Br J Urol* 69:141-143, 1992.
45. Murray KH, Nurse DE, Mundy AR: Detrusor behavior following implantation of the Brantley Scott artificial urinary sphincter for neuropathic incontinence, *Br J Urol* 61:122-128, 1988.
46. Diokno AC, Hollander JB, Alderson TP: Artificial urinary sphincter for recurrent female urinary incontinence: indications and results, *J Urol* 138:778-780, 1987.
47. Appell RA: Techniques and results in the implantation of the artificial urinary sphincter in women with type III stress urinary incontinence by a vaginal approach, *Neurourol Urodyn* 7:613, 1988.
48. Raz S, Sussman EM, Erickson DB, et al: The Raz bladder neck suspension: results in 206 patients, *J Urol* 148:845-850, 1992.
49. German KA, Kynaston H, Weight S, Stephenson TP: A prospective randomized trial comparing a modified needle suspension procedure with the vagina/obturator shelf procedure for genuine stress incontinence, *Br J Urol* 74:188-190, 1994.
50. Jarvis GJ: Surgery for genuine stress incontinence, *Br J Obstet Gynaecol* 10[illegible]:371-374, 1994.
51. Stanton SL, Williams JE, Ritchie D: The colposuspension operation for urinary incontinence, *Br J Obstet Gynaecol* 83:890-895, 1976.
52. Marshall VF, Marchetti AA, Krantz KE: The correction of stress incontinence by simple vesicourethral suspension, *Surg Gynecol Obstet* 88:509-512, 1949.
53. Zimmern PE, Hadley HR, Leach GE, Raz S: Female urethral obstruction after Marshall-Marchetti-Krantz operation, *J Urol* 138:517-520, 1987.
54. Walters MD: Retropubic repair of urethral incontinence. In Kursh ED, McGuire EJ, editors: *Female urology,* Philadelphia, 1994, Lippincott.
55. Raz S, Albo ME: A new approach in the treatment of urethral incontinence: the anterior vaginal wall sling, *Issues in Incontinence* 3:2, 1996.
56. Stricker P, Haylen B: Injectable collagen for type 3 female stress incontinence: the first 50 Australian patients, *Med J Aust* 158:89-91, 1993.

Chapter 26

Urge Incontinence

Said A. Awad, Jerzy B. Gajewski

Urge incontinence refers to involuntary urine loss that is preceded by a strong and sudden desire to void. Patients frequently may say, "I have to hurry to the bathroom and sometimes I leak urine before I can get there." Older patients often may say, "Sometimes I seem to have no warning and I can't get to a bathroom." In some instances pain and discomfort may trigger voiding. The underlying disorder may be neurogenic (stroke, spinal cord injury, multiple sclerosis) or nonneurogenic (bladder outlet obstruction, stress incontinence, or idiopathic). In this chapter we mainly discuss nonneurogenic urge incontinence.

Pathophysiology

Nonneurogenic urge incontinence can be classified as sensory or motor urge incontinence. It is well established that distinction between these two groups is sometimes very difficult, and there is a lot of overlap. There is also a suggestion that the underlying mechanism is the same.[1] Nevertheless, this classification will help to understand the syndrome at the clinical level.

Sensory Urge Incontinence

Sensory urge incontinence is caused by hypersensitivity of the urethra or the bladder so that it causes a strong desire to void at low urine volume. Occasionally it can also cause a constant feeling to urinate. This sensation may or may not be relieved by voiding. Several conditions may cause an increase in bladder sensory output, that is, acute or chronic cystitis, interstitial cystitis, bladder stones, or bladder cancer. Very often, however, the underlying condition is unknown. Unless there is a definite cause of bladder hypersensitivity there are almost no objective tests to confirm diagnosis, which may rely on subjective patient perception of the symptoms. Patients who develop a fibrotic bladder after radiation, chronic infection, or chronic catheterization also tend to have low compliance. In these patients the bladder wall is stiff and cannot accommodate urine volume and a steady increase in bladder pressure eventually leads to urgency, pain, and the triggering of voiding.

Motor Urge Incontinence

Symptomatic presentation of motor urge incontinence is similar to sensory urge incontinence. The diagnosis can usually be supported by urodynamic findings of detrusor contractions. Involuntary detrusor contractions without sign of neurologic disease is referred to as *detrusor instability.* Detrusor instability in men is usually associated with bladder outlet obstruction caused by benign prostatic hypertrophy (BPH) or bladder neck dysfunction. The association of urge incontinence with anatomic stress incontinence has been also well documented.[2] Incontinence caused by bladder instability that is not associated with bladder outlet obstruction, anatomic stress incontinence, or bladder disorders can be labeled "idiopathic detrusor instability" and occurs more often in women. Whether the detrusor muscles themselves constitute the primary trigger for the contraction[3,4] or whether it is a primary neurogenic event[5] remains uncertain. Some instances of detrusor instability may be accompanied by an impaired contractility of the detrusor muscle, which may aggravate the problem.

In a small group of patients detrusor contraction is triggered by urethral instability.[6,7] In this condition, the speed and strength with which the urethra contracts and relaxes increases significantly.[8] During the relaxation phase, not only does urethral occlusion pressure drop, but the bladder is deinhibited as well, and detrusor contraction is triggered, resulting in incontinence.

CLINICAL PRESENTATION

Symptoms vary from patient to patient, but the common clinical picture usually includes frequency, urgency, and urge incontinence. Some patients can also have obstructive symptoms. Nocturia may or may not be part of the urge incontinence syndrome. It is unclear why at night some patients have decreased sensory output from the bladder and no nocturia whereas others have increased sensory output. In elders there might be an increase in urine output at night leading to nocturia. Enuresis is an uncommon presentation with this condition and indicates rather sleep disturbances or neurogenic lesion. Clinically it is sometimes very difficult to distinguish sensory from motor urge incontinence, and very often both coexist. Stress incontinence may coexist with urge incontinence, and in some cases it may also be an underlying cause.[9] It is sometimes difficult to differentiate between urge and stress incontinence from the history alone, since both may be provoked by physical stress or sudden movement. Also, other symptoms may obscure the clinical picture. Suprapubic pain or discomfort may indicate bladder infection or interstitial cystitis. Perception from the bladder is a very subjective feeling, and a patient's depiction of symptoms can be inaccurate. Several studies showed that a particular symptom is not diagnostic of a particular bladder condition.

Some patients have associated bowel complaints like irritative bowel syndrome. Also, many patients are emotionally unstable,[10] and it is not clear if it is primary or secondary to the bladder symptoms.

EVALUATION

The evaluation of urge incontinence begins with a thorough history and physical examination, involving urologic, gynecologic, and neurologic assessment with regard to urinary function. Further information from a patient's "voiding diary" and postvoid residual and urine leak tests, which can be part of the clinical assessment, will help to confirm the nature and extent of the problem. One then proceeds to specific laboratory tests such as urinalysis, urine culture, and serum creatinine. According to this information, the need for additional tests and specialized studies can be assessed.

The *voiding diary* objectively records the patient's voiding pattern and documents episodes of incontinence. A simple form to enter time, voiding volume, and incontinence episodes is most commonly used. This chart offers reliable information about a patient's symptoms; however, its diagnostic value is limited.[11] Several portable leak-recording devices are now on the market to help patients record episodes of incontinence. Such devices are particularly useful for patients who have trouble understanding or sensing episodes of incontinence. One can estimate the volume of urine loss by the number of pads used daily or can calculate more precisely by weighing the wet pads.

The *postvoid residual* is a measure of the volume of urine left in the bladder after voiding. Sometimes this can be estimated by palpating the bladder but is more precisely measured using suprapubic ultrasonography or bladder catheterization. An increased residual may be responsible for urge or overflow incontinence and reflects a decrease in detrusor contractility, which may be neurogenic, idiopathic, or secondary to bladder outlet obstruction. For practical purposes, a residual over 100 ml, or more than one third of the voiding volume, can be considered abnormal.

The *urine leak test* is performed to confirm the presence of stress incontinence at an office visit. The patient, with full bladder, is asked to cough while standing. Observable urine leakage constitutes a positive test. In most cases, this simple test is enough to confirm stress incontinence, but in 5% to 10% it will not reveal urine leakage, possibly because the tension of the sphincter muscles is abnormally increased during the test. It is important to make sure that the urine leakage is related to increased abdominal pressure and not to a detrusor contraction induced by coughing, which would cause urine to leak several seconds after the stress event and does not stop when the coughing ceases. Presence of the stress incontinence does not automatically exclude urge incontinence. In 40% of patients, stress and urge incontinence coexist. In many instances stress incontinence may lead to development of urge incontinence.

If any doubt remains after this test, more thorough urodynamic investigation is warranted. Although some of these tests are highly specific and sensitive, results must always be viewed in the context of the patient's clinical picture.

Urinalysis with or without a urine culture and sensitivity should be done to rule out infections before more specialized urodynamic tests are performed.

Urodynamic Tests

Uroflow is a useful screening test mainly to evaluate bladder outlet obstruction. Consistently low flow rates generally indicate a bladder outlet obstruction but may also indicate decreased detrusor contractility.

Cystometrogram (CMG) provides information about bladder sensation, maximum cystometric capacity, detrusor compliance, and bladder stability. Although the test is very simple and is performed frequently, interpreting results requires some expertise. CMG can be performed using either gas or liquid to fill the bladder, with different interpretive criteria applying to each. *Bladder sensation* is assessed when one records the volumes at which the patient first becomes aware of filling and then of bladder fullness. Although with low- and medium-speed liquid cystometry (10 to 50 ml/min) the bladder fills faster than it would physiologically, it has an insignificant effect on bladder sensation in most patients. A hypersensitive bladder, with or without incontinence, may indicate urinary tract infection, interstitial cystitis, idiopathic sensory urgency, or a neurogenic bladder. *Maximum cystometric capacity* (MCC) is a bladder volume at which either a strong urge to void occurs, further filling becomes extremely painful, or urethral leakage with detrusor contraction occurs. In our opinion, a volume of MCC under 300 ml usually indicates a hypersensitive bladder. Because gas fills the bladder much faster than liquid does, the volume of first sensation and bladder capacity will be lower with the former type of cystometry. *Detrusor compliance* is defined as the change in volume over the change in pressure. Compliance inversely correlates to the speed of the bladder filling and is usually lower in a urodynamic setting than during normal physiologic filling. The increase in bladder pressure during the filling phase of CMG should not exceed a range of 10 to 15 cm H_2O (at a MCC of 500 ml). Conditions like chronic bladder infections, radiation cystitis, or neurogenic bladder can cause decreased compliance, sometimes to the point of incontinence. *Bladder instability* refers to an involuntary detrusor contraction that occurs during the filling phase in patients without neurologic conditions. Detrusor hyperreflexia describes an involuntary detrusor contraction in the presence of neurologic disease. The International Continence Society (ICS)[12] defines a detrusor contraction as an increase in bladder pressure of more than 15 cm H_2O. In everyday practice, however, even contractions of less than 15 cm H_2O, referred to as "subthreshold," may be considered meaningful. Evidence of detrusor instability on CMG confirms a diagnosis of urge incontinence. Sometimes techniques such as having the patient cough, sneeze, stand up, or jump can trigger a detrusor contraction and unveil instability. To overcome some of the drawbacks of the urodynamic lab environment, the concept of "ambulatory urodynamic study" evolved.[13] A portable transducer/recorder connected to a small bladder catheter records bladder pressure during ambulatory activities. Initial studies showed an increased rate of detection of detrusor instability with this technique in comparison to laboratory urodynamics tests. The clinical importance of this finding remains to be seen, since some of the detected detrusor contractions were not associated with any symptoms.[14]

Electromyography (EMG) of the external sphincter is used to record striated muscle activity and could be useful to assess the possibility of sudden sphincter relaxation syndrome. In this case a detrusor contraction is preceded by a sudden decrease in EMG activity. It is also useful in determining detrusor sphincter dyssynergia when obstruction associated with detrusor instability is suspected.

Urethral pressure profile (UPP) records intraluminal pressure through the entire length of the urethra. Normal UPP curves differ between men and women. The UPP values of maximum urethral closure pressure (MUCP) and functional urethral length (FUL) are used most often. These tend to be lower in patients with stress incontinence. However the specificity and sensitivity of the test appear very low. Nonetheless, extremely low values of MUCP (under 20 cm H_2O) indicate probable damage to the intrinsic property of the sphincter (type III stress incontinence), and extremely high values (more than 200 cm H_2O) point to a possible bladder outlet obstruction. The leak point pressure test, now under development, may provide a more objective means of assessing the competence of the urethra. The value of this test is primarily in detecting type III incontinence.

Voiding cystourethrogram (VCUG) is a fluoroscopy test to assess bladder neck and urethral function (external sphincter) during filling and voiding phases. It can be used to measure the descent of the bladder neck and calculate the vesicourethral angle in the work-up of stress incontinence. This study can also be used to confirm detrusor-sphincter dyssynergia (DSS) or dysfunctional voiding in case of unclear EMG results.

Pressure-flow study simultaneously records the voiding detrusor pressure and the rate of urinary flow. Detrusor pressure is then plotted against flow rate. This is the only test able to provide information about detrusor contractility. It also reveals the extent of a bladder outlet obstruction. It is particularly useful in investigating men with incontinence and obstructive voiding and women with persistent or renewed incontinence after surgical treatment. Pressure-flow study can be combined with VCUG and videourodynamic study for very complicated cases of incontinence. It requires very sophisticated and expensive equipment, and there is considerable controversy in the literature over the value of this test in routine clinical practice.

Ultrasonography, in the forms of transabdominal, transvaginal, transperineal (translabial), and transrectal sonography, has recently been introduced to assess the severity of a case of stress incontinence. These diagnostic procedures await clinical acceptance.

Cystoscopy allows for a visual assessment of the bladder, bladder neck, and urethra. Obvious causes of bladder hyperactivity such as cystitis, stone, and tumor can be easily diagnosed. It is important here to point out the association between incontinence and interstitial cystitis because it is easy enough to miss interstitial cystitis and attribute irritative bladder symptoms to stress incontinence or instability. The incontinence may, in fact, prevent the bladder from becoming full enough to cause the pain usually associated with cystitis. Cystoscopy with adequate hydrodistension should be performed when there is even minimal suspicion of interstitial cystitis, because failure to diagnose this disease has therapeutic and prognostic implications.[15]

TREATMENT

Correctable causes of urge incontinence like bladder outlet obstruction, cystitis, or a stone should obviously be treated first before other options are contemplated.

Conservative

Behavioral therapy. Bladder retraining is considered by some to be the most effective conservative treatment. It is based on the premise that bladder instability is an effect of frequent voiding. The patient is asked to increase slowly the intervals between voiding until a 3- to 4-hourly pattern is achieved. Long-term results, however, are only in the range of 50%.[16]

In patients with high volume instability a voiding schedule every 2 to 3 hours may prevent uninhibited detrusor contractions and incontinence. It is especially useful in an elderly patient who has problems with mobility and reaching the bathroom on time.[17,18]

Biofeedback is another conservative treatment[19] highly dependent on the patient's compliance. After the patient is connected to the urodynamic device that transmits visual or auditory signals of detrusor contractions, he or she is then asked to inhibit conscientiously these contractions. The patient learns how to recognize and then how to inhibit these contractions during everyday activities. Although initial results were encouraging, the long-term results are uncertain. Pelvic muscle exercises are mainly indicated for stress incontinence but were also found to decrease bladder instability. Again there is a problem with long-term compliance. Vaginal stimulation has been used extensively in Europe[20] with less popularity in North America. The basis of this treatment is to evoke pelvic muscle contraction, which inhibits voiding reflex through central action. Maximal pelvic floor stimulation was effective up to 1 year in 50% of the treated patients.[21] Some women find this treatment unpleasant and difficult to perform. Hypnotherapy has been also suggested with some subjective responses but is not often used.[22] Acupuncture was tried but only with limited success.

Pharmacotherapy.[23] The indications for pharmacologic treatment should be viewed in the context of the patient's global clinical picture. Since urge incontinence is mainly attributable to bladder overactivity, anticholinergic and antispasmodic drugs are the first line of pharmacologic treatment. When a new drug is tried, the patient must be carefully followed to monitor the drug's effectiveness and watch for signs of adverse reactions. Although each patient will respond to a drug slightly differently, several general contraindications and potential adverse reactions should be kept in mind. Smooth muscle relaxants and anticholinergics should not be given to patients with obstructive uropathy, bowel obstruction, ulcerative colitis, narrow-angle glaucoma, myasthenia gravis, or severe cardiovascular disease. Dryness of the mouth is a common side effect. Patients may become less alert when taking anticholinergics and should be cautioned about the potential hazards of driving or operating dangerous machinery.

Oxybutynin chloride (Ditropan) has anticholinergic, antispasmodic, and anesthetic properties. Dosage ranges from 2.5 mg PO OD to 5 mg qid. For elderly patients, the recommended dosage is lower than 5 mg PO OD. Intravesical approach has been suggested with good symptomatic response and fewer side effects.[24]

Propantheline bromide (Pro-Banthine) is a cholinergic receptor competitor. Usual dosage ranges from 7.5 mg PO OD to 15 mg PO qid. Higher dosages (up to 30 mg PO qid) are advised if absorption in the digestive tract is incomplete.

Dicyclomine chlorhydrate (Bentylol) has both a musculotropic and anticholinergic effect on smooth muscles. The Dospan formulation provides continuous-release medication. Dosages up to 80 mg PO OD in three or four doses can be used.

Flavoxate hydrochloride (Urispas) is a papaverine-like antispasmodic with some anticholinergic and anesthetic properties. Usual dosages range from 200 mg PO tid or qid up to 1200 mg/day. There is a low incidence of side effects. It is recommended for the elderly and patients who have trouble tolerating other drugs.

Imipramine chlorhydrate (Tofranil, Apo-Imipramine) is a tricyclic antidepressant with anxiolytic, anticholinergic, direct musculotropic, and adrenergic properties. It also has mild anesthetic and antihistamine effects. It inhibits the norepinephrine reuptake at presynaptic nerve terminals. The most common indications include enuresis and voiding dysfunction arising from supraspinal lesions or dysfunction. Dosage should be increased gradually to about 25 mg tid, but a dosage of up to a maximum of 200 mg/day can be used if necessary. Imipramine should not be given along with monoamine oxidase inhibitors.

Belladonna/opium suppositories have analgesic, anticholinergic, and antispasmodic properties. Because of their potential addictiveness, they should be used only over the short term, such as to control pain and bladder spasm after bladder or prostate surgery. One suppository is used every 3 to 4 hours as necessary.

New groups of drugs like receptor-specific (muscarinic) blockers, potassium-channel opener (Cromakalim), or new calcium-channel blockers are under investigation but are not yet used in clinical practice.

Surgical Treatment

Patients who failed conservative treatment may benefit from surgical intervention. This treatment, however, should not be undertaken without consideration given to the balance between the risk of surgery versus benefit of the treatment to the patient. Bladder and urethra dilatation has been used quite extensively as an initial treatment with variable results. This is easy to do during diagnostic cystoscopy. Exactly how it works is not clear. At least some temporary relief was achieved in patients with interstitial cystitis, urethral syndrome, or similar conditions. Increase in mast cell concentration in the detrusor has been considered to be a primary cause of symptoms in interstitial cystitis. Degradation of the mast cells by bladder or urethral distension has been attributed to the improvement in the symptoms. Phenol injection has been used with only limited success because of the risk of dangerous side effects.[25] Selective sacral cryoneurolysis was successfully used with good short-term results.[26] Mean duration of effect was 5 months. Long-term results, however, are uncertain. Sacral foramen nerve stimulation is a new treatment for detrusor instability. It has a 60% to 70% success rate.[27] Patients are subjected initially to temporary sacral foramen nerve stimulation through a percutaneously placed electrode. If the patient responds well to temporary sacral foramen nerve stimulation, a permanent implant is offered. The exact mechanism of the electrical modulation is not yet well defined, but activation of the spinal interneurons or beta-adrenergic neurons, which inhibit bladder activity, has been postulated.

Ileocystoplasty is one of the valuable alternative treatments of detrusor instability, with a success rate of 60%.[28] An ileal (or colonic) patch is anastomosed to the bladder after the bladder ("clam") is split.[29] Bladder capacity increases and instability decreases.[30] Long-term consequences of this surgery, especially a risk of developing carcinoma of the ileal patch,[31] still remain unclear. Increased bowel problems after such procedures should also be kept in mind. Many patients have also increased mucus production by the patch in the bladder and recurrent urinary tract infections, and 30% to 40% will need intermittent self-catheterization at least once daily.

Detrusor myomectomy "autoaugmentation" is an alternative surgical technique for the treatment of the bladder instability.[32] Limited numbers of patients and short-term follow-up study in published series makes this procedure still experimental.[33] Clinical application remains to be seen.

Urinary diversion is an ultimate surgical intervention for desperate patients who failed conservative or less invasive surgical treatments. Particular effort should be made to weigh advantages versus disadvantages of this procedure. Sometimes a particular patient's situation, such as extreme obesity or social or economic situation, might have a critical role in making a decision. There are several options: ileoconduit, continent diversion, or orthotropic bladder replacement.

Summary

The pathophysiology of urge incontinence still remains unclear and several questions remain to be answered. Is sensory urge incontinence different from motor incontinence? What is the so-called idiopathic urge incontinence? Why do some patients not respond to the conservative treatment? Until these questions are answered we will be struggling to manage patients with urge incontinence on a trial-and-error basis.

References

1. Coolsaet BLRA, van Duyl WA, van Os-Bossagh P, De Bakker HV: New concepts in relation to urge and detrusor activity, *Neurourol Urodyn* 12:463-471, 1993.
2. McGuire EJ, Savastano JA: Stress incontinence and detrusor instability/urge incontinence, *Neurourol Urodyn* 4:313-316, 1985.
3. Cucchi A: Bladder contractility and idiopathic detrusor instability in males, *Neurourol Urodyn* 13:627-635, 1994.
4. Del Carro U, Riva D, Comi GC, et al: Neurophysiological evaluation in detrusor instability, *Neurourol Urodyn* 12:455-462, 1993.
5. Petros PEP, Ulmsten U: Bladder instability in women: a premature activation of the micturition reflex, *Neurourol Urodyn* 12:235-239, 1993.
6. Low JA: Urethral behaviour during the involuntary detrusor contraction, *Acta Obstet Gynaecol Scand* 128:32-42, 1977.
7. Ulmsten U, Henriksson L, Iosif S: The unstable female urethra, *Am J Obstet Gynecol* 144:93-97, 1982.
8. Wise BG, Cardozo LD, Cutner A, et al: Prevalence and significance of urethral instability in women with detrusor instability, *Br J Urol* 72:26-29, 1993.
9. Awad SA, Gajewski JB, Katz NO, Acker-Roy K: Final diagnosis and therapeutic implications of mixed symptoms of urinary incontinence in women, *Urology* 39:352-357, 1992.
10. Hafner RJ, Stanton SL, Guy J: A psychiatric study of women with urgency and urge incontinence, *Br J Urol* 49:211-214, 1977.
11. Larsson G, Abrams P, Victor A: The frequency/volume chart in detrusor instability, *Neurourol Urodyn* 10:533-543, 1991.
12. Abrams P, Blaivas JG, Stanton SL, Andersen JT: The standardisation of terminology of lower urinary tract function, *Scand J Urol Nephrol* 114(suppl) 5-19, 1988.
13. Webb RJ, Ramsden PD, Neal DE: Ambulatory monitoring and electronic measurement of urinary leakage in the diagnosis of detrusor instability and incontinence, *Br J Urol* 68:148-152, 1991.
14. Webb RJ, Griffiths CJ, Ramsden PD, Neal DE: Measurement of voiding pressures on ambulatory monitoring: comparison with conventional cystometry, *Br J Urol* 65:152-154, 1990.
15. Awad SA, MacDiarmid S, Gajewski JB, Gupta R: Idiopathic reduced bladder storage versus interstitial cystitis, *J Urol* 148:1409-1412, 1992.
16. Holmes DM, Stone AR, Bary PR, et al: Bladder training: 3 years on, *Br J Urol* 55:660-664, 1983.
17. McLish DK, et al: Bladder training in older women with urinary incontinence: relationship between outcome and changes in urodynamic observation, *Obstet Gynecol* 77(2):281-286, 1991.
18. Sogbein SK, Awad SA: Behavioural treatment of urinary incontinence in geriatric patients, *Can Med Assoc J* 127:863, 1982.
19. Cardozo LD, Stanton SL, Hafner J, Allan V: Biofeedback in the treatment of detrusor instability, *Br J Urol* 50:250-254, 1978.
20. Primus G: Detrusor inhibition by intravaginal stimulation of the pudendal nerve: experience in idiopathic detrusor hyperactivity, *Aktuel Urol* 23:70-72, 1992.
21. Eriksen BC, Bergmann S, Eik-Nes SH: Maximal electrostimulation of the pelvic floor in female idiopathic detrusor instability and urge incontinence, *Neurourol Urodyn* 8:219-230, 1989.
22. Freeman RM, Boxby K: Hypnotherapy for incontinence caused by detrusor instability, *Br Med J* 284:1831-1832, 1982.
23. Wein AJ: Practical uropharmacology, *Urol Clin North Am* 18:269-281, 1991.
24. Massad CA, Kogan BA, Trigo-Rochau FE: The pharmacokinetics of intravesical and oral oxybutynin chloride, *J Urol* 148:595-597, 1992.
25. Chapple CR, Hampson SJ, Turner-Warwick RT, Worth PH: Subtrigonal phenol injection: how safe and effective is it? *Br J Urol* 68:483-486, 1991.
26. Awad SA, Flood HD, Acker KL, Clark AJ: Selective sacral cryoneurolysis in the treatment of patients with detrusor instability/hyperreflexia and hypersensitive bladder, *Neurourol Urodyn* 6:307-315, 1987.

27. Thon WF, Schmidt RA, Jonas U, Tanagho EA: Neurostimulation of voiding dysfunctions, *Aktuel Urol* 22:41-44, 1991.
28. McInerney PD, Harris SA, Pritchard A, Stephenson TP: Night studies for primary diurnal and nocturnal enuresis and preliminary results of the clam ileocystoplasty, *Br J Urol* 67:42-43, 1991.
29. Mundy AR, Stephenson TP: "Clam" ileocystoplasty for the treatment of refractory urge incontinence, *Br J Urol* 57:641-646, 1985.
30. Bramble FJ: The treatment of adult enuresis and urge incontinence by enterocystoplasty, *Br J Urol* 54:693-696, 1982.
31. Nurse DE, Mundy AR: Assessment of the malignant potential for cystoplasty, *Br J Urol* 64:489-492, 1989.
32. Cartwright PC, Snow BW: Bladder auto-augmentation: partial detrusor excision to augment the bladder without use of bowel, *J Urol* 142:1050-1053, 1989.
33. Stöhrer M, Kramer A, Goepel M, et al: Bladder auto-augmentation: an alternative for enterocystoplasty: preliminary results, *Neurourol Urodyn* 14:11-23, 1995.

Chapter 27 Mixed Urinary Incontinence

Pat O'Donnell

Mixed incontinence is often a complex bladder and urethral dysfunction that results in loss of voluntary bladder control. The voluntary control of the elimination of urine by the body is one of the most important functions that determines the quality of life any individual can experience in our society. The loss of that function results in changes that affect essentially every aspect of a person's life. Mixed incontinence is one of the most common types of incontinence in patients presenting to their primary care physician and represents one of the most perplexing management problems for clinicians treating patients who have loss of bladder control. Any long-term treatment decision must be made by the patient and physician with as accurate information as is possible about the specific bladder dysfunction involved. This requires using the best current technology available so that the patient can consider the risks and benefits in realistic terms as these factors apply to the specific lifestyle of that person.

Conditions such as bladder noncompliance or neurologic diseases that significantly alter the resting pressures of the bladder can present a threat to long-term survival resulting from deteriorating renal function. However, for most people who suffer from urinary incontinence, treatment of incontinence does not prolong survival, and quality of life is the major issue involved in the management decision. The compromise in quality of life caused by urinary incontinence is perceived very differently among people. Both the characteristics and the severity of incontinence as well as the particular lifestyle of the person are important in assessment of the great effect of incontinence on the daily activities of the patient. For example, a woman whose occupation involves strenuous activity or a woman who derives enormous enjoyment from playing tennis may have a major compromise in lifestyle from mild stress incontinence, whereas a similar person having a more sedentary lifestyle may experience much less compromise in lifestyle from the same level of incontinence. Similarly, people who have mild urge incontinence with associated frequency and nocturia will often experience a much greater compromise in lifestyle than a person with mild stress incontinence having the same severity of involuntary urine loss without the annoying problems of urgency, frequency, and nocturia.

Mixed urinary incontinence is present when a patient has symptoms consistent with stress incontinence and also has symptoms consistent with urge incontinence. Since stress incontinence is extremely rare in men in the absence of previous prostate or pelvic surgery, mixed urinary incontinence occurs primarily in women. However, mixed incontinence is often seen in men who have postprostatectomy incontinence. Mixed incontinence is usually more difficult to manage than either stress or urge incontinence alone. Treatment of mixed incontinence is usually complicated by the combination of symptoms of stress and urge incontinence, which can vary considerably in the severity of either component. The category of mixed incontinence seems justifiably separate from stress or urge incontinence, since the combination of symptoms seems to represent a somewhat different clinical entity with many levels of complexity. Because of the interaction between these symptoms, the management of mixed incontinence is often more complicated than the management of the stress component and the urge component separately. In patients who have mixed incontinence, the stress component and urge component clinically seem to aggravate or worsen the other.

As described in other sections, the bladder and urethra function as a physiologic unit to provide storage of urine and reflexly interact with one another. Therefore, in a patient who is being treated for the stress component or urge component of mixed incontinence, the physician is actually managing a separate clinical entity that comprises the combination of both symptoms. For example, it is well known that in patients who have mixed incontinence, surgery that effectively corrects the stress component will eliminate or improve the urge component in a very high percentage of patients.[1,2] The mechanism of the improvement in the urge component of mixed incontinence after successful surgery for stress incontinence is unclear. However, the changes in both stress and urge incontinence after successful surgery for stress incontinence demonstrates the close interaction of the two components as a clinical entity.

The coexistence of symptoms of stress incontinence and urge incontinence often makes it difficult for the physician and the patient to determine which component is predominantly contributing to the patient's loss of bladder control. The reason is that both urge and stress components appear to be contributing simultaneously to the symptoms experienced by the patient. It is the combined symptom complex that results in mixed incontinence. Since the objective measurements used in the evaluation of mixed incontinence involves measurement of each component separately, it is clinically necessary to refer to the characteristics of the stress component or urge component separately in the evaluation and treatment of the patient.

If one considers mixed incontinence as a clinical problem in which stress incontinence and urge incontinence are simultaneously involved in the symptoms that the patient experiences, it is easier to appreciate the complexity of the patient's history, the urodynamic studies, and the patient's response to different therapies. Since there are endless combinations of severity of either component interacting with the other among different patients, the symptoms can present a confusing clinical picture to the physician. Therefore, it is sometimes extremely difficult for the physician to determine on the basis of a clinical history alone the possible cause of incontinence in patients with symptoms of mixed incontinence. In patients with mixed incontinence compared with patients who have symptoms of stress incontinence only, the urodynamic studies become even more essential to determine the functional abnormalities present in the bladder and urethra as well as the interaction between them. It is the assessment of these more complex patients that the capabilities of the urodynamic laboratory become critical in the successful diagnosis and treatment of the patients who have mixed incontinence.

Incontinence History

Stress Incontinence

In patients who have mixed incontinence, the incontinence history is extremely important in allowing one to initially identify the complicated management problem from the patient who is less complicated.[3] For example, a young woman with mild stress incontinence and no other significant complicating factors in her voiding history will likely experience some mild symptoms of urgency with an occasional or rare episode of urge incontinence. The presence of both symptoms of stress and urge incontinence in this patient represents an uncomplicated case of mixed incontinence and will likely respond well to either surgical or nonsurgical therapy. In this patient, a successful surgical procedure that eliminates the symptoms of stress incontinence will almost always also eliminate the symptoms of urgency and urge incontinence without further treatment.

At the other end of the range of complexity is the patient whose stress component of mixed incontinence is caused by significant intrinsic sphincter deficiency (ISD) with a coexisting severe component of urge incontinence. The history of this complicated patient is often one of a woman who changes absorbent pads many times during the day. Also, it is sometimes unclear to the patient when an episode of incontinence occurs or what causes it to occur. A patient with this history may be an older woman who has had previously failed surgical procedures for incontinence. However, it can occur in younger women who have never had surgery. The occasional younger woman without previous surgery who has mild urge incontinence and is subsequently found to have ISD presents a constant diagnostic problem. Without a complete evaluation, the component of ISD will not be identified, and a conventional suspension procedure is unlikely to be successful over the long term. For incontinent patients like these, every detail of the history can be helpful. In the patient who has complicated mixed incontinence, the interaction between the urethra, bladder, and modulating neurologic centers are involved in producing the symptoms. Therefore the physician must evaluate every aspect of the history, physical exam, urodynamics, radiographic evaluation, and endoscopic examination to understand the pathophysiology involved in each patient. The management decisions in these patients are sometimes extremely difficult, and a complete evaluation is critical for a long-term successful continence outcome of treatment.[4]

Urge Incontinence

In the treatment of mixed incontinence, the role of urge incontinence in the management of patients who also have stress incontinence has been controversial to some extent for decades. Many clinical studies show that the results of surgery for stress incontinence have a poor continence outcome when preoperative urge incontinence is present.[5,6] Other studies show that successful surgical correction of stress incontinence results in relief of symptoms of urge incontinence in most of the patients.[7,8] Most physicians would agree that it is extremely important to completely evaluate urge incontinence in any patient with mixed incontinence to successfully manage the patient. Also many physicians believe that the clinical history is the most reliable and most valid source of information about urge incontinence for a patient who has mixed incontinence.[9] The presence or absence of detrusor instability during filling cystometry is somewhat controversial in establishing the role of urge incontinence in the diagnosis and prognosis of a patient with mixed incontinence.[10] The primary reason for the controversy is that some patients who have a clinical history of urge incontinence may have a stable bladder during filling cystometry and other patients without a clinical history of urge incontinence may have an unstable bladder. Therefore many physicians believe that patients who have a clear clinical history of urge incontinence are probably having involuntary bladder contractions regardless of whether it can be demonstrated during filling cystometry.

If one assumes that the clinical history of urge incontinence represents involuntary detrusor contractions that occur during daily activities of the patient, the clinical history would be essential in determining the severity as well as the characteristics of the urge incontinence. Standardized questionnaires with an urge incontinence scale are not commonly used in clinical practice. Awad et al. classified urge incontinence as grades I, II, and III based on frequency, nocturia, urgency, and urge incontinence in patients with mixed incontinence.[11] Although this classification is extremely useful in the assessment of patients with mixed incontinence, further research is needed in delineating the clinical attributes and relative significance of each symptom in defining the characteristics and severity of urge incontinence. Ideally a questionnaire would need to provide a symptom score that is predictive of treatment outcome. This would allow the primary care physician to evaluate the urge component of mixed incontinence to identify patients for further study and establish a basis for long-term therapy.

The classification described by Awad et al. is an extremely helpful clinical guide to assessment of the severity of urge incontinence in patients who have mixed incontinence. When the physician interviews the patient, every detail of the history can be useful to determine the severity of the urge component of mixed incontinence. For example, the number of times the patient experiences nocturia each night is usually an event that has a significant influence on the quality of life of the patient and something that the patient can remember quite well. Therefore the information about nocturia can be considered relatively reliable in most patients. Also the incidence and characteristics of urge incontinence associated with nocturia is something the patient can usually describe in detail. Therefore the patient who says, "I have to hurry to the bathroom at night, and occasionally I will leak a few drops before I get there" is considerably different from the patient who says, "When I get up to go to the bathroom, it gushes out before my feet hit the floor almost every time." For many patients who have mixed incontinence, the complexity of the management problem is determined by the severity of the problem of urge incontinence. Therefore the physician must make the best clinical assessment possible of the severity of the urge component in patients who have mixed incontinence.

Physical Examination

The physical examination of the patient with mixed incontinence is primarily focused on the assessment of the stress incontinence component. The physical examination of the patient with stress incontinence is described in further detail in the chapters on both physical examination and stress incontinence. Of particular importance in the examination of the patient with mixed incontinence is the determination of the presence or absence of urethral mobility. In patients who have failed previous surgery for stress incontinence, an assessment on the physical exam of scarring around the urethra is important in the event that a surgical approach to management is eventually considered. If scarring around the urethra is present on examination, the patient needs to be carefully evaluated for bladder outlet obstruction. Outlet obstruction from previous incontinence surgery is often a factor in the cause of urge incontinence in women with mixed incontinence. Assessment of bladder outlet obstruction requires urodynamic evaluation with pressure-flow studies as described in other sections.

The absence of hypermobility on physical examination would be suggestive that the cause of the stress incontinence component is not anatomic. This is especially true if the patient has failed previous surgical procedures for treatment of incontinence. Patients who have failed previous incontinence surgery who do not have hypermobility on physical examination are likely to have intrinsic sphincter deficiency (ISD) as the cause of the stress component, and any consideration of surgical management will usually involve either intraurethral injections or a urethral sling procedure. Even in this group of patients, ISD needs to be confirmed on urodynamic studies before therapy is planned.

Patients who have a history of mixed incontinence and hypermobility on physical examination need urethral function studies to determine if ISD is present or absent, since the physical exam does not contribute to the diagnosis in the same way as the patient with a fixed urethra. It is important to determine if the patient with mixed incontinence has ISD as the stress component, since the long-term treatment and the continence outcome are likely to be different from that in the patient without ISD.

Urodynamic Studies

On the initial routine urinary flow study in patients who have mixed incontinence, the flow rate is usually normal with no residual urine. However, a low flow rate (<15 ml/sec) is sometimes associated with bladder outlet obstruction, which can be a factor in the urge component. Also, an elevated residual urine (>50 ml) can be a contributing factor to urge incontinence, as well as being associated with overflow incontinence.

The cystometric evaluation of patients with mixed incontinence is focused primarily on capacity, compliance, and stability. A small functional capacity of the bladder may be associated with urge incontinence preoperatively and persistent irritative symptoms postoperatively.[11] Compliance is an extremely important measure of bladder function in patients with mixed incontinence.[12] Bladder noncompliance is a very serious disorder that can cause mixed incontinence. This important clinical problem is further described in the chapter on bladder noncompliance. Failure to recognize bladder noncompliance in the patient with mixed incontinence will almost certainly result in failure of therapy as well as present a risk for deterioration of function of the upper urinary tract.

In patients who have a history of mixed incontinence, detrusor instability (DI) is a urodynamic finding that is associated with urge incontinence. Since many patients who have a history of urge incontinence do not have DI on routine urodynamic studies and some patients who have DI do not have a history of urge incontinence, the role of DI in the management of patients with urge incontinence has been controversial.[8,13] Compared with routine cystometry, provocative testing or ambulatory monitoring will show a higher incidence of DI in patients with a history of urge incontinence.[7,14] Therefore the diagnosis of DI is somewhat dependent on the cystometric technique used to identify DI. Since all patients who have a clear history of urge incontinence probably have an unstable bladder or at least an unstable urethra at the moment of experiencing urge incontinence, the relative difficulty involved in eliciting an unstable detrusor contraction during urodynamic studies probably indicates the relative severity of the underlying problem of detrusor stability. Patients who demonstrate DI on routine cystometry may have a greater problem maintaining bladder stability than those who do not demonstrate unstable activity. Therefore, in patients who have a significant urge component of mixed incontinence, the treatment outcome is likely to be better in patients who have a stable bladder than in those with DI on routine urodynamic testing.

Patients who have mixed incontinence will have some degree of urethral sphincteric incompetence. In patients with a significant component of urge incontinence, the stress component may not be apparent from the incontinence history. Therefore identifying the severity of the stress component of mixed incontinence will require urodynamic studies with measurement of urethral function. Objective measurement of urethral function using the urethral pressure profile and leak point pressures are utilized to assess the presence and severity of sphincteric incompetence. The urodynamic measurement of urethral function not only will assess the severity of urethral dysfunction but also will identify patients who have ISD. The techniques and interpretation of these urethral function studies are described in other chapters of the text. It is imperative to recognize that one cannot assume that a patient has only urge incontinence without urethral function studies to demonstrate that urethral function is normal and mixed incontinence is not present. Again, it is emphasized that mixed incontinence appears to be a clinical entity that is more complex than the combined components of both urge and stress incontinence.

Endoscopic Examination

Urethroscopy can be extremely important in the evaluation of the patient with mixed incontinence. One can evaluate the mobility of the urethra during resting and straining. The endoscopic assessment of hypermobility is an important correlate of the physical examination and radiographic evaluation to establish the presence or absence of hypermobility.

The clinical concept of ISD that is so much a part of our current management strategy of stress incontinence was originally described in the most severe form as an endoscopic observation called a "lead pipe" urethra. Since we have much more clinical experience with ISD at the present time, we are able to make endoscopic observations about urethral function that are much more subtle than a "lead pipe." For example, the mucosal appearance of the urethra contributes significantly to our assessment of severity and selection of treatment of patients who have ISD. In elderly women where ISD is much more common,[14,15] the endoscopic appearance of the urethral mucosa and coaptation of the mucosa is invaluable in the clinical evaluation of the urethra. Detrusor hyperactivity as a component of mixed incontinence is also much more common in the elderly and may occur during bladder filling while endoscopy is being performed.

The endoscopic appearance of the bladder is also important in the evaluation of the patient with mixed incontinence. The presence and severity of trabeculation of the bladder may indicate the long-term effects that urge incontinence has had on the bladder. Any abnormal areas on the mucosa of the bladder should be considered for biopsy, since carcinoma in situ of the bladder can cause irritative bladder symptoms including urge incontinence.

Treatment of Mixed Incontinence

As described previously, the clinical management of mixed incontinence is usually more complex than the separate treatment of each component of stress and urge incontinence. Because of the wide range in severity of combinations of stress and urge incontinence among patients, each patient is unique in the clinical management. In the treatment of mixed incontinence, the severity and complexity of the combined stress and urge incontinence problem is usually more important in determining the outcome of treatment than the modality selected for management.[16] The patient with mild stress incontinence and associated mild urge incontinence will usually respond well to both surgical and nonsurgical therapy. In contrast, the patient with severe urge incontinence and type III stress incontinence (ISD) is an extremely difficult management problem.

It is a reasonable consideration in the initial management of complicated mixed incontinence to treat the urge component with behavioral therapy, pharmacologic therapy, electrical stimulation, or a combination of these therapies.[17,18] Following a trial of conservative therapy, the physician can determine to some extent the responsiveness of the urge component in the patient to nonsurgical therapy. Again, it is important to recognize that as long as a component of stress incontinence exists, it is not possible to adequately determine treatment response to urge incontinence, since stress incontinence is part of the problem of urge incontinence in patients who have mixed incontinence. Likewise, a therapeutic improvement in urge incontinence after nonsurgical therapy may also result in an improvement in symptoms of stress incontinence.

If the stress component of mixed incontinence is amenable to surgical therapy, it is a reasonable consideration to treat the stress incontinence surgically and manage the residual urge incontinence postoperatively. The reason for this approach is that in most patients the symptoms of urge incontinence will completely resolve or significantly improve after successful surgery for stress incontinence. However, the symptoms of urge incontinence usually do not resolve immediately and may persist for 3 to 6 months postoperatively even though the symptoms of stress incontinence have resolved.

Type III stress incontinence (ISD) is unlikely to respond to nonsurgical therapy in most patients. If hypermobility is not present in patients with mixed incontinence, intraurethral injection therapy for treatment of stress incontinence may be successfully combined with nonsurgical therapy for management of urge incontinence. In these patients, intraurethral injection therapy has a major advantage of not producing prolonged obstruction of the urethra. In patients who have mixed incontinence with type III stress incontinence and hypermobility, intraurethral injections are currently not indicated, and a urethral sling procedure is probably the best long-term choice for management of the stress incontinence.[19] The problem of the sling procedure in these patients is that temporary outlet obstruction is common after placement of a urethral sling. In most patients, the problem of temporary outlet obstruction is managed relatively easily with clean intermittent self-catheterization. In patients who have complicated mixed incontinence, the temporary outlet obstruction usually aggravates the underlying urge incontinence, often resulting in severe bladder spasms postoperatively. In many cases, the patient may be unable to void without clean intermittent catheterization and at the same time may have frequent episodes of incontinence because of bladder spasms. Fortunately, this complicated postoperative course resolves in most patients when the outlet obstruction from the sling resolves. Symptomatic outlet obstruction after a urethral sling procedure usually resolves within a few weeks in most patients,[20,] though it can persist for many months in some patients. The long-term continence results of the sling procedure in these extremely complicated patients are very good, but the patient and physician need to be prepared for a potentially complicated postoperative course during the short term. Long-term nonsurgical therapy may be required postoperatively in some patients with mixed incontinence to control persistent symptoms of urge incontinence, though these symptoms eventually resolve in most patients over time. Fortunately the complicated patient with mixed incontinence is relatively uncommon and is most often seen after multiple previous unsuccessful surgical procedures for treatment of incontinence.

SUMMARY

Mixed incontinence occurs when symptoms of stress incontinence and urge incontinence coexist in the same patient. Since stress incontinence rarely occurs in men in the absence of previous prostate or pelvic surgery, mixed incontinence primarily occurs in women. Clinically, mixed incontinence appears to be more complex than the combined components of stress and urge incontinence for many patients. When patients have mixed incontinence, the stress component appears to aggravate the urge component, and the urge component seems to worsen the stress component. Successful treatment of the stress component can significantly improve the urge component in most patients. However, in patients with severe mixed incontinence surgical procedures that produce bladder outlet obstruction can increase the symptoms of urge incontinence after surgery. Fortunately, outlet obstruction related to surgical procedures to correct incontinence usually resolves over time. Unfortunately, in some patients who present with mixed incontinence, outlet obstruction from previous surgery that failed to resolve may be a major factor in the cause of the urge component.

Because the cause of mixed incontinence is often complex, most physicians use conservative therapy initially, which includes behavioral therapy, pharmacologic therapy, electrical stimulation, or a combination of therapy. If the stress incontinence component is attributable to intrinsic sphincter deficiency (ISD), the management is much more complicated, since ISD is unlikely to respond well to conservative management. If the urge component of mixed incontinence can be managed satisfactorily, the quality of life of the patient is significantly improved even though the patient may still experience stress incontinence. Urge incontinence is often more distressing and usually compromises quality of life more than stress incontinence. Although a surgical approach to the stress component of mixed incontinence may have a prolonged and complicated course in some patients, the long-term outcome is usually very good. It is reasonable to manage these patients conservatively to determine the level of continence that can be achieved and to determine the effect that the residual incontinence has on the quality of life of the patient. The decision to have surgery for the patient with severe complicated mixed incontinence needs to be based on a clear understanding of the potential postoperative problems as well as the long-term benefits. Also, the patient needs to have a personal commitment to achieving the best long-term continence outcome possible, which often requires surgery for treatment of stress incontinence and may require nonsurgical treatment of residual urge incontinence postoperatively in some patients.

The clinical management of mixed incontinence needs to be based on the most complete evaluation possible of both the bladder and urethra. In patients who have complicated combinations of stress and urge incontinence, both surgical and nonsurgical therapy may be required in combination to achieve the best long-term continence results possible. In these complicated patients, a long-term commitment to continence by the physician, patient, and family of the patient is extremely important for the most successful outcome possible to be achieved.

REFERENCES

1. Ramon J, Mekras JA, Webster GD: The outcome of transvaginal cystourethropexy in patients with anatomical stress urinary incontinence and outlet weakness, *J Urol* 144:106-109, 1990.
2. Langer R, Ron-El R, Bukovsky I, Caspi E: Colposuspension in patients with combined stress incontinence and detrusor instability, *Eur Urol* 14:437-439, 1988.
3. Lee RA: Recurrent stress incontinence of urine: preoperative assessment and surgical management, *Clin Obstet Gynecol* 19:3:661-671, 1976.
4. McGuire EJ: Identifying and managing stress incontinence in the elderly, *Geriatrics* 45:44-52, 1990.
5. Sand PK, Bowen LW, Ostergard DR, et al: The effect of retropubic urethropexy on detrusor stability, *Obstet Gynecol* 71:6:818-822, 1988.
6. Arnold EP, Webster JR, Loose H, et al: Urodynamics of female incontinence: factors influencing the results of surgery, *Am J Obstet Gynecol* 15:805-813, 1973.
7. Couillard DR, Webster GD: Detrusor instability, *Urol Clin North Am* 22(3):593-612, 1995.
8. McGuire EM: Bladder instability in stress incontinence, *Neurourol Urodyn* 7:563, 1988.
9. Petros PP, Ulmsten U: Urge incontinence history is an accurate predictor of urge incontinence, *Acta Obstet Gynecol Scand* 71:537-539, 1992.
10. McGuire EJ, Lytton B, Kohorn E, Pepe V: The value of urodynamic testing in stress urinary incontinence, *J Urol* 124:256-258, 1980.
11. Awad SA, Gajewski JB, Katz NO, Acker-Roy K: Final diagnosis and therapeutic implications of mixed symptoms of urinary incontinence in women, *Urology* 39(4)352-357, 1992.
12. McGuire EJ: Urodynamic evaluation of stress incontinence, *Urol Clin North Am* 22(3):551-555, 1995.
13. McGuire EJ, Savastano JA: Stress incontinence and detrusor instability, *Neurourol Urodyn* 4:313, 1985.
14. Webb RJ, Ramsden PD, Neal DE: Ambulatory monitoring and electronic measurement of urinary leakage in the diagnosis of detrusor instability and incontinence, *Br J Urol* 68:148-152, 1991.
15. Horbach NS, Ostergard DR: Predicting intrinsic urethral sphincter dysfunction in women with stress urinary incontinence, *Obstet Gynecol* 84(2):188-192, 1994.
16. Raz S, Sussman EM, Erickson DB, et al: The Raz bladder neck suspension: results in 206 patients, *J Urol* 148:845-850, 1992.
17. Koonings PP, Bergman A. Urethral pressure changes in women with detrusor instability: bladder or urethral pathologic process? *Urology* 37(6):540-542, 1991.
18. Karram MM, Bhatia NN: Management of coexistent stress and urge urinary incontinence, *Obstet Gynecol*73:(1):4-7, 1989.
19. Blaivas JG, Jacobs BZ: Pubovaginal fascial sling for the treatment of complicated stress urinary incontinence, *J Urol* 145:1214-1218, 1991.
20. McGuire EJ, O'Connell HE: Surgical treatment of intrinsic urethral dysfunction, *Urol Clin North Am* 22(3):657-664, 1995.

Chapter 28

Intrinsic Sphincter Deficiency

Mike J. Kennelly, Edward J. McGuire

Urinary continence against abdominal pressure as an expulsive force is normally achieved by action of the vesical neck and proximal portion of the urethra. In males, this segment of the urethra, which passively resists abdominal pressure, includes the vesical neck, prostatic urethra, and the short segment of urethra (approximately 1 cm long) from the distal verumontanum to the onset of the higher pressure area of the so-called external sphincter or membranous urethra. In females, this segment is the proximal 1 to 1.5 cm of urethra from the bladder outlet to the midurethral high-pressure zone, or "external sphincter." Abnormalities of urethral sphincteric behavior are divisible into two broad groups. These are abnormalities of urethral support resulting in urethral hypermobility and abnormalities of urethral closure, which may or may not be associated with hypermobility. When urethral hypermobility is present, a normally closed sphincter unit may still leak under the influence of increased abdominal pressure. This is the most common type of stress incontinence in women.[1] Intrinsic sphincter deficiency exists when detrusor pressures and proximal urethral pressures are isobaric, or nearly so. In patients with loss of functional closure of the bladder neck and proximal portion of the urethra, leakage generally occurs at low to very low abdominal pressures.[1,2] In instances where urethral hypermobility occurs, abdominal pressures required to cause leakage are higher.[3] Although intrinsic sphincter deficiency and urethral hypermobility may exist independently, many patients with incontinence suffer from both abnormalities.

The true incidence of intrinsic sphincter deficiency is unknown. Previous reports of the incidence of intrinsic sphincter deficiency identified by a precise fluorourodynamic technique in patients selected for urodynamic evaluation before stress incontinence surgery indicates that those patients presenting with primary stress incontinence and no previous operative therapy have a low incidence (6% to 9% percent) of intrinsic sphincter deficiency.[4,5] On the other hand, those who failed one or more operative procedures have a much higher incidence of intrinsic sphincter deficiency as a contributing cause or the sole cause of stress incontinence.[5] Intrinsic sphincter deficiency is much more common in elderly women than in younger women. Women with new-onset stress incontinence after 70 years of age almost invariably suffer from some component of intrinsic sphincter deficiency.[4]

The failure rate for standard vesicourethral suspension procedures varies from 5% to as much as 60%.[6] A major cause of operative failure is poor function of the intrinsic sphincter.[5] Bladder neck and proximal urethral suspension procedures reliably treat stress urinary incontinence associated with urethral hypermobility, but these are unreliable in the presence of intrinsic sphincter deficiency alone or in concert with urethral hypermobility. Moreover, the recent introduction of injectable agents with relatively narrow indications makes precise identification of the specific cause of stress urinary incontinence in an individual patient even more relevant.

PATHOPHYSIOLOGY

Factors responsible for normal intrinsic sphincter closure include smooth muscle contractility, integrity of the periurethral fascia, normal innervation, and mucosal seal factors, which include mucosal turgor and thickness, and the vascularity of the urethra. In females the rugated mucosal folds and the well-vascularized submucosal cushion are hormonally sensitive. Estrogen promotes proliferation and maturation of urethral epithelium and submucosal vasculature.[7] Estrogen, in addition, enhances mucosal secretion, which increases the surface tension and the mucosal seal effect within the urethra. The spongelike rich vascular tissue in the area of the submucosa is surrounded by smooth muscle, fibroelastic tissue, and the periurethral fascia, which supports and helps to coapt the intrinsic sphincter mechanism.

There is currently no general agreement on all the neural processes that subserve the function of the urethra as a sphincter. Motor innervation that drives closure of the intrinsic sphincter is chiefly derived from the intermediolateral cell columns of the thoracolumbar area. These fibers traverse the sympathetic chain. At the level of the third and fourth lumbar vertebrae, the preganglionic nerves ramify around the inferior mesenteric ganglion. These ramified fibers, which constitute the superior hypogastric plexus, cross the common iliac arteries and pelvic brim to become part of the inferior hypogastric plexus and ultimately supply the intrinsic sphincter. Although closure of the bladder neck and proximal urethra is vitally important for passive continence, the precise relationship between the component parts of the inferior hypogastric plexus, which include neural elements derived from the thoracolumbar sympathetic outflow as well as the sacral parasympathetic outflow, is at present unknown. Lack of closure of the internal sphincter with resultant incontinence can be achieved by prolonged administration of alpha-adrenergic blocking agents and is associated with specific neural entities, namely, myelodysplasia, T12 to L1 spinal cord injury, and peripheral neural injuries associated with radical hysterectomy, or abdominal perineal resection. In addition spinal cord infarction can induce total loss of intrinsic sphincter function.[8-10]

Intrinsic sphincter deficiency (where the bladder and proximal urethra are isobaric) results in leakage driven by abdominal pressure as an expulsive force. Critical to understanding the pathophysiology of intrinsic sphincter deficiency is the observation that abdominal pressure and detrusor pressure are (as far as the urethra is concerned) completely different expulsive forces.[3] Urethral resistance to bladder muscular contractility, or pressures exerted on the urinary bolus by contractile activity, or the vesicoelastic properties of the detrusor during filling are resisted by that part of the urethra manifesting the highest intraluminal closing pressure at the instant the detrusor forces are brought to bear on the urethra. Normally the highest intraluminal urethral pressures are recorded in the external sphincter high pressure zone.[12] Except in disease states, the internal sphincter is neurologically linked to detrusor behavior. When a detrusor is quiescent in the storage mode, the internal sphincter is closed. When the detrusor contracts, the internal sphincter opens. Lack of internal sphincter opening occurs only in a few conditions, including benign prostatic hypertrophy, but also in detrusor areflexia where there is no neural mechanism to provide for intrinsic sphincter opening with detrusor activity. On the other hand, abdominal pressure is resisted passively by closure of the intrinsic sphincter mechanism from the bladder neck to the external sphincter. This part of the urethra lies within the abdominal cavity, and normally abdominal pressure does not have a differential effect on the bladder, but influences both the bladder and the urethra equally and simultaneously. Hypermobility of the urethra contributes to the development of urinary leakage by allowing the dislocation of the urethra from the pressure influence of the abdominal cavity.

Intrinsic sphincter deficiency is a condition where the proximal urethra and bladder are isobaric. In effect the continence line moves down the urethra to the external sphincter. Because the external sphincter is at the margin of the abdominal cavity, abdominal pressure excursions then become an expulsive force. This occurs because abdominal pressure has a differential effect on the bladder that has incorporated the proximal portion of the urethra (in a hydraulic sense) and the area of the urethra compressed by the external sphincter. In circumstances where the sphincter from the bladder neck to the external sphincter is always open, as occurs in myelodysplasia, after radical prostatectomy, in certain cases of spinal cord injury, and in women with type III stress incontinence, leakage will be induced at low to very low abdominal pressures, even if there is a normal external (striated) urethral sphincter function.[11] That observation is the basis for the idea that the external sphincter is not an effective resistive force to abdominal pressure in the absence of a functional intrinsic sphincter. Patients with myelodysplasia are especially illustrative of this relationship, since external sphincter pressure in these individuals is often normal and can be, in fact, higher than pressures recorded in age-matched normal individuals.[8] This results in a situation where an areflexic detrusor faces relatively high urethral resistance, which in turn can result in altered bladder compliance and back-pressure effects on the upper urinary tract. Despite this relationship urinary leakage can be induced across the open nonfunctional proximal parts of the urethra at low abdominal pressures. In a study of myelodysplastic children, when the abdominal pressure required to cause leakage was compared with the bladder pressure required to do the same (and cause leakage), there was no correlation between the two values individually or collectively.[3]

Specific Etiology

Neural Causes

The motor innervation of the intrinsic sphincter is chiefly derived from the thoracolumbar sympathetic nervous system. It has been demonstrated experimentally and clinically that intrinsic sphincter deficiency can result from a central or peripheral sympathetic neural injury.[13-16] Sacral rhizotomy involving S1 through S5, however, does not result in loss of intrinsic sphincter function despite loss of "external sphincter" function.[17]

Myelodysplasia, the Shy-Drager syndrome, spinal cord infarction, spinal cord tumors located within the thoracolumbar sympathetic area, and peripheral neural lesions can cause intrinsic sphincter deficiency. Myelodysplasia is associated with an 85% incidence of nonfunction of the internal sphincter, from the bladder neck to the external sphincter. Myelodysplasia is associated with an open, nonfunctional internal sphincter mechanism, an areflexic bladder, and variable function of the external sphincter.[18] The Shy-Drager syndrome, an uncommon degenerative disorder resulting in atrophy of the cerebellum, brainstem, peripheral autonomic ganglia, and the thoracolumbar sympathetic neurons, also causes intrinsic sphincter deficiency. Spinal cord infarction with loss of the thoracolumbar sympathetic cell mass is associated with intrinsic sphincter deficiency as are T12 spinal cord injuries. In addition, peripheral neural injuries incurred at the time of radical extirpative pelvic surgery can be associated with transient or permanent intrinsic sphincter deficiency.

Prior Pelvic Surgery

The majority of women who are found to have intrinsic sphincter deficiency will have had prior antiincontinence or pelvic surgery.[19] Previous surgery on the urethra, vagina, or bladder neck may damage the structural elements within the intrinsic sphincter, and previous gynecologic or general surgical procedures may damage the peripheral sympathetic innervation of the urethra. The precise association between prior antiincontinence surgery and the development of intrinsic sphincter deficiency is debated. There is no question that intrinsic sphincter deficiency is often identified as a problem after failure of a previous operative procedure to resolve urinary stress incontinence.[5] It may be that there is a causal association between the previous surgery and the development of intrinsic sphincter deficiency, but that has not been proved. Prospective studies indicate that patients with intrinsic sphincter deficiency will fail standard suspension operations and therefore these patients might be selected for operative failure. Other surgical procedures including urethral diverticulectomy or urethrotomy or transurethral resection of prostate or radical prostatectomy can result in intrinsic sphincter deficiency, leading to urethral leakage at low abdominal pressures.[20]

Prostatectomy

The most common cause of male stress urinary incontinence, which is virtually always related to intrinsic sphincter deficiency, is a simple or radical prostatectomy. The incidence of incontinence after an open simple prostatectomy or transurethral prostatic resection is low. The incidence of incontinence after radical prostatectomy is reported to range from 2.5% to 87%.[20-23] Intrinsic sphincter deficiency is the reason for stress incontinence after any type of prostatectomy, though detrusor instability may be (rarely) the sole cause of incontinence.[24] More commonly intrinsic sphincter deficiency coexists with detrusor instability, which may even be caused by that intrinsic sphincter deficiency. Normally, after transurethral resection or open prostatectomy, function of the internal sphincter is lost from the bladder neck to the verumontanum. Continence is maintained by closure of the approximately 1 cm area from the distal verumontanum to the "external sphincter."[24]

After radical prostatectomy some continence function may be the result of preservation of the bladder neck, but the critical area of function against abdominal pressure is the residual urethra above the pelvic floor. That is the urethra between the pelvic diaphragm and the anastomotic suture line at the bladder neck. If the area does not function because of the lack of length or lack of coaptation, urinary stress incontinence will occur.

Other Factors

Estrogen deficiency has been implicated as a factor in intrinsic sphincter deficiency, since anecdotally estrogen administration in patients who are estrogen depleted does result in improved continence function. Trials of estrogen therapy have concentrated on postmenopausal patients who have stress incontinence. The mechanisms involved in stress incontinence in most postmenopausal patients would preclude effective therapy by estrogens, since the major reason for incontinence in this group is urethral hypermobility related to the lack of urethral support.[19] On the other hand, when estrogens have been given to patients who demonstrate intrinsic sphincter deficiency and profound estrogen deficiency together with a lack of urethral hypermobility, they have been effective.[25] Long-term catheter drainage may induce total urethral dysfunction in females, and often this follows a pattern of larger and larger catheters required to seal a less and less effective urethra, followed by development of constant urinary leakage through what amounts to a conduit.[26]

Diagnosis

History

A history of incontinence related to increased abdominal pressure is important. In men after prostatectomy, incontinence occurs in the upright position with coughing or straining. This is excellent evidence for intrinsic sphincter deficiency even if the history is also compatible with detrusor instability.[24] In women, grade III incontinence, or incontinence that occurs without any association with activity, is often associated with intrinsic sphincter deficiency. Female patients who experience no improvement or worsening of incontinence after previous operative procedures for stress incontinence often have intrinsic sphincter deficiency.[25] Patients with previous extirpative pelvic surgery or radiation therapy, elderly patients with new-onset stress incontinence, and patients with neurologic disease should be suspected of intrinsic sphincter deficiency. Alpha-adrenergic blocking agents taken for protracted periods may result in intrinsic sphincter deficiency in susceptible individuals, but this is not a common cause for that problem.

Physical Examination

In males the upright position is used and the bladder should be filled to a reasonable volume (at least 200 ml) before testing. The patient is asked to do a Valsalva maneuver or cough while the urethral meatus is visualized. Any leakage in a male induced by coughing or the Valsalva maneuver is evidence of intrinsic sphincter deficiency. The only other condition that can result in this occurrence is a poorly compliant bladder. A cystometrogram is thus essential so that one can be sure that a poorly compliant bladder does not produce a situation where detrusor pressure results in an isobaric bladder and urethra at some point during bladder filling, which will result in leakage at low abdominal pressures.

In females it is useful to gauge the extent of urethral hypermobility. A well-supported urethra that shows no hypermobility with the Valsalva maneuver or coughing but nevertheless leaks is presumptive evidence of intrinsic sphincter deficiency. However, the classic supine pelvic exam position is not the most effective position to elicit urinary leakage or to determine mobility. Forces acting on the urethra, such as the weight of the abdominal viscera combined with the height of the fluid column within the bladder, are brought out by the upright position. In patients where no leakage can be demonstrated in the supine position a repeat evaluation with the patient upright should be done with the same maneuvers (that is, Valsalva maneuver and cough).

Urodynamic Evaluation Without Video Studies

The first basic urodynamic evaluation in males or females with incontinence should be a cystometrogram to determine detrusor pressure responses to filling. This is an important variable, since any leakage produced in patients with stress incontinence occurs at some measurable total bladder pressure. The detrusor component of the total bladder pressure is vitally important. A poorly compliant bladder that generates pressure as a result of volume will make even a very good urethra look as though it suffers from intrinsic sphincter deficiency. Therefore in both males and females a baseline cystometrogram to document normal detrusor storage of urine to normal capacity is important. A bladder that does not store urine normally, that is, with a pressure less than 12 cm H_2O at capacity, may contribute to urethral leakage. This is an additional risk factor that must be considered in patients subjected to procedures to increase urethral resistance to abdominal pressure. If detrusor pressure is part of the expulsive force, the patient will not be benefited by an operative procedure on the urethra, and instead treatment must be directed at the abnormal detrusor response to filling.

Leak Point Pressure Testing

Detrusor leak point pressure. The detrusor leak point pressure test is designed to establish the relationship between the detrusor and the outlet. With the patient supine, the bladder is filled until leakage occurs across the urethra. This may be as a result of a reflex bladder contraction, or as a result of an areflexic increase in detrusor pressure as a result of volume increments. This kind of testing is useful in neurologic disease processes where the interrelationship of the detrusor and the outlet are vitally important to upper tract integrity. The detrusor leak point pressure, however, has no bearing on function of the urethra vis-à-vis abdominal pressure or intrinsic sphincter deficiency. Typically the detrusor leak point pressure describes the relationship between the detrusor and the external sphincter high-pressure zone.[8,18]

Abdominal Leak Point Pressure. The abdominal leak point pressure is a measure of the ability of the intrinsic sphincter mechanism to oppose abdominal pressure. The bladder capacity is determined by a cystometrogram. Leak point pressure testing is by convention and is done at 200 ml in adults. In children, the test volume (half bladder capacity) is determined by the cystometrogram.

The bladder is filled with the patient supine using a 10 Fr catheter of some variety. A urodynamic catheter is best, but any catheter can be used. Catheter diameters greater than 10 Fr result in falsely high leak point pressures. To do the leak point pressure test, the patient is placed in the upright position with the catheter maintained in the bladder. The patient is asked to do as vigorous a Valsalva maneuver as possible while the pressure in the bladder is recorded and noted at the instant of leakage. If the Valsalva maneuver fails to induce leakage and repetitive coughing is necessary to induce leakage, the leak point pressure will be high.

Pitfalls of Leak Point Pressure Testing. The detrusor pressure component must be controlled by registration of the detrusor response to filling from zero volume to the test volume, since the detrusor pressure contributes to the total bladder pressure responsible for leakage. Detrusor storage pressure should be normal for accurate interpretation of the leak point pressure findings.

Genital prolapse in females involving any portion of the vagina: anterior vagina (cystocele formation), vaginal apex (enterocele formation), or posterior vaginal wall (enterocele or rectocele) all adversely influence leak point pressure testing. Genital prolapse results in dissipation of abdominal pressure forces and artificially inflates the leak point pressure. Reduction of genital prolapse and maintenance of that reduction by a sponge stick or some other device should be done, and the leak point pressure testing repeated. Patients with genital prolapse who have severe intrinsic sphincter deficiency may not have clinical stress incontinence symptoms until the genital prolapse is reduced.[27]

Partial urethral coaptation or sealing of a rigid narrow-caliber urethra is possible, particularly in males with postprostatectomy incontinence, with a 10 Fr catheter. If no leakage is induced around the 10 Fr catheter, the 10 Fr catheter should be removed and the Valsalva maneuver or coughing repeated to document the effect of the catheter and the presence of stress incontinence.

Videourodynamics Assessment

The most precise method to diagnose intrinsic sphincter deficiency is by videourodynamics. The leak point pressure testing technique described above was derived from observations made during thousands of videourodynamic studies. Normal function of intrinsic sphincter maintains a closed bladder neck so that in the upright position no contrast is seen in the urethra. Normally videourodynamics show the base of the bladder to be flat and located just at or above the pubic symphysis. With intrinsic sphincter deficiency, some contrast medium may be seen in the open bladder neck and proximal portion of the urethra in the absence of a detrusor contraction.[1,2] In this case, the urethra no longer functions as a sphincter with respect to abdominal pressure. Leakage can occur without any motion of the bladder base and urethra at low to very low abdominal pressures (Fig. 28-1). Patients with a wide-open contrast-filled proximal urethra associated simply with the upright position, at moderate bladder volumes, generally have excellent external sphincter mechanisms.[9] Good external sphincter closure results in the columnization of contrast medium in the proximal area of the urethra and ease of diagnosis on an upright cystogram. Patients with total sphincter deficiency involving both the external sphincter and the internal sphincter may have a radiographic appearance that is less dramatic because there is no resistance in the urethra at any point; the contrast medium does not seem to appear in the urethra despite steady-state leakage. Moreover, intrinsic sphincter deficiency does not require a patulous ('wide-open') internal sphincter from the bladder neck to the external sphincter. The diagnosis of intrinsic sphincter deficiency is basically determined by the amount of abdominal pressure required to cause leakage.[24,25] In women, if leakage occurs at pressures less than 90 cm H_2O, some degree of intrinsic sphincter deficiency exists.[3] Ancillary information is necessary to determine whether this is pure intrinsic sphincter deficiency or intrinsic sphincter deficiency coexisting with urethral hypermobility. Patients with hypermobility typically leak at pressures above 100 cm H_2O (Fig. 28-2).

Urethral pressure profiles (UPP) and EMG determinations can result in information that has some importance in individual cases of stress incontinence. Urethral pressure profilometry,

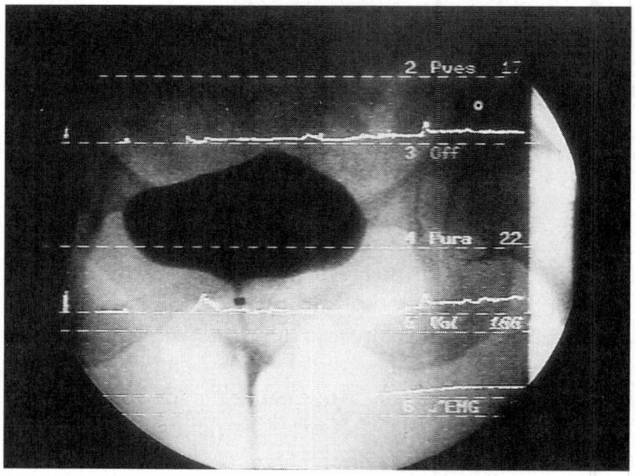

FIG. 28-1 *Upright videourodynamic study in a patient with intrinsic sphincter deficiency. Simultaneous bladder (P_{ves}) and urethral (P_{ura}) pressures are measured. The precise point is identified by the square radiopaque marker. Notice the open nonfunctional internal sphincter. At a volume (Vol) of 166 ml, the patient demonstrates urinary leakage at a low abdominal pressure of 17 cm H_2O.*

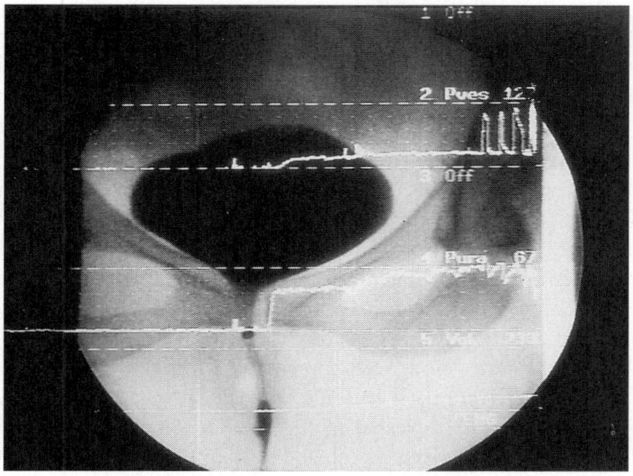

FIG. 28-2 *Upright videourodynamic study in a patient with urethral hypermobility. Notice the descent of the proximal portion of the urethra and opening of the bladder neck. At a volume (Vol) of 233 ml, the patient demonstrates urinary leakage at a high abdominal pressure (P_{ves}) of 127 cm H_2O.*

however, typically concentrates on measurement of pressures in the high-pressure zone. These are only indirectly related to the ability to the urethra to oppose abdominal pressure.[3] Although EMG abnormalities have been recorded in patients with stress incontinence, the exact type of stress incontinence associated with these patients has not been identified with a standard videourodynamic technique. Although EMG abnormalities and perhaps UPP abnormalities are related to urethral hypermobility (since integrity of the striated muscle of the pelvic floor contributes to urethral support), there are no data on UPP and abdominal leak point pressure that show any correlation between those two variables.

Endoscopy provides information on the character on the urethral wall and its coaptation and is occasionally a reasonable substitute for fluoroscopy in the investigation of the character of the intrinsic sphincter. Used with leak point pressure testing, urethroscopy is helpful.

TREATMENT

The objective of treatment of intrinsic sphincter deficiency is to gain closure, or coaptation, of the urethra as close to the bladder outlet as possible. It is feasible to gain closure of the internal sphincter without changing the detrusor pressure required to induce voiding or leakage.[11,28] Since the relationship between the detrusor and the urethra (or the detrusor pressure required to cause leakage or voiding) is critically important to upper tract function, a procedure that closes the urethra without changing the detrusor pressure required to cause leakage or induce voiding is desirable.

Surgical procedures directed at the creation of a normally functioning internal sphincter involve reconstructive techniques such as the Young-Dees-Leadbetter and the Kropp urethral reimplantation, or replacement procedures such as the Tanagho procedure, which uses an anterior bladder wall flap to create a neourethra. Neourethral construction has also been described using ileum, appendix, and ureter.[29-31] In addition to these procedures, mechanical urethra-compression devices including the artificial sphincter, pubovaginal sling, puboprostatic sling in males, and the vaginal wall sling have been used. In addition, injectable agents can be used to treat intrinsic sphincter deficiency in certain well-defined instances.[32-35] Nonsurgical therapies such as biofeedback, electrical stimulation, and pharmacologic therapy are not so effective.[36] Only very rarely are alpha-adrenergic agents effective as treatment for intrinsic sphincter deficiency. Patients with congenital absence of the internal sphincter do not respond to alpha-adrenergic agents at all.[18]

Bladder Neck Reconstruction

Bladder neck reconstruction techniques are typically used for patients with severe anatomic or embryologic genitourinary defects such as bladder exstrophy, epispadias, and myelomeningocele. The Young-Dees-Leadbetter operation has been used for many years with variable success rates.[31] The Tanagho procedure has not been widely used but incorporates an anterior bladder flap that is reconstructed to serve as a proximal urethral sphincter with a reported success rate as high as 80%.[31] A reimplantation of the urethra underneath the mucosa and in front of the bladder muscular mass described by Kropp results in a urethra that is as effective in opposition to detrusor expulsive forces as abdominal expulsive forces is.[31] The procedure is effective in inducing continence, but it must be combined with augmentation cystoplasty to avoid the changes in compliance that invariably accompany elevated urethral resistance in patients with neurogenic vesical dysfunction.

Artificial Urinary Sphincters

Artificial urinary sphincters provide urethral compression that is variable and allows patients to reduce urethral pressure during voiding. Patients who are candidates for artificial sphincter implantation should have good bladder capacity and compliance and no uninhibited bladder contractility. In males the most effective position for placement of the artificial sphincter is the bladder neck. Where that is impossible (after radical prostatectomy or transurethral prostatectomy resection) bulbous urethral placement is necessary. An extra-abdominal position of the artificial sphincter, about the bulbous urethra, reduces its mechanical efficiency. Coapted pressures must be relatively high in this area because all changes in abdominal pressure are expulsive forces. That is not the case when the artificial sphincter is placed about the bladder neck, within the abdominal cavity. Total dryness with an artificial urinary sphincter placed in the bulbous urethra may not be achievable in some 20% to as many as 40%.

Use of artificial sphincters in females had been limited because of the perceived high complication rate particularly after multiple previous operative procedures.[32] Despite reports of erosion and difficulty with artificial sphincter function some workers have reported excellent results in women.[33] Artificial sphincters raise abdominal leak point pressures very substantially when placed about the intrinsic part of the sphincter, but because they are also effective against detrusor pressure when the cuff is inflated, they may result in the development of poor compliance, particularly in neurogenic bladders.[37]

Pubovaginal Slings

Many variations of the pubovaginal sling technique have been reported. Muscle, autogenous fascia, rectus fascia, bladder, and fascia lata, as well as synthetic materials and the vaginal wall, have been used to provide support of the urethra. Slings support the urethrovesical junction, and they seem to be somewhat dynamic in that they result in high local closing pressure at the moment of an increase in intra-abdominal pressure. A sling is, however, a vector force, and it will not close effectively a very patulous urethra. Most reported series where autogenous fascia is used, including rectus fascia or fascia lata, are associated with a cure rate of 82% to 95%.[28,34,35] Spontaneous erosion has not been a problem with autogenous fascia, though prolonged urinary retention has. Synthetic materials used as slings carry a much higher risk of infection and erosion, but similar efficacy has been achieved.[38,39] Pubovaginal slings raise local urethral closing pressure by 2 to 10 cm H_2O. In most individuals detrusor pressures required to induce voiding are not inordinately elevated after sling procedures. There has been no recorded patient with a pubovaginal sling who developed poor compliance resulting in upper tract changes.[11]

Injectable Bulking Agents

Injectable agents such as polytetrafluoroethylene, collagen, and autologous fat have been used to improve intrinsic sphincteric function. These coapt the proximal urethra as close as possible to the bladder outlet. Injectable agents can improve urethral sphincter efficiency dramatically, raising the abdominal leak point pressure substantially, without inducing any change in urethral closing pressure profile values, or the detrusor pressure required to cause leakage (or induce voiding).[40,41] In women the indication for injectable agents is persistent intrinsic sphincter deficiency without urethral hypermobility associated with leak point pressures less than 65 cm H_2O. Typically these patients are older and are not good candidates for open operative procedures. In men the indication is intrinsic sphincter deficiency persistent for more than 1 year. The primary advantage of injectable agents is the ability to inject under local anesthesia with minimal associated side effects and complications.

Polytetrafluoroethylene (Polytef, Teflon, Urethrin). Injection of polytetrafluoroethylene (PTFE) micropolymer particles into the proximal portion of the urethra stimulates the ingrowth of fibroblasts, which help bind the particles in the tissue and produce urethral coaptation as well. PTFE is not approved in the United States because of concerns about local and distal migration of PTFE (nodes, lungs, and brain).[42] PTFE has been used over the last 20 years outside the United States, and no significant clinical complication secondary to distal migration has been reported.[43]

Collagen (Contigen). Contigen (C.R. Bard, Inc., Atlanta, Ga.) is a purified bovine dermal collagen that is cross-linked with glutaraldehyde. Cross-linking the collagen has been shown to decrease the antigenicity and render it nearly resistant to fibroblast-secreted collagenases. Pathologic studies show minimal foreign-body reaction and gradual replacement of bovine collagen with native collagen over 9 to 19 months.[44] The University of Michigan experience with collagen and female intrinsic sphincter deficiency shows an 83% cured, greatly improved, or improved rate at a mean 46-month follow-up study. Seventeen out of 42 women (40%) were cured with a mean 2.3 injections (total mean collagen used, 15 ml) and experienced a mean increase in abdominal LPP of 68.0 cm H_2O. Collagen injections for intrinsic sphincter deficiency are safe and effective and appear durable.

Autologous Fat. Before FDA approval of Contigen, periurethral fat injections were used to treat intrinsic sphincter deficiency. Autologous fat is harvested from the abdominal wall by liposuction and then injected periurethrally under local anesthesia. Blaivas reported a 70% cured or improved status at 12 months mean follow-up period in 42 women with intrinsic sphincter deficiency.[45] Autologous fat injections appear to be cost effective and initial reports are promising therapy, but long-term results are lacking.

The various procedures described attest to the lack of an ideal method to treat intrinsic sphincter deficiency that should be simple, reliable, and incur minimal morbidity. All procedures effectively increase intrinsic sphincter efficiency as assessed by abdominal LPP, yet some therapies also increase urethral closing pressure. Any increase in urethral closure pressure can raise mean bladder pressure. Procedures that increase urethral closing pressures such that intrinsic bladder pressure is higher at the time of leakage are likely to gradually induce a change in bladder compliance and potentially risk upper tract function.[37,46] Of all the treatments of intrinsic sphincter deficiency, the injectable bulking agents induce the least change in urethral closing pressure, whereas artificial sphincters induce the greatest change.

References

1. McGuire EM, Lytton B, Pepe V, et al: Stress urinary incontinence, *Obstet Gynecol* 47:255, 1976.
2. Blaivas JG, Salinas J: Type III stress urinary incontinence: the importance of proper diagnosis and treatment, *Surg Forum* 35:472, 1984.
3. McGuire EJ, Fitzpatrick CC, Wan J, et al: Clinical assessment of urethral sphincter function, *J Urol* 150:1452-1454, 1993.
4. McGuire EJ: Adult female urology. In Yalla SV, McGuire EJ, Elbadawi A, Blaivas JG, editors: *Neurology and urodynamics: principles and practice,* New York, 1988, Macmillan.
5. McGuire EJ: Urodynamic findings in patients after failure of stress incontinence operations. In Zinner NR, Sterling AM, editors: *Female incontinence,* New York, 1980, Liss.
6. Jarvis GJ: Stress incontinence. In Mundy DR, Stephenson TP, Wein AJ, editors: *Urodynamics: principles, practice and application,* Edinburgh, 1994, Churchill Livingstone.
7. Bhatia NN, Bergman A, Karram MM: Effects of estrogen on urethral function in women with urinary incontinence, *Am J Obstet Gynecol* 160:176, 1989
8. McGuire EJ, Woodside JR, Borden TA, et al: Prognostic value of urodynamic testing in myelodysplatic patients, *J Urol* 126:205, 1981.
9. McGuire EJ: Combined radiographic and manometric assessment of urethral sphincter function, *J Urol* 118:632, 1977.
10. McGuire EJ, Noll F, Maynard F: A pressure management system for the neurogenic bladder after spinal cord injury, *Neurourol Urodyn* 10:223-230, 1991.

11. McGuire EJ: Active and passive factors in urethral continence function, *Int Urogynecol J* 3:54-60, 1992.
12. Awad SA, Downie JW: Relative contributions of smooth and striated muscles to the canine urethral pressure profile, *Br J Urol* 48:347, 1976.
13. Woodside JR, McGuire EJ: Urethral hypotonicity after suprasacral spinal cord injury, *J Urol* 121:783, 1979.
14. Bannister R, Oppenheimer DR: Degenerative diseases of the nervous system associated with autonomic failure, *Brain* 95:457, 1972.
15. Salinas JM, Berger Y, De La Roche RE, Blaivas JG: Urologic evaluation in the Shy-Drager syndrome, *J Urol* 135:741, 1986.
16. McGuire EJ: Urodynamic evaluation after abdominal perineal resection and lumbar intervertebral disc herniation, *Urology* 6:63, 1975.
17. McGuire EJ, Wagner F Jr: The effects of sacral denervation on bladder and urethral function, *Surg Gynecol Obstet* 144:343-346, 1977.
18. Wang SC, McGuire EJ, Bloom DA: A bladder pressure management system for myelodysplasia: clinical outcome, *J Urol* 140:1499-1502, 1988.
19. McGuire EJ, Lytton B, Kohorn EI, Pepe V: The value of urodynamic testing in stress urinary incontinence, *J Urol* 124:256, 1980.
20. Nanninga JE, O'Connor VJ Jr.: Suprapubic and retropubic prostatectomy. In Walsh PC, Gittes RF, Perlmutter AD, Stamey TA, editors: *Campbell's urology,* ed 5, Philadelphia, 1986, Saunders.
21. Rudy DC, Woodside JR, Crawford ED: Urodynamic evaluation of incontinence in patients undergoing modified Campbell radical retropubic prostatectomy: a prospective study, *J Urol* 132:708, 1984.
22. Walsh PC, Jewett AJ: Radical surgery for prostatic cancer, *Cancer* 45:1906, 1980.
23. Leach GE, Yun SK: Post-prostatectomy incontinence: part I. The urodynamic findings in 107 men, *Neurourol Urodyn* 11:91, 1992.
24. Gudziak MR: Assessment of urethral sphincter function after prostatectomy. In McGuire EJ, Bloom D, Catalona W, Lipshultz L, editors: *Advances in urology,* St Louis, 1995, Mosby.
25. McGuire EJ: Urethral dysfunction. In Kursh ED, McGuire EJ, editors: *Female urology,* Philadelphia, 1994, Lippincott.
26. McGuire EJ, Savastano JA: Comparative urologic outcome in females with spinal cord injury, *J Urol* 135:730-731, 1986.
27. McGuire EJ, Gardy M, Elkins T, DeLancey JO: The treatment of incontinence with pelvic prolapse, *Urol Clin North Am* 18(2):349-353, 1991.
28. McGuire EJ, Wang CC, Usitalo H, Savastano J: Modified pubovaginal sling in female children with myelodysplasia, *J Urol* 135:94-96, 1986.
29. Leadbetter GW Jr: Surgical reconstruction for complete urinary incontinence: a 10- to 22-year followup, *J Urol* 133:205, 1985.
30. Tanagho EA: Bladder neck reconstruction for total urinary incontinence: ten years of experience, *J Urol* 321:1215, 1981.
31. Kropp KA: Urethral lengthening and reimplantation. In Lytton B, Catalona W, Lipshultz L, McGuire EJ, editors: *Advances in urology,* St Louis, 1989, Mosby.
32. Light JK, Scott FB: Management of urinary incontinence in women with the artificial urinary sphincter, *J Urol* 134:476, 1985.
33. Appell RA: Techniques and results in the implantation of artificial urinary sphincter in women with type III stress incontinence by a vaginal approach, *Neurourol Urodyn* 7:613, 1988.
34. McGuire EJ, Bennett CJ, Konnak JA, et al: Experience with pubovaginal slings for urinary incontinence at University of Michigan, *J Urol* 138:525, 1987.
35. Raz S, Siegel AL, Short JL, et al: Vaginal wall sling, *J Urol* 141:43, 1989.
36. Burgio KL, Stutzman RE, Engel BT: Behavioral training for post-prostatectomy urinary incontinence, *J Urol* 141:303, 1989.
37. Connor JP, Perlmutter AD, Kroovand LR: Long term effects of artificial urinary sphincter on bladder function and upper urinary tract morphology, *J Urol* 153(suppl):Abst. 200, 1995.
38. Stanton SL, Brindley GS, Holmes DM: Silastic sling for urethral sphincter incompetence in women, *Br J Obstet Gynaecol* 92:747, 1985.
39. Horbach NS, Blanco JS, Ostergard DR, et al: A pubourethral sling procedure with Polytetrafluoroethylene for the treatment of genuine stress incontinence in patients with low urethral closure pressure, *Obstet Gynecol* 71:648, 1988.
40. Appell RA: Injectables for urethral incompetence, *World J Urol* 8:208, 1990.
41. Wan J, McGuire EJ, Bloom DA, Ritchey ML: The treatment of urinary incontinence in children using glutaraldehyde cross-linked collagen, *J Urol* 148:127-130, 1992.
42. Malizia AA, Reiman HM, Meyers RP, et al: Migration and granulomatous reaction after periurethral injection of polytef (Teflon), *JAMA* 251:3277, 1984.
43. Leonard MP, Canning DA, Epstein JI, et al: Local tissue reaction to the subureteric injection of glutaraldehyde cross-linked bovine collagen in humans, *J Urol* 143:1209, 1990.
44. Kennelly MJ, et al: Long-term results of endoscopic injection of GAX-collagen for the treatment of intrinsic sphincter deficiency, 73rd Annual South Central Section of the American Urological Association, Vancouver, B.C., abstract, August 1994.
45. Blaivis JG, et al: Periurethral fat injection for sphincteric incontinence in women, AUA 89th annual meeting, San Francisco, Calif., Abstract 755, May 1994; Baltimore, American Urological Association.
46. Ghoniem EM, Bloom DA, McGuire EJ, Stewart KL: Bladder compliance in meningomyelocelic children, *J Urol* 141:1404, 1989.

Chapter 29 Raz Suspension Procedure

Pat D. O'Donnell

The Raz urethral suspension procedure is one of the most commonly used surgical procedures for treatment of stress urinary incontinence in women. The Raz procedure[1] originated from the modified Pereyra[2] urethral suspension procedure and involves transvaginal lateral dissection of urethral support, lateral placement of permanent sutures in the urethropelvic ligament as well as endopelvic fascia and vaginal wall, and direct finger guidance of the ligature carrier through the prevesical space. The Raz procedure has a short operative time, rapid recovery with a short hospital stay, and excellent continence results with minimal complications.

Vaginal needle suspension procedures that do not involve dissection of the lateral urethral attachments do not allow suture placement at the bladder neck under direct vision. This appears clinically to be a significant advantage of the Raz procedure compared with the nondissected needle suspension procedures. The Raz procedure along with the modified Pereyra procedure has become the preferred urethral suspension procedure among many surgeons for uncomplicated patients who require surgery for the management of stress incontinence.[3] However, one of the problems of the Raz procedure has been differences in success among clinicians who routinely perform the operation.[4-9] Like many operative procedures that have differences in success rates reported, the surgical outcome is often dependent on the selection of patients for the procedure, the definition of successful outcome, and differences in techniques among surgeons.

Clinical Perspective

Over the past decade, many surgeons who routinely perform incontinence procedures have acquired extensive experience with the Raz procedure, which has resulted in better clinical outcomes. Also, many physicians who have completed residency training programs in the recent past have had significant experience with the modified Pereyra procedure and the Raz procedure, and that has made this approach to the surgical management of stress incontinence a preferred clinical treatment for even more surgeons than in the past. As with any urethral suspension procedure for treatment of stress urinary incontinence, the success of the Raz procedure over the past decade has been improved by changes in patient selection based on routine assessment of intrinsic function of the urethra.

One of the most important concepts that has evolved over the past decade in patient selection for urethral suspension procedures in the treatment of stress urinary incontinence has been the preoperative identification of those patients who have intrinsic sphincter deficiency (ISD). This group of patients, originally classified by McGuire as having type III stress incontinence, have a high failure rate after any type of urethral suspension procedure.[10]

After the initial description of the Raz procedure, enthusiasm for the procedure led many clinicians to utilize the operative technique for almost all patients having surgery for urinary incontinence. Before the concept of ISD became well recognized, failures of urethral suspension procedures in patients having stress urinary incontinence were more common. Postoperative evaluation of patients who failed the Raz procedure often showed surgical correction of the anatomic problem, whereas clinically such patients had persistent stress urinary incontinence. These experiences among many clinicians resulted in wide acceptance of the concept of ISD and the opinion that patients who have ISD should be managed with a urethral sling procedure rather than a Raz urethral suspension procedure.

With the use of the leak point pressure (LPP) measurement of intrinsic urethral function, it has been possible to identify those patients with intrinsic sphincter deficiency preoperatively. This has resulted in most physicians modifying their approach to the surgical management of stress urinary incontinence by utilizing a pubovaginal sling procedure for management of those patients with significant ISD. Many surgeons continue to use a Raz urethral suspension procedure for those patients who have stress incontinence without ISD because of the short operating time, low morbidity, short hospitalization, and clinical success of the procedure. The preoperative identification of patients who have ISD and the utilization of a urethral sling procedure for the surgical management of those patients has significantly improved the surgical results of the Raz urethral suspension procedure by selecting patients for the operation who have a favorable outcome. This preoperative selection has eliminated many of the patients who were at risk for failure of the Raz suspension procedure.[11]

Another difficult problem in the selection of patients for a Raz urethral suspension procedure has been associated urge incontinence. In the early years of surgery for stress incontinence in women, many clinicians believed that coexisting urge urinary incontinence was a contraindication to performing a urethral suspension procedure. Subsequently it was found by McGuire that correction of stress urinary incontinence resulted in resolution of urge urinary incontinence in most patients.[12] The surgical management of patients who have a component of urge urinary incontinence has allowed surgery to be successful for many patients who would otherwise not have been considered candidates for surgery. However, there are some patients who have urge incontinence preoperatively in whom the urge component does not resolve postoperatively after a Raz procedure.[7] In addition, there are occasional patients who develop urge urinary incontinence after a Raz urethral suspension procedure who did not have it preoperatively. Therefore persistent urge incontinence after a Raz urethral suspension procedure in patients with preexisting urge incontinence has resulted in a lower success rate of the operation compared with results in patients who do not have preexisting urge incontinence.

As with any operative procedure, there are differences in operative technique among surgeons. The modified Pereyra procedure and the Raz procedure have been done for many years, and the operative techniques have been well described. Detailed technical descriptions with illustrations have appeared in numerous textbooks on incontinence surgery.[2,13-17] Although the Raz procedure is usually not difficult to perform in the uncomplicated patient, many of the technical aspects of the surgical procedure are sometimes difficult to conceptualize. Therefore, among surgeons who perform the Raz procedure routinely, there is considerable variation in the specific techniques of performing the procedure. Most of these differences among surgeons are minor personal variations that do not significantly influence the outcome of the procedure. However, there are some aspects of the operative techniques that can alter the outcome of the procedure. Therefore differences among surgeons may account for some of the variation that is seen in the results of the Raz suspension procedure.

Operative Technique

Many physicians currently completing residency programs have significant experience in performing the Raz procedure. However, many common technical difficulties are encountered by physicians learning the Raz procedure, and they are described in this section. The operative technique involved in performing the Raz procedure requires confidence and experience in vaginal surgery. Concepts of vaginal surgery do not seem to naturally follow surgical experience in other areas. Therefore, without some previous experience in vaginal surgery, the pelvic anatomy and the surgical approach to the Raz procedure can sometimes be confusing. The three-dimensional concepts of vaginal surgery are not so easy to understand as surgery in other areas. For this reason, it is more difficult for the surgeon to apply the technical concepts from descriptions of the Raz procedure in textbooks as well as those demonstrated in detailed technical illustrations to the actual performance of the procedure.

The operative technique for the Raz procedure actually begins with patient selection. Usually a Raz procedure is easier to perform in a patient who has not had previous surgery for urinary incontinence. Also, a Raz urethral suspension procedure is unlikely to be successful in a patient who has intrinsic sphincter deficiency. In addition, a patient with normal bladder function usually will have a much better surgical result than a patient with abnormal bladder function. If the history, the physical exam, the radiographic exam, the endoscopic exam, and the urodynamic studies indicate uncomplicated type II genuine stress incontinence, the patient is likely to have an excellent continence outcome with minimal morbidity after a Raz urethral suspension procedure.

As with any urethral suspension procedure, it is not only important to be precise in the operative technique, but also important to avoid anything technically that could result in a complication or a poor outcome. Sometimes very simple things can compromise the outcome of an operative procedure. With the Raz procedure, for example, on the day of surgery it is an important consideration to recheck the urine to be sure that it is free of infection. The interval between preoperative testing and surgery can occasionally be long enough that a urinary tract infection can develop. Although that is an unlikely occurrence, the presence of a urinary tract infection at the time of surgery can significantly alter the postoperative course and the success of the operation.

When the Raz procedure is performed, the patient is placed in the lithotomy position. It is very important to carefully position the patient, since there are occasional patients who will experience troublesome postoperative paresthesias in one or both lower extremities. It may be possible that the use of specialized stirrups can decrease the risk of this complication. Also, a shorter operating time appears to decrease the risk of postoperative paresthesias. In the event that a postoperative paresthesia does occur, the patient and physician can be reasonably sure it will spontaneously resolve within approximately 6 weeks. The potential for this problem to have permanent residual effects after vaginal procedures is mentioned here to emphasize the importance of positioning the patient for surgery.

The vaginal incision shown in Fig. 29-1 is a simple straight incision along the anterior crease in the vaginal epithelium that is present laterally on either side of the vagina. Although an inverted U-shaped incision described by Raz can be used also, the objective of the incision is to provide access to the lateral attachments of the urethra, and the exact location of the incision does not appear to be critical. For example, a midline incision is often used when a cystocele repair also is performed. The next step is to separate the vaginal wall and expose the urethropelvic ligament (Fig. 29-2). Once the urethropelvic ligament has been identified, a critical step in the Raz procedure is to perforate the urethropelvic ligament at exactly the correct location near its attachment to the pubis. The separation of the urethropelvic ligament from the pubic bone should not be done with blunt finger dissection. The separation needs to be done with the dissecting scissors by perforation of the urethropelvic ligament at precisely the right place, since the location of the perforation of the urethropelvic ligament determines the dissection plane of the lateral urethral attachments.

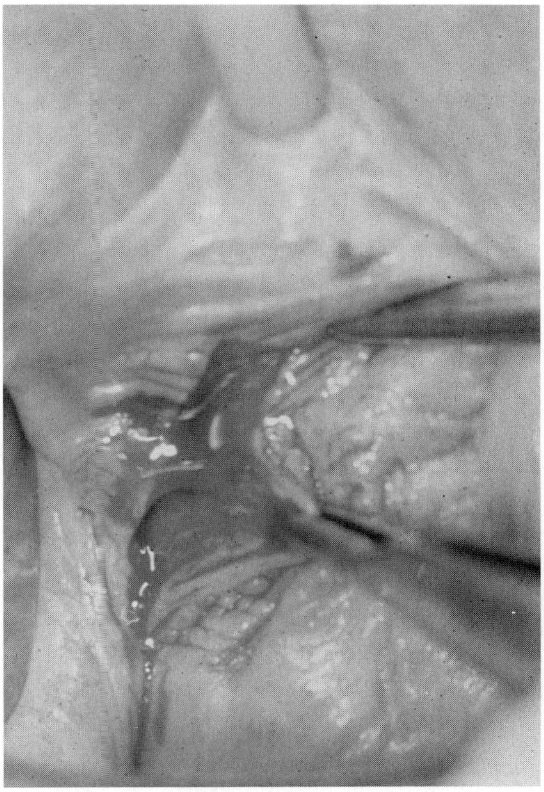

FIG. 29-1 *The incision in the vaginal epithelium can be a simple straight incision along the lateral anterior surface on each side of the vagina. A midline incision can be used when a cystocele repair is being done along with the Raz procedure. The Foley catheter in the urethra can be seen at top, and the indentation in the vaginal wall of the pubococcygeus muscle can be seen adjacent to the incision in the vaginal epithelium.*

One of the common problems encountered by surgeons without experience in performing the Raz urethral suspension procedure involves the pubococcygeus muscle. The pubococcygeus muscle attaches to the pubic bone lateral to the urethra. The dissection of the urethropelvic ligament must be done medially to the attachment of the pubococcygeus muscle, otherwise the pubococcygeus muscle will be incorporated into the suspension. However, it is extremely important that the urethropelvic ligament is separated from its attachments as laterally as possible away from the urethra to provide tissue for anchoring the suspension sutures. The anchoring suture through the endopelvic fascia, the urethral pelvic ligament, and the vaginal wall needs to be as far laterally as possible away from the urethra to avoid any alteration in urethral function. Therefore the separation of the urethropelvic ligament from its lateral attachments is a critical step because it determines the tissue available for suture placement and the subsequent outcome of the procedure.

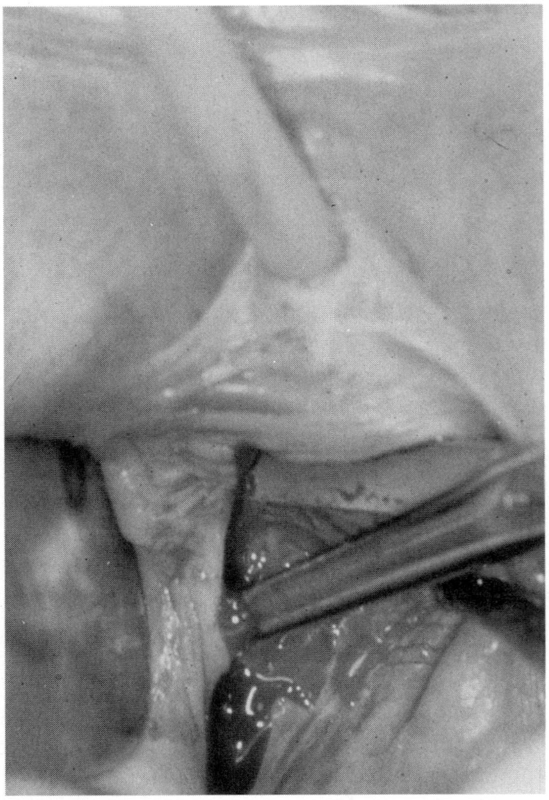

FIG. 29-2 *The dissecting scissors can be used to separate the vaginal epithelium off the vaginal wall laterally and to separate the vaginal wall away from the urethropelvic ligament.*

If the perforation through the urethropelvic ligament is too far laterally, the pubococcygeus muscle will be incorporated into the suspension. That means that when the suspension sutures are tied the entire levator complex will be pulled anteriorly and minimal anatomic change will occur at the bladder neck. If the urethropelvic ligament perforation is performed too far medially, there will not be enough tissue to anchor the suspension sutures. That means that the suspension sutures are more likely to pull out. Also, the suspension sutures are more likely to be placed too close to the urethra resulting in postoperative urethral obstruction or postoperative irritative symptoms because of the suture placement altering urethral function.

By placing the index finger in the initial incision through the vaginal epithelium, one can palpate the striated ligamentous attachment of the pubococcygeus muscle to the pubic bone. By sliding the tip of the scissors just under the pubic bone immediately medial to the insertion of the pubococcygeus muscle, one can remain medial to the pubococcygeus muscle and preserve the most lateral attachments of the urethropelvic ligament. Spreading of the tips of the dissecting scissors at this anatomic position will separate the urethropelvic ligament from its most lateral attachments. If striated skeletal muscle is visible anywhere along the medial surface of the incision at any time during the operative procedure, it means that part of the pubococcygeus muscle is present medially and the muscle has been separated.

The location of the pubococcygeus muscle is shown in Fig. 29-3, where it has been dissected from surrounding tissues both medially and laterally. It is apparent in this dissection of the pubococcygeus muscle the amount of space that is lateral to it, and it would not be difficult to extend the vaginal dissection of the Raz procedure lateral to this muscle. In Fig. 29-4 the blunt dissection, which is routinely performed with the index finger, is lateral to the pubococcygeus muscle, and such a position is incorrect. The prevesical space can be entered by perforation of the endopelvic fascia from a position that is too far lateral, which will allow the surgeon to believe that the position is correct. It is extremely important for the blunt dissection that is usually done with the index finger to be medial to the pubococcygeus muscle as shown in Fig. 29-5 while retaining all the connective tissue possible of the endopelvic fascia and urethropelvic ligament on the urethra side of the dissection for anchoring the sutures.

If part of the pubococcygeus muscle is present medially along the urethropelvic ligament, it will be incorporated in the suspension sutures as they are placed in the endopelvic fascia, urethropelvic ligament, and vaginal wall. When this occurs, the upward tension on the sutures pulls anteriorly on the pubococcygeus muscle and impedes the high retropubic fixation of the bladder neck. In addition, it places a significant tension on the pubococcygeus muscle, which may result in an anterior displacement of the perineal body. This can create a ridge in the posterior vagina that subsequently may result in dyspareunia. Also, anterior displacement of the perineal body may be a factor in postoperative pelvic pain problems that occasionally occur after the Raz urethral suspension procedure.

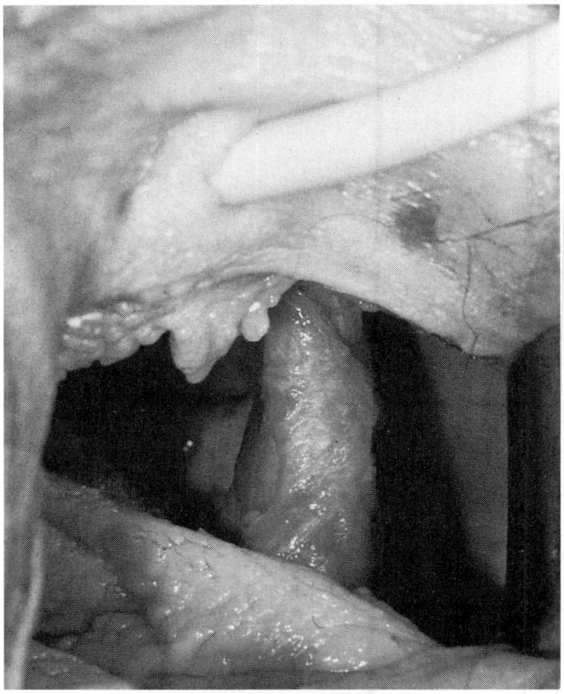

FIG. 29-3 *In this patient having a Raz procedure, the pubococcygeus muscle was dissected away from surrounding vaginal tissue. The location of the muscle relative to the urethra is well demonstrated in this dissection.*

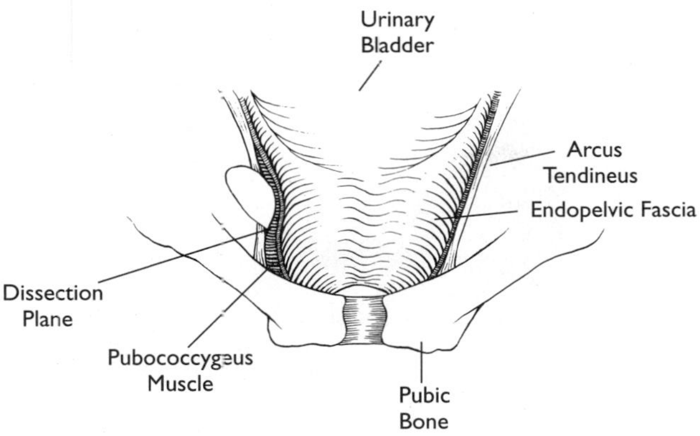

FIG. 29-4 *View from the pelvis of the location of finger dissection that the surgeon must avoid. The pubococcygeus muscle is located medial to the vaginal dissection plane when one needs to be medial to the muscle. Also, in this illustration, the dissection plane is medial to the arcus tendineus when the surgeon needs to be lateral to it.*

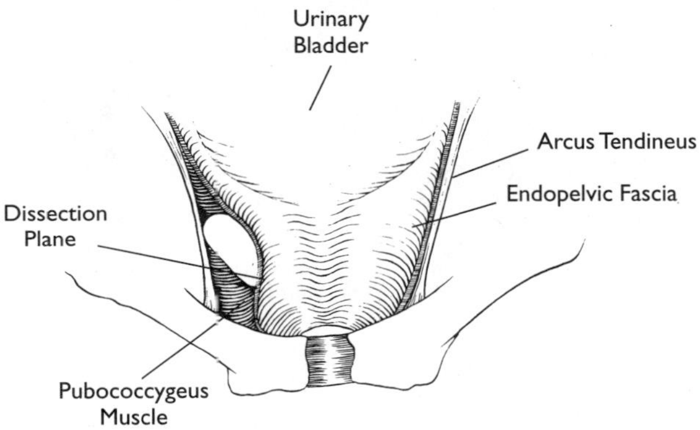

FIG. 29-5 *Dissection plane medial to the pubococcygeus muscle where the surgeon needs to be. The dissection continues laterally to perforate the endopelvic fascia lateral to the arcus tendineus.*

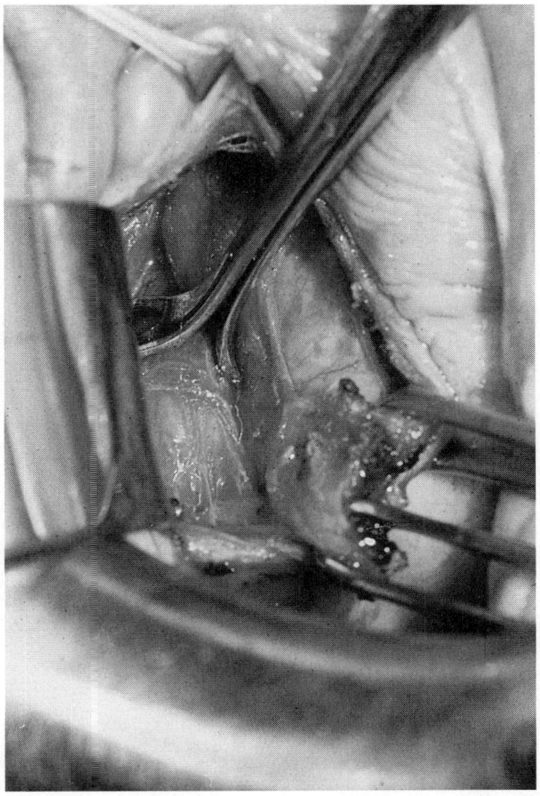

FIG. 29-6 *Same patient as shown in Figs. 29-1 and 29-2. A Babcock clamp is placed around the pubococcygeus muscle to show the lateral location of the muscle in the vaginal dissection. The Allis clamps are placed on the vaginal epithelium. The vaginal wall is located just above the lower Allis clamps with the urethropelvic ligament above it. There is no evidence of striated muscle on the medial side of the incision demonstrating the desired location of the vaginal perforation into the prevesical space relative to the pubococcygeus muscle.*

The key to avoiding problems from the pubococcygeus muscle is the identification of the striated ligamentous attachments to the pubic bone before the urethropelvic ligament is perforated. If the urethropelvic ligament is perforated just beneath the pubic bone immediately medial to the attachment of the pubococcygeus, one can easily dissect the urethral attachments away from the muscle using blunt index finger dissection without difficulty. The pubococcygeus muscle is easily visible along the lateral surface of the vaginal incision and no skeletal muscle should be present medially in the entire vaginal dissection (Fig. 29-6). It is also extremely important to be in the proper dissection plane to avoid bleeding. Almost always, any excessive bleeding that occurs during a Raz procedure is an indication that one is not in the correct dissection plane. Previous surgical procedures may result in relatively intense scarring as well as anatomic planes that are difficult to delineate. If anatomic planes cannot be identified because of scarring from previous surgery, the Raz procedure can sometimes be extremely difficult to perform. Intense scarring from previous surgery can usually be palpated on physical examination preoperatively, and a sling procedure is usually a much better choice in these patients.

Once the vaginal dissection has been completed in the Raz procedure, medial retraction of the vaginal epithelium will show each layer including the perivesical fat, endopelvic fascia, urethropelvic ligament, vaginal wall, and vaginal epithelium, as shown in Fig. 29-7. An Allis clamp can be placed on the endopelvic fascia, the urethropelvic ligament, and the vaginal wall with the vaginal epithelium well outside the clamp (Fig. 29-8). The spiral suture needs to be placed as far laterally to the urethra as possible and still have excellent anchoring in tissue (Figs. 29-9 and 29-10). It is preferable for the spiral suture to begin just proximally to the bladder neck and extend to the proximal or middle portion of the urethra. In this way, the suspension suture will provide a high retropubic fixation of the bladder neck[18] and support to the midurethra without urethral obstruction. Also, lateral placement of the sutures in relationship to the urethra is much less likely to result in either obstruction or irritation to the urethra that might result in postoperative urge urinary incontinence. High retropubic fixation of the bladder neck without

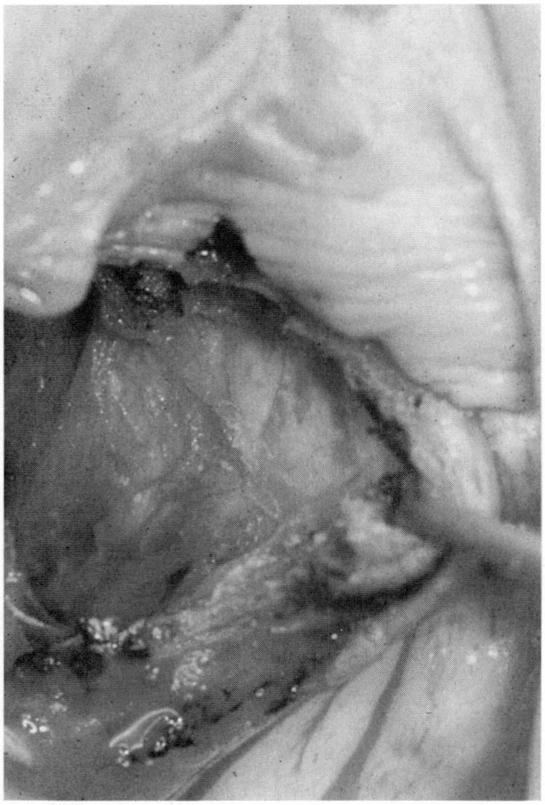

FIG. 29-7 *An Allis clamp is on the vaginal epithelium medially. The urethra is located at top. The endopelvic fascia, urethropelvic ligament, and vaginal wall are often difficult to specifically delineate when the vaginal epithelium is taut, as shown.*

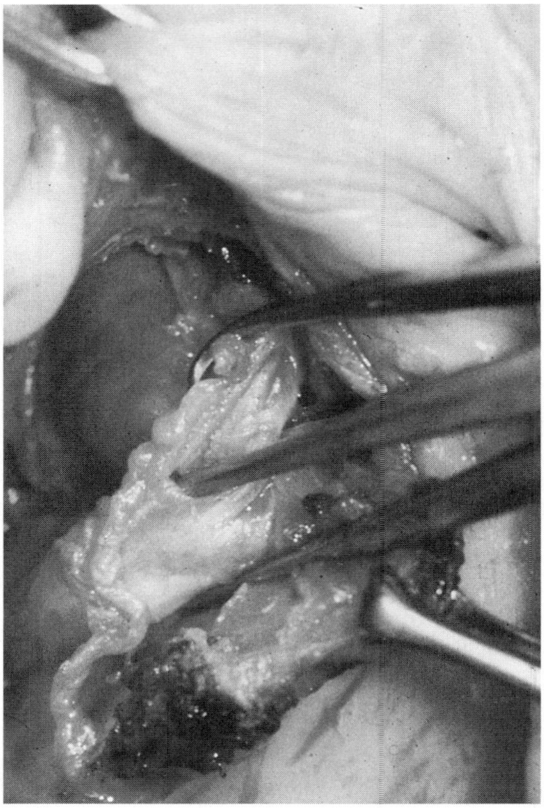

FIG. 29-8 *When the endopelvic fascia, urethropelvic ligament, and vaginal wall are grasped with an Allis clamp, it is easy to see the different layers that were not so apparent in Fig. 29-7 of the same patient. The upper and lower Allis clamps contain the edge of the vaginal epithelium. The bladder can be seen above the two Allis clamps holding the urethropelvic ligament.*

overcorrection of the urethral axis will achieve the anatomic, functional, and continence result that is the clinical objective of the Raz procedure.[19]

After the suspension sutures are placed laterally to the urethra, a small suprapubic incision is made just above the pubic bone. A ligature carrier is passed adjacent to the pubic bone under direct finger guidance into the vaginal area, and the ligatures are transferred to the suprapubic position.

Postoperative pain syndromes in the suprapubic area because of the suspension sutures are a common problem after a Raz urethral suspension procedure. Fortunately, these pain syndromes usually resolve spontaneously within 3 months after surgery. The bone-fixation technique described by Leach[20] significantly reduces this problem (Fig. 29-11). The sutures are actually placed in the rectus fascia as it attaches to the pubic bone. A single-prong ligature carrier is used when the bone-fixation technique is utilized. It is important to pass the ligature carrier immediately adjacent to the pubic bone so that the fixation of the suspension suture occurs at the same point that it exits the rectus fascia as it comes anteriorly from the vagina.

One of the most frequently asked questions about the Raz procedure is how tight should the sutures be tied. Unfortunately this is difficult to determine because it varies among patients. For example, in patients with significant hypermobility and an easy vaginal dissection with well-placed sutures, overcorrection of the urethra can be done with a relatively mild amount of tension on the sutures. On the other hand, patients who have less mobility and stronger attachments of the urethra and bladder will require more tension to achieve high retropubic fixation without overcorrection of the urethral axis. Therefore it becomes a clinical judgment on the part of the surgeon at the time of the operative procedure regarding where the most appropriate anatomic location of the bladder neck should be. High retropubic fixation of the bladder neck without significant overcorrection of the urethral axis occurs with considerable differences among patients in the amount of tension applied to the suspension sutures.

Another problem that may occur in the patient who has significant hypermobility is a loss of normal attachment of the urethra to the pubis. In patients who have anatomic incontinence, there is considerable variation in the attachment of the urethra to the pubic bone. When there is a loss of normal attachment, excessive tension on the suspension sutures will result in the urethral meatus disappearing behind the pubic bone. Should clean intermittent self-catheterization be considered postoperatively, it is extremely difficult for these patients to learn to perform self-

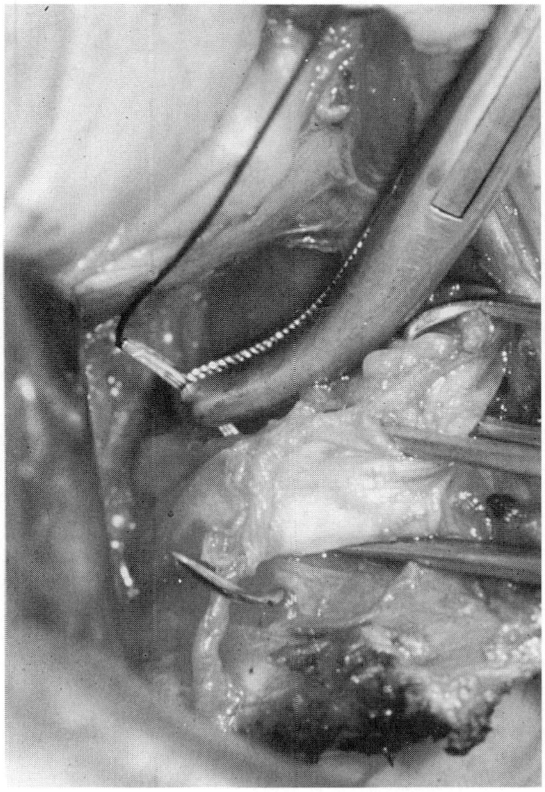

FIG. 29-9 *Adjacent to the tip of the needle holder, the endopelvic fascia is barely visible traversing in front of the needle. The urethropelvic ligament is contained in the Allis clamps. The needle can be seen leaving through the vaginal wall below the urethropelvic ligament. The edge of the vaginal epithelium can be seen below the exit site of the needle. The suture material used is no. 1 Prolene.*

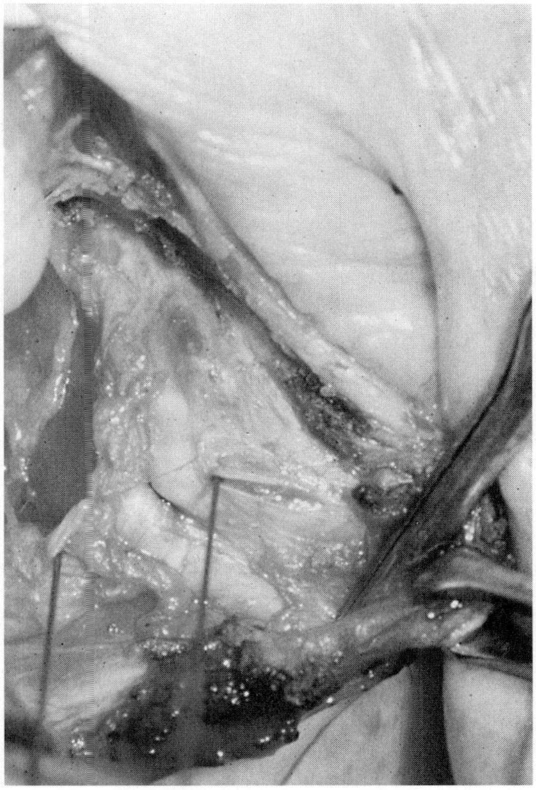

FIG. 29-10 *The spiral suture is shown through the endopelvic fascia with the separated edge seen just above the suture. The strong urethropelvic ligament has a white appearance where the spiral suture is placed. The vaginal wall is not well seen, and the vaginal epithelium is contained in the Allis clamp. The urethral meatus appears just outside the top right.*

catheterization. Again, these patients require clinical judgment on the part of the surgeon to determine the amount of tension to be placed without compromising the long-term anatomic position of the urethra as well as the success of the operation.

Another important postoperative problem to avoid is a suprapubic wound infection. Often, patients having a Raz urethral suspension procedure are obese, and obesity complicates wound management. It is difficult to operate in the vagina and suprapubic area simultaneously without potential contamination of the suprapubic wound. It is extremely important to take extra time to make sure that there are no bleeding sites present in the suprapubic wound. A small suction catheter placed in the wound as shown in Fig. 29-12 is a consideration for eliminating dead space and fluid collection. This drain is easily managed and usually can be removed within 24 hours. If suprapubic wound infections have been a problem for a surgeon who performs transvaginal suspension procedures, use of the suction catheter for the suprapubic incision is a technique to consider.

One of the postoperative problems associated with a Raz suspension procedure is transient urinary retention. Transient urinary retention after a Raz suspension procedure is more common than with suprapubic procedures such as the Burch procedure.[21] Transient urinary retention can be managed with a suprapubic catheter placed at the time of surgery or it can be managed with clean intermittent self-catheterization postoperatively. A urethral Foley catheter usually can be removed within 24 hours, and clean intermittent self-catheterization can be begun without problems in most uncomplicated patients who have a Raz procedure.[22] The advantage of clean intermittent self-catheterization is that it makes patients in control of their own postoperative care. Problems of the suprapubic catheter becoming obstructed at an inconvenient time of day or an inconvenient location is eliminated. Also the patient is able to perform her own residual urine measurement. In this way, the patient becomes catheter free at the earliest possible time. In the event that the patient is unable to void for an extended period of time, clean intermittent self-catheterization is tolerated much better over time than a suprapubic catheter for most patients. The disadvantage of clean intermittent self-catheterization is that it requires approximately 30 minutes of skilled nursing instruction and sometimes considerably longer in difficult patients. Some physicians advocate teaching clean intermittent self-catheterization preoperatively. However, preoperative teaching of clean intermittent self-catheterization may not be necessary, since some patients may not require catheterization postoperatively. Also, the position of the urethra may have changed enough fol-

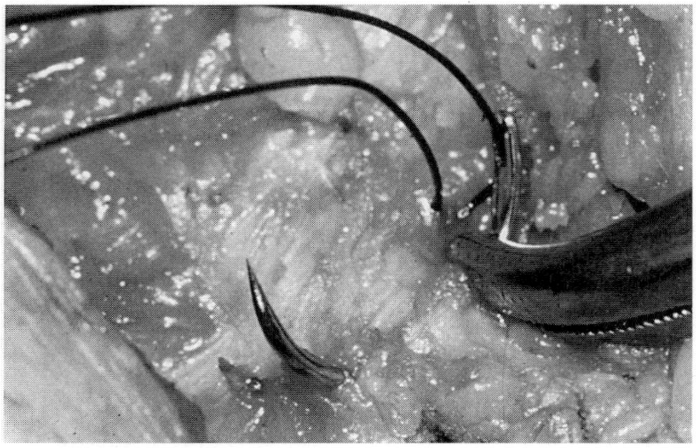

FIG. 29-11 *A hernia repair needle is used to anchor the suture in the connective tissue over the medial edge of the pubic bone. The entrance point of the anchoring suture needs to be at the same point that the suture exits the rectus fascia from the vagina. A small amount of this tough tissue provides excellent anchoring of the suture without danger of nerve entrapment. Anatomic failure of needle suspension procedures are almost always from the vaginal suture placement and rarely from the suprapubic suture placement regardless of the technique used.*

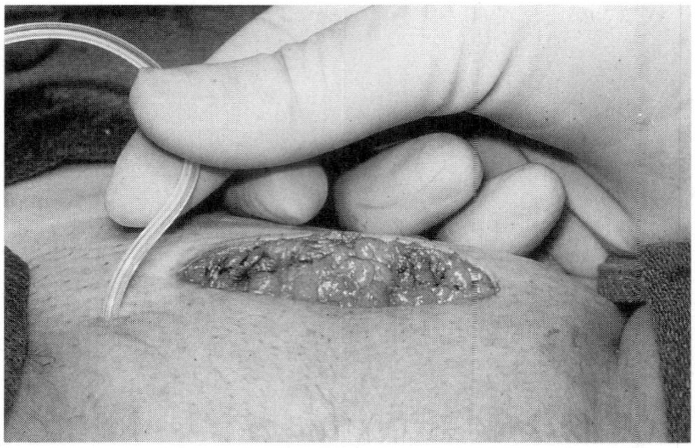

FIG. 29-12 *The use of a very small suction catheter in the suprapubic wound of obese patients is a consideration that may be of some benefit in reducing suprapubic wound problems in these patients. This can be removed in less than 24 hours after surgery in most patients.*

lowing the operative procedure that the patient will require teaching again. If a patient has transient urinary retention postoperatively and clean intermittent self-catheterization is the preferred way the patient can empty the bladder, the motivation of the patient to learn is usually high at that time, and the teaching time is often relatively short.

Uncomplicated patients having a Raz urethral suspension procedure are usually able to leave the hospital within 24 hours after the operation. In uncomplicated patients, the Raz urethral suspension procedure requires approximately 30 minutes to 1 hour to perform. Patients who are obese or have had previous surgery may require a considerably longer operating time and usually are unable to leave the hospital as quickly as the uncomplicated patient. Also, patients who are elderly or have significant comorbid conditions are usually unable to leave the hospital as quickly as the uncomplicated patient. Because the risk of incontinence surgery is higher in older women, the Raz urethral suspension procedure is frequently used in this group because of the low morbidity and the excellent continence results in such a group.[23,24]

SURGICAL RESULTS

Patient selection is a key factor in obtaining excellent continence results with a Raz procedure. Appropriate patient selection requires as complete evaluation as possible for the surgeon to be confident of the type of incontinence that the patient has and the characteristics of the incontinence problem that each particular patient has. In properly selected patients, one can expect excellent continence results in more than 90% of patients having a Raz procedure at 1 year after surgery.[7,23] The long-term results of the procedure are less clear because of differences in patient selection and long-term continence-outcome measures.

Although the Raz suspension procedure has been advocated for some patients who have had previous failed incontinence operations, those patients need to be evaluated very carefully.[25-28] Most importantly, any patient who has had previous incontinence surgery that failed needs to be evaluated for intrinsic sphincter deficiency and coexisting bladder dysfunction. Even in those patients who have anatomic incontinence after previously failed urethral suspension procedures, the technical difficulty of a Raz suspension procedure is unpredictable. Often, a subsequent Raz suspension procedure can be done almost as if no previous surgery had occurred. In other cases, scarring can be extremely intense and significantly complicates the operative procedure. Although most studies indicate that the results in patients with previously failed incontinence procedures are similar to those patients who have not had previous surgery, these studies are primarily from centers where larger numbers of previously operated patients are routinely reoperated.[28] In most patients who have failed previous urethral suspension procedures, a urethral sling procedure is usually a much better choice for surgical management.

SUMMARY

The Raz urethral suspension procedure is an excellent operation for women who have genuine stress incontinence with hypermobility, normal bladder function, no previous incontinence surgery, and no evidence of ISD. In these patients, the operative procedure is short, the hospitalization is short, and the results are excellent. In patients who have more complicated incontinence, the results of the Raz procedure have been reported to be good in these patients also. However, the complexity of the operative procedure can increase significantly in some of these patients who have failed previous incontinence procedures. For this reason, these patients should be evaluated very carefully before a Raz procedure is recommended. Because the incidence of intrinsic sphincter deficiency is high in patients who have failed previous incontinence procedures, the clinician needs to be especially careful to evaluate these patients for the presence of ISD. In previously operated patients who have recurrent incontinence and marginal urethral function by leak point pressure determination, a urethral sling should be considered as the primary operative procedure because of a much better success of sling procedures in patients with ISD compared with urethral suspension procedures.

REFERENCES

1. Raz S: Modified bladder neck suspension for female stress incontinence, *Urology* 17:82-85, 1981.
2. Pereyra AJ, Lebherz TB: The revised Pereyra procedure. In Buchsbaum HJ, Schmidt JD, editors: *Gynecologic and obstetric urology,* Philadelphia, 1978, Saunders.
3. Cornella JL, Ostergard DR: Needle suspension procedures for urinary stress incontinence: a review and historical perspective, *Obstet Gynecol Surv* 45:805-816, 1990.
4. Korman HJ, Sirls LT, Kirkeno AK: Success rate of modified Pereyra bladder neck suspension determined by outcomes analysis, *J Urol* 152:1453-1457, 1994.
5. Bosman G, Vierhout ME, Huikeshoven FJ: A modified Raz bladder neck suspension operation: results of a one to three years follow-up investigation, *Acta Obstet Gynecol Scand* 72:47-49, 1993.
6. Karram MM, Angel O, Koonings P, et al: The modified Pereyra procedure: a clinical and urodynamic review, *Br J Obstet Gynaecol* 99:655-658, 1992.
7. Raz S, Sussman EM, Erickson DB, et al: The Raz bladder neck suspension: results in 206 patients, *J Urol* 148:845-850, 1992.
8. Shah PJ, Holder PD: Comparison of Stamey and Pereyra-Raz bladder neck suspensions, *Br J Urol* 64:481-484, 1989.
9. Bergman A, Ballard CA, Koonings PP: Comparison of three different surgical procedures for genuine stress incontinence: prospective randomized study, *Am J Obstet Gynecol* 160:1102-1106, 1989.
10. McGuire EJ, Lytton B, Kohorn EI, Pepe V: The value of urodynamic testing in stress urinary incontinence, *J Urol* 124:256-258, 1980.
11. Koonings PP, Bergman A, Ballard CA: Low urethral pressure and stress incontinence in women: risk factor for failed retropubic surgical procedure, *Urology* 36:245-248, 1990.
12. McGuire EJ, Lytton B: Pubovaginal sling procedure for stress incontinence, *J Urol* 119:82-84, 1978.
13. Leach GE, O'Donnell P, Raz S: Needle urethral-vesical suspension procedures. In Raz S, editor: *Female urology,* Philadelphia, 1983, Saunders.
14. Raz S, Little NA, Juma S: Female urology. In Walsh PC, Retik AB, Stamey TA, Vaughan ED, editors: *Campbell's urology,* ed 6, Philadelphia, 1992, Saunders.
15. Raz S: Surgical therapy for urinary incontinence. In Raz S, editor: *Atlas of transvaginal surgery,* Philadelphia, 1992, Saunders.
16. Nitti VW, Bregg KJ, Raz S: Surgical management of incontinence in elderly women. In O'Donnell P, editor: *Geriatric urology,* Boston, 1994, Little, Brown.
17. Erickson DE, Sussman ER, Raz S: Endoscopic urethropexy. In Kursh E, McGuire E, editors: *Female urology,* Philadelphia, 1994, Lippincott.
18. Lam TC, Hadley HR: Surgical procedures for uncomplicated ("routine") female stress incontinence, *Urol Clin North Am* 18:327-337, 1991.
19. Leach GE, Yip CM, Donovan BJ: Mechanism of continence after modified Pereyra bladder neck suspension: prospective urodynamic study, *Urology* 29:328-331, 1987.
20. Leach GE: Bone fixation technique for transvaginal needle suspension, *Urology* 31:388, 1988.
21. Bhatia NN, Bergman A, Karram M: Changes in urethral resistance after surgery for stress urinary incontinence, *Urology* 34:200-204, 1989.
22. Forneret E, Leach GE: Cost-effective treatment of female stress urinary incontinence: modified Pereyra bladder neck suspension, *Urology* 25:365-367, 1985.
23. Golomb J, Goldwasser B, Mashiach S: Raz bladder neck suspension in women younger than sixty-five years compared with elderly women: three years' experience, *Urology* 43:40-43, 1994.
24. Nitti VW, Bregg KJ, Sussman EM, Raz S: The Raz bladder neck suspension in patients 65 years old and older, *J Urol* 149:802-807, 1993.
25. Ramon J, Mekras J, Webster GD: Transvaginal needle suspension procedures for recurrent stress incontinence, *Urology* 38:519-522, 1991.
26. Holschneider CH, Solh S, Lebherz TB, Montz FJ: The modified Pereyra procedure in recurrent stress urinary incontinence: a 15-year review, *Obstet Gynecol* 83:573-578, 1994.
27. Wheelahan JB: Long-term results of colposuspension, *Br J Urol* 65:329-332, 1990.
28. Leach GE, Raz S: Modified Pereyra bladder neck suspension after previously failed anti-incontinence surgery: surgical technique and results with long-term follow-up, *Urology* 23:359-362, 1984.

Chapter 30 Nondissected Needle Suspension Procedures

Ross A. Rames

When patients are considering the surgical treatment options for management of stress incontinence, the physician who is counseling the patient about the different surgical procedures needs to present the nondissected needle suspension choices to the patient with as much information about them as possible. For many patients who have urinary incontinence, either concomitant medical problems or patient preference often makes a nondissected needle suspension procedure the most appropriate treatment option. Compared with a suprapubic operation, a major consideration for nondissected needle suspension procedures is interoperative and perioperative morbidity. Bladder neck suspension for stress urinary incontinence was originally accomplished through a large abdominal incision and retropubic dissection. The bladder neck and urethra were then suspended in the manner of Marshall-Marchetti- Krantz,[1] Burch,[2] or the obturator shelf procedure.[3] The desire for less morbidity spurred the development of the needle suspension procedures. Essentially two types are performed today: a Raz "dissected" technique and the "nondissected" bladder neck suspensions. In this chapter we discuss the principles of the nondissected needle suspension (NDNS) procedure, its origins, patient selection, technical aspects, reported efficacy, complications, and new developments.

PRINCIPLES

Nondissected needle suspension procedures differ from retropubic vesicourethropexy procedures in that they utilize small abdominal skin incisions, the rectus fascia remains intact, and there is no retropubic dissection performed before suspension of the bladder neck. They differ from the Raz modification of needle suspension that mobilizes the bladder neck and proximal portion of the urethra retropubicly through a vaginal incision. In NDNS procedures, polypropylene sutures and bolsters in the anterior vaginal wall support the bladder neck to correct genuine stress urinary incontinence (Fig. 30-1). Finally the suspension is anchored to the rectus fascia or alternatively the pubic bone.

ORIGIN

In 1959 Armand Pereyra introduced a technique to restore support and elevation to the bladder neck and urethra without a large abdominal incision or retropubic dissection.[4] A new instrument (Fig. 30-2) was used to pass stainless steel wires from the anterior vaginal wall to the suprapubic area. After tying, the wires would cut through the periurethral tissues leaving a scar to support the repair.

From this procedure the commonly used techniques of needle suspension have evolved. The two most commonly performed NDNS procedures proposed by Stamey and Gittes are described here.

PATIENT SELECTION

Successful correction of stress incontinence depends on patient selection as well as operative technique. Patients with bladder neck hypermobility who leak urine during increases in abdominal pressure have genuine stress urinary incontinence (GSUI) and are appropriate candidates for NDNS procedures.[5]

A complete medical history and physical examination is obtained with prior obstetric history, pelvic surgery, irradiation, or neurologic injury being noted. Pad counts and a voiding diary are used to quantify incontinence. Episodes associated with coughing, straining, and sneezing are consistent with GSUI. Incontinence preceded by the unsuppressible urge to void (urge incontinence) may indicate detrusor instability and is best handled with nonsurgical treatment. Instability coexisting with GSUI usually resolves after suspension of the bladder neck.[5] Severe incontinence (4 to 6 pads per day), advanced age, and failure of previous suspension procedures are associated with intrinsic sphincter dysfunction, and more extensive urodynamic evaluation should be considered.[6] A thorough urodynamic evaluation is essential in this group of patients, especially patients who have failed previous incontinence surgery, to determine if intrinsic sphincter deficiency is present. In those patients who have intrinsic sphincter deficiency to any significant extent, NDNS procedures should not be considered as a treatment option because of the high likelihood of failure.

Pelvic examination plays a critical role in selecting patients for NDNS procedures. After voiding, the patient is placed in the dorsal lithotomy position, and the condition of the external genitalia and vaginal epithelium is noted. Stress maneuvers are repeated with the half-speculum removed and then placed anteriorly to examine for uterine prolapse, rectocele, and enterocele. Finally, a careful bimanual examination of the vaginal and rectal vault is performed.

Intravenous urography or renal ultrasonography are not routinely obtained but are desirable in patients with significant detrusor dysfunction, large cystoceles, or history of previous pelvic surgery. Laboratory evaluation includes serum electrolytes, prothrombin time/partial thromboplastin time (PT/PTT), complete blood cell count (CBC), urinalysis, and urine culture. Patients who have anatomic incontinence with associated cystoceles should have the cystocele repaired at the time the urethral suspension procedure is performed.

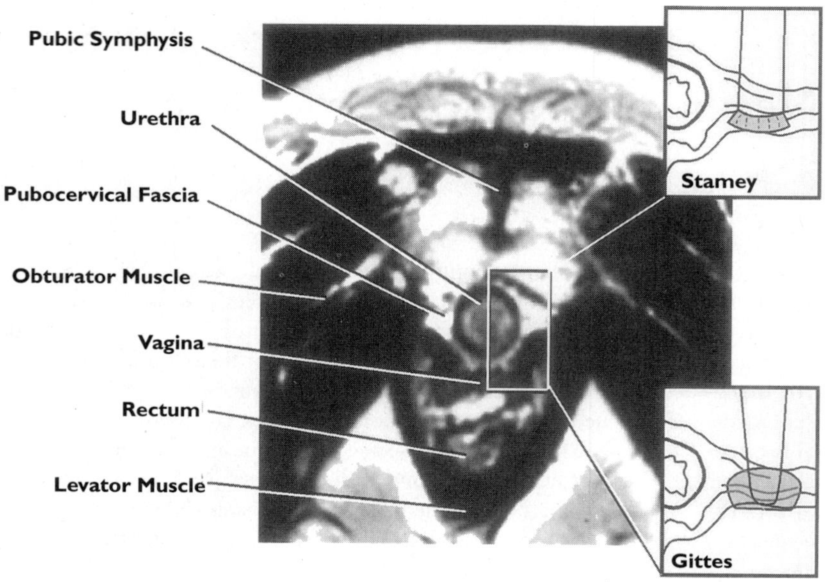

FIG. 30-1 *Magnetic resonance imaging scan of female pelvis at the level of the bladder neck.* Insets *demonstrate placement of bolsters in suspension procedures.*

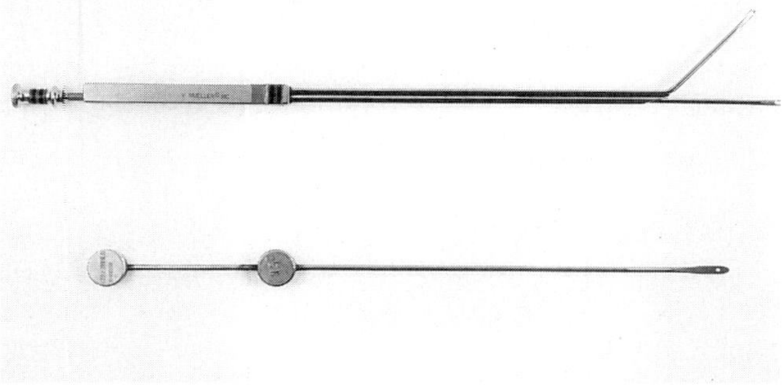

FIG. 30-2 *Pereyra needle with trochar and angled cannula* (top, *V. Mueller, McGaw Park, Ill.). Stamey needle* (bottom, *Greenwald Surgical, Lake Station, Ind.).*

Patient Preparation

Most patients undergo a trial of conservative therapy before considering surgical repair. Medications, Kegel exercises, behavior modification, and bladder training may obviate the need for surgical intervention. Postmenopausal women with vaginal atrophy undergo estrogen replacement for at least 1 month before the surgery.

Nondissected needle suspensions are generally performed with the patient presenting to the ambulatory surgery suite on the day of surgery. A Fleet enema is administered with adequate time allowed for evacuation of the rectum. Prophylactic intravenous cephalosporins and thromboembolic compression hose are routine. General, regional, or local anesthesia is used depending on patient preference and medical condition.

The patient is placed in the dorsal lithotomy position with the thighs relatively low to keep the abdomen flat and the buttocks off the edge of the table enough to accommodate a weighted posterior vaginal retractor. Well-padded Allen stirrups and careful positioning help prevent nerve injury.

The Stamey Procedure

Introduced in 1973,[7] the Stamey procedure employs a knit Dacron buttress to support the periurethral tissues near the vesical neck and intraoperative cystoscopy to assure correct placement of sutures.

Two-centimeter skin incisions are made on either side of the midline at the upper border of the pubic symphysis. Dissection is carried down to the rectus fascia, and the incisions are packed with gauze sponge.

After placement of a weighted posterior vaginal retractor, the anterior vaginal wall is infiltrated with injectable saline just beneath the epithelium to aid in dissection. A transverse superficial incision through the epithelium is made with a no. 15 blade scalpel midway between the bladder neck and the meatus and then extended deeper into the vagina laterally to create a U-shaped flap. The epithelium is dissected from the underlying urethra and periurethral tissues using curved scissors and Bonney forceps. The correct plane is identified when a relatively bloodless, white, shiny layer of fascia is exposed with the scissor tips just below the epithelium. Dissection is carried out until the areas lateral to the bladder neck on each side of the catheter balloon are exposed (Fig. 30-3, *A*). The posterior vaginal retractor is then removed.

A Stamey needle (Fig. 30-2; Greenwald Surgical, Lake Station, Ind.) is introduced into the suprapubic incision, and the rectus fascia is perforated just above the pubic symphysis. Straight Stamey needles suffice; however, I prefer needles with 15-or 30-degree angles at the tip. The top of the pubic bone is gently probed with the needle until the space of Retzius is entered. With the needle tip angled down behind the pubic bone, the needle is advanced parallel to the posterior surface of the pubic symphysis while the surgeon's nondominant index finger is placed beside the bladder neck within the vaginal incision. The urethral catheter is held in the palm with minimal tension, anchoring the balloon at the bladder neck and creating the landmark used to identify the bladder neck. The needle tip is positioned more vertically, palpated on the tip of the index finger, and then guided alongside the vesical neck as it perforates the periurethral tissues and enters the vagina (Fig. 30-3, *B*).

At that point a cystoscope with a 70-degree lens is inserted and directed toward the ipsilateral bladder neck. At the urethrovesical junction, slight medial pressure on the suprapubic end of the Stamey needle should indent the ipsilateral vesical neck. If it fails to do so, the needle may have been placed too far laterally. One should inspect the bladder and urethra to ensure that the needle has not perforated these structures. If the needle passes through the bladder wall but does not perforate the mucosa, an indentation is seen without the needle being pushed medially, or the glare of the needle beneath the mucosa may be seen. If this occurs, the needle is withdrawn into the retropubic space and passed again in a more lateral position.

Once correct needle position has been obtained, a no. 2 polypropylene suture is passed through the eye of the Stamey needle and drawn up into the suprapubic incision. Both ends of the suture are secured with hemostats, and the Stamey needle is reintroduced through the rectus fascia 1 cm lateral to the original insertion site. With digital localization, the needle tip is brought out 1 cm lateral to the first vaginal exit site, and cystoscopy is again performed. The posterior retractor is replaced, and the vaginal end of the suspension suture is passed through a 1 cm long tube of 5 mm knitted Dacron arterial graft and then through the eye of the needle (Fig. 30-3, *C*). The suture and the needle are drawn back up into the suprapubic wound, and the ends are secured with a hemostat. With the Dacron tube grasped lengthwise with an Allis clamp, the ends of the suture in the suprapubic area are elevated as the Dacron buttress is guided into place in the vaginal incision. The procedure is repeated on the contralateral side.

With the posterior weighted retractor removed, the 30-degree lens is used to observe the bladder neck. The mucosa should be circular and slightly agape at rest. Then coapt with gentle upward tension on the suspension sutures. Paradoxical opening may be seen in the presence of periurethral fibrosis from previous vesical neck suspensions, and repositioning of a suspension suture may be required.

After irrigation with an antibiotic solution, the vaginal incision is closed with a running 3-0 chromic suture to assure complete coverage of the bolsters. The suprapubic incisions are irri-

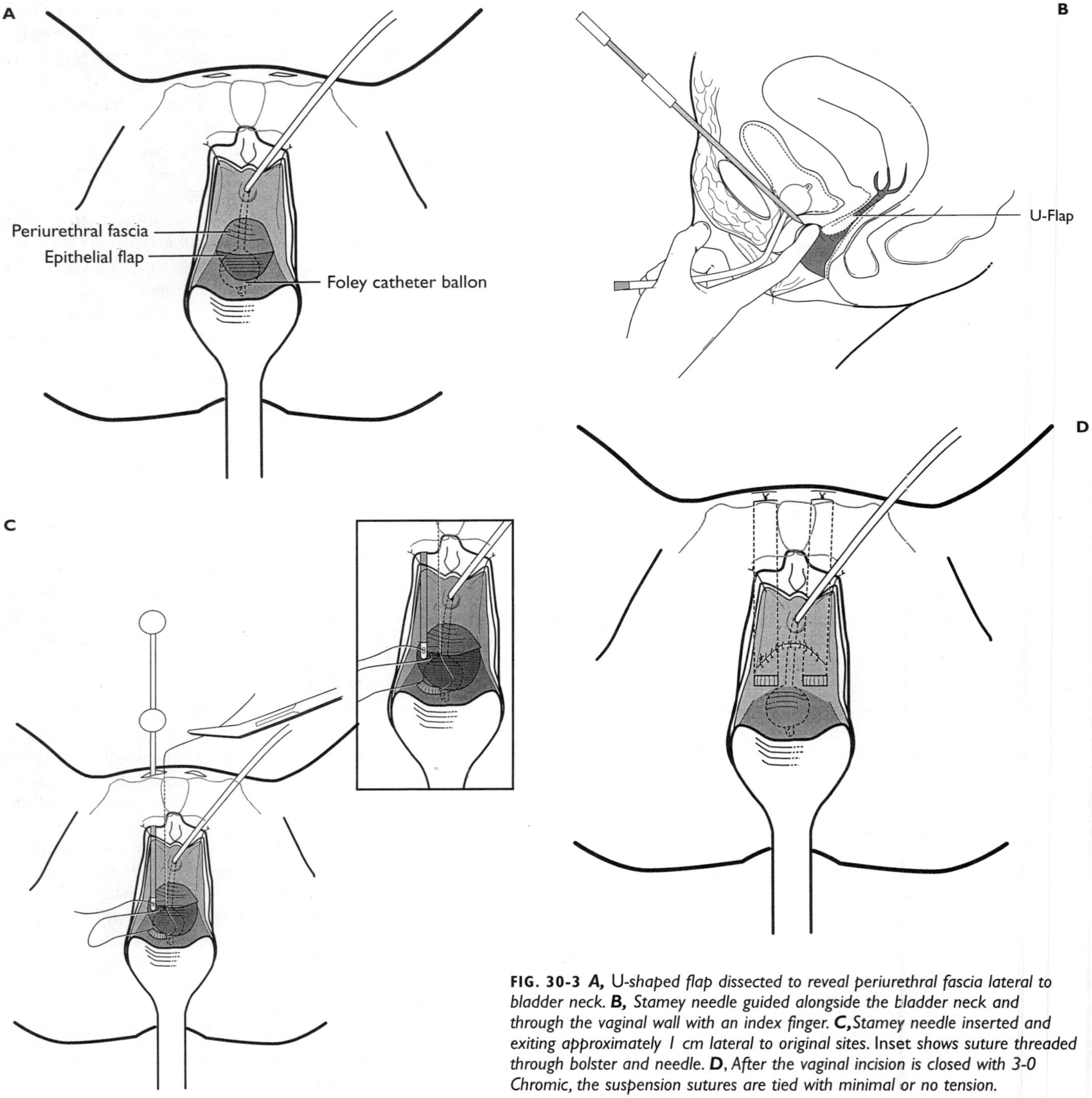

FIG. 30-3 ***A,*** *U-shaped flap dissected to reveal periurethral fascia lateral to bladder neck.* ***B,*** *Stamey needle guided alongside the bladder neck and through the vaginal wall with an index finger.* ***C,*** *Stamey needle inserted and exiting approximately 1 cm lateral to original sites. Inset shows suture threaded through bolster and needle.* ***D,*** *After the vaginal incision is closed with 3-0 Chromic, the suspension sutures are tied with minimal or no tension.*

gated, the bladder is emptied, and the suspending sutures are elevated until taut. Tension is released, and both sutures are tied so that the knots lie flat on the rectus fascia (Fig. 30-3, D). Care is taken to avoid slippage of the knot that would create any additional tension. The skin is closed with 4-0 Vicryl (polyglactin 910) subcuticular sutures, and a dressing is applied.

The Stamey endoscopic suspension procedure is used by many physicians with very good results for treatment of stress urinary incontinence. However, many urologists have discontinued the Stamey procedure for many reasons. The placement of the sutures is determined by the eventual position of the ligature carrier, which is passed without direct vision. This results in a wide variation of location of the suspension sutures relative to the bladder neck. A very small amount of tissue is enclosed in the loop of suture adjacent to the bladder neck, and pullthrough of sutures in vaginal tissue that is compromised to begin with is fairly common. Fortunately the Stamey procedure does not involve extensive dissection and subsequent repairs are relatively easy to perform, since scarring is minimal after that technique. Another problem related to suture placement involves placement of the suture in the midurethra level without suspension at the bladder neck level. A midurethral suture may result in obstruction of the urethra at the midurethral level without correction of stress incontinence. If the suture is placed too close to the urethra, it may contribute to postoperative irritative symptoms of increased frequency and urgency. However, in patients who have genuine stress incontinence with anatomic changes of the bladder and urethra, the Stamey procedure is still a commonly used operative technique for treatment of these patients.

The Gittes Procedure

Originally described in 1987,[8] the Gittes procedure uses no incisions in the anterior vaginal wall and small suprapubic skin punctures. Subsequent modifications include a small suprapubic skin incision to tie the suspension sutures directly onto the rectus fascia. A no. 15 blade scalpel is used to make a small puncture just above the suprapubic fat pad and lateral to the midline. A Stamey needle is passed through the rectus fascia just above the pubic symphysis and advanced immediately behind the pubic bone. With a fingertip in the vagina and the Foley balloon on slight traction, the bladder neck is palpated. Direct the needle just lateral to the bladder neck by manipulating it from above and palpating the tip from below (Fig. 30-4, *A*). When the tip of the Stamey needle is palpable at the anterior vaginal wall, its position is confirmed visually, and it is advanced through the vaginal epithelium and out the introitus. This may be facilitated by intermittent placement of a posterior vaginal retractor. The end of a no. 2 polypropylene suture is passed through the eye of the Stamey needle (Fig. 30-4, *B*), and drawn back up into the suprapubic area, and hemostats are placed on both ends of the suture.

The needle is reinserted into the skin puncture, and the rectus fascia is perforated 1 to 2 cm lateral to the original insertion site. The Stamey needle is advanced behind the pubic bone until the tip is palpable. The second vaginal exit site should be 1.5 to 2 cm distal to the first exit site and should yield elevation of the bladder neck with gentle upward tension. Placement too far distally or laterally results in tethering, and successful bladder neck elevation is unlikely. Medial placement can result in compression or perforation of the bladder or the urethra. Once the needle is advanced out the introitus the posterior retractor is replaced, and the vaginal end of the suture is passed through a Mayo free needle. Several helical full-thickness bites incorporating epithelium and pubocervical fascia are placed between the first and second needle perforation sites (Fig. 30-4, *C*). This has been referred to as the autologous buttress by Gittes and becomes incorporated into the underlying vaginal tissues. The vaginal free end of the suture is then passed through the eye of the Stamey needle and drawn up into the suprapubic area. After the ends of the suture are secured with a hemostat, gentle upward traction should produce elevation of the bladder neck and anterior vaginal wall (Fig. 30-4, *D*). The procedure is repeated on the contralateral side. Cystourethroscopy is then carried out with a 30-degree and 70-degree telescope. Both orifices are observed to confirm efflux of urine. If suture material is visible, that portion is removed and repositioned.

The sutures are tied down into the suprapubic puncture sites under slight tension that is relieved as the suture cuts through the underlying fat. The edges of the skin punctures are grasped with forceps, pulled upward to eliminate inversion and to bury the knots, and a dressing is applied.

Postoperative Care

A vaginal pack is seldom needed but may be placed at surgery if desired. Postoperative discomfort usually responds to oral analgesics.

On the day after surgery the urethral catheter is removed, and the patient is instructed to void without straining. Postvoid residuals are checked, and if they are greater than 50 ml, the patient is discharged with instructions to record voided volumes and postvoid residuals by self-catheterization or suprapubic tube. When residuals are consistently below 50 ml and the patient is voiding comfortably, residuals are no longer measured. A follow-up examination at 1 week includes checking skin and vaginal wounds. Suprapubic tubes are removed if no voiding problems are present. Symptoms of urgency and frequency are sometimes attributable to the suprapubic tube and resolve after removal. If one assumes no new problems, the patient is seen again at 1 month and thereafter on an as-needed basis.

Results

There is a divergence of success rates in the literature, owing in part to what is defined as "success." Although some define success as absolute absence of urine leakage, others include patients who no longer wear pads.

Reported success rates after the Stamey procedure range from 56% to 91% in the first few years after surgery.[7,10] Similar results are found after the Gittes modification, with dryness attained in 87% to 91%.[8,11]

How do NDNS procedures compare to their more invasive retropubic vesicourethropexy counterparts? Side-by-side comparisons are few, but nearly equivalent outcome has been found when the Stamey procedure has been compared to the MMK procedure (61% dry versus 57%).[6] When the Stamey procedure was compared to the vaginal-obturator shelf suspension over a mean follow-up time of 2 years, continence was achieved in 58% versus 70%.[12] At 1 year, one study revealed cure of stress incontinence in 92.5% of patients after the Burch procedure and 84% in those who underwent a Stamey suspension.[13]

Compounding difficulty in assessing various types of repair is the durability of successful outcomes. In one series, 26% of failures occurred after 2 years.[14] Indeed, a recent study with relatively long follow-up (mean 41.5 months) showed that although 68.3% of patients who underwent a Stamey procedure were improved only 39.4% remained dry at all times.[15] Long-term follow-up of 9 to 17 years shows cure rates of 66% to 90% for retropubic suspension procedures.[16,17]

Briefly summarized, all NDNS techniques enjoy good success rates initially. Although retropubic cystourethropexies seem to offer more durable success rates, NDNS procedures offer reduced circumoperative morbidity and the advantages of an outpatient procedure with rapid return to daily activities.

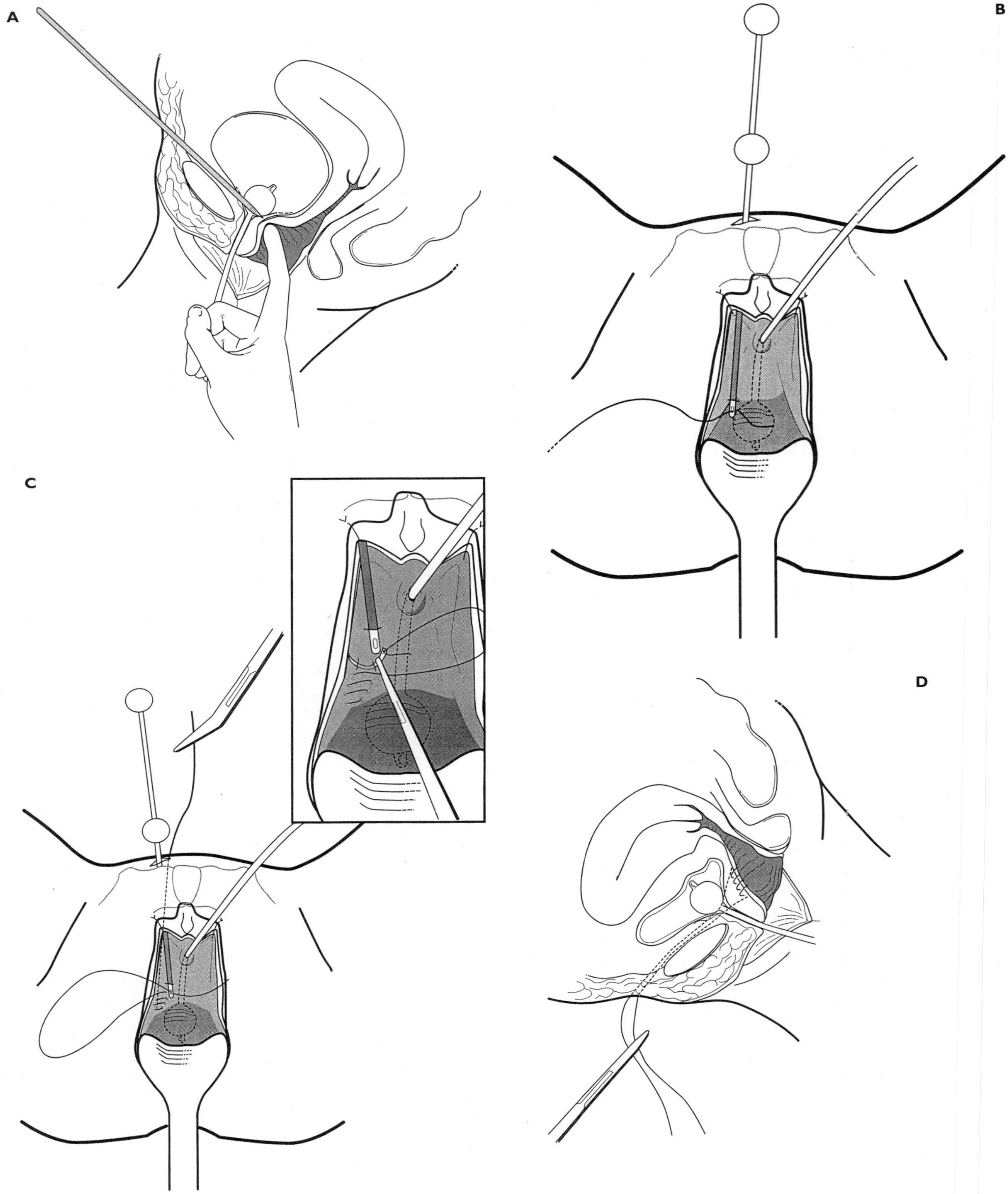

FIG. 30-4 ***A,*** *The needle tip is guided from the retropubic space, alongside the bladder neck, and out the vaginal wall.* ***B,*** *A no. 2 polypropylene suture is threaded through the eye of the Stamey needle and then drawn back through the suprapubic incision.* ***C,*** *After placement of several full-thickness helical sutures between needle exit sites* (inset), *the suture is threaded into the Stamey needle and drawn back through the suprapubic puncture site.* ***D,*** *Gentle upward traction elevates and supports the bladder neck.*

Complications

Complications associated with NDNS include bleeding, infections, failure to attain continence, voiding dysfunction, buttress erosion, and persistent discomfort.

Bleeding is less common than during retropubic procedures, and the need for transfusion is rare.[6,9] Wound infection is unusual, since the use of monofilament nylon suspension sutures began. Most series report rates between none and 2%; however, it has been as high as 12%.[8-10] Management with drainage, removal of suture and Dacron bolstering material, and antibiotics usually results in prompt resolution. Patients often remain continent with one suspension suture left in place. Osteitis pubis is seldom seen but has been reported.[18]

Failure to attain continence may be secondary to (1) misplacement of sutures, (2) suture breakage, (3) erosion of sutures and buttress material through the pubocervical fascia, and (4) the presence of intrinsic sphincter dysfunction or detrusor instability. Failures usually occur early but can occur years after surgery. Misplaced sutures may fail to support the bladder neck or, if they perforate or impinge upon the bladder, result in discomfort, irritable voiding symptoms, infection, and bladder stone formation. Suture breakage is minimized by careful handling of the suture with instruments at the ends only. Delayed erosion occasionally presents with suture and bolster material within the bladder and is usually managed by endoscopic removal.[10,19,20]

Voiding dysfunction in the form of urinary retention develops in approximately one third of patients.[21] As a group, most patients with postoperative voiding problems improve within 1 to 3 months, and very few require long-term intermittent catheterization. Persistent incomplete emptying or irritable voiding symptoms may be attributable to obstruction from "hypersuspension." Urodynamic evaluation of these patients with pressure-flow studies can show high detrusor pressure with a low flow rate, but low flow with low or normal detrusor pressure is seen as well. If retention persists, takedown of the suspension and resuspension without tension usually results in resolution.[22]

Persistent suprapubic discomfort may be attributable to suture placement through mobile muscle and fascia or impingement on the ilioinguinal nerve. If conservative management with antiinflammatories and observation fail, suture removal under local anesthesia should be performed.

New Developments

Nondissected needle suspension of the bladder neck continues to evolve with accruing experience. Although much was made of the appropriate amount of tension placed on the suspension sutures at the inception of these procedures, most authors now recommend no or minimal tension to reduce the incidence of suture erosion and bladder outlet obstruction. Sutures originally placed laterally above the pubic bone may have resulted in a higher incidence of protracted discomfort. They are now placed at or near the midline or fixed to the bone.

A recent modification of NDNS introduced by Benderev in 1992[23] has stimulated the development of new instrumentation[24] (Fig. 30-5). A disposable suture carrier (Vesica, Microvasive/Boston Scientific Corp., Watertown, Mass.) is used to incorporate pubocervical fascia lateral to the bladder neck and urethra in a large Z-stitch. The suspension sutures are fixed to an anchor placed in the pubic bone and tied without tension by use of a removable spacer. The procedure is performed on an outpatient basis with minimal requirements for postoperative analgesia. Although still early in follow-up study, results thus far are encouraging.[25]

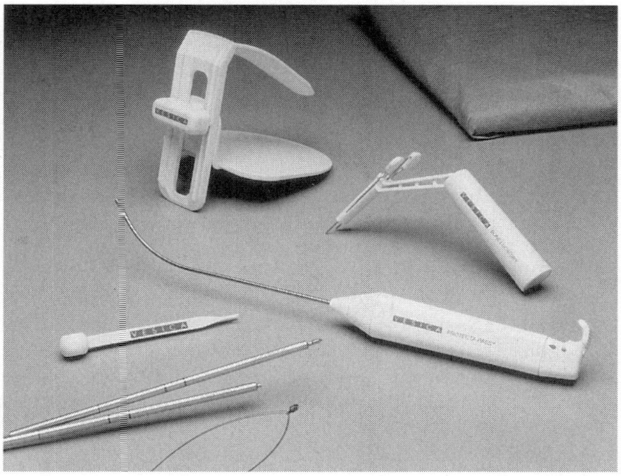

FIG. 30-5 *Vesica percutaneous bladder neck suspension kit with disposable suture carrier, bone anchors/suture, bone locator, suture spacer, and posterior retractor.* (Courtesy Microvasive/Boston Scientific Corp., Watertown, Mass.

Conclusions

Nondissected needle suspension of the bladder neck is an effective method to correct genuine stress urinary incontinence in women. It accomplishes this with minimal morbidity, brief or no hospitalization, and rapid return to normal activity. Efforts to improve technique and enhance success continue. The result is an enhanced quality of life for our patients who regain a sense of self-control and resume social functions they previously avoided.[26]

References

1. Marshall VF, Marchetti AA, Krantz KE: The correction of stress incontinence by simple vesico-urethral suspension, *Surg Gynecol Obstet* 88:509, 1949.
2. Burch JC: Urethrovaginal fixation to Cooper's ligament for correction of stress incontinence, cystocele, and prolapse, *Am J Obstet Gynecol* 81:281-290,1961.
3. Richardson AC, Lyon JB, Williams NL: A new look at pelvic relaxation, *Am J Obstet Gynecol* 126:568, 1976.
4. Pereyra AJ: A simplified surgical procedure for correction of stress incontinence in women, *West J Surg Obstet Gynecol* 67:223, 1959.
5. McGuire EJ, Lytton B, Kohorn EI, Pepe V: The value of urodynamic testing in stress urinary incontinence, *J Urol* 124:256, 1980.
6. Spencer JR, O'Connor VJ Jr, Schaeffer AJ: A comparison of endoscopic suspension of the vesical neck with suprapubic vesicourethropexy for treatment of stress urinary incontinence, *J Urol* 137:411, 1987.
7. Stamey TA: Endoscopic suspension of the vesical neck for urinary incontinence, *Surg Gynecol Obstet* 136:547, 1973.
8. Gittes RF, Loughlin KR: No-incision pubovaginal suspension for stress incontinence, *J Urol* 138:568, 1987.

9. Loughlin KR, Whitmore WF, Gittes RF, Richie JP: Review of an 8-year experience with modifications of endoscopic suspension of the bladder neck for female stress urinary incontinence, *J Urol* 143:44, 1990.
10. Stamey TA: Urinary incontinence in the female: the Stamey endoscopic suspension of the vesical neck for stress urinary incontinence. In Walsh PC, Retik AB, Stamey TA, Vaughan ED, editors: *Campbell's urology,* ed 6, Philadelphia, 1992, Saunders.
11. Morales A, Van Cott GF: The Gittes procedure as an improved simplification of current techniques for vesical neck suspensions, *Surg Gynecol Obstet* 167:243, 1988.
12. German KA, Kynaston H, Wright S, Stephenson TP: A prospective randomized trial comparing a modified needle suspension procedure with the vagina/obturator shelf procedure for genuine stress incontinence, *Br J Urol* 76:188, 1994.
13. Mundy AR: A trial comparing the Stamey bladder neck suspension procedure with colposuspension for the treatment of stress incontinence, *Br J Urol* 55:687, 1983.
14. Rodriguez R, Partin AW, Mostwin JL, Kavoussi LR: Long-term follow-up of surgically treated stress urinary incontinence, *Proc American Urological Association 90th annual meeting,* Las Vegas, Nevada, Apr. 23-28, 1995.
15. Knispel HH, Klan R, Siegmann K, Miller K: Results with the Stamey procedure in 251 consecutive patients with genuine urinary stress incontinence, *Proc American Urological Association 90th annual meeting,* Las Vegas, Nevada, Apr. 23-28, 1995.
16. Riggs JA: Retropubic cystourethropexy: a review of two operative procedures with long-term follow-up, *Obstet Gynecol* 68(1):98, 1986.
17. Herbertsson G, Iosif CS: Surgical results and urodynamic studies 10 years after retropubic colpourethrocystopexy, *Acta Obstet Gynecol Scand* 72:298, 1993.
18. Wheeler JS Jr: Osteomyelitis of the pubis: complication of a Stamey urethropexy, *J Urol* 151:1638, 1994.
19. Weiss RE, Cohen E: Erosions of buttress following bladder neck suspension, *Br J Urol* 69:656, 1992.
20. Jarvis GJ: Letter to the editor, *Br J Urol* 70:695, 1992.
21. Green DF, McGuire EJ, Lytton B: A comparison of endoscopic suspension of the vesical neck versus anterior urethropexy for the treatment of stress urinary incontinence, *J Urol* 136:1205, 1986.
22. Webster GD, Kreder KJ: Voiding dysfunction following cystourethropexy: its evaluation and management, *J Urol* 144:670, 1990.
23. Benderev TV: Anchor fixation and other modifications of endoscopic bladder neck suspension, *Urology* 4(5) 409, 1992.
24. Benderev TV: A modified percutaneous outpatient bladder neck suspension system, *J Urol* 152:2316, 1994.
25. Rackley RR, Winters JC, Cohen TD, Appell RA: Use of a bone anchoring needle suspension for genuine stress urinary incontinence, *Proc American Urological Association 90th annual meeting,* Las Vegas, Nevada, Apr. 23-28, 1995.
26. Elia G, Kraemer J, Bergman A: Personality changes after anti-incontinence operations in women, *Int Urogynecol J* 5:141, 1994.

Chapter 31 Intraurethral Injections

Rodney A. Appell, Jack Christian Winters

Urinary incontinence may originate at the level of the bladder or the urethra. In evaluating patients for the use of intraurethral injections as a treatment of urinary incontinence, it is essential to identify the cause or causes of incontinence to recommend appropriate therapy. Intraurethral injections benefit patients with incontinence occurring at the level of the urethra. Incontinence occurring at the level of the urethra may be caused by anatomic displacement of a normally functioning urethra (anatomic genuine stress urinary incontinence) in females or intrinsic incompetence of the urethral closure mechanism (intrinsic sphincteric dysfunction) in females or males. Patients with intrinsic sphincteric dysfunction (ISD) commonly have had a previous surgical procedure on or near the urethra, a sympathetic neurologic injury, or myelodysplasia. Female patients with genuine stress urinary incontinence have normal urethral function but hypermobility of the bladder neck and proximal urethra resulting from a deficiency in pelvic support. These patients benefit from a bladder neck elevation and stabilization. Patients with ISD have poor urethral function and require procedures to increase outflow resistance. Bladder neck suspension procedures will fail in these patients because of the poor urethral function, and these patients require pubovaginal sling procedures, artificial urinary sphincters, or periurethral injections.

In patients with ISD, the presence or absence of anatomic support will assist in directing future management. At present, patients with a lack of anatomic support (hypermobility) and ISD do best undergoing sling procedures or artificial urinary sphincters. Patients with a fixed, well-supported urethra in association with ISD are excellent candidates for periurethral injection. During the multicenter investigation of collagen in the treatment of ISD, the patients selected with anatomic (type II) incontinence did not fare well.[1,2] Therefore the recommendation currently is to perform intraurethral or periurethral injections on patients with a poorly functioning urethra (ISD) and good anatomic support. However, recent data indicate that intraurethral injections may be used for selected patients with anatomic stress urinary incontinence.[3]

Evaluation and Patient Selection

When one is obtaining a history from patients with urinary incontinence, it is important to elucidate whether previous surgery has been performed or an underlying neurologic disorder exists. Also, the activity precipitating urinary leakage is important. Patients who leak in the supine position, have bedwetting, or leak with a sensation of urinary urgency do not have genuine stress urinary incontinence and need to be investigated for bladder or intrinsic sphincteric deficiency. In females, the physical examination is essential to ascertain if concomitant urogenital prolapse and urethral hypermobility are present. The

Q-Tip test is used, with an angle of greater than 30 degrees signifying urethral hypermobility.[4]

Urodynamic studies are performed to evaluate possible bladder causes of incontinence (instability, decreased contractility, overflow) and to evaluate urethral function. Tests of urethral function may be performed using leak point pressures or urethral pressure profiles. An abdominal leak point pressure (P_{abd}) is the abdominal pressure required to drive urine through the urethra. This corresponds to urethral opening pressure, and low urethral opening pressure implies minimal urethral resistance and poor urethral function. Therefore low abdominal leak point pressures are required to elicit leakage per urethra in patients with ISD. The abdominal leak point pressure (Valsalva leak point pressure, VLPP) is obtained with the patient straining while the bladder is filled at incremental volumes of 50 ml beginning at 150 ml and followed to 300 ml. The patient is asked to strain, and the pressure at which urine leaks through the sphincteric mechanism is recorded. Leakage can be identified either by direct vision or by radiofluoroscopic assessment of contrast during a videourodynamic procedure. VLPP of less than 60 cm H_2O signifies poor or absent urethral function. These measurements have been shown to correlate with urethral pressure profiles and are less variable and easier to perform.[5] Videourodynamics are urodynamic studies performed with radiographic analysis of the bladder. The presence of an open bladder neck with the bladder at rest in the absence of a detrusor contraction implies the presence of ISD. Patients who have undergone multiple surgical procedures, have mixed incontinence, or have neurogenic bladders benefit greatly from videourodynamic procedures. At present, the ideal patient for periurethral injections is a patient with poor urethral function, normal bladder capacity, and good anatomic support. Patients with minimal hypermobility and high leak point pressures or elderly, less active females with anatomic incontinence may be considered for periurethral injections as well; however, it is wise to reserve this therapy for patients in this population who represent a surgical risk or have a more limited mobility.

Contraindications to periurethral injections include active urinary tract infection, untreated detrusor instability, and known hypersensitivity to the injected agent. Patients who are to have intraurethral injection of collagen must undergo skin testing 1 month before the procedure to determine if hypersensitivity to the material is present.[6] In the glutaraldehyde cross-linked (Gax) collagen multicenter trial, 4% of the female patients exhibited hypersensitivity during skin testing, whereas only 1% of males exhibited hypersensitivity.[7]

Injectable Materials

The ideal material for periurethral injection is one that is easily injected, is biocompatible, and causes little or no inflammatory reaction. Also the substance should elicit no immunogenic response. There should be no migration of the injected material, and it should maintain its bulking effect for a long period of time. Many agents have been used as injectables for urinary incontinence ranging from sclerosing agents to autologous blood.[8,9] Currently the most widely used agent is cross-linked bovine collagen. Collagen (Contigen) received United States Food and Drug Administration approval for the treatment of ISD in male and female patients in September 1993. Autologous fat has gained acceptance in patients who demonstrated hypersensitivity to collagen, although results have not been as satisfactory.[10] Polytetrafluoroethylene (PTFE) paste has recently been removed from the United States marketplace because of concerns over its migration and safety,[11] despite being proved as an effective method of treatment for urinary incontinence with no reports of untoward sequelae in human beings.[12] These agents may be injected safely under local anesthesia, allowing potential use in patients considered poor surgical risks.

PTFE Paste (Urethrin)

PTFE paste (Urethrin) is a sterile mixture of PTFE micropolymer particles, glycerin, and polysorbate. PTFE particles stimulate an ingrowth of fibroblasts at the injection site, become encapsulated, and produce a permanent bolstering effect.[12] These particles elicit a chronic foreign-body reaction with granuloma formation. Documented evidence of particle migration and granuloma formation have raised concerns about the use of this material.[11]

Autologous Fat

As a periurethral bulking agent, fat has several advantages: it is readily available, biocompatible, and easily obtainable. Fat integrates as a graft, but a significant portion of the injected material is reabsorbed and replaced by inflammation and fibrosis with connective tissue producing the final bulk effect.[10] The high degree of absorption is the major limitation in using fat as an injectable agent. There is no evidence of migration of the injected fat particles.

Glutaraldehyde Cross-Linked Bovine Collagen (Contigen)

Glutaraldehyde cross-linked bovine collagen (Contigen) is both biocompatible and biodegradable. It is a sterile, nonpyrogenic bovine dermal collagen cross-linked with glutaraldehyde and dispersed in a phosphate-buffered physiologic saline solution. The cross-linking process improves the integrity of the material for the injection. A minimal inflammatory response has been associated with the injection of collagen, and no granuloma formation or foreign body reaction is present. Also no foreign body reaction occurs. Contigen begins to degrade in approximately 12 weeks, but in this period of time neovascularization and the deposition by fibroblasts of host collagen occurs within the implant. The collagen completely degrades within 10 to 19 months.[13] There are no reports of particle migration of the collagen material.[1-]

Silicone Polymers

Macroplastique and Bioplastique are textured silicone macroparticles suspended within a hydrogel. The hydrogel is rapidly absorbed by the host tissue, but the macroimplant becomes fixed in position by encapsulation. The particle size is greater than 100 μ, which inhibits migration.[15] Henly et al. compared migratory and histologic tendencies of solid silicone macrospheres to smaller silicone particles in dogs.[15] Nuclear imaging revealed small particles dissipated throughout the lung, kidney, brain, and lymph nodes at 4 months. One episode of large-particle migration to the lung occurred without associated inflammation; an x-ray analysis confirmed that the particles were silicone. Initial clinical trials demonstrate the potential of this substance for the treatment of ISD and genuine stress incontinence; however, migration has been documented to be a problem with even large-particle injections, and the use of this material will likely be limited in the United States.[16]

TECHNIQUE OF INJECTION

The technique of injection of material is not difficult, but it is essential to perform precise placement of the material to ensure an optimal result. The injection can be performed either suburothelially through a needle placed directly through a cystoscope (transurethral injection) or periurethrally with a spinal needle inserted percutaneously and positioned in the urethral tissues in the suburothelial space for observing the manipulation cystoscopically.[17]

Males are injected predominantly by the transurethral approach, and females are injected by either transcystoscopic implantation of a needle into the suburothelium[18] or by placement of a spinal needle inserted percutaneously along the wall of the urethra while the delivery of the material is being observed directly by urethroscopy.[17] Also, indirect visualization by ultrasonography has been described as useful in the precise localization of the injection.[19] Recently Neal et al.[20] have introduced a technique to facilitate periurethral needle placement utilizing methylene blue mixed with local anesthesia enabling the surgeon to place the implant more accurately. There is certainly a learning curve with any technique chosen that ultimately results in using less injectable material to attain continence. We first describe the technique of injection in males and females employing collagen because this is currently the most widely used injectable substance. After this description we make additional comments concerning the alterations of techniques in the injection of other injectable materials.

The Male Patient

The male patient is positioned in the semilithotomy position, and 2% lidocaine jelly is placed intraurethrally and left in place 10 minutes before instrumentation. Cystourethroscopy with a zero-degree lens is employed. The injectable material is then delivered suburothelially by way of a transcystoscopic injection needle under direct vision. This is performed in a circumferential matter employing four-quadrant needle placements, whereby the needle is advanced suburothelially into four quadrants and the material is injected until a mucosal bleb is created in each quadrant. Gradually, after circumferential injection is employed, the urethral mucosa coapts itself in the midline (Fig. 31-1).

In cases of ISD occurring after radical prostatectomy surgery, a short segment of urethra remains above the external sphincter. If visualization of this urethra is difficult, the needle may be placed at the level of the external sphincter and advanced to ensure deposition of the material proximal to the external

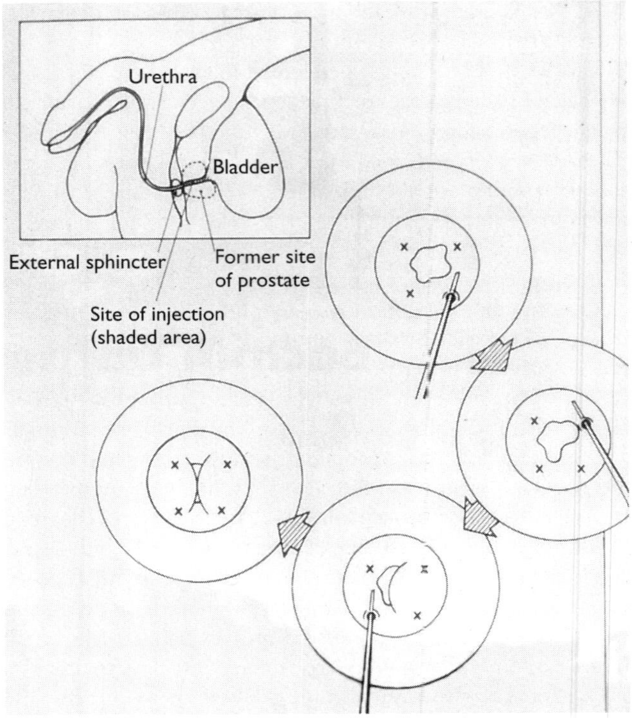

FIG. 31-1 *Transurethral injection in males.*

sphincter. It is important to note that the material should not be injected directly into the external sphincter because this can cause pudendal nerve spasm.

Injection is more difficult in patients with post–radical prostatectomy incontinence resulting from the short segment of urethra above the level of the external sphincter and extensive scarring, which usually occurs in this area after surgery. To ensure optimal placement of the material proximal to the external sphincter and at the level of the bladder neck, antegrade injections employing either a flexible cystoscope,[21] a small ureteroscope with a 5 Fr working port,[22] or a commercial PFTE injector[23] may be performed through a small suprapubic punch cystotomy. This technique allows more precise localization of the bladder neck and urethra above the level of the external sphincter. In addition, it facilitates injection of the material in more supple, less scarred tissue near the bladder neck (Fig. 31-2). Although only in very early clinical trials, this technique seems to facilitate more precise injection of material generating improved results with the use of less material (Fig. 31-3). It is our opinion that this technique represents an exciting new method of collagen implantation in the male and should be considered in any male patient not achieving adequate success by way of a transurethral approach.

The Female Patient

Women may be injected by way of a transcystoscopic technique[18] or a periurethral approach.[17] We prefer the periurethral approach because it minimizes intraurethral bleeding and

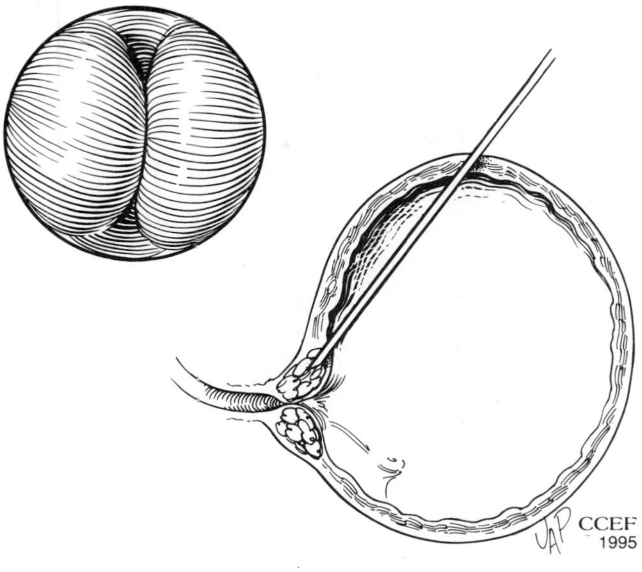

FIG. 31-2 *Antegrade injection by cystotomy.*

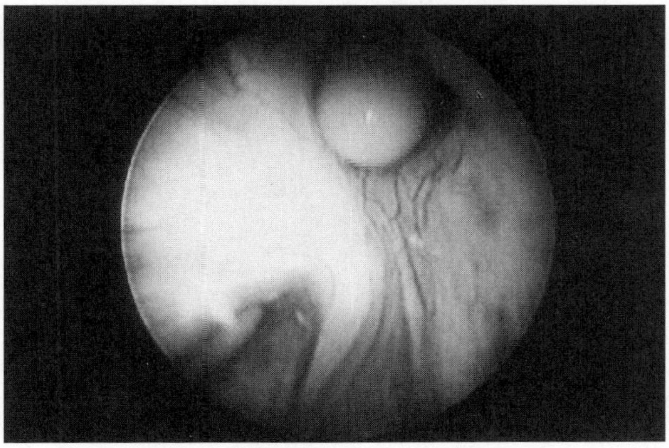

FIG. 31-3 *Endoscopic view during antegrade injection.*

extravasation of the injectable substance. With either approach, the woman is placed in the lithotomy position, the introitus is anesthetized with 20% topical benzocaine, and the urethra is anesthetized with topical 2% lidocaine jelly. After this, a local injection of 1% plain lidocaine is performed periurethrally at the 3 and 9 o'clock positions using 2 to 4 ml on each side.

Panendoscopy is performed with a zero- or 30-degree lens, and a 22-gauge spinal needle with the obturator in place is positioned periurethrally at the 4 or 8 o'clock position with the bevel of the needle directed toward the lumen. The needle is then advanced into the urethral muscle in the lamina propria in an entirely suburothelial plane. Once the needle is positioned in the lamina propria it usually advances with very little force. The needle may also be placed at the 6 o'clock position, and again needle placement is fully observed endoscopically. Bulging of the tip of the needle against the lining of the urethra is observed during advancement of the needle to ensure its proper placement. When the needle tip is properly positioned just below the bladder neck, the material is injected until swelling is visible on each side creating the appearance of occlusion of the urethral lumen. Once the urethra is approximately 50% occluded, the needle is removed and reinserted on the opposite side, and additional material is injected until the urethral mucosa is coapted in the midline creating the endoscopic appearance of two lateral prostatic lobes (Fig. 31-4).

The technique and approaches chosen for the injection of PTFE for urinary incontinence are similar to the Contigen injection, except for the depth of penetration of the needle. As stated previously, the needle placement for the injection of Contigen is suburothelially just behind the urethra mucosa. However, if the needle is placed too superficially for PFTE injection, the material may perforate and extrude into the urethral lumen, which can be problematic because the PFTE is sometimes difficult to remove. Therefore, when one is performing a PFTE injection, the needle is inserted at a 45-degree angle to allow deposition of the material 2 cm below the urethral mucosa.[24] This allows for the adequate bulk-enhancing effect minimizing the possibility of a perforation and extrusion of the injected Teflon into the urethra.

The technique of injection of autologous fat is divided into two phases: (1) harvesting the fat and (2) periurethral injection of the fat. There are multiple variations existing in the technique to harvest autologous fat ranging from aspiration with a large-bore needle to liposuction.[25,26] The authors use the Tulip fat harvesting and injection system to obtain autologous fat. An injection cannula is used to inject a lactated Ringer's/lidocaine injection solution into the subcutaneous fat. After this, a liposuction cannula is inserted into a 60 ml syringe that is locked in the suction position. With a gentle rocking motion to and fro through the infiltrated lower abdomen, 20 to 30 cc of fat is obtained. A 60 ml transferring adapter adds additional saline solution to the syringe, and with a rocking motion the fat is cleansed with saline. The bloody saline is discarded, and the process is repeated until the saline is clear. This provides golden brown fat. The syringe is placed upright, and the fat is allowed to settle. The excess saline is discarded, and the fat is then transferred to a Luer-Lok syringe for periurethral injection through an 18-gauge needle. The second phase of autologous fat injection is similar to the injection of collagen in both needle placement and depth of needle placement.

Postoperative Care

Perioperative antibiotic coverage is continued for 3 days after the procedure. Most patients are able to void easily after the procedure; however, if retention does develop, clean intermittent catheterization is begun with a 12 or 14 Fr catheter. Indwelling catheters are to be avoided in patients undergoing collagen and fat injection because they promote molding of the material around the catheter. Although usually unnecessary, if long-term catheterization is needed, suprapubic cystotomy should be performed in these patients.

Patients are contacted 2 weeks after the procedure to determine their continence status. Repeat injections are scheduled 1 month later as necessary.

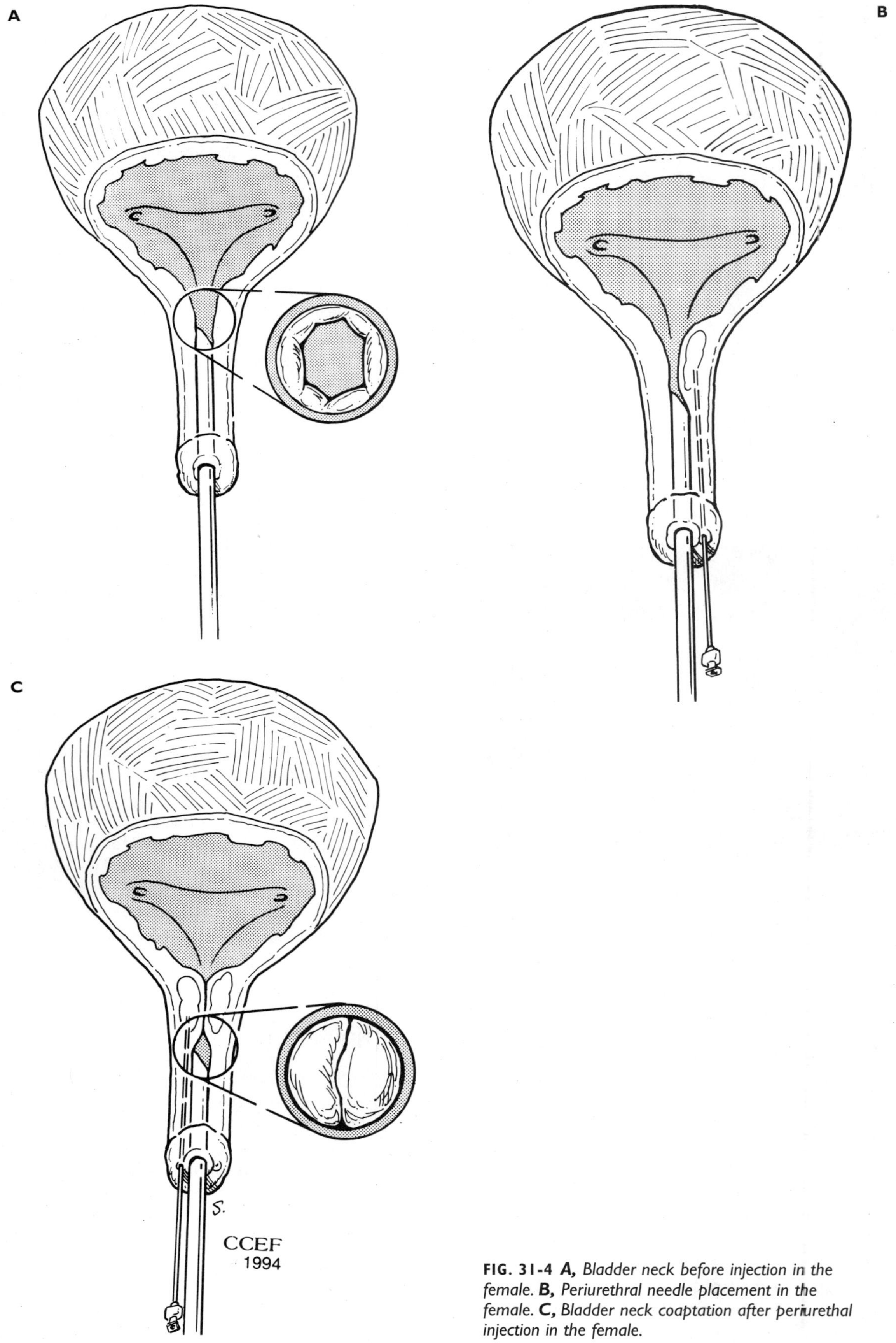

FIG. 31-4 ***A,*** *Bladder neck before injection in the female.* ***B,*** *Periurethral needle placement in the female.* ***C,*** *Bladder neck coaptation after periurethral injection in the female.*

Results

The first clinical trial of collagen in humans for urinary incontinence was performed by Shortliffe et al. in 1989.[27] Of patients with incontinence, 16 males and 1 female underwent injection. Nine of 17 experienced cure or improved symptoms, and no granuloma or distant migration of the collagen material was noted in two patients who died of causes unrelated to the collagen injection. Three hundred and six patients evaluated by urodynamic testing underwent collagen implantation in the multicenter North American Study group.[7] In 137 female patients with ISD, 96.4% were dry 1 year later. In 17 patients with hypermobility of the sphincteric complex, 82.3% were improved or dry. Of the 134 patients with postprostatectomy incontinence, 89.6% were dry or improved 1 year later. Females with ISD required approximately 2.5 injections with an average of 24.3 ml of collagen, whereas men with ISD required 3.9 injections with an average of 51.3 ml of collagen. Stricker and Haylen[28] noted an 82% success rate of the injection of collagen in the first 50 Australian patients to receive this therapy. Although the success and efficacy of collagen implantation for females with ISD have been reproduced in several series, debate exists about the efficacy of collagen material in patients with type II, or anatomic, stress urinary incontinence. A recent study by Herschorn et al.[3] reported equal success rates among patients with type II, or anatomic, stress incontinence and patients with ISD; however, the number of injections and the amount of material injected were higher in patients with anatomic urinary incontinence. It has also been documented that elderly female patients with anatomic incontinence do well with the injections of collagen material.[29]

With respect to the application of autologous fat injection for urinary incontinence, the male patients with prior prostatectomy demonstrate poor results, as do women with hypermobility of the sphincteric complex. Of the 12 patients with ISD, 83% were improved subjectively, but this improvement rate appeared to drop precipitously at 1 year.[30] Therefore, although autologous fat injections seem to work reasonably well for ISD, the long-term follow-up study needs to be assessed because it appears that autologous fat undergoes a rapid rate of reabsorption attributable to its high water content. At the ninetieth annual meeting of the American Urological Association held in Las Vegas in April 1995, several conclusions concerning Contigen were reached, including that the only difference between female patients with ISD versus those with hypermobility when treated with Contigen as a primary treatment modality is the requirement for greater volumes of Contigen in ISD patients than those with hypermobility alone. Another consensus was that retreatment is usually successful in females when dryness had been previously achieved, if relapse did occur. Unfortunately the results in men have not been so optimistic, especially in those treated after radiation or bladder neck contracture. Stothers et al.[31] have concluded that Contigen is a less cost-effective means of treatment than the artificial urinary sphincter in males.

Efficacy and safety of PTFE has been reviewed by the Department of Technology Assessment of the American Medical Association,[32] and the conclusion reached was that PTFE is a reasonably effective treatment for incontinence but the safety of the product is uncertain. A study is currently taking place to evaluate the safety and efficacy of PTFE when compared with Contigen.

Complications

The perioperative complications associated with periurethral injections are uncommon. The rate of urinary retention in patients undergoing PTFE injections is approximately 20% to 25%.[12] In the multicenter United States clinical trial of Contigen injections, transient retention developed in approximately 15% of patients.[7] Irritative voiding symptoms develop in approximately 20% of patients after the injection of PTFE but resolve after several days.[33] With Contigen, only 1% of patients experienced irritative voiding symptoms and 5% developed a urinary tract infection.[7] Patients following PTFE injections have noted the development of fever with negative blood cultures and urine cultures at a rate of 25%. This usually resolves after several days and probably indicates a mild allergic response.[12] Regardless of the material, the use of periurethral injections has proved to be safe, eliciting only minor complications. All complications are rapid to resolve, and a serious long-term complication from the use of periurethral injections has yet to be reported.

Summary

In the properly selected patient, periurethral injections offer excellent treatment results for patients with ISD. Patients with no anatomic hypermobility and ISD appear to be the most satisfactory candidates for periurethral injections. Contigen is the most widely used injectable, since it has been shown to be both biocompatible and biodegradable. There are no reports of particle migration with this material, and repeat injections can be performed safely under local anesthesia. Autologous fat is an alternative in periurethral injection, particularly in patients who have had positive skin tests to the collagen material.

The treatment response in females with these procedures is similar to surgical procedures to correct ISD, and the complications are minimal. However, in males the success rate of intraurethral injections does not approach that of the artificial urinary sphincter up to now.

In selected elderly and less mobile female patients with anatomic incontinence, recent data indicate that collagen may be useful in this patient population. The use of periurethral injections certainly has a role in the treatment of ISD in the properly selected patient and allows treatment of incontinence in patients who are poor surgical candidates and may be denied other forms of therapy.

References

1. Appell RA: Injectables for urethral incompetence, *World J Urol* 8:208, 1990.
2. McGuire EJ, Appell RA: Transurethral collagen injection for urinary incontinence, *Urology* 43:413, 1994.
3. Herschorn S, Radomski SB, Steele DJ: Early experience with intraurethral collagen injections for urinary incontinence, *J Urol* 148:1797, 1992.
4. Crystle C, Charme LS, Copeland WE: Q-tip test for stress urinary incontinence, *Obstet Gynecol* 38:313, 1971.
5. Appell RA: Valsalva leak point pressure (LPP) versus urethral pressure profile (UPP) in the evaluation of intrinsic sphincteric deficiency (ISD). Presented at the American Urogynecology Society annual meeting, Toronto, 1994.
6. Appell RA: Periurethral collagen injection for female incontinence, *Prob Urol* 5:134, 1990.

7. Bard CR: PMAA submission to US Food and Drug Administration for IDE #G850010, 1990.
8. Sachse H: Treatment of urinary incontinence with sclerosing solutions, indications, results and complications, *Urol Int* 15:225, 1963.
9. Appell RA: The periurethral injection of autologous blood. Presented at the American Urogynecology Society annual meeting, Toronto, 1994.
10. Santarosa R, Blaivas J: Building continence with periurethal fat injections, *Contemp Urol* 5:96, 1993.
11. Malizia AA Jr, Reiman HM, Myers RP, et al: Migration and granulomatous reaction after periurethral injection of polytef (teflon), *JAMA* 251:3277, 1984.
12. Politano V: Periurethral polytetrafluorethylene injection for urinary incontinence, *J Urol* 127:439, 1982.
13. Stegman SJ, Chu S, Bensch K Armstrong R: A light and electron microscopic evaluation of Zyderm collagen and Zyplast implants in aging human facial skin: a pilot study, *Arch Dermatol* 123:1644, 1987.
14. Remacle M, Marbaix E: Collagen implants in the human larynx: pathologic dissemination of two cases, *Arch Otolaryngol* 245:203, 1988.
15. Henly DR, Barrett DM, Weiland TL, et al: Particulate silicone for use in periurethral injections: local tissue effects and search for migration, *J Urol* 153:2039, 1995.
16. Press S, Badlani G: Injection therapy for urinary incontinence, *AUA Update Series,* vol 14, lesson 2, Baltimore, 1995, American Urological Association.
17. Appell RA: Collagen injection therapy for urinary incontinence, *Urol Clin North Am* 21:177, 1994.
18. O'Connell HE, McGuire EJ: Transurethral collagen therapy in women, *J Urol* 154:1463-1465, 1995.
19. Kageyama S, Kawabe K, Suzuki K, et al: Collagen implantation for post prostatectomy incontinence: early experience with a transrectal ultrasonographically guided method, *J Urol* 152:1473, 1994.
20. Neal D Jr, Lahaye M, Lowe D: Improved needle placement technique in periurethral collagen injection, *Urology* 45:865, 1995.
21. Klutke C: Personal communication, Dearborn, Mich., 1995.
22. Pintauro W: Personal communication, Stamford, Conn., 1995.
23. Winters JC, Appell RA: Antegrade collagen injections in males, *Urology,* (In press).
24. Stanisic T, Jennings CE, Miller JI: Polytetrafluoroethylene injection for post prostatectomy incontinence: experience with 20 patients during three years, *J Urol* 146:1575, 1991.
25. Cervigni M, Panei M: Periurethral autologous fat injection for Type III stress urinary incontinence, *J Urol* 149(Part 2):403A, 1993.
26. Ganibathi K, Leach GE: Periurethral injection techniques, *Atlas Urol Clin North Am* 2:101, 1994.
27. Shortliffe LMD, Freiha FS, Kessler R, et al: Treatment of urinary incontinence by the periurethral implantation of glutaraldehyde cross-linked collagen, *J Urol* 141:538, 1989.
28. Stricker P, Haylen B: Injectable collagen for type 3 female stress incontinence: the first 50 Australian patients, *Med J Aust* 158:189, 1993.
29. Faerber GJ: Endoscopic collagen injection therapy for elderly women with Type I stress urinary incontinence, *J Urol* 153(Part 2):527A, 1995.
30. Santarosa RP, Blaivas JG: Periurethral injection of autologous fat for the treatment of sphincteric incontinence, *J Urol* 151:607, 1994.
31. Stothers L et al: A cost-effective and utility analysis of the artificial urinary sphincter and collagen injection in the treatment of post-prostatectomy incontinence, *J Urol* 153(Part 2):112A, 1995.
32. Cole HM, editor: Diagnostic and therapeutic technology assessment (DATTA), *JAMA* 269:2975, 1993.
33. Schulman C, Simon J, Wespes E, Germeau F: Endoscopic injection of teflon for female urinary incontinence, *Eur Urol* 9:246, 1983.

Chapter 32

Retropubic Suspension Procedures

Sherif R. Aboseif, Emil A. Tanagho

Leakage of urine in association with stress was initially described by Sir Eardley Holland late in the last century. Most authors at that time believed that stress incontinence was the result of a defect in the internal urethral meatus and the bladder sphincter. Accordingly, early attempts to cure this condition focused either on closure of the urethra with creation of a new channel[1] or on narrowing of the urethra and bladder neck by placement of a catgut suture around the upper two thirds of the urethra with a catheter in place.[2,3] Later, most authors realized that the sphincteric mechanism itself remains intact in stress incontinence and that the abnormality lies in the anatomic displacement and mobility of the vesicourethral junction; simply correcting this anatomic defect will restore sphincteric function. Subsequently this concept stimulated the development of various suspension procedures.

Abdominal suspension for the correction of stress urinary incontinence was first reported in 1923 when Bonney described ventrofixation of the bladder.[4] Despite this early report, abdominal procedures—in which the urethrovesical segment is repositioned into the pelvis by attachment of the vaginal wall lateral to the urethra and the bladder neck to structures in the retropubic area—did not really attract the interest of surgeons until Marshall, Marchetti, and Krantz published their report in 1949.[5] Their procedure was initially described to correct stress incontinence in males after abdominoperineal resection of the colon. Later, they successfully applied the same procedure to female patients with sagging of the bladder neck and stress incontinence. Although the basic concept of the Marshall-Marchetti-Krantz (MMK) procedure was very attractive because it successfully restored the anatomic defect, it had two main disadvantages. First, placement of heavy suture material in the periurethral tissue and possibly the urethral wall itself is extremely damaging to its delicate muscular structure, which constitutes the main element of the sphincteric mechanism. If this is done, scarring of the urethral musculature is inevitable, with permanent intrinsic weakness of the sphincteric mechanism as the outcome. In addition, including the periurethral tissue in the suspension sutures (and pulling it upwards to the symphysis) carries the risk of urethral compression and strangulation against the back of the pubic bone with varying degrees of postoperative obstruction and volumes of residual urine. Secondly, fixing the sutures to the periostium of the pubic bone is sometimes very difficult and carries the risk of osteitis pubis. These two considerations stimulated many investigations for further modifications.

Burch recommended the use of Cooper's ligament as an alternative point of anterior fixation.[6,7] This is a strong thick band of fibrous tissue that runs along the superior ramus of the pubis. Colpocystourethropexy, described by Tanagho,[8] is similar to the techniques of Burch and Murnaghan[9] with respect to anterior fixation; however, the latter did not describe the exact suture position in relation to the vaginal wall. We believe that placement of the sutures in the anterior vaginal wall is one of the most important steps of the procedure. They should include full thickness and should be placed as far laterally as technically possible, avoiding the delicate urethral musculature and the periurethral tissue. Our approach has been based on the rationale that the less one interferes with the sphincteric mechanism the better. The main goal of surgery is to restore the normal anatomic position and mobility and to provide adequate support to the vesicourethral segment.

Anatomic and Physiologic Background

Interest in female urinary incontinence has grown as a result of the increased appreciation of the pathophysiologic factors contributing to it. This expanding knowledge of the anatomy and function of the continence mechanism should underlie the rationale for any operative corrective procedure.

Urethral Musculature

The female urethra is a muscular tube about 4 cm long from the internal to the external meatus. Its structure, in particular that of the smooth and striated muscles and the continence mechanism, has been the subject of considerable debate. Histologically the urethra has three main elements that theoretically contribute to sphincteric function: the smooth muscular structure; abundant collagenous tissue, which firmly binds the fibers of this smooth musculature; and a well-developed sleeve of striated muscle fibers, which are maximally condensed around the midportion of the urethra.

Urethral Smooth Muscle. In the female the smooth musculature of the urethra extends throughout its entire length. Although it was previously believed that the smooth muscles of the bladder and the urethra were distinct,[10,11] Tanagho and Smith[12,13] clearly demonstrated in anatomic studies that the urethra and bladder have the same embryologic origin and their musculature is directly continuous. The smooth musculature of the urethra is composed of two main coats. The inner longitudinal coat is a direct continuation of the inner longitudinal coat of the detrusor. This is a relatively thick layer, formed of very delicate muscle bundles, in contradistinction to the coarse arrangement on the bladder side. Its muscle bundles are firmly bound together by dense, compact collagen tissue and elastic fibers. The outer coat consists of semicircular fibers that likewise are a direct continuation of the outer longitudinal layer of the detrusor. The semicircular muscle fibers, also known as the sling fibers, are oriented at various degrees of obliquity, looping around the urethra and then turning back toward the bladder.[14] The thickness of this outer semicircular coat is constant throughout the length of the urethra, though it may be slightly heavier in the proximal than in the most distal third. It is the semicircular fibers that are responsible both for the sphincteric function and for the role of the smooth muscle component in developing urethral resistance. Innervation of the urethral smooth musculature is mainly by the parasympathetic autonomic nervous system. The sympathetic system controls the rich vascular bed of the urethra and not the urethral smooth muscle proper.[15]

Collagen. Collagen forms a major component of the urethra, occupying more of the tissue mass than the smooth muscle does.[16] It firmly binds the smooth muscle in both the longitudinal and the circular layers. The collagen associated with the circular muscle fibers is considered an important component of passive closure of the urethra, especially because it requires no energy to maintain tone.

External Urethral Sphincter. A sleeve of striated skeletal muscle fibers encircles the midurethral segment as it traverses the pelvic floor to gain exit at the external meatus. Although embryologically related to the musculature of the pelvic floor, these fibers are anatomically separate—a differentiated segment of the cloacal sphincter, which gives each of the urethral, vaginal, and anal orifices its own specialized sphincteric function. The striated sphincter consists of bundles of circularly oriented fibers maximal in bulk at the midurethral level (the high-pressure zone in urodynamics[15]), forming more or less a complete ring with the median raphe in the midline posteriorly.

Periurethral Striated Musculature

The periurethral striated musculature is composed of the levator ani (pubococcygeus) and the deep transverse perineal muscle. The pubococcygeus, composed of the most medial fibers of the levator muscle, abuts the urethra as it runs from the pubis past the lateral walls of the vagina to the coccyx. It is not attached to the urethra but passes on either side. The deep transverse perineal muscle consists of two portions: the urethral compressor and the urethrovaginal sphincter, which extends along the sides of the urethra and the vagina to enclose them. Innervation of the external urethral sphincter and the periurethral striated musculature is somatic through S2-3 spinal nerves. Juenemann et al. have shown that the branches to the external urethral sphincter begin quite proximally before the pudendal nerve reaches the ischiosacral ligament.[17]

Histologically the striated muscle fibers can be classified into two main groups: slow-twitch and fast-twitch. The former are small-diameter muscle fibers, rich in acid-stable myosin adenosine triphosphatase, and possessing numerous mitochondria. On contraction, they attain a low amplitude, which they can sustain for a relatively long time. They constitute about 35% of the overall striated muscle mass. The fast-twitch fibers constitute the remaining 65%. Detailed study of the histochemical characteristics of these fibers has revealed two different subgroups: fast-twitch fatigable fibers (50%) and an intermediate type that is fatigue-resistant (15%). The mixture of the muscle fibers accounts for the varied contribution of the striated sphincter to the continence mechanism. The slow-twitch fibers are needed for sustained tonus, whereas the fast-twitch fibers serve for emergency (stress). The presence of fast-twitch fatigue-resistant fibers provides the combination of these two properties in an effective way—high amplitude sustained for a longer time.

The intrinsic striated muscles together with the smooth involuntary muscles constitute the intrinsic sphincteric mechanism. This is supported and held in place by multiple ligaments, fascial attachments, and, more importantly, a muscularly active pelvic floor that acts as an indirect sphincteric mechanism.

Anatomy of the Space of Retzius

To understand the anatomy of urethral support and of retropubic bladder suspension, one should be familiar with the anatomy of the space of Retzius. When the bladder is pulled backward and the loose areolar tissue is removed, the inner surface of the symphysis pubis can be seen in the midline with the paired pubourethral ligaments on either side, suspending a complex aponeurotic plate to either side of the symphyseal midline. The plate is continuous with the endopelvic fascia. The latter forms a condensation along both side walls extending from the inner surface of the pubic bone to the ischial spine. This is known as the arcus tendineus fasciae pelvis. A second tendinous arc (the arcus tendineus musculi levatoris ani), from which the ileococcygeus muscle takes its origin, begins near the top of the pubic rami and passes diagonally down toward the ischial spine to fuse with the arcus tendineus fasciae pelvis. In the midline between the pubourethral ligaments, the deep dorsal vein of the clitoris courses beneath the endopelvic fascia. Along the pelvic sidewall, the obturator foramen with the obturator nerve and vessels can be seen. Along the superior ramus of the pubis, the horizontal fibers of Cooper's ligaments are apparent. Proper identification of this ligament is important in placement of the sutures during retropubic suspension.

Pathophysiology

It is generally agreed that genuine urinary stress incontinence is primarily an anatomic disturbance (Fig. 32-1) that lessens the effectiveness of the sphincteric control mechanism, which in itself is essentially normal. However, pelvic floor weakness and the lack of appropriate support to the vesicourethral segment undermine its functional capability. Correcting the anatomic abnormality, that is, the pelvic floor weakness, and restoring the normal relationship of the vesicourethral segment to the surrounding structures will restore the functional integrity of the sphincteric mechanism. These facts are well recognized by most investigators in the field. Realizing them sets the guidelines to be applied in devising any surgical approach to correction. Since the development of modern surgical techniques, the goal has been singular (correcting the anatomic abnormality), but the means of achieving it have been multiple and diverse. Some people favor retropubic approaches; others, the vaginal route. The variety of procedures by either approach most likely reflects uncertainty about the exact mode of action of any of them. Although there is a progressive interest in the easiest, least traumatic approach, what seems easier technically may not have lasting value.

A

B

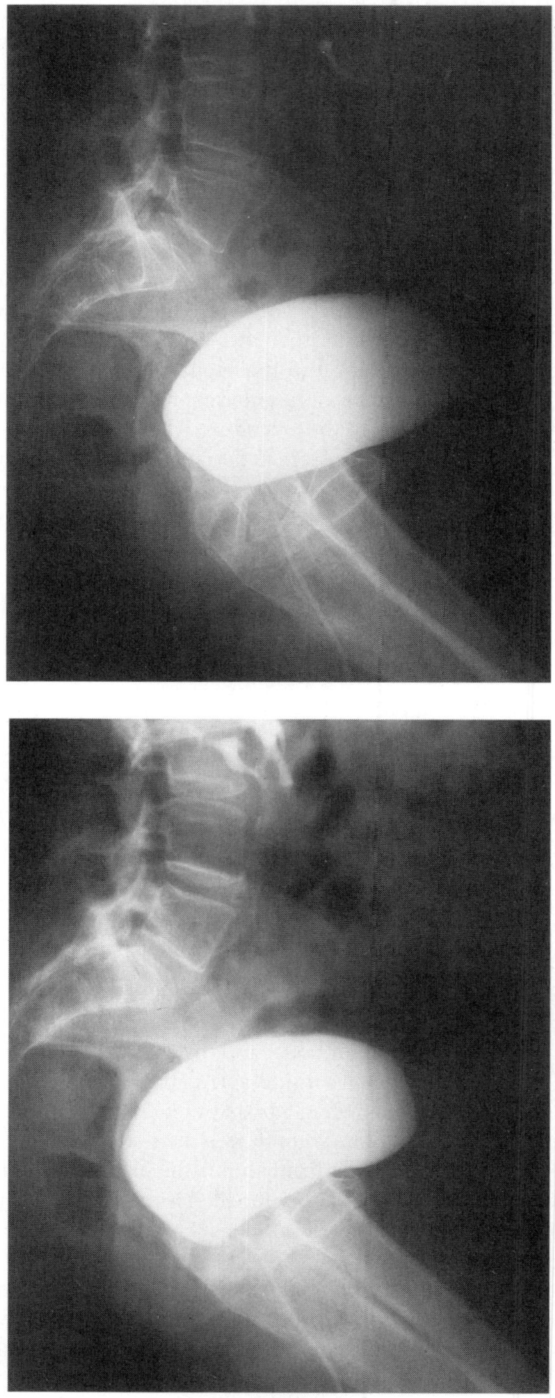

FIG. 32-1 *In this patient at rest the low vesicourethral junction,* ***A,*** *is exacerbated with straining,* ***B.***

Vaginal Approaches

Vaginal approaches have the advantages of being simple, with a shorter hospitalization and rapid recovery. However, usually they rely on nonabsorbable sutures to hold the vesicourethral junction in position. Our belief is that one cannot rely on suture material to maintain suspension. The sutures won't break, but neither will they maintain the immediate postoperative position. They will gradually give way in response to the degree of tension to which they are subjected and ultimately hold at a level dictated by the degree of resilience of the tissue they should be supporting. An attempt to create a fibrotic reaction with the vaginal exposure is feasible but is not so efficient as the retropubic approach. Several techniques have been applied vaginally: the Pereyra technique,[18] the Stamey endoscopic suspension,[19] and the Raz vaginal suspension.[20] All apply essentially the same principal with some modifications in the details in an attempt to effect more accurate positioning and greater durability. Bergman et al.[21] reported a prospective randomized comparison of three different suspension procedures: anterior colporrhaphy, modified Pereyra vaginal suspension, and the Burch retropubic suspension. The cure rate was defined by strict clinical and urodynamic criteria. Their results revealed a significantly higher cure rate with Burch urethropexy than with the Pereyra technique and anterior colporrhaphy at 1 year's follow-up study (87% versus 70% and 69%, respectively). It is important to remember that, even if vaginal procedures have been shown to be feasible in patients with no previous retropubic pelvic surgery these are very difficult in recurrent cases where the bladder neck is scarred and fixed below the level of the pubic bone. It is very hard to believe that any suture, regardless of the tension applied, could mobilize all the scarred tissue. Suturing simply creates compression against the fixed urethra and results in obstruction. Numerous urodynamic studies confirm this. In these situations, the retropubic approach will allow for sharp dissection to enable the bladder neck to be mobilized freely and elevated to an appropriate position.

Retropubic Approaches

Since the initial description of bladder neck suspension by Marshall et al. in 1949,[5] the suprapubic approach has been widely used to correct female stress incontinence. The high success rate, the durability of the response, and the fact that most urologists are familiar with the anatomy of the retropubic space have made this approach very popular. This has prompted numerous modifications, the most significant being the Burch procedure,[7] Turner Warwick's approach,[22] Richardson's,[23] and Tanagho's[8] colpocystourethropexy. All of these procedures share one basic principle: to suspend and stabilize the bladder neck and the proximal urethra in a retropubic position, taking advantage of the tough vaginal wall and using it as a hammock behind the vesicourethral segment to lift and support it. The retropubic approach has many advantages over other approaches. It provides direct visualization of the anatomic abnormality; under direct control, free mobilization can be easily accomplished, and all retropubic and perivaginal fat can be removed, permitting very firm postoperative adherence and fixation to ensure a permanent repair. One should respect the vesicourethral segment itself and avoid any dissection or mobilization in the midline in an attempt to preserve its very delicate musculature. This was one of the main modifications from the original technique described by Marshall et al., who recommended the placement of two or three sutures through the lateral wall of the urethra deep into the adjacent vaginal wall junction. These sutures carry the risk of damaging the urethral sphincteric mechanism or its nerve supply. Adequate support can usually be achieved by fixation of the tough vaginal wall to Cooper's ligament with sutures placed so far lateral as to leave a wide retropubic space for limited urethral mobility without urethral compression. Recently, Goodno and Powers reported a good success rate with their 7 years' experience with fixing the vaginal sutures to the abdominal wall fascia.[24] Although this might be a good alternative, the use of Cooper's ligament, which is readily available, as an anterior fixation point is very reliable.

With widespread use of laparoscopic surgery, extraperitoneal laparoscopic retropubic suspension has been reported by many authors.[25-27] Several techniques have been described for suspension including the use of nonabsorbable mesh bands that are attached to the vagina and Cooper's ligament with titanium staples.[28,29] All advocates of laparoscopy cite the advantages of short hospitalization, minimal postoperative pain, and early recovery. In addition, it can achieve the same therapeutic result as traditional open surgery. Short-term results are certainly encouraging; however, long-term durability is still to be seen. Most authors claim that one of the main advantages of laparoscopic surgery is that it requires minimal retropubic dissection, but others believe that this is probably a disadvantage because the scarring and fibrosis that develop after retropubic dissection are more responsible than the sutures for keeping the bladder and the urethra suspended in proper anatomic position.

Surgical Technique

Position and Preparation

The patient is placed in a low lithotomy position with the legs slightly abducted in Allen stirrups. The vagina, perineum, and abdomen are sterilely prepped and draped to permit easy access to the lower abdomen and vagina. A 22 Fr 5 ml Foley catheter is passed into the urethra and kept in the sterile field. One dose of intravenous antibiotic (second-generation cephalosporin) is given circumoperatively and continued over the first 24 hours as prophylaxis

Dissection of the retropubic space. The retropubic space is exposed through a Pfannenstiel or midline incision. Staying close to the back of the pubic bone, the surgeon's hand is introduced into the retropubic space, and the bladder and the urethra are gently pushed downward, exposing the urethrovesical junction and the anterior vaginal wall. This step is critically important and can be extremely difficult after previous surgical intervention. In such a situation, adhesions are usually dense, and the anterior bladder wall frequently is displaced downward and adheres to the back of the pubic bone. Unless the anterior bladder wall is freed and pulled upwards, one will not be able to expose the urethra and the urethrovesical junction. Proper identification of the urethrovesical junction is facilitated by palpation of the balloon of the Foley catheter at the bladder neck.

Primary Cases

Once the retropubic space is entered and the urethra is dropped downward with the anterior vaginal wall, no dissection should be done in the midline over the urethra. Whatever amount of tissue is covering it should be left undisturbed. In this way the delicate musculature of the urethra is protected from any possibility of surgical trauma. Attention should be directed to the anterior vaginal wall on either side of the urethra, again easily identified with the catheter in place. Most of the overlying fat should be cleared away to permit future firm adherence to any tissues brought into contact with it. This area is extremely vascular, having a rich thin-walled venous plexus that should be avoided as much as possible. After most of the fat is peeled off, the vesicourethral junction becomes more apparent. Again one can facilitate this step by palpating the Foley balloon or, even better, by partially distending the bladder and defining the rounded lower margin of the anterior bladder wall as it meets the anterior vaginal wall. No dissection should be done at the urethrovesical junction itself because, at that point, all the detrusor muscle fibers are moving downward to encircle the urethra, and every effort should be made to protect them from trauma. More laterally, however, the inferior margin of the bladder is identified and mobilized upward. Placing fingers in the vagina facilitates this dissection and also is essential to determine the extent of the needed mobilization and freeing of the anterior vaginal wall.

Repeat Cases

If previous retropubic repairs have been performed, exposure of the retropubic space becomes extremely difficult with dense adhesions from the anterior bladder wall and urethra to the symphysis pubis. Nevertheless, it is in such circumstances that the dissection must be impeccable if good results are to be achieved. These adhesions should be taken down sharply until the anterior bladder wall, urethra, and vagina are free and mobile. Utmost care must be taken not to lacerate or damage urethral or vesical musculature. If identification of the inferior margin of the bladder is difficult, one should consider opening the bladder; a finger inside the cavity helps to define its lower limit for easier dissection and mobilization.

Sutures

When mobilization has been completed, two fingers of the left hand should be placed in the vagina, lifting the anterior vaginal wall upward and forward. This will confirm adequate mobility and will lift the vesicourethral segment to a normal position. In addition, it will assist in complete mobilization of the retropubic space and better definition of the vesicourethral angle for proper placement of the sutures. Absorbable suture material (such as no. 1 Maxon) on an atraumatic needle is generally recommended. Nonabsorbable sutures are not necessary because sutures are meant to last only long enough for fibrosis, scarring of opposed tissues, and adhesions from extensive retropubic dissection to develop and fix the tissues in the properly suspended position. Its continuing fixation and support are going to be dependent on this rather than on the suture material holding it in place.

Positioning the sutures is an important step in the procedure, second only to proper mobilization. The sutures should be placed as far laterally as technically possible in the anterior vaginal wall. Two sutures are placed on either side parallel to the urethra. The distal suture is placed first, opposite to the middle part of the urethra. The proximal suture is the most important and is placed just below the reflection of the anterior bladder wall at the level of the urethrovesical junction yet far laterally from it. In placing these sutures, one should take a good bite in the vaginal wall parallel to the urethra, taking full thickness but sparing the mucosa and being guided by the vaginal finger at the appropriate sites (Fig. 32-2). All four sutures are placed into the vagina and left with their needles attached before being placed anteriorly. This area is extremely vascular, and visible vessels should be avoided if possible. If excessive bleeding occurs, it can be controlled by underrunning with figure-of-eight sutures. Bleeding commonly stops

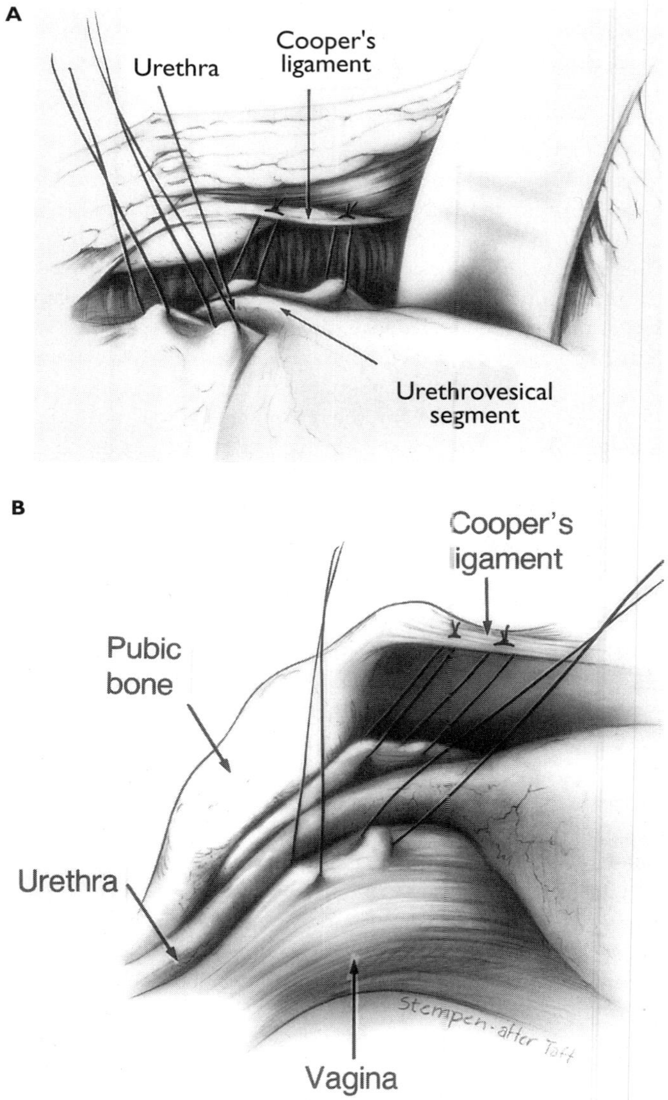

FIG. 32-2 ***A,*** *Diagram of retropubic space after mobilization of anterior vaginal wall and placement of sutures, two on either side and far lateral from the midline. Distal sutures are opposite the middle portion of the urethra, and proximal sutures are at the end of the vesicourethral junction. Sutures are attached to Cooper's ligament.* ***B,*** *Side view of suture placement with one side tied. Anterior vaginal wall is acting as a broad sling supporting and lifting the vesicourethral segment, yet the urethra is free in the retropubic space.*

once these fixation sutures are finally tied. Stanton has suggested placing the vaginal sutures slightly differently.[30] He recommends placing four sutures on each side: one suture distal to the bladder neck, one at the level of the bladder neck, and two proximally along the side of the bladder. The vaginal sutures are pulled straight upwards and attached to Cooper's ligament. The distal sutures are placed first, followed by the proximal sutures, which are placed in the same ligament but slightly laterally.

Once all sutures are placed, with the operator's fingers in the vagina lifting it upward and forward, the assistant ties the distal sutures and then the proximal ones. In tying the sutures one does not have to be concerned about whether the vaginal wall site of the suture meets Cooper's ligament, but one should not overdo the tension on the vaginal wall. The suture is approximated as close as the supporting fingers in the vagina feel it to be safe. There should be no tension on the sutures beyond that governed by the fingers lifting the vaginal wall. After the four sutures are tied, the vaginal fingers will feel immediately how much the vaginal wall is lifted upward and forward, carrying with it the vesicourethral segment. However, the latter is still free in the retropubic space (Fig. 32-3). One can easily insert two fingers between the pubic bone and the urethra. The urethra is in no way compressed against the bone. Again, it is the fibrosis and scarring that develop rather than the suture material that will hold the tissues in place. A drain is usually left in the retropubic space lateral to the sutures, and the wound is closed. The catheter is changed to a 16 Fr 5 ml Foley.

Postoperative Care

In addition to routine postoperative measures, some authors recommend keeping the patient on bed rest for 5 days with the catheter in place. Voiding after removal of the catheter is generally free, without problems of urinary retention or residual urine. If for any unexpected reason the patient has to strain to void, the catheter is reinserted for a few more days. This has been noted mostly in patients with an atonic bladder that did not demonstrate any detrusor activity in preoperative urodynamic studies. Postoperative activity is restricted for 3 to 4 months and gradually built up to the normal individual level.

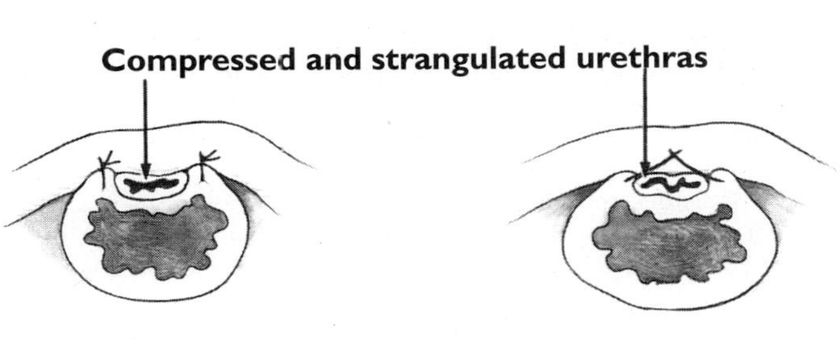

FIG. 32-3 Upper, *Cross-section shows the urethra free in the retropubic space with the anterior vaginal wall lifting and supporting it.* Lower, *The urethra is compressed and strangulated against the pubic bone when vaginal sutures are applied close to the urethra and then fixed to the symphysis pubis.*

Clinical Outcome

Our technique has been uniformly successful in primary cases. It has also been effective in patients who have experienced repeated previous failures when preoperative urodynamic evaluation has identified adequate sphincteric muscular activity. Poor results have been limited to those patients with intrinsic damage to the sphincteric mechanism from previous surgical attempts that traumatized and scarred the urethral musculature. In these situations, one is dealing with a noncompliant urethral segment. These patients cannot be regarded as having purely anatomic stress incontinence. The component of significant intrinsic sphincteric muscular damage may make them candidates for other approaches such as a sling procedure, artificial sphincter, or bladder neck reconstruction.

In our experience with retropubic suspension, this repair has been very durable with a long-term success rate as good as the short-term rate. Indeed, in our experience, once the surgical repair has been maintained for 6 months, it will hardly ever deteriorate, even with pregnancy and vaginal delivery. This has also been the experience of many other investigators who reported both short- and long-term results with a follow-up time ranging from 4 months to 10 years (Table 32-1). (Caveat: Most of these studies are limited by the lack of preoperative and postoperative objective urodynamic criteria to establish both the diagnosis and the cause of failure.)

Several studies looked at different preoperative factors that might allow one to predict the outcome of retropubic suspension procedures: age, parity, hormonal status, previous hysterectomy or antiincontinence surgery, and preoperative urodynamic findings (detrusor instability, functional urethral length, and maximal ure-

Table 32-1 **Long-term Results after Burch Colposuspension**

Series	Number of Patients	Success Rate (%)	Follow-up (Years)
Burch[7]	143	93	1 - 5
van Geelen et al.[31]	33	75.8	5 - 7
Ericksen et al.[32]	76	71	5
Feyereisl et al.[33]	87	81.6	5 - 10
Abu-Heija[34]	88	88	4
Vinagre et al.[35]	227	90	4
Lim et al.[36]	113	80	2 - 5
Gillion and Stanton[37]	35	88	3 - 5
Galloway et al[38]	50	84	1 - 6
Lose et al.[39]	80	63	4 mo – 6 yr
Rydhström and Iosif[40]	30	86	3
TOTAL	**962**	**81.7**	

thral closure pressure). Most authors believe that previous urinary incontinence surgery and maximal urethral closure pressure less than 20 cm H_2O greatly increase the risk of surgical failure. The presence of detrusor instability in addition to the genuine stress incontinence may also affect the success rate; however, in about 60% to 70% of patients with incontinence of mixed cause, detrusor instability resolves after urethropexy. Advanced age has been associated with a lower rate of cure in some studies,[41] but other studies have shown cure rates not significantly related to age, hormonal status, body weight, or previous hysterectomy.[32,33,42]

COMPLICATIONS

Detrusor Instability

Detrusor instability is a recognized postoperative complication that can develop in a previously stable bladder after successful surgery for stress incontinence, particularly the retropubic procedure. The pathophysiologic mechanism of this phenomenon is not clearly understood. It may be neurogenic and result from disruption of the autonomic innervation of the bladder,[43] or it may be obstructive and result from excessive urethral elevation or compression. Vierhout and Mulder,[44] in a review of six studies with a total of 396 patients who underwent Burch colposuspension, found an average incidence of detrusor instability of 17% (range 5% to 27%). Most cases can be controlled by anticholinergic medication, though a small but significant number will be resistant, and urinary incontinence may continue despite the successful correction of the anatomic defect.

Genital Prolapse and Enterocele

Genital prolapse and enterocele are relatively common complications after retropubic suspension. They were first reported by Burch,[7] who found that 7.6% of his patients developed enterocele a few years after the procedure; Langer et al. later reported an incidence of 13.6%.[45] Wiskind et al. reviewed the incidence of postoperative genital prolapse after Burch colposuspension and reported a rate of 26.7%.[46] They did not find any correlation between the patient's age, parity, weight, menopausal status, prior pelvic surgery, and the incidence of prolapse. The only risk factor identified was the presence of a large cystocele. The exact mechanism is not clear (whether attributable to disruption of the vaginal axis or to an intrinsic weakness of the pelvic floor).

Urinary Retention and Voiding Dysfunction

The complication of urinary retention and voiding dysfunction is more commonly seen after the MMK procedure because of placement of the sutures too close to the urethra. When these sutures are pulled upward, they will compress the urethra against the pubic bone, resulting in varying degrees of obstruction.[47] In our colpocystourethropexy, we usually don't encounter this complication except in patients with atonic or flaccid bladder.

Osteitis Pubis

Osteitis pubis is a painful inflammation of the periosteum of the pubic bone and occurs in about 2.5% of cases of the MMK procedure. The exact cause is not clear (an infectious process, trauma, or impaired circulation within the vessels of the pubic bone).

REFERENCES

1. Baker Brown I: Clinical lectures on some diseases of women remedial by operation, *Lancet* 1:263, 1864.
2. Kelly HA: Incontinence of urine in women, *Urol Cutan Rev* 17: 291, 1913.
3. Kelly HA, Dumm WM: Urinary incontinence in women without manifest injury to the bladder, *Surg Gynecol Obstet* 18:444, 1914.
4. Bonney V: On diurnal incontinence of urine in women, *J Obstet Gynecol Br Emp* 30:358, 1923.
5. Marshall VF, Marchetti AA, Krantz KE: The correction of stress incontinence by simple vesicourethral suspension, *Surg Gynecol Obstet* 88:509, 1949.
6. Burch JC: Urethrovaginal fixation to Cooper's ligament for correction of stress incontinence, cystocele and prolapse, *Am J Obstet Gynecol* 81:281, 1961.
7. Burch JC: Cooper's ligament urethrovesical suspension for stress incontinence, *Am J Obstet Gynecol* 100:764, 1968.
8. Tanagho EA: Colpocystourethropexy: the way we do it, *J Urol* 116:751, 1976.
9. Murnaghan GF: Colposuspension in the management of stress incontinence, *Br J Urol* 47:236, 1975
10. Hutch JA: The internal urethral urinary sphincter: a double loop system, *J Urol* 105:375, 1971.
11. Donker PJ, Droes JThPM, van Ulden BM: Anatomy of the musculature and innervation of the bladder and urethra. In Williams DI, Chisholm GD, editors: *Scientific foundations of urology,* London, 1976, Heinemann.
12. Tanagho EA, Smith DR: Anatomy and function of the bladder neck, *Br J Urol* 38:54, 1966.
13. Tanagho EA, Smith DR: Mechanism of urinary continence. 1. Embryologic, anatomic and pathologic considerations, *J Urol* 100:640, 1968.
14. Tanagho EA: The anatomy and physiology of micturition, *Clin Obstet Gynecol* 5:3, 1978.
15. Tanagho EA, Meyers FH, Smith DR: Urethral resistance: its components and implications. I. Smooth muscle component, *Invest Urol* 7:139, 1969
16. Hickey DS, Phillips JI, Hukins DWL: Arrangement of collagen fibers and muscle fibers in the female urethra and their implications for the control of micturition, *Br J Urol* 54:556, 1982.
17. Juenemann KP, Lue TF, Schmidt RA, Tanagho EA: Clinical significance of sacral and pudendal nerve anatomy, *J Urol* 139:74, 1988.
18. Pereyra AJ: A simplified surgical procedure for the correction of stress incontinence in women, *West J Surg Obstet Gynecol* 67:223, 1959.
19. Stamey TA: Endoscopic suspension of the vesical neck for urinary incontinence, *Surg Gynecol Obstet* 136:547, 1973.
20. Raz S: Modified bladder neck suspension for female stress incontinence, *Urology* 18:82, 1981.
21. Bergman A, Koonings PP, Ballard CA: Primary stress urinary incontinence and pelvic relaxation: prospective randomized comparison of three different operations, *Am J Obstet Gynecol* 161:97, 1989.
22. Turner-Warwick R: The Turner-Warwick vagino-obturator shelf VOS urethral repositioning procedure. In Abrams P, Gingell JC, editors: *Controversies and innovations in urological surgery,* Berlin, 1988, Springer-Verlag.
23. Richardson AC, Edmond PB, Williams NL: Treatment of stress urinary incontinence due to paravaginal fascial defect, *Obstet Gynecol* 57:357, 1981.
24. Goodno JA Jr, Powers TW: Modified retropubic cystourethropexy. II. *Am J Obstet Gynecol* 166:1678, 1992.
25. Riza ED, Deshmukh AS: A laparoscopic-assisted extraperitoneal bladder neck suspension: an initial experience, *J Laparoendosc Surg* 4:319, 1994

26. Liu CY: Laparoscopic treatment for genuine urinary stress incontinence, *Baillieres Clin Obstet Gynecol* 8:789, 1994.
27. Sanchez de Bajadoz E, Jimenez Garrido A, Gutierrez de la cruz JM, Vara Thorbeck C: [Extraperitoneal laparoscopic urethropexy], *Arch Espanol Urol* 47:415, 1994.
28. von Theobald P, Barjot P, Liegeois P, et al: [Laparoscopic colposuspension by the Burch technique by celioscopy], *Presse Méd* 23:1301, 1994.
29. Ou CS, Presthus J, Beadle E: Laparoscopic bladder neck suspension using hernia mesh and surgical staples, *J Laparoendosc Surg* 3:563, 1993.
30. Hodgkinson CP, Stanton SL: Retropubic urethropexy or colpo-suspension. In Stanton SL, Tanagho EA, editors: *Surgery of female incontinence,* Berlin, 1980, Springer-Verlag.
31. van Geelen JM, Theeuwes AG, Eskes TK, Martin CB Jr: The clinical and urodynamic effects of anterior vaginal repair and Burch colposuspension, *Am J Obstet Gynecol* 159:137, 1988.
32. Eriksen BC, Hagen B, Eik-Nes SH, et al: Long-term effectiveness of the Burch colposuspension in female urinary stress incontinence, *Acta Obstet Gynecol Scand* 69:45, 1990.
33. Feyereisl J, Dreher E, Haenggi W, et al: Long-term results after Burch colposuspension, *Am J Obstet Gynecol* 171:647, 1994.
34. Abu-Heija AT: Long-term results of colposuspension operation for genuine stress incontinence, *Asia Oceania J Obstet Gynaecol* 20:179, 1994.
35. Vinagre M, Pardo H, Roa E, de la Fuente S: Colposuspension in the treatment of stress urinary incontinence: long-term yield, *Rev Chil Obstet Ginecol* 56:284, 1991.
36. Lim PH, Brown AD, Chisholm GD: The Burch colposuspension operation for stress urinary incontinence, *Singapore Med J* 31:242, 1990.
37. Gillion G, Stanton SL: Long-term follow up of surgery for urinary incontinence in elderly women, *Br J Urol* 56:478, 1984.
38. Galloway NT, Davies N, Stephenson TP: The complications of colposuspension, *Br J Urol* 60:122, 1987.
39. Lose G, Jorgensen L, Mortensen SO, et al: Voiding difficulties after colposuspension, *Obstet Gynecol* 69:33, 1987.
40. Rydhström H, Iosif CS: Urodynamic studies before and after retropubic colpourethrocystopexy in fertile women with stress urinary incontinence, *Arch Gynecol Obstet* 241:201, 1988.
41. Kjølhede P, Rydén G: Prognostic factors and long-term results of the Burch colposuspension: a retrospective study, *Acta Obstet Gynecol Scand* 73:642, 1994.
42. Gillion G, Engelstein D, Servadio C: Risk factors and their effect on the results of Burch colposuspension for urinary stress incontinence, *Israel J Med Sci* 28:354, 1992.
43. Cardozo L.D, Stanton SL, Williams JE: Detrusor instability following surgery for genuine stress incontinence, *Br J Urol* 51:204, 1979.
44. Vierhout ME, Mulder AF: De novo detrusor instability after Burch colposuspension, *Acta Obstet Gynecol Scand* 71:414, 1992.
45. Langer R, Ron-El R, Newman M, et al: Detrusor instability following colposuspension for urinary stress incontinence, *Br J Obstet Gynecol* 95:607, 1988
46. Wiskind AK Creighton SM, Stanton SL: The incidence of genital prolapse after the Burch colposuspension, *Am J Obstet Gynecol* 167:399, 1992.
47. Zimmern PE Hadley HR, Leach GE, Raz S: Female urethral obstruction after Marshall-Marchetti-Krantz operation, *J Urol* 138:517, 1987.

Chapter 33

Anterior Vaginal Wall Sling

Shlomo Raz, Lynn Stothers, A. Chopra

The vaginal wall sling is a surgical technique for treatment of stress urinary incontinence in women who have both anatomic incontinence and intrinsic sphincter deficiency. The surgical concept that leads to the development of this technique includes: (1) a need to correct a defect of midurethral support, (2) the application of anatomic principles of the levator musculature as it envelopes the urethra just distal to the pubourethral ligaments. The anterior vaginal wall sling involves construction of a urethral sling from the anterior vaginal wall and underlying fascia, which provides both compression and support for the midportion of the urethra and the bladder neck.

ANATOMY

Support of the bladder and anterior vaginal wall is primarily the function of the levator musculature and its associated fascial attachments. The levator muscle is shaped like a bowl and creates a floor for the pelvis. A hiatus is present for the rectum, vagina, and urethra. A view of the levator as seen from an abdominal view is shown in Fig. 33-1.

The levator muscle is composed of two groups of muscles; the pubococcygeus and the iliococcygeus. The pubococcygeus originates from the pubic bone and anterior portion of the tendinous arc. It extends posteriorly to its insertion at the median raphe between the rectum and the coccyx. The iliococcygeus originates from the tendinous arc of the obturator and inserts into the anococcygeal ligament and the lateral aspect of the coccyx.

A central hiatus in this muscle group, the levator hiatus, allows passage of the urethra, vagina, and rectum. The location of the insertion of the levator musculature onto the inferior margin of the pubis should be noted. It is this insertion point that is included in the anterior vaginal wall sling. The fascia of the levator musculature has both an abdominal side and a vaginal side. As such, this fascia forms a sandwich conceptually, covering the bladder and urethra. Both the abdominal and vaginal layers come together to insert into a common location, which is the tendinous arc of the obturator. The abdominal side of the levator fascia is commonly referred to as the endopelvic fascia. The vaginal side is called the urethropelvic fascia at the level of the urethra and the vesicopelvic fascia at the level of the bladder.

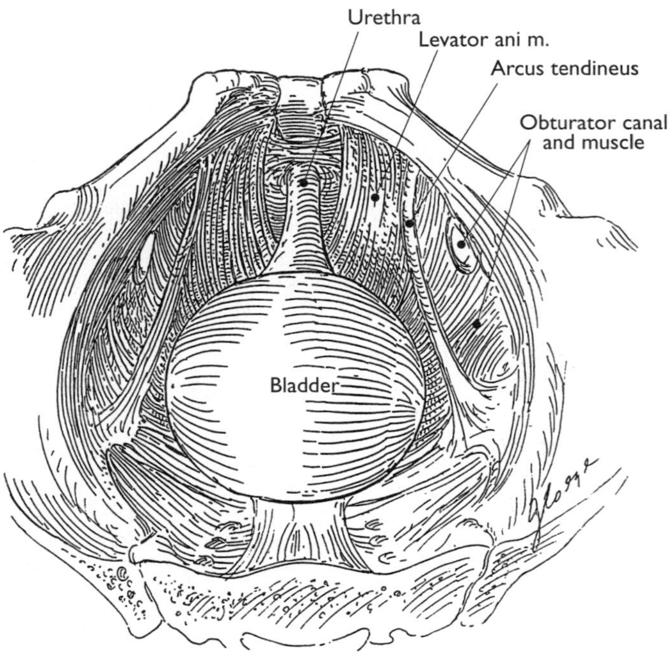

FIG. 33-1 *Abdominal view of the pelvic anatomy. The levator and coccygeus muscles support the pelvic viscera. The medial edges of the levator muscles fuse posteriorly, but anteriorly they form a hiatus for the passage of the urethra, vagina, and rectum. The pubococcygeal segment of the levator complex originates in the tendinous arc, a thickening of the obturator fascia.* (From Walsh PC, Retik AB, Stamey TA, Vaughan ED, editors: *Campbell's urology,* ed 6, Philadelphia, 1992, Saunders.)

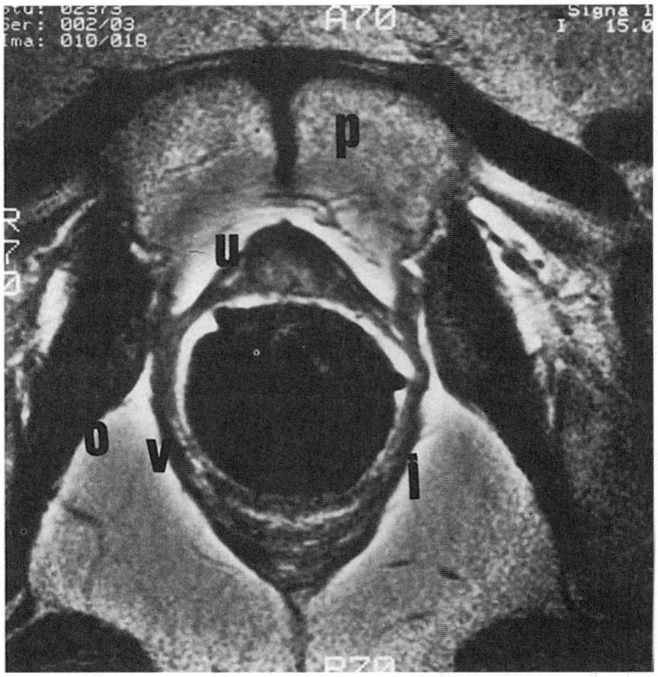

FIG. 33-2 *Magnetic resonance imaging of the urethropelvic ligament. The vagina* (in black) *is round and distended by an intravaginal coil. The urethropelvic ligament is seen stretching from the urethra to the tendinous arc (insertion site of the levator muscle to the obturator fascia).* l, *Levator muscle;* o, *obturator muscle;* p, *pubic bone;* u, *urethra;* v, *vaginal wall distended by coil.* (From Raz S: *Atlas of transvaginal surgery,* Philadelphia, 1992, Saunders.)

The levator fascia has several significant condensations that provide support. The *pubourethral ligaments* suspend the midurethra from the undersurface of the pubic bone. The *urethropelvic ligament* surrounds the urethra from the external meatus to the bladder neck. The urethropelvic ligament is exposed during dissection in preparation to form the anterior vaginal wall sling. Magnetic resonance imaging clearly demonstrated the urethropelvic ligament as shown in Fig. 33-2. The *cardinal ligaments* extend laterally from the cervix and upper vagina and anchor these structures to the pelvic sidewall. The *uterosacral ligaments* attach to the posterolateral cervix and extend to the periosteum of the fourth sacral vertebra. It is important to remember that conceptually all these ligaments are regions or specialized condensations of the same fascia—the levator fascia—which through its various ligamentous regions provides support to the urethra, bladder and cervix.

ANATOMIC CLINICAL CORRELATES

Anatomic incontinence results from loss of pelvic support of the bladder neck and urethra through several factors including birth trauma, posthysterectomy status, lack of estrogen, pelvic denervation, congenital weakness, or aging. A combination of factors frequently coexist in a single patient. In patients who have anatomic incontinence, the physical examination and videourodynamic testing reveal hypermobility of the bladder neck and urethra with increases in abdominal pressure. Video and MRI studies may reveal a further defect, which includes separation of the urethra from the symphysis pubis.

The diagnosis of intrinsic sphincter dysfunction (ISD) is based on a combination of factors including history, physical examination, voiding cystourethrogram, urethral pressure profile, and leak point pressure. In contrast to anatomic incontinence, intrinsic sphincter dysfunction (ISD) may be apparent when the bladder neck and proximal urethra are open at rest, in the absence of detrusor contraction. The urethra may be radiologically closed, but the patient may have ISD, as evidenced by a well-supported bladder neck and urethra that leaks with small increases in abdominal pressure. The cause of ISD may be multifactorial including damage to the sphincter mechanism from multiple prior surgeries, radiation, direct trauma, or neurologic dysfunction.

SURGICAL TECHNIQUE

As a basic principle, a sling can be created by the use of autologous fascial strips (rectus fascia, fascia lata, and so forth), by burying vaginal mucosa, or by the use of permanent sutures placed into the periurethral supporting structures. The anterior vaginal wall sling makes use of the latter concept and uses the patient's normal surrounding anatomic features to construct a hammock of support. The surgical goals of the anterior vaginal wall sling are (1) to provide elastic support to the urethra and (2) to create a strong hammock of vaginal wall and underlying tissues to provide a backboard to increase coaptation and support.

The patient is placed in the dorsal lithotomy position. The vagina and lower abdomen are prepared with an iodine scrub. A weighted vaginal speculum and labial retraction sutures are used for exposure. A suprapubic tube using the Lowsley retractor and urethral catheter are placed. After saline infiltration of the anterior vaginal wall tissues to facilitate dissection, two longitudinal incisions are made in the anterior vaginal wall (Fig. 33-3). Dissection is carried out over the glistening periurethral fascia with the Metzenbaum scissors. The attachment of the urethropelvic fascia to the tendinous arc of the obturator is identified. With the curved Mayo scissors, the retropubic space is entered at the level of the tendinous arc (Fig. 33-4). Any adhesions encountered in the retropubic space are divided by means of a combination of blunt and sharp dissection (Fig. 33-5). The urethropelvic ligament is exposed.

Two no. 1 Prolene (polypropylene) sutures are placed on each side during creation of the anterior vaginal wall sling. The first no. 1 Prolene suture includes the vesicopelvic fascia, the urethropelvic ligament, and the anterior vaginal wall without epithelium. The arc of the needle should include a large area of tissue in both the vesicopelvic fascia and the urethropelvic ligament. With a forceps in the retropubic space the second no. 1 Prolene suture is placed. This suture includes the levator ani musculature as it inserts onto the midurethral segment, the medial edge of the urethropelvic ligament, and the anterior vaginal wall without epithelium. Placement of these sutures is depicted in Fig. 33-6. To obtain an adequate amount of levator tissue one must place the needle deep into the retropubic space, and the levator musculature is included as it inserts onto the pubic bone as shown in Fig. 33-1. The levator should be visualized on the arc of the needle. When the anterior vaginal wall without epithelium is taken, the arc of the needle should not cross the midline but should include a generous amount of tissue.

A stab incision in the lower abdomen is made 1 to 1.5 cm anterior to the symphysis pubic. Blunt dissection with a clamp should expose the rectus fascia. The double-pronged needle is

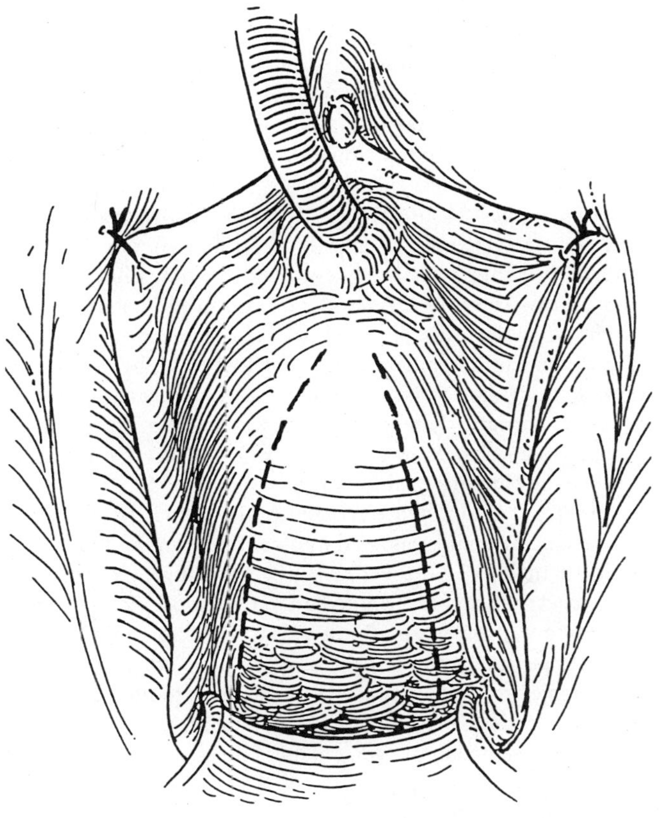

FIG. 33-3 *Incisions for the anterior vaginal wall sling. Retraction is aided by the weighted speculum posteriorly and lateral silk retraction sutures in the labia.* (From Raz S: *Atlas of transvaginal surgery*, Philadelphia, 1992, Saunders.)

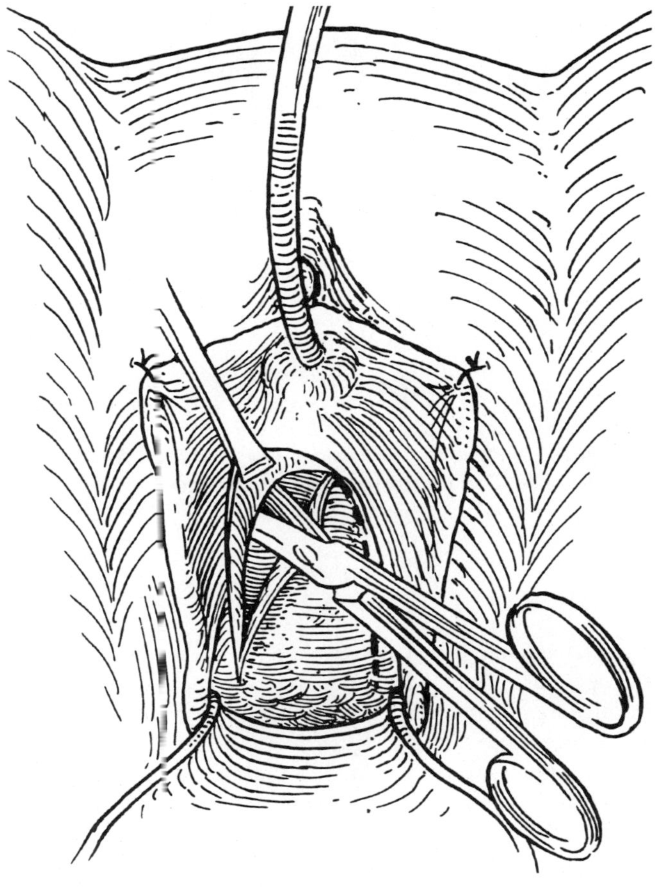

FIG. 33-4 *The Metzenbaum scissors are used to dissect over the glistening surface of the periurethral fascia. The retropubic space is entered using the curved Mayo scissors, with the scissors pointed toward the ipsilateral shoulder of the patient. This maneuver results in entering of the retropubic space and exposes the urethropelvic ligament, which will be incorporated in the Prolene (polypropyline) sutures.* (From Raz S: *Atlas of transvaginal surgery*, Philadelphia, 1992, Saunders.)

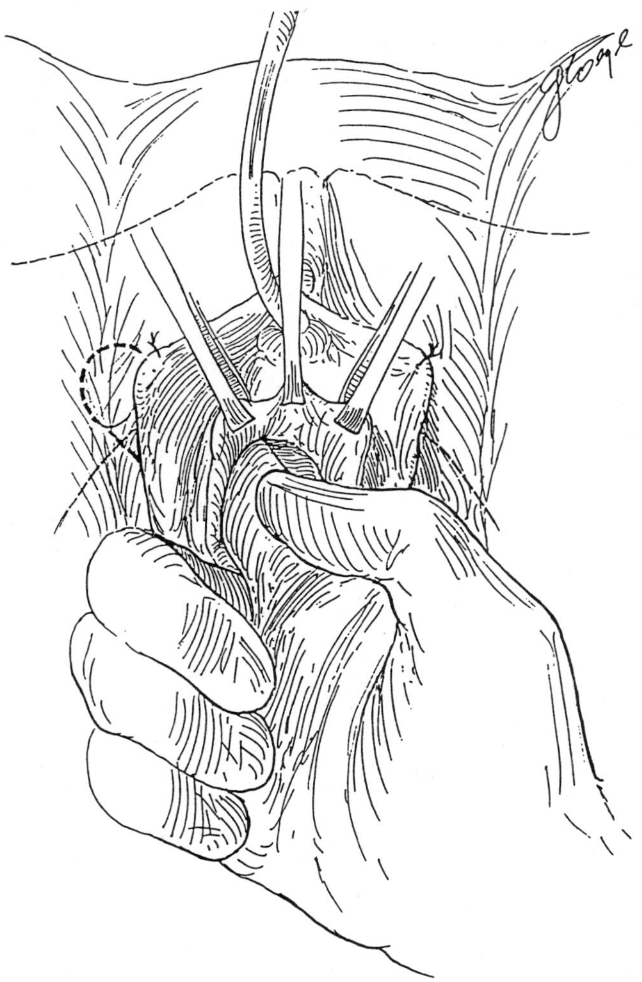

FIG. 33-5 *A finger is inserted into the retropubic space and adhesions or previous sutures are palpated. Adhesions or prior suture material are then divided by use of a combination of sharp and blunt dissection.* (From Raz S: *Atlas of transvaginal surgery*, Philadelphia, 1992, Saunders.)

passed, scratching the symphysis into the retropubic space onto the operator's finger, which is placed into the retropubic space through the vaginal incision. Under fingertip control the needle is advanced through the vaginal incision, and the ends of the Prolene suture are passed through the eyes of the needle. One then transfers the suture to the lower abdomen by pulling the needle. When all four sutures have been transferred to the lower abdominal stab incision, cystoscopy is carried out. The patient is given indigo carmine, and blue efflux should be noted from both ureteral orifices. The location of the suprapubic catheter is noted, and the side walls of the bladder and trigone are inspected to ensure that no suture has passed within the bladder. The urethral Foley catheter is then replaced, and the anterior vaginal wall incisions are closed with a running and locking absorbable suture. A vaginal pack covered with sulfonamide cream is placed and the suspension sutures are tied down without undue tension. The suprapubic wound is closed with a subcuticular 4-0 absorbable suture and Steri-Strip tapes. Both the suprapubic tube and the urethral catheter are placed to straight drainage.

This procedure is currently performed on an outpatient. Within 24 hours the vaginal pack and urethral catheter are removed. The suprapubic tube is clamped and placed in slight traction to prevent leakage around the tube. The patient is asked to void through her urethra and to check her own postvoid residual urines. Oral antibiotics, stool softeners, and oral analgesics are given to the patient to use after discharge. Antibiotics are continued while the suprapubic tube is in place. The suprapubic catheter is removed once the postvoid residuals are consistently less than 2 ounces.

In contrast to other techniques for formation of a sling, no vaginal flaps are created, no transverse incision is made over the urethral area or the area of the bladder neck, and no vaginal tissue is buried. The advantage of this technique lies in its simplicity, avoidance of a laparotomy, short hospital stay, lateral placement of permanent nonreactive sutures, and the ability to correct grade I and grade II cystocele. It is important to note that the technique relies on healthy, well-vascularized supporting tissues.

Measuring Outcome After Incontinence Surgery

There currently exists a voluminous literature on both the surgical and nonsurgical treatment for stress urinary incontinence. A significant problem in the review of this literature is evident when one begins to examine the various ways in which we measure the outcome of our treatment. For example, success outcome of therapy has been defined by various authors as less than one episode of incontinence per week, less than one episode of incontinence per day, use of no pads per day, less than 2 wet pads per day, complete dryness at 3, 6, or 12 months after therapy, and so forth. It is immediately evident that it is impossible to make valid comparisons of treatments from within and between institutions when such discrepancies in measurement exist. Recent advances in clinical epidemiology have lead to sophisticated validation processes for clinical outcome scores. Such outcome scores are particularly relevant to the treatment of stress incontinence because the aim of therapy is based on the ability to improve the patient's quality of life.

The SEAPI incontinence classification system is a scoring system designed for and validated in incontinent individuals.[1] The system is analogous to the TNM system for tumor staging and each aspect of the score is graded between 0 and 3. *Zero* indicates no symptom, problem, or abnormality, and 1, 2, and 3 are correspondingly increasing severity of symptoms. When applicable, both a subjective and an objective score can be graded separately for a given patient. Five domains are covered by the SEAPI score and are represented in the score name: *S* for stress activity related incontinence, *E* for emptying ability, *A* for anatomy, *P* for protection, and *I* for inhibition. The score is shown in Appendixes E and F at the end of the text.

Various other methods of measuring outcomes of stress incontinence therapies reported in the literature. The Pyridium (phenazopyridine HCl) pad test and quantitative weighing of

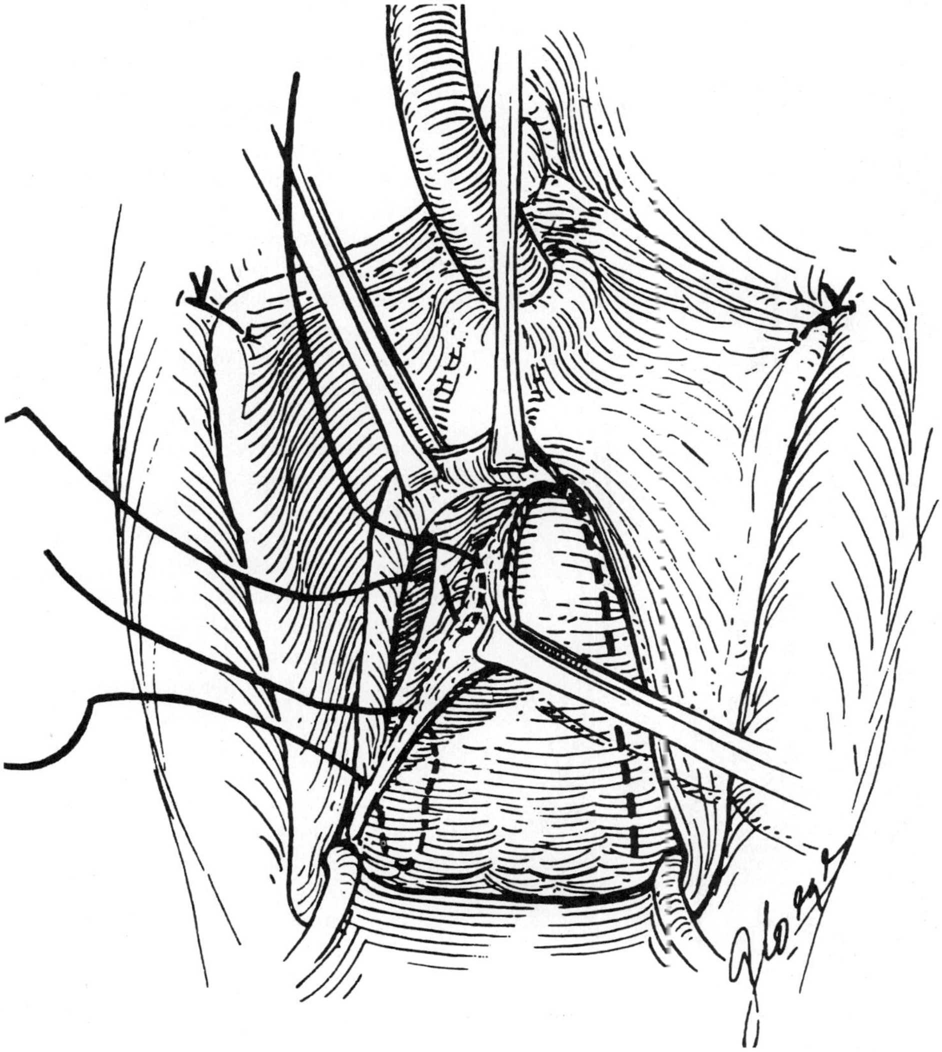

FIG. 33-6 *Placement of the Prolene sutures on one side of the dissection is shown. The first suture is placed at the level of the bladder neck. This suture includes the vesicopelvic fascia, the urethropelvic ligament, and the anterior vaginal wall without epithelium. Notice that the entire arc of the needle should be utilized to incorporate a significant amount of the vesicopelvic fascia and the urethropelvic ligament in the suture. The second Prolene suture is placed at the midurethral level. This suture includes the levator musculature, the edge of the urethropelvic ligament, and the anterior vaginal wall without epithelium. Allis clamps should be used to facilitate exposure. After placement of the contralateral sutures, the Prolene sutures are transferred through the retropubic space with the use of the double-pronged needle carrier.* (From Raz S: *Female urology*, Philadelphia, publication pending, Saunders.)

pads to detect urinary leakage has been compared by Wall et al.[2] In this study 23 normal volunteers without stress urinary incontinence (SUI) were compared to 18 urodynamically proved stress-incontinent females. The accuracy of the qualitative pad test with Pyridium staining was compared to the quantitative pad weight to detect the presence of SUI in the two groups. The authors found that in the group with stress incontinence all 18 had positive Pyridium pad tests and positive pad weight gains of over 1 g. However, 52% of healthy volunteers had a positive Pyridium pad test. The mean pad weight gain in the volunteer group was 0.1 g. Therefore the Pyridium pad test had a high false-positive rate in continent volunteers and would be misleading as an outcome measure if pad-weighing tests were not performed. This emphasizes the need for common outcome measures when reporting the results of therapy for patients with stress incontinence.

RESULTS

One hundred thirty-seven females underwent the sling procedure between June of 1992 and June of 1994 at our institution.[3] Preoperative evaluation included lateral cystography, videouro-

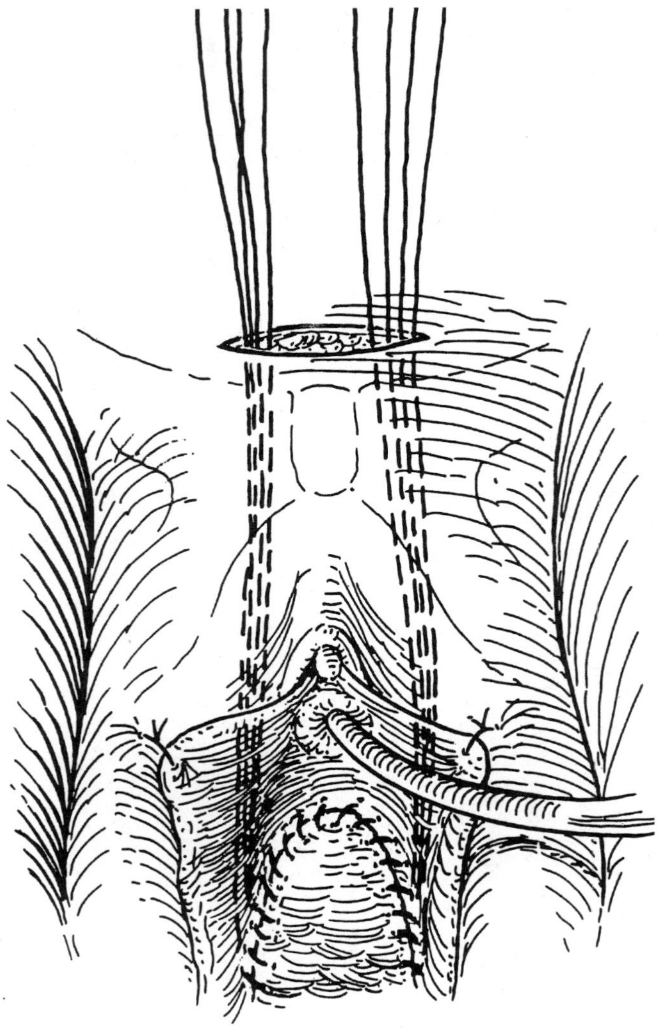

FIG. 33-7 *Diagram showing the Prolene sutures transferred through the lower abdominal stab incision. The vaginal wall should be closed with a running, locking, polyglycolic acid suture and a vaginal pack placed before the Prolene sutures are tied down. The Prolene sutures are carefully tied over the rectus fascia, without undue tension.* (From Raz S: *Female urology,* Philadelphia, publication pending, Saunders.

dynamics, cystoscopy, quality of life measures, and SEAPI incontinence classification (see above). Postoperative outcome measures were prospectively assigned on a 6-monthly basis by a third party and included SEAPI, quality-of-life scores, and assessment of any complications. Statistics were applied using SPSS* computer software to create regression models for outcome variables of interest.

The median follow-up time is 11 months (range 3 to 24 months). Age ranged from 32 to 81 years. Three patients were lost to follow-up study. Of the 134 evaluable, 91 had intrinsic sphincter dysfunction (ISD) and 42 anatomic incontinence (AI). Overall, 54% of patients had undergone an average of 2.5 prior procedures for stress incontinence. Associated urgency incontinence was common preoperatively and was seen clinically in 47% of patients. One hundred twenty-nine patients were considered cured at last follow-up examination and had clinical SEAPI scores of S0-1, E0, A0, P0-1. Five of 134 patients were considered failures, having late recurrent incontinence that was unrelated to instability and required further therapy. Time to failure comparing ISD and AI patients was modeled by use of Kaplan-Meier survival curves, and the logrank test showed no significant difference between groups ($p > 0.05$). Conditional logistic regression covariates revealed no significant predictive factors for postoperative failures. Seven percent of patients developed renewed instability. Preoperative patient age was the only predictive factor of renewed instability identified by the logistic regression model ($p < 0.05$). Preoperative and postoperative within-patient changes of quality-of-life scores were statistically significantly different for patients with both ISD and AI.

SUMMARY

A better understanding of the pelvic anatomy through the advent of magnetic resonance imaging has led to modifications of standard bladder neck suspension procedures for the treatment of stress incontinence. The initial results of the anterior vaginal wall sling indicate that continence was achieved in patients with both ISD and AI. Further follow-up study will be required to establish the longevity of these results. Currently the procedure may be safely performed in outpatients with low morbidity and a high degree of acceptance by each patient.

*SPSS is a registered trademark of SPSS Inc., 444 North Michigan Ave., Chicago, Ill.

REFERENCES

1. Raz S, Erickson DR: SEAPI QMM incontinence classification system, *Neurourol Urodyn* 11:187-199, 1992.
2. Wall LL, Wang K, Robson I, Stanton SL: The Pyridium pad test for diagnosing urinary incontinence: a comparative study of asymptomatic and incontinent women, *J Reprod Med* 35(7):682-684, 1990.
3. Stothers L, Chopra A, Raz S: Vaginal wall sling for anatomic incontinence and intrinsic sphincter damage: efficacy and outcome analysis, *J Urol*, 153:525A, 1995.

Chapter 34 Pubovaginal Sling Procedure

E. Ann Gormley, Edward J. McGuire

The use of a pubovaginal sling for the treatment of urinary incontinence was first described in 1907 by Von Giordano.[1] After a variety of modifications the procedure became known as the Goebell-Stoeckel-Frangenheim operation.[2-4] Initially slings were fashioned from muscle including the pyramidalis, gracilis, levator ani, rectus, and bulbocavernosus. Price described the first fascial sling in 1933.[4] He used a strip of fascia lata and passed the fascia beneath the urethra from a suprapubic approach fixing the ends of the sling to the rectus muscles. In the 1940s Millen, a urologist, and Aldridge, a gynecologist, described the creation of slings using paired strips of rectus fascia.[5,6] Millen looped the strips under the urethra and then tied them together over the top of the urethra, whereas Aldridge sutured the strips together underneath the urethra. Aldridge noted that one of the advantages of the procedure the way he did it was the automatic compression of the urethra when the rectus muscle contracted during coughing or straining.[6] Now some 50 years later we continue to take advantage of the same mechanical advantage, particularly for the patient with poor resting closure of the intrinsic proximal sphincter. We now recognize that a standard suspension operation does not close an open proximal urethra whereas a sling can both coapt the proximal urethra and restore the bladder neck to its correct anatomic position.

Diagnosis of Stress Urinary Incontinence

Stress urinary incontinence is leakage of urine in association with an increase in abdominal pressure such as that associated with coughing, lifting, exercise, or laughing. The diagnosis of stress urinary incontinence therefore rests on the demonstration of urethral urinary leakage associated with an increase in abdominal pressure. An important part of the assessment of stress urinary incontinence is measurement of the amount of abdominal pressure required to cause leakage. A normally functioning intrinsic urethral sphincter prevents urethral loss of urine with any rise in abdominal pressure. Patients with anatomic stress urinary incontinence which is due to urethral movement will leak at relatively high abdominal pressure. A patient with an intrinsic sphincter that closes poorly will leak at low (<60 H_2O) abdominal pressure.[7] Incontinence associated with intrinsic sphincteric dysfunction has been called type III stress urinary incontinence, or intrinsic sphincter deficiency. Intrinsic sphincter deficiency was initially described in women who had failed one or more operations for stress incontinence.[8,9] The patient with intrinsic sphincter deficiency will often report that the prior procedure not only did not help their incontinence but also appeared to make it worse. Intrinsic sphincteric deficiency associated with prior operative failure has been attributed to urethral and periurethral scarring and fibrosis, though this has never been documented pathologically. Intrinsic sphincter deficiency may also be neural in origin as in individuals with myelodysplasia, sacral agenesis, and T12 spinal cord injury. In these conditions there is usually loss of proximal urethral sphincter closing function but preservation of external sphincter function. Other causes include radiation or alpha-adrenergic receptor blockers. Approximately 10% of women who present with stress incontinence will have intrinsic sphincter deficiency with no predisposing factors.[10] These women are typically older and describe a sudden onset of severe incontinence.

Patient Selection

Traditionally slings have been used for patients with intrinsic sphincteric dysfunction. In addition to those patients who demonstrate a defect in proximal urethral sphincter function there are individual circumstances that favor the use of a sling because of the strength and durability of that procedure. Among these relative indications are a very obese patient, a patient with poor paravaginal tissue, a patient who enjoys extreme physical activity such as gymnastics, and patients with chronic pulmonary conditions especially severe asthma, or progressive chronic obstructive pulmonary disease. Blaivas and others have suggested that for the experienced pelvic surgeon the pubovaginal sling offers the best chance for long-term cure of stress incontinence from either intrinsic sphincter deficiency or urethral hypermobility.[11] A sling is a very reasonable treatment option for the woman with anatomic stress incontinence provided that she is willing to perform intermittent catheterization in the postoperative period. Slings may also be used to effect complete closure of a damaged or nonfunctional urethra in combination with augmentation cystoplasty and construction of an abdominal neourethra or an ileovesicostomy. A sling is a suitable procedure for patients of any age provided that the patient or caregiver can provide intermittent catheterization should that be required. The procedure has been used for patients ranging in age from 10 to 83 years.

A potential candidate for the procedure must demonstrate reasonable bladder storage ability (compliance). Poor compliance may potentially be exacerbated by the increased urethral resistance provided by the sling. Although it is very unusual for this to occur, it is better preoperatively to be as certain as possible that the bladder stores a reasonable volume at low pressure. A sling is not an effective barrier to bladder pressure as an expulsive force and leakage driven by bladder pressure will recur at progressively lower bladder volumes after the sling procedure. In those situations where poor compliance coexists with poor urethral resistance a sling must be combined with some treatment that either reduces bladder pressure or enlarges bladder capacity.

The relationship between stress incontinence, urge incontinence, and an unstable detrusor is complex. Some 30% of patients with videourodynamically identified stress incontinence will have both urge incontinence and demonstrable detrusor instability during a filling cystometrogram (CMG).[9,12] Another 20% to 30% of women with videourodynamically proved stress incontinence will also complain of urge incontinence. In this group the filling CMG will not demonstrate any detrusor overactivity; that is, they will have a perfectly normal CMG. Additionally, some patients with no symptoms of urge incontinence will, on a filling CMG, demonstrate uninhibited detrusor contractions. The CMG therefore is not a method to establish or confirm the diagnosis of "urge incontinence." A patient with objectively established stress incontinence and a normal CMG is not necessarily a better operative candidate than a patient with stress and urge incontinence with or without a CMG that shows detrusor instability.

Seventy percent of patients with both stress and urge incontinence are relieved of both conditions by an operation that cures their stress incontinence.[12] To complicate matters, about 2% to 6 % of all patients undergoing any operation for stress incontinence will develop, early, usually transient, de novo urge incontinence.[13] In patients with persistent urge incontinence after surgery, including those who develop the problem de novo, treatment with drugs or occasionally operative methods may be required. The nonoperative treatment of urge incontinence associated with severe stress incontinence is almost never effective and is probably not worthwhile. In other words, women with intrinsic sphincter deficiency and urge incontinence will not benefit from anticholinergic therapy in lieu of surgery or injection therapy.

PATIENT EVALUATION

History

The onset, frequency, severity, and pattern of incontinence should be sought as well as any associated symptoms such as frequency, dysuria, urgency, or nocturia. One may quantify incontinence by asking the patient if she wears pads and how often the pads are changed. Patients with intrinsic sphincter deficiency will often be very wet with minimal activity. Obstructive symptoms, such as a feeling of incomplete emptying, hesitancy, straining, or weak stream, may coexist with incontinence particularly in patients with previous bladder suspension, cystoceles, or poor detrusor contractility. Response to previous treatments, including drugs, should be noted. Patients should be asked regarding symptoms of pelvic prolapse such as recurrent urinary tract infection, a sensation of vaginal fullness or pressure, or the observation of a bulge in the vagina. All incontinent patients should be asked about bowel function and neurologic symptoms.

Important features of the past history include previous gynecologic or urologic procedures, neurologic problems, and past medical problems. A list of the patient's current medications, including use of over-the-counter medications, should be obtained. A knowledge of the patient's social history, including the type of physical exercise she does or would like to do, may also be important.

Physical

A physical examination is performed with emphasis on the abdominal, pelvic, and rectal examination and a neurologic assessment. The condition of the vaginal mucosa and the degree of urethral mobility is determined. A simple pelvic examination with the patient supine is sufficient to determine if the urethra moves with straining or coughing. The degree of movement is not so important as the determination of whether movement occurs. Urethral leakage with straining in the supine position is seen in many patients with intrinsic sphincter deficiency. The presence of associated vaginal prolapse should also be noted. The pelvic exam is repeated in the upright position in the search for a cystocele, rectocele, enterocele, or uterine prolapse. These conditions, when identified, should be repaired at the same time as the sling is done.

Postvoid residual

A postvoid residual (PVR) should be measured when the patient is catheterized for urodynamics. A normal PVR is less than 50 ml, and a PVR in excess of 200 ml is abnormal. A significant PVR urine may reflect either bladder outlet obstruction or poor bladder contractility. The only way to distinguish outlet obstruction from poor contractility is with urodynamic testing.

Urodynamics

Urodynamic testing is used to accurately diagnose the patient's incontinence. A cystometrogram allows one to assess bladder behavior during filling. Normally bladder pressure remains flat during filling. If bladder pressure rises incrementally during filling, a diagnosis of poor compliance is made. Poor bladder compliance makes the assessment of bladder neck and urethral function difficult, since the rise in bladder pressure and accompanying leakage may occur before stress incontinence can be provoked. Poor compliance and poor urethral function may coexist.

When urethral resistance is very low, leakage may occur during filling, and bladder urine storage function may appear to be good when it is in fact poor. A Foley catheter with the balloon inflated and pulled down to occlude the bladder neck may be required for an accurate assessment of the ability of the bladder to store urine at low pressures.[14]

The most common abnormality of bladder function is detrusor overactivity that causes urge incontinence. Detrusor overactivity is defined as the inability to suppress involuntary detrusor contractions during filling.[15] As noted earlier, a cystometrogram may fail to demonstrate any detrusor overactivity in a patient who has urge incontinence by history. Other patients with no history of urge incontinence will have uninhibited detrusor contractions during filling. Any patients with symptoms of urge incontinence by history should be presumed to have urge incontinence. The purpose of urodynamics in the patient with stress incontinence is not to diagnose detrusor overactivity but to diagnose the type of stress incontinence and to ensure that the patient has a reasonable, safe, bladder capacity. The diagnosis of stress incontinence is best made with measurement of the abdominal pressure required to induce urinary loss (the abdominal leak point pressure) or fluoroscopy. Measurement and interpretation of abdominal leak point pressure is addressed Chapter 13.

Fluoroscopy may also be used to distinguish between hypermobility of the urethra or intrinsic sphincter dysfunction that is manifest by an open fixed bladder neck at rest. Anatomic incontinence must be distinguished from intrinsic sphincter incontinence, since the treatment for each is potentially different.

Detrusor Function and Stress Incontinence Surgery

Patients with significant residual urine volumes preoperatively, not attributable to a cystocele, are not likely to be able to empty their bladder after a sling procedure. Patients who void habitually by straining will not be able to void in that manner after the procedure, since the sling raises the abdominal leak point pressure to infinity. Some women with severe stress incontinence never void by a detrusor contraction, since they can easily leak or void by barely increasing their abdominal pressure. After a sling procedure some of these women may be able to relearn to void by a detrusor contraction, but there is no way to predict this on an individual basis.[8] Preoperative assessment of detrusor function is further complicated by the fact that many patients who normally do void by a detrusor contraction will fail to develop one in the urodynamic testing situation. Therefore even a crude assessment of detrusor power and strength, which requires a bladder contraction, often cannot be done. It is, however, quite reasonable to use a sling for patients with poor or absent detrusor contractile function provided that the patient can do intermittent catheterization and is willing to do that indefinitely.

Difficult Cases

A patulous urethra surrounded by dense fibrotic tissue may not be completely closed by a sling because a sling provides a vector force only against the back of the urethra. There is a risk that the tension necessary to close a fibrotic urethra could result in obstruction or erosion. In some of these cases the sling will prevent stress incontinence. On fluoroscopic urodynamics the sling can be seen to be driven into the urethra securely closing it. Unfortunately, when the patient is relaxed, minimal motion, such as bending forward, can produce urinary leakage. In these cases once the urethra is partly closed and immobile as a result of the sling, collagen can be injected with excellent results.

The patient who has had an indwelling catheter for a long period of time and has a very wide patulous urethra with associated tissue loss may be better served by a formal urethral closure and construction of a continent abdominal stoma or an ileovesicostomy.[9]

Preoperative Preparation

All patients are told that intermittent catheterization will be required and must be mastered before discharge. They are told that there is a small risk of permanent retention requiring lifelong catheterization. If there is any question about a patient's ability to do intermittent catheterization, such a patient is taught the technique preoperatively. Preoperative teaching of intermittent catheterization also facilitates early discharge.

A clear urinalysis or a sterile urine culture is required before surgery. Patients are admitted through the same-day facility. A second-generation parental cephalosporin is given circumoperatively.

Surgical Technique

The basic sling procedure has undergone many modifications since the description by Lytton and McGuire in 1978.[8] At present a combined abdominal and vaginal approach is used. The procedure takes about 30 minutes if there are two surgical teams and less than 50 minutes with one operator. Patients are placed in the dorsal lithotomy position with the feet supported by Allen stirrups. An 18 Fr Foley catheter is placed and the balloon overfilled with 10 ml. A weighted vaginal speculum is placed into the vagina, and an Allis clamp is placed just inferior to the urethral meatus to elevate the anterior vaginal wall, which is then infiltrated with normal saline solution to aid in the dissection (Fig. 34-1). The bladder neck is identified by palpation of the catheter balloon. A midline incision is made about 4 to 5 cm in length, from the area of the midurethra to the bladder neck. The vaginal wall is sharply dissected off the underlying periurethral fascia, which is visible as a glistening white surface. If dissection is carried out in the plane between the periurethral fascia and the vaginal wall, it is relatively bloodless, and inadvertent entry into the bladder or urethra is prevented. The vaginal wall is dissected

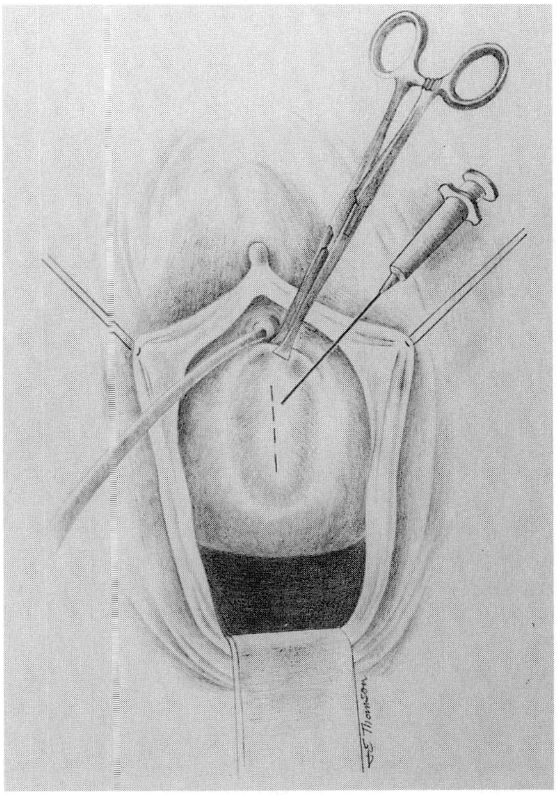

FIG 34-1 *The anterior vaginal wall is infiltrated with normal saline solution to facilitate dissection between the vaginal mucosa and the periurethral fascia*

laterally toward the ischium. The pubocervical fascia is perforated sharply on either side to the urethra, gaining entry into the retropubic space (Fig. 34-2). Perforation of the pubocervical fascia and subsequent blunt dissection frees the attachment of the vagina from the tendinous arc, allowing free motion of the urethra and the fascial envelope that contains it. Blunt dissection with the index finger is used to create a tunnel for the sling into the retropubic space toward the rectus muscle bellies.

A transverse suprapubic incision is made and carried down to the rectus fascia, which is opened in the direction of the skin incision (Fig. 34-3). The fascia is lifted off the rectus muscle bellies inferiorly and superiorly, and a strip of fascia measuring 1.5 cm by 4 to 8 cm is taken from either the upper or lower leaf. The ends of the sling are sutured with several bites of no. 0 polypropylene suture to trap all the fibers of the sling. The suture is tied down on the sling, and the needle is removed with the sutures being left as long as possible. The suprapubic operator then retracts the lateral border of the rectus muscle just above the insertion into the symphysis toward the midline. A triangular opening in the abdominal musculature is visualized to permit easy access to the retropubic space in an area where no previous operative scarring has occurred. Retropubic tunnels are developed in continuity with the previous vaginal dissection. A long curved clamp, such as a Crawford, is passed through the retropubic tunnel from above downward guided by the vaginal operator's index finger. The nose of the clamp is kept in constant contact with the posterior surface of the symphysis to avoid inadvertent puncture of the bladder (Fig. 34-4). Once a Crawford clamp has been passed on both sides, the bladder is checked for injury by irrigation of the Foley catheter with saline. A bladder injury is suspected if blood is seen. The sutures on either end of the sling are grasped in the Crawford clamp, and the sling is gently pulled into the retropubic space bilaterally (Fig. 34-5). This seats the sling at the bladder neck in the correct position, since the entry points into the retropubic space

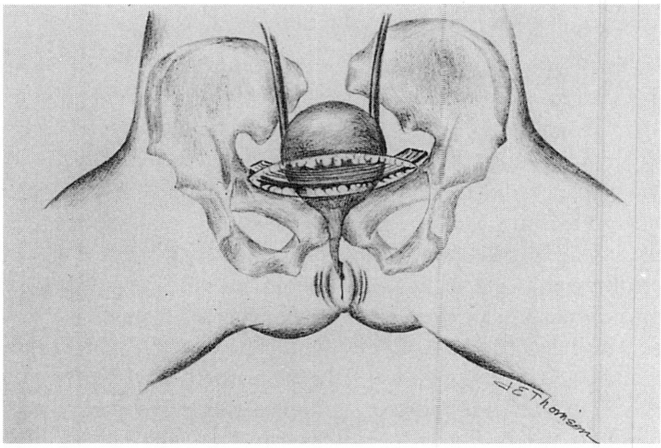

FIG. 34-3 *A strip of rectus fascia is obtained through a suprapubic incision.*

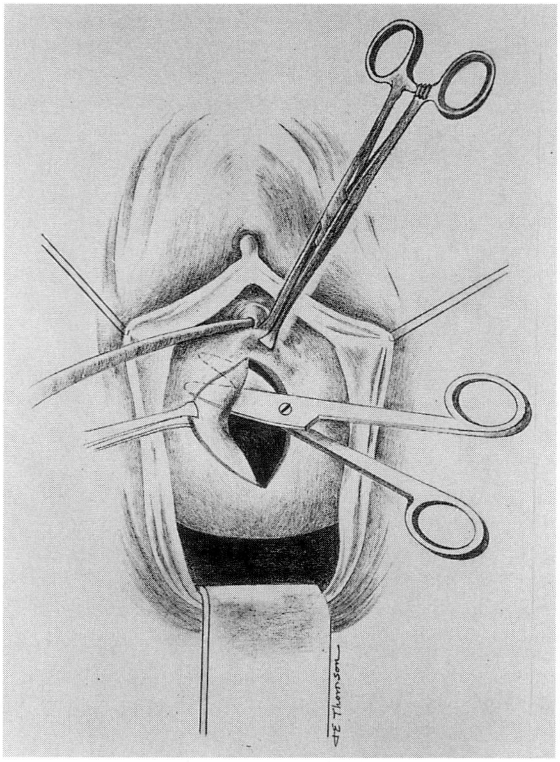

FIG. 34-2 *The retropubic space is entered from below by perforation of the pubocervical fascia.*

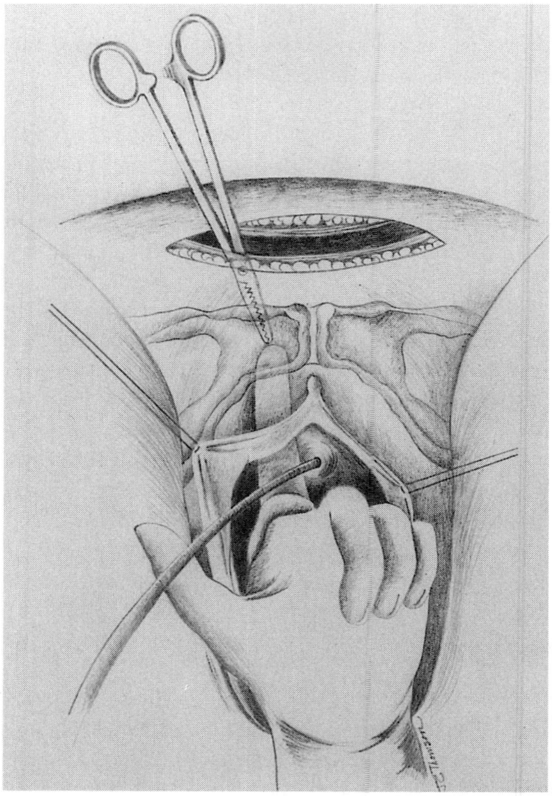

FIG. 34-4 *A Crawford clamp is passed through the retropubic tunnel. Bimanual palpation is used, and the clamp is kept in contact with the symphysis.*

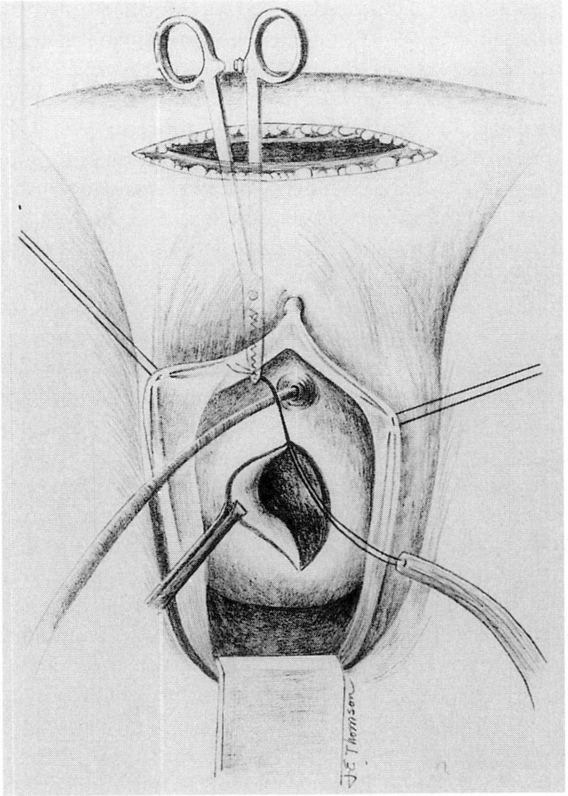

FIG. 34-5 *The sling suture is grasped, and the sling is pulled up into the retropubic tunnel.*

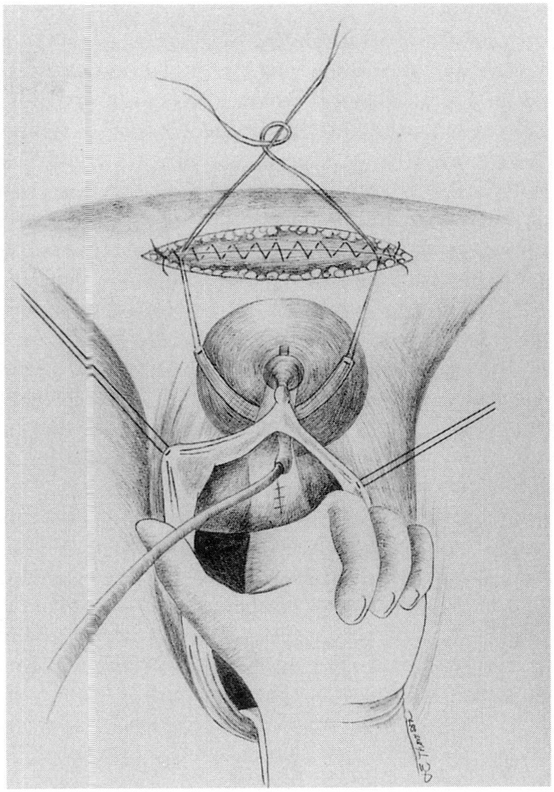

FIG. 34-6 *The sling tension is assessed by palpation. The sling is then loosely tied.*

are just at the bladder neck and proximal end of the urethra. The sling can move upward neither toward the trigone nor toward the urethral meatus. At this point the sling is sutured to the periurethral fascia with a no. 000 Vicryl (polyglactin 910) or similar suture to prevent dislocation and to spread the bearing surface of the fascia on the urethra as widely as possible.

Two small defects are made in the inferior leaf of the rectus fascia, and the sling sutures are brought through these small defects. The abdominal fascia is closed with no. 0 Prolene (polypropyline) or no. 0 Vicryl and the vaginal wound is closed with no. 000 chromic or similar suture. The vaginal wound is difficult to close once the sling has been tied. The sling tension is adjusted so that gentle traction on the Foley catheter does not result in inferior and posterior urethral mobility (Fig. 34-6). The sling is secured when the two sutures are tied to each other, loosely, above the rectus fascia. The subcutaneous tissues and skin are closed, and the vaginal vault is packed.

Sling Tension

To avoid prolonged postoperative retention the surgeon ties the sling loosely, enabling him or her to place two or three fingers between the knot of the sling and the rectus fascia. There is no objective way to measure sling tension intraoperatively that has prognostic value either in terms of achieving continence or in preventing the long-term use of intermittent catheterization. Previously we applied tension to the sling in an effort to increase urethral pressure beneath the sling by 6 to 10 cm.[8] This method required considerable time and had no predictive value. Others have described filling the bladder with fluid and then adjusting the sling tension so that compression of the full bladder does not result in leakage. This is considerable overkill because a sling does not have to impede the expulsive force of bladder pressure. A sling that does prevent leakage from high bladder pressure is more likely to lead to loss of bladder compliance. The purpose of a sling is to oppose abdominal pressure, and that can be achieved by a sling that barely closes the urethra. Coaptation may be assessed endoscopically, however doing so ensures neither absence of incontinence nor freedom from retention.

Postoperative Care

The vaginal pack is removed 6 to 24 hours postoperatively. Patients are encouraged to drink, eat, and walk. As soon as the patient is mobile and reasonably comfortable, the Foley catheter is removed. This usually occurs on the first postoperative day. When the catheter is removed, patients are encouraged to attempt voiding frequently. They are told not to strain to void because straining will tighten the sling. They are asked to catheterize if they cannot void. Catheterization is performed at least every 3 to 4 hours and any time the patient is uncomfortable. The patient is advised to keep the total bladder volume below 500 ml. If the patient was not taught intermittent catheterization preoperatively, she is catheterized by the nurses who begin the process of teaching intermittent catheterization as soon as the Foley catheter is removed. When the patient can do intermittent catheterization independently, she is discharged. In general this occurs on the second postoperative day. A patient who has performed intermittent self-catheterization preoperatively is often ready for discharge on the first postoperative day. Intermittent catheterization schedules are individualized and are adjusted as the patient's voiding ability improves. The ability to void large amounts does not indicate a low residual; therefore the patient is asked to record both her voided volume and postvoid residual volume. The patient ceases catheterization once successive residuals are 60 to 70 ml or less. Patients are advised to self-catheterize any time they feel that they haven't emptied. Intermittent catheterization is performed using a 14 Fr catheter. A catheter coudé (elbowed catheter) is easier for some patients to use because the shape of the catheter coudé facilitates passage of the catheter when the bladder is very full and the sling is tighter than it would be at rest. The catheter coudé also prevents trauma to the posterior urethral wall. Every patient, even if she can void to completion postoperatively, is expected to and does learn intermittent catheterization. Occasionally a patient may develop retention if the patient overdistends her bladder despite having previously achieved low residuals. It is very useful to have the patient in a position to handle this problem herself should this happen once she has been discharged.

Complications

Complications include inadvertent malposition of the sling within the urethra or bladder, wound infection, pain related to the sling or sling sutures, prolonged retention, and potential erosion of the sling into the urethra. Inadvertent malposition of the sling is associated with bleeding during the operation and should prompt cystoscopy. If the periurethral fascia is violated during the initial vaginal dissection, there is increased bleeding, and the risk of immediate urethral injury is increased. Immediate urethral injury is rare, with there being none reported in the literature.

Inadvertent injury to the bladder occurs from the passage of the Crawford clamp and is suspected if bleeding is noted when the catheter is irrigated. A bladder injury from the Crawford clamp will be located at the upper lateral aspect of the anterior bladder wall. Once the Crawford clamp has been passed a subsequent time cystoscopy should be performed with the Crawford clamp in situ. Visualization of a clamp in the bladder is very dramatic, whereas it is possible to miss seeing a piece of suture peeking through a small hole. If the bladder is entered, it is drained for a period of 5 to 7 days rather than the standard 1- to 2-day period. Practically this complication is most likely to occur in patients with a past history of urinary extravasation, patients incontinent after pelvic fractures, or those who have failed retropubic procedures in the past.

Wound infections are a potentially serious complication because they may involve the polypropyline suture. If this occurs, the foreign material is removed through a small suprapubic incision under local anesthesia. To safeguard against causing incontinence the procedure is not performed until 10 to 12 weeks postoperatively. Fortunately no patient who has required removal of her sutures has been made incontinent.

Patients often complain of a pulling sensation in either inguinal area for 1 to 5 weeks after the procedure. This is usually transient and is often relieved by infiltration of long-acting local anesthetic. If the pain persists and prevents normal activity, removal of the suspension sutures above the rectus fascia will resolve the problem. These patients also do not redevelop stress incontinence.

Prolonged urinary retention can be troublesome. It usually occurs because a sling, which prevents leakage, provides too much resistance for a relatively poorly contractile bladder to overcome. In some instances it is possible to reduce sling tension by having the patient bend forward from the hips to void. Attempting to void in the upright position accomplishes the same thing. A full urodynamic investigation is warranted if retention or troublesome urge incontinence or any variety of incontinence develops or persists after a sling. First the ability of the urethra to resist abdominal pressure is determined. If that is satisfactory, the next step is to determine whether the sling causes obstruction. Obstruction is assessed by measurement of bladder pressure during voiding. When this measurement is made, the external sphincter must be demonstrably relaxed and the proximal urethra open. Voiding pressures greater than 30 cm H_2O are abnormal in a female and indicative of obstruction. Pressures of less than 30 cm H_2O may be reflective of obstruction in a bladder with poor contractility. Precise identification of obstruction in such a bladder is impossible with clinically available urodynamic equipment. If a bladder contraction cannot be elicited during urodynamics, obstruction cannot be assessed. Since management consists in relieving sling tension, it is comforting to have objective evidence of obstruction, though this is not always possible. Takedown of a sling is accomplished by the same steps in the initial preparation for placement of the sling, that is, the transvaginal mobilization of the urethra within its envelop of fascia until urethral mobility has been obtained.

Urethral erosion, though fairly common with slings made of synthetic material, has not been reported with autogenous fascial slings to our knowledge.

Conclusion

The pubovaginal sling procedure generally results in success rates of 92% to 95%.[9,16] The results are durable with sustained successes after 5 to 10 years. The small numbers of patients who are dissatisfied have either urge for or difficulty in emptying. The majority of patients, including some who are dissatisfied, would have the procedure again because of the considerable improvement in their stress incontinence.

References

1. Ridley JH: The Goebel-Stoeckel sling operation. In Mattingly RF, Thompson JD, editors: *TeLinde's operative gynecology,* Philadelphia, 1985, Lippincott.
2. Goebell R: Zur operativen Besorigung der angeborenen incontinentia vesicae, *Z Urol Gynäk* 2:187, 1910.
3. Miller NF: Surgical treatment of urinary incontinence in the female, *JAMA* 98:628, 1932.

4. Price PB: Plastic operations for incontinence of urine and of feces, *Arch Surg* 26: 1043, 1933.
5. Aldridge AA: Transplantation of fascia for relief of urinary stress incontinence, *Am J Obstet Gynecol* 44:398, 1942.
6. Millen T: Stress incontinence in women. In Millen T, editor: *Retropubic urinary surgery,* Baltimore, 1947, Williams and Wilkens.
7. McGuire EJ, Fitzpatrick CC, Wan J, et al: Clinical assessment of urethral sphincter function, *J Urol* 150:1452,1993.
8. McGuire EJ, Lytton B: Pubovaginal sling procedure for stress incontinence, *J Urol* 119:82, 1978.
9. McGuire EJ, Bennett CJ, Konnak JA, et al: Experience with pubovaginal slings for urinary incontinence at the University of Michigan, *J Urol* 138:525, 1987.
10. McGuire EJ: Abdominal procedures for stress incontinence, *Urol Clin North Am* 12:285, 1985.
11. Blaivas JG: Pubovaginal sling. In Kursh ED, McGuire EJ, editors: *Female urology,* Philadelphia, 1994, Lippincott.
12. McGuire EJ Lytton B, Kohorn EI, et al: The value of urodynamic testing in stress urinary incontinence, *J Urol* 124:256, 1980.
13. McGuire EJ, Savastano JA: Stress incontinence and detrusor instability/urge incontinence, *Neurourol Urodyn* 4:313, 1985.
14. McGuire EJ, Woodside JR, Borden TA, et al: Prognostic value of urodynamic testing in myelodysplastic patients, *J Urol* 126:205, 1981.
15. International Continence Society: Standardization of terminology of lower urinary tract function, *Neurourol Urodyn* 7:403, 1988.
16. Gormley EA, Bloom DA, McGuire EJ, Ritchey ML: Pubovaginal slings for the management of urinary incontinence in adolescent females, *J Urol* 152:822, 1994.

Chapter 35 Urethrolysis

Harris E. Foster, Jr, Edward J. McGuire

The choice of a method of treatment for stress urinary incontinence (SUI) involves many factors. These include the severity and type of the SUI, the presence or absence of detrusor instability, and the goals of both patient and physician. Patients with more severe SUI are usually more likely to seek treatment. Furthermore, the presence of mixed incontinence requires an assessment of the severity of each type before one decides on definitive therapy. Finally, urinary incontinence is generally a quality-of-life issue, requiring that patients actively participate in the choice of treatment. Recent attention has focused on various nonsurgical and minimally invasive techniques to manage SUI. Such methods may include but are not exclusive to pelvic floor exercises and suburethral injectable substances. Although verbal instruction is often sufficient to correctly perform pelvic floor exercises, in some patients, other adjuncts, such as weighted vaginal cones and biofeedback, are beneficial.[1,2] Suburethal injection with collagen, polytetrafluoroethylene (Teflon), and fat is an attempt to increase bladder neck coaptation in the absence of urethral hypermobility.[3-5] These methods become very attractive to many patients with SUI because of their minimal invasiveness and low associated risks. Their efficacy however, in particular the cure rates and duration of response, are quite variable thereby tempering some enthusiasm.

Despite significant advances in the nonsurgical and minimally invasive methods of treating SUI, clearly the mainstay of therapy is the surgical bladder neck suspension. Many surgical techniques exist to adequately support the bladder neck and the proximal part of the urethra in the retropubic space. These can be subdivided into retropubic urethropexies and transvaginal needle suspensions. The former procedures are the classic Marshall-Marchetti-Krantz (MMK) suspension and the Burch colposuspension, differing in placement of the sutures in the periurethral tissues and in the supporting structures to which they are attached.[6,7] An additional advantage of these procedures is their ability to be simultaneously performed with other intra-abdominal operations. The Burch procedure also allows simultaneous correction of mild to moderate cystoceles. In an attempt to reduce postoperative morbidity and improve cosmetic results, transvaginal procedures have become popular. Small prepubic or suprapubic incisions are used to tie the suspension sutures over the rectus fascia, in contrast to low-midline or Pfannenstiel incisions mandated for the retropubic procedures. Common transvaginal needle suspensions include those described by Peyrera, Stamey, Gittes, and Raz.[8-11] Additional advantages to these surgical approaches include the ability to simultaneously correct coexistent vaginal prolapse such as cystocele, enterocele, rectocele, and uterine prolapse. Recently interest has developed in the laparoscopic approach for bladder neck suspension. Both transperitoneal and extraperitoneal approaches have been used, the latter being preferable in most instances. Early experiences have demonstrated this technique to be similarly successful in the short term when compared to standard approaches.[12] In general, with all bladder neck suspension procedures, success rates in the range of 75% to 85% can be expected.[13,14] Choice of surgical procedure depends on experience and preference of the physician, presence of a coexisting disorder, and the patient's desire.

The preoperative identification of intrinsic sphincter deficiency (ISD) by either an open bladder neck on cystography, decreased or absent proximal urethral closing pressure on urethral pressure profile, or Valsalva leak point pressure less than 60 cm H_2O precludes the use of standard bladder neck suspension procedures in most instances. Surgical treatment of ISD generally requires the use of suburethral sling procedures or placement of an artificial urinary sphincter. The former procedure enjoys the most popularity and allows utilization of either rectus fascia, tensor fasciae latae, in situ vaginal epithelium, or prosthetic material (that is, Goretex) as the suburethral sling. Although suburethral slings support the urethra in a way similar to that of standard bladder neck suspensions, an additional and arguably more important mechanism is mild compression of the urethra resulting in mucosal coaptation of the internal sphincter complex. Use of the artificial urinary sphincter in females requires its placement around the bladder neck and the proximal portion of the urethra. During the bladder storage phase, an inflated cuff provides resistance to urinary outflow and inadvertent urine loss. The major drawbacks to using the artificial sphincter in females are difficult placement, infection, and mechanical failure. Reported success rates for the suburethral sling procedures and artificial urinary sphincter are excellent ranging from 85% to 95%.[14]

Complications of Surgical Management of Stress Incontinence

The most common complications after surgical attempts to correct SUI are persistent SUI, continuous or de novo detrusor instability, and urethral obstruction. Persistent SUI generally results from either incorrect placement of the suspension sutures, poor periurethral and perivesical support tissues, or undiagnosed intrinsic sphincter deficiency.[15] Occasionally resumption of vigorous physical activity in the early postoperative period can either tear the suspending sutures from the supporting structures or break the sutures themselves. Restriction of physical activity therefore is usually recommended for 6 to 8 weeks. Use of nonabsorbable material for the suspending sutures may reduce failure secondary to early resumption of vigorous physical activity.

Postoperative detrusor instability is difficult to predict and can occur despite a flawlessly performed procedure.[16,17] Many patients present to the physician with mixed urinary incontinence, that is, stress and urgency, though the stress component may be predominant. Classic teaching dictated that eradication of the detrusor instability with anticholinergic agents before surgical correction of the SUI was mandatory. It is now believed, however, that urethral hypermobility itself or a nonfunctioning proximal portion of the urethra allowing entrance of urine into the posterior portion of the urethra at rest can precipitate involuntary bladder contractions. Therefore surgical correction of SUI, despite the concomitant existence of detrusor instability, is a reasonable option in this subset of patients. As expected though, some will continue to suffer from urgency incontinence notwithstanding the successful correction of their SUI. Furthermore, a smaller number of patients may develop de novo detrusor instability. Although correction of SUI is the primary goal of the surgeon, the continued presence of urinary incontinence, albeit secondary to detrusor instability, is still considered a treatment failure when viewed from the patient's perspective.

Successful surgical bladder neck suspension or suburethral sling procedure requires that the urethra be adequately suspended in the retropubic space or that there be sufficient compression of the nonfunctioning proximal portion of the urethra to prevent involuntary loss of urine. Since the primary goal of the procedure is to eradicate the existing SUI, the tendency when placing and tying the suspension sutures therefore is to overcorrect the problem. Overcorrection of urethral hypermobility or of ISD however can result in undue compression of the urethra against the undersurface of the symphysis pubis causing an anatomic obstruction to the bladder outlet. The clinical sequelae that follow generally manifest as frank urinary retention or chronic incomplete voiding requiring either continued indwelling catheter drainage or intermittent self-catheterization.

Prevention of urethral obstruction following these surgical procedures requires adequate but not overaggressive application of tension when one is tying the suspension sutures. As expected, certain procedures may be more likely to result in urethral obstruction than others based on the technique utilized. Procedures where the suspension sutures are placed laterally to the urethra and bladder neck (retropubic urethropexy and transvaginal needle suspension) would be expected to result in less obstruction compared to those that involve placement of tissue underneath the urethra (suburethral slings). Furthermore, since retropubic urethropexies involve tying the suspension sutures to either the symphysis pubis or Cooper's ligament, there would be less expected variation between procedures. On the other hand, in most transvaginal needle suspension procedures, the suspension sutures are tied over the rectus fascia, a technique that leaves more room for variation, thereby at least in theory increasing the possibility of obstruction. Experience has taught that minimal to no tension is required when suburethral slings are tied, since the mere presence of tissue underneath the urethra is all that is required to provide adequate support and proximal urethral coaptation during transient increases in intra-abdominal pressure. On the other hand, a properly functioning artificial urinary sphincter placed around the bladder neck compresses the urethra only during the storage phase and is deflated just before micturition to provide an unobstructed outlet. Urethral obstruction resulting in urinary retention is therefore uncommon after artificial urinary sphincter insertion. This absence of urethral compression during micturition practically eliminates the risk of urinary retention and furthermore significantly reduces the risk of postoperative detrusor instability related to outlet obstruction. It is for the above reasons that some prefer the artificial sphincter to suburethral slings for the treatment of female ISD.

Although application of excessive tension represents the most common cause of urethral obstruction after surgical correction of SUI, occasional cases may occur after incorrect placement of the suspension sutures. When both anterior and posterior walls of the urethra are incorporated in the suspension sutures, compression and impingement on the urethral lumen may result, eventuating in bladder outlet obstruction. Reported rates of urethral obstruction range from 1% to 20% after retropubic urethropexies, transvaginal needle suspensions, and pubovaginal slings.[18-21]

Diagnosis of Urethral Obstruction

The diagnosis of urethral obstruction after surgical correction of SUI can be relatively straightforward in many instances but less obvious in others. Clearly the patient who was voiding without difficulty and with low postvoid residuals before surgery and is unable to void postoperatively probably suffers from urethral obstruction. Instances where incomplete voiding and urgency incontinence coexist, however, can represent more complex issues such as detrusor hypocontractility and detrusor instability. Therefore the diagnosis of urethral obstruction, particularly the less distinct cases, may require some diligence in patient evaluation. These include the medical history, physical examination, and various diagnostic procedures such as endoscopy, urodynamics, and radiographic studies. Because de novo urethral obstruction is uncommon in the average female patient, clearly those who present with either urinary retention or incomplete bladder emptying after surgical correction of SUI are highly suspicious for obstruction. In general, since many patients will experience temporary voiding dysfunction after surgical correction of SUI, it is reasonable to wait at least 2 to 3 months before definitive therapy is undertaken.

The medical history is likely to elicit frank urinary retention or incomplete voiding in many patients. Associated irritative voiding symptoms such as urgency, urge incontinence, frequency, and nocturia are also common in our experience (Table 35-1). Other less prevalent symptoms may include pain, persistent stress urinary incontinence, recurrent urinary tract infection, decreased force of stream, dysuria, postvoid dribbling, and double voiding. In most patients, the poor bladder emptying is managed with either an indwelling catheter (Foley or suprapubic) or intermittent self-catheterization. Urethral obstruction is most likely to occur in the immediate period after surgical correction of SUI but can have delayed onset. The duration between initial operative procedure and presentation of symptoms can range from 2 months to 35 years.

Physical examination of the patient suspected of having urethral obstruction should be focused but not limited to the perineum. The most common finding is a fixed urethra in a high retropubic position. Other findings on physical examination may include a cystocele, which is a common sequela of chronic bladder outlet obstruction, or foreign-body granuloma from local reaction to the suspension suture or pledget. Since many patients may also have a coexisting disorder, during the physical examination one should assess for enterocele, rectocele, and uterine prolapse, since correction of these abnormalities can be performed at the time of urethrolysis. A limited neurologic examination should be included to search for signs of occult neurologic disease that could be suggestive of poor bladder function. These signs include reduced or absent reflexes mediated by the sacral cord (bulbocavernosus), gait abnormalities, visual disturbances, poor anal sphincter tone, and decreased perineal sensation.

Table 35-1 Presenting symptoms by order of saliency

Symptom	Number (percentage)
Irritative voiding	34 (71%)
Urgency/urge incontinence	32 (67%)
Inability/incomplete voiding	29 (60%)
Frequency	13 (27%)
Nocturia	11 (23%)
Pain	10 (21%)
Stress urinary incontinence	9 (19%)
Recurrent urinary tract infections	8 (17%)
Other (decreased force of stream, dysuria, postvoid dribbling, double voiding)	6 (13%)

Endoscopic evaluation of the lower urinary tract with cystoscopy may add useful information in the diagnosis of urethral obstruction. Excluding diagnoses such as a penetrating permanent suture, bladder tumor and bladder stones represent its main usefulness. The urethra is found to be in a high fixed retropubic position, similar to the findings on physical examination of the pelvis. In general, however, the urethral lumen has a of normal caliber. If an aberrant penetrating suture is identified, endoscopic incision of the suture is often possible and may eliminate both the obstruction and associated irritative symptoms.

Urodynamic evaluation of the patient with suspected urethral obstruction should in most instances result in the appropriate diagnosis. Although not formally a urodynamic study, postvoid residual (PVR) urine measurement provides an indirect assessment of bladder contractility and urethral outlet resistance and therefore should be a part of every examination. The presence of an elevated postvoid residual urine indicates either an impaired detrusor contraction or an impediment to urine outflow related to increased urethral resistance. In the patient who has recently undergone surgical correction of SUI in the absence of preoperative voiding difficulties, the finding of an elevated PVR would in most instances be suggestive of the presence of urethral obstruction. The urodynamic studies most useful in diagnosing urethral obstruction include cystometry, uroflowmetry, and pressure-flow study. Cystometry may but not always demonstrate involuntary bladder contractions secondary to the bladder outlet obstruction. Cystometric evidence of reduced bladder capacity is also not uncommon and often correlates with the patient's symptoms. Uroflowmetry will in general reveal a prolonged voiding time and a decrease in the maximum and mean urinary flow rate. Pressure-flow studies remain the standard urodynamic evaluation to assess for the presence of urethral obstruction. Maximum detrusor voiding pressure at 40 cm H_2O in the presence of a decreased urinary flow rate is pathognomonic (Fig. 35-1). If fluoroscopy is utilized during urodynamic evaluation, a hypersuspended, immobile urethra is often identified, and frequently a cystocele is demonstrated.

Important in assessing the patient with possible urethral obstruction in whom there is either an elevated postvoid residual urine or frank urinary retention is the elimination of detrusor hyporeflexia or areflexia. This is significant because the choice of treatment, that is, whether to attempt surgical correction, depends on the presence of urethral obstruction and an active detrusor muscle. Maximum detrusor pressures during voiding and pressure-flow studies provide the most effective means of differentiating detrusor contractility abnormalities from obstruction of the urethra. To obtain the necessary information from these studies, the patient is required to void in the urodynamic laboratory. Such voiding for some patients is difficult to impossible because of the artificial nature of this setting. This inability to void prevents acquisition of important data. In fact, 64% of patients were unable to void during the urodynamic evaluation in a study published by the authors.[22] This also occurred in [illegible]0% of patients in a study by Nitti and Raz, all of whom had a successful surgical outcome.[23] Furthermore, many physicians who regularly treat patients with stress urinary incon-

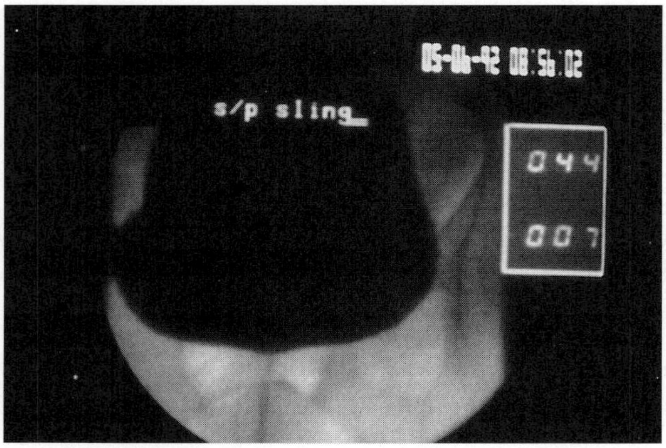

FIG. 35-1 *Videourodynamic study demonstrating elevated voiding pressure, normal external sphincter relaxation, and poor opening of vesical neck.* (From Foster HE, McGuire EJ: Management of urethral obstruction with transvaginal urethrolysis, *J Urol* 150:1448, 1993.

tinence may not possess advanced urodynamic equipment. In the above instances, that is, either inability to void during urodynamic study or absence of advanced urodynamic equipment, utilization of other diagnostic procedures, such as those previously mentioned, has to be combined with clinical judgment in deciding whether urethral obstruction is present and if surgical correction should be attempted.

Surgical Treatment of Urethral Obstruction

Once the diagnosis of urethral obstuction has been comfortably established, surgical management is generally required to eliminate the obstructive process. In rare instances where there is incomplete emptying or urinary retention and no evidence of detrusor instability, some patients may prefer continued intermittent catheterization to another surgical procedure. In general, however, most patients prefer an attempt at correcting the outlet obstruction. Choices for surgical correction include removal of the suspending sutures or dissection of the urethra from the surrounding fibrous tissue. Removal of the suspending sutures is a feasible option but is generally limited to the early postoperative period before permanent fixation of the urethra in the retropubic space by fibrous tissue. Removal of one or both suspending sutures in the early postoperative period however risks recurrent urethral hypermobility and stress urinary incontinence.

Adequate release of the urethra from surrounding obstructive fibrous tissue generally requires urethrolysis. This procedure, which can be performed either retropubically or transvaginally, involves sharp dissection of the urethra from its high retropubic position. The goal of the procedure is to release the urethra from the obstructing fibrous tissue yet maintain adequate support so that continence is preserved. For reasons not unlike those that separate retropubic urethropexies from needle suspensions, the transvaginal route for urethrolysis is much preferred over the retropubic approach. The transvaginal approach is less morbid and allows simultaneous correction of coexisting vaginal abnormalities. Transvaginal urethrolysis was first described in 1984 by Leach and Raz to release the urethra from surrounding periurethral tissue in preparation for a repeat needle suspension procedure.[24] Use of transvaginal urethrolysis to specifically manage urethral obstruction after surgical bladder neck suspension was then reported by Zimmern et al. with further studies by McGuire et al., Foster and McGuire, and Nitti and Raz.[22,23,25]

Transvaginal urethrolysis can be performed through virtually any anterior vaginal wall incision. Choice of incision depends on surgeon preference and whether a simultaneous procedure will be performed. We prefer a midline incision from midurethra to bladder neck; however, an inverted-U incision can provide similar if not better exposure. Dissection of the vaginal wall off the underlying periurethral fascia is then performed, often facilitated by preinjection of the submucosa with sterile saline or lidocaine with epinephrine. The dissection then proceeds bilaterally, lateral to the urethra and up to the endopelvic fascia. This fascia is then perforated with the dissecting scissors allowing entrance into the retropubic space. The index finger is inserted into this opening in the fascia, extending it proximally and distally using blunt dissection. Anterior attachments from the urethra to the symphysis pubis are left intact in an attempt to maintain urethral support and prevent recurrent SUI. Intermittent traction placed on the Foley catheter should demonstrate resumption of previously absent urethral movement. Additional vaginal procedures can then be performed, the vaginal wall closed in standard fashion, and a vaginal pack inserted. Despite adequate lysis of the urethra from this periurethral fibrotic process, recurrence of obstruction may occur. In secondary urethrolysis procedures, therefore, it is sometimes desirable to surround the urethra with protective tissue such as a Martius labial fat pad.

Postoperative management after transvaginal urethrolysis is generally uncomplicated. The Foley catheter and vaginal pack can usually be removed on the morning after surgery unless other simultaneous procedures or patient care demand otherwise. Intermittent self-catheterization should be performed to measure postvoid residuals. It is not uncommon for the postvoid residual to remain elevated in the early postoperative period because of temporary urethral edema. Patients can generally be discharged home in the afternoon after the day of surgery.

Results

Successful transvaginal urethrolysis should usually result in near-total to complete bladder emptying after micturition, absence of de novo detrusor instability, and maintenance of continence in situations of increased intra-abdominal pressure. Zimmern et al. evaluated 13 patients with urodynamically proved urethral obstruction following Marshall-Marchetti-Krantz procedure.[18] These patients underwent transvaginal urethrolysis and resuspension resulting in 12 of the 13 patients (92%) returning to a normal voiding pattern with decreased postvoid residuals. Thirteen more patients were reported on by McGuire et al. who developed urethral obstruction after retropubic urethropexy in six, needle suspension in four, and pubovaginal sling in three.[25] Only two patients underwent simultaneous resuspension and 10 of 13 (77%) were defined as cured without stress incontinence. A follow-up report from the same institution by the authors evaluated 48 patients almost equally divided between the three suspension procedures, demonstrating a slightly lower cure rate of 65% with only five having undergone resuspension.[22] This lower success rate may be related to the larger proportion of patients with urethral obstruction after pubovaginal sling. In fact, a successful outcome was achieved more often in patients with urethral obstruction after retropubic urethropexy and needle suspension than after pubovaginal sling; 71%, 63%, and 50% respectively. It is also important to note that no patients developed postoperative stress incontinence after transvaginal urethrolysis. Recent reports by Dmochowski et al. and Nitti and Raz achieved similar success rates of 75% and 80%, respectively, with simultaneous bladder neck resuspension.[23,26]

These data indicate that transvaginal urethrolysis may be an effective procedure to correct urethral obstruction following procedures designed to cure SUI. Success rates in the range of 50% to 92% can be expected, varying based on the type of procedure that resulted in the obstruction. It appears that the patient with urethral obstruction following retropubic urethropexy can expect the best chance for improvement, followed by those who have undergone needle suspensions and finally those who use pubovaginal slings. Whether or not resuspension should be performed in all patients at the time of urethrolysis is debatable. Clearly the patient with concomitant recurrent SUI and urethral obstruction should be resuspended. For the remainder of patients the decision is less clear. A review of the literature may indicate that better results may be obtained when resuspension is performed. The fact that resuspension will be performed may provide the surgeon with more confidence when dissecting the urethra from surrounding fibrous tissue since fear of producing recurrent SUI would be reduced. Recurrence of SUI however has not been a problem in our experience. It therefore becomes an issue of the individual surgeon's preference and experience.

Summary

In conclusion, urethral obstruction is a well-recognized complication of surgical procedures designed to correct SUI. Although the most common cause of urethral obstruction is overaggressive application of tension when one is tying the suspension sutures, incorrect placement of the sutures resulting in occlusion of the urethra can also occur. Presenting symptoms usually occur early but can also be delayed and often include frank urinary retention or incomplete bladder emptying requiring an indwelling catheter or intermittent self-catheterization. Irritative voiding symptoms are very common secondary to the effects of obstruction on the detrusor muscle. Other possible presenting symptoms include pain, recurrent urinary tract infections, decreased force of stream, and hesitancy. Diagnosis can at times be made with the medical history and physical examination; however endoscopy, urodynamics, or radiographic studies are often needed for confirmation. Transvaginal urethrolysis is the most effective procedure to correct urethral obstruction after surgical repair of SUI.

References

1. Burgio KL, Robinson C, Engel BT: The role of biofeedback in Kegel exercise training for stress urinary incontinence, *Am J Obstet Gynecol* 154:58, 1986.
2. Moore K, Metcalfe JB: Effectiveness of vaginal cones in treatment of urinary incontinence, *Urol Nurs* 12:69, 1992.
3. Herschorn S, Radomski SB, Steele DJ: Early experience with intraurethral collagen injections for urinary incontinence, *J Urol* 148:1797, 1992.
4. Politano VA, et al: Periurethral Teflon injections for urinary incontinence, *J Urol* 111:180, 1994.
5. Santarosa RP, Blaivas JG: Periurethral injection of autologous fat for the treatment of sphincteric incontinence, *J Urol* 151:607, 1994.
6. Marshall VF, Marchetti AA, Krantz KE: The correction of stress incontinence by simple vesicourethral suspension, *Surg Gynecol Obstet* 88:509, 1949.
7. Burch JC: Urethrovaginal fixation to Cooper's ligament for the correction of stress incontinence, cystocele and prolapse, *Am J Obstet Gynecol* 81:281, 1961.
8. Pereyra AJ: Simplified surgical procedure for the correction of stress urinary incontinence in women, *West J Surg* 67:223, 1959.
9. Stamey TA: Endoscopic suspension of the vesical neck for urinary incontinence, *Surg Gynecol Obstet* 136:547, 1973.
10. Gittes RF, Loughlin KR: No-incision pubovaginal suspension for stress incontinence, *J Urol* 138:568, 1987.
11. Raz S: Modified bladder neck suspension for female stress incontinence, *Urology* 17:82, 1981.
12. McDougall EM, Klutke CG, Cornell T: Two-year follow-up of the transvaginal (VBNS) and laparoscopic (LBNS) bladder neck suspension for anatomic stress urinary incontinence, *J Urol* 153:356A, 1995.
13. Pow-Sang JM, Lockhart JL, Suarez A, et al.: Female urinary incontinence: preoperative selection, surgical complications and results, *J Urol* 136:831, 1986.
14. Urinary Incontinence Guideline Panel: Urinary incontinence in adults: clinical practice guideline, AHCPR Pub. No. 92-0038, Rockville, Md., March 1992, Agency for Health Care Policy and Research, Public Health Service, U.S. Department of Health and Human Services.
15. Lockhart JL, Tirado A, Morillo G, Politano VA: Vesicourethral dysfunction following cystourethropexy, *J Urol* 128:943, 1982.
16. McGuire EJ, Lytton B, Kohorn EI, Pepe V: The value of urodynamic testing in stress urinary incontinence, *J Urol* 124:256, 1980.
17. Kelly MJ, Zimmern PE, Leach GE: Complications of bladder neck suspension procedures, *Urol Clin North Am* 18:339, 1991.
18. Zimmern PE, Hadley HR, Leach GE, Raz S: Female urethral obstruction after Marshall-Marchetti-Krantz operation, *J Urol* 138:517, 1987.
19. McDuffie RW Jr, Litin RB, Blundon K: Urethrovesical suspension (Marshall-Marchetti-Krantz): experience with 204 cases, *Am J Surg* 141:297, 1981.
20. Spencer JR, O'Conor VJ Jr: Comparison of procedures for stress urinary incontinence, AUA Update Series, vol 6, lesson 28, Baltimore, 1987, American Urological Association.
21. McGuire EJ, Lytton B: Pubovaginal sling procedure for stress incontinence, *J Urol* 119:82, 1989.
22. Foster HE, McGuire EJ: Management of urethral obstruction with transvaginal urethrolysis, *J Urol* 150:1448, 1993.
23. Nitti VW, Raz S: Obstruction following anti-incontinence procedures: diagnosis and treatment with transvaginal urethrolysis, *J Urol* 152:93, 1994.
24. Leach GE, Raz S: Modified Pereyra bladder neck suspension after previously failed anti-incontinence surgery: surgical technique and results with long-term follow-up, *Urology* 23:359, 1984.
25. McGuire EJ, Letson W, Wang S: Transvaginal urethrolysis after obstructive urethral suspension procedures, *J Urol* 142:1037, 1989.
27. Dmochowski RR et al.: Urethrolysis to relieve outlet obstruction after prior incontinence surgery, *J Urol* 151:420A, 1994.

Chapter

36 Artificial Urinary Sphincter

Kevin T. Stone, Ananias C. Diokno

The artificial urinary sphincter has completely changed the quality of life for thousands of people who have had urinary incontinence that could not be successfully managed by any other treatment approach. The artificial urinary sphincter was one of the initial successful applications of a prosthetic implant in management of problems of the genitourinary system.

Foley is credited for introducing the first artificial urinary sphincter in 1947.[1] The device consisted of an inflatable cuff, made of latex, that was placed around the corpus spongiosum just distal to the penoscrotal junction. It was connected by tubing to a valve and syringe that were kept by the patient in his trouser pocket. The cuff was inflated to prevent incontinence and deflated to empty the bladder. Unfortunately, pressure necrosis and infections occurred, which led to fistulas and other unmanageable complications.

The modern artificial urinary sphincter was introduced by Scott and co-workers in 1973.[2] This device, called AMS721, was made of silicone rubber and consisted of three major components: the reservoir, an occlusive cuff, and two pumps. The reservoir contained fluid used to activate the device and was implanted in the prevesical space. The cuff encircled the bulbous urethra or the vesical neck and the inflate and deflate pumps were placed in each hemiscrotum or labium (Fig. 36-1).

Experience with this initial prosthesis was favorable with an overall success rate of 60% to 70%.[3] Most of the complications and failures encountered with this device were attributable to urethral erosion and infection. Other problems that could be repaired included mechanical failures such as tube kinks, valvular failure, and device leakage.

Although the device was fairly successful, there were clearly areas for improvement. Over the next 10 years, through the efforts of American Medical Systems (Minnetonka, Minn.) and several urologists active in implanting the artificial urinary sphincters, the device was constantly modified in an effort to simplify the design, improve reliability, and reduce the complication and reoperation rates. In 1983, American Medical Systems (AMS) introduced the latest artificial urinary sphincter model, the AMS800 (Fig. 36-2). This model has been very successful and has changed very little over the past 12 years. The modifications that have been made, however, appear to have significantly improved the durability and reliability of this artificial urinary sphincter. The current device is constructed of a wear-resistant, biocompatible silicone elastomer and consists of three components all connected by special kink-resistant color-coded silicone tubing: a soft, pliable, dip-coated silicone cuff that is placed around the urethra or bladder neck, a seamless pressure-regulating balloon placed in the prevesical space of Retzius and a pump placed in the scrotum or labia majora with a flow resistor that acts to slow cuff refill, allowing adequate voiding time, and a deactivation button that when engaged prevents cuff refill altogether (Fig. 36-3). This button is located on the cephalad portion of the pump mechanism (easily palpated through the skin). By squeezing it, one can move a poppet valve to a position such that no fluid can be transferred. Reactivation is accomplished with a sharp squeeze on the pump that releases the poppet. An important point in sphincter deactivation is that some fluid in the pump is necessary to unseat the poppet valve. To accomplish this, we generally allow the pump to refill to the point where a shallow dimple is palpable before deactivating the device. This feature was an important addition to the artificial urinary sphincter in that Furlow showed that deactivation for 6 to 8 weeks after implantation (to allow for periurethral swelling to decrease and tissue healing) decreased the incidence of infection and erosion with artificial urinary sphincters.[4] The ability to deactivate a sphincter is also an important feature when the patient requires Foley catheter drainage or undergoes instrumentation, events that increase the risk for cuff erosion or infection. In these situations the cuff should *always* be emptied, and then the device be deactivated (as described above).

The AMS800 system is fluid filled and works hydraulically. The occlusive force of the cuff is determined by the pressure of a regulating balloon, and the balloon is manufactured so that precalibrated reservoirs are available in different pressure ranges: 51-60, 61-70, 71-80, and 81-90 cm H_2O. The intra-abdominal prevesical location of the reservoir also permits the transmission of abdominal pressure changes to the cuff, helping reduce leakage with straining maneuvers.[5] The patient squeezes the pump to empty the cuff, transferring fluid to the regulating balloon. As

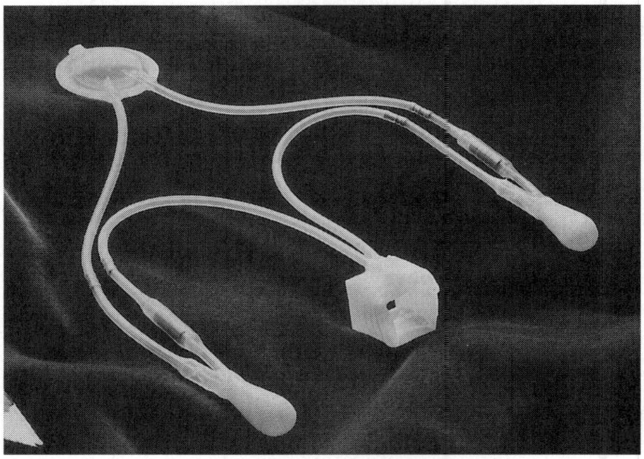

FIG. 36-1 *AMS Sphincter 721 Urinary Prosthesis, an artificial urinary sphincter.* (Courtesy American Medical Systems, Minnetonka, MN.)

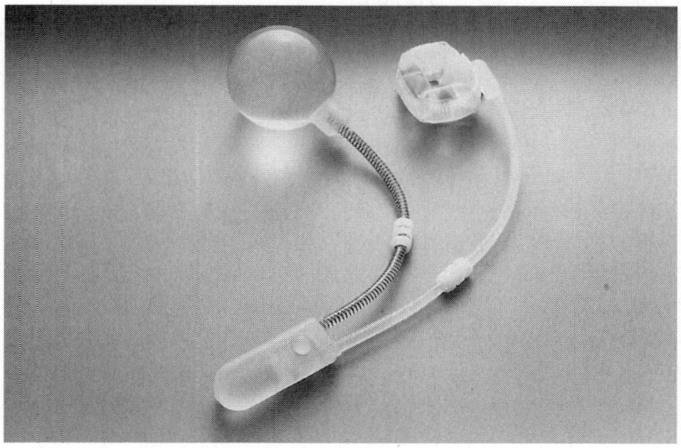

FIG. 36-2 *AMS Sphincter 800 Urinary Prosthesis, an artificial urinary sphincter.* (Courtesy American Medical Systems, Minnetonka, MN.)

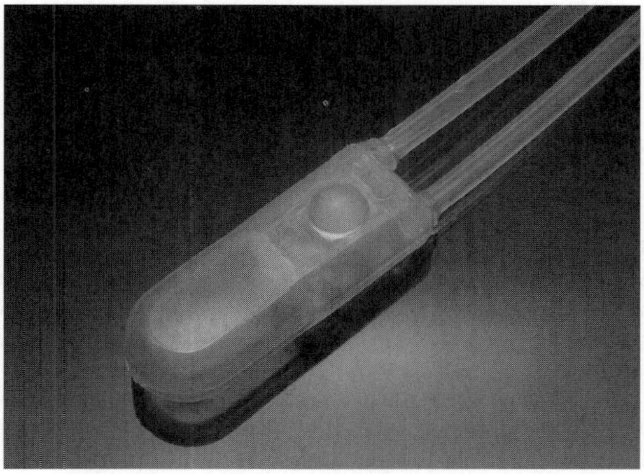

FIG. 36-3 *AMS Sphincter 800 Urinary Prosthesis, with artificial urinary sphincter pump and deactivation button.* (Courtesy American Medical Systems, Minnetonka, MN.)

the cuff empties, the occlusive force on the urethra is removed, and the patient can void. Resistors in the pump mechanism delay cuff refill for approximately 2 to 3 minutes, allowing the patient adequate time to empty his/her bladder.

Indications and Patient Selection for Artificial Urinary Sphincter Implantation

Most patients who are considered for implantation of an AUS fall into one of five groups: neuropathic bladder dysfunction (mainly congenital), postprostatectomy incontinence, failed antistress incontinence surgery, congenital anomalies, and trauma.

Before considering an incontinent patient for AUS implantation, one must realize that an AUS is treatment for incontinence because of sphincteric incompetence and only that.[5,6] Thus the importance of preoperative evaluation cannot be overemphasized. The history of urinary incontinence should be delineated to determine its cause. Physical examination should include a neurologic examination to identify neuropathologic disturbances. During this evaluation particular attention should be paid to the patient's upper extremity motor skills. Physical examination should define or confirm the clinical impression as to the type of incontinence present. Urinary tract infection should be ruled out and eradicated. In addition, the cause of such infection should be elucidated, since recurrent infection in the presence of the prosthesis may lead to prosthesis infection. Appropriate urodynamic testing should be done to document not only the mechanism of incontinence, but also the state of detrusor function. Ideal candidates for the artificial urinary sphincter are patients with irreversible sphincteric dysfunction and normal detrusor function. Extensive experience with this device has shown that areflexia and hyperreflexia are not absolute contraindications. However, before any implantation, appropriate provisions should be made to ensure that the bladder can be emptied regularly and that hyperreflexia can be suppressed. Ideal bladder capacity should be $\geq$ 400 ml with pressures of <40 cm H_2O. Failure to identify bladder function problems could lead to elevated bladder storage pressures and upper tract and renal deterioration in the presence of an artificial urinary sphincter. One can treat incomplete bladder emptying by performing a flap urethroplasty at the time of sphincter implantation as advocated by Scott et al.[7] or with intermittent self-catheterization,[8,9] both of which have been shown to be compatible with the AUS implant. Hyperreflexic or hypertonic bladder may be managed with anticholinergics, and if this is not effective, bladder augmentation with bowel segments has been successful with the artificial urinary sphincter.[10,11] If hyperreflexia can be controlled with drugs or other means, implantation of a sphincter is feasible. Otherwise, urge incontinence will persist and upper tract deterioration could occur.

Currently our work-up includes a detailed history and physical examination including neurologic and pelvic examination with postvoid residual urine determination. If intrinsic sphincter deficiency is suspected, patients then undergo an extensive evaluation. All patients undergo flexible cystoscopy with particular attention paid to bladder neck and sphincteric function during provocative maneuvers. In females, bladder neck with sphincteric incompetence and the presence or absence of a hypermobile vesical neck can be evaluated endoscopically. In males endoscopic evaluation can also identify bladder neck with sphincteric incompetence as well as other potential urethral disorders (contracture, stricture, and so forth). Special attention should be directed to the distal bulbous urethra, the area in the urethra where the cuff is usually implanted to assure that there are no signs of scarring, false passage, or strictures. In women, a bimanual examination should be performed at the time of urethroscopy to ascertain the thickness of the bladder neck and proximal area of the urethra in relation to the vaginal wall thickness, since dissection of these area is critical at the time of implantation. After cystoscopy, patients undergo urodynamic testing, including a cystometrogram, for evaluation of bladder instability or hyperreflexia, bladder capacity and sensation, and urethral pressure profilometry to demonstrate the relationship between bladder and urethral pressures with stress. Another technique that has gained recent prominence and can yield useful information is the measurement of the leak point pressure (LPP). Finally, sphincter candidates undergo static and dynamic cystography to elicit information about bladder neck and urethral anatomy. Patients considered for implantation of artificial sphincters must demonstrate evidence of type III stress urinary incontinence, or intrinsic sphincter deficiency (ISD).

The most common reason for insertion of an artificial urinary sphincter in adult males is for postprostatectomy incontinence. It is recommended that artificial urinary sphincter implantation be delayed for at least 6 months after the prostatectomy to allow time for possible spontaneous resolution. Insertion of the artificial sphincter in males can be performed at essentially two sites: the vesical neck and the bulbous urethra. For postprostatectomy incontinence, however, we recommend placement of artificial urinary sphincters only at the bulbous urethra site primarily because of the significant postoperative changes at the bladder neck in these patients. In male children the indication is generally for incontinence secondary to neurogenic dysfunction, most commonly caused by myelomeningocele. Generally in these patients the sphincter should be placed at the bladder neck. These patients may need to receive intermittent self-catheterization and may be nonambulatory. It is believed that the bladder neck position is more compatible with intermittent straight catheterization. Also, if these patients are nonambulatory, they will be in seated positions for long periods of time. A bulbar urethral position is of concern in this situation because it would theoretically expose the cuff to extended periods of pressure increasing the risk for erosion and infection. Potential problems with bladder neck placement in prepubertal males and subsequent prostate growth disrupting AUS function have not been reported. When one is implanting sphincters in children, it is advised to use conservative measures for management of incontinence initially and delay AUS insertion until at least 6 years of age to allow for anatomic, emotional and social maturation.[12]

SURGICAL TECHNIQUE

The most common indication for an AUS in adult men is postprostatectomy incontinence, and the bulbous urethra is the preferred site for cuff placement. A midline perineoscrotal incision is used, the bulbospongiosus muscle is separated to expose the urethra (Fig. 36-4), and the cuff size is determined. A transverse suprapubic incision is made for reservoir placement (Fig. 36-5), pump placement (Fig. 36-6), and tubing connections (Fig. 36-7). A 60 to 70cm H_2O pressure reservoir is the preferred AMS800 AUS pressure for a bulbous urethral cuff. The reservoir should contain 20 ml of isosmotic contrast with the system activated and equilibrated.

In children and females, a suprapubic approach is usually used, and the cuff is placed at the bladder neck (Fig. 36-8). A 6 to 8 cm cuff is used in most females, and an 8 to 14 cm cuff is used in males. Also, a vaginal approach to placement of the AUS is an option in females. Again, the AUS is deactivated at the time of surgery to be activated at a later time.

The long-term continence results of the AUS are not only dependent on proper patient selection, but also very dependent on the surgical technique. Placement of the AUS needs to be performed by a physician who has experience with the device in an environment having experience with the technique.

RESULTS WITH THE AMS800 ARTIFICIAL URINARY SPHINCTER

Since the development of the AMS721 sphincter in 1973, numerous modifications of the device and insertion techniques have gradually improved the effectiveness of the artificial urinary sphincter and reduced the reoperation and complication rates.

As stated, the AMS800 artificial urinary sphincter should be utilized only in well-defined situations of urinary incontinence. The most frequent indications are for patients with neurogenic dysfunction (most commonly myelodysplasia), postprostatectomy incontinence in men and intractable stress incontinence in

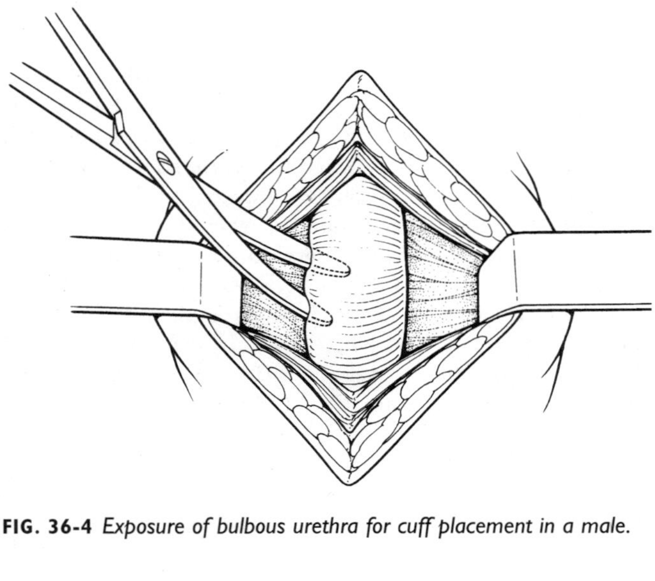

FIG. 36-4 *Exposure of bulbous urethra for cuff placement in a male.*

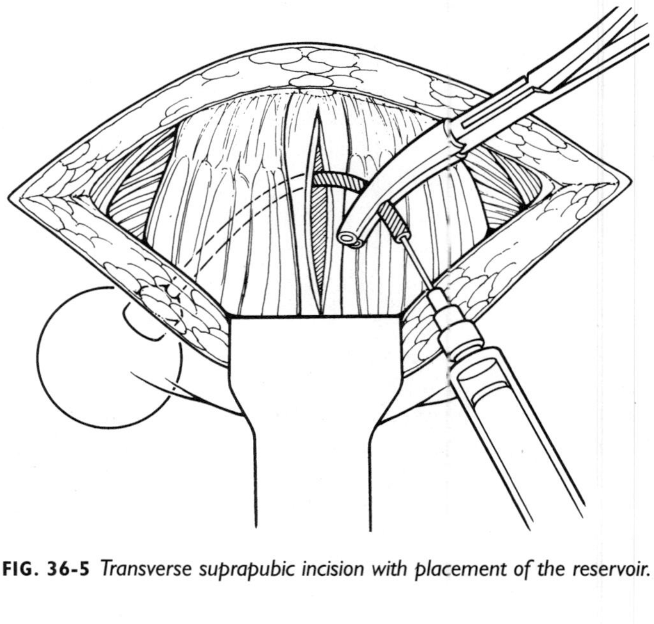

FIG. 36-5 *Transverse suprapubic incision with placement of the reservoir.*

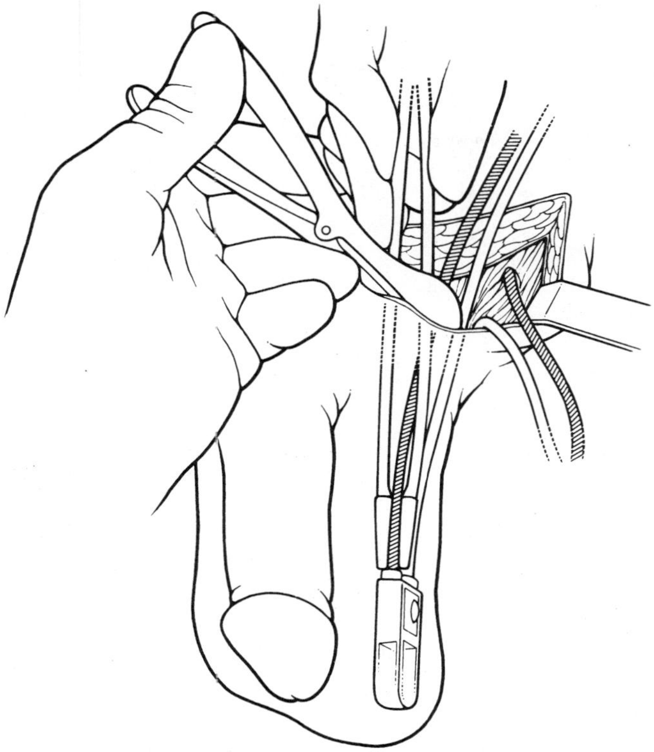

FIG. 36-6 *Scrotal placement of the pump through suprapubic incision.*

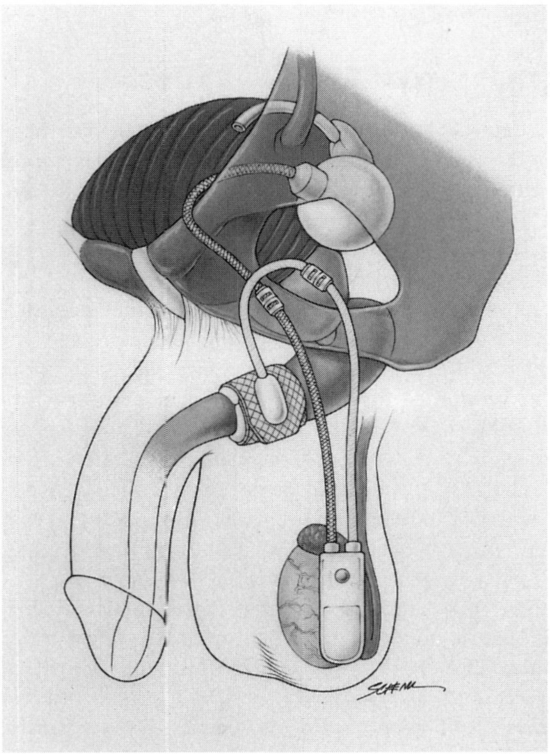

FIG. 36-7 *Cuff, pump, and reservoir in place with tubing connections completed.*

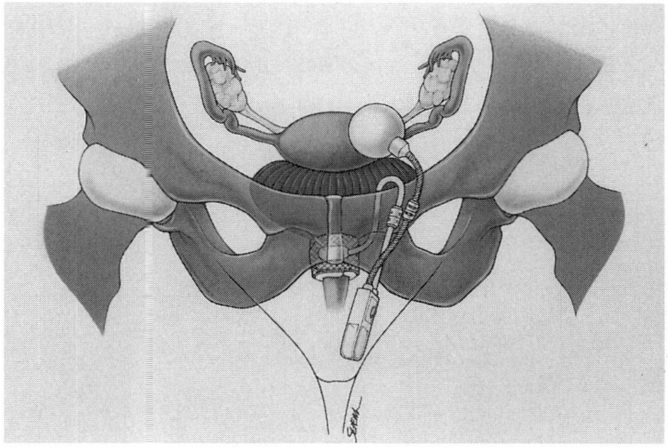

FIG. 36-8 *Cuff, pump, and reservoir in place with tubing connections completed for a suprapubic placement of an artificial urinary sphincter at the bladder neck in a female.*

females. When implanting the AUS in children or patients with neurologic or congenital urinary dysfunction, one must keep in mind that these patients often have complex genitourinary problems requiring complex management procedures. In addition, they may have other medical and neurologic problems that make them more susceptible to complications.

Despite the added considerations during insertion of the artificial urinary sphincter in children and patients with congenital urinary incontinence, successful results have been achieved (Table 36-1). Barrett et al. reported good continence in 80% of their patients (young adults and children) after a mean of 43 months.[12] Bosco et al. reported their experience with 36 patients after a follow-up time of 5 years or more.[13] This group reported an overall success rate of 84% at 2 years and 62% at 5 years.[14] Mouriquand and Mollard reported on 39 patients with a mean follow-up time of 5 years. In their series, 16 patients were reported to have a good result with no complications, and 12 additional patients were considered to have a good result after a second operation. Eleven patients in this group were considered failures for various reasons.[15] Because myelodysplastic patients have variable degrees of neurogenic dysfunction, thorough evaluation of the bladder capacity and function preoperatively are necessary, and the patients must be followed closely postoperatively to monitor the bladder and upper tract function. Often these patients require an augmentation. We believe that this possibility should be determined before implantation and be performed if possible before AUS insertion. In 1988, Strawbridge et al. reported good results with artificial urinary sphincters used with augmentation cystoplasty in 18 patients.[10] In that series all patients were continent, 15 required intermittent self-catheterization, and three patients were able to void abdominally. Complications with the AUS occurred in five patients and in two with the cystoplasty.[10] Gonzalez et al. also demonstrated the effectiveness of the AUS with an augmentation cystoplasty because this group reportedly achieved a continence rate of 87%.[11] Obviously, when the AUS is in place in conjunction with augmentation, the patient must be vigilant about emptying reg-

Table 36-1 Results in Children with Congenital Dysfunction

STUDY	NUMBER OF PATIENTS	DRY (NO PADS)	SOCIALLY CONTINENT (SATISFACTORY)	REOPERATIONS
Bellioli et al.*	37	59% (22)	90% (33)	19 (14)
Light and Scott†	132	70% (92)	89% (105)	48 (38)
Churchill et al.‡	44	64% (28)	91% (40)	NA
O'Flynn and Thomas§	44	91% (40)	96% (42)	NA (23)
Mouriquand and Mollard‖	39	NA	72% (28)	NA (23)
Bosco et al.¶	36	56% (20)	69% (25)	25 (22)
Barrett et al.#	59	NA	94% (55)	24 (24)

*Belloli G, Campobasso P, Mercurella A: *J Pediatr Surg* 27:1461, 1992.
†Light JK, Scott FB: *Br J Urol* 56:54, 1984.
‡Churchill BM, Gilmour RF, Khoury AE, McLoria GA: *J Urol* 138:1116, 1987.
§O'Flynn KJ, Thomas DG: *Br J Urol* 67:155, 1991.
‖Mouriquand PE, Mollard P: *Scand J Nephrol Suppl* 141:28, 1992.
¶Bosco PJ, Bauer SB, Colodny AH, et al: *J Urol* 146:396, 1991.
#Barrett DM, Parulkar BG, Kramer SA: *Urology* 42:431, 1993.

ularly to prevent overdistension and rupture of the bladder augmentation, and again these patients need to be monitored closely by their physicians. Finally, in the management of incontinence in these patients one must realize that the primary goal is renal preservation, and incontinence control should not overshadow this.

By far and away most experience has been accumulated on adult males and females in whom the AUS has been implanted for the problem of intrinsic sphincter deficiency. Generally, male type III urinary incontinence occurs after prostatectomy, and results with the AUS in this group have been very successful. In 1988, Marks and Light reported on 37 patients, 95% of whom achieved socially acceptable levels of incontinence and 81% of whom were completely dry. This group suffered three erosions (9%) and two infections (5%) and required four revisions 11%.[20] Gundian and colleagues from the Mayo Clinic reported on their experience with 96 patients, 83% of whom had incontinence requiring ≤2 pads/day. This group of patients also reported a 90% satisfaction rate.[17] Finally Malloy et al. reported a 76% complete continence rate in 42 males in whom the AMS800 device was implanted[18] (Table 36-2).

Because of increased technical demands with AUS insertion in females, there is more concern with long-term reliability and potential problems. Female AUS results, however, are impressive when one considers that these patients have devastating incontinence and have usually undergone several unsuccessful incontinence procedures before artificial sphincter insertion (Table 36-3). A report by Scott in the *Urologic Clinics of North America* demonstrated improvement in female AUS success rates as his techniques and the sphincter itself were improved. His early experience between 1972 and 1978 with 38 females met with an overall success rate of 69%. From 1978 to 1984 with second-generation devices and more surgical experience his success rate improved to 84%. Of these patients 92% were socially continent.[19] Parulkar and Barrett have reported good continence rates in 70.8% of their female patients after a mean follow-up time of 41 months.[20] Noll and Schreiter reported on 106 females (80 patients have been followed for at least 1 year) with an 86.3% complete continence rate. However, they report the need for reoperation in nearly 56% of their patients.[21] Recently, Webster et al. reported on 24 women implanted with artificial urinary sphincters between 1982 and 1990. Ninety-two percent had considerable improvement requiring no pads.[22] And Appell while using his transvaginal approach reported 100% dryness on all 34 of his patients, 19 of whom have had the device at least 3 years. Appell reports infections or erosions in only 3 cases.[23]

We have met with similar success. Upon review of our long-term data (>2 years) with insertion of the AMS800 artificial sphincter in 46 females we found 70% to be completely continent and 92% to have incontinence requiring no more than one pad per day. Our overall reoperation rate is 26%, and we have seen four erosions. Average follow-up time for this group of patients is now >5 years.[24]

POSTOPERATIVE FOLLOW-UP

Because the artificial sphincter is a prosthetic device, the patient who receives an AUS and the physician who implants it must be committed postoperatively to regular follow-up and care. Both must also be willing to deal with potential infections and mechanical problems that can arise and accept the possibility that reoperations may be required.

Our postoperative care routine begins in the operating room soon after the device is implanted. The device is tested while the patient is still under an anesthetic. Once successful cycling has been accomplished the cuff is opened. The pump is allowed to refill until a slight dimpling is palpable, and then the device is deactivated. If the device is deactivated immediately after opening, the cuff reactivation may be extremely difficult, in that some fluid is needed in the pump to unseat the poppet used to deactivate the cuff. The patient is then taken from the operating room with a Foley catheter that remains for 24 hours.

After removal of the Foley catheter, the patient is again incontinent because the sphincter is deactivated in the open position. All patients are aware of this preoperatively. Our patients remain in the hospital postoperatively for 2 or 3 days to receive intravenously 48 hours of antibiotics and on discharge are orally maintained on 7 to 10 days of antibiotics. During the patient's stay, the abdominal (and perineal) wounds are inspected daily, and the pump position is checked. Patients are instructed as to

Table 36-2 **Male Results**

Study	Number of patients	Dry (no pads)	Socially continent (satisfactory)	Reoperations
Marks and Light*	37	81% (30)	95% (35)	9 (9)
Gundian et al.†	96	NA	90% (86)	64 (37)
Malloy et al.‡	42	76% (32)	85% (36)	8 (8)

NA, Not applicable.
*Marks JL, Light JK: *J Urol* 142:302, 1989..
†Gundian JC, Barrett DM, Parulkar BG: *J Urol* 142:1459, 1989.
‡Malloy TR, Wein AJ, Carpiniello VL: *Urology* 33:274, 1989.

Table 36-3 **Female Results**

Study	Number of patients	Dry (no pads)	Socially continent (satisfactory)	Reoperations
Appell*	34	100% (34)	100% (34)	3 (3)
Noll and Schreiter†	80	86% (69)	86% (69)	62 (38)
Parulkar and Barrett‡	24	71% (17)	83% (20)	16 (12)
Light and Scott§	39	NA	92% (36)	21 (14)
Stone et al.‖	54	59% (32)	78% (50)	18 (14)
Webster et al.¶	24	92% (22)	100% (24)	8 (4)

*Appell RA: *Neurourol Urodyn* 7:613, 1988.
†Noll F, Schreiter F: *Urologe* 30(5):294, 1991.
‡Parulkar BG, Barrett DM: *Surg Gynecol Obstet* 171:131, 1990.
§Light JK, Scott FB: *J Urol* 134:476, 1985.
‖Stone KT, Diokno AC, Mitchell BA: *J Urol* 153(suppl):433A, 1995.
¶Webster GD, Perez LM, Khoury JM, Timmons SI: *Urology* 39:499, 1992.

pump position and encouraged to check position at least once daily and apply light traction as needed. We believe that this may help maintain pump position during scarring and healing and also help get the patient familiar with manipulating the device.

At 6 weeks postoperatively the patient returns for a follow-up exam and pump activation. At this time the patient is reinstructed on the use of the device and given a trial run. If a patient can successfully use the device, he or she is followed regularly (or more frequently if problems arise) at least once a year.

Potential Problems

Potential problems with the implantation or insertion of an artificial urinary sphincter can be classified under three general headings—infection, erosion, and mechanical malfunction. In general, a prosthesis that is carefully and properly placed will provide significant continence, and incontinence or changes in the patient's voiding habits or symptoms indicate a problem. Infections generally occur because of a breech in sterile technique or because the device has been colonized secondarily because of bacteremia. Signs and symptoms of an infection are erythema, tenderness, and swelling over a component or the entire device. In this scenario we will try a prolonged course of antibiotics. However, if infection persists, we recommend removal of the entire device, a course of antibiotics, and then replacement of the artificial urinary sphincter when signs of infection are gone (usually after 3 months). At the time the cuff is removed, if it is at a bladder neck position, an omental flap may be mobilized and wrapped around the urethra to maintain a plane for subsequent cuff placement.[25] To limit infections and complications careful attention to sterile technique and use of circumoperative antibiotics are a must.

Erosions can occur at any time and are generally attributable to a combination of factors. This complication is usually heralded by infection around the sphincter and recurrent incontinence. Additional signs that may indicate a possible erosion are pain in the perineum, swelling around the cuff, bloody urethral discharge, and gross hematuria. Irritative voiding symptoms may also be present.[26] Early erosions are most commonly secondary to insertion problems, with violation of the urethra during dissection being the most significant contributing factor. When this occurs and is recognized, it has been recommended that the urethra be repaired and attempt at AUS insertion be abandoned at that time. We have found, however, that in some instances, if minor urethral defects can be repaired and a new or different plane is established, the AUS may still be placed. If not, a silicone implant or omental flap may be inserted temporarily to maintain any developed plane for delayed insertion of the AUS cuff.[12] The incidence of erosion has decreased significantly since the introduction of delayed activation[4] and the AMS800 model. Motley and Barrett reported an erosion incidence of 18% before the advent of delayed activation and an incidence of 1.3% with delayed activation techniques.[26]

Late erosions may be caused by infection but in our experience are most commonly caused by catheter trauma. The usual scenario is that a catheter is inserted and left indwelling for an extended period without deactivation of the device with the cuff empty. Erosion and subsequent infection occur because of ischemia produced by the pressurized cuff squeezing the urethra against a rigid Foley catheter for a prolonged period of time. It is important to note that as the number of patients with artificial urinary sphincters increases the potential that a urologist or primary care physician will be involved in the care of an AUS patient is increasing. Because of this *it is imperative that all care providers be aware of the need to deactivate an artificial urinary sphincter if a Foley catheter is to be left indwelling.* To prevent potential problems patients are thoroughly educated about the care of their device and instructed to notify anyone about to place a catheter or to instrument the urinary tract that an AUS is in place. We also recommend that patients carry some sort of medical identification. *Again, if a patient is to be catheterized and the catheter is left indwelling, the AUS must be pumped (cuff deflated) and deactivated in this position* (as described previously). For a one-time in-and-out catheterization, deactivation is not necessary, *but the cuff must be pumped open.* Diagnosis of an erosion can be confirmed by cystoscopy and retrograde urethrography, and in general principle, erosions should be treated with removal of the entire AUS.

The third major category of sphincter dysfunction comprises mechanical problems. Leaks are the most common problem in our experience. A leak can occur in the balloon, pump, or tubing, or most commonly in the cuff, and this problem usually manifests with recurrent incontinence. This particular complication, however, appears to have decreased with improvements in the cuff design. The current cuff has a coated urethral contact side to decrease friction and a uniform circular configuration for uniform pressure transmission around the urethra. Leaks can be diagnosed by means of a plain film of the abdomen if a contrast medium is used in the system. A loose cuff caused by pressure atrophy of the urethra under the cuff may be the most common problem if the device is functioning intact. This can be successfully managed with cuff resizing and replacement. A device malfunction may also be manifested by failure to open the cuff with pumping or failure of reinflation after opening. This is often secondary to inadvertent deactivation or malfunction of the pump, kinking or clogging of the tubing (usually with blood or debris during insertion), or loosening of the cuff because of improper cuff insertion. To avoid mechanical problems, meticulous care is necessary when one is filling and connecting the components. All components and tubing should be securely connected as indicated in the instructions.

Another issue that may need to be addressed in patients with artificial urinary sphincters is with sexual function. Most data seem to indicate that sexual function is not affected in females or males except for males who have a sphincter in the bulbar urethral position. In this circumstance, the male patient will generally have retrograde ejaculation. Also of importance, in pregnant females, strong consideration should be given to elective cesarean section to avoid excess pressure or trauma to the bladder neck and device possible during vaginal delivery. In this situation a urologist familiar with AUS function should be involved with the case.

CONCLUSIONS

Clearly the use of the artificial urinary sphincter should be part of the armamentarium in the management of refractory incontinence caused by intrinsic sphincter deficiency for every urologist. The current device, the AMS800, has proved successful and effective in the short and long term. Meticulous care in the patient work-up preoperatively and during insertion is necessary, however, if maximum success is to be met. Proper indications for insertion are type III urinary incontinence caused by intrinsic sphincter deficiency. This should be well documented with endoscopic, urodynamic, or videofluoroscopic evaluation. All patients and their families should be well educated about potential outcomes and problems, particularly given that the device is a prosthesis.[27] Before implantation the patient's ability to use the sphincter from a physical and motivational standpoint should be thoroughly assessed.

Because of the risks for infection, erosion, and mechanical malfunction, extreme attention to detail and meticulous surgical technique are required during insertion. Finally, to meet with continued success after insertion, the patients must be monitored closely as long as the device is in place. Patients and physicians should be aware of signs of potential problems, changes in voiding habits, or signs of voiding dysfunction or infection. We also recommend that they carry a medical identification card to identify them as having an AUS in case of an emergency. If a catheter is to be placed, the device should first be deactivated, and if the patient becomes pregnant or undergoes any abdominal surgery, a urologist with knowledge of AUS insertion and function should be available to assist in patient circumoperative management. With careful preoperative evaluation, intraoperative technique, and postoperative follow-up, problems can be dealt effectively if they arise, and incontinent patients can achieve a significant improvement in their quality of life.

REFERENCES

1. Foley FB: An artificial urinary sphincter, *J Urol* 50:250, 1947.
2. Scott FB, Bradley WE, Timm GW: Treatment of urinary incontinence by implantable prosthetic sphincter, *Urology* 1:252, 1973.
3. Diokno AC, Taub ME: Experience with the artificial urinary sphincter at Michigan, *J Urol* 116:496, 1976.
4. Furlow WL: Implantation of a new semiautomatic artificial genitourinary sphincter: experience with primary activation and deactivation in 47 patients, *J Urol* 126:741, 1981.
5. Light JK: The artificial urinary sphincter in children, *Urol Clin North Am* 12:103, 1985.
6. Mundy AR: Artificial urinary sphincters, *Br J Urol* 67:225, 1991.
7. Scott FB, et al: Implantation of an artificialurinary sphincter for urinary incontinence, *Contemp Surg* 18:11, 1981.
8. Diokno AC, Sonda LP: Compatibility of genitourinary prostheses and intermittent self-catheterization, *J Urol* 125:659, 1981.
9. Barrett DM, Furlow WL: Incontinence, intermittent self- catheterization and the artificial genitourinary sphincter, *J Urol* 132:268, 1984.
10. Strawbridge LR, Kramer SA, Castillo OA, Barrett DM: Augmentation cystoplasty and the artificial genitourinary sphincter, *J Urol* 142:297, 1989.
11. Gonzalez R Nguyen DH, Koleilat N, Sidi AA: Compatibility of enterocystoplasty and the artificial urinary sphincter, *J Urol* 142:502, 1989.
12. Belloli G, Campobasso P, Mercurella A: Neuropathic urinary incontinence in pediatric patients: management with artificial sphincter, *J Pediatr Surg* 27:1461, 1992.
13. Bosco PJ, Bauer SB, Colodny AH, et al: The long-term results of artificial urinary sphincters in children, *J Urol* 146:396, 1991.
14. Light JK, Scott FB: The artificial urinary sphincter in children, *Br J Urol* 56:54, 1984.
15. Churchill BM, Gilmour RF, Khoury AE, McLorie GA: Biological response of bladders rendered continent by insertion of artificial sphincter, *J Urol* 138:1116, 1987.

16. Marks JL, Light JK: Management of urinary incontinence after prostatectomy with the artificial urinary sphincter, *J Urol* 142:302, 1989.
17. Gundian JC, Barrett DM, Parulkar BG: Mayo Clinic experience with use of the AMS800 artificial urinary sphincter for urinary incontinence following radical prostatectomy, *J Urol* 142:1459, 1989.
18. Malloy TR, Wein AJ, Carpiniello VL: Surgical success with AMS M800 GU sphincter for male incontinence, *Urology* 33:274, 1989.
19. Scott FB: The use of the artificial sphincter in the treatment of urinary incontinence in the female patient, *Urol Clin North Am* 12(2):305, 1985.
20. Parulkar BG, Barrett DM: Application of the AS-800 artificial sphincter for intractable urinary incontinence in females, *Surg Gynecol Obstet* 171:131, 1990.
21. Noll F, Schreiter F: The AS800 artificial sphincter for the treatment of female incontinence. *Urologe* 30(5):294, 1991.
22. Webster GD, Perez LM, Khoury JM, Timmons SL: Management of type III stress urinary incontinence using artificial urinary sphincter, *Urology* 39:499, 1992.
23. Appell RA: Techniques and results in the implantation of the artificial urinary sphincter in women with Type III stress urinary incontinence by vaginal approach, Neurourol Urodyn 7:613, 1988.
24. Stone KT, Diokno AC, Mitchell BA: Just how effective is the AMS 800 artificial urinary sphincter: results of a long-term followup in females, *J Urol* 153(suppl):433A, 1995.
25. Nurse DE, Mundy AR: One hundred artificial sphincters, *Br J Urol* 61:318, 1988.
26. Motley RC, Barrett DM: Artificial urinary sphincter cuff erosion: experience with reimplantation in 38 patients, *Urology* 35:215, 1990.
27. Diokno AC, Lapides J: *Urinary incontinence and genitourinary prostheses,* New York, 1970, Harper & Row, Chapter 19.

Chapter 37

Complications of Incontinence Surgery

Brett A. Trockman, Gary E. Leach

When surgery is indicated for the treatment of urinary incontinence, the concerns of the patient are usually related to the long-term success of surgery and complications of the operative procedure. Although urinary incontinence has a devastating effect on the quality of life of an individual, it is not a life-threatening disorder. Even though the results of surgery are excellent in most cases, it is extremely important for the patient to appreciate the potential problems associated with surgery so that the patient and family members are comfortable through the postoperative course and recovery process. Complications of incontinence surgery can result from patient selection based on incomplete information, incomplete evaluation that could more clearly define the problem, a decision to perform a procedure that may not be the best surgical approach for that particular patient, and specific surgical technique events that compromise the outcome of the surgery.

Urinary incontinence is a major social and medical problem resulting in immense morbidity for the patient.[1] Involuntary loss of urinary control is usually secondary to bladder dysfunction or incompetence of the bladder neck and the proximal portion of the urethra. Although bladder dysfunction can often be successfully controlled with behavioral modification or pharmacologic therapy, surgical therapy is often required to correct incontinence associated with abnormal bladder outlet resistance. In general, these procedures are very effective and are associated with few significant complications. However, since these procedures are elective, a careful discussion of the prevention, recognition, and treatment of complications associated with incontinence surgery is warranted. The following discussion is based on a review of the literature and our experience at a large tertiary care center specializing in urinary incontinence.

FEMALE INCONTINENCE SURGERY

Patient Selection and Evaluation

Proper patient selection and evaluation is critical to both maximizing the success rate and minimizing the complications of incontinence procedures. All patients considered for incontinence surgery should undergo a thorough clinical evaluation including appropriate radiographic and urodynamic testing when indicated.

A careful history documenting all lower urinary tract symptoms and past gynecologic and urologic history is required. A thorough pelvic examination should be performed to assess the degree of bladder neck and urethral hypermobility and to evaluate for coincidental vaginal disorders including cystocele, rectocele, urethral diverticula, uterine decensus and vaginal vault prolapse. Although complex urodynamic testing is not always needed in the evaluation of uncomplicated stress urinary incontinence associated with urethral hypermobility, demonstration of involuntary loss of urine simultaneous with increased abdominal pressure is mandatory before one performs bladder neck suspension surgery. Complete urodynamic testing and additional radiologic imaging may also be needed in selected cases.

Stress incontinence. Stress urinary incontinence associated with pelvic floor relaxation (type II stress incontinence) is the most common type of surgically correctable female incontinence. With pelvic floor relaxation, the proximal urethra and bladder neck become hypermobile rendering them incompetent during stress maneuvers. Some form of bladder neck suspension is the most effective treatment for type II stress incontinence. Many types of transabdominal and transvaginal procedures have been described to elevate and support the bladder neck and proximal urethra.

A more severe form of stress urinary incontinence has also been recognized and is known as intrinsic sphincter deficiency

(ISD), or type III stress urinary incontinence. Recently, improved understanding of ISD has led to heightened clinical awareness of this condition. Patients with type III stress urinary incontinence have an intrinsic deficiency of urethral closure usually resulting in pronounced urethral incompetence and severe incontinence. Most of these patients have a history of prior incontinence surgery, radiation, or neurologic abnormalities that may have functionally damaged the urethra, although about 10% of women with intrinsic sphincteric deficiency have no identifiable predisposing cause. Type III stress urinary incontinence is classically described as occurring in a fixed, rigid, "pipestem urethra"; however, intrinsic sphincteric deficiency may also occur in the presence of urethral hypermobility. When stress incontinence is demonstrated in the absence of urethral hypermobility, intrinsic sphincteric deficiency should be suspected. ISD is usually diagnosed by history, physical examination, and urodynamic testing including leak point pressure determination. A videourodynamic evaluation may also allow identification of an open proximal urethra in the absence of a bladder contraction highly suggestive of ISD. Since a routine bladder neck suspension is unlikely to correct ISD, a high clinical suspicion for intrinsic sphincteric deficiency along with appropriate urodynamic testing is needed to make the diagnosis preoperatively. The most widely accepted treatment for ISD is a pubovaginal sling procedure. Artificial urinary sphincters have also been successfully implanted for the treatment of female ISD.[2-5] More recently, periurethral injection therapy with collagen[6,7] or autologous fat[8,9] has been introduced as a minimally invasive means to treat type III stress incontinence. Although repeat injections may be required and long-term results are not yet available, periurethral injection therapy appears to be a feasible alternative treatment for female ISD.

Bladder dysfunction. Women with both stress urinary incontinence and symptoms of detrusor instability including urinary frequency, urgency, and urge incontinence present a difficult clinical situation. In our experience, about two thirds of patients treated for type II stress urinary incontinence also reported a component of urge incontinence preoperatively.[10] In these patients, urodynamics may be useful to document the presence of detrusor instability. Unfortunately, even in patients with severe symptoms of urgency and urge incontinence, uninhibited detrusor contractions are frequently not detected under routine urodynamic testing conditions. Ambulatory urodynamics have been proposed to more accurately assess bladder function; however, artifacts and other technical problems have prevented ambulatory urodynamics from gaining widespread clinical acceptance.

Most importantly, the prognostic significance of the preoperative presence of detrusor instability on the outcome of female incontinence surgery is unclear. When patients present with mixed stress and urge incontinence, the clinician must ascertain the relative contribution of both the stress and urge symptoms. Clearly, patients with symptoms of detrusor instability alone should not be treated with incontinence surgery directed at increasing outlet resistance. Our review of 125 patients undergoing modified Pereyra bladder neck suspension with mean 10-year follow-up time[10] (and a large series by McGuire et al.[11] with a shorter follow-up time after incontinence surgery) did not reveal the preoperative presence of urodynamically documented detrusor instability to be a significant negative prognostic factor. However, other series have suggested that preoperative, urodynamically documented detrusor instability has a negative effect on results after female incontinence surgery.[12-14] Unfortunately, none of these conflicting studies has definitively resolved this issue. Without a well-designed prospective study, the true effect of detrusor instability on outcome after female incontinence surgery remains unknown. Until this issue is resolved, the clinician must rely on clinical judgment and experience when planning the treatment of women with mixed incontinence.

In our practice, patients with predominant symptoms of urgency and urge incontinence with or without urodynamically documented detrusor instability are initially managed with behavioral therapy or pharmacologic therapy, or both. When the patient remains significantly bothered by symptoms of stress incontinence after control of symptoms of detrusor instability, surgery is offered. When significant symptoms of detrusor instability persist despite behavioral and pharmacologic therapy, surgery is offered to correct a major component of stress incontinence only after careful patient counseling that detrusor instability symptoms may persist or even be exacerbated postoperatively. In our experience, about half of patients with uncontrolled symptoms of detrusor instability preoperatively have similar or exacerbated instability symptoms after stress incontinence surgery.

Approach and Procedure Selection

The experience of the surgeon and the presence of associated vaginal or pelvic disorder should be the most important considerations when planning incontinence surgery. Selection of an inappropriate approach may increase the likelihood of both intraoperative and postoperative complications. Patients with routine type II stress urinary incontinence and no other significant vaginal or pelvic disorder may be safely treated with any form of transvaginal or transabdominal bladder neck suspension. No single procedure has been conclusively shown to be superior; although anterior repair is believed to be the least effective.[15]

In patients with combined pathologic states, the appropriate approach and procedure selection are essential to minimize complications and improve outcome. For example, patients with a large cystocele treated with the retropubic Marshal-Marchetti-Krantz or Burch suspension procedures are at risk for postoperative outlet obstruction secondary to a persistent cystocele.[16] Patients with a large cystocele are best served by a transvaginal cystocele repair and transvaginal bladder neck suspension or pubovaginal sling procedure. Similarly, patients with the combined problem of type II stress incontinence and a urethral diverticulum are best managed with a combined transvaginal diverticulectomy and bladder neck suspension. Simultaneous hysterectomy has been proposed to improve success rates after bladder neck suspension,[17] although in our experience and that of others[18,19] simultaneous hysterectomy and bladder neck suspension has not been advantageous. To avoid unnecessarily increasing the complexity and potential morbidity of incontinence surgery, it is our practice to perform simultaneous hysterectomy only when a coincidental uterine disorder exists or advanced uterine prolapse is present. The choice of abdominal versus transvaginal hysterectomy should dictate the approach to bladder neck suspension.

Intraoperative Complications

Bladder and urethral injuries. Except for periurethral injection therapy, bladder and urethral injuries can occur with all types of female incontinence surgery. Risk of this complication is increased in patients who have previously undergone incontinence or pelvic surgery. Scarring from previous surgery may obliterate normal planes of dissection increasing the risk of injury to the bladder and urethra during the course of repeat incontinence procedures. During transabdominal bladder neck suspensions, these injuries usually occur during dissection of the retropubic space to gain exposure of the bladder neck and anterior portion of the urethra. Parnell et al. reported a 7% incidence of urinary perforation among 114 women with a history of prior incontinence surgery undergoing Marshall-Marchetti-Krantz bladder neck vesicourethropexy.[20] Lee et al. advocated intentional cystotomy at the time of Marshall-Marchetti-Krantz vesicourethropexy to aid in the prevention and recognition of bladder injury during dissection and suture placement.[21] Prompt recognition and repair of any bladder injuries that occur during transabdominal bladder neck suspension procedures should prevent any significant sequalae. When the injury is large, placement of a suprapubic tube and postoperative retropubic drainage should be considered. Transvaginal incontinence procedures offer a more direct approach to dissection of the bladder neck and urethra and avoid an extensive retropubic dissection, thus decreasing the risk of significant cystotomy.

Bladder perforation is not uncommon during performance of the Stamey and Gittes transvaginal needle suspension procedures.[19,22] These minor injuries occur during the passage of the suspension needle. Performing the needle passage with the bladder on drainage decreases the chance of bladder penetration. After needle passage, careful cystoscopic examination of the entire bladder, especially the anterolateral bladder walls where perforation is most likely to occur, is recommended. Perforation should be suspected when bladder drainage is bloody or a blood clot is noted on the bladder wall. When suture material is noted with the bladder, the suture should be removed and needle passage repeated. Nonrecognition of a penetrating suture can lead to stone formation and chronic infection and should be considered in any patient with recurrent urinary tract infections after incontinence surgery.[16]

The modified Pereyra bladder neck suspension allows fingertip control of needle passage thus minimizing the risk of bladder perforation during needle passage. Leach and Raz reported no intraoperative bladder perforations in 54 women with a history of prior incontinence procedures undergoing the Raz modification of the modified Pereyra bladder neck suspension.[23] When a cystotomy does occur during vaginal incontinence surgery, the cystotomy can usually be safely repaired transvaginally before the planned procedure is completed.[24] In some cases, placement of a suprapubic tube to ensure optimal bladder drainage may also be advisable.

Urethral injuries are less common during incontinence procedures but may occur during dissection of a urethra severely scarred and fixed from previous surgery. Urethral injuries should be immediately repaired once recognized intraoperatively. When the urethral closure is tenuous, a Martius labial fat pad graft may be utilized to reinforce the repair.[25] An unrecognized urethral injury or inadequate repair of any urethral violation is likely to result in a urethrovaginal fistula.[26]

Ureteral injuries. Ureteral injuries are an uncommon but serious complication of incontinence surgery. Ureteral injuries most commonly occur with the Marshall-Marchetti-Krantz and Burch colposuspensions.[16,27] Erikson reported a 1% incidence of unrecognized ureteral obstruction after Burch colposuspension.[28] Although ureteral injury after transvaginal bladder neck suspension is extremely rare,[16] we have recently treated a patient referred with a ureterovaginal fistula that developed several days after a modified Pereyra bladder neck suspension. This injury probably occured during placement of the suspension suture in the medial edge of the perforated endopelvic fascia, also known as the urethropelvic ligament. Routine use of intravenous indigo carmine and direct or cystoscopic visualization of efflux from the ureteral orifices aids in the intraoperative recognition of ureteral injury during incontinence surgery. Ureteral injury noted postoperatively should be managed using standard endoscopic, percutaneous, or open surgical techniques.

Bleeding. Although venous bleeding arising from the rich perivesical, periurethral, and perivaginal venous complexes is often encountered during incontinence surgery, serious hemorrhage rarely occurs. The incidence of significant pelvic or vaginal hematomas is less than 3% in most series.[16] Venous oozing can usually be controlled by direct compression or vaginal packing. One can usually manage significant venous bleeding that occurs during the anterior vaginal dissection of a Burch colposuspension by placing figure-of-eight suspension sutures through the anterior vaginal wall and securing them to Cooper's ligament to both tampon the bleeding and complete the suspension.[16]

When performing modified Pereyra bladder neck suspension, on can minimize the bleeding by dissecting in the correct plane directly on the white shiny inner surface of the anterior vaginal wall. Infiltrating the anterior vaginal wall with saline solution facilitates development of this relatively avascular plane. Troublesome bleeding that does occur during transvaginal incontinence surgery is usually indicative of the wrong plane of dissection. Techniques helpful to obtain hemostasis include use of a headlight and adequate retraction to maximize visualization and allow identification and control of the open vessels with figure-of-eight sutures. When the offending vessels cannot be visualized to allow direct control, timely completion of the procedure and placement of a vaginal pack are usually sufficient to control the bleeding. In the rare case in which hemorrhage cannot be controlled with routine measures, Katske and Raz[29] described placing a Foley catheter with a 30 ml balloon into the vagina, placing packing around the catheter, and inflating the balloon to tampon the bleeding.

Nerve injury. Nerve injury is a possible complication of incontinence surgery especially when patients are positioned in the dorsolithotomy position. Injury of the common peroneal nerve can result from direct compression of the nerve between the fibular neck and the supporting leg brace. Injury to the femoral, saphenous, obturator, sciatic, and tibial nerves can also occur and may be related to excessive flexion and external rotation of the hips during positioning.[16] Once positioning-related neurologic injuries have been recognized, appropriate neurologic and physical medicine consultation should be obtained. First-degree injuries (neurapraxia) usually resolve within 1 to 6 weeks, whereas second-degree injuries (axonotmesis) usually resolve within 2 to 6 months.[16]

A nerve-entrapment syndrome has also been recognized after transvaginal needle suspension procedures. Small sensory branches of the ileoinguinal and genital branch of the genitofemoral nerve medial to the inguinal ring that are usually not visible are at risk for this injury.[16] Patients suffering from this complication experience pain radiating down the medial aspect of the thigh or a pulling sensation over the groin and suprapubic areas. This type of postoperative pain has been noted in 8% to 16% of patients undergoing various transvaginal needle suspension procedures.[16,30,31] One can minimize the risk of this complication by passing and anchoring the sutures to the fascia or pubic tubercle as medial as possible to avoid entrapping the lateral nerve branches. In our experience, the use of the bone-fixation technique to anchor the suspension sutures to the pubic tubercle has decreased the incidence of this postoperative pain syndrome.[32]

Postoperative Complications

Urinary retention. Temporary urinary retention frequently occurs after incontinence surgery regardless of the approach. A 27% incidence of immediate urinary retention has been reported after the Marshall-Marchetti-Krantz procedure.[20] Kelly et al.[33] reported that 44% of 114 women undergoing modified Pereyra bladder neck suspension experienced transient elevation of postvoid residual urine volumes (>100 ml) necessitating postoperative intermittent self-catheterization. The majority of postoperative urinary retention resolves within 1 to 2 weeks after bladder neck suspension procedures but is usually more prolonged after pubovaginal sling procedures.

Immediate postoperative urinary retention can be managed by replacement of the urethral Foley catheter and repeatition of voiding trials until adequate emptying is demonstrated. However, this method of management often results in multiple office visits for voiding trials and may be associated with significant catheter-related patient discomfort or urinary tract infection. Another option for management of postoperative retention is intraoperative placement of a suprapubic tube through which residual urine volumes can be checked postoperatively. We prefer to manage postoperative retention with clean intermittent self-catheterization. All patients are instructed in the technique of self-catheterization preoperatively with the option of intraoperative suprapubic tube placement reserved for those patients who are unable to master the technique. After a voiding trail on the first postoperative day, patients in retention or with postvoid residuals greater than 100 ml are reinstructed in self-catheterization technique. The patient then continues to perform self-catheterization until low residual urine volumes are obtained.

Permanent urinary retention is rare after bladder neck suspension procedures but is reported in approximately 5% of patients undergoing pubovaginal sling procedures.[34,35] Chronic retention after incontinence procedures is usually the result of oversuspension of the bladder neck and the proximal portion of the urethra creating outlet obstruction. Patients with elevated postvoid residuals preoperatively or other evidence of myogenic decompensation of the bladder may be at risk for prolonged or permanent retention after incontinence surgery. Indeed, in some patients with acontractile bladders or sacral arc denervation and associated stress incontinence, permanent retention may be the desired outcome of the surgery; thus continence is achieved and the patient can perform chronic intermittent catheterization. When undesired chronic urinary retention occurs after transvaginal needle suspension procedures and urodynamic evaluation has demonstrated adequate bladder contractility, cutting one or both suspension sutures may relieve the obstruction often with preservation of continence.[36,37] When the proximal part of the urethra and the bladder neck are clearly fixed in a high obstructed position, transvaginal urethrolysis may be required to treat the obstruction, with resuspension being performed by use of laterally placed sutures tied with minimal tension.[38] Raz et al. reported the return of normal voiding in 19 (66%) of 29 patients with iatrogenic outlet obstruction and elevated postvoid residuals or retention treated with urethrolysis.[39]

Immediate urinary incontinence. Urinary incontinence occurring immediately after incontinence surgery has several possible causes including persistent stress urinary incontinence, overflow incontinence, detrusor instability with associated urge incontinence, or urinary fistula.[16] Causes of immediate failure after bladder neck suspension include improper location of suture placement resulting in inadequate urethral support or obstruction; suture breakage, or "pull through," from the anchoring tissue; and improper procedure selection in patients with intrinsic sphincter deficiency. Overflow incontinence results from unrecognized postoperative retention and should be managed with fluid restriction and intermittent self-catheterization.

Detrusor instability. Significant symptoms of urgency and frequency can be persistent after incontinence surgery or develop de novo. Some authors have reported that greater than 50% of women with persistent or recurrent incontinence after incontinence surgery have unstable bladders.[13,40] In our review of 125 women after modified Pereyra bladder neck suspension with a mean 10-year follow-up time,[10] 64% of women with a known component of urge incontinence preoperatively reported urge incontinence at follow-up time and 16% reported de novo urge incontinence. Importantly, the presence of significant irritative symptoms at follow-up was correlated with decreased patient satisfaction. In our experience (as well as that of Blaivas et al.[35]), postoperative urgency and urge incontinence is also a major cause of patient dissatisfaction after pubovaginal sling procedures.

Iatrogenic outlet obstruction should be considered in patients with exacerbated or de novo postoperative urgency symptoms after incontinence surgery. Periurethral suspension suture placement or tying the sutures with excessive tension may result in iatrogenic outlet obstruction and symptoms of bladder instability (Fig. 37-1). Both the pubovaginal sling procedure and the Stamey transvaginal bladder neck suspension achieve continence by the induction of outlet obstruction and therefore may induce postoperative bladder instability. In contrast, Leach et al. have

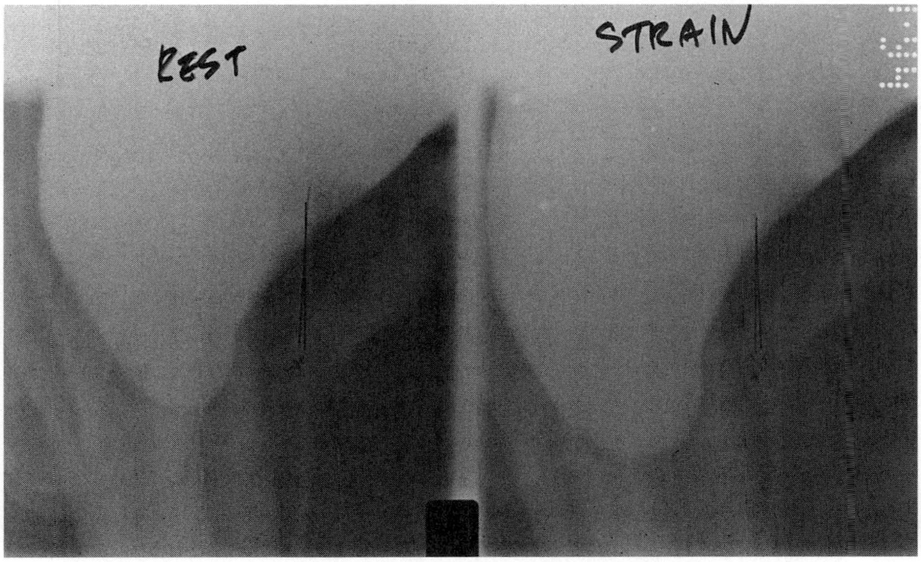

FIG. 37-1 *Patient with urethral obstruction after needle suspension. Notice the hyperelevated fixed urethra and associated cystocele.*

demonstrated that the lateral suspension suture placement used in the modified Pererya bladder neck suspension corrects stress incontinence without inducing outlet obstruction.[41] When outlet obstruction has been identified by videourodynamics and pressure-flow analysis as the cause of postoperative bladder instability, urethrolysis should be considered to relieve the obstruction.[39,42] Unfortunately, the cause of postoperative irritative symptoms is frequently impossible to clearly define. Management of these patients is difficult because the majority do not respond to standard behavioral and anticholinergic therapy.[16]

Wound infections. Wound infection rates among the various incontinence procedures range from 2% to 16%. Factors that may increase the risk of wound infection include reoperations, use of synthetic materials, diabetes, and obesity.[16] True retropubic abscess formation is rare after incontinence surgery. We have achieved a wound infection rate of less than 3% by routinely confirming the sterility of the urine preoperatively, use of an antiseptic abdominal scrub and vaginal douche the evening before and the morning of surgery, and the circumoperative administration of broad-spectrum antibiotic prophylaxis.

Osteitis pubis. Osteitis pubis is an uncommon usually self-limited complication of incontinence surgery. Most cases have been reported after the Marshall-Marchetti-Krantz cystourethropexy with a cited incidence of 1% to 10%.[20,21,43,44] The symptoms of osteitis pubis usually become apparent several weeks to months after the offending surgery, although we recently treated a patient presenting with osteitis pubis 9 years after undergoing a Raz transvaginal bladder neck suspension. Patients usually report significant pubic pain, often resulting in a waddling gait. Low-grade fever may also be present.[45] Radiographic abnormalities of the symphysis are usually seen 2 to 4 weeks after the onset of symptoms.[45] The plain radiograph findings range from a mild separation to a generalized moth-eaten appearance of the symphysis pubis (Fig. 37-2). Since not all cases of osteitis show abnormalities on plain radiographs,[20] a bone scan may be required to confirm the diagnosis.

The cause of osteitis pubis is not known but may be related to trauma, infection, and impaired circulation to the symphysis.[45,46] Since the etiology of osteitis pubis is not definitively known, treatment is supportive usually including heat, antibiotics, and anti-inflammatory agents. In rare debilitating cases unresponsive to conservative therapy, wedge resection of the symphysis pubis may be required.[47] True osteomyelitis is even less common than osteitis pubis and frequently requires open débridement of the infected bone as well as a long course of intravenously administered antibiotics.[45]

Enterocele formation. Enterocele formation may be a late complication of both transabdominal and transvaginal bladder neck suspension with a reported incidence of 5% to 17%.[34,48,49] Patients with symptomatic enteroceles usually describe a both-

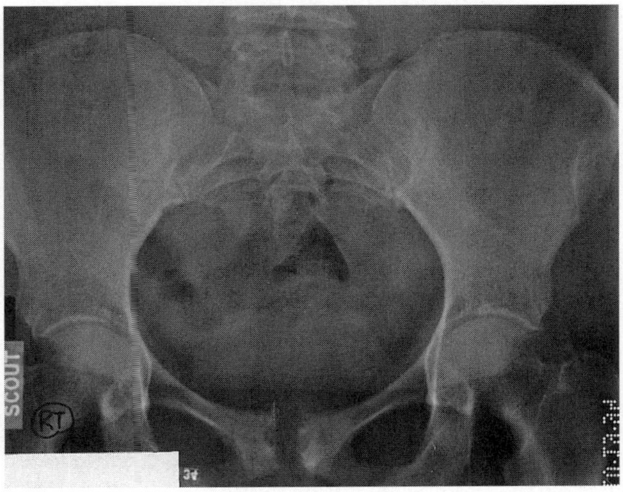

FIG. 37-2 *Plain film of the pelvis demonstrating separation and irregularity of the pubic symphysis typical of osteitis pubis.*

ersome sensation of vaginal pressure or fullness. Most enteroceles occur in patients who previously have undergone hysterectomy and may be associated with vaginal vault prolapse. After bladder neck suspension, the anterior bladder wall is elevated changing the vaginal axis and facilitating the formation of an enterocele through the separated remnants of the uterosacral and cardinal ligaments. Symptomatic enteroceles should be repaired transvaginally or transabdominally, and any associated vault prolapse should be repaired simultaneously with a vaginal vault suspension.

Artificial urinary sphincter placement. The intraoperative and late complications associated with artificial urinary sphincter placement in females are similar to those that occur after artificial urinary sphincter placement in males. These complications are discussed in detail in the following section on male incontinence surgery. Although most investigators have reported using the transabdominal approach for artificial urinary sphincter placement in females,[2,3] others have reported similar results and complication rates using a transvaginal approach.[50]

MALE INCONTINENCE

Like incontinence in females, male incontinence results from abnormalities in bladder or sphincteric function or a combination of both of these problems. In contrast to women, abnormalities in bladder outlet resistance rarely occur in the absence of neurologic abnormalities or a history of prior pelvic trauma, or urethral or prostatic surgery. With the advent of prostate specific antigen screening to detect prostate cancer, the number of radical prostatectomies performed has dramatically increased. Subsequently the unfortunate complication of postprostatectomy incontinence has increased as well. Although some authors have suggested that sphincteric insufficiency alone is responsible for postprostatectomy incontinence,[51] in our experience[52] as well as that of others[53] the majority of men with postprostatectomy incontinence do not suffer from sphincteric insufficiency alone, but most have a significant component of concomitant bladder dysfunction. In men with postprostatectomy incontinence, detailed urodynamic testing is needed to determine the contribution of bladder dysfunction, sphincteric insufficiency, or both, to the inability to store urine. Treatment should be directed by the results of the urodynamic testing. When present, bladder dysfunction should be controlled pharmacologically before surgical intervention to correct sphincteric insufficiency. Placement of an artificial urinary sphincter (AUS) around the bulbar urethra is the standard treatment for postprostatectomy stress incontinence with normal bladder pressures. Initial continence rates of about 80% can be expected after AUS placement in well-selected patients.[2] Unfortunately, the results of periurethral injection therapy for the correction of postprostatectomy sphincteric insufficiency have been disappointing.[54,55]

With appropriate patient selection, circumoperative care, and surgical technique, AUS placement can be accomplished with minimal morbidity. Utmost care should be taken to minimize the risk of infection during prosthetic surgery for incontinence. The sterility of the urine should be confirmed preoperatively, and all patients should receive broad-spectrum circumoperative antibiotic prophylaxis. We also routinely instruct all patients to perform an antiseptic scrub of the lower abdomen, genitals, and perineum the evening before and the morning of surgery and shave patients in the operating room. When one is implanting an AUS, the urethral dissection must be performed meticulously to avoid inadvertent urethral injury, especially in patients with a history of prior pelvic radiation. We routinely perform intraoperative perfusion sphincterometry to identify any unrecognized urethral injury and document appropriate function of the AUS.[56] This simple technique may also be performed in the office setting when one is evaluating patients with persistent or recurrent incontinence after AUS placement.

One performs perfusion sphincterometry by placing an 8 Fr pediatric Foley catheter in the meatus and inflating the balloon slightly in the fossa navicularis until the urethra is occluded. We routinely use a 51 to 60 cm H_2O pressure-regulating ballon; therefore a bag of sterile saline stained with indigo carmine is raised until the fluid level at the top of the bag is 51 cm above the level of the cuff. The sterile fluid is then infused through the catheter. Once the urethral segment between the closed cuff and occluded meatus is filled with fluid, infusion should stop. The pump is then squeezed several times so that the cuff is opened and infusion is allowed to resume. The interval until the cuff reinflates and infusion again stops is noted. The cuff reinflation time is usually between 3 and 5 minutes. Once the reinflation time has been documented, the height of the bag is slowly raised until fluid begins to drip through the drip chamber. The height at which fluid begins to drip through the drip chamber represents the cuff-closure pressure and should be recorded within the range of the pressure-regulating balloon (51 to 60 cm H_2O). When one is performing perfusion sphincterometry intraoperatively, a white gauze should be placed at the cuff site before beginning the infusion of the stained sterile saline. After completion of the perfusion study the gauze is carefully inspected for any evidence of blue staining, which would indicate the presence of an unrecognized urethral injury.

Late complications associated with AUS placement include mechanical failure, prosthetic infection, or recurrent incontinence. Fortunately, improvements of the AUS device have resulted in a decreased incidence of mechanical failure. The latest AMS-800 device has been estimated to have a reliability rate of 95% over a 36-month period, with most failures related to fluid leak from the cuff or pump-assembly failure.[57] However, even with use of the latest models, about 20% to 35% of adult patients undergoing AUS insertion require reoperation and revision for mechanical failures or surgical problems such improper cuff size or pump migration.[58] Over extended follow-up study, the revision rate is undoubtedly higher. Cuff erosion or infection has been reported in 8% to 13% of adults undergoing implantation of the late-model AUS.[2,58-61] Patients with a history of prior urethral surgery or radiation therapy are at increased risk for cuff erosion because of compromised vascularity of the urethra.[4] Unfortunately, many cases of erosion are associated with inappropriate urethral catheterization through an activated, closed cuff. Cuff erosion necessitates removal of at least the cuff and usually the entire device, since, even in the absence of frank infection, colonization of the other components can occur via the pseudocapsule enveloping the device. Similarly, infection of any one component of the AUS usually necessitates removal of the entire device. Reimplantation after adequate treatment of any infection and allowance for the urethra to heal has been successful in the majority of patients.[62]

Recurrent incontinence after AUS insertion can occur for a variety of reasons including high-pressure bladder dysfunction, mechanical failure, cuff erosion, or urethral atrophy at the cuff site. Fig. 37-3 provides an algorithm for the evaluation of incontinence after AUS placement. In our experience, use of this logical sequence of testing allows clear definition of the cause of the incontinence and thus facilitates appropriate therapy.

The importance of assessing the patient for high-pressure bladder dysfunction cannot be overstated. Abnormal compliance or detrusor instability may have been overlooked preoperatively or developed after AUS insertion. The high-pressure bladder dysfunction may result in incontinence and an increased risk of cuff erosion, vesicoureteral reflux, and hydronephrosis.[63,64] These serious complications associated with high-pressure bladder dysfunction have been well documented in pediatric patients with neurogenic bladder dysfunction, such as myelomeningocele, treated with AUS placement.[64]

Radiographic evidence for fluid loss from the system using plain radiographs of the contrast medium–filled reservoir or reservoir volume determinations using ultrasonography necessitate exploration of the device. When the exact site of the leak can be definitively localized, only the defective component should be replaced. Webster et al. have recommended the use of electrical testing to determine the site of the fluid leak.[65] When the exact location of the leak is unclear, the entire device should be replaced.

Commonly, incontinence associated with decreased closure pressure as determined by perfusion sphincterometry is secondary to urethral atrophy. In our practice, we have attempted to delay or prevent the development of urethral atrophy by routine use of the low-pressure 51 to 60 cm H_2O pressure-regulating balloon. Urethral atrophy is usually treated by moving the cuff site more distally to a more normal segment of the urethra. Some authors have recommended treatment of incontinence secondary to urethral atrophy by simply increasing the pressure of the reservoir with or without decreasing the cuff size and without moving the cuff site.[65,66] However, we rarely use this approach because of concern that increasing the pressure exerted on the already atrophied urethra may increase the long-term risk of cuff erosion.

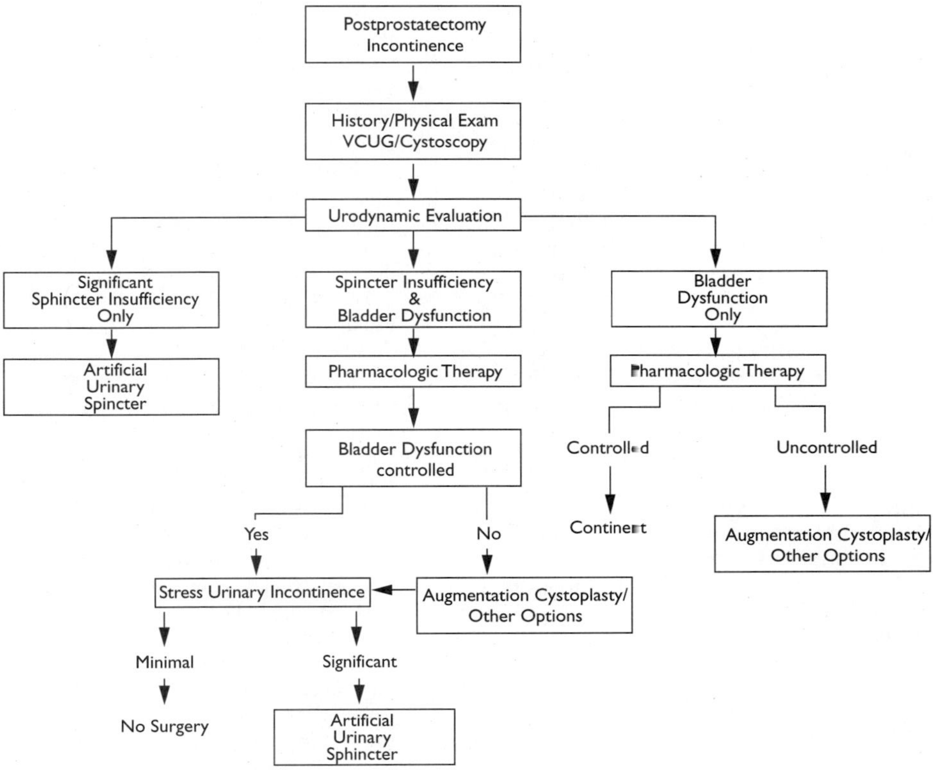

FIG. 37-3 *Algorithm for evaluation of incontinence after artificial urinary sphincter placement.*
(From Leach GE: *J Urol* 138:529, 1987.)

REFERENCES

1. Department of Health and Human Services. Public Health Service, Agency for Health Care Policy and Research: *Clinical practice guideline: urinary incontinece in adults*, Washington, D.C., 1992.
2. Scott FB: The artificial urinary sphincter: experience in adults, *Urol Clin North Am*, 16(1):105, 1989.
3. Webster GD, Perez LM, Khoury JM, Timmons SL: Management of type III stress urinary incontinence using artificial urinary sphincter, *Urology* 39(6):499, 1992.
4. Duncan HJ, Nurse DE, Mundy AR: Role of the artificial urinary sphincter in the treatment of stress incontinence in women, *Br J Urol* 69:141, 1992.
5. Diokno AC, Hollander JB, Anderson TP: Artificial urinary sphincter for recurrent female urinary incontinence: indications and results, *J Urol* 138:778, 1987.
6. Appell RA et al: Updated multicenter study on the GAX-collagen for female type III stress urinary incontinence [abstract], *J Urol* 147(suppl):279A, 1992.
7. Herschorn S et al: Long-term followup of intraurethral collagen for stress incontinence [abstract], *J Urol* 153(suppl):433A, 1995.
8. Ganabathi K, Leach GE: Periurethral injection techniques, *Atlas Urol Clin North Am* 2(1):101, 1994.
9. Santarosa RP, Blaivas JG: Periurethral injection of autologous fat for the treatment of sphincteric incontinence, *J Urol* 151:607, 1994.
10. Trockman BA, Leach GE, Hamilton J, et al: Modified Pereyra bladder neck suspension: 10 year mean follow up in 125 patients, *J Urol* 154(5):1841, 1995.
11. McGuire E, Savastono JA: Stress incontinence and detrusor instability/urge incontinence, *Neurourol Urodyn*, 4:313, 1985.
12. Lose G, Jørgensen L, Johnsen A: Predictive value of detrusor instability index in surgery for female urinary incontinence, *Neurourol Urodyn* 7:141, 1988.
13. Lockhart JL, Tirado A, Morillo G, Politano VA: Vesicoureteral dysfunction following cystourethropexy, *J Urol* 128:943, 1982.
14. Stanton SL, Cardozo L, Williams JE, et al: Clinical and urodynamic features of failed incontinence surgery in the female, *Obstet Gynecol* 51:515, 1978.
15. Creighton SM, Stanton SL: Comparison of surgical techniques, *Curr Opin Obstet Gynecol* 2:585, 1990.
16. Kelly MJ, Zimmern PE, Leach GE: Complications of bladder neck suspension procedures, *Urol Clin North Am* 18(2):339, 1991.
17. Green TH Jr: Urinary stress incontinence: differential diagnosis, pathophysiology, and management, *Am J Obstet Gynecol* 122:368, 1975.
18. Stanton SL, Cardozo L: Results of the colposuspension operation for incontinence and prolapse, *Br J Obstet Gynecol* 86:693, 1979.
19. Stamey TA: Endoscopic suspension of the vesical neck for urinary incontinence in females, *Ann Surg* 192:465, 1980.
20. Parnell JP, Marshal VF, Vaughn ED: Management of recurrent urinary stress incontinence by the Marshall-Marchetti- Krantz vesicourethroplasty, *J Urol* 132:912, 1984.
21. Lee RA, Symmonds RE, Goldstein RA: Surgical complications and results of modified Marshall-Marchetti-Krantz procedure for urinary incontinence, *Obstet Gynecol* 53:447, 1979.
22. Gittes RF, Loughlin KR: No-incision pubovaginal suspension for stress incontinence, *J Urol* 138:568, 1987.
23. Leach GE, Raz S: Modified Pereyra bladder neck suspension after previously failed anti-incontinence surgery, *Urology* 23:359, 1984.
24. Hadley RH, Myers RC: Complications of vaginal surgery: does unintentional cystotomy result in vesicovaginal fistula? *Proc Western Section American Urological Association,* p. 32, Scottsdale, Ariz., 1989, the Association.
25. Leach GE: Urethrovaginal fistula repair with Martius labial fat pad graft, *Urol Clin North Am* 18(2):409, 1991.
26. Zimmern P, Schmidbauer CP, Leach GE, et al: Vesicovaginal and urethrovaginal fistulae, *Semin Urol* 4:24, 1986.
27. Persky L, Guerriere K: Complications of Marshal-Marchetti-Krantz urethropexy, *Urology* 8:469, 1976.
28. Erikson BG: Long-term effectivenes of colposuspension in stress incontinence. In *Electrostimulation of the pelvic floor in female urinary incontinence,* Trondheim, Norway, 1989, p. 37.
29. Katske FA, Raz S: Use of Foley catheter to obtain transvaginal tamponade, *Urol Urotech* p. 8, May 1987.
30. Diaz DL, Fox BM, Walzak MP, Nieh PT: Endoscopic vesicourethropexy: experience and complications, *Urology* 24:321, 1984.
31. Kelly MJ, Leach GE: Longterm results of bladder neck suspension procedures, *Probl Urol* 5(1):94, 1991.
32. Leach GE: Bone fixation technique for transvaginal needle suspension, *Urology* 31:388, 1991.
33. Kelly MJ, Knielsen K, Bruskewitz R, et al: Symptom analysis of patients undergoing modified Pereyra bladder neck suspension for stress urinary incontinence: pre- and postoperative findings, *Urology* 37(3):213, 1991.
34. Raz S, Little NA, Juma S: Female urology. In Walsh PC, Retik AB, Stamey TA, Vaughn ED Jr, editors: *Campbell's urology,* ed 6, vol 3, Philadelphia, 1992, Saunders.
35. Blaivas JG, Jacobs BZ: Pubovaginal fascial sling for the treatment of complicated stress urinary incontinence, *J Urol* 145:1214, 1991.
36. Jones DJ, Shah PJR, Worth PHL: Modified Stamey procedure for bladder neck suspension, *Br J Urol* 63:157, 1989.
37. Morales A, VanCott GF: The Gittes procedure as an improved simplification of current techniques for vesical neck suspensions, *Surg Gynecol Obstet* 167:243, 1988.
38. Zimmern PE, Hadley HR, Leach GE, Raz S: Female urethral obstruction after Marshall-Marchetti-Krantz operation, *J Urol* 138:517, 1987.
39. Nitti VW, Raz S: Obstuction following anti-incontinence procedures: diagnosis and treatment with transvaginal urethrolysis, *J Urol* 152:93, 1994.
40. Webster GD, Sihelnik SA, Stone AR: Female urinary incontinence: the incidence, identification, and characteristics of detrusor instability, *Neurourol Urodyn* 3:235, 1984.
41. Leach GE, Yip C-M, Donovan BJ: Mechanism of continence after modified bladder neck suspension, *Urology* 23:359, 1984.
42. Dmochowski RR et al: Urethrolysis to relieve outlet obstruction after prior incontinence surgery [abstract], *J Urol* 151(suppl):420A, 1994.
43. McDuffie RW, Litin RB, Blundun KE: Urethrovesical suspension (Marshall-Marchetti-Krantz), *Am J Surg* 141:297, 1981.
44. Peters WA, Thornton WN: Selection of the primary operative procedure for stress incontinence, *Am J Obstet Gynecol* 137:923, 1980.
45. Burns JR, Gregory JG: Osteomyelitis of the pubic symphysis after urologic surgery, *J Urol* 118:803, 1977.
46. Steinback HL, Petrakis NL, Gilfillan RS, Smith DR: The pathogenesis of osteitis pubis, J Urol 74:840, 1955.
47. Grace JN: Wedge resection of the symphysis pubis for the treatment of osteitis pubis, *J Bone Joint Surg* 71A(3):358, 1989.
48. Stanton SL: The colposuspension operation for urinary incontinence, *Br J Obstet Gynaecol* 83:890, 1976.
49. Symmonds RE et al: Posthysterectomy, enterocele, and vaginal vault prolapse, *Obstet Gynecol* 140:852, 1976.
50. Hadley R: Long-term follow up (2-5 years) of transvaginally placed artificial urinary sphincters by an experienced surgeon [abstract], *J Urol* 153(suppl):432A, 1995.
51. Mostwin JL: Editorial: Urinary incontinence, *J Urol* 153:352, 1995.
52. Leach GE, Yip C-M, Donovan BJ: Post-prostatectomy incontinence: the influence of bladder dysfunction, *J Urol* 138:574, 1987.
53. Goluboff ET, Chang DT, Olsson CA, Kaplan SA: Urodynamics and the etiology of post prostatectomy incontinence: the initial Columbia experience, *J Urol* 153:1034, 1994.
54. McGuire EJ, Appell RA: Transurethral collagen injection for urinary incontinence, *Urology* 43:413, 1994.
55. Gill HS, Payne CK: Experience with collagen injection therapy in men with urinary incontinence [abstract], *J Urol* 153(suppl):277A, 1995.

56. Leach GE: Incontinence after artificial urinary sphincter placement: the role of perfusion sphincterometry, *J Urol* 38:529, 1987.
57. Barret DM, Furlow Wl: Artificial urinary sphincter in children. In Kelalis PP, King LR, Belman, editors: *Clinical pediatric urology,* vol 1, ed 2, Philadelphia, 1985, Saunders.
58. Mitchell ME et al: Augmentation cystoplasty implantation of artificial urinary sphincter in men and women and reconstruction of the dysfunctional urinary tract. In Walsh PC, Retik AB, Stamey TA, Vaughn ED Jr, editors: *Campbell's urology,* ed 6, vol 3, Philadelphia, 1992, Saunders.
59. Marks JL, Light JK: Management of urinary incontinence after prostatectomy with the artificial urinary sphincter, *J Urol* 142:302, 1989.
60. Fishman IJ, Shabsigh R, Scott FB: Experience with the artificial urinary sphincter model AS 800 in 148 patients, *J Urol* 141:307, 1989.
61. Gundian JC, Barrett DM, Parulkan BG: Mayo Clinic experience with use of the AMS 800 artificial sphincter for urinary incontinence following radical prostatectomy, *J Urol* 142:1459, 1989.
62. Motley RC, Barrett DM: Artificial urinary sphincter cuff erosion, experience with reimplantation in 38 patients, *Urology* 35(3):215, 1990.
63. Bitsch M, Nerstrøm H, Nordling J, Hald T: Upper urinary tract deterioration after implantation of artificial urinary sphincter, *Scand J Urol Nephrol* 24:31, 1990.
64. Bauer SB, Reda EF, Colodny AH, Retik AB: Detrusor instability, a delayed complication in association with the artificial sphincter, *J Urol* 135:12 2, 1986.
65. Kreder KJ, Webster GD: Evaluation and management of incontinence after implantation of the artificial urinary sphincter, *Urol Clin North Am* 1[illegible](2):375, 1991.
66. Martins FE, Boyd SD: Artificial urinary sphincter in patients following major pelvic surgery and/or radiotherapy: are they less favorable candidates? *J Urol* 153:1188, 1995

Chapter 38 Biofeedback Therapy

Patricia A. Burns

Disorders of urinary bladder control affect millions of people of all ages. Many of these people desperately want and need treatment but are not candidates for surgery, prefer a nonsurgical alternative, have failed pharmacologic therapies, have already failed surgery, or have failed other nonsurgical treatment such as pelvic muscle exercises. Biofeedback is a very specific treatment that can restore bladder control by altering the balance in centers that modulate the mechanisms of continence. Swartz et al.[1] defines the process of applied biofeedback as the "utilization of electromechanical instruments to accurately measure, process and feed back to persons information about neuromuscular and autonomic activity both normal and abnormal in the form of analog or binary, auditory and /or visual feedback signals." The International Continence Society defines biofeedback as a behavioral treatment modality for incontinence used to teach acquisition of pelvic muscle contractions and voluntary inhibition of detrusor contractions.

Biofeedback Research

Stress Incontinence

In the late 1940s Andrew Kegel developed the first vaginal perineometer used in a biofeedback treatment for urinary incontinence.[2] This early biofeedback device consisted of a vaginal chamber attached to a manometer that measured pelvic muscle contractions and provided visual feedback. Kegel's initial study of the effectiveness of biofeedback therapy for stress incontinence effectively resulted in 90% reduction in symptoms of urine loss.[3] Despite these promising results, further studies were not conducted until the late 1970s. Shepherd[4] treated 11 community-dwelling women with genuine stress incontinence using visual biofeedback as compared to a nontreatment control group. Ninety-one percent ($n = 10$) showed improvement or were cured in the biofeedback group, whereas only 55% ($n = 6$) had similar results without visual reinforcement. Burgio's[5] study of 19 stress-incontinent women succeeded in reducing the frequency of incontinent episodes an average of 82% after receiving bladder-sphincter biofeedback. Baigis-Smith et al.[6] studied 54 male and female subjects 60 to 86 years of age with symptoms of stress, urge and complex types of incontinence. Pelvic muscles exercises were augmented by the use of biofeedback, habit training, and relaxation techniques. Biofeedback was given through the use of a clinical perineometer that used light-emitting diodes and an adjustable speaker that provided both visual and audio biofeedback. Fifty percent of the subjects demonstrated a 90% improvement. Burns et al.[7] conducted a randomized, controlled clinical trial of biofeedback treatment in women with stress and mixed incontinence using an electronic vaginal perineometer with biofeedback provided through the visual line graph display of the pelvic muscle contractions. Subjects in the biofeedback group had a 61% reduction in symptoms with a 9% increase in urine losses in the control group.

Urge Incontinence

Biofeedback has also been used to treat motor urge incontinence or detrusor instability. Biofeedback techniques for the suppression of uninhibited detrusor contractions require the use of a transurethral bladder catheter and a rectal pressure monitor. The bladder catheter measures increases in intravesical pressure indicative of uninhibited contractions. The rectal catheter measures and subtracts the intra-abdominal pressure component of the bladder pressure measurements. Patients view the graphic tracing of the intrabladder measures and learn to sense these contractions and institute a pelvic muscle contraction to overcome the contractions. Burgio[5] in an uncontrolled study demonstrated an 88% reduction in incontinence episodes in elderly men with urge incontinence who participated in an average of four ½-hour biofeedback training sessions.

Cardoza[8] treated 27 female patients with four to eight biofeedback training sessions by means of cystometry converted into auditory and visual stimuli of changes in bladder pressure. Eighty-one percent of the patients either reported improvement in symptoms or no longer exhibited detrusor contractions on cystometry. Kjolseth et al.,[9] using bladder filling and pressure measurements with visual stimuli in the form of lighted lamps, taught their adult and child patients to suppress detrusor contractions by tensing the pelvic musculature. Treatment sessions varied with the mean number of trainings, 2.2 in the adults and 3.3 in the children. In the 15 child subjects, 60% had a pronounced improvement. Of the seven adult subjects only two showed a moderate treatment effect. O'Donnell[10] treated 20 male patients with urge incontinence over 65 years of age using 1-hour sessions twice weekly for 5 weeks. The mean number of incontinent episodes was decreased from 5.1 to 2.0 per day after treatment.

Clinical Procedures

The clinical procedures in biofeedback treatment for urinary incontinence can be divided into three sessions: initial, middle, and terminal. The following section describes the biobehavioral procedures provided by a primary health care provider.

Initial Session

In the initial session the provider should determine the extent of the patient's urine loss problem. This incontinence history taking can be supplemented and standardized by means of a urinary-symptom questionnaire. A complete medical examination should be performed with an extensive evaluation of the genitourinary and neurologic systems.

Discuss the rationale and procedure for using biofeedback as a treatment for urinary incontinence. Many people view biofeedback as a mysterious process. As a biofeedback therapist you can explain to the patient that their bodily activities give them very little feedback or information about their function. The equipment used for biofeedback obtains distinct information on the patient's pelvic muscle activity and strength.

Demonstrate and hold a practice session of the biofeedback techniques. After discussing the rationale for the biofeedback procedure we then set up the biofeedback equipment and perform a demonstration. For the demonstration, we place patch electrodes on our forearm and contract and relax the forearm muscles. We demonstrate how increasing and relaxing the muscles changes the line graph on the computer screen and its corresponding auditory changes. Finally, we assist the patient in a practice session using the vaginal or rectal probe or patch electrodes.

Establish procedures for recording urine loss symptoms. The patient is instructed in how to keep a record of his or her daily voiding, urine losses, and at-home practice sessions. The therapist records the electromyograph readings. In addition, a graph of the patient's weekly urine losses and electromyograph readings provides a visual patient progress record. The records also provide documentation for the clinical records of the patient.

Set up a specific treatment plan with the type of procedures and the goals and results that will be sought during the therapy program. A videotape containing the following areas is presented to each client: (1) prevalence of the problem, (2) pelvic organ and muscle anatomy, (3) progressive pelvic muscle exercise program, (4) individualized exercise schedule, and (5) instructions for diary keeping. A separate pamphlet describes the electromyograph equipment electromyography concept, and the biofeedback procedure (Appendix G at the end of the text).

Middle Sessions

Once a program has been designed and initiated, the goals for the middle treatment sessions for biofeedback are focused on evaluation of the client's home practice, symptoms, and overall treatment progress.

Home practice. The patient's urinary diaries are reviewed at each visit to determine effectiveness of the behavioral therapy and document progress. Is there a change in the frequency of symptoms? Is there a pattern in the symptoms—are they related to certain activities or time of day (that is, nocturia)? During this review it is important to give praise and encouragement to enhance success.

Biofeedback procedure. A quiet, comfortable environment should make the patient feel isolated from the surroundings and able to concentrate on the biofeedback technique. The first step in the biofeedback procedure is to have the patient relax his or her pelvic muscles and observe the electromyographic or manometric activity as it is displayed on the computer screen. The treatment sessions are essentially training sessions that strive to increase the strength and endurance of the pelvic muscles.

Initially, the therapist should have the patient identify the pelvic muscles during a rectal or pelvic examination. The patient should be instructed to contract the pelvic muscles around the examiner's fingers while relaxing the abdominal, thigh, and buttock muscles.

Electromyography of pelvic muscle activity is accomplished by use of skin surface electrodes or a vaginal or rectal probe. To perform biofeedback the therapist should use two channels on the electromyograph machine: one channel for measuring pelvic muscle activity and the second channel to measure abdominal activity.

The first channel displays pelvic muscle activity through the placement of active surface electrodes around the anus at the 10 o'clock and 2 o'clock positions with the ground lead placed on a bony prominence (such as the iliac crest).

The second channel displays the abdominal muscle activity through two active electrodes placed 1 inch apart just below the umbilicus. Again, a ground electrode is placed on a convenient bony prominence.

A second method of biofeedback utilizes manometry or pressure biofeedback by means of an intravaginal or intrarectal device. The advantage to using pressure manometry is the fact that as the patients contract their pelvic muscles the device or sensor produces a resistive pressure that gives feedback to the patient of his or her success in contracting the muscle. Similar to the above procedure, a second channel using surface electrodes measures abdominal activity. The main disadvantage in using this method is the fact that patients need to purchase a personal vaginal or rectal probe, whereas surface electrodes are disposable, convenient, and easily used, especially in a home setting.

Practice sessions. The goal of practice sessions is to have the patient practice biofeedback skills and develop strength and endurance. Because biofeedback requires effort, the sessions should not overtax the patient. The *first criterion* used to judge the appropriateness of the session is to obtain a statement from the patient as to how long he or she can practice successfully. The *second criterion* is the patient's record of success. If the patient's performance begins to deteriorate after 15 minutes or less there is no therapeutic advantage to continuing. In general, the initial sessions are shorter than subsequent sessions. Initially, the therapist may need to have weekly or twice-weekly sessions to assist the patient in identifying and isolating the pelvic muscles. Thereafter, session interval times may be increased incrementally as the patient shows progress and symptom improvement.

Patients with symptoms of *urge incontinence* can also be taught to contract the pelvic floor muscles voluntarily. In addition, their treatment is aimed at providing bladder pressure biofeedback and learning voluntary inhibition of detrusor contraction during bladder filling with sterile water. Patients with urge incontinence learn how to contract pelvic floor muscles in response to urgency or any rise in bladder pressure as they view the electromyographic display of their intrabladder pressure (that is, contractions) and learn to sense and subsequently inhibit those contractions. They also receive abdominal pressure feedback (through either a rectal pressure catheter or circumanal surface electrodes) so that they learn how to keep the abdominal muscles relaxed when they sense the urge to void. The timing and length of biofeedback sessions vary as 1-hour sessions once or twice weekly for 1 to 2 months.[5,10]

Treatment progress. A goal should be set for each biofeedback session to enable the clinician to evaluate the success of the patient's effort. The goal set by the clinician should be high enough to motivate the individual but low enough to ensure a high probability of success. Usually the goals are set very low to allow the patient time to learn the biofeedback operation and how to contract the pelvic muscles in an appropriate manner (learning curve). The goal should then be altered on the basis of past performance; increased when performance is excellent, held constant when performance is adequate, and decreased when performance is poor.

Elimination of biofeedback. A final goal in biofeedback therapy is to enable the client to perform pelvic muscle exercises without the need of the biofeedback equipment. Once the patient has reached a successful level of functioning, practice without biofeedback is accomplished by initiation of alternating periods with or without feedback during a training session. As training progresses, the periods without feedback can be gradually increased. Initially the sessions without feedback might be only a few minutes long. The length of time that this elimination training requires will depend on the success of the patient.

Terminal and Follow-up Sessions

Termination usually comes as the result of a joint decision between the clinician and the patient. Clinical visits are spaced farther and farther apart, and the patient's symptoms and performance are evaluated for any regression or increase in symptoms. Generally, 1-month follow-up examinations should be adequate to determine any important changes as a result of the termination of treatment. Thereafter, 3-month follow-up exams to determine the lasting effects of the treatment are generally sufficient.

Biofeedback Equipment

Biofeedback equipment is chosen by the clinician on the basis of cost and ease of application (that is, home versus office use).

In order for biofeedback equipment to be effective both pelvic and abdominal muscle activities should be monitored. These measurements can be accomplished through a two-channel system. Multichannel systems can allow for pressure and electromyographic measurements as well as abdominal measurements, thereby providing the clinician with multiple methods of biofeedback. Multiple avenues of measurement are effective in treating patients with urge incontinence where monitoring of bladder pressure and sphincter and abdominal muscle activity composes the treatment protocol.

A few examples of the multiple types of EMG biofeedback equipment are presented in this section. Fig. 38-1 depicts the Myoexorciser III dual-channel device connected to a personal computer through a software interface. Dual-channel devices allow the clinician to monitor through the secondary EMG channels the activity of the abdominal, buttock, or other muscles that the patient is using to substitute for the pelvic muscles. In addition, the personal-computer interface allows the clinician to archive an unlimited amount of session data, thereby providing the clinician the ability to quantify the treatment progress objectively.

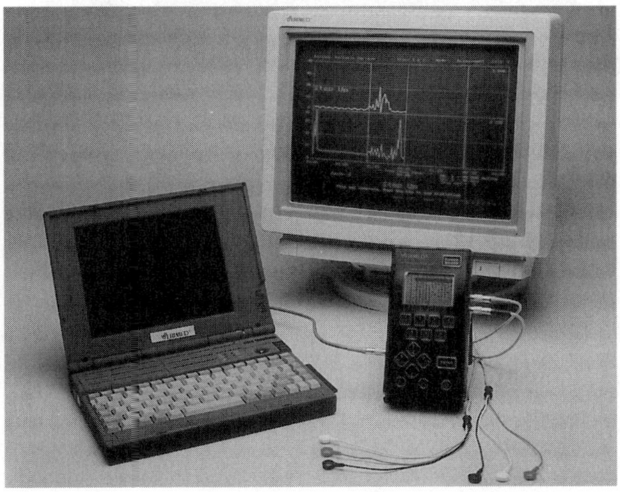

FIG. 38-1 *The Myoexorciser III dual-channel biofeedback unit.* (Courtesy xxx.)

The Myoexorciser II and perineometer is a single-channel EMG device used for home usage (Fig. 38-2). In conjunction with the vaginal sensor (perineometer) the Myoexorciser II can augment regular, clinical treatment sessions with a home exercise program designed specifically to meet the patient's requirements. In addition, the Myoexorciser II records and stores quantified statistics regarding each home treatment session, allowing the therapist to both ensure compliance with the home treatment program and track patient progress objectively.

As shown in Fig. 38-3, InCare Medical Products offer the PRS9500 Pelvic Floor Therapy System for the treatment of female urinary incontinence. This system allows the treatment of patients using EMG or pressure biofeedback and electrical stimulation. Vaginal, anal, and surface sensors are available. InCare also offers home units, which allow patients to continue their pressure biofeedback or electrical stimulation therapy at home.

Another equipment example, found in Fig. 38-4, is the Orion Continence System with a video-interactive home trainer. This is a dual-channel EMG system that uses an internal microprocessor and firmware display cartridges. It may also be used with an external computer and optional software. The trainer plugs into any cable-ready television. Both vaginal and rectal EMG sensors are available (shown on the right and left units respectively).

SUMMARY

As described in this chapter, there are many different aspects to biofeedback treatment. Biofeedback research comparing and testing the differences between pressure and electromyograph activity as a biofeedback mechanism has not been conducted. Therefore the biofeedback therapist needs to determine empirically the appropriate mechanism for his or her client. Rates of improvement in patients vary with the type and severity of incontinence and should be fully evaluated before therapy initiation as a method of individualizing treatment.[7] Lastly, accurate and complete treatment data are necessary for each patient to validate progress and ensure appropriate medical records for each patient.

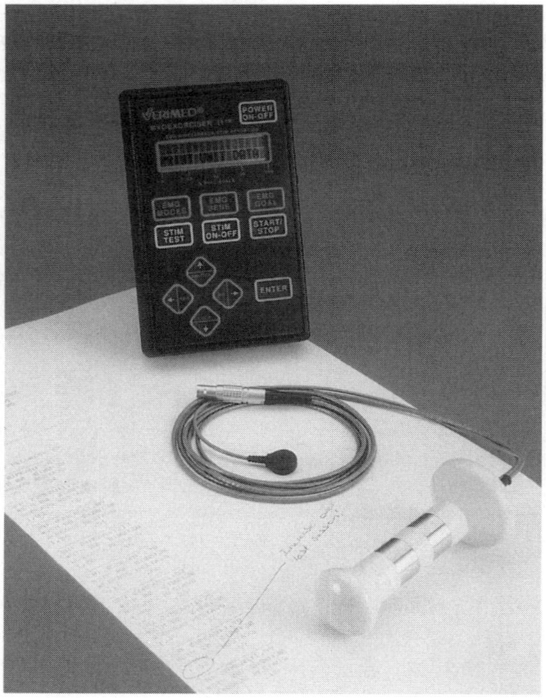

FIG. 38-2 *The Myoexorciser II single-channel home biofeedback unit.* (Courtesy xxx.)

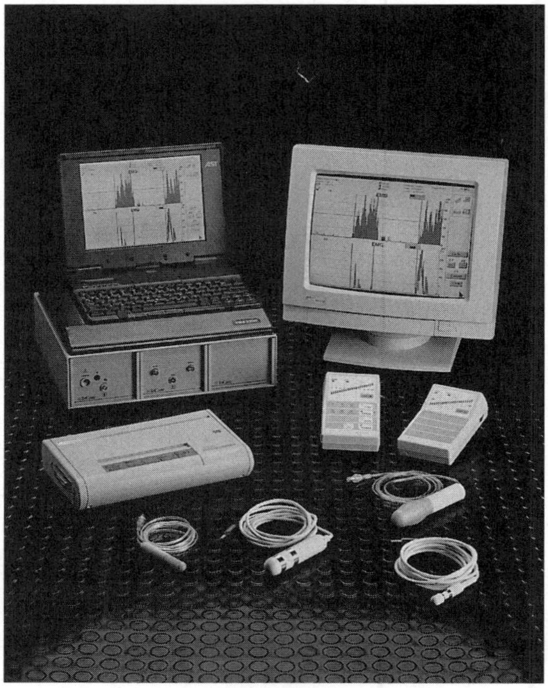

FIG. 38-3 *The PRS9500 Pelvic Floor Therapy System.* (Courtesy InCare Medical Products.)

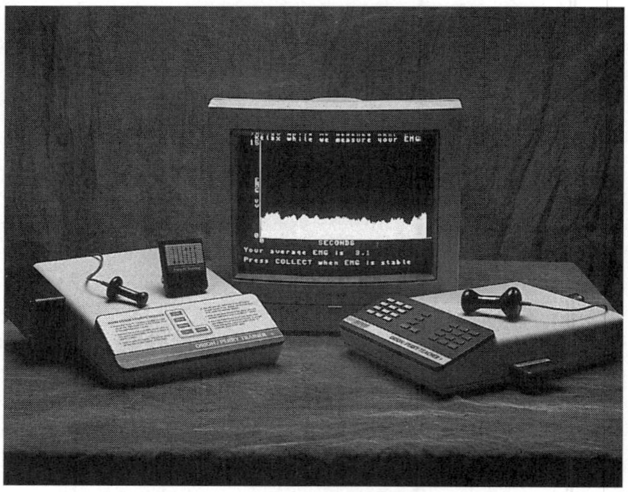

FIG. 38-4 *The Orion Continence System.* (Courtesy Orion Medical Products, Inc., Wheeling, Ill.)

REFERENCES

1. Swartz MS: *Biofeedback: a practitioner's guide,* New York, 1987, The Guilford Press.
2. Kegel AH: Progressive resistance exercise in the functional restoration of the perineal muscles, *Am J Obstet Gynecol* 56:238, 1948.
3. Kegel A: Stress Incontinence of women: physiological treatment, *J Int Coll Surg* 25:434, 1956.
4. Shepherd AM: Treatment genuine stress incontinence with a new perineometer, *Physiotherapy* 69(4):113, 1983.
5. Burgio KL, Whitehead WE, Engel BT: Urinary incontinence in the elderly, *Ann Intern Med* 104:507, 1985.
6. Baigis-Smith J, Smith DA, Rose M, Newman DK: Managing urinary incontinence in community-residing elderly persons, *Gerontologist* 29(2):229-233.
7. Burns PA, Pranikoff K, Nochajski TH, et al: A comparison of effectiveness of biofeedback and pelvic floor exercise treatment of stress incontinence in older community dwelling women, *J Gerontol Med Sci* 48(4):M167-M174, 1993.
8. Cardozo LD, Abrams PD, Stanton SL, Feneley RC: Idiopathic bladder instability treated by biofeedback, *Br J Urol* 50:521-523, 1978.
9. Kjolseth D, Madsen B, Knudsen LM, et al: Biofeedback treatment of children and adults with idiopathic detrusor instability, Scand J Urol Nephrol 28:243-247, 1994.
10. O'Donnell PD: Biofeedback therapy technique for treatment of urinary incontinence, *Urology* 37(5):432-436, 1991.

Chapter 39 Pharmacologic Therapy

Denise A. Nigro, Alan J. Wein

The basis for uropharmacology lies in an understanding of the autonomic innervation and the anatomy of the lower urinary tract. Many of the drugs employed in the treatment of lower urinary tract dysfunction have been chosen for theoretically similar modes of action elsewhere in the body. Unfortunately, the majority of drugs used for the treatment of urinary incontinence are not site specific. Thus therapy may be limited by significant side effects of the drugs.

Normal storage of urine requires accommodation of increasing volumes of urine at a low intravesical pressure, a bladder outlet that is closed at rest and remains so during increases in intra-abdominal pressure, and absence of involuntary bladder contractions.[1] Pharmacologic therapy for urinary incontinence, then, is focused on restoring one or a combination of these factors.Most therapeutic agents discussed, then, can be classified according to the primary site of action—bladder or bladder outlet[2] (see box). Aberrations from the normal state will lead to failure of the lower urinary tract to function properly. Involuntary contractions are most commonly seen in association with neurologic disease or after neurologic injury. They may also be associated with inflammatory or irritative processes in the bladder wall, or bladder outlet obstruction. Involuntary contractions may even be idiopathic. Decreased compliance during filling results from any process that destroys the viscoelastic properties of the bladder wall. Purely sensory urgency can also account for storage failure. This can be associated with an inflammatory, infectious, neurologic, psychologic, or idiopathic process. A fixed decrease in outlet resistance may result from a variety of insults to the innervation or the structural elements of the smooth or striated sphincter, neurologic disease or injury, surgical or other mechanical trauma, or aging. Classic stress urinary incontinence in the female implies failure of the normal transmission of increases in intra-abdominal pressure to the area of the bladder neck and proximal portion of the urethra. This may be attributable to changes in anatomic features or related to a decrease in the reflex striated sphincter contraction associated with increases in intra-abdominal pressure.

None of the agents discussed can completely restore normal lower urinary tract function. Quite often, success can be achieved with a combination of pharmacologic agents and behavior modification. One must also keep in mind that scientific evaluation of the results obtained using any of these methods of therapy is complicated by the effect of placebo in any condition generally characterized by subjective symptoms.[3,4]

Therapeutic Agents

INCREASE CAPACITY
Anticholinergic agents
Musculotropic relaxants
Calcium antagonists
Potassium channel openers
Prostaglandin inhibitors
Beta-adrenergic agonists
Tricyclic antidepressants
Dimethyl sulfoxide
Bromocriptine
Polysynaptic inhibitors

INCREASE OUTLET RESISTANCE
Alpha-adrenergic agonists
Tricyclic antidepressants
Beta-adrenergic antagonists
Estrogen

REDUCE URINE VOLUME
Antidiuretic hormone

INHIBITING BLADDER CONTRACTILITY

Anticholinergic Agents

A major portion of the neurohumoral stimulus for physiologic bladder contraction is acetylcholine-induced stimulation of postganglionic parasympathetic cholinergic receptor sites on bladder smooth muscle. Atropine and atropine-like agents will therefore depress involuntary bladder contractions of any cause.[5] In such patients the volume to the first involuntary contraction will generally be increased, with a proportionate reduction in symptomatology.[6-8] Although the threshold volume for an involuntary contraction may be increased, the "warning time" may not, and thus urge incontinence may still occur unless therapy is combined with timed voiding or a toileting regimen. The effect of the antimuscarinic agents on intravesical pressure during filling in patients who exhibit only decreased compliance has not been well studied. Outlet resistance, as reflected by urethral pressure measurements, does not seem to be affected by anticholinergic therapy. Although the antimuscarinic agents can produce significant clinical improvement in patients with involuntary bladder contractions and the associated symptoms, only partial inhibition generally results. In many animal models, atropine only partially antagonizes the bladder response to pelvic nerve stimulation and the bladder strips to field stimulation. Atropine does completely inhibit the response of bladder smooth muscle to exogenously administered acetylcholine. This phenomenon is called "atropine resistance" and may be caused by release of a noncholinergic excitatory neurotransmitter.[9]

Atropine sulfate is available as a 0.5 mg tablet; it and all related belladonna alkaloids are well absorbed from the gastrointestinal tract. Atropine has almost no detectable central nervous system effects at clinically administered dosages.[10] It has a half-life of 4 hours. Lack of selectivity is a major problem. All the antimuscarinic compounds tend to affect parasympathetically innervated organs in the same sequence, with generally larger dosages required to depress bladder activity than required to alter salivary, bronchial, nasopharyngeal, and sweat secretions. Scopolamine (hyoscine) is another belladonna alkaloid; it has prominent central depressive effects at low dosages, probably because of greater penetration of the blood-brain barrier. Hyoscyamine sulfate (Levsin, Levsinex) inhibits the effects of acetylcholine on structures innervated by postganglionic cholinergic nerves; it does not act on autonomic ganglia. This preparation is rapidly absorbed and is available in capsule, sublingual, elixir, and timed-release forms. Although it is used extensively for irritable bowel complaints, no comparative studies have been conducted on bladder efficacy. The usual adult dose is 0.125 to 0.250 mg orally or sublingually every 4 hours. The timed-release capsules are administered 0.375 mg orally twice daily. Atropine compounds can be administered intravesically, though the exact dosing regimen has not been determined.[11]

Propantheline bromide (Pro-Banthine) is the traditional oral agent used to produce an antimuscarinic effect in the lower urinary tract. The usual adult oral dosage is 15 to 30 mg every 4 to 6 hours. Higher doses may be necessary to achieve the desired clinical effect. Propantheline is a quaternary ammonium compound. Since these are poorly absorbed from the gastrointestinal tract,[10] oral administration in the fasting state, rather than with or after meals, is preferable from the standpoint of bioavailability. There seems to be little difference between the antimuscarinic effects of propantheline on bladder smooth muscle and those of other antimuscarinic agents such as glycopyrrolate, isopropamide, hyoscyamine, anisotropine, methylbromide, and others. Some,like glycopyruvate, have a more convenient dosing schedule.

The potential side effects of all antimuscarinic agents include inhibition of salivary secretion (dry mouth), decreased sweating (heat stroke), blockade of the ciliary muscle of the lens to cholinergic stimulation (blurred vision for near objects), tachycardia, drowsiness, and inhibition of gut motility. Those agents that possess some ganglionic blocking activity may also cause orthostatic hypotension and impotence at high dosages. Antimuscarinic agents are generally contraindicated in patients with narrow-angle glaucoma and should be used with caution in patients with significant bladder outlet obstruction because complete urinary retention may be precipitated.

Musculotropic Relaxants

Musculotropic relaxants are direct-acting smooth muscle depressants. They act directly on smooth muscle at a site that is "metabolically distal" to the cholinergic receptor mechanism. All the following agents relax smooth muscle in vitro by a papaverine-like activity and possess varying degrees of acetylcholinergic and local anesthetic properties. There is still a question as to how much of their clinical efficacy is attributable simply to their atropine-like effect. If any of these agents do exert a clinically significant inhibitory effect independent of an antimuscarinic action, there exists a therapeutic rationale for combining their use with that of a relatively pure anticholinergic agent.[12]

Oxybutynin chloride (Ditropan) is a moderately potent anticholinergic agent with a strong independent musculotropic relaxant activity and local anesthetic activity. This agent is effective in treating bladder hyperactivity of many different types.[13,14] In a prospective random study of 34 patients with voiding dysfunction secondary to multiple sclerosis, Gajewski and Awad[15] found that 5 mg of oxybutynin orally administered tid produced a good response more frequently than 15 mg of propantheline tid. They concluded that oxybutynin was more effective in the treatment of detrusor hyperflexia in patients with multiple sclerosis than propantheline was. Holmes et al.[16] compared oxybutynin and propantheline bromide in a small group of women with detrusor instability. The experimental design was a randomized crossover trial with a patient-regulated variable-dosage regimen. Of the 23 women in the trial, 14 reported subjective improvement with oxybutynin compared with 11 treated with propantheline bromide. Both drugs significantly increased the maximum cystometric capacity and reduced the maximum detrusor pressure on filling. The only significant objective difference in the two drugs was a greater increase in the maximum cystometric capacity in those patients treated with oxybutynin. The mean total tolerated daily dosage of oxybutynin was 15 mg (range 7.5 to 30 mg) and that of propantheline was 90 mg. On the other hand, oxybutynin has been shown to be no more effective than placebo coupled with scheduled toileting in treating incontinence in an elderly population with detrusor hyperactivity. Zorzitto et al.[17,18] showed similar results with oxybutin and propantheline in a double-blind placebo-controlled trial among incontinent geriatric institutionalized patients.

Intravesical instillation is an appealing alternative for drug delivery. Madersbacher and Jilg[19] reviewed such usage and presented data on 13 patients with complete suprasacral cord lesions on clean intermittent catheterization. One 5 mg tablet was dissolved in distilled water, and the solution was instilled into the bladder. Of the 10 patients who were incontinent, 9 remained dry for 6 hours. For the group, the changes in bladder capacity and maximal detrusor pressure were significant. Blood levels after an oral dosage rose to 7.3 ng/ml within 2 hours and then precipitously dropped to slightly less than 2 ng/ml at 4 hours. After intravesical administration, the blood levels rose gradually to a peak of about 6.2 ng/ml at 3½ hours, but the level at 6 hours was still greater than 4 ng/ml, and at 9 hours was still between 3 and 4 ng/ml. These data raise the question of whether the intravesically applied drug acts locally or systemically. Although the occurrence of significant systemic side effects seems to be less with intravesical treatment, some patients will still experience the adverse effects of oxybutynin chloride.[20]

The recommended adult oral dosage of oxybutynin is 5 mg tid to qid. Intravesical dosage is 5 mg dissolved in 10 to 30 ml of distilled water. The solution is instilled 2 or 3 times per day with a catheter and left in place until the next scheduled catheterization. The potential side effects of oxybutynin chloride are antimuscarinic ones.

Dicyclomine hydrochloride (Bentyl) reportedly possesses a direct relaxant effect on smooth muscle in addition to having an antimuscarinic action.[21] An oral dosage of 20 mg tid in adults has been reported to increase bladder capacity in patients with detrusor hyperreflexia.[22] We have used 20 to 30 mg tid to qid. The potential side effects are also antimuscarinic.

Flavoxate hydrochloride (Urispas) is another compound that has a direct inhibitory action on smooth muscle in addition to anticholinergic and local analgesic properties.[23] The elderly population, however, does not seem to benefit from use of flavoxate hydrochloride. This correlates with the in vitro effects noted by Briggs et al.[24] The recommended adult dosage is one to two tablets tid or qid. As with all agents in this group, a short clinical trial may be worthwhile. Reported side effects are rare and primarily anticholinergic.

Calcium Antagonists

Calcium is well established as a messenger between extracellular stimuli and the intracellular environment and is involved in excitation contraction coupling in striated, cardiac, and smooth muscle.[25,26] Interference with calcium inflow or intracellular calcium release or concentration are each a potential means for bladder smooth muscle relaxation.[27] Calcium antagonists have been shown to effectively inhibit bladder contraction induced by these mechanisms in animal and in human smooth muscle strips. This has led to the development of clinical agents that combine calcium-antagonist activity with an antimuscarinic action. The calcium antagonist nifedipine is an effective inhibitor of contraction in human and guinea pig bladder muscle.[28-30] It is also capable of completely blocking the noncholinergic portion of the contraction produced by electric field stimulation in rabbit bladder.[31] Nifedipine more effectively inhibits potassium-induced than carbachol-induced contraction in rabbit bladder strips. At low concentrations it has mainly an antimuscarinic action, whereas at higher concentrations a calcium-antagonist effect becomes evident. In vitro experiments have shown that these two effects are additive with regard to bladder contractility. More recent experiments have confirmed the inhibitory effect of the calcium antagonists nifedipine, verapamil, and diltiazem on a variety of experimental models of spontaneous and induced activity using bladder muscle strip and whole bladder preparation.[32,33] Andersson et al.[30] showed that nifedipine effectively and selectively inhibits the nonmuscarinic part of the contraction whereas other calcium antagonists cause pronounced depression of both the total and nonmuscarinic part of the contraction. This finding indicates probable differences between various calcium-channel blockers with respect to their effects on electrically induced bladder muscle contraction. These results were used as support for the view that, given the phenomenon of "atropine-resistant" contractions in rabbit and human bladders, a combined calcium-channel blocker and antimuscarinic agent might more effectively control bladder hyperactivity.

Nifedipine is also effective in pretreatment against the development of autonomic hyperreflexia and as therapy during an acute episode. For prophylaxis, 10 mg orally 30 minutes before examination has been successful. Sublingual administration of 10 mg can relieve acute symptoms.

Terodiline had been marketed in Europe since 1986 for the treatment of hyperreflexia and bladder instability. Terodiline can completely inhibit the response of the rabbit bladder to electric field stimulation.[30] At low concentrations it seems to have mainly an antimuscarinic action in vitro, whereas at higher concentrations a calcium-antagonist effect becomes evident. There have been several randomized and blinded studies on the inhibitory action of terodiline on bladder hyperactivity, and these have shown clinical effectiveness.[34] Peters et al.[35] reported the results of a multicenter study that ultimately included data from 89 patients (of an original 128), comparing terodiline and placebo in women with motor urge incontinence. The authors concluded that terodiline was more effective than placebo but noted that this was much more apparent on a subjective assessment of effect than on an objective assessment of cystometric and micturition data. Tapp et al.[36] reported on a double-blind placebo study, using dosage titration of 70 women with urodynamically proved detrusor instability and bladder capacities of less than 400 ml. Sixty-two percent of the 34 women in the terodiline group considered themselves improved, as opposed to 38% unchanged. Of the 36 women in the placebo, 42% considered themselves improved, 47% unchanged, and 11% worse, a statistically significant response in favor of terodiline with regard to improvement rate. Micturition variables of daytime frequency, daytime incontinence episodes, number of pads used, and average voided volumes were all statistically in favor of terodiline. Absolute value changes were small (such as daytime incontinence episodes that changed in placebo from 2.5 to 1.9 per day and 3.7 to 1.6 for terodiline). Urodynamic data, though showing a trend in favor of terodiline in each parameter, showed no statistically significant differences in any category. The incidence of anticholinergic side effects was higher in the drug group, with 29% of the terodiline patients and 11% of the placebo patients complaining of dry mouth and 20% of the terodiline patients but none of the placebo patients complaining of blurred vision.

Terodiline is almost completely absorbed from the gastrointestinal tract and has a low serum clearance, with a half-life of around 60 hours. The recommended initial dose in adults is 25 mg bid. This is reduced to 12.5 mg bid in geriatric patients and children. More common side effects seen with calcium antagonists (hypotension, facial flushing, headache, dizziness, abdominal discomfort, constipation, nausea, rash, weakness, and palpitations) had not been seen in placebo-controlled studies with terodiline: its reported side effects were primarily those consequent to its anticholinergic properties. After reports of cardiac arrhythmia among patients using terodiline in England and on the European continent, clinical investigations in the United States were suspended by the Food and Drug Administration in 1991. A letter to the *British Medical Journal* in August 1991 first described an atypical rapid ventricular arrhythmia, torsades de pointes, in a patient using terodiline.[42] Confirmation of this complication and subsequent deaths secondary to ventricular fibrillation associated with terodiline have been reported.[37]

Potassium-Channel Openers

By increasing potassium efflux and causing membrane hyperpolarization, potassium-channel openers relax various types of smooth muscle in vitro.[29] There are some suggestions that the bladder instability associated with intravesical obstruction and detrusor hypertrophy might be secondary to supersensitivity to depolarizing stimuli. Thus the potassium-channel openers are an attractive alternative for the treatment of detrusor instability in such circumstances. With these agents, the contractile ability produced by voluntary initiation of micturition is unaltered.[38] Pinacidil is a compound that inhibits spontaneous myogenic contractions and contractile responses induced by electrical field stimulation and carbachol in isolated human detrusor and in normal and hypertrophied rat detrusor.[39] A preliminary study with this agent in a double-blind crossover format showed no effect on bladder symptoms with dosages sufficient to decrease both standing systolic and diastolic blood pressures. Symptom status in nine patients with detrusor instability and bladder outlet obstruction was unchanged.[40]

Nurse et al.[41] reported on the use of cromakalim, another potassium-channel opener, in 17 patients with refractory detrusor instability or hyperreflexia. The patients had stopped other drug therapy because of intolerable side effects. Six out of 16 patients who completed the study showed a decrease in frequency and an increase in voided volume. Long-term follow-up study has not been possible, since the drug was withdrawn after reports of adverse effects of high dosages in animal toxicologic studies. Further experimental and clinical trials with potassium-channel openers for the treatment of detrusor hyperactivity states are awaited.

Prostaglandin Inhibitors

Prostaglandins have been described as having multiple actions on the bladder and urethra. Potential roles exist in the development of bladder contractility or tension during filling, in the contractile response during emptying of bladder smooth muscle, and even in the maintenance of urethral tone during the storage phase of micturition, as well as in the release of this tone during the emptying phase.[1] Other mechanisms of action in the lower urinary tract have been suggested.[42] Andersson et al.[29] implied possible sensitization of sensory afferent nerves by prostaglandins, increasing afferent input at a given degree of bladder filling and progressing to the point of triggering involuntary contractions at a small bladder volume. There are multiple mechanisms by which prostaglandin synthesis inhibitors might decrease bladder contractility in response to various stimuli; however, objective evidence that this can occur is scant. Cardozo et al.[43] reported on the effects of 50 mg tid of flurbiprofen, a prostaglandin synthetase inhibitor, on 30 women with detrusor instability. In a double-blind placebo study, it was concluded that the drug did not abolish involuntary bladder contractions or abnormal bladder activity but delayed the intravesical pressure rise to a greater degree of distension. Forty-three percent of the patients experienced side effects: nausea, vomiting, headache, indigestion, gastric distress, constipation, and rash. Cardozo et al.[43] reported symptomatic improvement in patients with detrusor instability given indomethacin in dosages of 50 to 200 mg daily. This was a short-term study with no cystometric data, and the drug was compared only with bromocriptine. The incidence of side effects was high (19 out of 32), though no patient had to stop treatment because of these. Prostaglandin synthetase inhibitors have proved useful in the treatment of other disorders.[44] Numerous prostaglandin inhibitors exist, most of which fall under the heading of nonsteroidal anti-inflammatory drugs. It should be remembered that these drugs can interfere with platelet function and may have adverse renal effects.[45]

Beta-Adrenergic Agonists

The presence of beta-adrenergic receptors in human bladder muscle has prompted attempts to increase bladder capacity with beta-adrenergic stimulation. Such stimulation can cause significant increases in the capacity of animal bladders. In vitro studies show a dosage-related relaxant effect of $beta_2$-adrenergic agonists on the bladder body of rabbits but little effect on the bladder base or the proximal portion of the urethra. Terbutaline, in oral dosages of 5 mg tid, has been reported to have a "good clinical effect" in some patients with urgency and urge incontinence but no significant effect on the bladders of neurologically normal humans without voiding difficulty.[46] Although these results are compatible with those in other organ systems (beta-adrenergic stimulation causes no acute change in total lung capacity on normal humans, whereas it does favorably affect patients with bronchial asthma), few adequate studies are available on the effects of beta-adrenergic stimulation in patients with detrusor hyperactivity. Lindholm and Lose.[47] used 5 mg tid of terbutaline in eight women with motor and seven with sensory urge incontinence. After 3 months of treatment, 14 patients claimed beneficial effects, and 12 became subjectively continent. In 6 of 8 patients, the detrusor became stable on cystometry. Interestingly, the volume of the first desire to void in the patients with originally unstable bladders increased from a mean of 200 to 300 ml, but the maximum cystometric capacity did not change. Nine patients had transient side effects, including palpitations, tachycardia, or hand tremor. In three patients, the side effects continued but were acceptable. In one patient the drug was discontinued because of severe adverse symptoms.

Tricyclic Antidepressants

By both decreasing bladder contractility and increasing outlet resistance, tricyclic antidepressants, particularly imipramine hydrochloride (Trofranil), can be useful agents for facilitating urine storage. Most data on the mechanisms of action of these drugs has been accumulated from central nervous system tissue and relate to the antidepressant properties of these agents. It is unknown whether these results apply to the lower urinary tract.

All tricyclic antidepressant agents possess varying degrees of at least three major pharmacologic actions: (1) central and peripheral anticholinergic effects at some but not all sites, (2) blockage of the presynaptic nerve ending reuptake of the amine neurotransmitters norepinephrine and serotonin, and (3) sedation, either through a central mechanism or by antihistaminic (H_1 receptors) properties.

Imipramine has prominent systemic anticholinergic effects but only a weak antimuscarinic effect on bladder smooth muscle. A strong direct inhibitory effect on bladder smooth muscle exists, and it is neither anticholinergic nor adrenergic. This may be attributable to a local anesthetic-like action at the nerve terminals or to a calcium-antagonist action.[48,49] Aside from the direct inhibitory effect on bladder smooth muscle, one might postulate a further decrease in bladder body contractility effected by a peripheral blockade of norepinephrine reuptake, since there is an increased concentration of beta-adrenergic over alpha-adrenergic receptors in the bladder body. The density of alpha receptors exceeds beta receptors in the bladder base and the proximal portion urethra. Thus an enhanced alpha-adrenergic effect in the smooth muscle is generally considered to be the mechanism whereby imipramine increases outlet resistance. Castleden et al.[50] began therapy in elderly patients with detrusor instability with a single 25 mg nighttime dosage of imipramine. This was increased every third day by 25 mg until the patient was continent, had side effects, or reached a dosage of 150 mg. Six of 10 patients became continent. In those who underwent repeated cystometry, bladder capacity increased by a mean of 105 ml, and bladder pressure at capacity decreased by a mean of 18 cm H_2O. Maximum urethral pressure increased by a mean of 30 cm H_2O. Some patients in this series became continent after only 3 to 5 days of therapy. Our usual adult dosage for voiding dysfunction is 25 mg qid; half that dosage is given in elderly patients because elimination has been shown to be prolonged. In our experience, the effects of imipramine on the lower urinary tract are often additive to those of atropine-like agents. A combination of imipramine and an antimuscarinic or an antispasmodic is sometimes useful for decreasing bladder contractility. If imipramine is used with an atropine-like agent, be aware that the anticholinergic side effects of the drugs may be additive.

Doxepin (Sinequan) is another tricyclic antidepressant, and it was found to have more potent antimuscarinic and musculotropic relaxant activity on in vitro rabbit bladder strips than other tricyclic compounds.[51] Lose et al.,[52] in a randomized double-blind crossover study of females with involuntary bladder contractions and frequency, urgency, or urge incontinence, found that doxepin caused a significant decrease in nighttime micturition frequency and nighttime incontinence episodes and a nearly significant decrease in urine loss. Increases in the cystometric parameters of first sensation and maximum capacity were noted. The dosage used was either a 50 mg bedtime dose alone or one in combination with a 25 mg dose in the morning. The number of daytime incontinence episodes decreased in both the doxepin and the placebo groups. Of 14 patients who stated a preference for doxepin, 12 claimed that they became continent during treatment, whereas two claimed improvement. The two patients who preferred placebo claimed improvement.

The most frequent side effects of the tricyclic antidepressants are those attributable to their systemic anticholinergic activity. These usually occur in the generally larger doses employed for antidepressant effects. Allergic phenomena are reported. Central nervous system side effects may include weakness, fatigue, parkinsonian effect, a fine tremor noted most in the upper extremities, a manic or schizophrenic picture, and sedation, probably from its antihistaminic effect. Antidepressants can be shown electrophysiologically and hemodynamically to have a depressant effect on the myocardium shortly after therapy is begun.[21] However, it has been pointed out that in the animal studies showing a direct myocardial depressant effect plasma concentrations in the toxic range for humans were present. Whether cardiotoxicity will prove to be a legitimate concern in patients receiving smaller dosages for lower urinary tract dysfunction remains to be seen and is a potential matter of concern. Consider consultation with an individual patient's internist or cardiologist before instituting such therapy in questionable situations. Tricyclic antidepressants can also cause excess sweating of obscure cause and a delay of orgasm or orgasmic impotence, the cause of which is likewise unclear. The use of imipramine is contraindicated in patients receiving monoamine oxidase inhibitors because severe central nervous system toxic effects, including hyperpyrexia, seizures, and coma can be precipitated. The potential side effects of the antidepressants may be especially significant for elderly persons, specifically weakness, fatigue, and orthostatic hypotension. If imipramine or any of the tricyclic antidepressants is to be prescribed for the treatment of voiding dysfunction, the patient should be thoroughly informed of the fact that this is not the usual indication for this drug and that potential side effects exist. These drugs should be discontinued gradually, especially in patients receiving high doses, to prevent adverse side effects (severe abdominal distress, nausea, vomiting, headache, lethargy, and irritability).

Dimethyl Sulfoxide

Dimethyl sulfoxide (DMSO) is a relatively simple, naturally occurring organic compound that has been used as an industrial solvent for many years. It has multiple pharmacologic actions (as being a membrane penetrant, antiinflammatory, local analgesic, bacteriostatic, diuretic, cholinesterase inhibitor, collagen solvent, and vasodilator) and has been used for the treatment of arthritis and other musculoskeletal disorders, generally in a 70% solution. The formulation for human intravesical use is a 50% solution. DMSO has not been shown to be useful in the treatment of detrusor hyperreflexia or instability in any patients with urgency and frequency without interstitial cystitis.

Polysynaptic Inhibitors. Baclofen can decrease outlet resistance secondary to striated sphincter dyssynergia and is often used in managing neurogenic outlet dysfunction. It has also been shown to be capable of depressing detrusor hyperreflexia secondary to a spinal cord lesion.[53] Taylor and Bates,[54] in a double-blind crossover study, reported baclofen to be very effective in decreasing daytime and nighttime urinary frequency and incontinence in patients with idiopathic instability. Cystometric changes were not recorded, and considerable improvement was also obtained in the placebo group. The intrathecal use of baclofen for treatment of detrusor hyperactivity is a potentially exciting area, and further reports are awaited. This mode of administration is FDA approved for treatment of skeletal muscle spasticity. In this way, potentially higher levels can be achieved in the cerebrospinal fluid with lower doses than would be required orally to reach the same effect.[55]

Increasing Capacity by Decreasing Sensory (Afferent) Input

The clinical implications of being able to defunctionalize pharmacologically at least some primary afferent neurons from the lower urinary tract are extraordinary. Such an action would be ideal for the treatment of sensory urgency. It could also be used to treat instability or hyperreflexia in a bladder with relatively normal viscoelastic properties in which the sensory afferents were the first limb in the abnormal micturition reflex. Maggi et al.[56,57] have written extensively about this type of potential pharmacologic treatment, specifically with reference to the properties of capsaicin. Capsaicin is the pungent ingredient in a variety of red peppers and a neurotoxic compound that causes initial excitation and then desensitization of thin type B sensory neurons, depleting their content of certain neuropeptides, including substance P. Patients experience a warm or burning sensation with intravesical administration of 100 ml of a 1 or 2 mmol/L solution of capsaicin dissolved in 30% alcohol. Follow-up urodynamic studies have shown an increased capacity and a decrease in maximum detrusor pressure.[58,59] Initial findings imply a greater effect on detrusor hyperreflexia and detrusor instability than on sensory urgency.[59] Despite the undesirable sequelae of the initial excitatory effects and potential adverse long-term outcome, this is an interesting concept that holds promise for future avenues of drug treatment.

Increasing Outlet Resistance

Alpha-Adrenergic Agonists

The bladder neck and proximal portion of the urethra contain a preponderance of alpha-adrenergic receptor sites, which, when stimulated, produce smooth muscle contraction.[60,61] This contraction alters the urethral pressure profile by increasing maximum urethral pressure (MUP) and maximum urethral closure pressure (MUCP). Various orally administered pharmacologic agents that produce alpha-adrenergic stimulation are available. Generally, outlet resistance is increased by a variable degree. Because of the potential side effects of all of these agents, they should be used with caution in patients with hypertension, cardiovascular disease, or hyperthyroidism.

Ephedrine is a sympathomimetic agent that causes the peripheral release of norepinephrine but also directly stimulates alpha- and beta-adrenergic receptors. The adult dosage is 25 to 50 mg orally qid. Some tachyphylaxis develops to its peripheral actions, probably as a result of depletion of norepinephrine stores. Pseudoephedrine (Sudafed) is a stereoisomer that is used for similar indications with similar precautions. The adult dosage is 30 to 60 mg qid, and the 30 mg dosage form is available as an over-the-counter drug in the United States. Diokno and Taub[62] reported a good to excellent result in 27 of 38 patients with sphincteric incontinence treated with ephedrine sulfate. Beneficial effects were achieved most frequently in those with minimal to moderate wetting; little benefit was achieved in patients with severe stress incontinence. Phenylpropanolamine hydrochloride shares the pharmacologic properties of ephedrine and is approximately equal in peripheral potency but causes less central neural stimulation. It is available in 25 and 50 mg preparations and 75 mg timed-release capsules and is a component of numerous proprietary mixtures marketed as appetite suppressants and for the treatment of nasal and sinus congestion (usually in combination with an antihistamine H_1 drug). Utilizing dosages of 50 mg tid, Awad et al.[63] found that 11 of 13 women and 6 of 7 men with stress incontinence significantly improved after 4 weeks of therapy. MUCP increased from a mean of 47 to 72 cm H_2O in patients with a full bladder. Using a capsule that contained 50 mg of phenylpropanolamine, 8 mg of chlorpheniramine (an antihistamine), and 2 mg of isopropamide (an anticholinergic), Stewart et al.[64] found that 18 of 77 women with stress urinary incontinence were completely cured with one sustained-release capsule bid. Twenty-eight patients were "much better," 6 were "slightly better," and 25 were not better. In 11 men with postprostatectomy stress incontinence, the respective numbers in the corresponding categories were 1, 2, 1, and 7. The formulation of Ornade has been changed, and each capsule of drug now contains only 75 mg of phenylpropanolamine and 12 mg of chlorpheniramine. Some authors have emphasized potential complications of phenylpropanolamine. Lasagna[65] has pointed out that prior reported blood pressure elevations were with a product that differed from American phenylpropanolamine and probably contained a different and much more potent isomer. He pointed out that even though a huge volume of phenylpropanolamine has been consumed for decongestant and anorectic purposes, the world literature has carried only a minimal number of possible toxic reactions, most of which have involved excessively high dosages in combination medications. Liebson et al.[66] found no cardiovascular or subjective adverse effects with dosages of 25 mg tid or a 75 mg sustained-release preparation.

Midodrin is a long-acting alpha-adrenergic agonist reported useful in the treatment of seminal emission and ejaculation disorders after retroperitoneal lymphadenectomy. Treatment with 5 mg bid for 4 weeks in 20 patients with stress incontinence produced a cure in one and improvement in 14.[67] MUCP rose by 8.3%, and the planometric index of the continence area on profilometry increased by 9%.

The bladder effects of imipramine have been discussed. On a theoretic basis, an increase in outlet resistance might be expected if an enhanced alpha-adrenergic effect were produced at the urethral level as a result of the inhibition of norepinephrine reuptake. Many clinicians have noted improvement in sphincteric incontinence in patients who were treated with imipramine primarily for reasons related to bladder hyperactivity but who had, in addition, some component of sphincteric incontinence. Gilja et al.[68] reported on 30 women with stress incontinence before and after treatment with 75 mg of imipramine in divided doses for 4 weeks. Twenty-one women subjectively reported continence. Mean MUCP increased (for the whole group) from 34.06 to 48.23 mm Hg.

Although some clinicians have reported spectacular cure and improvement rates for sphincteric incontinence with agents that produce an alpha-adrenergic effect in the urethra, our own experience coincides with those who report that treatment with such agents often produces some improvement but rarely total dryness in patients with severe or even moderate stress incontinence. A clinical trial is certainly worthwhile, especially with pelvic floor physiotherapy and biofeedback.

Beta-Adrenergic Antagonists

Theoretically, beta-adrenergic blocking agents might be expected to "unmask," or potentiate, an alpha-adrenergic effect, thereby increasing urethral resistance. Gleason et al.[69] reported success in treating certain patients with stress urinary incontinence with propranolol. Oral dosages of 10 mg qid were used. The beneficial effect became manifest only after 4 to 10 weeks of treatment. Cardiac effects occur rather promptly after administration of this drug. The hypotensive effects do not usually appear so rapidly, though it is difficult to explain such a long delay in the onset of therapeutic effect on this basis. Kaisary[70] also reported success with propranolol in treating stress incontinence. Although such treatment has been suggested as an alternative treatment to alpha-adrenergic agonists in patients with sphincteric incontinence hypertension, few if any subsequent reports of such efficacy have appeared. Others have reported no significant changes in urethral profile pressures in normal women after beta-adrenergic blockade.[71] The major potential side effects of the propranolol are related to its therapeutic beta-blocking effects. Heart failure may develop, as well as an increase in airway resistance. Asthma is a clear contraindication to its use. Abrupt discontinuation may precipitate an exacerbation of anginal attacks and rebound hypertension.[72]

Estrogen

Much attention has been paid to the innervation and autonomic responses of the smooth muscle of the uterus. Estrogen has been found to affect many of these properties, including excitability, neuronal influences on the muscle, receptor density and sensitivity, and transmitter metabolism, especially in adrenergic nerves. The urethra and trigone are embryologically related to the uterus. Significant work has also been done on the effects of estrogen hormones on the lower urinary tract. Hodgson et al.[73] reported that the sensitivity of the rabbit urethra to alpha-adrenergic stimulation was estrogen dependent. Castration caused a decreased sensitivity, and treatment with low levels of estrogen reversed this. Levin et al.[74] have shown that parenteral estrogen administration can change the alpha-adrenergic receptor content and the autonomic innervation of the lower urinary tract of immature rabbits. A pronounced increase in the density of adrenergic receptors in the bladder body, though not the base, occurred. Larsson et al.[75] reported that estrogen treatment of the isolated female rabbit urethra caused an increased sensitivity to norepinephrine. The mechanism was postulated to be related to a more than twofold increase in the density of alpha-adrenergic receptor number and was suggested to be attributable to a selective increase in the number of alpha-$_2$ postjunctional (not the classic alpha-$_2$ prejunctional receptor) adrenoceptors. Callahan and Creed[76] reported that pretreatment with estrogen of oophorectomized dogs and wallabies did increase sensitivity of urethral strips to alpha-adrenergic stimulation, but this did not occur in the rabbit or guinea pig. Bump and Friedman[77] reported that estrogen replacement, but not testosterone, enhances the urethral sphincter mechanism in the castrate female baboon by effects that were unrelated to skeletal muscle. They added that these effects might be related not only to changes in the urethral smooth musculature but also to changes in the urethral mucosa, submucosal vascular plexus, and connective tissue.

Estrogen therapy certainly seems capable of facilitating urinary storage in some postmenopausal female patients. Whether this effect is related to just changes in the autonomic innervation or receptor content or function of the smooth muscle, to estrogen binding sites, or to changes in the nonmuscular elements of the urethral wall has not been settled.[78] Batra et al.[79] have shown that low dosages of estradiol and estratriol increased blood perfusion into the urethra (and also the vagina and uterus) of oophorectomized mature female rabbits. After menopause, urethral pressure profiles normally decrease somewhat, and this decrease is generally conceded to be related in some way to decreased estrogenic levels.[80] Whether the actual changes occur in smooth muscle, blood circulation, the supporting tissues, or the "mucosal seal mechanism" is still largely a matter of speculation. Raz et al.[81] found that a daily dosage of 2.5 mg of conjugated estrogen (Premarin) improved stress incontinence and increased urethral pressures in postmenopausal patients. These effects were attributed to muscosal proliferation with a consequently improved "mucosal seal effect" and to enhancement of the alpha-adrenergic contractile response of urethral smooth musculature to endogenous catecholamines. Schreiter et al.[82] reported similar benefits after 10 days of treatment with daily divided dosages of 6 mg of estriol. They presented evidence also that there were effects of 4 mg daily dosages of estradiol and 8 mg daily doses of estriol on 30 women with an average age of 61 years, 24 of whom had stress urinary incontinence. Small but statistically significant changes occurred in the MUP (59 to 63 cm H_2O), functional urethral length (25 to 28 mm), and actual urethral length (36 to 39 mm). There was no correlation between subjective or objective improvement, 9 experienced subjective improvement only, and 6 experienced neither subjective nor objective improvement. There was no correlation between subjective or objective improvement and the urodynamic measurements. However, of 18 patients in whom pressure transmission to the urethra was recorded during cough, 7 improved. All of these had subjective improvement, and 5 were shown to be objectively dry. Rud[80] suggested that it is hard to believe that the small changes in urodynamic measurements, even though statistically significant, were directly related to resumption of continence and noted that the increased pressure transmission ratio might be attributable to factors outside the urethra—either in the striated musculature of the pelvic floor or in the periurethral vasculature or supporting tissues. He also studied profilometry during the menstrual cycle in six women. There was no change in any profilometry values during the menstrual cycle and no correlation between estrogen levels and MUP. It may be, as has been suggested, that at physiologic levels estrogen has little influence on urodynamic measurements related to continence and that only pharmacologic dosages cause urodynamically significant changes. Pharmacologic doses of estrogen might also alter responses to other exogenous autonomic agents, particularly alpha-adrenergic ones, as the previously mentioned laboratory experiments would indicate.

More recently, Beisland et al.[83] carried out a randomized open, comparative crossover trial in 20 postmenopausal women with urethral sphincteric insufficiency. Both phenylpropanolamine, 50 mg orally bid and estriol vaginal suppositories, 1 mg daily, increased the maximum urethral closure pressure and the continence area on profilometry significantly. Phenylpropanolamine was clinically more effective than estriol but not sufficiently to obtain complete continence. With combined treatment, however, 8 patients became completely continent, 9 were considerably improved, and only 1 patient remained unchanged. Two patients dropped out of the study because of the side effects. Bhatia et al.[84] used 2 mg daily of conjugated estrogen vaginal cream for 6 weeks in 11 postmenopausal women with stress incontinence. Six were cured or improved significantly. Favorable response was correlated with increased closure pressure and increased pressure transmission. Walter et al.[85] concluded, in a randomized double-blind placebo study of 28 postmenopausal women, that estriol and phenylpropanolamine were effective treatment for stress incontinence. Based on subjective assessment, combined treatment was more effective than treatment with each drug separately, but the enhanced effect seemed very moderate compared to the effect of phenylpropanolamine alone. Cardozo[86] in a review article has concluded that "there is no conclusive evidence that oestrogen even improves, let alone cures, stress incontinence," though it "apparently alleviates urgency, urge incontinence, frequency, nocturia and dysuria." The potential benefits of estrogen treatment must be carefully considered in the light of data showing that unopposed estrogen therapy significantly increases the risk of developing endometrial cancer.[87,88] Adding a progestogen to the regimen may reduce this risk close to the normal range.[89,90,91] Regarding other sex hormone–related cancers, there may be a significant increased risk of developing breast or ovarian cancer after long-term use of even estrogen-progestin combination therapy.[90,92] At the very least, if a beneficial effect on the lower urinary tract is achieved by a regimen that uses estrogen alone or in combination with other therapy, the lowest maintenance dosage possible should ultimately be used: a dosage hopefully below that used for general replacement therapy in menopausal and postmenopausal women. Estrogen therapy should be frequently reevaluated, especially if the patient has a family or personal history of any of these cancers, is obese, or has or had late onset of menopause[93] Consultation with an oncologist is always helpful for patients who have a prior personal history of a sex hormone–related cancer.[94]

REDUCE URINE VOLUME

The synthetic antidiuretic hormone peptide analog 1-(3-mercaptopropionic acid)-8-D-arginine vasopressin (desmopressin, DDAVP) alters renal water conservation and has shown long-term efficacy and safety only in the management of patients with diabetes insipidus. Desmopressin has been used to treat primary enuresis.[95,96] Administration is convenient by nasal spray at bedtime, and suppression of urine production lasts for 7 to 10 hours. Side effects during long-term use do no appear to cause depression of endogenous antidiuretic hormone secretion. Overingestion of water could potentially cause water intoxication and hyponatremia. The drug has been associated with rises in blood pressure on initial use and should be used with caution in patients with hypertension and coronary artery disease. With high dosages, transient headache, nausea, nasal congestion, rhinitis, flushing, and mild abdominal cramps have been reported.

REFERENCES

1. Wein AJ, Levin RM, Barrett DM: Voiding function: relevant anatomy, physiology and pharmacology. In Gillenwater JY, Grayhack JT, Howards ST, Duckett JW, editors: *Adult and pediatric urology*, ed 2, St. Louis, 1991, Mosby.
2. Barrett D, Wein AJ: Voiding dysfunction: diagnosis, classification and management. In Gillenwater JY, Grayhack JT, Howards ST, Duckett JW, editors: *Adult and pediatric urology*, ed 2, St. Louis, 1991, Mosby.
3. Turner JA, Deyo RA, Loeser JD, et al: The importance of placebo effects in pain treatment and research, *JAMA* 271:1609-1614, 1994.
4. Carter R, Aitchinson MA: Placebo responses in the treatment of urge incontinence, *Int Urogynecol* 4:229-231, 1993.
5. Kolta MG, Wallace LJ, Gerald MC: Age related changes in sensitivity of rat urinary bladder to autonomic agents, *Mech Ageing Dev* 27:183, 1984.
6. Jensen D JR: Uninhibited neurogenic bladder treated with prazosin, *Scand J Urol Nephrol* 15:229, 1981c.
7. Jensen D Jr: Altered adrenergic innervation in the uninhibited neurogenic bladder, *Scand J Urol Nephrol* 60:61, 1981b.
8. Jensen D Jr: Pharmacological studies of the uninhibited neurogenic bladder, *Acta Neurol Scand* 64:175, 1981a.
9. Andersson K-E: Pharmacology of lower urinary tract smooth muscles and penile erectile tissues, *Pharmacol Rev* 45:253-308, 1993.
10. Brown JH: Atropine, scopolamine and related antimuscarinic drugs. In Gilman AG, Rall TW, Nies AS, Taylor P, editors: *Goodman and Gilman's The pharmacological basis of therapeutics*, ed 8, New York, 1990, Pergamon Press.
11. Ekström B, Andersson K-E, Mattiasson A: Urodynamic effects of intravesical instillation of atropine and phentolamine in patients with detrusor hyperactivity, *J Urol* 149:155-158, 1993.
12. Levin RM, Staskin D, Wein AJ: The muscarinic cholinergic binding kinetics of the human urinary bladder, *Neurourol Urodyn* 1:221, 1982.

13. Moisey C, Stephenson T, Brendler C: The urodynamic and subjective results of treatment of detrusor instability with oxybutynin chloride, *Br J Urol* 52:472, 1980.
14. Hehir M, Fitzpatrick JM: Oxybutynin and the prevention of urinary incontinence in spina bifida, *Eur Urol* 11:254, 1985.
15. Gajewski JB, Awad JA: Oxybutyunin versus propantheline in patients with multiple sclerosis and detrusor hyperreflexia, *J Urol* 135:966, 1986.
16. Holmes DM, Monty FJ, Stanton SL: Oxybutynin versus propantheline in the management of detrusor instability: a patient regulated variable dose trial, *Br J Obstet Gynaecol* 96:607, 1989.
17. Zorzitto ML, Holliday PJ, Jewett MA, et al: Oxybutynin for geriatric urinary dysfunction: a double-blind placebo controlled study, *Age and Ageing* 18:195, 1989.
18. Zorzitto ML, Jewett MA, Fernie GR, et al: Effectiveness of propantheline bromide in the treatment of geriatric patients with detrusor instability, *Neurourol Urodyn* 5:133, 1986.
19. Madersbacher H, Jilg G: Control of detrusor hyperreflexia by the intravesical instillation of oxybutynin hydrochloride, *Paraplegia* 19:84, 1991.
20. Kasabian NG, Vlachiotis JD, Lais A, et al: The use of intravesical oxybutynin chloride in patients with detrusor bypertonicity and detrusor byperreflexia, *J Urol* 151:944-945, 1994.
21. Wein AJ: Voiding dysfunction: neurogenic or non-neuorgenic? *AUA Update Series* 7(23):178-183, Baltimore, 1988, American Urological Association.
22. Fischer C, Diokno A, Lapides J: The anticholinergic effects of dicyclomine hydrochloride in uninhibited neurogenic bladder dysfunction, *J Urol* 120:328, 1978.
23. Jonas U, Petri E, Kissal J: The effect of flavoxate on hyperactive detrusor muscle, *Eur Urol* 5:106, 1979.
24. Briggs RS, Castleden CM, Asher MJ: The effect of flavoxate on uninhibited detrusor contractions and urinary incontinence in the elderly, *J Urol* 123:656, 1980.
25. Stull JT, Kamm KE, Taylor DA: Calcium control of smooth muscle contraction, *Am J Med Sci* 31:241-245, 1988.
26. Ebashi S, Mikawa T, Kuwayama H, et al: Calcium regualtion in smooth muscle. In Siegman MJ, Somlyo AP, Stephens N, editors: *Regulation and contraction of smooth muscle,* New York, 1987, Alan R. Liss.
27. Levin RM, Hypolite J, Ruggieri MR, et al: Effects of muscarinic stimulation on intracellular calcium in the rabbit bladder: comparison with metabolic response, *Pharmacology* 39:69-77, 1989.
28. Forman A, Andersson K, Henriksson L, et al: Effects of nifedipine on the smooth muscle of the human urinary tract in vitro and in vivo, *Acta Pharmacol Toxicol* 43:111, 1978.
29. Andersson K-E, Andersson PO, Fovaeus M, et al: Effects of pinacidil on bladder muscle, *Drugs* 36(suppl 7):41, 1988.
30. Andersson K-E, Fovaeus M, Morgan E, et al: Comparative effects of five different calcium channel blockers on the atropine resistant contraction in electrically stimulated rabbit urinary bladder, *Neurourol Urodyn* 5:579, 1986.
31. Husted S, Andersson KE, Sommer L, et al: Anticholinergic and calcium antagonistic effects of terodilene in rabbit urinary bladder, *Acta Pharmacol Toxicol* 146(suppl 1):20, 1980.
32. Finkbeiner AE: Effect of extracellular calcium and calcium blocking agents on detrusor contractility: an in vitro study, *Neurourol Urodyn* 2:245, 1983.
33. Malkowicz SB, Wein AJ, Brendler K, Levin RM: Effect of diltiazem on in vitro rabbit bladder function, *Pharmacology* 31:24, 1985.
34. Ouslander JG, et al: Effects of terodiline on urinary incontinence among older non-institutionalized women, *J Am Geriatr Soc* 41:915-922, 1993.
35. Peters D and the Multicenter Study Group: Terodiline in the treatment of urinary frequency and motor urge incontinence: a controlled multicenter trial, *Scand J Urol Nephrol* 87(suppl):21, 1984.
36. Tapp A, Fall M, Norgaard J, et al: Terodiline: a dose titrated, multicenter study of the treatment of idiopathic detrusor instability in women, *J Urol* 142:1027, 1989.
37. Connolly MJ, Astridge PS, White EG, et al: Torsades de pointes ventricular tachycardia and terodilene, *Lancet* 338:344, 1991.
38. Malmgren A, Andersson KE, Andersson PO, et al: Effects of cromkalin and pinacidil on normal and hypertrophied rat detrusor in vitro, *J Urol* 143:828, 1990.
39. Fovaeus M, Andersson KE, Hedlund H: The action of pinacidil in the isolated human bladder, *J Urol* 141:637, 1989.
40. Hedlund H, Mattiasson A, Andersson KE: Lack of effect of pinacidil on detrusor instability in men with bladder outlet obstruction, *J Urol* 143:369A, 1990.
41. Nurse DE, Restorick JM, Mundy AR: The effect of cromakalim on the normal and hyperreflexic human detrusor muscle, *Br J Urol* 68:27, 1991.
42. Downie JW, Karmazyn M: Mechanical trauma to bladder epithelium liberates prostanoids which modulate neurotransmission in rabbit detrusor muscle, *J Pharmacol Exp Ther* 230:445, 1984.
43. Cardozo LD, Stanton SL, Robinson H, Hole D: Evaluation of flurbiprofen in detrusor instability, *Br Med J* 280:281, 1980.
44. Chan WY: Prostaglandins and nonsteroidal anti-inflammatory drugs in dysmenorrhea, *Am Rev Pharmacol Toxicol* 23:131, 1983.
45. Brooks PM, Day RO: Non-steroidal anti-inflammatory drugs: differences and similarities, *N Engl J Med* 324:1716, 1991.
46. Norlen L, Sundin T, Waagstein F: Beta-adrenoceptor stimulation of the human urinary bladder in vivo, *Acta Pharmacol Toxicol* 43:5, 1978.
47. Lindholm P, Lose G: Terbutaline (Bricanyl) in the treatment of female urge incontinence, *Urol Int* 41:158, 1986.
48. Raezer DM, Benson GS, Wein AJ, et al: The functional approach to the management of the pediatric neuropathic bladder: a clinical study, *J Urol* 117:649, 1977.
49. Tulloch AGS, Creed KE: A comparison between propantheline and imipramine on bladder and salivary gland function, *Br J Urol* 51:359, 1979.
50. Castleden CM, George CF, Renwick AG, Asher MJ: Imipramine: a possible alternative to current therapy for urinary incontinence in the elderly, *J Urol* 125:218, 1981.
51. Levin RM, Wein AJ: Comparative effects of five tricyclic compounds on the rabbit urinary bladder, *Neurourol Urodyn* 3:127, 1984.
52. Lose G, Jorgensen L, Thunedborg P: Doxepin in the treatment of female detrusor overactivity: a randomized double-blind crossover study, *J Urol* 142:1024, 1989.
53. Kiesswetter H, Schober W: Lioresal in the treatment of neurogenic bladder dysfunction, *Urol Int* 30:63, 1975.
54. Taylor MC, Bates CP: A double-blind crossover trial of baclofen: a new treatment for the unstable bladder syndrome, *Br J Urol* 51:505, 1979.
55. Bushman W, Steers WD, Meythaler JM: Voiding dysfunction in patients with spastic paraplegia: urodynamic evaluation and response to continuous intrathecal baclofen, *Neurourol Urodyn* 12:163-170, 1993.
56. Maggi CA, Barbank G, Santicoli P, et al: Cystometric evidence that capsaicin sensitive nerves modulate the afferent branch of micturition reflex on humans, *J Urol* 142:150, 1989.
57. Maggi CA: Capsaicin and primary afferent neurons: from basic science to human therapy? *J Auton Neuro Syst* 33:1, 1991.
58. Fowler CJ, Beck RO, Gerrard S, et al: Intravesical capsaicin for treatment of detrusor hyperreflexia, *J Neurol Neurosurg Psychiatry* 57:169-173, 1994.
59. Barbanti G, Maggi CA, Beneforti P, et al: Relief of pain following intravesical capsaicin inpatients with hypersensitive disorders of the lower urinary tract, *Br J Urol* 71:686-691, 1993.
60. Wein AJ, Levin RM, Barrett DM: Voiding function: relevant anatomy, physiology and pharmacology. In Gillenwater JY, Grayhack JT, Howards SS, Duckett JW, editors: *Adult and pediatric urology,* St Louis, 1987, Mosby.

61. Steers WD: Physiology of the urinary bladder. In Walsh PC, Retik AB, Stamey TA, Vaughan ED, editors: *Campbell's urology,* Philadelphia, 1992, Saunders.
62. Diokno A, Taub M: Ephedrine in treatment of urinary incontinence, *Urology* 5:624, 1975.
63. Awad SA, Downie J, Kiruluta H: Alpha adrenergic agents in urinary disorders of the proximal urethra: I. Stress incontinence, *Br J Urol* 50:332, 1978.
64. Stewart B, Borowsky L, Montague D: Stress incontinence: conservative therapy with sympathomimetic drugs, *J Urol* 115:558, 1976.
65. Lasagna L: Phenylpropanolamine and blood pressure, *JAMA* 253;2491, 1985.
66. Liebson L, Bigelow G, Griffiths RR, Funderbuck M: Phenylpropanolamine: effects on subjective and cardiovascular variables at recommended over-the-counter dose levels, *J Clin Pharmacol* 27:685, 1987.
67. Kiesswetter H, Hennrich F, Englisch M: Clinical and urodynamic assessment of pharmacologic therapy of stress incontinence, *Urol Int* 38:58, 1983.
68. Gilja I, Radej M, Kovacic M, Parazajades J: Conservative treatment of female stress incontinence with imipramine, *J Urol* 132:909, 1984.
69. Gleason D, Reilly R, Bottaccini M, Pierce MJ: The urethral continence zone and its relation to stress incontinence, *J Urol* 112:81, 1974.
70. Kaisary AU: Beta adrenoceptor blockade in the treatment of female stress urinary incontinence, *J d'Urologie* (Paris) 90:351, 1984.
71. Donker P, van der Sluis C: Action of beta adrenergic blocking agents on the urethral pressure profile, *Urol Int* 31:6, 1976.
72. Hoffman BB, Lefkowitz RJ: Adrenergic receptor antagonists. In Gilman AG, Rall TW, Nies AS, Taylor P, editors: *Goodman and Gilman's The pharmacological basis of therapeutics,* ed 8, New York, 1990a, Pergamon Press.
73. Hodgson BT, Dumal S, Bolling DR, Helsch CM: Effect of estrogen on sensitivity of rabbit bladder and urethra to phenylephrine, *Invest Urol* 16:67, 1978.
74. Levin RM, Jacobowitz D, Wein AJ: Autonomic innervation of rabbit urinary bladder following estrogen administration, *Urology* 17:449, 1981.
75. Larsson B, Andersson KE, Batra S, et al: Effects of estradiol on norepinephrine-induced contraction, alpha adrenoreceptor number and norepinephrine content in the female rabbit urethra, *J Pharmacol Exp Ther* 229:557, 1984.
76. Callahan SM, Creed KE: The effects of estrogens on spontaneous activity and responses to phenylephrine of the mammalian urethra, *J Physiol* 358:35, 1985.
77. Bump RC, Friedman CL: Intraluminal urethral pressure measurements in the female baboon: effects of hormonal manipulation, *J Urol* 136:508, 1986.
78. Batra SC, Losif CS: Female urethra: a target for estrogen action, *J Urol* 129:418, 1983.
79. Batra S, Bjellin L, Sjörgren C et al: Increases in blood flow of the female rabbit urethra following low dose estrogens, *J Urol* 136:1360, 1986.
80. Rud T: Urethral pressure profile in continent women from childhood to old age, *Acta Obstet Gynecol Scand* 59:331, 1980.
81. Raz S, Ziegler M, Caine M: The role of female hormones in stress incontinence, *Proceedings of 16th Congress of Société* International d'Urologie, vol 1, Amsterdam, 1973, Doin, pp. 397-402.
82. Schreiter F, Fuchs P, Stockamp K: Estrogenic sensitivity of alpha receptors in the urethral musculature, *Urol Int* 31:13, 1976.
83. Beisland HO, Fossberg E, Moer A, et al: Urethral sphincteric insufficiency in postmenopausal females: treatment with phenylpropanolamine and estriol separately and in combination, *Urol Int* 39:211, 1984.
84. Bhatia NN, Bergman A, Karrom MM: Effects of estrogen on urethral function in women with urinary incontinence, *Am J Obstet Gynecol* 160:176, 1989.
85. Walter S, Kjaergaard B, Lose G, et al: Stress urinary incontinence in postmenopausal women treated with oral estrogen (estriol) and an alpha adrenergic stimulating agent (phenylpropanolamine): a randomized double-blind placebo controlled study, *Inter Urogynecol J* 1:74, 1990.
86. Cardozo L: Role of estrogens in the treatment of female urinary incontinence, *J Am Geriatr Soc* 38:326, 1990.
87. Grady D, Gebretsadik T, Kerlikowske K, et al: Hormone replacement therapy and endometrial cancer risk: a meta-analysis, *Obstet Gynecol* 85(2):304-13, 1995.
88. Brinton LA, Hoover RN: Estrogen replacement therapy and endometrial cancer risk: unresolved issues. The Endometrial Cancer Collaborative Group, *Obstet Gynecol* 81(2):265-71, 1993.
89. Samsioe G: The endometrium: effects of estrogen and estrogen-progestogen replacement therapy [Review], *Int J Fertil Menopausal Stud* 39(suppl 2):84-92, 1994.
90. Hulka BS: Links between hormone replacement therapy and neoplasia [Review], *Fertil Steril* 62(6 Suppl 2):168s-175s, 1994.
91. McGonigle KF, Karlan BY, Barbuto DA, et al: Development of endometrial cancer in women on estrogen and progestin hormone replacement therapy, *Gynecol Oncol* 55(1):126-32, 1994.
92. Barrett-Connor E: Hormone replacement and cancer [Review], *Br Med Bull* 48(2):345-55, 1992.
93. Nason FG, Nelson BE: Estrogen and progesterone in breast and gynecologic cancers: etiology, therapeutic role, and hormone replacement [Review], *Obstet Gynecol Clin North Am* 21(2):245-70, 1994.
94. Birkhauser M: Hormone replacement therapy and strogen-dependent cancers [Review], *Int J Fertil Menopausal Stud* 39(suppl 2):99-114, 1994.
95. Nørgaard JP, Rittig S, Djurhuus JC: Nocturnal enuresis: an approach to treatment based on pathogenisis, *J Pediatr* 114:705, 1989.
96. Rew DA, Rindle JSH: Assessment of the safety of regular DDAVP therapy on primary nocturnal enuresis, *Br J Urol* 63:352, 1989.
97. Brading A: Physiology of bladder smooth muscle. In Torrens M, Morrison JFB, editors: *The physiology of the lower urinary tract,* London, Berlin, New York, 1987, Springer Verlag.

Chapter 40 Electrostimulation

Christopher K. Payne

Electrostimulation (ES) was first used to treat urinary incontinence by Caldwell in 1963.[1] He developed electrodes that were permanently implanted into the pelvic floor and controlled by radiofrequency. The initial encouraging results lead to noninvasive approaches such as the "electric pessary" reported on by Alexander et al.[2] and similar devices from other investigators in the early 1970s. The last 20 years have produced an enormous variety of techniques (and terminology) using ES in treating urinary incontinence; this diversity presents a real impediment to the typical clinician trying to evaluate this form of therapy. The fact that many experts in the field disagree about some of the fundamental issues and that some investigators have reported contradictory results has lead many clinicians to dismiss ES altogether. Although electrostimulation has thus far failed to win a leading role in the treatment of urinary incontinence, there is a substantial body of research attesting to its efficacy. This chapter provides a practical overview of the rationale for electrostimulation, a summary of the published clinical data, and recommendations for use in routine clinical settings. For those who are interested in exploring the science behind electrostimulation, refer to the work of Magnus Fall,[3,4] William de Groat,[5] and Stanislav Plevnik.[6]

PHYSIOLOGY

The anatomy and physiology of continence are reviewed in greater detail in the chapters in Part 2 but are summarized again here as an introduction to the theory behind electrostimulation. There are at least three mechanisms of continence that might be beneficially influenced by electrostimulation: the structural support of the urethra and bladder neck, the resting and active closure of the proximal urethra, and the inhibition of reflex bladder contractions. The first two mechanisms primarily have to do with treatment of stress incontinence and the latter with urge incontinence and bladder instability.

The female patient with anatomic stress urinary incontinence (AI) has impaired support of the bladder neck and urethra. Bladder neck support comes from the levator muscle and its overlying fascial condensations, primarily the urethropelvic ligament (UPL). The bladder neck and proximal portion of the urethra are circumferentially covered with muscle and fascia, with fascia attaching laterally to the tendinous arc of the pelvis. In the nulligravid female this support is dense; no descent of the bladder neck and urethra occurs with cough and strain. In the stress-incontinent female the support is lax; the bladder neck rotates posteriorly and inferiorly with abdominal pressure. Normal support acts like a Chinese finger trap—when abdominal force is applied, the supporting structures are stretched under tension, and the tension on the ligaments closes the urethra. In addition, reflex contraction of the pelvic floor muscles occurs with increased intraabdominal pressure, and this contributes to urethral closure. In stress-incontinent patients, the abdominal pressure is inefficiently transferred to the urethra, and closure is incomplete. The majority of the support comes from the UPL and can be corrected only through surgery; however, part of the bladder neck support is attributable to the pelvic floor musculature, and this portion can conceivably be augmented through electrostimulation. In addition, strong active or reflex contraction of these muscles can compensate (to some degree) for lax ligamentous support. For example, it is not uncommon to examine a multiparous female and find significant urethral hypermobility in the absence of any clinical incontinence. Thus simple structural support is not the whole story in stress incontinence.

The urethral seal is a second mechanism of continence. Passive coaptation and closure is primarily attributable to the rich, spongy vascular submucosal layer of the urethra. It is difficult to assess the integrity of this mechanism; urethral pressures measured during profilometry correlate poorly with continence. However, some of the urethral closure is caused by resting tone of the striated muscle (a third of the total closure pressure as measured by Rud[7]). Electrostimulation might increase the bulk and tone of this muscle and thus, at least theoretically, improve the resting urethral seal.

The third continence mechanism that can be manipulated with conservative therapy is bladder inhibition. In a small child, urination occurs by reflex whenever a critical bladder volume is reached. Bladder wall mechanoreceptors trigger reflex micturition with filling; coordination of voiding is mediated through the pons and the sacral spinal cord. Continence is achieved when a child gains the ability to inhibit these spontaneous bladder contractions. In the adult, urgency incontinence occurs when the ability to inhibit the bladder is lost. Most inhibitory stimuli to the bladder are cortical in origin, and so classic suprasacral neurologic injuries lead to an unstable (hyperreflexic) bladder. However, detrusor instability is very commonly seen in older women without neurologic lesions. The cause of these cases is unclear but may have to do with loss of local inhibitory pathways. There are some local pelvic reflexes that control and coordinate lower urinary tract function. Afferent autonomic nerves from the rectum, vagina, and genitals and afferent somatic nerves from the lower extremities and pelvic floor muscles synapse in the sacral spinal cord and are inhibitory to the bladder parasympathetic afferents. The delicate balance between the positive-feedback loop that produces complete bladder emptying and the reflexes that inhibit such contractions can easily be disturbed, leading to bladder instability and urgency incontinence.

There is significant evidence for denervation of the pelvic floor in incontinent women; this may be caused by childbirth or other pelvic trauma, surgery, hormonal factors, or aging. Pudendal nerve latency has been demonstrated to be prolonged by vaginal delivery[8] and by vaginal surgery[9] for prolapse (but not by retropubic operations). Patients with stress urinary incontinence have been shown to have prolonged pudendal nerve latency periods when compared to continent controls,[10,11] and similar findings are present in patients with fecal incontinence.[12] Decreased anal sphincter motor unit fiber density has been demonstrated in stress-incontinent women compared to normal controls.[13] Evidence of pelvic floor denervation injury and subsequent reinnervation was seen on electromyograph in women after a first vaginal delivery.[14] Finally, biopsy specimens taken from the pubococcygeus muscle at the time of surgery for genital prolapse or stress incontinence were compared to specimens taken from asymptomatic controls.[15] Histologic evidence for denervation in the study group was found, limited to the posterior portion of the muscle.

Individually these studies are interesting; taken together, they present a compelling case for the role of nerve injury in female urinary incontinence. It is reasonable to consider these abnormalities to be potentially reversible, or at least treatable, since the nerve supply in these patients is only compromised, not totally disrupted. It is theorized that ES may result in reinnervation or electrical reorganization of the pelvic floor. If so, ES may be the most physiologic treatment for many incontinent patients.

Mechanics

Electrostimulation has been used for stress urinary incontinence, urge incontinence, urgency and frequency, and painful bladder syndromes. In each case, the attempt is made to alter lower urinary tract function by stimulation of the sacral autonomic or somatic nerves. In most cases vaginal or anal probes are employed. Patch electrodes have been used on the skin to stimulate the underlying peripheral nerves of the lower extremities, the dorsal nerve of the penis, and the clitoral nerve. Two main types of stimulation have been used: long-term, or chronic, ES and acute maximal functional electrostimulation (AMFES), or, simply, maximal stimulation. Chronic stimulation is delivered below the sensory threshold; the patient is instructed to use the device "as much as possible," which usually translates into 6 to 12 hours per day. The treatment usually lasts several months. Pelvic muscle contractions are not elicited during stimulation. The introduction of maximal stimulation is attributed to Godec and Cass.[16] In this technique a higher-intensity stimulus (the maximum tolerable without pain) is used for short periods, 15 to 30 minutes, at intervals of one to three times per week. Adjustable current is mandatory and is set at a level that is sensed but is not unpleasant. A pelvic muscle contraction should be visible during stimulation. The success of maximal stimulation has led to the development of home ES units, which undoubtedly represent the future of this treatment modality. Electrostimulation current is pulsed; this means that short bursts of stimulation are alternated with rest. The ratio of stimulation time to rest time is called the "duty cycle." A typical duty cycle is in the range of 1:2. Most systems have used 9- or 12-volt batteries. In both forms of ES the frequency is chosen based on the patient's clinical diagnosis as discussed below. Low frequencies (about 10 Hz) are used for instability, and high frequencies (50 Hz) for stress incontinence. In mixed incontinence, two strategies have been employed—a compromise setting of about 20 Hz or delivering both low- and high-frequency stimuli. Single-probe home units are now commercially available and can be programmed to deliver either high-frequency, low-frequency, or mixed stimulation. The optimal settings are unknown but probably not of critical importance, since there is general agreement on these basic points. Other ES treatment methods include faradism and interferential therapy. Faradism is quite similar to the maximal stimulation programs used today; short bursts of cycled stimulation are given to produce a pelvic floor contraction and the patient is instructed to try to augment the contraction. There are few published data on this technique. Interferential therapy involves setting up two competing currents using surface electrodes. These higher-frequency currents "interfere" with each other and produce low-frequency stimulation in the area of interest. It has primarily been employed in the treatment of stress incontinence with promising results[17,18] but has also been used in hyperreflexia.[19] It is somewhat cumbersome and not readily adaptable to home use. Unless future studies demonstrate a clear advantage against maximal stimulation it is unlikely to play an important treatment role.

Electrostimulation is used in the treatment of stress urinary incontinence to improve the function of the intrinsic urethral and levator musculature. These include both smooth and striated muscle fibers of three types—one with slow contraction and two with faster contractions. Although the primary mechanism of action is always proposed as direct stimulation of the pudendal efferent nerves, all clinical ES is at suboptimal conditions compared to a laboratory setting, and most experts agree that some of the muscular response to stimulation is through local reflex pathways. The majority of the nerve fibers supplying the muscle of the urethra operate at relatively high frequencies, 50 to 100 Hz. This is the rationale for use of higher frequencies in the treatment of pure stress incontinence.

What happens to the muscle after stimulation is much less clear. It has been proposed that the effect of stimulation is simply to increase the bulk of the levator. It has also been proposed that stimulation increases the proportion of fast-twitch fibers and thus the ability of the muscle to respond to a sudden increase in intra-abdominal pressure; on the other hand, it has been suggested that the stimulus increases the number and strength of slow-twitch fibers and thus improves the resting urethral closure. Another theory is that after a course of electrostimulation there is improved recruitment of levator muscle fibers with nonstimulated reflex and voluntary contractions. All of these theories can be considered as pelvic floor "reeducation" as opposed to the simple bulking effect on the levator. It would obviously be extremely difficult to prove or disprove any of these theories, and, in fact, basic urodynamic measurements after stimulation have usually revealed no significant change. Although the optimal method of stimulation is still to be elucidated, there is general agreement on the use of high-frequency stimuli in the treatment of stress incontinence.

In the treatment of urgency incontinence and bladder instability the goal is to increase the inhibitory stimulus to the bladder by stimulating afferent sacral nerves of the pelvic organs or lower extremities. As discussed above, these nerves synapse in the sacral micturition center where they provide a inhibitory stimulus to the efferent pelvic nerve. The sacral afferent nerves, particularly the autonomic nerves of the pelvic organs, tend to be poorly (A-delta, A∂) or unmyelinated (C) fibers, which conduct current at a slow rate of 5 to 20 Hz.[19] Thus in the treatment of bladder instability and hyperreflexia the strategy has been to use low-frequency stimulation, which has generally been applied to the pudendal nerve afferents through vaginal or rectal probes. However, equally good results have been demonstrated with a stimulus of the clitoris, glans penis, and posterior tibial nerve. Frequencies below about 10 Hz are more likely to be sensed as painful, and so this is the typical frequency employed in treating instability. The ultimate, long-term effect of such an inhibitory stimulus has always been difficult to visualize. If a chronic, "carry-over" effect of electrostimulation for instability exists, it may depend on some type of reorganization of the sacral micturition center that results in facilitation of existing bladder inhibition. Plevnik[6] argues that stimulation can lead to "re-activation of lost functional patterns (re-education)." This may be true, but definitive proof is lacking.

Electrostimulation in Clinical Practice

Patient Selection

There are few contraindications to the use of electrostimulation. There is general agreement that a patient with complete denervation of the pelvic floor will not respond to treatment. Many patients will not accept treatment with vaginal or anal probes, and this produces a selection bias inherent in most studies. It is even more problematic when one is considering the use of home units because many patients will allow a treatment with a vaginal probe to be performed by a nurse or a doctor but will not agree to insert the device themselves as required for home use. Severe genital prolapse or significant vaginal shortening usually prevents the use of vaginal electrodes, but mild prolapse has not been a significant problem. The patient with stress incontinence and a low-pressure urethra has been considered to be a poorer candidate for stimulation than other patients, but three investigators have reported at least some success in this group.[20-22] It seems unlikely that a fixed, radiated urethra or a heavily scarred urethra will respond to ES, but many elderly women have very low urethral pressures without an obvious cause, and they should not be excluded from treatment. A small study of cognitively impaired nursing home patients showed no benefit, and this group must be considered to be unlikely to respond in the absence of other data.[23] The available data would indicate that the best candidates may be younger patients with mild to moderate incontinence. However, motivated patients of any age and degree of incontinence can be offered ES, and unmotivated patients are difficult to treat.

One major problem in reviewing literature on incontinence is the lack of data presented on the pretreatment status of the patients enrolled. This problem occurs particularly when noninvasive forms of therapy are being examined, since one major advantage of such treatments is that exact urodynamic classification is not required. For academic purposes it would be ideal if all patients would be completely classified by both clinical history and urodynamics with a system such as Shlomo Raz's SEAPI scale, both before and after treatment.[24] This scale would optimally allow for critical evaluation of a patient's response to therapy and might enable investigators to predict which patients will respond to a particular treatment. As the clinical results of electrostimulation are reviewed, we find that the patients are often not urodynamically classified, and this limits our ability to interpret the data. For the purposes of this chapter, only English-language studies since 1980 and reports that classify patients by the type of incontinence have been included. Data published in abstract form only have not been included.

Clinical Results

Stress urinary incontinence. Table 40-1 presents the data on chronic electrostimulation for stress incontinence. The best study is that of Eriksen,[28] using a dual vaginal-anal electrode, which demonstrated an initial 68% response rate with 47% of the overall group becoming dry. The results were largely maintained over a long-term follow-up study. It is disconcerting to see that Leach[27] failed to reproduce the good results previously obtained by others using a device called Incontan. The trial was ruined by mechanical failures and patient intolerance because of pain. As with any other medical therapy, electrostimulation equipment should be demonstrated to be effective and reliable in multiple centers before a device is generally endorsed.

Table 40-2 summarizes the use of maximal electrostimulation for stress incontinence. Of a total of 237 patients enrolled in these studies 43 (18%) became dry and another 81 (34%) had significant improvement. There is significant variation in the length of the treatment given by these investigators, and many of the patients, particularly those who were receiving office-based therapy, were probably undertreated. The study by Sand et al.[34] is the only published placebo-controlled study of ES and showed an unquestionable superiority of the treatment arm. There are no trials that directly compare chronic to maximal therapy, but it seems likely that daily use of home units for maximal stimulation will produce results comparable to chronic stimulation.

Urgency incontinence, instability, and hyperreflexia. The results of chronic and maximal ES for urgency incontinence are presented in Tables 40-3 and 40-4 respectively. There have simply not been any studies of the chronic type of stimulation with adequate numbers of patients and adequate follow-up done in the last 15 years to draw firm conclusions. It is particularly frustrating that the excellent results reported by McGuire et al.[34] using the simple technique of TENS stimulation to the posterior tibial nerve distribution have not been followed up by any other investigators. Patch electrodes are more acceptable to many patients (particularly men) than vaginal and anal ES probes are, and the cost is comparable. This would be a very acceptable treatment for many patients with difficult neurogenic bladder problems if these results were reproducible.

Excluding Vereecken's[37] study, which examined only the acute urodynamic effects of stimulation, 361 patients were enrolled in studies of maximal electrostimulation. Almost all

Table 40-1 Chronic Electrostimulation for Stress Incontinence

Author	Year	Study design	Enrolled	Dropout	Subjective response: Dry	Subjective response: Improved	Objective response: UDS	Pad test	Follow-up time
Krauss and Lilien[25]	1981	After prostatectomy with perineal patches	9		4	3	No change in urethral pressure profile	None	—
Fall[26]	1984	Females: vaginal electrode	10		6	2	None	None	>6 months
Leach and Bavendam[27]	1989	Females: anal electrode	23	67% in 3 months		6% response in overall group	No change in responders	None	None
Eriksen and Eik-Nes[28]	1989	Women awaiting surgery using vaginal-anal electrode	55		26	12	Stress profile improved	None	2 years

UDS, Ultra-Doppler sonography.

Table 40-2 Maximal Electrostimulation for Stress Incontinence

Author	Year	Study design	Enrolled	Dropout	Subjective response: Dry	Subjective response: Improved	Objective response: UDS	Pad test	Follow-up time
Plevnik et al.[29]	1986	Females: home stimulation with vaginal electrode	80		25	13	None	None	1 year
Plevnik et al.[29]	1986	Postprostatectomy home stimulation with anal electrode	12		3	1	None	None	1 year
Jonasson et al.[30]	1990	Consecutive females using vaginal electrode	17			8	No change	6 of 17 are >50% improved	6 months
Esa et al.[31]	1991	Men and women using anal electrode	7		1	2	1 of 6 tested had improved urethral closure	None	None
Bent et al.[32]	1993	Females using vaginal electrode	14		1	9	Minimal change in urethral profile	Slight improvement	None
Caputo et al.[21]	1993	Females using vaginal electrode	19			15	17 improved by voiding diary	None	6 months in 40%
Schiøtz[22]	1994	Women awaiting surgery using vaginal electrode	53	2	6	17 "much" 16 "slightly"	Static urethral pressure profile	Pronounced improvement	1 year
Sand et al.[33]	1995	Female: placebo and vaginal electrode	35	7	7	16	Voiding diary: 13 improved	None	None

UDS, Ultra-Doppler sonography.

had documented detrusor instability (not only symptomatic urgency), and several studies included neurogenic patients. Seventy-seven (20%) became dry, and 134 (37%) were significantly improved. It is not possible to determine if there is a different response between patients with symptomatic urgency, detrusor instability, and detrusor hyperreflexia, though it would seem logical that these are progressively more difficult problems to treat. It is also not possible to determine how many patients will maintain their response once the short-term treatment is completed. In the few studies that have followed patients for more that 1 year after treatment the majority of patients do seem to have a "carry-over" effect with improved continence.

Table 40-3 Chronic Electrostimulation for Urge Incontinence

Author	Year	Study design	Enrolled	Dropout	Subjective response: Dry	Subjective response: Improved	Objective response: UDS	Pad test	Follow-up time
McGuire et al.[34]	1983	Idiopathic instability; posterior tibial nerve	8		7	0	Not stated	None	None
McGuire et al.[34]	1983	Hyperreflexia; posterior tibial nerve	8		5	3	Not stated	None	None
Nakamura et al.[35]	1984	Acute study only; male urge incontinence; dorsal nerve of the penis	22		N/A	N/A	Capacity increased 10 of 22; DI suppressed 7 of 10	N/A	N/A
Nakamura et al.[35]	1984	Acute study only; female urge incontinence; clitoral nerve	10		N/A	N/A	Capacity increased 1 of 10; DI suppressed 1 of 3	N/A	N/A
Fall[26]	1984	Females idiopathic instability; vaginal electrode	20		9	9	None	None	>6 months
Vodusek et al.[36]	1986	Acute study only; suprasacral spinal cord lesions; pudendal nerve	10		N/A	N/A	Capacity >> during stimulus, all patients; 3 of 10 respond after stimulus	N/A	N/A
Leach and Bavendam[27]	1989	Female instability; hyperreflexia; anal electrode	5	67% in 3 months		6% response in overall group	No change in responders	None	None

DI, Detrusor instability;
N/A, Not applicable;
UDS, Ultra-Doppler sonography.

Mixed incontinence. The few studies that clearly delineate treatment of patients with both stress incontinence and detrusor instability are listed in Table 40-5. Obviously it is uncommon to cure these difficult patients but, if we exclude Leach's poor results with the Incontan, a respectable 58% of 109 patients were dry or significantly improved after treatment with ES.

Conclusions

Electrostimulation is an effective therapy for the majority of patients with urinary incontinence. Unfortunately, there are more questions about the application of ES than there are answers. There are few studies directly comparing ES to any other treatment and few that define the long-term results. Until adequate studies are done the clinician will have to be guided by personal bias and patient preference. As with all incontinence therapy, the guiding principle is that treatment should be delivered in as simple, inexpensive, and effective a way as possible and in the most expedient fashion. The cost and effectiveness of ES must be considered in comparison to the available alternatives including pelvic floor exercises, biofeedback, medications, and surgery.

The role for ES in the treatment of pure stress incontinence seems to be rather limited. Electrostimulation has not been demonstrated to be superior to pelvic floor exercises or biofeedback with vaginal cones and is clearly significantly more expensive. Randomized studies with appropriate numbers of patients and adequate follow-up study would be welcomed. The cure rate of ES is far below that of surgery, and periurethral injection therapy is another alternative that is simple, safe, and effective for a large number of stress-incontinent females. It is my opinion that electrostimulation is primarily useful in treating those patients who are unable to perform a proper Kegel exercise after a few minutes of instruction in the office. These patients do not improve without some formal training, and electrostimulation is comparable in cost to physical therapy or office biofeedback. Vaginal cones are still a cheaper and effective option for many of these patients.

Electrostimulation offers the most benefit to the patient with pure urgency or mixed incontinence. Although medications are available, many patients find them to be intolerable at effective doses. Surgery can cure the stress component of the incontinence but may exacerbate the urgency. Bladder augmentation and surgical neuromodulation are the only effective alternatives for pure urgency incontinence, and many patients simply are not able to tolerate procedures of this magnitude. It seems clear that ES is significantly underutilized in this patient population. More work is needed to define the optimal method of stimulation and to delineate the parameters for patient selection.

Table 40-4 Maximal Electrostimulation for Urge Incontinence

Author	Year	Study design	Enrolled	Dropout	Subjective response: Dry	Subjective response: Improved	Objective response: UDS	Pad test	Follow-up time
Vereecken et al.[37]	1984	Paraplegics; anal electrode; acute study only	15		N/A	N/A	Instability suppressed in 11 of 15	N/A	None
Plevnik et al.[29]	1986	Female idiopathic instability	67		20	14	None	None	1 year
Plevnik et al.[29]	1986	Postprostatectomy instability	12		6	2	None	None	1 year
Nakamura et al.[38]	1987	Urge incontinence; perianal-anal electrode	21	8	8	5	2 of 6 with DI suppressed	N/A	None
Ericksen et al.[39]	1989	Females: idiopathic instability; vaginal-anal electrode	48		25	16	21 "cured"; 13 "improved"		15 months
Fossberg et al.[40]	1990	Consecutive patients with instability; vaginal-anal electrode	91	17	8	32	Small improvement in CMG capacity	None	6 weeks
Jonasson et al.[30]	1990	Consecutive patients with instability; vaginal electrode	20			14	No change	13 of 20 are >50% improved	6 months
Esa et al.[31]	1991	Urge incontinence; anal electrodes	41		17 dry or satisfied	9 "fair"	No correlation between CMG and subjective result	None	None
Zollner-Nielsen and Samuelsson[41]	1992	Consecutive females with instability-hyperreflexia; vaginal-anal electrode	21			16 cured or improved	Voiding diaries with increased volumes	None	None
Bent et al.[32]	1993	Females: idiopathic instability; vaginal electrode	10		1	6	CMG unchanged	Slight improvement	None
Caputo et al.[21]	1993	Females: idiopathic instability; vaginal electrode	30		7	19	22 improved by voiding diary	None	6 months in 40%

DI, Detrusor instability;
CMG, Cystometrogram;
N/A, Not applicable;
UDS, Ultra-Doppler sonography.

References

1. Caldwell KPS: The electrical control of sphincter incompetence, *Lancet* 2:174-175, 1963.
2. Alexander S, Rowan D: Electrical control of urinary incontinence by radio implant, *Br J Surg* 55:358-364, 1968.
3. Fall M, Lindstrom S: Electrical stimulation: a physiologic approach to the treatment of urinary incontinence, *Urol Clin North Am* 18(2):393-407, 1991.
4. Fall M, Lindstrom S: Functional electrical stimulation: physiological basis and clinical principles, *Int Urogynecol J* 5:296-304, 1994.
5. de Groat WC: Neurophysiology of the pelvic organs. In Rushton DN, editor: *Handbook of neuro-urology,* New York, 1995, Marcel Dekker.
6. Plevnik S, Janez J, Vodusek DB: Electrical stimulation. In Krane RJ, Siroky MB, editors: *Clinical neuro-urology,* Boston, 1991, Little, Brown.
7. Rud T, Andersson KE, Asmussen M, et al: Factors maintaining the intraurethral pressures in women, *Invest Urol* 17(4):343-347, 1980.
8. Sultan AH, Kamm MA, Hudson CN: Pudendal nerve damage during labour: prospective study before and after childbirth, *Br J Obstet Gynaecol* 101:22-28, 1994.

Table 40-5 Electrostimulation for Mixed Incontinence

Author	Year	Study design	Enrolled	Dropout	Subjective response: Dry	Subjective response: Improved	Objective response: UDS	Pad test	Follow-up time
Fall[26]	1984	Females: chronic stimulation; vaginal electrode	10		3	7	None	None	>6 months
Plevnik et al.[29]	1986	Females: home stimulation with vaginal electrode	51		14	10	None	None	1 year
Leach and Bavendam[27]	1989	Females: chronic stimulation; anal electrode	7	67% in 3 months		6% response in overall group	No change in responders	None	None
Bent et al.[32]	1993	Females: maximal stimulation; vaginal electrode	21		0	11	Unchanged	Unchanged	None
Caputo et al.[21]	1993	Females: maximal stimulation; vaginal electrode	27			18	19 improved by voiding diary	None	6 months in 40%

UDS, Ultra-Doppler sonography.

9. Benson JT, McClellan EJ, Pillai-Allen AV: Bulbocavernosus reflex study in asymptomatic females, *Int J Urogynecol* 4(6):403, Abstract #65, 1993.
10. Snooks, SJ, Badenoch DF, Tiptaft RC, Swash M: Perineal nerve damage in genuine stress urinary incontinence, *Br J Urol* 57:422-426, 1985.
11. Smith ARB, Hosker GL, Warrell DW: The role of pudendal nerve damage in the aeticlogy of genuine stress incontinence in women, *Br J Obstet Gynaecol* 96:29-32, 1989.
12. Snooks SJ, Swash M: Abnormalities of the innervation of the urethral striated sphincter musculature in incontinence, *Br J Urol* 56:401-405, 1984.
13. Anderson RS: A neurogenic element to urinary genuine stress incontinence, *Br J Obstet Gynaecol* 91:41-45, 1984
14. Allen RE, Hosker GL, Smith ARB, Warrell DW: Pelvic floor damage and childbirth: a neurophysiological study, *Br J Obstet Gynaecol* 97:770-779, 1990.
15. Gilpin SA, Gosling JA, Smith ARB, Warrell DW: The pathogenesis of genitourinary prolapse and stress incontinence of urine: a histological and histochemical study, *Br J Obset Gynaecol* 96:15-23 1989.
16. Godec C, Cass A: Acute electrical stimulation for urinary incontinence, *Urology* 12(3):340-342, 1978.
17. Dougall DS: The effects of interferential therapy on incontinence and frequency of micturition, *Physiotherapy* 71(3):135-136, 1985.
18. Olah KS: The conservative management of patients with symptoms of stress incontinence: a randomized, prospective study comparing weighted vaginal cones and interferential therapy, *Am J Obstet Gynecol* 162(1):87-92, 1990.
19. Van Poppel H, Ketelaer P, Van DeWeerd A: Interferential therapy for detrusor hyperreflexia in multiple sclerosis, *Urology* 25(6):607-612, 1985.
20. Sand PK: Pelvic floor stimulation (PFS) treatment of the low pressure urethra, *Int J Urogynecol* 4(6):403, 1993.
21. Caputo RM, Benson JT, McClellan E: Intravaginal maximal electrical stimulation in the treatment of urinary incontinence, *J Reprod Med* 38(9):667-671, 1993.
22. Schiotz HA: One month maximal electrostimulation for genuine stress incontinence in women, *Neurourol Urodyn* 13:43-50, 1994.
23. Lamhut P, Jackson TW, Wall LL: The treatment of urinary incontinence with electrical stimulation in nursing home patients: a pilot study, *J Am Geriatr Soc* 40:48-52, 1992.
24. Raz S, Erickson DR: SEAPI QMM incontinence classification system, *Neurourol Urodyn* 11:187-199, 1992.
25. Krauss DJ, Lilien OM: Transcutaneous electrical nerve stimulator for stress incontinence, *J Urol* 125:790-793, 1981.
26. Fall M: Does electrostimulation cure urinary incontinence? *J Urol* 131:664-667, 1984.
27. Leach GE, Bavendam TG: Prospective evaluation of the incontan transrectal stimulator in women with urinary incontinence, *Neurourol Urodyn* 8:231-235, 1989.
28. Eriksen BC, Eik-Nes SH: Long-term electrostimulation of the pelvic floor: primary therapy in female stress incontinence? *Urol Int* 44:90-95, 1989.
29. Plevnik S, et al: Short-term electric stimulation: home treatment for urinary incontinence, *World J Urol* 4:24-26, 1986.
30. Jonasson A, Larsson B, Pschera H, Nylund L: Short-term maximal electrical stimulation: a conservative treatment of urinary incontinence, *Gynecol Obstet Invest* 30:120-123, 1990.
31. Esa A, Kiwamoto H, Sugiyama T, et al: Functional electrical stimulation in the management of incontinence: studies of urodynamics, *Int Urol Nephrol* 23(2):135-141, 1991.
32. Bent AE, Sand PK, Ostergard DR, Brubaker LT: Transvaginal electrical stimulation in the treatment of genuine stress incontinence and detrusor instability, *Int Urogynecol J* 4:9-13, 1993.
33. Sand PK, Richardson DA, Staskin DR, et al: Pelvic floor electrical stimulation in the treatment of genuine stress incontinence: a multicenter, placebo-controlled trial, *Am J Obstet Gynecol* 173(1):72-79, 1995.
34. McGuire EJ, Shi-Chun Z, Horwinski ER, Lytton B: Treatment of motor and sensory detrusor instability by electrical stimulation, *J Urol* 129:78-79, 1983.
35. Nakamura M, Sakurai T: Bladder inhibition by penile electrical stimulation, *Br J Urol* 56:413, 1984.
36. Vodusek DB, Light JK, Libby JM: Detrusor inhibition induced by stimulation of pudendal nerve afferents, *Neurourol Urodyn* 5:381-389, 1986.

37. Vereecken RL, Das J, Grisar P: Electrical sphincter stimulation in the treatment of detrusor hyperreflexia of paraplegics, *Neurourol Urodyn* 3:145-154, 1984.
38. Nakamura M, Sakurai T, Sugao H, Sonoda T: Maximum electrical stimulation for urge incontinence, *Urol Int* 42:285-287, 1987.
39. Eriksen BC, Bergmann S, Eik-Nes: Maximal electrostimulation of the pelvic floor in female idiopathic detrusor instability and urge incontinence, *Neurourol Urodyn* 8:219-230, 1989.
40. Fossberg E, Sørensen S, Ruutu M, et al: Maximal electrical stimulation in the treatment of unstable detrusor and urge incontinence, *Eur Urol* 18:120-123, 1990.
41. Zollner-Nielsen M, Samuelsson SM: Maximal electrical stimulation of patients with frequency, urgency and urge incontinence, *Acta Obstet Gynecol Scand* 71:629-631, 1992.

Chapter 41

Vesicovaginal Fistulas

Nabil K. Bissada

The first documented occurrence of vesicovaginal fistula occurred about 4000 years ago. An extensive urinary fistula was found by Professor Derry of Cairo in the mummy of a woman called Henhenit, who was one of the ladies of the court of King Mentuhotep II of the Eleventh Dynasty in Egypt around 2050 B.C.[1-3] The first documented medical reference to management is the Ebers Egyptian papyrus dated at 1550 B.C. and describes a possible vesicovaginal fistula warning physicians against attempting to cure it. The next documented medical reference to urinary fistulas was that of Avicenna (Ibn Sina, died in AD 1037), who recognized that urinary incontinence in women may be attributable to a fistula after difficult labor. He also described the condition as incurable. The first reference in European literature to urinary fistulas in women was made by Platter in 1597.[1] During the next 100 years, several clear descriptions of urinary fistulas occurring after difficult labor appeared together with descriptions of surgical treatment that consistently failed.[4] The first known description of a scientific approach to management was that of Hendrick van Roonhuyse of Amsterdam in 1663.[5] The Swiss physician Johann Fatio described two successful fistula repairs using van Roonhuyse's technique in 1675 and 1684.

Many attempts at fistula closure followed. However, successful cases were rare. Over many decades the principles of treatment slowly began to emerge. Catheter drainage was mentioned more frequently. Access to the fistula, both for diagnosis and treatment, was improved by the knee-elbow, knee-chest, lithotomy, and prone positions. Suture materials changed from bird's quills to linen, silk, and "nonreactive metal." In 1852, Sims published his classic article on the treatment of vesicovaginal fistula, ushering in an era of great interest in the problem.[6] Sims's associates, Bozeman and later Emmett, contributed their own improvements.[7,8] Other important landmarks included the introduction of abdominal approach to fistula repair by Trendelenburg in 1890 and by von Dittel in 1893 and the transperitoneal transvesical approach by Felix Leguen of Paris in 1914.[4] The concept of placing grafts of new tissue between the genital and urinary tracts was advanced by Martius[9] and Garlock[10] in 1928.

The era of "fistula specialists" started with the eloquent contributions of Mahfouz of Cairo.[1,11,12] His work stimulated many great surgeons who devoted their skills to the treatment of urinary fistulas. Notable among these are Moir[13-15] in Oxford, Lawson[16-18] in West Africa, and the Hamlins[19] in Addis Ababa, Ethiopia.

Etiology

There are four causes of vesicovaginal fistula:

Obstetric injury. The usual mechanism of obstetric fistulas is slough injury after prolonged pressure during obstructed labor. Trauma sustained at the time of difficult operative delivery may play a role in many patients. In developed countries, most of the fistulas caused by obstetric trauma occurred before 1940.[20-22] In developing countries where hospitals and obstetric care are not readily available, obstetric complications remain the leading cause of genitourinary fistulas.[4,23-30]

Surgical trauma. Surgical trauma is the most common cause of fistulas in developed countries where modern maternity care has largely eliminated obstetric fistulas. The majority of these fistulas result from gynecologic surgery.[28,31-34]

Radiation therapy. A significant number of fistulas were previously associated with radiation treatment for gynecologic malignancy.[32,35-37] With recent improvements in instrumentation, dosimetry, fractionation, and understanding of radiobiology, there has been a decrease in the incidence of fistulas secondary to radiotherapy alone.[31,32]

Pelvic malignancy. Fistula formation may occur spontaneously in very advanced pelvic malignancy. More frequently, it occurs after radiation therapy for pelvic malignancy, either alone or combined with surgery.[23,35] The combination of radiation therapy and hysterectomy increases the fistula rate dramatically.[38-42]

Clinical Presentation

The classic presentation of a urinary fistula is continuous urinary incontinence. Urinary leakage may occur immediately after the initiating event, or it may be delayed for several days or even a few weeks. Immediate leakage after operation probably represents unrecognized perforation or laceration of the urinary tract. Slightly delayed leakage, between the second and tenth days postoperatively, is often the result of varying degrees of trauma and precarious placement of clamps or sutures followed by devascularization and necrosis, with delayed development of the fistula. Complications, such as infection and hematoma formation may contribute to local compression, devascularization, and necrosis. Radiation-induced vesicovaginal fistulas are much more delayed, occurring weeks to years after radiotherapy and therapeutic pelvic manipulation.[34]

The degree of urinary leakage is related to the size and location of the fistula. With very small fistulas, urine leakage may be minimal, and the patient may also be able to void normal quantities. However, normal voiding in addition to continuous leakage is more characteristic of patients with unilateral ureterovaginal fistulas. Patients with incontinence caused by urethrovaginal fistulas usually have leakage immediately after the trauma or, if they had an indwelling Foley catheter, after catheter removal.

Diagnosis

The aim of the diagnostic evaluation is not only to establish the diagnosis of genitourinary fistula but also to determine the precise anatomic situation, that is, exact number, site, and location of the fistula (or fistulas), its relationship and proximity to ureteral orifices or bladder neck, and the presence of associated conditions, such as rectovaginal fistula. The presence and adequacy of vaginal access, mobility, and tissue vasculature are assessed. In addition, the upper tracts should be evaluated.[43]

In our experience, an excretory urogram (intravenous pyelogram) and careful pelvic examination, together with endoscopy under anesthesia or under adequate sedation, are usually adequate for the evaluation of patients with vesicovaginal fistula. This is assisted at the time of pelvic examination by the placement of a Foley catheter in the bladder and by filling the bladder with normal saline solution while the vagina is being inspected.

Almost all ureterovaginal fistulas requiring treatment are associated with an abnormal intravenous pyelogram, usually with some degree of obstruction of the involved upper urinary tract unilaterally or bilaterally.[23,44] In the presence of upper tract abnormality, retrograde urography should be done at the time of pelvic examination and endoscopy.

Timing of Surgical Repair

There is general agreement that if the injury is discovered intraoperatively or within the first 24 to 48 hours of surgery immediate repair should be performed. A fistula diagnosed several days to weeks postoperatively is accompanied by significant edema and inflammation, rendering repair more difficult. This has prompted many surgeons to delay definitive surgical intervention for about 3 months.[33] This delay, however, adds considerably to patient suffering. Several authors have questioned the necessity for such delay in patients with clean iatrogenic (gynecologic) fistulas.[33,44,45] In an attempt to enhance resolution of inflammatory changes and decrease the waiting period before surgical correction, some authors have used corticosteroids.[28,45-47] Others found this to be unnecessary and advocate early repair in most patients with gynecologic fistulas. On the other hand, some small fistulas may close spontaneously on catheter drainage (after fulguration of the edges unless the fistula is of recent onset).[16-18,20,31,32,48-52] Accordingly it is reasonable to treat very small fistulas with fulguration and catheter drainage for 3 to 6 weeks (or catheter drainage alone for those of recent onset). In patients with obstetric fistulas, we prefer to delay definitive repair for 3 months.

Since radiation-induced fistulas generally undergo subtle enlargement, periodic assessment of the diameter of the defect is warranted, and repair should be contemplated 6 to 12 months after stabilization of the defect size.[32,34,35,53] Occasionally earlier repair is possible by wide excision of the fistula and bridging of the defect by nonradiated tissues.[54]

Preoperative Management

When definitive management has to be delayed, the patient has to deal with the continuous urinary leakage and its unpleasant sequelae including odor and perineal, vulvar, and vaginal irritation. As stated previously, patients with very small vesicovaginal fistulas may be managed initially with fulguration and catheter drainage. Catheter drainage also reduces or eliminates leakage in such patients. In the presence of a large defect the catheter is generally ineffective. Some patients may be managed by an intravaginal urinary collecting device. Such collecting devices have been described as early as the late 1700s by French physicians.[5] More recently, a modification of the Tassette menstrual cup was advocated for this purpose.[55,56] If this is not practical, frequent washing and changing of pads helps to keep a healthy perineal area.

Before definitive management of a vesicovaginal fistula, we generally discontinue Foley catheter or any intravaginal collecting device. We treat any urinary tract infection, use frequent sitz baths and apply Premarin (conjugated estrogens) cream to the vulva and outer portion of the vagina. If there is severe irritation, we also apply antimicrobial antifungal cream. This regimen has generally resulted in rapid resolution of vulvar and perineal inflammation.

Surgical Repair

The majority of uncomplicated vesicovaginal fistulas are accessible by the vaginal approach, which is associated with less postoperative discomfort and a shorter hospital stay than other methods; however, some high-vault fistulas with extensive scarring and giant, complex, and combined fistulas (such as vesicoureterovaginal fistulas) require abdominal or combined vaginal and abdominal approach.

Technique of Vaginal Repair

The patient is placed in the exaggerated lithotomy position. If exposure is not optimal because of a narrow vagina, it may be improved by a Schuchardt or a generous posterolateral relaxing incision before placement of the weighted vaginal retractor.[25,33] The labia minora are sewn laterally to facilitate exposure. If the ureteral orifices are close to the fistula, ureteric catheters are placed cystoscopically before the repair. A punch suprapubic catheter is also placed. A longitudinal vaginal incision is made so that it surrounds the fistula and extends sufficiently, proximally, and distally. Only 1 to 2 mm of fistulous margin, if any, needs to be excised.[23,34] In fact, closure is possible without any excision of the bladder edge of the fistulous tract.[57,58] The lateral vaginal flaps are mobilized. If the patient has a hypermobile urethra, a transvaginal bladder neck suspension is performed before repair of the fistula.[32,59,60] A pubovaginal sling procedure may also be performed if necessary. The bladder is closed transversely with 3-0 polyglycolic acid (Dexon) suture. A second muscular layer closure may be used extending beyond the margins of the initial layer. The endopelvic fascia is closed longitudinally in the midline, at a right angle to the initial closure. Finally the vaginal mucosa is approximated. In addition, for most fistulas, we prefer to utilize a bulbocavernosus fibrofatty flap (Martius) that is interposed between the bladder and the vaginal closure.

As stated previously, the transabdominal approach is suitable for high-vault fistulas with extensive scarring, for giant vesicovaginal or vesicourethrovaginal fistulas, and for complex fistulas associated with ureteric or bowel involvement.[61-63]

Technique of Abdominal Repair

The patient is positioned in a modified lithotomy position to allow simultaneous abdominal and vaginal access. A midline suprapubic incision is made. The anterior bladder wall and the dome are mobilized. The bladder is opened in the midline. The ureters are catheterized. The bladder incision is extended to the fistula, which is circumscribed and excised. Only about a 2 mm margin needs to be excised. Large stay sutures on the uterine fundus help in traction and exposure. The bladder wall is separated from the vagina. The vaginal defect is closed vertically with 2-0 Dexon continuous suture. Omentum is then brought down to completely cover the vaginal closure. The distal margin of the omental graft is anchored with several 3-0 polyglycolic acid sutures to the anterior vaginal wall beyond the repair site. If the omentum does not easily reach the fistula site without tension, it may be mobilized from the greater curvature of the stomach by use of the gastroepiploic artery. Although many surgeons limit the indications of use of omental interposition graft, I believe that the advantages of its use are such that we use it routinely for all patients undergoing transperitoneal transvesical fistula repair. The omentum supplies neovascularity and separates the urinary and vaginal closures, enhances the healing potential, and minimizes the risk of recurrence.[34,64-66]

After securing the position of the omentum, the urinary bladder is closed with a continuous 2-0 polyglycolic acid suture. In the presence of extensive scarring around the fistula, a bladder wall flap obtained posterosuperiorly to the fistula may be advanced to cover the diseased area to accomplish more reliable healing.[67] I generally leave both a suprapubic tube and a urethral Foley catheter to drain the bladder.

When the vesicovaginal fistula incorporates the ureter or ureteric orifice or is associated with a ureterovaginal fistula, transabdominal repair is necessary. The ureter is reimplanted simultaneously with repair of the vesicovaginal fistula. If unilateral tension-free antireflux reimplantation is not possible, a unilateral vesicopsoas hitch is used to allow tension-free ureteroneocystostomy. The ipsilateral bladder flap is sutured to the psoas. The contralateral bladder wall is mobilized. The posterior bladder wall is then approximated, and the bladder is closed after placement of a suprapubic Malecot catheter. In patients with vesicovaginal fistula associated with bilateral ureteric involvement, either one side is reimplanted as described above, whereas the other ureter is managed by a transureteroureterostomy, or alternatively both ureters are reimplanted together into the same bladder flap. I believe that standard bilateral reimplantation in patients with extensive vesicoureterovaginal fistula puts excessive tension on the bladder repair and should be avoided.[23,34]

Postoperative Care

Adequate postoperative care is essential for successful repair of vesicovaginal fistulas. Any increase in intravesical pressure during the healing process must be avoided. Catheter care must ensure unimpeded drainage by avoidance of kinking and catheter occlusion from hematuria, mucus, or urinary sediment. Generous fluid intake is ensured (initially by intravenous fluids and later orally). Urinary output is monitored. The Foley catheter is removed about 3 to 5 days postoperatively, whereas bladder drainage by the suprapubic tube is maintained for a minimum of 2 weeks in simple fistula repair and up to 6 weeks in complicated repairs.

Antimicrobial therapy is used for the first 5 days. It is then stopped until the time of removal of the suprapubic tube. Urine cultures are performed 3 days before removal of the suprapubic tube, and the appropriate antibiotic (guided by results of culture and sensitivity) is started before removal of the catheter and is maintained for 3 days.

Occasionally, after removal of the ureteric stents, the patient may experience fever or flank pain. An excretory urogram or radioisotope renal scan is performed to rule out ureteric obstruction. Antibacterial treatment is also started after urine is collected for culture and sensitivity. If ureteric obstruction is present, which is rare, percutaneous nephrostomy is performed without further manipulation. Two to three weeks later, one ensures the absence of ureteric obstruction by performing a nephrostomogram before removing the percutaneous nephrostomy tube.

Urinary leakage in the postoperative period may be attributable to bladder spasms and should be managed by appropriate anticholinergics. Rectal suppositories of belladonna and opium are also helpful. Vaginal examination or manipulation should be avoided in the postoperative period to prevent additional trauma. Patients are instructed to avoid sexual intercourse for 12 weeks after the repair. If the patient has continued leakage during the convalescence, catheter drainage is instituted. If successful in eliminating leakage, it is maintained for 4 to 6 weeks.

MANAGEMENT OF RADIATION-INDUCED VESICOVAGINAL FISTULAS

In patients who have received preoperative radiation therapy and develop vesicovaginal fistula after radical surgery, the fistula may be repaired in standard fashion as described previously, provided that the tissues are well vascularized. The placement of intervening nonirradiated tissue between the bladder and vaginal closure is emphasized.

When the fistula occurs as a result of radiation necrosis, local tissues are most often unsuitable for repair. They almost never close spontaneously. The surrounding tissues are fibrotic and inelastic and have poor vascularity as a result of radiation-induced endarteritis. Successful repair requires increasing vascularity at the fistula site by mobilizing vascular pedicles. Several vascular pedicles were used for this purpose.* These include the gluteus maximus, adductor longus, gracilis, sartorius, rectus abdominis, pubococcygeus, bulbocavernosus muscle–labial fat pad, and gastric and omental flaps.

Before attempting repair, recurrent malignancy must be ruled out by biopsy. As stated previously, repair must be delayed in most patients long enough to allow demarcation and slough of necrotic tissue and stabilization. Most radiation-induced vesicovaginal fistulas that are suitable for primary repair and are not associated with ureteral or bowel involvement may be repaired vaginally. This has the advantage of obviating the need for bowel manipulation in a previously irradiated field if an abdominal approach is used. Currently, with a vaginal approach, the most frequently used tissues for interposition are the Martius flap and the gracilis muscle.[34,53] If it is necessary to use an abdominal approach, the omentum or omental and gastric flaps are the most suitable for interposition.[53,54,73]

Martius Flap Technique

The Martius flap is our preferred technique because of its simplicity and effectiveness.[34,53,74] A generous episiotomy at the 5 or 7 o'clock position may be necessary. This divides the pubococcygeus, transverse perineal, and a portion of the levator ani. Once adequate exposure has been obtained, the fistula is excised, and the bladder and vaginal walls are mobilized. The mobilization needs to be more generous than in nonirradiated fistulas to allow closure without tension. The bladder is closed with 3-0 polyglycolic acid sutures. After that, the skin of the medial aspect of the contralateral labium majus is incised vertically from the level of the mons pubis to the lower third of the labium. The skin edges are retracted and the bulbocavernosus muscle and its labial fat pad are exposed and dissected (Fig. 41-1, *A*). The combined fat pad and muscle are divided high at the level of the mons pubis to provide sufficient length to reach and cover the fistula without tension (Fig. 41-1, *B*). A tunnel is then formed under the skin between the labium majus and the fistula, through the lateral vaginal wall. The tunnel must be wide enough to prevent compression of the blood supply to the pedicle. The flap is passed through the tunnel and placed over the closed bladder defect. The flap is placed to completely cover the bladder closure and is anchored in place with 3-0 polyglycolic acid sutures (Fig. 41-1, *C*). The vaginal mucosa is then closed over the pedicle. If there is no adequate vaginal mucosa to close the defect, the graft will become completely epithelialized. Alternatively, the defect may be bridged with a myocutaneous flap.

The episiotomy is then closed with absorbable sutures after a small Penrose drain is placed. The labial incision is also closed with absorbable sutures after a small Penrose drain is placed. The drains are removed 48 hours postoperatively. The bladder is decompressed with a suprapubic tube as well as an indwelling urethral Foley catheter for 3 to 4 weeks. The patient is instructed to avoid sexual intercourse for 3 months.

*31,38,39,53,54,68-72.

Gracilis Muscle Flap Technique

Some authors advocate the use of gracilis muscle brought from one or both sides[75,76] for interposition between bladder and vaginal closures. The technique is similar to that described above except for the use of the gracilis muscle instead of a Martius flap An incision is made overlying the course of the gracilis muscle. The muscle flap is developed. The gracilis is divided at the medial femoral condyle and is dissected free in a cephalad direction. The blood supply is encountered about 8 to 10 cm from its origin and should not be disturbed. A tunnel is developed between the thigh and the fistula site. The distal end of the muscle flap is passed through the tunnel and anchored to the pubocervical fascia along the opposite margin of the defect with 3-0 polyglycolic acid sutures so that the muscle completely covers the bladder closure. Vaginal closure is performed as described above.

Combined Gastric and Omental Segments Technique

Through a long midline transperitoneal approach, the bladder is exposed. The bladder is opened in the midline, and the ureters are catheterized. The bladder incision is extended to the fistula. A generous excision of the fistula is performed to remove not only apparent nonvascularized or necrotic tissue but also all fibrotic tissue. If the vagina is greatly scarred, it may be impossible to close without tension. In this case the gap may be bridged with the omental segment.[54] The stomach, omentum, and gastroepiploic vessels are inspected. It is crucial to ensure adequate blood supply to the segments by routine testing of the patency of the left and right gastroepiploic vessels before selecting the side to be used as a pedicle for the gastric and omental segments.[77] The gastric segment is outlined on the anterior and posterior walls with the base at the greater curvature. The segment is separated from the stomach, and the stomach continuity is reestablished. The omental flap is also isolated. The gastroepiploic vessels are mobilized off the stomach to create an adequate pedicle. The combined stomach and omentum segments are based on the same pedicle and are brought down to the site of the fistula. The omental patch is used either to bridge the vaginal defect or as an interposition between the vaginal closure posteriorly and the gastrocystoplasty anteriorly. The gastric segment is sutured to the bladder and replaces the posterior bladder wall. The anterior bladder wall is approximated. The bladder is drained with a suprapubic tube and an indwelling urethral catheter for 3 to 4 weeks. Indwelling ureteric catheters are optional.

Results of Repair of Radiation-Induced Vesicovaginal Fistulas

Although the cure of radiation-induced vesicovaginal fistula is not so good as in nonirradiated cases, 33% to 50% percent of women with radiation-induced vesicovaginal fistula could be cured. These results can be improved by careful selection. In our

A

B

C

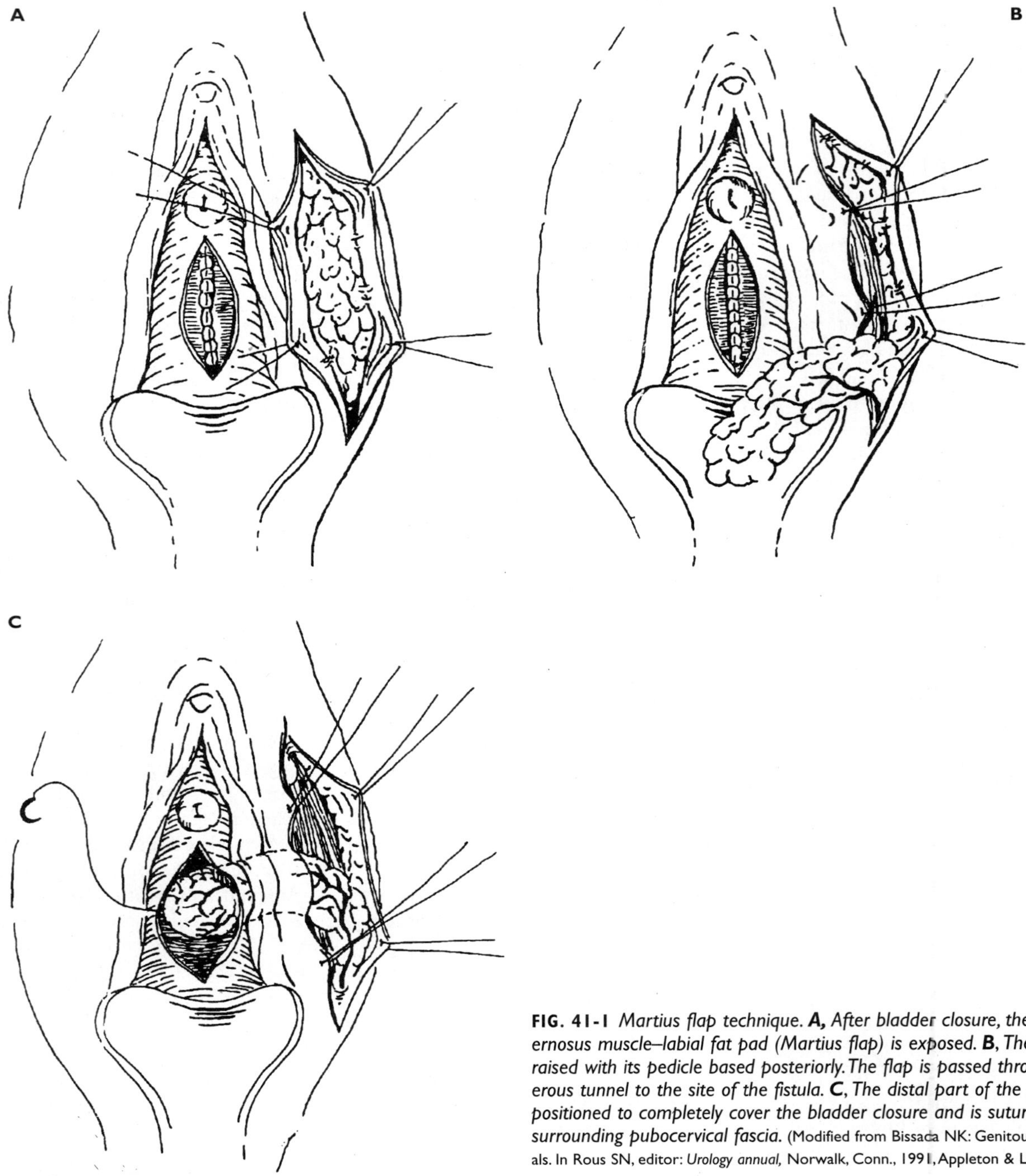

FIG. 41-1 *Martius flap technique.* ***A,*** *After bladder closure, the bulbocavernosus muscle–labial fat pad (Martius flap) is exposed.* ***B,*** *The flap is raised with its pedicle based posteriorly. The flap is passed through a generous tunnel to the site of the fistula.* ***C,*** *The distal part of the flap is positioned to completely cover the bladder closure and is sutured to the surrounding pubocervical fascia.* (Modified from Bissada NK: Genitourinary fistulas. In Rous SN, editor: *Urology annual,* Norwalk, Conn., 1991, Appleton & Lang.)

experience successful closure was eventually accomplished in 9 of 10 patients managed by primary repair, 8 of whom were managed successfully with 1 attempt.

URINARY DIVERSION

Some patients with radiation fistulas are not suitable for primary repair but could be managed by urinary diversion. The risk of using irradiated lower ureter and bowel for diversion must be considered in these patients. I prefer a transverse colon conduit as the most suitable for conduit diversion.[78] For continent urinary diversion I have utilized the Charleston pouch initially in these patients.[79] However, currently we recommend a nonradiated gastrocolic pouch when continent diversion is performed in patients with radiation-induced vesicovaginal fistulas.[80]

Some patients will be unsuitable for any surgical management. These must be managed with supportive nonoperative palliative measures. Our experience in managing 30 patients with radiation-induced vesicovaginal fistulas indicates that these patients represent a heterogeneous group and that careful assessment, proper selection, timing, and choice of appropriate surgical procedures are crucial. However, with adherence to these guidelines, most of these patients can be managed satisfactorily.[53]

Management of Isolated Urethrovaginal or Bladder Neck Fistulas

Continence in females mainly depends on the bladder neck and uppermost portion of the urethra.[81,82] In fact, in patients with distal urethral diverticulum, an intentional urethrovaginal fistula has been created without producing incontinence, provided that the bladder neck mechanism is intact.[83] However, since a considerable proportion of urethrovaginal fistulas result from operations that were primarily designed to improve urinary incontinence, it is important that reconstructive surgery be directed not only toward the closure of the fistula and reapproximation of the urethral defect but also to incorporation of appropriate procedures to ensure continence.

Limited Bladder Neck or Proximal Urethral Fistulas

Although the repair is more difficult in limited bladder neck or proximal urethral fistulas because of the limited mobility of the bladder neck and the proximal portion of the urethra that is often accentuated by the scarring and fibrosis resulting from previous surgical manipulation, I prefer a vaginal approach for limited (small) bladder neck or proximal urethral fistulas without ureteric involvement. The technique is similar to that described for vaginal repair of vesicovaginal fistulas with some modification.

A longitudinal vaginal incision starts a few centimeters proximal to the fistula, circumscribes the fistula, and then extends distally to near the urethral meatus. The lateral vaginal flaps are mobilized. The bladder neck defect is then closed longitudinally with 3-0 polyglycolic acid sutures. The endopelvic fascia is reapproximated. The reapproximation of the endopelvic fascia should extend superiorly for 2 cm to allow adequate plication. If it is believed that a bladder neck suspension or a pubovaginal sling procedure is indicated, it is performed at this time before vaginal closure. If tissue vascularity is not optimal, the interposition of a bulbocavernosus fibrofatty pad, as described before, is performed.

Extensive Urethrovaginal Fistulas

In more extensive urethrovaginal fistulas with loss of urethral floor, the bladder neck may be involved. If sufficient urethral roof is available, one may assume that sufficient contractile properties are retained to allow creation of a small-caliber urethra.[32] An incision begins 1 to 2 cm proximally to the fistula at the midline and bifurcates distally along the junction of the residual urethral roof and the vaginal mucosa to the site of the proposed external urethral meatus. Mobilization of the residual urethra should be limited to avoid additional injury. Only adequate mobilization to allow tension-free closure is required. Lateral vaginal mucosal flaps are mobilized, and the urethral floor is closed. Adjacent supporting tissues are plicated, and the vaginal mucosal margins are closed. The interposition of a bulbocavernosus fibrofatty pad, as described before, may be advantageous especially when there is question about vascularity. If a tension-free closure of the vaginal mucosa is in doubt, a labial skin flap, or a perineal flap may be used.[32,84,85]

Management of Giant Vesicovaginal and Vesicourethrovaginal Fistulas

Giant fistulas are defined as those with a diameter greater than 5 cm.[61] These are best repaired transperitoneally as described before. In our experience, if the fistula is confined to the bladder with or without ureteric involvement and there is adequate remaining bladder tissue, the success rate has been excellent irrespective of the size of the fistula.[62] When the bladder capacity is greatly reduced but the bladder neck and urethra are intact, there are two alternatives: either to proceed with standard fistula repair as outlined above and then use detubularized bowel to increase the bladder capacity (vascularized intestinocystoplasty),[86-92] or to use a vascularized patch of bowel (usually ileum or stomach in irradiated cases) to replace the posterior bladder wall.[93] Both of these alternatives have been satisfactory in our experience.

Giant vesicourethrovaginal fistulas with extensive urethral, bladder neck, and trigonal damage are among the most difficult urologic situations to manage.[1,19,94,95] Even in expert hands and with multiple operations, reported success rates varied from minimal to about 50%.[1,57,94] Most failures were eventually managed with urinary diversion. Fortunately these fistulas are seldom of gynecologic cause and only represent a minority of obstetric fistulas.[57,61]

Although giant vesicourethrovaginal fistulas may be closed readily with a combined abdominal and vaginal approach, most patients have remained incontinent after closure because of sphincteric inadequacy. A vaginal wall flap to replace a damaged urethra has been unsatisfactory in our experience. Others agree that this procedure alone is unsatisfactory. Blaivas performed a simultaneous vaginal flap urethral reconstruction and an antiincontinence procedure in 10 patients.[96] Although several patients subsequently required additional procedures, satisfactory results were eventually obtained in nine patients. In our experience, urethra-lengthening procedures using vaginal mucosa as well as vesicourethropexy have also been unsatisfactory in this situation. The incorporation of a Tanagho anterior bladder tube[97,98] in the management of patients with giant vesicourethrovaginal fistula has been satisfactory in our experience.[61-63] An overall continence rate of 75% was achieved. Patients who had no prior suprapubic procedures seem to benefit more from this procedure; 83% of them were continent. It must be realized, however, that despite of attainment of continence in the majority of patients most of those with giant obstetric fistulas and extensive urethral damage did not regain normal voiding and many required intermittent catheterization. The voiding dysfunction in these patients seems similar to that encountered after extirpative pelvic visceral surgery,[99-102] and indicates that the extensive vesicourethral tissue loss that is a prerequisite for the occurrence of giant vesicourethrovaginal fistula in these patients is associated with variable degrees of denervation.[62]

Technique of Simultaneous Neourethral Reconstruction and Closure of Fistula

A midline suprapubic incision is made, and the retropubic space is developed by dissection just posterior to the periosteum. The vesicourethral junction is identified, and an anterior bladder flap (3 cm long and 2.5 cm wide) is outlined by four stay sutures. The flap is raised to expose the fistula. The ureters are catheterized with 5 or 8 Fr feeding tubes. The fistula is excised, and the bladder is separated completely from the urethra and slightly mobilized upwards. The vagina is then repaired with a continuous suture of 2-0 polyglycolic acid. A pedicle graft of omentum is then brought down to completely cover the vaginal closure and is anchored in position. The bladder flap then is rolled into a tube around a 12 Fr catheter, with the two edges brought together with 4-0 polyglycolic acid interrupted sutures. The 12 Fr catheter is then replaced by a 8 or 10 Fr Foley catheter passed through the meatus, then through the neourethra into the bladder. The catheter is secured by a no. 1 nylon suture, which is passed through the dome of the bladder and brought out suprapubically. The two ureteral catheters and a Malecot catheter are brought out through the dome of the bladder. The apex of the trigone is sutured to the base of the flap, and the bladder closure is completed on either side. The distal end of the neourethra is sutured to the remaining urethra or to the vaginal introitus if the urethra is destroyed completely. The new bladder neck is suspended by two sutures of no. 1 polyglycolic acid between the anterior bladder wall close to the base of the tube and the rectus sheath. A Penrose drain is placed, and the wound is closed. The two ureteric catheters are removed 10 days postoperatively. The urethral stent is left for 4 weeks, and the suprapubic tube is removed a few days later.

In patients with greatly reduced bladder capacity but with healthy anterior bladder wall judged to be adequate for neourethral construction, the procedure may be combined with augmentation intestinocystoplasty as outlined above. Likewise, patients who have had the procedure but remain with quite small bladder capacity, resulting in intractable frequency and incontinence, will benefit from augmentation cystoplasty. These patients usually require intermittent catheterization to empty their bladder.

References

1. Mahfouz N: Urinary fistulae in women, *Br J Obstet Gynaecol* 64:23, 1957.
2. Derry DE: Note on five pelves of women of the eleventh dynasty in Egypt, *Br J Obstet Gynaecol* 42:490, 1935.
3. Englebach R, Derry DE: Mummification, *Ann Service Antiquité de l'Egypte* 41:233, 1942.
4. Zacharin RF: *Obstetric fistula,* New York, 1988, Springer-Verlag.
5. Miller NF: Treatment of vesicovaginal fistulas, *Am J Obstet Gynecol* 30:675, 1935.
6. Sims JM: On the treatment of vesico-vaginal fistula, *Am J Med Sci* 23:59, 1852.
7. Bozeman N:. Vesico-vaginal fistules: comparative analysis of different surgical methods: results, American and European, *Am J Med Sci* 60:100, 1870.
8. Emmett TA: A memoir of Dr. James Marion Sims, *NY Med J* 39:1, 1884.
9. Martius H: Die operative Wiederherstellung der vollkommen fehlenden Harnröhre und des Schliessmuskels derselben, *Zentralbl Gynäkol* 52:480, 1928.
10. Garlock JH: The cure of an intractable vesicovaginal fistula by the use of a pedicled muscle flap, *Surg Gynecol Obstet* 47:255, 1928.
11. Mahfouz N: Urinary and rectovaginal fistulae in women, *Br J Obstet Gynaecol* 36:581, 1929.
12. Mahfouz N: Urinary fistulae in women, *Br J Obstet Gynaecol* 37:566, 1930.
13. Moir JC: J. Marion Sims and the vesico-vaginal fistula: then and now, *Br Med J* 2:773, 1940.
14. Moir JC: Vesicovaginal fistulae: review of 100 consecutive cases, *Lancet* 1:57, 1954.
15. Moir JC: Vesicovaginal fistula: thoughts on the treatment of 350 cases, *Proc R Soc Med* 59:1019, 1966.
16. Lawson JB: Birth canal injuries, *Proc R Soc Med* 61:368, 1968.
17. Lawson J: The management of genito-urinary fistulae, *Clin Obstet Gynecol* 5:209, 1978.
18. Lawson J: Vesical fistulae into the vaginal vault, *Br J Urol* 44:623, 1972.
19. Hamlin RHJ, Nicholson EC: Reconstruction of urethra totally destroyed in labor, *Br Med J* 2:147, 1969.
20. Judd ES: The operative treatment of vesicovaginal fistulae, *Surg Gynecol Obstet* 30:447, 1920.
21. Massee JS, Welch JS, Pratt JH, et al: Management of urinary vaginal fistula: 10 year survey, *JAMA* 190:902, 1964.
22. Hedlund H, Lindstedt E: Urovaginal fistulas: 20 years of experience with 45 cases, *J Urol* 137:926, 1987.
23. Bissada NK, McDonald DJ, Raham FR, et al: Acquired obstetric and gynecologic urinary fistulas, *King Faisal Spec Hosp Med J* 4:223, 1984.
24. Russell CS: *Vesico-vaginal fistulas and related matters,* Springfield, Ill., 1962, Charles C Thomas.
25. Keettek WC: Vesicovaginal and urethrovaginal fistula revisited, *Obstet Gynecol* 72:307, 1988.
26. Elkins TE, Drescher C, Martey JO, et al: Vesicovaginal fistula revisited, *Obstet Gynecol* 72:307, 1988.
27. Fu SG, Shen QE: Operative treatment of female urinary fistulas: report of 405 cases, *Chin Med J* 92:263, 1979.
28. Symmonds RE: Incontinence: vesical and urethral fistulas, *Clin Obstet Gynecol* 27:499, 1984.
29. Vanderputte SR: Obstetric vesicovaginal fistulas: experience with 89 cases, *Ann Soc Belg Med Trop* 65:303, 1985.
30. Arrowsmith SD: Genitourinary obstruction in obstetric fistulas, *J Urol* 152:403-406, 1994.
31. Lee RA, Symmonds RE, Williams TJ: Current status of genitourinary fistulas, *Obstet Gynecol* 72:313, 1988.
32. Podratze KC, Symmonds RE, Hagen JV: Vesicovaginal fistulae, *Bail Clin Obstet Gynecol* 1:414, 1987.
33. Blandy JP, Badenoch DF, Fowler CG, et al: Early repair of iatrogenic injury to the ureter or bladder after gynecological surgery, *J Urol* 146:761-765, 1991.
34. Bissada NK: Genitourinary fistulas. In Rous SN, editor: *Urology annual,* vol 5, Norwalk, Conn., 1991, Appleton & Lang, pp. 115.
35. Buchsbaum HJ, Schmidt JD, editors: *Gynecologic and obstetric urology,* Philadelphia, 1978, Saunders.
36. Villasanta V: Complications of radiotherapy for carcinoma of the uterine cervix, *Am J Obstet Gynecol* 114:717, 1972.
37. Cushing RM, Tovell HM, Leigner LM: Major urologic complications following radium and x-ray therapy for carcinoma of the cervix, *Am J Obstet Gynecol* 101:750, 1968.
38. Boronow RC: Repair of the radiation-induced vaginal fistula utilizing the Martius technique, *World J Surg* 10:237, 1986.
39. McCall ML, Bolten KA: *Martius' gynecological operations,* Boston, 1956, Little, Brown, p. 327.
40. O'Quinn AG, Fletcher GH, Wharton JT: Guidelines for conservative hysterectomy after irradiation, *Gynecol Oncol* 9:68, 1980.

41. Kottmeier HL: Complications following radiation therapy in carcinoma of the cervix and their treatment, *Am J Obstet Gynecol* 88:854, 1964.
42. Boronow RC: Urologic complications secondary to radiation alone or radiation and surgery. In Delgado G, Smith JP, editors: *Management of complications in gynecologic oncology,* New York, 1982, John Wiley & Sons.
43. Lagundoye SB, Bell D, Gill G, et al: Urinary tract changes in obstetric vesicovaginal fistulae: a report of 216 cases studied by intravenous urography, *Clin Radiol* 27:531, 1976.
44. Goodwin WE, Scardino PT: Vesicovaginal and ureterovaginal fistulas: a summary of 25 years of experience, *J Urol* 123:370, 1980.
45. Persky L, Herman G, Guerrier K: Non-delay in vesicovaginal fistula repair, *Urology* 13 273, 1979.
46. Collins CG, Collins JH, Harrison BR, et al: Early repair of vesicovaginal fistula, *Am J Obstet Gynecol* 111:524, 1971.
47. Collins CG, Pent D, Jones FB: Results of early repair of vesicovaginal fistula with preliminary cortisone treatment, *Am J Obstet Gynecol* 80:1005, 1960.
48. O'Conor VJ Jr: Review of experience with vesicovaginal fistula repair, *J Urol* 123:367, 1980.
49. Alonso Gorrea M, Fernandez Zuaza J, Mompo Sanchis JF, et al: Spontaneous healing of ureterovesicovaginal fistulas, *Eur Urol* 11:341, 1985.
50. O'Conor VJ: Non-surgical closure of vesicovaginal fistula, *TransAmer Assoc Genito-urinary Surg* 31:255, 1938.
51. Molina LR, Lynne CM, Politano VA: Treatment of vesicouterine fistula by fulguration, *J Urol* 141:1422-1423, 1989.
52. Stovsky MD, Ignatoff JM, Blum MD, et al: Use of electrocoagulation in the treatment of vesicovaginal fistulas, *J Urol* 152:1443-1444, 1994.
53. Bissada NK: Management of radiation-induced vesicovaginal fistula. In Jewett MAS, editor: *Urologic complications of pelvic surgery and radiotherapy,* Pittsburgh, Penn., 19xx, Medical Media.
54. Bissada SA, Bissada NK: Repair of active radiation-induced vesicovaginal fistula using combined gastric and omental segments based on the gastroepiploic vessels, *J Urol* 147:1368, 1992.
55. Redman JF, Baker JJ: Favorable experience with an intravaginal urinary collection device, *Obstet Gynecol* 42:912, 1973.
56. Leiter E, Brendler H: An intravaginal urinary collecting device, *J Urol* 98:410, 1967.
57. Zimmern PE, Hadley HR, Staskin DR, et al: Genitourinary fistulae: vaginal approach for repair of vesicovaginal fistulae, *Urol Clin North Am* 12:361, 1985.
58. Hadley HR, Zimmern PE, Raz S: Transvaginal repair of vesicovaginal fistula, *Proc Western Section Am Urol Assoc,* Reno, Nevada, 1984, Abstract 102.
59. Leach GE, Raz S: Vaginal flap technique: a method of transvaginal vesicovaginal fistula repair. In Raz S, editor: *Female urology,* Philadelphia, 1983, Saunders.
60. Raz S: Modified bladder neck suspension for female stress incontinence, *Urology* 17:82, 1981.
61. Bissada NK, McDonald D: Management of giant vesicovaginal and vesicourethrovaginal fistulas, *J Urol* 130:1073, 1983.
62. Bissada NK, Morcos RR: Voiding patterns and urinary control after repair of giant vesicovaginal and vesicourethrovaginal fistulas and neourethral construction, *Neurourol Urodyn* 5:321, 1986.
63. Bissada NK: Current management of complex urinary fistulae in women, *Proc Intern Soc Urol,* 21st congress, Buenos Aires, Argentina, 1988, abstract no. 319.
64. Baines REM, Orford HJL, Theron JLL: The repair of vesicovaginal fistulae by means of omental slings and grafts, *S Afr Med J* 50:959, 1976.
65. Turner-Warwick R: Urinary fistulae in the female. In Walsh PC, Gittes RF, Perlmutter AD, Stamey TA, editors: *Campbell's urology,* vol 3, ed 5, Philadelphia, 1986, Saunders.
66. Turner-Warwick R: The use of omental pedicle graft in urinary tract reconstruction, *J Urol* 116:341, 1976.
67. Gil-Vernet JM, Gil-Vernet A, Campos JA: New surgical approach for treatment of complex vesicovaginal fistula, *J Urol* 141:513-545, 1989.
68. Boronow RC, Rutledge F: Vesicovaginal fistula, radiation and gynecologic cancer, *Am J Obstet Gynecol* 111:85, 1971.
69. Bastiaanse NA, Van B: Bastiaanse's method for surgical closure of very large irradiation fistula of the bladder and rectum. In Youssef AF, editor: *Gynecological urology,* Springfield, Ill., 1960, Charles C. Thomas.
70. Graham JB: Vaginal fistulas following radiotherapy, *Surg Gynecol Obstet* 120 1019, 1965.
71. Byron RL, Ostergard DR: Sartorius muscle interposition for the treatment of the radiation-induced vaginal fistula, *Am J Obstet Gynecol* 104:104, 1969.
72. Stirnemann H: Treatment of recurrent recto-vaginal fistula by interposition of a glutaeus maximus muscle flap, *Am J Proctol* 20:52, 1969.
73. Kiricuta I, Goldstein AMB: The repair of extensive vesicovaginal fistulas with pedicled omentum: a review of 27 cases, *J Urol* 108:724, 1972.
74. Hoskins WJ, Park RC, Long R, et al: Repair of urinary fistulas with bulbocavernosus myocutaneous flaps, *Obstet Gynecol* 63:588, 1984.
75. Obrink A, Bunne G: Gracilis interposition in fistulas following radiotherapy for cervical cancer: a retrospective study, *Urol Int* 33:370, 1978.
76. Patil U, Waterhouse K, Laungani G: Management of 18 difficult vesicovaginal and urethrovaginal fistulas with modified Ingleman-Sundberg and Martius operations, *J Urol* 123:653, 1980.
77. Bissada SA, Bissada NK: Choice of gastroepiploic vessels for gastrocystoplasty, *J Urol* 148:101, 1992.
78. Bissada NK: The current status of supravesical urinary diversion and bladder substitution. In Rous SN, editor: *Urology annual,* New York, 1993, Norton, pp. 69-99.
79. Bissada NK: New continent ileocolonic urinary reservoir: Charleston Pouch with minimally altered in-situ appendix stoma, *Urology* 41:524-526, 1993.
80. Kaczmarek T, Bissada NK: New continent urinary reservoir with gastric tube outlet: experimental and clinical experience, *J Urol* 153:242A, 1995.
81. DeLancey JOL: Structural aspects of urethrovesical function in the female, *Neurourol Urodyn* 7:509, 1988.
82. Gosling JA: The structure of the female lower urinary tract and pelvic floor, *Urol Clin North Am* 12:207, 1985.
83. Spence HM, Duckett JW Jr: Diverticulum of the female urethra: clinical aspects and presentation of a simple operative technique for cure, *J Urol* 104:432, 1970.
84. Hendren WH: Construction of female urethra from vaginal wall and a perineal flap, *J Urol* 123:657, 1980.
85. Wang Y, Hadley HR: The use of rotated vascularized pedicle flaps for complex transvaginal procedures, *J Urol* 149:590-592, 1993.
86. Goodwin WE, Winter CC: Technique of sigmoidocystoplasty, *Surg Gynecol Obstet* 108:370, 1959.
87. Goodwin WE, Turner RD, Winter CC: Results of ileocystoplasty, *J Urol* 80:461, 1958.
88. Gittes RF: Bladder augmentation procedures. In Libertino J, editor: *Reconstructive urologic surgery: pediatric and adult,* Philadelphia, 1976, Saunders.
89. Thuroff JW, Alken O, Engelmann U, et al: The Mainz pouch (mixed augmentation ileum and zecum) for bladder augmentation and continent urinary diversion, *Eur Urol* 11:152, 1985.
90. Thuroff JW, Alken P, Riedmiller H, et al: 100 cases of Mainz pouch: continuing experience and evolution, *J Urol* 140:283, 1988.
91. Seddon JM, Best L, Bruce AW: Intestinocystoplasty in treatment of interstitial cystitis, *Urology* 10:431, 1977.

92. Goldwasser B, Webster GD: Augmentation and substitution enterocystoplasty, *J Urol* 135:215, 1986.
93. Podratz KC, Angerman NS, Symmonds RE: Complications of ureteral surgery in the non-radiated patient. In Delgado G, Smith JP, editors: *Management of complications in gynecologic oncology,* New York, 1982, Wiley.
94. Benchekroun A, Lakrissa A, Tazi A, et al: Vesicovaginal fistulae (450 cases), *Proc Intern Soc Urol,* San Francisco, Calif., 1982, abstract no. 427.
95. Khanna S: Posterior bladder flap plasty for repair of vesicourethrovaginal fistula, *J Urol* 147:656-657, 1992.
96. Blaivas JG: Vaginal flap urethral reconstruction: an alternative to the bladder flap neourethra, *J Urol* 141:542-545, 1989.
97. Tanagho EA, Smith DR, Meyers FH, et al: Mechanism of urinary continence. II. Technique for surgical correction of incontinence, *J Urol* 101:305, 1969.
98. Tanagho EA: Bladder neck reconstruction for total urinary incontinence: ten years of experience, *J Urol* 125:321, 1981.
99. McGuire EJ: Urodynamic evaluation after abdominal-perineal resection and lumbar intervertebral disk herniation, *Urology* 6:63, 1975.
100. Blaivas JG, Barbalias GA: Characteristics of neural injury after abdominoperineal resection, *J Urol* 129:84, 1983.
101. Seski JC, Diokno AC: Bladder dysfunction after radical abdominal hysterectomy, *Am J Obstet Gynecol* 128:643, 1977.
102. Yalla SV, Andriole GL: Vesicourethral dysfunction following pelvic visceral ablative surgery, *J Urol* 132:503, 1984.

Chapter 42 Pelvic Prolapse and Lower Urinary Tract Dysfunction in Females

Mickey M. Karram, John R. Miklos, Eddie H.M. Sze

Urinary incontinence in women is often associated with a wide range of loss of support of the urethra, bladder, and other pelvic organs. Usually patients who have both urinary incontinence and loss of support of other pelvic organs are very concerned about long-term treatment decisions involving both problems. The role of the physician initially is to help the patient understand the interaction of genitourinary prolapse with incontinence and to help the patient make a decision about the long-term management.

The cause of genitourinary prolapse is a failure of the fibromuscular support system to confine the pelvic organs within the pelvic cavity. This loss of support often results in visceral prolapses, voiding difficulties, and sexual dysfunction in females. The anatomic proximity of the internal female genital organs to the lower urinary tract makes it easy to understand how pelvic organ prolapse can affect bladder and urethral function.

Anatomic variations among patients in the genital tract can have a profound effect on the urinary tract system. A common example of this would be the patient who had a large cystourethrocele and, after surgical correction of the cystourethrocele, experienced the development or unmasking of underlying stress incontinence. It has been long appreciated that both urinary incontinence and voiding difficulty may be attributable to causes other than defective anatomic support. Thus the link between anatomic support and bladder function is very important but certainly not absolute, but it makes the evaluation and management of these patients often complex.

Although in the past decade we have witnessed advances in both the understanding and treatment of prolapse coexisting with urinary tract dysfunction, surprisingly up to now there has still been a lack of prospective data on the relationship between prolapse and lower urinary tract dysfunction.

Anatomy of Pelvic Support

The pelvic floor is composed primarily of muscular and fascial structures that lie at the bottom of the abdominal cavity and close the canal within the bony pelvis. In this position, it must act as a supportive layer that prevents the abdominal and pelvic organs from falling through the opening within the bony pelvis.[1] The pelvic floor has been described as having several layers of support.[2] However, it is the combination of connective tissue (that is, endopelvic fascia) and striated muscles (that is, pelvic diaphragm) that is responsible for the bulk of normal support.[3]

The uterus and upper part of the vagina are supported above the pelvic diaphragm to the pelvic wall by the upper portion (level I) of the endopelvic fascia. These structures are identified surgically as the cardinal and uterosacral ligaments. The midportion of the endopelvic fascia (level 2) attaches the vagina to the arcus tendineous fasciae pelvis and superior fascia of the levator ani muscles. Similarly, the posterior vaginal wall and endopelvic fasciae (rectovaginal fascia) form the restraining layer that prevents the rectum from protruding forward. In the distal part of the vagina (level III), the vaginal wall is directly attached to surrounding structures[4] (Fig. 42-1).

In a normally functioning pelvis the levator ani muscles are always contracting keeping the pelvic floor closed and allowing minimal tension on the endopelvic fascia.[5-7] The fascia simply suspends the organs in their position above the levator ani muscles. The interaction between pelvic floor muscles and fascia is critical to proper pelvic floor support and function. If the pelvic floor muscles are damaged or relaxed for a prolonged period of time, increases in intra-abdominal pressure and gravity can maximize tension and damage the endopelvic fascia. Endopelvic fascia defects in conjunction with a poorly functioning levator ani result in genital prolapse.

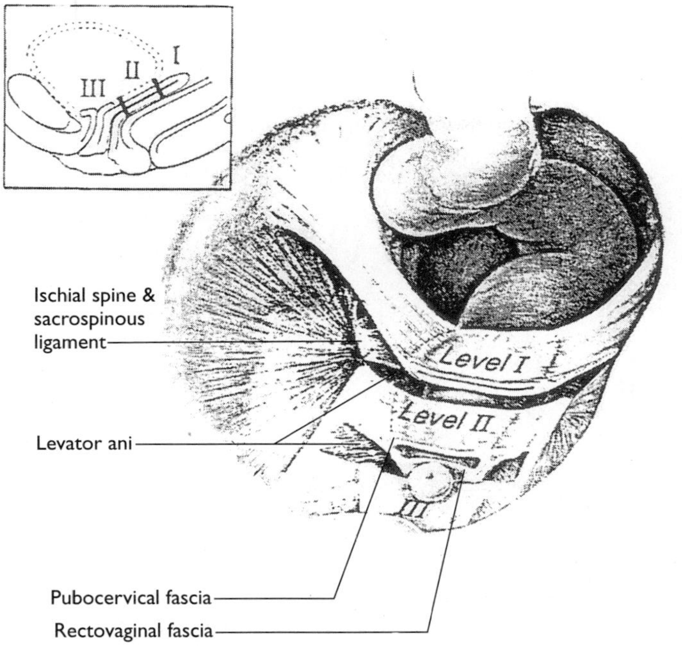

FIG. 42-1 *Levels of support of the upper and middle portions of the vagina. In level I (suspension), endopelvic fasciae suspend the vagina from lateral pelvic walls. Fibers of level I extend both vertically and posteriorly toward sacrum. In level II (attachment), the vagina is attached to arcus tendineus fasciae pelvis and superior fascia of levator ani muscles.* (From Delancey JO: *Am J Obstet Gynecol* 166:1717, 1992.)

Incidence of Pelvic Organ Prolapse

The true incidence of genital prolapse is unknown because milder degrees of prolapse may be asymptomatic and therefore unknown to the patient and ignored by the physician. The incidence also varies with parity, age, and race. Estimates indicate that 50% of parous women have some degree of genital prolapse but that only 10% to 20% of these cases are significant enough to cause symptoms. Prolapse is more common in whites and less common in Asians and African Americans. Unfortunately there are no good studies that have looked at the incidence of various types of prolapse and their correlation to lower urinary tract dysfunction. Likewise, the natural history of pelvic prolapse is unknown and has resulted in vague indications for operative intervention.

Etiology of Prolapse

For many years it was believed that stretching of the endopelvic fascia was the mechanism by which prolapse develops. This concept has never been supported by any data, and new observations indicate that prolapse develops because structures break away from each other. The supportive structures, which have already been mentioned, attach the vagina and uterus to the pelvic sidewalls. As long as the pelvic floor muscles are closing the pelvic floor, there is minimal stress on the fascia and ligaments. Damage to the levator ani muscles will, however, open the pelvic floor, and thus the ligaments and fascia will have to support the vagina and uterus without assistance of the pelvic musculature. Breaks in the fascia will allow the walls of these various organs to prolapse downwards.

Why certain women develop pelvic organ prolapse and others do not is not fully understood. Factors that have been shown to contribute to the development of these various conditions include damage that occurs at childbirth, deterioration with aging, and loss of levator strength because of either neural damage with chronic straining or metabolic disease that affects muscle function. Also women who have a long-term increase in abdominal pressure because of either chronic obstructive lung disease or work activities that require prolonged lifting or exertion will be at high risk. There is also a subgroup of patients who must have an inherent weakness in these muscles and ligaments even though they have no predisposing factors but will present at relatively early stages of life with advanced prolapse. The last subgroup of patients who are at high risk to develop prolapse are those who undergo reconstructive pelvic surgery resulting in alteration of the vaginal axis or failure to have reattached important structures that are detached at the time of surgery.[7] Examples of this would be failure to have reattached the cardinal uterosacral ligament complex to the vaginal apex at the time of vaginal hysterectomy. If this is not performed, the patient will certainly be at great risk for the development of enterocele and vaginal vault prolapse. Also patients who undergo anterior vaginal wall suspensions, such as a retropubic urethropexy, are at high risk for posterior vaginal wall defects in the form of enterocele and rectocele,[8] just as patients who undergo vaginal vault suspension operations such as sacrospinous ligament fixation or abdominal sacral colpopexy are at high risk for anterior vaginal wall defects.[9,10]

Types of Prolapse

Traditionally prolapse has been named according to the organ lying closest to the vagina that is prolapsed (Fig. 42-2). Prolapse of the anterior vaginal wall can occur in one of four areas. Loss of urethral support distal to the urethrovesical crease results in a urethrocele. This will manifest as flattening of the urethrovesical crease with descent of the lower anterior vaginal wall. Detachment of the pubocervical fascia from the arcus tendineous fasciae pelvis or the pelvic side wall results in a displacement cystocele or a paravaginal defect that can occur unilaterally or bilaterally. If this attachment breaks, the lateral crease falls below its normal line of attachment to the pelvic sidewall, which runs between the inferior edge of the pubic symphysis and the ischial spine. The detached vaginal sulcus descends downward, and such a descent causes the urethra and bladder to prolapse. Transverse defects that result from avulsion of the pubocervical fascia from its attachment to the cervix or vaginal cuff will cause the bladder base to dissect downward. Distension or midline cystocele results from a central defect in the pubocervical fascia. The vaginal epithelium over the prolapsed bladder appears thin and shiny with loss of rugae. These four defects may present in an isolated fashion or in combination with each other[11,12] (Fig. 42-3).

The cervix is normally situated in the upper third of the vagina. The location of the cervix in relation to the vagina is used to gauge the degree of uterine prolapse. Contrary to popular

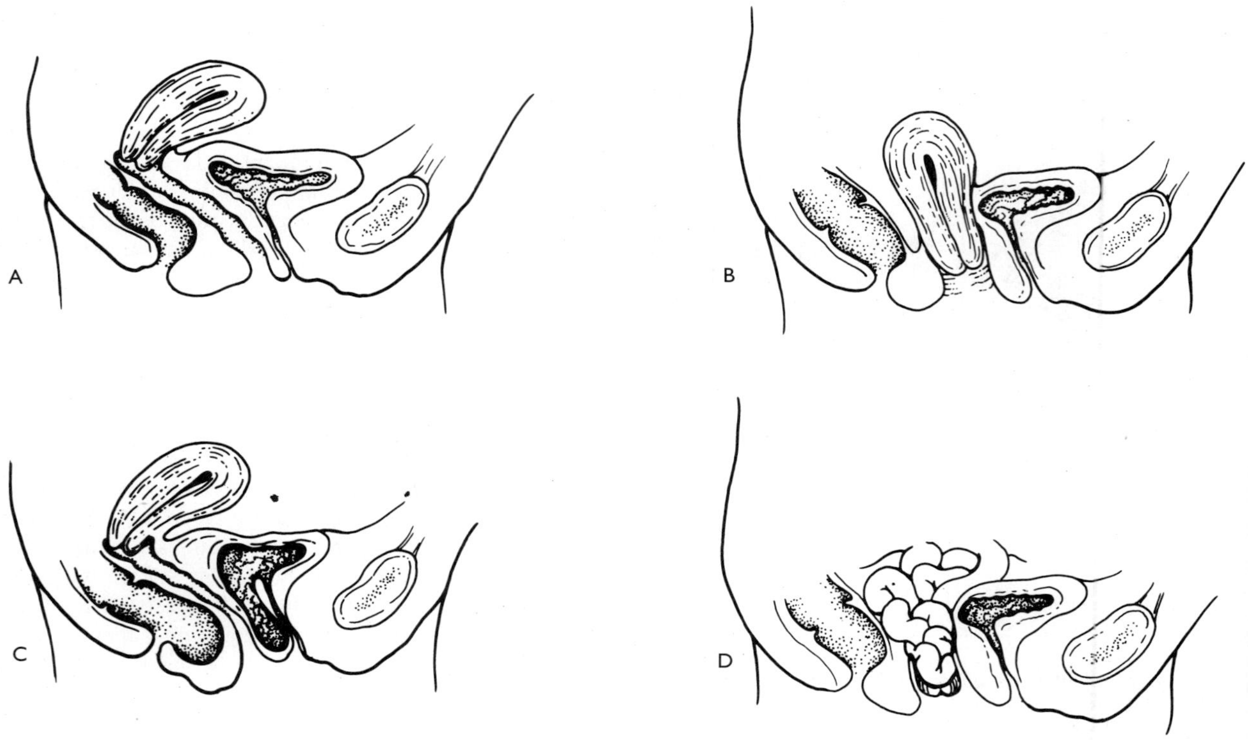

FIG. 42-2 *Types of prolapse.* ***A,*** *Pelvic organs with normal support.* ***B,*** *Uterine prolapse with good support of anterior and posterior vaginal walls.* ***C,*** *Cystocele and rectocele with good uterine support.* ***D,*** *Posthysterectomy vault prolapse with enterocele.*

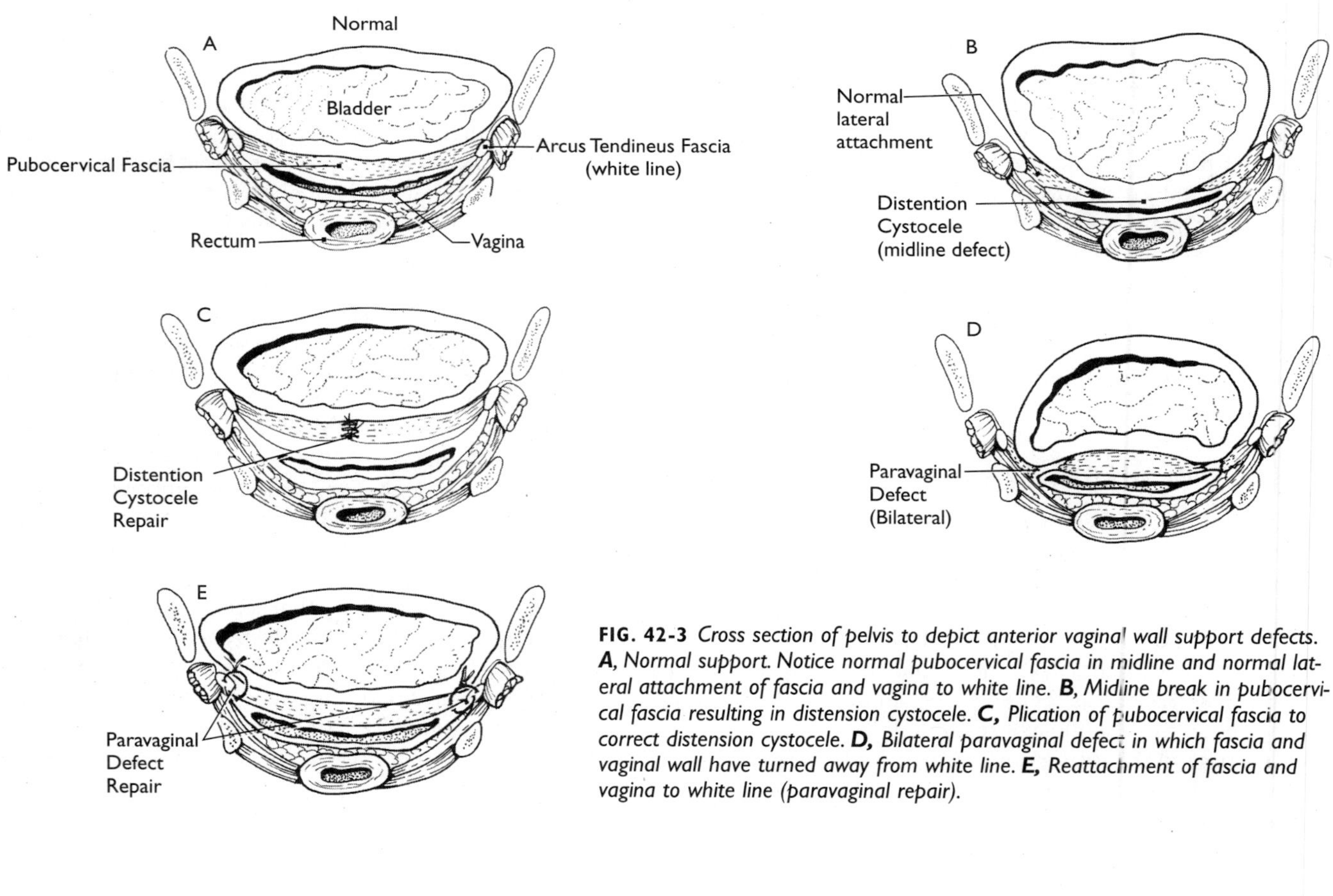

FIG. 42-3 *Cross section of pelvis to depict anterior vaginal wall support defects.* ***A,*** *Normal support. Notice normal pubocervical fascia in midline and normal lateral attachment of fascia and vagina to white line.* ***B,*** *Midline break in pubocervical fascia resulting in distension cystocele.* ***C,*** *Plication of pubocervical fascia to correct distension cystocele.* ***D,*** *Bilateral paravaginal defect in which fascia and vaginal wall have turned away from white line.* ***E,*** *Reattachment of fascia and vagina to white line (paravaginal repair).*

belief, uterine descensus is the result and not the cause of vaginal vault prolapse. The term "procidentia" is used to describe complete prolapse of the uterus outside of the body (Fig. 42-4).

Two distinctly different defects, that is, rectocele and enterocele, can occur in the posterior vaginal wall. A rectocele is caused by a defect in the rectovaginal fascia and manifests as a bulge in the posterior vaginal wall. In contrast, a pseudorectocele is caused by detachment of the perineal body resulting in the illusion of a bulge in the vaginal wall. The posterior cul-de-sac normally is located at or above the ischial spine. Enterocele is a herniation of the cul-de-sac peritoneum with or without intraperitoneal contents into the fascial layers between the vagina and the rectal walls. The size of the enterocele may range from a small bulge in the posterior fornix to a large posterior vaginal wall defect that protrudes beyond the introitus. There are four types of enterocele. A congenital enterocele occurs secondarily to incomplete fusion of the peritoneum between the anterior vaginal wall and the posterior rectal wall. Pulsion enterocele develops from chronic increases in intra-abdominal pressure, and traction enterocele is secondary to uterovaginal prolapse. Iatrogenic enterocele develops after surgical procedures that distort the normal horizontal vaginal axis toward the vertical, such as a retropubic urethropexy.

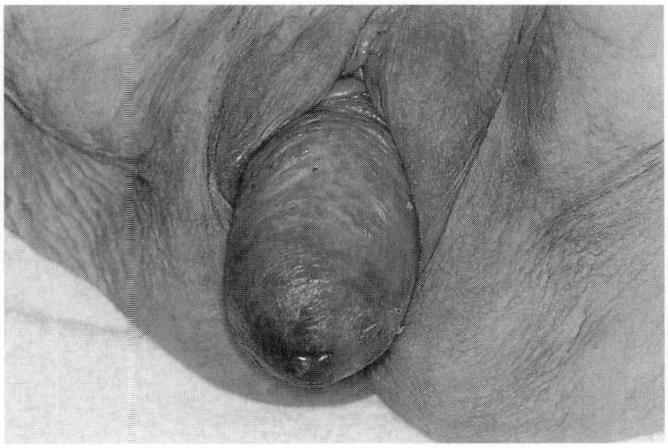

FIG. 42-4 *Complete uterine procidentia with complete inversion of anterior and posterior vaginal walls.*

Grading of Prolapse

One of the major deficiencies in the management of patients with pelvic organ prolapse is the lack of a simple, accurate, and uniformly accepted grading system to record aspects of pelvic support. The absence of such a system prevents longitudinal evaluation of patients and comparison of therapeutic outcomes from different institutions. Although several classification systems have been proposed, each has its own deficiencies and none has been universally accepted. In 1980 Beecham proposed a classification that divided rectocele, enterocele, uterine or vaginal cuff prolapse, and cystocele with or without urethrocele into three degrees.[13] The evaluation for prolapse was performed without straining or having traction applied to any structure. A first-degree prolapse describes a pelvic support defect that has descended just proximal to the vaginal introitus. When the protrusion is at or just beyond the vaginal introitus, the defect is classified as a second-degree prolapse, whereas a third-degree prolapse extends past the introitus. This system is simple to use; however, there are several deficiencies that limit its usefulness. These include failure to examine the patient under stress conditions that may cause one to fail to identify all pelvic support defects, and the grading system is imprecise and misleading in regard to the description of the extent of prolapse because it uses the nonspecific introitus as a reference point. Because of the numerous possible combinations of pelvic support defects, this system is extremely difficult if not impossible to use for population studies.

Baden and Walker introduced the halfway system classifying pelvic organ relaxation.[14] This system allows one to assess each of the six potentially defective sites (urethra, bladder, uterus or cuff, cul-de-sac, rectum, and perineum) in relation to the hymen while the patient is straining. Although the system corrects some of the deficiencies associated with the system proposed by Beecham, it is still relatively imprecise and difficult to use in population studies.

In 1994 the International Continence Society (ICS) drafted a document on the Standardization of Terminology of Female Organ Prolapse and Pelvic Floor Dysfunction. This quantitative system gives a precise description of an individual woman's pelvic support by the measurement of six precisely identified anatomic landmarks from the hymen. Since many variables of the examination techniques may influence findings in patients with pelvic organ relaxation, the ICS system also required investigators to specify the conditions and the instrument used during the examination. In addition, patients are also assigned a stage, according to the most severe portion of the prolapse, after the full extent of the protrusion has been demonstrated. Although various descriptions and definitions used in this system and its reproducibility have not been validated by any reliable studies, it addresses many of the deficiencies present in the previously proposed systems and is the most comprehensive system to describe female pelvic organ prolapse ever introduced.

Symptoms Associated with Prolapse

Patients who have descent of any portion of the vagina beyond the hymen will commonly complain of protrusion and pressure. The downward force that this pressure creates puts tension on the fascia and ligaments that normally support the vagina and may result in pain. This pain is usually characterized by the patient as occurring in the groin or in the lower back and is relieved when the prolapse is reduced or when she lies down. In addition, friction of the prolapse against clothing may cause ulceration of the vaginal mucosa as well as bleeding (Fig. 42-5).

Other more specific symptoms will depend on the type and severity of the prolapse. A woman with anterior vaginal wall relaxation to the middle or even lower portion of the vagina may very well be asymptomatic from her prolapse but may complain of stress incontinence if the urethrovesical junction is poorly supported. As the prolapse progresses and descends to or beyond the introitus, the patient's stress incontinence may improve or even disappear because of a kinking effect. It has been demonstrated that women with such severe cystoceles have preferential

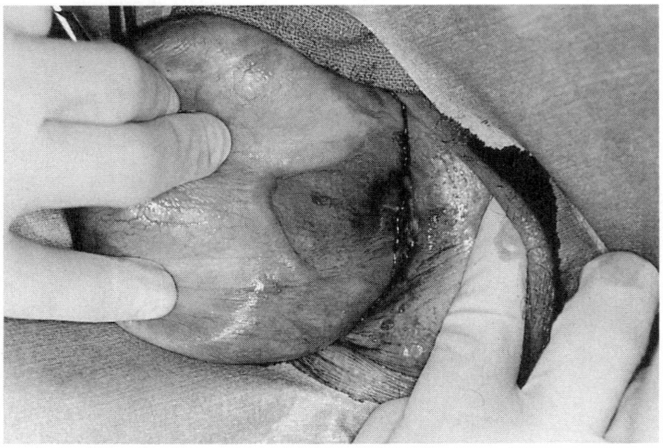

FIG. 42-5 *Large vaginal ulcer secondary to long-standing vaginal prolapse.*

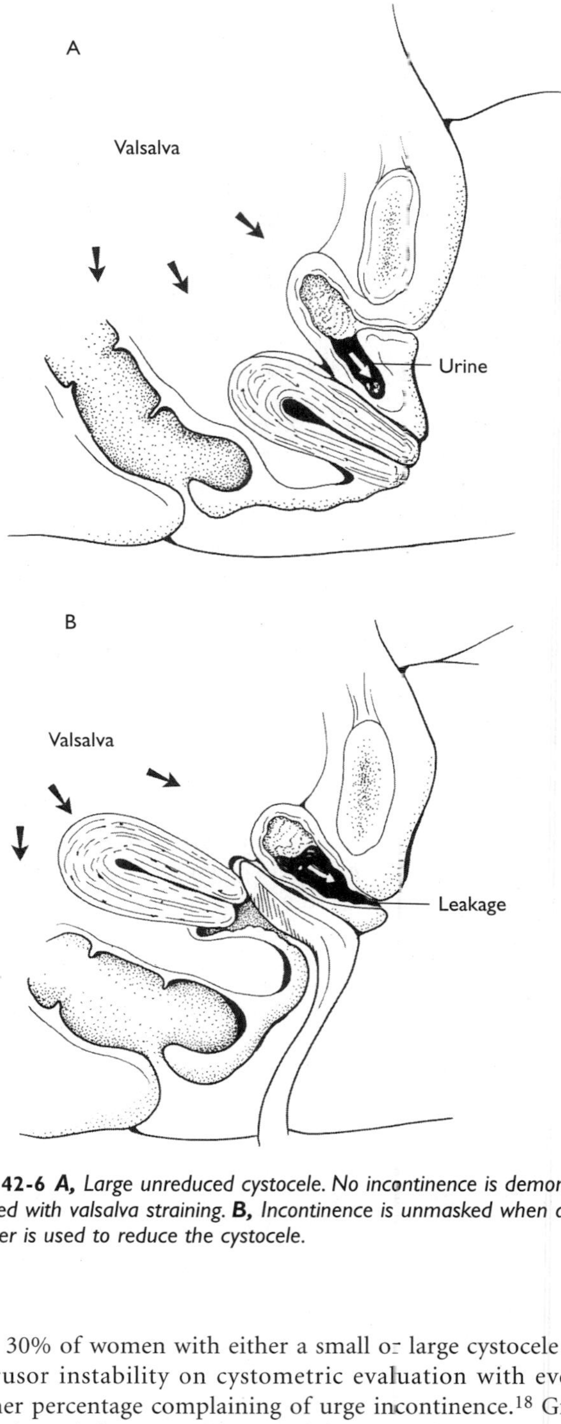

FIG. 42-6 ***A,*** *Large unreduced cystocele. No incontinence is demonstrated with valsalva straining.* ***B,*** *Incontinence is unmasked when a barrier is used to reduce the cystocele.*

transmission of rapid increases in abdominal pressure to the urethra compared to the bladder when the prolapse is protruding; in other words the anatomic distortion created by the prolapse is protective of any stress incontinence. However, when the prolapse is reduced and a barrier is used to limit descent of the bladder posterior and superior to the urethrovesical junction, urine loss may be observed in a significant percentage of women[15,16] (Fig. 42-6). Thus, if the prolapse is reduced by surgical repair in which preferential support to the bladder neck is not obtained, the underlying defect in the continence mechanism may suddenly be revealed. A cystocele may also improve urethral closure by pushing against the urethra improving its closure during a cough, or it may act as a shock absorber by dampening sudden increases in bladder pressure. In this scenario urine is pushed into the cystocele by a cough or sneeze, rather than spurting out the urethra. No matter what the mechanism, the possibility of stress incontinence developing after prolapse repair must always be anticipated.

Certain women with advanced pelvic prolapse mostly secondary to a cystocele will have totally normal voiding on subjective questioning as well as on objective uroflow studies. However, a certain percentage will have obstructed voiding as demonstrated by symptoms of hesitancy, frequency, and a feeling of incomplete emptying as well as a large postvoid residual and a slower obstructed uroflow pattern. Normal women void by a combination of urethral relaxation and detrusor contraction. If a patient has difficulty emptying her bladder, she probably voids with abdominal straining and does not have an adequate detrusor contraction during voiding. These patients are at high risk to have continued voiding dysfunction after appropriate repair of their prolapse and should be warned about this and possibly be taught intermittent self-catheterization.

The association between genital prolapse and an overactive detrusor, whether it be instability or hyperreflexia, has recently been the subject of investigation. A recent study noted that 41% of women with severe prolapse had uninhibited bladder contractions on cystometry.[17] They also showed that in two out of nine patients placing a vaginal pessary was associated with resolution of the detrusor contractions. Grady et al. noted that 30% of women with either a small or large cystocele had detrusor instability on cystometric evaluation with even a higher percentage complaining of urge incontinence.[18] Grady also showed that vaginal repair of the cystocele was associated with an 87% resolution of symptoms of urge incontinence.[18] The mechanism by which prolapse may produce detrusor overactivity may be external compression that could lead to a sensory stimulus in the urethra similar to that described by Chalfin and Bradley and is relieved when the prolapse is reduced.[19] This does not explain all cases of detrusor overactivity with prolapse but probably explains the cases that are relieved by reduction of the prolapse when some sort of a barrier or surgical correction is used.

There are few specific symptoms related to prolapse of the uterus, the vaginal apex, or an enterocele. These patients usually complain of the previously mentioned generalized symptoms. Lower urinary tract symptoms in the form of frequency and urgency may be present and are probably related to the pressure of the prolapse on the bladder base. Also large prolapses of the uterus and posterior vaginal wall may produce voiding dysfunction and mask underlying stress incontinence.

The most common symptom associated with a rectocele is difficulty emptying the rectum. With bearing down, stool is pushed into the rectocele, and many women have to manually depress the posterior vaginal wall to facilitate defecation. Many elderly women will complain of constipation that may be attributable to factors unrelated to the presence of a rectocele. Thus it is important to counsel these patients properly before surgical correction.

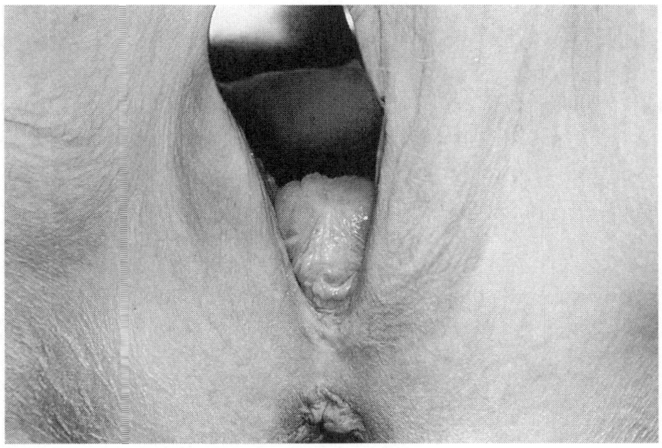

FIG. 42-7 *Retractor placed anteriorly to visualize posterior vaginal wall.*

Diagnosis of Pelvic Support Defects

The diagnosis of pelvic organ prolapse is made on physical exam. The most important aspect of this exam is to evaluate every segment of the pelvic floor. This should include the entire anterior vaginal wall, the vaginal apex or uterus, the upper portion of the posterior vaginal wall, and the distal portion of the posterior vaginal wall, as well as the perineum and an assessment of the introitus. The initial exam should be performed with the patient in a supine position, straining maximally. If the examiner is able to see the full extent of the prolapse and believes that this is truly depicting the maximal degree and grade of the prolapse, the examination can be completed in the supine position. If the patient is not able to strain sufficiently in the supine position so that the prolapse is seen in its largest extent, examination in the standing position is mandatory. This is an extremely important point because it is only when the prolapse can be seen in its fullest extent that all the various elements can be appropriately evaluated. For example, a patient may have a large cystocele that is seen when the patient strains in the supine position. She may also have a small enterocele that will be recognized only with continuous straining and displacement of the cystocele. This examination is best performed with use of either a posterior half of a vaginal speculum or a Sims speculum. The anterior and posterior vaginal walls should be separately examined by retraction of the opposite wall with the vaginal speculum (Figs. 42-7 and 42-8). Examination of the anterior vaginal wall should attempt to establish the status of urethral support. This is most easily accomplished when a lubricated Q-tip is placed into the bladder and is slowly withdrawn until a slight amount of resistance is felt; this position is the anatomic site of the urethrovesical junction. The patient is then asked to strain maximally, and a deflection of greater than 30 degrees is consistent with hypermobility of the bladder neck.[20] If a cystocele is present, an attempt should be made to determine if it is caused by a midline defect in the pubocervical fascia or by separation of the fascia from its normal attachments to the pelvic side wall.

If the uterus is present, the location of the cervix is used to gauge the severity of uterine prolapse. Also an attempt should be made to determine the length of the cervix. Not infrequently, cervical elongation may occur in patients with prolapse. In these cases, the uterine corpus may lie in a normal position. This is important to know preoperatively because a vaginal hysterectomy on a patient with a greatly elongated cervix can be challenging even to the experienced vaginal surgeon. If surgery for stress incontinence is being contemplated, hysterectomy should also be performed if uterovaginal prolapse is present. If the uterus appears to be well supported on exam, one should test its support by grasping the cervix with a tenaculum and applying gentle traction. A well-supported uterus should not descend below the hymen.

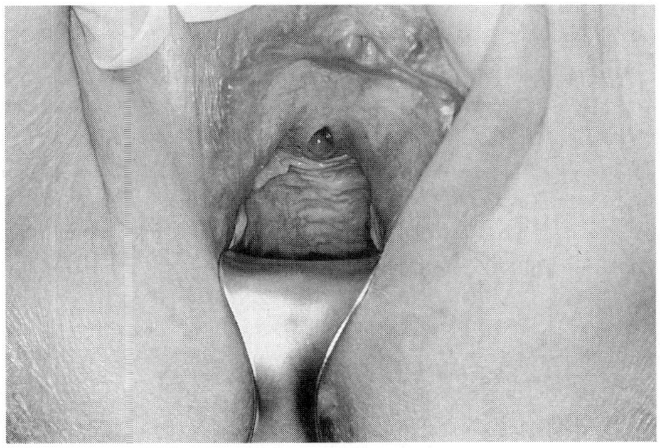

FIG. 42-8 *Retractor placed posteriorly to visualize anterior vaginal wall.*

If the patient has had a previous hysterectomy, apical or vaginal vault support needs to be assessed. If the vaginal vault descends to the hymen and reconstructive surgery is planned, a vaginal vault suspension procedure will usually need to be performed.

Evaluation of posterior vaginal wall defects can at times be challenging, since it is very difficult to distinguish a high rectocele from an enterocele. The distinction between these two conditions is best made on rectovaginal examination performed in the standing position. With the index finger in the rectum and the thumb in the vagina, the examiner determines whether small bowel or a peritoneal sac can be palpated between the rectum and the vagina. If a sac or bowel can be palpated, an enterocele is present, whereas if the bulge is created by a sacculation in the anterior rectal wall, a high rectocele is present. It is imperative to determine if an enterocele is present preoperatively because, when the patient is supine and anesthetized, the ability to palpate the enterocele sac may be lost. Obviously failure to identify and properly correct an enterocele at the time of reconstructive pelvic surgery will lead to an unacceptably high surgical failure rate.

DIAGNOSTIC TESTING

The evaluation of lower urinary tract symptoms in the face of pelvic organ prolapse can be a challenging endeavor. All patients should have a urinalysis and culture (when appropriate) to rule out urinary tract infection. The vagina should be grossly inspected for signs of atrophy because atrophy may cause irritative bladder symptoms, which are easily resolved by application of local estrogen cream.

All patients with advanced or symptomatic pelvic organ prolapse who are contemplating surgical correction should undergo an assessment of their lower urinary tract. This should include the determination of a postvoid residual urine. An elevated postvoid residual urine may produce recurrent urinary tract infections and rarely upper urinary tract damage. As a minimum, the bladder should be filled in a retrograde fashion, and provocative maneuvers such as coughing and straining should be performed with and without reduction of the prolapse. For testing purposes, the prolapse can be reduced with either a pessary or the posterior half of a speculum. The reduction maneuver should attempt to duplicate what the planned surgery will accomplish. When reduction techniques are used to limit visceral descent, 41% to 47% of women with severe prolapse will have occult genuine stress incontinence uncovered.[17,34] Results of reduction tests have been used to determine if a formal urethropexy should be performed at the time of prolapse surgery. In reality, we do not believe that the incidence of occult genuine stress urinary incontinence in such patients is nearly as high as barrier studies have predicted. This is probably attributable to an overcorrection of the prolapse by the barrier or retractor causing stretching of the anterior vaginal wall and thus artificially inducing stress incontinence. The wide range in the estimated prevalence of occult genuine stress incontinence attests to the fact that barrier testing is far from standardized. In reality, probably only 15% to 20% of patients with advanced prolapse will have occult genuine stress incontinence, and these are the patients for whom formal urethropexy will be most beneficial. Even if barrier studies fail to reveal occult stress incontinence and anterior colporrhaphy is going to be performed, the surgeon should pay special attention to providing preferential support to the bladder neck.[22]

Whenever possible, subtracted cystometry should be performed with the prolapse reduced to assess bladder compliance and rule out an overactive detrusor as the cause for urinary incontinence. Pressure-flow studies may be helpful in predicting which patients are at high risk for postoperative voiding dysfunction and even retention. This is of particular benefit in patients who present with elevated postvoid residual urine. Based on the presence or absence of a detrusor contraction during voiding, these patients can be appropriately counseled and possibly be taught intermittent self-catheterization preoperatively.[23,24]

Two studies have noted that approximately 50% of passive urethral pressure can be eliminated with barrier reduction of a large prolapse.[15,25] Some patients demonstrate complete or nearly complete elimination of measurable urethral closure pressure with reduction. These situations are concerning because the prolapse may be masking severe intrinsic sphincter deficiency. This deficiency should further be suspected when prolapse reduction with a subjectively full bladder results in continuous leakage or leakage with a very low leak point pressure. Patients who are at high risk for intrinsic sphincter deficiency are those who have had previous anterior vaginal wall surgery or retropubic urethropexy and those who have received pelvic radiation. These patients will usually complain of severe incontinence if a pessary can be successfully maintained. In these situations, the procedure of choice is an obstructive type of operation, such as a suburethral sling.[26] Another option that can be utilized, especially in elderly patients, would be to stabilize the urethral axis at the time of prolapse surgery and perform injections of periurethral bulk-enhancing agents postoperatively if incontinence occurs.[28]

THE EFFECTS OF HYSTERECTOMY ON THE LOWER URINARY TRACT

The role of hysterectomy at the time of stress incontinence surgery has long been debated. There are no data to support that routine hysterectomy improves the outcome of surgery for stress incontinence. If the uterus is well supported and there are no gynecologic problems, hysterectomy need not be performed. Many women with urinary incontinence will have some degree of uterine prolapse, and assuming child bearing has been completed, hysterectomy should be strongly encouraged.

There are few data to support the belief that simple hysterectomy has a detrimental effect on lower urinary tract function. The few studies that have attempted to evaluate this have concluded that urinary tract dysfunction that appears after hysterectomy is almost always present before the hysterectomy but may have been overshadowed by the more distressing symptoms for which the hysterectomy was performed.[28] It is, however, possible that hysterectomy can potentially damage some elements important for pelvic support and over time this may lead to the development of stress incontinence. Radical hysterectomy has been shown to have an effect on the lower urinary tract probably secondary to injury to the autonomic nerve supply of the bladder and urethra. Most commonly, this initially produces voiding dysfunction or even retention caused by a temporary paralysis.[29]

MANAGEMENT

Except in rare situations, urinary incontinence and pelvic organ prolapse are both quality-of-life issues. Thus the risk of therapy must be based on the patient's wishes and desires. Unfortunately, nonsurgical options for the management of prolapse are very limited. All postmenopausal patients should be placed on estrogen replacement therapy unless a strong contraindication exists. We prefer initially to utilize local estrogen cream (2 g per night) in the vagina for 6 weeks to 3 months. We also like to give estrogen locally for at least 6 weeks before any reconstructive pelvic surgery. If the patient has not previously had a hysterectomy, progesterone must also be given either in a continuous or a cyclic fashion. Estrogen therapy has been shown to improve mild to moderate degrees of prolapse and will commonly make a mildly symptomatic patient asymptomatic. Estrogen has also been noted to improve irritative bladder symptoms, such as frequency and urgency and urge incontinence. Contrary to previously held beliefs, estrogen has not been shown to improve stress incontinence.[30,31]

The only other mode of nonsurgical therapy is the use of a vaginal pessary. This can allow the patient to eliminate the morbidity associated with severe pelvic organ prolapse without undergoing the cost and risk of surgical repair. The placement of a vaginal pessary can be used as a permanent treatment of pelvic relaxation or as a temporary treatment while the patient is awaiting surgery. As has been mentioned, the pessary can also be used in the diagnostic evaluation of women with uterovaginal prolapse to determine if they have incompetent urethral sphincteric function when the vagina is reduced. Finally, the pessary has been used successfully in several studies to treat genuine stress incontinence because it can support the bladder neck during strenuous activity, coughing, or straining.[32,33] Recently a vaginal pessary has been devised specifically for supporting the bladder neck in patients with stress incontinence.[34] Numerous pessaries are marketed for various types of prolapse. We have preferred the use of ring pessaries with or without support because these are easily inserted, have minimal reaction with the vagina, and can be left in place for up to 3 months. The main complications to pessary use are vaginal skin erosion and vaginal infections. These problems can generally be managed easily by removal of the pessary until the abrasions heal. Vaginal infections respond well to douching or to a course of antibiotic therapy. If patients with a pessary are not seen at regular intervals or if the pessary is forgotten by the patient, pessary impaction or chronic vaginal infection can occur, leading to more severe alteration, and ultimately damage to the bladder or rectum.

Many vaginal and abdominal operations have been described to correct the various anatomic defects. The goals of reconstructive pelvic surgery should be to correct all anatomic defects in a site-specific fashion and maintain or restore visceral and sexual function. In the majority of cases surgery is done on an elective basis. All medical problems should be evaluated or controlled before one considers surgical correction. Treatment of the vaginal mucosa with topical estrogen helps improve the pliability of the tissue before surgery. Also, estrogen helps in treating or reducing the size of vaginal ulcers. Any suspicious ulcers should be biopsied to rule out malignancy.

Advanced age should not be considered a contraindication to surgery for advanced prolapse. Even patients with disabling medical conditions that have contraindications for general anesthesia can be operated on with good success under intravenous sedation, with a pudendal block, and intravenous infiltration of an anesthetic agent.[35]

It has previously been emphasized that when a patient has advanced prolapse occult stress incontinence must be looked for. It must also be emphasized that before one performs surgery for stress incontinence, occult prolapse must be looked for and corrected if present. This is extremely important when one is contemplating a urethropexy for stress incontinence because these operations predispose the patient to the development of posterior vaginal wall defects in the form of rectocele and enterocele. If these defects are present and not corrected at the time of surgery, they can commonly become much more prominent postoperatively. Some pelvic surgeons believe that routine obliteration of the cul-de-sac should be performed at the time of retropubic urethropexy. Anterior vaginal wall prolapses are best managed based on the type of defect present. Midline or distension types of cystoceles can be managed by anterior colporrhaphy with plication of pubocervical fascia in front of the defect. Displacement cystoceles are probably best managed by paravaginal repair, which can be performed transvaginally or more commonly retropubically.[12,36] If stress incontinence caused by hypermobility of the bladder neck coexists with cystocele, urethropexy should also be performed. If no stress incontinence is present, a simple plication of the urethrovesical junction should be performed to provide preferential support to the bladder neck.[22]

Prolapse of the vaginal vault can be managed by a vaginal or abdominal route. Although many different operations have been described to suspend the prolapsed vaginal vault, most surgeons would prefer to use a posterior structure with the hope of laying the vagina into the hollow of the sacrum. This has commonly been the sacrospinous ligament when a vaginal route is utilized and the longitudinal ligament of the sacrum when an abdominal procedure is performed. Both of these operations can predispose a patient to significant anterior vaginal wall prolapse and stress incontinence because the vaginal axis is altered in a posterior direction.

Enteroceles can also be corrected by a vaginal or abdominal route. The abdominal correction of an enterocele involves the placement of concentric pursestring sutures as described by Moskowitz or the approximation of the serosa of the sigmoid colon to the posterior vaginal wall as was described by Halban. Also simple plication of the uterosacral ligaments will help support the vaginal cuff and obliterate the cul-de-sac.[37] Transvaginally the enterocele is best corrected by complete dissection of the peritoneal sac off the vagina, entrance into the peritoneal sac, excision of the sac, and closure of the defect at the neck of the hernia. When a vaginal hysterectomy is performed and a deep cul-de-sac is noted, a McCall culdoplasty should be performed.[37] This will obliterate the cul-de-sac, support the vaginal cuff, and increase the length of the posterior vaginal wall. Some pelvic surgeons believe that this should routinely be performed at the time of vaginal hysterectomy.

A rectocele is best repaired through the vagina by plication of the rectovaginal fascia in front of the prolapsed anterior rectal wall. Some pelvic surgeons also like to plicate the inner aspects of the levator muscles across the midline. A perineorrhaphy is almost always necessary in a patient with long-standing prolapse because the prolapse will very commonly create a gaping introitus that will still be present after the prolapse is corrected.

Obliterative procedures, such as colpocleisis and colpectomy, should be used only as a last resort to cure prolapse, since the women will not be left with a functional vagina. These operations are commonly used in elderly patients who are a relatively poor surgical risk and who otherwise would have no other treatment options. Obliterative procedures can be performed safely and quickly under local or regional anesthesia with minimal blood loss.

In summary, pelvic organ prolapse and voiding dysfunction will very commonly coexist in females. These problems should be routinely looked for and evaluated. Each condition should be individually managed in the most appropriate fashion.

References

1. DeLancey JOL: Anatomy and biomechanics of genital prolapse, *Clin Obstet Gynecol* 36(4):897, 1993.
2. DeLancey JOL, Richardson AC: Anatomy of genital support. In *Urogynecologic surgery,* Gaithersburg, Md., 1992, Aspen.
3. DeLancey JOL, Richardson AC: Anatomy of genital support. In *Female pelvic floor disorders,* New York, 1992, Norton.
4. DeLancey JOL: Anatomic aspects of vaginal eversion after hysterectomy, *Am J Obstet Gynecol* 166:1717, 1992.
5. Nichols DH, Milley PS, Randall CL: Significance of restoration of normal vaginal depth and axis, *Obstet Gynecol* 36:251, 1970.
6. Parks AG, Porter NH, Melzak J: Experimental study of the reflex mechanism controlling muscles of the pelvic floor, *Dis Colon Rectum* 5:407, 1962.
7. Bonney V: The principles that should underlie all operations for prolapse, *Br J Obstet Gynaecol Br Emp* 41:669, 1934.
8. Burch JC: Cooper's ligament urethrovesical suspension for stress incontinence: nine years' experience—results, complications, technique, *Am J Obstet Gynecol* 100:764, 1968.
9. Addison WA, Timmons MC: Abdominal approach to vaginal eversion, *Clin Obstet Gynecol* 36:995, 1993.
10. Shull BL, Capen CV, Riges MW, Kuehl TJ: Preoperative and postoperative analysis of site-specific pelvic support defects in 81 women treated with sacrospinous ligament suspension and pelvic reconstruction, *Am J Obstet Gynecol* 166:1764, 1992.
11. Goff BH: The surgical anatomy of cystocele and urethrocele with special reference to the pubocervical fascia, *Surg Gynecol Obstet* 87:725, 1948.
12. Richardson AC, Lyons JB, Williams NL: A new look at pelvic relaxation, *Am J Obstet Gynecol* 126:568, 1976.
13. Beecham CT: Classification of vaginal relaxation, *Am J Obstet Gynecol* 136:957, 1980.
14. Baden WF, Walker TA: Genesis of the vaginal profile, *Clin Obstet Gynecol* 15:1048, 1972.
15. Bump RC, Rantz TA, Hurt WG: The mechanism of urinary incontinence in women with severe uterovaginal prolapse: results of barrier studies, *Obstet Gynecol* 72:291, 1988.
16. Bhatia N, Bergman A: Pessary test in women with urinary incontinence, *Obstet Gynecol* 65:220, 1985.
17. Rosenzweig BA, Pushkin S, Blumenfeld D, Bhatia N: Prevalence of abnormal urodynamic test results in continent women with severe genitourinary prolapse, *Obstet Gynecol* 79:539, 1992.
18. Grady M, Kozminski M, Delancey J, et al: Stress incontinence and cystoceles, *J Urol* 145:1211, 1991.
19. Chalfin SA, Bradley WE: The etiology of detrusor hyperreflexia in patients with intravesical obstruction, *J Urol* 127:938, 1982.
20. Karram MM, Bhatia N: The Q-tip test: standardization of the technique and its interpretation in women with urinary incontinence, *Obstet Gynecol* 71:807, 1988.
21. Davila CW, Ostermann KV: The bladder neck support prosthesis: a nonsurgical approach to stress incontinence in adult women, *Am J Obstet Gynecol* 171:206, 1994.
22. Walters MD: Pelvic organ prolapse: cystocele and rectocele. In Walters MD, Karram MM, editors: *Clinical urogynecology,* St. Louis, 1993, Mosby.
23. Bhatia N, Bergman A: Urodynamic predictability of voiding following incontinence surgery, *Obstet Gynecol* 63:85, 1984.
24. Lose G, Jorgensen T, Mortensen SO, et al: Voiding difficulties after colposuspension, *Obstet Gynecol* 69:33, 1987.
25. Bergman A, Loonings PP, Ballard CA: Predicting postoperative urinary incontinence development in women undergoing operation for genital prolapse, *Am J Obstet Gynecol* 158:117, 1988.
26. Karram MM, Bhatia N: Patch procedure: modified transvaginal fascia lata sling for recurrent or severe stress urinary incontinence, *Obstet Gynecol* 75:451, 1990.
27. Winters JC, Appell R: Periurethral injection of collagen in the treatment of intrinsic sphincter deficiency in the female patient, *Urol Clin North Am* 22:673, 1995.
28. Griffith-Jones MD, Jarvis GJ, McNamara HM: Adverse urinary symptoms after total abdominal hysterectomy: fact or fiction? *Br J Urol* 67:295, 1991.
29. Wake CR: The immediate effect of abdominal hysterectomy in intravesical pressure and detrusor activity, *Br J Obstet Gynaecol* 87:901, 1980.
30. Walter S, Wolf H, Barlebo H, et al: Urinary incontinence in postmenopausal women treated with estrogens: a double blind clinical trial, *Urol Int* 33:135, 1978.
31. Wilson PP, Faragher B, Butler B, et al: Treatment with oral piperazine oestrone sulphate for genuine stress incontinence in postmenopausal women, *Br J Obstet Gynaecol* 94:568, 1987.
32. Bhatia N, Bergman A, Gunning J: Urodynamic effects of a vaginal pessary in women with urinary stress incontinence, *Am J Obstet Gynecol* 147:876, 1983.
33. Cardozo LD, Stanton SL: Evaluation of female urinary incontinence device, *Urology* 13:398, 1979.
34. Wall LL, Hewitt JK: Urodynamic characteristics of women with complete posthysterectomy vaginal vault prolapse, *Urology* 44:336, 1994.
35. Miklos JR, Sze EHM, Karram MM: Vaginal correction of pelvic organ relaxation using local anesthesia, *Obstet Gynecol* 86:922, 1995.
36. Shull BL, Benn SL, Kuehl TJ: Surgical management of prolapse of the anterior vagnal segment: an analysis of support defects, operative morbidity, and anatomic outcome, *Am J Obstet Gynecol* 171:1429, 1994.
37. Karram MM, Walters MD: Pelvic organ prolapse: enterocele and vaginal vault prolapse. In Walters MD, Karram MM, editors: *Clinical urogynecology,* St. Louis, 1993, Mosby.

Chapter 43 Interstitial Cystitis

Deborah R. Erickson

Interstitial cystitis (IC) is a multifactorial syndrome characterized by pelvic and perineal discomfort, urinary frequency, or urgency. The symptoms vary greatly in severity, and mild cases usually do not progress to the severe form. Thus it may be more appropriate to use a different name, such as lower urinary tract hypersensitivity, for mild cases. Incontinence is not a typical feature of IC, but the two conditions can occur together, and some of the symptoms may overlap.

Since IC is multifactorial, several types of treatments are used. Treatment response is quite variable. Conservative therapy is successful for some patients, whereas others require more invasive procedures and treatments. Many aspects of diagnosis and treatment are still controversial. This chapter is an attempt to provide a balanced, practical approach to patients with IC. Special considerations for incontinent IC patients are also described.

Etiology

No definite cause has been found for IC, but several theories have been proposed. It is likely that different patients have different causes. At this time the most commonly discussed theories include (1) a defect in the bladder epithelial permeability barrier, (2) an allergic or autoimmune process, (3) an infection by a fastidious organism, (4) changes in bladder innervation, and (5) bladder ischemia (possibly analogous to reflex sympathetic dystrophy).

Evaluation

NIDDK Criteria

The National Institute of Diabetes and Digestive and Kidney Diseases (NIDDK) has established criteria for entering patients into IC research studies. The original criteria[1,2] were later revised; the current criteria are listed in the box below.[2,3] The purpose of these criteria is to improve uniformity among patients in research studies. This requires that the criteria be restrictive, and in some cases they may exclude patients who truly have IC. Therefore these criteria are not meant for clinical use in deciding whether to treat an individual patient for IC. The usual clinical practice is to treat the patient for IC when the symptoms are characteristic and a thorough evaluation reveals no other cause. Individual practitioners vary in their evaluation of IC, but most use an approach similar to the one described below.

Initial Evaluation

History. The classic history for IC is pelvic or perineal pain, worse when the bladder is full and relieved (temporarily) by voiding. Since holding urine is painful, urinary frequency and nocturia ensue. However, not all patients have this classic history. Some patients describe pain increased by voiding, dysuria, urgency rather than pain, or a constant urge to void, with or without frequency and nocturia. Some of these variations are suggestive of a problem other than IC. For example, urgency may be attributable to detrusor instability, and dysuria with postvoid pain is suggestive of a urethral diverticulum.

Additional questions may indicate other possible sources for the patient's symptoms. These include back pain, neurologic symptoms, flank pain (suggestive of a distal ureteral stone), hematuria, bowel disturbances, and the relationship of the pain to eating, bowel movements, physical activities, and the menstrual cycle. IC pain is typically worse just before menstruation, whereas endometriosis is typically worse during menstruation. Pelvic floor dysfunction, which often responds well to physical therapy, should be considered if the patient complains of dyspareunia, pain with bowel movements, or obstructive voiding symptoms.

A baseline reference for planning conservative therapy should include questions about voiding habits, fluid intake (type and quantity), contraception and hygiene practices, dietary habits,

NIDDK Criteria for Interstitial Cystitis

INCLUSION CRITERIA (BOTH MUST BE PRESENT)

1. Pain associated with the bladder or urinary urgency
2. Hunner's ulcer or glomerulations after bladder distension

EXCLUSION CRITERIA

1. Bladder capacity of greater than 350 ml on awake cystometry using either a gas or liquid filling medium
2. Absence of an intense urge to void with the bladder filled to 100 ml of gas or 150 ml of water during cystometry, using a fill rate of 30 to 100 ml/min
3. The demonstration of phasic involuntary bladder contractions on cystometry using the fill rate described above
4. Duration of symptoms of less than 9 months
5. Absence of nocturia
6. Symptoms relieved by antimicrobials, urinary antiseptics, anticholinergics, or antispasmodics
7. A frequency of urination, while awake, of less than eight times per day
8. A diagnosis of bacterial cystitis or prostatitis within a 3-month period
9. Bladder or ureteral calculi
10. Active genital herpes
11. Uterine, cervical, vaginal, or urethral cancer
12. Urethral diverticulum
13. Cyclophosphamide or any type of chemical cystitis, tuberculous cystitis, or radiation cystitis
14. Benign or malignant bladder tumors
15. Vaginitis
16. Age less than 18 years

and whether eating certain foods exacerbates the symptoms.[4] If the patient also has incontinence, the appropriate questions should be asked. These are described in other chapters in this book. After taking the focused history, a complete medical, surgical, medication, and allergy history is indicated. This may identify other possible extravesical causes for the symptoms and is useful for planning appropriate treatment.

Physical examination. The main goals of examination are to identify other possible causes for the symptoms and to help with deciding the initial treatment approach. The back should be checked for curvature, clues of occult spinal dysraphism, or costovertebral angle tenderness. The abdominal exam is usually normal in IC, except that some patients have suprapubic tenderness. However, the exam may reveal masses, hernias, or tenderness to be suggestive of other causes for the symptoms. Neurologic exam is focused on the S2 to S4 segments and lower extremities unless the history is suggestive of other areas of neurologic disease.

The most revealing examination in female IC patients is the pelvic exam. Lack of estrogen, as evidenced by atrophic skin changes, may contribute to vaginal pain, dysuria, dyspareunia and stress incontinence. Vulvovaginitis (from herpes, yeast, *Trichomonas* protozoa, *Gardnerella* bacteria, and so forth) may also cause dysuria and pain. Idiopathic vulvovestibulitis may be a single condition or may accompany IC; the usual findings are erythema and tenderness to touch on the posterior fourchette. Treatment of these conditions is beyond the scope of this chapter, but excellent references are available.[5-7]

After inspection, different areas should be palpated through the vagina, while one is asking the patient if palpation reproduces her symptoms. In classic IC, pain is reproduced by palpation of the bladder. Pelvic floor dysfunction may accompany IC or be the primary condition; this is suspected if the levator ani muscles are tight or tender to palpate. The urethra should also be palpated to check for a mass, tenderness, or expression of pus. These findings are suggestive of a urethral diverticulum. Finally, the patient's ability and strength in pelvic floor exercises should be addressed. If stress incontinence is present, this is a good opportunity to teach or reinforce the correct technique.

Genital prolapse by itself is not usually relevant to the symptoms of IC but may coexist and may be relevant if incontinence is also associated. Evaluation and treatment of genital prolapse is covered in other chapters of this book.

Rectal exam should assess for other sources of perineal pain (ulcers, fissures), sphincter tone, strength of voluntary contraction, and presence of pelvic masses. Rectovaginal and bimanual exams may reveal masses or implants suggestive of endometriosis. Inspection of the cervix and the taking of a Papanicolaou smear are also essential; some urologists do this themselves, whereas others recommend that a primary care practitioner or gynecologist perform the test.

In male patients the genitourinary exam is not usually helpful for diagnosing IC but is essential to evaluate for other disorders such as meatal stenosis, penile skin lesions, epididymitis, testicular masses, or hernias. A digital prostate exam is important to check for cancer, but prostate tenderness is nonspecific and may indicate IC, prostatitis, or pelvic floor dysfunction. If prostate secretions are expressed, microscopic examination and culture are helpful in evaluating prostatitis.[8]

Other initial studies. Urinalysis, urine culture, and urine cytologic features are recommended to evaluate irritative voiding symptoms. Also, patients who complain of urinary frequency should have a postvoid residual checked. This can be done by catheterization or office ultrasonography, or included in other studies such as an intravenous urogram or voiding cystourethrogram.

Decision Making After Initial Evaluation

If the above evaluation reveals no serious pathologic condition, conservative therapy may be offered. Some patients with mild symptoms may decline any treatment after being reassured that no dangerous disorder was found. Others may find that increased hydration, urinary alkalinization, changes in hygiene habits, and dietary changes are sufficient to resolve the symptoms.[3,4,9] If the main complaints are urgency and frequency but pain is not severe, the symptoms may respond well to a course of behavior therapy with timed, progressively increasing voiding intervals.[9,10]

If the history and examination are suggestive of pelvic floor dysfunction, the mainstay of treatment is pelvic floor reeducation by a physical therapist or nurse practitioner experienced in pelvic floor dysfunction. Adjunctive treatments include sitz baths and possibly oral muscle relaxants. Low-dose diazepam is commonly used. However, I prefer low-dose baclofen (10 mg two to four times a day), which is usually effective and has less abuse potential than benzodiazepines have.

When should more invasive tests be performed? Opinions vary, but general guidelines include the following: (1) if symptoms do not respond to conservative therapy, (2) if initial symptoms are so severe that the patient needs more immediate treatment, (3) if any abnormalities are found in the initial examination or urine studies, (4) if incontinence accompanies IC-like symptoms, and (5) if there are male patients, most will require further evaluation for obstructed voiding. (On the other hand, anatomic urethral obstruction is extremely rare in women without prior antiincontinence surgery and urethral dilatation is very rarely indicated.) The use of invasive procedures in the evaluation of IC-like symptoms is described next.

Intravenous Urogram

Intravenous urogram (IVU) is definitely indicated if the patient has hematuria, a history of recurrent infections, and back or flank pain. In other patients, the IVU will probably be normal. However, distal ureteral stones may cause urinary frequency and urgency without back pain. Since stones can be definitively treated, the practitioner should have a low threshold for obtaining an IVU.

Urodynamic Studies

Urodynamic studies are especially helpful for male patients or for women whose symptoms include incontinence, obstructive voiding complaints, or severe urgency. The rationale and techniques of urodynamic studies are given in other chapters. This chapter provides a description of the findings relevant to IC. Postvoid residual is usually normal in IC. If it is elevated, suspect an additional problem such as detrusor weakness, anatomic bladder outlet obstruction, or voiding dysfunction (neurogenic or nonneurogenic).

The cystometric findings characteristic of IC are an intense urge to void with up to 150 ml of water filling and a capacity of up to 350 ml limited by discomfort. Compliance may be normal or decreased. Detrusor instability is not typical for IC (in fact, it is an NIDDK exclusion criterion). If cystometry reveals that the symptoms of pain and urgency are associated with a detrusor contraction, treatment is directed toward relieving detrusor instability. On the other hand, IC and detrusor instability may coexist as separate entities. In this case, the patient will probably need separate therapies because no single treatment is effective for both conditions.

Cystoscopy

Cystoscopy under local anesthesia is usually normal in IC. However, under general or regional anesthesia, cystoscopy with bladder distension helps with diagnosis and sometimes relieves symptoms. (Symptom relief usually lasts 6 to 9 months, but individual patients vary.)

If regional anesthesia is used, the level should be above T8 because pain with bladder distension may be carried by sympathetic pathways. After preliminary cystoscopy, the bladder is distended to 80 cm of water pressure for 1 to 2 minutes. The usual finding in IC is multiple submucosal hemorrhages ("glomerulations"). The significance of glomerulations is unclear but may be related to chronic underfilling of the bladder. Mucosal cracking may also be seen. The classic finding, Hunner's ulcer, is seen in a minority of patients, so its absence does *not* exclude the diagnosis of IC.

Bladder capacity under anesthesia can range from very small (30 to 60 ml) to over 1000 ml. A normal capacity under anesthesia does not rule out IC. The main significance is that the awake capacity will always be less, and so patients with small anesthetic capacities may have persistent frequency even if pain can be resolved.

During cystoscopy under anesthesia, multiple cold-cup biopsy specimens are recommended. They are not helpful for the diagnosis of IC by itself because biopsy findings of IC are nonspecific. However, biopsies may reveal an alternate cause for the symptoms, such as carcinoma in situ or eosinophilic cystitis.

TREATMENT

Goals

If conservative treatment fails, a wide variety of oral and intravesical medications can be used. The usual course of IC is that symptom flares will alternate with periods of remission. The majority of treatments are helpful in maintaining remission but do not provide acute relief during flares. Treatments that may help during flares include intravesical local anesthetics, transcutaneous electrical nerve stimulation (TENS), or, in severe confirmed cases, narcotics (see below).

Oral Treatments

A wide variety of oral treatments for IC have been recommended. Patients should be informed that none of these drugs is Food and Drug Administration (FDA) approved to treat IC. Most are approved for treating other conditions. Most of these drugs require at least 2 to 3 months to achieve a good effect. The usual plan is to start with the most innocuous and to try others if the initial trials fail. The drugs used most commonly include the following:

Hydroxyzine. An antihistamine. Start with 10 mg PO qhs and work up as tolerated to 50 to 75 mg PO qhs. The main side effect is sleepiness, but for most patients this problem improves over time.[2,11]

Amitriptyline. A tricyclic antidepressant that, in low doses, acts on the pain transmission pathways and may also stabilize mast cells. Start with 10 mg PO qhs and work up as tolerated to 50 to 100 mg qhs. The main side effects are sleepiness and weight gain. The therapeutic effects may be additive with hydroxyzine.[2,9,12]

Doxepin. Similar to amitriptyline but less sedating and more potent at stabilizing mast cells. The usual dose is 50 to 75 mg a day.

Klonopin. A benzodiazepine anticonvulsant that is especially helpful for neuropathic ("stabbing, shooting") kinds of pain. The usual dose is 0.5 mg bid. Effects may be additive with tricyclics. Side effects include central nervous system depression (especially if combined with alcohol or other CNS-depressing drugs). Patients must be warned not to discontinue the drug abruptly. Liver function tests and complete blood counts should be monitored.

Elmiron. An oral analog of heparin, believed to improve the bladder epithelium's function as an impermeable barrier. The drug is pending FDA approval in the United States but can be obtained on "compassionate use" protocols from Baker Cummins Pharmaceuticals, Miami, Fla.[2,9,13-15]

Nifedipine. A calcium-channel blocker that may work by improving bladder blood flow, altering nerve conduction, or suppressing the immune system. The usual dose is 30 to 60 mg per day by extended-release tablets. The main side effects include orthostatic hypotension, dizziness, or lower leg swelling.[2,16]

A blocker histamine (H_2) receptors may be additive with hydroxyzine. The usual dose is 300 mg bid. The main side effects are drug interactions (by affecting microsomal enzyme systems).[17]

Mexiletine. An oral analog of lidocaine, now being used by chronic pain specialists to treat may types of pain. Experience with IC patients is limited at this time, but use of this drug seems reasonable.

Nalmefene. An opioid agonist-antagonist, currently on trials for IC but not yet FDA approved.[2]

Narcotics. If other measures fail and the patient has debilitating pain, narcotics may be very helpful for returning to a more normal lifestyle. The drugs with the lowest abuse potential are methadone and sustained-release forms of morphine (such as MS Contin). Around-the-clock dosing is usually more effective than as-needed dosing. Narcotics should not be used unless the patient has objective findings (such as glomerulations or biopsy-proved inflammation) to confirm the diagnosis of IC and all other measures have failed. Collaboration with pain management specialists may be very helpful.

Intravesical Treatments

A variety of intravesical treatments can be offered. Most can be instilled by the patient at home, which decreases the expense of office visits and increases the patient's control over the disease.

Dimethyl sulfoxide. Dimethyl sulfoxide (DMSO) is the only drug currently approved by the FDA for treating IC. Its functions include antiinflammatory, analgesic, vasodilatation, dissolution of collagen, and induction of cellular differentiation. The usual course is use of Rimso-50, one bottle weekly for 6 weeks. Maintenance treatments at monthly or bimonthly intervals may be beneficial. Some patients find instillation painful. In my experience, one can avoid this by first instilling 10 ml of 1% lidocaine, waiting a few minutes, draining it out (to avoid having DMSO "carry" the lidocaine systemically), and then instilling the DMSO. A complete blood count and liver and kidney function tests should be done every 6 months if DMSO is used chronically.[2,9,18]

Heparin. Heparin is a sulfated glycosaminoglycan used to improve the bladder epithelial barrier function. Alone, the usual dose is 10,000 units in 10 ml of saline solution or water, three times a week. It can also be combined in cocktails. Intravesical heparin is not systemically absorbed, but the prothrombin time, partial thromboplastin time, and platelet count should be checked 2 to 4 weeks after therapy is started to rule out an idiosyncratic reaction or thrombocytopenia.[2,19]

Lidocaine. Surprisingly, instilling lidocaine into the bladder does not always relieve the pain of IC. Possible explanations are that (1) in chronic pain, new nerve fibers appear, and such fibers are unresponsive to lidocaine; (2) pathways within the spinal cord are responsible for pain signals; and (3) the pH may be too acid for lidocaine to enter cells. The last problem can be solved when one mixes 1 ml of 8.4% sodium bicarbonate with 10 ml of lidocaine. When lidocaine does relieve pain, a low dose (10 ml of 1% lidocaine) may be used two or three times a day as needed for flares, or as part of a multiagent cocktail. Bupivacaine is another choice, but at this time lidocaine has more extensive documentation that systemic absorption does not occur after intravesical administration.[20-24]

Steroids. Various steroid preparations have been used, but no study has compared the various forms or doses with regard to efficacy in IC.

Cromolyn sodium. Nasalcrom, a mast cell stabilizer, benefits some patients, but the ideal dosage schedule has not been established.[25] One would expect the best results in patients with mast cells on bladder biopsy, but this issue has not been addressed in the literature.

Multiagent cocktails. Many variations have been described. One example is as follows: bupivacaine 30 ml, heparin 10,000 units, hydrocortisone sodium succinate (Solu-Cortef) 100 mg, sodium bicarbonate 48 mEq, gentamicin 80 mg, given either weekly or biweekly for 6 doses.[24]

Other Treatments for IC

Transcutaneous electrical nerve stimulation (TENS) is helpful for some patients.[2,9] However, chronic use may diminish its effectiveness. Therefore it is best used as an as-needed treatment for flares.

Surgical treatment (bladder augmentation, urinary diversion) is only rarely indicated.[2] In addition to the usual complications associated with these procedures, IC has unique potential problems. One is that symptoms may return in the diverted segment.[26] Another is that pain may be related to peripheral or spinal nerve changes rather than to the bladder itself; thus symptoms may persist after surgery.[27]

Treatment of Interstitial Cystitis Plus Incontinence

The treatments for IC and incontinence differ. The usual course is to get the IC pain under control first and then address the incontinence.

As described in other chapters in this book, the usual treatments for stress incontinence are pelvic floor exercises, alpha-adrenergic receptor drugs, estrogens, or surgery. Exercises will not harm IC patients; in fact, they can be beneficial, especially as part of therapy for pelvic floor dysfunction. However, it may be painful to use a vaginal probe or device during flares. Estrogens are unlikely to increase IC symptoms and may even be beneficial in some cases. Alpha-adrenergic receptor drugs occasionally exacerbate IC symptoms.

IC is not a contraindication to anti–stress incontinence surgery. However, since the pathophysiologic characteristics of IC are unknown and some cases do begin after surgery, the patient must be warned about possible IC-symptom exacerbation. It would also be prudent to avoid dissection around the subtrigonal nerves.

For urge incontinence, the usual treatments are behavior therapy (prolonged voiding intervals), pelvic floor exercises, anticholinergic drugs, or augmentation cystoplasty as a last resort. Behavior and exercise therapies may also benefit IC as long as pain does not preclude therapy. Anticholinergic drugs usually do not exacerbate IC, and in some cases they may be beneficial by stabilizing mast cells or decreasing bladder spasms. The risks of augmentation cystoplasty for urge incontinence are described in other chapters. In IC there is the additional risk that symptoms may remain unchanged or even become worse.

Summary

Since interstitial cystitis is multifactorial, symptoms vary greatly and so do treatment options. The most important aspect of evaluation for IC is to rule out other causes for the symptoms. Treatment is tailored to the individual patient. If conservative therapy fails, drugs (oral or intravesical) should be tried in a stepwise manner, depending on the patient's preference, usually starting with the most innocuous. For most treatments the goal of therapy is to maintain remission. Very few (except transcutaneous electrical nerve stimulation and intravesical lidocaine) provide rapid relief. Surgery should be undertaken rarely and with great caution because of its inherent risks, including persistent or recurrent symptoms. The majority of patients can achieve satisfactory relief with orally or intravesically administered drugs.

References

1. Gillenwater JY, Wein AJ: Summary of the NIDDK workshop on interstitial cystitis, *J Urol* 140:203-206, 1988.
2. Hanno PM, editor: Diagnosis of interstitial cystitis, *Urol Clin North Am* 21:63-66, 1994.

3. Harris MM: *Interstitial cystitis,* NIH pub no 94-3220, Bethesda, Md., 1994, National Kidney and Urologic Diseases Information Clearinghouse.
4. Bavendam TG: A common sense approach to lower urinary tract hypersensitivity in women, *Contemp Urol* 4:25-40, 1992.
5. Reed BD, Eyler A: Vaginal infections: diagnosis and management, *Am Fam Phys* 47:1805-1818, 1993.
6. Kreiger JN: Vaginitis syndromes: a practical approach to diagnosis and treatment, AUA Update Series, vol 9, Lesson 21, Baltimore, Md., 1990, American Urological Association.
7. Turner MLC, Marinoff SC: Vulvar diseases, *Dermatol Clin North Am* 10: 1992.
8. Schwager EJ: Treatment of bacterial prostatitis, *Am Fam Phys* 44:2137-2141, 1991.
9. Chalker R, Whitmore KE: *Overcoming bladder disorders,* New York, 1990, Harper and Row.
10. Parsons CL, Koprowski PF: Interstitial cystitis: successful management by increasing urinary voiding intervals, *Urology* 37:207-212, 1991.
11. Theoharides TC: Hydroxyzine for interstitial cystitis, *J Allergy Clin Immunol* 91:686-687, 1993.
12. Hanno PM, Buehler J, Wein AJ: Use of amitriptyline in the treatment of interstitial cystitis, *J Urol* 141:846-848, 1989.
13. Parsons CL, Mulholland SG: Successful therapy of interstitial cystitis with pentosanpolysulfate, *J Urol* 138:513-516, 1987.
14. Fritjofsson A, Fall M, Juhlin R, et al: Treatment of ulcer and nonculcer interstitial cystitis with sodium pentosanpolysulfate, *J Urol* 138:508-512, 1987.
15. Holm-Bentzen M, Jacobsen F, Nerstrøm B, et al: A prospective double-blind clinically controlled multicenter trial of sodium pentosanpolysulfate in the treatment of interstitial cystitis and related painful bladder disease, *J Urol* 138:503-507, 1987.
16. Fleischmann JD, Huntley HN, Shingleton WB, Wentworth DB: Clinical and immunological response to nifedipine for the treatment of interstitial cystitis, *J Urol* 146:1235-1239, 1991.
17. Seshadri P, Emerson L, Morales A: Cimetidine in the treatment of interstitial cystitis, *Urology* 44:614-616, 1994.
18. Pérez-Marrero R, Emerson LE, Feltis JT: A controlled study of dimethyl sulfoxide in interstitial cystitis, *J Urol* 140:36-39, 1988.
19. Parsons CL, Housley T, Schmidt JD, LeBow D: Treatment of interstitial cystitis with intravesical heparin, *Br J Urol* 73:504-507, 1994.
20. Asklin B, Cassuto J: Intravesical lidocaine in severe interstitial cystitis, *Scand J Urol Nephrol* 23:311-312, 1989.
21. Pode D, Zylber-Katz E, Shapiro A: Intravesical lidocaine: topical anesthesia for bladder mucosal biopsies, *J Urol* 148:795-796, 1992.
22. Thrasher JB, Peterson NE, Donatucci CF: Lidocaine as a topical anesthetic for bladder biopsies, *J Urol* 145:1209-1210, 1991.
23. Heffernan JP, Matthews RD, Sands JP, Nolan JF: Perioperative serum bupivacaine levels after topical bladder anesthesia for bladder biopsy, *Anesth Analg* 77:402-403, 1993.
24. Whitmore KE: Multiagent intravesical cocktail as instillation therapy for management of interstitial cystitis, NIH Research Symposium on Interstitial Cystitis, Bethesda, Md., Jan 9, 1995.
25. Edwards L, Bucknall TE, Makin C: Interstitial cystitis: possible cause and clinical study of sodium cromoglycate, *Br J Urol* 58:95-96, 1986.
26. McGuire EJ, Lytton B, Cornog JL: Interstitial cystitis following colocystoplasty, *Urology* 2:28-29, 1973.
27. Baskin LS, Tanagho EA: Pelvic pain without pelvic organs, *J Urol* 147:683-686, 1992.

Chapter 44 Postprostatectomy Incontinence

Peter G. Hammerer, Hartwig Huland

Prostatectomy performed for benign prostatic hyperplasia is the second most common type of surgery in men.[1] Approximately 1% of patients who undergo transurethral resection of the prostate suffer from a significant degree of postprostatectomy incontinence.[2-4] Prostate cancer is the most commonly diagnosed cancer in American men and is the second leading cause of cancer death in this group. In the United States approximately 244,000 new prostate cancer cases will be diagnosed in 1995.[5] There are four main treatment options for early-stage prostate cancer,[6-8] which include radical prostatectomy, radiation therapy, hormone treatment, and expectant management (watchful waiting). There has been a sharp increase in the rate of radical prostatectomies throughout the United States and Europe in recent years.[9] Most urologists believe that no treatment for localized prostate cancer provides a higher probability for complete cure of disease than radical prostatectomy.[10]

The most common complications after radical prostatectomy include incontinence, impaired sexual function, and urethral stricture. The estimates of these risks vary widely in the published literature.[11-15] With technical advances in the anatomic approach to radical retropubic prostatectomy, severe incontinence has become an increasingly rare complication; however, some studies that are based on patient-reported morbidity continued to report high rates of postprostatectomy incontinence.[16]

Definition of Incontinence

Postprostatectomy incontinence is a major social, medical, and economic problem. The definition of incontinence varies in the published literature. A fully continent patient should maintain full urinary control postoperatively. Even during severe coughing or sneezing no urinary dripping should occur. The following two different types of incontinence can be distinguished.[17]

Stress Incontinence

Stress incontinence means loss of urine during any physical exertion that tends to elevate intra-abdominal pressure. According to the International Continence Society it is defined as involuntary loss of urine when the measured intravesical pressure exceeds the measured maximum urethral pressure.[17]

Urge Incontinence

Urge incontinence is defined as involuntary loss of urine associated with a strong desire to void. In motor urge incontinence, it may be associated with increased motor activity of the detrusor, as in an unstable bladder. In sensory urge incontinence, it may be associated with increased bladder sensation.[17]

Quantification of Incontinence

To quantify the degree and incidence of incontinence after prostatectomy, patients can be asked to give a count of the number of pads required on a daily basis to control urinary leakage. However, patients have a wide range of tolerance to leakage. Some patients with urinary incontinence who should wear pads do not, whereas other patients will wear a pad even at the risk of loosing a drop of urine once in a while. For more accurate information urine absorption in the pad can be calculated by the weight of the used pad.[18]

Timing of Return of Continence

Postoperative incontinence improves in the year after surgery.[19] Immediately after removal of the Foley catheter almost all patients are incontinent. Therefore final determination of the patient's postoperative continence is usually made after 12 months.[20] In a recent report from our own group we could show that 3 months after radical prostatectomy the complete continence rate according to urodynamic criteria was 44.1%, 74.7% after 6 months, and 83.8% after 12 months.[20,21] Similar results were reported from Stanford University when postoperative continent patients were analyzed. Seventy-one percent of patients who completely recovered urinary continence after radical prostatectomy regained continence within 3 months after prostatectomy, an additional 22% regained continence between 3 and 6 months postoperatively, 4% recovered continence between 6 and 12 months, and only 3% recovered continence sometime after the first postoperative year.[14]

Anatomy of the Prostate and the Urethral Sphincter Mechanism

In 1724 Santorini[22] described the anatomy of the prostate and the urethral sphincter muscle. Johannes Müller[23] performed extensive dissections and descriptions of the prostate and the striated muscle urethral sphincter system 100 years later. His findings of the rectal neuroinnervation of the penis was the groundwork for the proof by Walsh and Donker[24] that these nerves could be saved and potency preserved in radical prostatectomy.

The modern concept of the prostate anatomy is based on McNeal's[25] findings. In contrast to Lowsley's[26] and Frank's[27] descriptions of the prostate, McNeal's description showed that the human prostate gland is made up of three glandular zones and one nonglandular region, the anterior fibromuscular stroma. The three distinct glandular regions arise from different segments of the prostatic urethra:

- Transition zone
- Peripheral zone
- Central zone

In the young adult prostate the transition zone constitutes about 5% of prostatic glandular tissue and is located on both sides of the prostatic urethra. It is in this zone that benign hyperplasia develops.[28] The transition zone is separated from the central and peripheral zones of the prostate by the surgical capsule. The peripheral zone comprises about 70% of the mass of the glandular prostate. It is located at the posterior and lateral aspects of the gland. Its ducts exit from the base of the verumontanum to the prostate apex. Most prostate carcinomas arise within the peripheral zone. The central zone is relatively resistant to disease processes and constitutes about 25% of prostatic glandular tissue in the young adult. It is situated around the base of the prostate, and the ejaculatory ducts pass through the central zone tissue to reach the verumontanum.

The peripheral zone is the most susceptible region to inflammation and the site of origin of most carcinomas,[29] but some cancers arise in the transition zone. These tumors are usually found in transurethral resection (TURP). Approximately 70% of all prostate cancers arise in the peripheral zone, 20% to 25% in the transition zone and 5% to 10% in the central zone.[29]

Urethral Sphincter Muscle

Internal Sphincter

The internal sphincter consists of smooth muscle fibers of the bladder neck and the proximal portion of the urethra.[30-32] It is also known as the "proximal sphincter," or "bladder neck sphincter." These smooth muscle fibers will increase resistance during bladder filling and storage and decrease resistance during voiding.

External Urethral Sphincter

The external urethral sphincter (also known as the "distal urethral sphincter") extends from the verumontanum to the bulbar urethra.[30,33,34] It can be subdivided into (1) the smooth muscle of the urethra between the prostatic apex and the urogenital diaphragm and (2) the intramural and extramural striated muscle of that area. It is composed of "slow-twitch" and "fast-twitch" fibers. The slow-twitch fibers are innervated by the autonomic system. These fibers are able to maintain tonus for prolonged periods.[30] The fast-twitch fibers may contribute to the interruption of the urinary stream; however, these muscle fibers have only a minimal contribution to passive continence. The ratio of smooth muscle to striated muscle decreases from the proximal to the distal portion of the urethral sphincter.[35] It appears that both the submucosal smooth muscle and the horseshoe shaped striated muscle contribute to the continence mechanism.[36]

Incontinence After Treatment for Benign Prostatic Hyperplasia

Benign prostatic hyperplasia (BPH) is the most common growth in men. As demonstrated by Berry et al.,[37] the size of the prostate increases with age. When there is BPH, obstructive symptoms such as the following may occur:

- Diminished urinary stream
- Hesitancy in initiating voiding
- Sensation of incomplete emptying of the bladder
- Urinary retention

These obstructive symptoms must be distinguished from irritative symptoms such as dysuria, frequency, and urgency.

There are few medical treatment agents available for benign prostatic hyperplasia, such as alpha$_1$-receptor blocker,[38] 5-alpha-reductase inhibitor,[39] and sitosterin.[40] However, if conservative management has failed, invasive procedures are necessary. The standard for the operative treatment of benign prostatic hyperplasia is transurethral resection of the prostate (TURP) or open suprapubic or retropubic prostatectomy.[41] Recently, techniques such as balloon dilatation,[42] laser treatment,[43] transurethral needle ablation (TUNA)[44] or transurethral vaporization of the prostate (TVP),[45] microwave therapy,[46] or transrectal high-intensity focused ultrasound[47] have become available.

Transurethral Resection of the Prostate

The goal of the resection is to excise the BPH tissue down to the surgical capsule. With a resectoscope the BPH tissue is resected, and the chips are evacuated. The verumontanum is the landmark denoting the distal boundary of the resection. After complete resection of the BPH tissue and evacuation of the prostatic chips a 22 or 24 French gauge catheter is inserted.

Although the incidence of urinary incontinence is relatively low, it is a known risk of surgery and the source of many malpractice suits. Approximately 1% of patients who undergo transurethral resection of the prostate suffer from postprostatectomy incontinence.[2-4] After TURP, the patient's continence is dependent on the distal continence mechanism. Most frequently damage to the distal urethral sphincter occurs anteriorly between the 10 and 2 o'clock positions.[48]

The resection should be limited at the verumontanum even if a small rim of adenoma is left behind. In Khan et al.'s report on 55 incontinent patients after TURP the verumontanum was absent in 2 patients.[49] Electrocoagulation of bleeding around the sphincter should be done carefully so that the distal continence mechanism is not injured by the cautery.

Fitzpatrick et al.[50] analyzed 68 patients with postprostatectomy incontinence. Sphincteric damage was responsible for incontinence in 47 out of 68 patients. However, detrusor instability was found in 45 of the 68 patients and was associated with sphincteric damage in 28 patients. Instability alone was present in 11 patients and associated with residual obstruction in 6 patients. They concluded that three factors are important for incontinence after transurethral prostate surgery:

- Sphincteric injury
- Bladder instability
- Bladder outlet obstruction

Suprapubic and Retropubic Prostatectomy

The suprapubic prostatectomy is the procedure by which the obstructing BPH tissue is removed through the cavity of the bladder after extraperitoneal incision of the superior wall.[51] It is also called "transvesical prostatectomy" to distinguish it from the transcapsular operation, which is usually spoken of as "retropubic prostatectomy."[52] In the early postoperative period urgency incontinence is common and improves dramatically in the first few weeks. Severe stress incontinence is extremely uncommon if one is careful in fracturing the urethral mucosa and removes the prostatic lobes individually.

Incontinence of urine after suprapubic prostatectomy is less common compared to perineal or even transurethral resection as reported by Nanninga et al.[53] They reported no permanent incontinence in their last 700 patients.

Laser Prostatectomy

A laser generates a monochromatic beam of light that can lead to coagulation, carbonization, or vaporization. The tissue effects depend on the power, the duration, and the wavelength of the laser.[54] The initial reports with laser technology have been encouraging, and in particular have documented the potential for significantly decreased morbidity using laser techniques when compared to standard transurethral resection of the prostate.[55] With the use of the neodymium:YAG laser no long-term incontinence was reported.[56] However, the efficiency and durability of laser treatment still remain controversial. Several additional new techniques to treat benign prostatic hyperplasia are available. Again, long-term evaluation of these procedures in properly controlled studies is necessary before the effect and the complication rate can be compared.

Incontinence After Treatment for Prostatic Carcinoma

The ideal candidate for radical prostatectomy is a patient with a life expectancy of more than 10 years who is in good health and has a tumor confined solely to the prostate.[57] These requirements limit the candidates for surgery to patients with clinical stages A2, B1, B2, or B3 (T1B-T2C N0 M0) disease.

Two different operative procedures are usually performed:

- Radical retropubic prostatectomy
- Radical perineal prostatectomy

Reiner and Walsh[58] developed an anatomic approach to the radical retropubic prostatectomy. Initially a technique for precise control of bleeding from the dorsal vein complex (Santorini's plexus) was developed to enable the surgeon to perform a more precise anatomic dissection, especially at the apex of the prostate. Subsequently the anatomy of the pelvic plexus and the branches that innervate the corpora cavernosa were identified, and modifications in the surgical technique were developed to enable the surgeon to preserve or widely excise the neurovascular bundles.[24] These observations allowed preservation of the cavernous nerves with the possibility of preserving sexual function in patients with localized prostate cancer. The anatomic approach to radical prostatectomy provided an almost bloodless field with excellent exposure, precise apical dissection to avoid injury to the pelvic floor musculature, preservation or wide excision of the neurovascular bundles, and an accurate sutured vesicourethral anastomosis with coadaptation of the mucosal surfaces.

Radical Perineal Prostatectomy

The advantages of perineal prostatectomy include easier access to the vesicourethral anastomosis.[59] There are some concerns regarding the perineal exposure. It does not allow simultaneous exposure of the pelvic lymph nodes.The limited access forces the surgeon to stay on the prostate, whereas the retropubic exposure allows approach to the prostate from the side walls of the pelvis. The limited view of the seminal vesicles deep within the operative field makes it necessary to enter Denonvilliers' fascia at the base of the prostate over the central zone to reach the walls of the ampullae and seminal vesicles, potentially creating positive surgical margins in patients with invasion of Denonvilliers' fascia.[60] Therefore perineal prostatectomy may create more useful margins than the radical retropubic prostatectomy operation would.

Technique of the Radical Retropubic Prostatectomy

The surgical technique of the radical retropubic prostatectomy (RRP) can be divided into different steps.[61]

- Pelvic lymphadenectomy
- Incision of endopelvic fascia
- Division of puboprostatic ligaments
- Division of dorsal vein complex
- Division of urethra
- Division of striated urethral sphincter
- Excision of neurovascular bundle or preservation of neurovascular bundle
- Division of bladder neck and excision of seminal vesicles
- Bladder neck closure and anastomosis

Based on the published literature, urinary incontinence occurs after radical prostatectomy with an incidence varying from 2.5% to 87%.[12-14,62] This variation might be attributable to different investigators' definitions of significant incontinence, time between radical surgery and assessment for incontinence, and different operative techniques (Table 44-1). In a survey of Medicare patients, at least one third of patients had incontinence significant enough to require the use of pads or clamps to deal with the wetness, an indication that incontinence may continue to be a common complication of RRP.[16]

Modification of Radical Retropubic Prostatectomy

Several technical modifications have been proposed in an attempt to maximize sphincteric competence after RRP. For postoperative continence, division of the dorsal vein complex, urethra, and striated urethral sphincter, and bladder neck closure and anastomosis might be the most important factors.

Anastomoses After Radical Prostatectomy

After removal of the prostate, different types of vesicourethral anastomoses are known.[35]

- Multiple simple sutures[12]
- Perineal traction sutures zone (vest anastomoses)[67]
- Combinations of simple sutures and vest anastomoses[59]
- No sutures[68]

With multiple simple sutures, mucosa-to-mucosa apposition will be established. However, with sutures tied too tightly, ischemia, edema, and inflammation with resulting fibrosis and decrease in functional urethral length will result. The vest anastomosis allows the absence of suture material at the vesicourethral junction with optimizing the urethral elasticity throughout the new continence zone.[67] The disadvantage is the risk of stricture because a mucosa-to-mucosa apposition is not guaranteed. For optimal continence, postoperative tissue reaction should be minimized and functional urethral length should be maximized without defection of any autonomic or symmetric nerve fibers.

Tubularization of the Bladder Neck

The benefit of tubularization of the bladder neck after radical prostatectomy for postprostatectomy continence is controversial.[69-72] No adequate urodynamic data are available to support a sphincteric role for the retubularized segment.[35,73]

In a urodynamic comparison between patients who underwent anterior bladder tubularization and patients after standard bladder neck reconstruction, a higher leak point pressure of 101 cm H_2O compared to 65 cm H_2O was found.[72] However, voiding pressure was also elevated relative to the control group. Two of the 14 patients had urinary retention after catheter removal.

Malizia et al.[68] reported a "double-continence technique" by blunt dissection of the bladder neck from the prostatic capsule exposing the prostatic urethra for approximately 1 cm. They reported favorable continence results with this technique. In contrast Klein[66] found no difference in postoperative continence in patients with reconstructed and unconstructed bladder neck.

Table 44-1 Continence Rate in Patients After Radical Prostatectomy

Author	Patients	Percentage continent	Percentage with stress incontinence	Percentage with total incontinence
Catalona and Basler[13]	435	94	6	
Ramon et al.[63]	398	95	5	0
Fowler et al.[16]	757	40		
Meyer-Moldenhauer[21]	211	83.8	15	1.2
Geary et al.[14]	456	80.1	14.7	5.2
Hautmann et al.[64]	191	80.8	16	3.2
Steiner et al.[65]	593	92		8
Klein[66]	83	88	11	1

Apical Dissection

During apical dissection two major goals should be achieved:

- Preservation of distal continence mechanism after the dorsal vein complex has been ligated.
- Avoidance of a positive surgical margin at the apex.

Myers developed a modified technique to maximize the length of a functional urethral sphincter to achieve a lower rate of postoperative incontinence.[74] He also described a longitudinal bunching technique of the deep venous complex that results in improved exposure of the prostate.[75] Recently Walsh et al.,[12] Stamey,[76] and others[13,66,77] described a modified apical dissection with incorporation of the Denonvilliers' fascia posterior to the urethra in the vesicourethral anastomosis. With this technique early continence was reported with 83% patients dry at 3 months.[66] However, unless precise data on the function of the continence mechanism by urodynamic or radiographic data are available we are guessing about which specific operative maneuver provides the best functional outcome.

A major concern about any modification in radical prostatectomy is the risk of compromising removal of prostate cancer tissue.[78] Reports on postprostatectomy incontinence should be judged in the light of positive margin rates. A low positive surgical margin rate should be considered as one of the major goals in radical prostatectomy.

Cryosurgical Ablation of the Prostate

Preliminary data are available on the results of cryosurgical ablation of prostate cancer.[79] Early results have shown promise, but long-term follow-up study is lacking. Most of the published studies emphasize technique and early biopsy results.[79,80] In a recent report by Cox et al.[81] the complication rate of this new procedure was greater than 50%. Urinary incontinence was reported in 17 of 63 patients (27%). It can be concluded that cryosurgical ablation of the prostate is an investigational procedure with a significant complication rate.

Evaluation of the Postprostatectomy Patient

Evaluation of the incontinent postprostatectomy patient includes history, physical examination, cystourethroscopy, radiographic evaluation of the bladder and urethra, transrectal ultrasonography of the anastomosis, and urodynamic studies. The history should determine the severity of incontinence as well as association with frequency, urgency, stress, nocturia, hesitancy, and the position and sensation of fullness. The urinary stream should be evaluated.

Patients reporting incontinence are asked how many pads are required daily to control urinary leakage.[18] The number of protective pads, penile clamps, external catheters, and procedures performed for urinary incontinence such as collagen or Teflon injection or implantation of an artificial urinary sphincter should be noted. If patients do not require pads, they should be considered as being continent. Patients should also be questioned regarding the caliber of the urinary stream. When patients reported narrowing of the stream, dilatation is usually performed by the passing of successive male urethral catheters. Whenever patients have a urethral dilatation or transurethral incision, they should be considered as having had a bladder neck stricture.

The time and type of prostatectomy should be evaluated. In patients with prostate cancer the postoperative prostate-specific antigen (PSA), as a predictor of cancer control, should be monitored.[82] Physical examination should include the abdominal wall. Postoperative hernias should be recognized. A neurologic examination including circumanal sensation and the bulbocavernosus reflex should be performed. Rectal palpation is necessary for assessment of anal tone and voluntary activity of the anal sphincter and evaluation of local recurrence after radical prostatectomy. Urine analysis should be performed to exclude urinary tract infection. Incontinent patients are more likely to have a urinary tract infection.

Cystourethroscopy

In patients with incontinence after treatments for benign prostatic hyperplasia the physician should search for the presence or absence of the verumontanum and residual BPH tissue or urethral strictures as well. Damage to the distal urethral sphincter can be noted by insufficient voluntary activity of the distal urethral sphincter. Urethral strictures can be identified. Pathologic states of the bladder such as low bladder capacity, trabeculation, or neoplasm can be seen.

Radiologic Evaluation

Radiologic evaluation of the lower urinary tract may include a retrograde urethrogram and a voiding cystourethrogram. The adequacy of the previous transurethral resection of the prostate and the level of continence can be identified with the patient in a standing position. The voiding cystourethrogram permits identification of bladder neck strictures, diverticula, residual urine, and vesicoureteral reflux.

Transrectal Ultrasonography

Transrectal ultrasonography of the vesicoureteral anastomosis and the urethral high-pressure zone allows assessment of the postoperative situation. In a recent report by Wassermann et al., the vesicourethral anastomosis was identified in every patient after radical prostatectomy. The urethral high-pressure zone, defined as the length of apposed walls of the bladder cuff and membranous urethra measured from the "vanishing point" of the bladder neck to the penile bulb in the sagittal plane, was identified in 9[illegible]% of the patients.[83]

Urodynamic Studies

For urodynamic studies in the postprostatectomy patient, uroflowmetry, filling cystometrography with electromyography of the external urethral sphincter, and a urethral pressure profile are performed.[17,84]

The urinary flow measures the voided volume, peak flow voiding time, and average flow. The filling cystometrogram describes bladder capacity, compliance, and sensory or motor bladder instability. The combined pelvic flow electromyogram provides an evaluation of detrusor sphincter dyssynergia. The urethral pressure profile is helpful in evaluating functional urethral length, the distal sphincter length, the urethral closure pressure, and usual closure pressure during voluntary contraction of the distal sphincter.

Mechanism of Postprostatectomy Incontinence

After prostatectomy the anatomic relations are altered. In patients with treatment for benign prostatic hyperplasia the internal sphincter system is removed (Fig. 44-1). In patients with localized prostate cancer who underwent radical prostatectomy the prostate, the seminal vesicles, and portions of the vasa deferentia, as well as the pelvic lymph nodes, have been removed. The bladder neck has been anastomosed to the membranous urethra. Functional urethral length is decreased (Fig. 44-2).

In the early postoperative period the bladder neck and anastomoses are edematous, a condition that results in a loss of elasticity. The bladder base has been mobilized and the vesical neck reconstructed. The disruption of pelvic nerve supply may affect normal urine storage and micturitional reflexes. The internal sphincter system has been destroyed; therefore postoperative continence is based on the distal sphincteric mechanism. Continence after prostatectomy is based on a balance between the pressures in the bladder during filling and during stress and the resistance of the distal sphincteric mechanism.

Three different etiologic groups can be differentiated:

1. Urethral insufficiency caused by sphincteric injury
2. Bladder dysfunction
3. Bladder outlet obstruction

Urethral Insufficiency

The urethral pressure responsible for a closed bladder outlet is contributed by at least the striated sphincteric element and perhaps by the smooth sphincteric element of the external urethral sphincter. Fluoroscopic studies indicate that the continence mechanism in the postprostatectomy patient may be located between the vesicourethral anastomosis and the distalmost extent of the striated external sphincter muscle.[73] The functional level of continence relative to the site of the intraoperative urethral anastomosis was studied by O'Donnell et al.[85] In eight patients an intraoperative hemoclip was placed at the site of the urethral anastomosis. The postoperative functional level of continence using a standing lateral cystogram was 9 mm distal to the site of the urethral anastomosis.

Urodynamic studies in postprostatectomy patients with urinary incontinence reported that sphincter damage was the sole cause of incontinence in 22% to 57%.[49,50,86,87] Leach et al.[86] divided the incontinent patients into two groups, those with cancer who underwent radical prostatectomy and those with benign disease who underwent transurethral resection or suprapubic prostatectomy. The cystometric findings revealed pure sphincteric insufficiency in 32% of the first group and 54% of the second group (Table 44-2).

Some studies indicate that the length of the coapting urethra after prostatectomy is important.[72,88,89] Hutch and Fisher[88] showed by lateral cystogram a membranous length of 0.7 to 1.6 cm in their five incontinent patients, compared to a membranous length of 2.6 to 3.4 cm in seven continent patients.

Urodynamic studies by Hellström et al.[89] and Presti et al.[70] indicated that urethral closure pressure and functional urethral length are the dominant factors that determine continence in the residual sphincter. Urethral pressure profilometry in severe incontinent patients revealed very low maximum closing pressure in the range of 35 to 40 cm H_2O and significant differences in functional urethral length (2.1 cm versus 3.6 cm) and maximal urethral closure pressure (39 cm H_2O versus 74 cm H_2O). Similar results were reported from our own group when urodynamic testing was performed before and after radical prostatectomy.[20] In incontinent men the postoperative measurement showed a significantly smaller functional profile length (2.15 + 1.03 cm versus 2.99 + 0.72 cm) and a lower maximum urethral closure pressure (51.3 + 12.7 cm H_2O versus 67.7 + 15.7 cm H_2O) compared to continent men. In a different study preoperative urodynamic testing to pre-

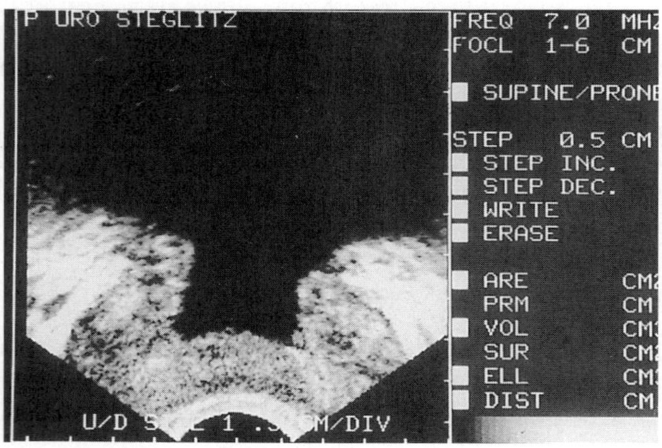

FIG. 44-1 *Transrectal ultrasonogram (TRUS) in a patient after transurethral resection (TURP) for benign prostatic hyperplasia (BPH), transverse view.*

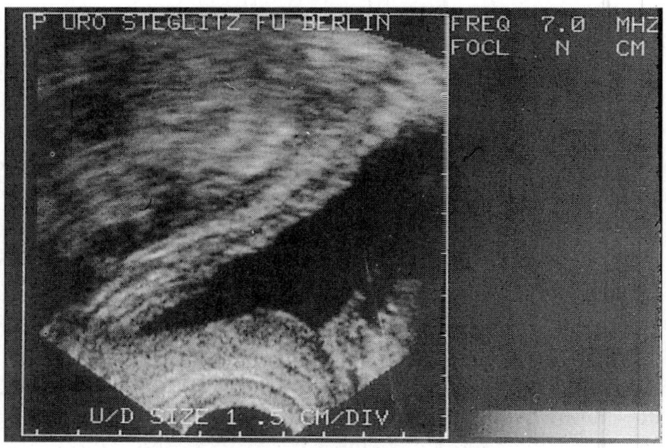

FIG. 44-2 *Transrectal ultrasonogram (TRUS) in a patient after radical prostatectomy, sagittal view.*

Table 44-2 Causes of Urinary Incontinence in Patients with Postprostatectomy Incontinence

	Detrusor instability	Detrusor instability and urethral insufficiency	Urethral insufficiency	Other causes
Khan[49] (N = 63)	31 (49%)	16 (25%)	14 (22%)	2 (3%)
Fitzpatrick et al.[50] (N = 68)	11 (16.2%)	26 (38.2%)	18 (26.5%)	13 (19%)
Leach et al.[86]	7 (18.5%)	16 (42%)	15 (39.5%)	
N = 25 CA	5 (20%)	12 (48%)	8 (32%)	
N = 13 BPH	2 (15%)	4 (31%)	7 (54%)	
Chao et al.[87] (N = 74)	3 (4%)	29 (39%)	42 (57%)	

BPH, Benign prostatic hyperplasia; *CA*, cancer.

dict continence after radical prostatectomy was performed in 86 men.[90] Men with preoperative high maximum urethral closure pressure (>80 cm H_2O) and long functional profile length (>3.2 cm) had a minimal risk of postprostatectomy incontinence.[90] We could not find a significant difference in bladder volume or compliance in continent versus incontinent patients.

Controversy still exists regarding the innervation of the external sphincter muscle. Narayan et al.[91] could show that innervation of the external urethral sphincter is received in part through special branches from the dorsal nerve of the penis, which are located 0.3 to 1.3 cm from the prostatic apex. Injury of these nerves may explain some features of urethral insufficiency caused by sphincteric injury.

Bladder Dysfunction

Bladder instability was found preoperatively in 45% of patients with bladder outlet obstruction.[92] Urinary tract infections, neurologic disorders, chronic retention, or radiation therapy may cause detrusor instability or hyperreflexia.[93] A persistent unstable bladder after prostatectomy may be explained by permanent residual damage of the bladder wall. It is important to diagnose detrusor instability preoperatively, since it is a common cause of postprostatectomy incontinence.

Studies by Jones and Schoenberg[94] in patients with BPH and age-matched controls indicate that some degree of instability may be associated with aging. Although some patients have persistent detrusor instability 6 months after surgery, this is not always the case. After TURP 62% of patients who suffered from detrusor instability associated with obstructive symptoms are cured, whereas 38% have persistent detrusor instability.[92] Persistent or acquired bladder dysfunction is an important cause of postprostatectomy incontinence, which occurs in up to 75% of patients.[49]

In the early postoperative period after prostatectomy, inflammation or irritation of the bladder wall may lead to involuntary bladder contractions. Changes in the elastic properties of the bladder wall may result in decreased compliance during filling, which can lead to postprostatectomy incontinence.

Constantinou and Freiha[95] found a substantial incidence of detrusor instability preoperatively in patients undergoing radical retropubic prostatectomy, which continued at least 2 years postoperatively. They found no statistically significant difference in maximum urethral closure pressure (94 cm H_2O versus 83 cm H_2O) or external sphincter length (3.6 cm versus 3.2 cm) in the 13 patients measured both preoperatively and postoperatively.

In a urodynamic study of 38 patients referred for evaluation of postprostatectomy incontinence, Leach et al.[86] reported a 60.5% bladder dysfunction rate as a major factor of incontinence. Of the studied patients, 42% had sphincteric insufficiency combined with bladder dysfunction. In 7 patients (18.5%) no evidence of sphincter insufficiency was found.

Foote et al.[96] reported urodynamic measurements in patients with incontinence 1 year after surgery for prostate cancer or benign prostatic hyperplasia. A low bladder compliance or detrusor instability was the significant criterion in most of these patients. In contrast, Chao and Mayo[84] reported detrusor instability alone as the sole cause of postprostatectomy incontinence in only 5 of 74 patients.

It can be concluded that detrusor instability and low bladder capacity contribute to early postprostatectomy incontinence. However most of the patients who complain of a constant dribbling or stress-induced incontinence may have sphincteric insufficiency.

Bladder Outlet Obstruction

Anastomotic strictures are a possible factor in the cause of urethral insufficiency. Chao and Mayo[87] analyzed 74 incontinent patients after radical retropubic or radical perineal prostatectomy. Anastomotic strictures were found in 26 of the patients and were an important factor in the cause of sphincteric weakness. Scarring of the anastomotic region may extend down into the urethral sphincter system and impair the closure mechanism, especially that provided by the submucosal vascular and elastic tissue. Dilatation of anastomotic strictures is often followed by sphincteric insufficiency.

Risk Factors for Postoperative Incontinence

The primary goal of radical prostatectomy is cancer control with low morbidity. However, certain risk groups may affect postoperative urinary incontinence:

- Age
- Nerve-sparing technique
- Prior transurethral resection of the prostate
- Prostate weight
- Neurologic disorders
- Unstable bladder
- Radiation therapy

Age

Normal aging will affect the lower urinary tract. It is our experience, confirmed by others, that younger men undergoing radical prostatectomy generally achieve continence more quickly than older men.[90,97,98] When we compared incontinence rates 6 months after radical prostatectomy in patients younger than 55 years to patients older than 75 years, the incontinence rate was zero versus 22.2% (p <0.001).[21,90] This observed phenomenon may not just be a function of age-related muscle atrophy, bladder instability may also be one of the possible mechanisms.

Steiner et al.[65] analyzed the impact of age and the return of urinary control. When patients were sorted by decade, urinary continence returned in 100% of the men less than 40 years of age, 98% in the 40 to 49 year age group, 91% in the 50 to 59 year age group, 92% in the 60 to 69 year age group, and 86% in the 70 to 76 year age group. In a recent analysis from Stanford University a similar trend toward increasing patient age with greater postoperative incontinence was seen.[14]

Nerve Sparing

O'Donnell and Finan[99] found a lower rate of incontinence after nerve-sparing radical retropubic prostatectomy with zero total incontinence and 6% stress incontinence compared to non–nerve sparing radical retropubic prostatectomy with 12% total incontinence and 18% stress incontinence. They found an increase in functional urethral length (2.3 cm versus 1.9 cm) and peak resting urethral pressure (46.5 cm H_2O versus 35.4 cm H_2O) in the nerve-sparing group and concluded that preservation of the pelvic nerves during radical prostatectomy played a major part in the functional preservation of urinary continence.

Steiner et al.[65] compared the results of patients with preservation of both neurovascular bundles to patients with preservation of only one neurovascular bundle and patients with excision of both neurovascular bundles. In the first group, continence was achieved in 94% of 328 patients compared to 92% of 228 patients. In patients with wide excision of both neurovascular bundles the continence rate was 81% of 37 patients. Although fewer patients were continent in the later group, no statistical significance was seen. Similar tendency toward a correlation of nerve bundles spared at radical prostatectomy with lower likelihood of incontinence was reported by Geary et al. and other investigators.[14,63,66]

Prior Transurethral Resection of the Prostate

Nichols et al.[100] reported on 26 patients who underwent radical prostatectomy after transurethral resection. Of their patients, 19% had total incontinence and 50% had stress incontinence. Bass et al.[101] reported similar incontinence rates in 36 patients who had had resection before radical prostatectomy. Of these patients 11% were totally incontinent and 39% were minimally incontinent. In a series by Lindner et al.[102] 38 of 143 patients treated with radical prostatectomy had previous transurethral resection of the prostate. In the patient group with prior TURP, minimal incontinence was 16.2% compared to 12.8%, and the rate of severe incontinence was 8.1% compared to 5%. They concluded that prior transurethral resection will slightly increase the postprostatectomy incontinence. In contrast Steiner et al.,[65] Catalona et al.,[13] and Ramon et al.[63] reported the same urinary continence rates in patients with history of transurethral resection of the prostate or open prostatectomy compared to patients with no history of previous prostate surgery. It is our experience that with the modern approach of the radical retropubic prostatectomy prior TURP does not affect postoperative continence.

Prostate Weight

The prostate weight was correlated to the postoperative incontinence rate by Steiner's careful analysis of postprostatectomy patients.[65] They found no significant difference in the mean prostate weight of men who were totally continent (50.9 g) compared to incontinent patients (53.7 g). In contrast our own group[20] found a significant correlation between prostate volume and continence in patients undergoing radical retropubic prostatectomy.

Radiation Therapy

Salvage radical prostatectomy after radiation therapy has been reported to be associated with higher urinary incontinence rates. Neerhut et al.[103] reported on 16 patients with persistent or recurrent prostate cancer after definitive radiotherapy who underwent salvage radical prostatectomy. They reported persistent urinary incontinence in 4 of 16 patients (25%) and anastomotic strictures in 4 patients. Similar results with an incontinence rate of 10% and vesical neck contracture of 17% were reported by Rainwater and Zincke.[104]

Neurologic Disease

Patients with Parkinson's disease have a high incidence of detrusor hyperreflexia as well as abnormalities of external sphincter control.[105] Staskin et al.[106] analyzed 36 patients with Parkinson's disease who underwent transurethral prostatectomy (TURP). The preoperative incontinence rate was 17% compared to postoperative incontinence rate of 28%. Abnormal voluntary sphincter control was associated with postoperative urinary incontinence. In patients with abnormal sphincter control 5 of 6 patients became incontinent compared to 1 of 24 patients with normal preoperative sphincter control. The risk of postprostatectomy incontinence arising after TURP in a parkinsonian patient was approximately 20%. The authors concluded that nonoperative management might be recommended whenever feasible.

Bladder Stability

Severe detrusor instability that persists after prostatectomy is an important cause of urinary incontinence. Therefore it is essential to investigate detrusor instability before surgery. Although spontaneous regression of detrusor instability occurs in the majority of patients with postprostatectomy incontinence, persisting detrusor instability can be extremely troublesome.[49,65]

CONCLUSION

In the majority of patients postprostatectomy incontinence is transitory and disappears within several months. It can be caused by urethral insufficiency attributable to sphincteric injury, bladder dysfunction, or bladder outlet obstruction. There may be a considerable overlap between these conditions; however, in most patients after radical prostatectomy who complain of constant dribbling or stress-induced incontinence urethral insufficiency is found.

References

1. Abrams PH: Investigations of postprostatectomy problems, *Urology* 15:209, 1980.
2. Habib NA, Luck RJ: Results of transurethral resection of the benign prostate, *Br J Surg* 70:218, 1983.
3. Meyhoff HH, Nordling J: Long-term results of transurethral and transvesical prostatectomy, *Scand J Urol Nephrol* 20:27, 1986.
4. Mebust WK, Holtgrewe HL: Current status of transurethral prostatectomy: a review of the AUA National Cooperative Study, *World J Urol* 6:194, 1989.
5. Wingo PA, Tong T, Boring S: Cancer statistics, 1995, *CA Cancer J Clin* 45:8-30, 1995.
6. Stamey TA, McNeal JE: Adenocarcinoma of the prostate. In Walsh PC, Retik AB, Stamey TA, Vaughan ED Jr, editors: *Campbell's urology,* ed 6, vol 3, Philadelphia, 1992, Saunders.
7. Schellhammer PF: Radiation for localized prostatic carcinoma, *Eur Urol* 27:26-27, 1995.
8. Johansson J-E, Adami H-O, Andersson S-O, et al: High 10-year survival rate in patients with early, untreated prostatic cancer, *JAMA* 267:2191-2196, 1992.
9. Lu-Yao GL, McLerran D, Wasson J, Wennberg JE: An assessment of radical prostatectomy, *JAMA* 269:2633-2636, 1993.
10. Frohmüller HGW, Theiss M: Long-term results of radical prostatectomy, *Eur Urol* 27:41-44, 1995.
11. Igel TC, Barret DM: Perioperative and postoperative complications from bilateral pelvic lymphadenectomy and radical retropubic prostatectomy, *J Urol* 137:1189-1191, 1987.
12. Walsh PC, Quinlan DM, Morton RA, Steiner MS: Radical retropubic prostatectomy: improved anastomosis and urinary continence, *Urol Clin North Am* 17:679-701, 1990.
13. Catalona WJ, Basler WJ: Return of erections and urinary continence following nerve sparing radical retropubic prostatectomy, *J Urol* 150:905-907, 1993.
14. Geary ES, Dendinger TE, Freiha FS, Stamey TA: Incontinence and vesical neck strictures following radical retropubic prostatectomy, *Urology* 45:1000, 1995.
15. Hammerer P, Hübner D, Gonnermann D, Huland H: Perioperative und postoperative Komplikationen der pelvinen Lymphadenektomie und radikalen Prostatektomie bei 320 konsekutiven Patienten, *Urologe* A 34:1-9, 1995.
16. Fowler FJ Jr, Barry MJ, Lu-Yao G, et al: Patient-reported complications and follow-up treatment after radical prostatectomy, the national Medicare experience: 1988-1990 (updated June 1993), *Urology* 42:622-629, 1993.
17. Bates G, Bradley WE, Glen E, et al: First report on the standardization of lower urinary tract function: procedures related to the evaluation of urine storage: cystometry, urodynamics, *Br J Urol* 48:39-42, 1976.
18. DuBeau CE, Resnick NM: Evaluation of the causes and severity of geriatric incontinence, *Urol Clin North Am* 18:243-256, 1991.
19. O'Donnell PD, Finan BF, Barnett T, Brookover T: Continence recovery following radical prostatectomy, *Neurourol Urodyn* 9(3):251-256, 1990.
20. Hammerer P, Schuler J, Gonnermann D, Huland H: Urodynamic parameters before and after radical prostatectomy, *J Urol* 149:235A, 1993.
21. Meyer-Moldenhauer WH: Risk factors for postprostatectomy incontinence, habilitation thesis, University of Hamburg, 1995.
22. Santorini GD: De virorum naturalibus. In *Observationes anatomicae,* Venice, 1724, Baptistam Recurti 173.
23. Müller J: *Über die organischen Nerven der erektilen männlichen Geschlechtsorgane des Menschen und der Säugetiere,* Berlin, 1836, F. Dummeler.
24. Walsh PC, Donker PJ: Impotence following radical prostatectomy: insight into etiology and prevention, *J Urol* 128:492, 1982.
25. McNeal JE: Regional morphology and pathology of the prostate, *Am J Surg Pathol* 49:347-357, 1968.
26. Lowsley OS: The development of the human prostate gland with reference to the development of other structures at the neck of the urinary bladder, *Am J Anat* 13:299, 1912.
27. Franks LM: Atrophy and hyperplasia in the prostate proper, *J Pathol Bacteriol* 63:617, 1954.
28. McNeal JE: Origin and evolution of benign prostatic enlargement, *Invest Urol* 15:340, 1978.
29. McNeal JE, Redwine EA, Freiha FS, Stamey TA: Zonal distribution of the prostatic adenocarcinoma: correlation with histologic patterns and direction of spread, *Am J Surg Pathol* 12:897-906, 1988.
30. Gosling JA, Dixon JS, Critchley HOD, Thompson SA: A comparative study of the human external sphincter and periurethral levator ani muscles, *Br J Urol* 53:35-41, 1981.
31. Oelrich TM: The striated urethral sphincter muscle in the male, *Am J Anat* 158:229-246, 1980.
32. Tanagho EA, Meyers FH, Smith DR: Urethral resistance: its components and complications. I. Smooth muscle component, *Invest Urol* 7:136-149, 1969.
33. Tanagho EA, Meyers FH, Smith DR: Urethral resistance: its components and complications. II. Striated muscle component, *Invest Urol* 7:195-205, 1969.
34. Elbadawi A, Schenk EA: A new theory of the innervation of bladder musculature. Part 4. Innervation of the vesicurethral junction and external urethral sphincter, *J Urol* 111:613-615, 1974.
35. Myers RP: Male urethral sphincteric anatomy and radical prostatectomy, *Urol Clin North Am* 18:211-214, 1991.
36. Steers WD: Physiology of the urinary bladder In Walsh PC, Retik AB, Stamey TA, Vaughan ED Jr, editors: *Campbell's urology,* ed 6, vol 1, Philadelphia, 1992, Saunders.
37. Berry SJ, Coffey DS, Walsh PC: The development of human benign prostatic hyperplasia with age, *J Urol* 132:474-479, 1984.
38. Lepor H: Role of long-acting selective alpha-1 blockers in the treatment of benign prostatic hyperplasia, *Urol Clin North Am* 17:651, 1990.
39. Finasteride Study Group: Finasteride (MK-906) in the treatment of benign prostatic hyperplasia, *Prostate* 22:291-299, 1993.
40. Berges RR, Windeler J, Trampisch HJ, Senge T: Randomized, placebo-controlled, double-blind clinical trial of beta-sitosterol in patients with benign prostatic hyperplasia, *Lancet* 345:1529-1532, 1995.
41. Mebust WK, Holtgrewe HL, Cockett ATK, et al: Transurethral prostatectomy: immediate and postoperative complications: a cooperative study of 13 participating institutions evaluating 3885 patients, *J Urol* 141:243-247, 1989.
42. Dowd JE, Smith JJ: Balloon dilation of the prostate, *Urol Clin North Am* 17:671, 1990.
43. Costello AJ, Bowsher WG, Bolton DM, et al.: Laser ablation of the prostate in patients with benign prostatic hypertrophy, *Br J Urol* 69:603, 1992.
44. Eardley I, Fitzpatrick J, Frick J, et al: TUNA therapy for symptomatic benign prostatic hyperplasia: a collaborative European trial, *J Urol* 153:533A, 1995.
45. Stewart SC, Benjamin D, Weil D, et al: Electro-vaporization of the prostate: a pilot study, *J Urol* 153:437A, 1995.
46. Linder A, Golomb J, Siegel Y, Lev A: Local hyperthermia of the prostate gland for the treatment of benign postatic hypertrophy and urinary retention: a preliminary report, *Br J Urol* 60:567-571, 1987.

47. Madersbacher S, Klingler HC, Schmidbauer CP, Marberger M: The impact of transrectal high intensity focused ultrasound on prostate obstruction in BPH assessed by pressure flow studies, *J Urol* 153:435A, 1995.
48. Turner-Warwick R: The sphincter mechanisms: their relation to prostatic enlargement and its treatment. In Hinman F Jr, editor: *Benign prostatic hypertrophy,* New York, 1983, Springer-Verlag.
49. Khan Z, Mieza M, Starer P, Singh VK: Post-prostatectomy incontinence, *Urology* 38:483-488, 1991.
50. Fitzpatrick JM, Gardina RA, Worth PHL: The evaluation of 68 patients with postprostatectomy incontinence, *Br J Urol* 51: 552-555, 1979.
51. Freyer PJ: A new method of performing prostatectomy, *Lancet* 1:774, 1900.
52. Millin T: Retropubic prostatectomy: new extravesical technique: report on 20 cases, *Lancet* 2:693, 1945.
53. Nanninga JB: Some aspects of striated urethral sphincter structure and function, *J Urol* 152:2321-2323, 1994.
54. Orihuela E, Motamedi M, Pow-Sang M, et al: Histopathological evaluation of laser thermocoagulation in human prostate: optimizing of laser irradiation for benign prostatic hyperplasia, *J Urol* 153:1531-1536, 1995.
55. Kabalin JN, Gill HS: Urolase laser prostatectomy in patients on warfarin anticoagulation: a safe treatment alternative for bladder outlet obstruction, *Urology* 42:738, 1993.
56. Kabalin JN, Gill HS, Bite G, Wolfe V: Comparative study of laser versus electrocautery prostatic resection: 18-month followup with complex urodynamic assessment, *J Urol* 153:94-98, 1995.
57. Frohmüller H, Wirth M: Selection criteria for radical prostatectomy with reference to long-term results, *Urologe* A 30:394-400, 1991.
58. Reiner WB, Walsh PC: An anatomical approach to the surgical management of the dorsal vein and Santorini's plexus during radical retropubic surgery, *J Urol* 121:198, 1979.
59. Paulson DF: Technique of radical perineal prostatectomy. In Skinner DG, Lieskovsky G, editors: *Diagnosis and management of genitourinary cancer,* Philadelphia, 1988, Saunders.
60. Villers A, McNeal JE, Redwine EA, et al: The role of perineural space invasion in the local spread of prostatic adenocarcinoma, *J Urol* 142:763-768, 1989.
61. Walsh PC: Radical retropubic prostatectomy. In Walsh PC, Retik AB, Stamey TA, Vaughan ED Jr, editors: *Campbell's urology,* ed 6, vol 3, Philadelphia, 1992, Saunders.
62. Rudy DC, Woodside JR, Crawford ED: Urodynamic evaluation of incontinence in patients undergoing modified Campbell radical retropubic prostatectomy: a prospective study, *J Urol* 132:708-712, 1984.
63. Vest SA: Radical perineal prostatectomy: modification of closure, *Surg Gynecol Obstet* 70:935, 1940.
64. Malizia AA, Banks DW, Newton E et al: Modified radical retropubic prostatectomy: double continence technique, *J Urol* 141:316A, 1989.
65. Hauri D: Urinary continence after radical prostatectemy: the urodynamic proof of an anatomical hypothesis, *Urol Int* 32:149-160, 1977.
66. Klein EA: Early continence after radical prostatectomy, *J Urol* 148:92-95, 1992.
67. Vest SA: Radical perineal prostatectomy: modification of closure, *Surg Gynecol Obstet* 70:935, 1940.
68. Malizia AA, Banks DW, Newton E, et al: Modified radical retropubic prostatectomy: double continence technique, *J Urol* 141:316A, 1989.
69. Hauri D: Urinary continence after radical prostatectomy: the urodynamic proof of an anatomical hypothesis, *Urol Int* 32:149-160, 1977.
70. Presti JC, Schmidt RA, Narayan PA, et al: Pathophysiology of urinary incontinence after radical prostatectomy, *J Urol* 143:975-978, 1990.
71. Breul J, Hofmann R, Block T, Hartung R: Tubularized neourethra for bladder neck reconstruction after radical prostatectomy: implications for urinary continence and bladder neck contracture (abstract 1046), *J Urol* 151:489A, 1994.
72. Steiner MS, Milam DF, Nashville TN: Urodynamic evaluation of patients who had a tubularized neourethra bladder reconstruction following radical retropubic prostatectomy, *J Urol* 153:383A (suppl), 1995.
73. Wein AJ: Editorial comment, *J Urol* 145:514, 1991.
74. Myers RP: Radical retropubic prostatectomy: balance between preserving urinary continence and achievement of negative margins, *Eur Urol* 27:32-33, 1995.
75. Myers RP: Improving the exposure of the prostate in radical retropubic prostatectomy: longitudinal bunching of the deep venous plexus, *J Urol* 142:1282, 1989.
76. Stamey TA: The Stanford radical retropubic prostatectomy, *J Urol* 145:49A-V-42, 1992.
77. Huland H: Morphologische Grundlagen zur radikalen Prostatektomie, *Urologe* A 30:61-369, 1991.
78. Stamey TA: Techniques for avoiding positive surgical margins during radical prostatectomy, *Atlas Urol Clin North Am* 2:37-51, 1994.
79. Miller RJ, Cohen JK, Merlotti LS: Percutaneous transperineal cryosurgical ablation of the prostate for the primary treatment of clinical Stage C adenocarcinoma of the prostate, *Urology* 44:170-174, 1994.
80. Onik GM, Cohen JK, Reyes GD, et al: Transrectal ultrasound-guided percutaneous radical cryosurgical ablation of the prostate, *Cancer* 72:1291-1299, 1993.
81. Cox RL, Crawford ED: Complications of cryosurgical ablation of the prostate to treat localized adenocarcinoma of the prostate, *Urology* 45:932-935, 1995.
82. Stamey TA, Kabalin JN, McNeal JE, et al: Prostate specific antigen in the diagnosis and treatment of adenocarcinoma of the prostate. II. Radical prostatectomy treated patients, *J Urol* 141:1076-1083, 1989.
83. Wassermann NF, Kapoor DA, Hildebrandt WC, et al: Transrectal US in evaluation of patients after radical prostatectomy. I. Normal postoperative anatomy, *Radiology* 185:361-366, 1992.
84. Bates G, Bradley WE, Glen E, et al: Fourth report on the standardization of the of terminology of lower urinary tract function: terminology related to neuromuscular dysfunction of the lower urinary tract, *Br J Urol* 53:333-335, 1981.
85. O'Donnell PD, Brookover T, Hewett M, Al-Juburi AZ: Continence level following radical prostatectomy, *Urology* 36:511-512, 1990.
86. Leach GE, Yip CM, Donovan BJ: Post-prostatectomy incontinence: the influence of bladder dysfunction, *J Urol* 138: 574-578, 1987.
87. Chao R, Mayo ME: Incontinence after radical prostatectomy: detrusor or sphincter causes, *J Urol* 154:16-18, 1995.
88. Hutch JA, Fisher R: Continence after radical prostatectomy, *Br J Urol* 40:62-67, 1968.
89. Hellström P, Lukkarinen O, Konturi M: Urodynamics in radical retropubic prostatectomy, *Scand J Urol Nephrol* 23:21, 1989.
90. Hammerer P, Dieringer J, Schuler J, et al: Urodynamic parameters to predict continence after radical prostatectomy, *J Urol* 145:292A, 1991.
91. Narayan P, Konety B, Aslam K, et al: Neuroanatomy of the external sphincter: implications for urinary continence preservation during radical prostatectomy, *J Urol* 153:337-341, 1995.
92. Andersen JT: Detrusor hyper-reflexia in benign infravesical obstruction, a cystometric study, *J Urol* 115:532, 1976.
93. Abrams P, Blaivas JG, Stanton SL, Andersen JT: The standardization of terminology of lower urinary tract function, *Scand J Urol Nephrol* 114(suppl):5, 1988.
94. Jones KW, Schönberg HW: Comparison of the incidence of bladder hyper-reflexia in patients with benign prostatic hypertrophy and age matched female controls, *J Urol* 133:425, 1985.
95. Constantinou CE, Freiha FS: Impact of radical prostatectomy on the characteristics of bladder and urethra, *J Urol* 148:1215-1220, 1992.
96. Foote J, Yun S, Leach GE: Postprostatectomy incontinence: pathophysiology, evaluation, and management, *Urol Clin North Am* 18:229-241, 1991.
97. Kerr LA, Zincke H: Radical retropubic prostatectomy for prostate cancer and the elderly and the young: complications and prognosis, *Eur Urol* 25:305-312, 1994.

98. Middleton AW Jr: Radical prostatectomy for carcinoma in men more than 69 years old, *J Urol* 138:1185-1188, 1987.
99. O'Donnell PD, Finan BF: Continence following nerve-sparing radical prostatectomy, *J Urol* 142:1227-1229, 1989.
100. Nichols RT, Barry JM, Hodges CV: The morbidity of radical prostatectomy for multifocal stage I prostatic adenocarcinoma, *J Urol* 117:83, 1977.
101. Bass RB, Barrett DM: Radical retropubic prostatectomy after transurethral prostatic resection, *J Urol* 124:495, 1980.
102. Lindner A, deKernion JB, Smith RB, Katske FA: Risk of urinary incontinence following radical prostatectomy, *J Urol* 129:1007, 1983.
103. Neerhut GJ, Wheeler T, Cantini M: Salvage radical prostatectomy for radiorecurrent adenocarcinoma of the prostate, *J Urol* 140:544, 1988.
104. Rainwater LM, Zincke H: Radical prostatectomy after radiation therapy for cancer of the prostate: feasibility and prognosis, *J Urol* 140:1455, 1988.
105. Pavlakis AJ, Siroky MB, Goldstein I, Krane RJ: Neurourologic findings in Parkinson's disease, *J Urol* 129:80, 1983.
106. Staskin DS, Vardi Y, Siroky MB: Post-prostatectomy continence in the parkinsonian patient: the significance of poor voluntary sphincter control, *J Urol* 140:17, 1988.

Chapter 45

Urinary Incontinence after Pelvic Surgery

Michael P. Aronson, Grannum R. Sant

Voiding dysfunction, including urinary incontinence, is a recognized complication of pelvic visceral ablative and reconstructive surgery.[1-3] As such, the primary care physician is liable to be faced with incontinent patients after major colorectal or gynecologic surgery. An understanding of the pathogenesis of incontinence after pelvic surgery as well as a patient-focused, cost-effective approach to diagnosis and treatment is essential.

Abdominoperineal resection (APR) is still the most frequent operation used in the treatment of rectal cancer, though mechanical stapling techniques, new anastomotic techniques (such as a coloanal anastomosis), and the use of adjuvant radiation and chemotherapy have increased the number of sphincter-saving and local excision procedures done for lower gastrointestinal tract cancer.[4] Improvements in the early diagnosis of rectal cancer, surgical technique, and postoperative care have increased the survival of patients undergoing major rectal surgery. Urinary incontinence occurring after gynecologic surgery such as radical hysterectomy, benign hysterectomy, or incontinence and prolapse surgery is not uncommon. Gynecologic surgical procedures deep in the female pelvis often involve dissection or extirpation of genital tract structures that are in intimate anatomic contact with the lower urinary tract. Anatomic support, neurologic and vascular supply, and the ureters, bladder, or urethra as well can be damaged resulting in postoperative urinary incontinence.[3,5] Urinary incontinence after gynecologic surgery is of multifactorial cause. However, whether attributable to stress urinary incontinence, detrusor instability, overflow incontinence, or extraurethral incontinence, it is all the same to the patient: leaking urine!

Although adequate tumor removal, organ removal, or cure of incontinence or prolapse is the primary goal of surgery, the functional outcomes and quality of life in patients after pelvic surgery are clearly important, particularly with respect to sexual function and voiding dysfunction.[5] To avoid postoperative disappointment, all patients undergoing major pelvic surgery should be counselled preoperatively regarding the risk of postoperative incontinence.

The cause of voiding symptoms after abdominoperineal resection, low anterior resection, and radical cancer surgery in women (such as radical hysterectomy) is multifactorial. In men with benign prostatic hyperplasia (BPH), bladder outlet obstruction from the enlarged prostate gland ("mechanical" obstruction) or increased sympathetic adrenergic tone in the prostatic smooth muscle and bladder neck ("dynamic" obstruction) can lead to obstructive voiding symptoms with or without urinary retention. Disturbances of the anatomic relationship between the bladder and sphincters as a result of the loss of posterior support (as after anteroposterior resection, posterior pelvic exenteration) can result in angulation deformities, clinical voiding difficulties, and incontinence in both sexes.

Lower Urinary Tract Innervation

Pelvic nerve damage with surgical denervation of the bladder and urethra is a major component of the postoperative voiding milieu after pelvic extirpative surgery.[7] The lower urinary tract—bladder and urethra—is innervated by the autonomic (parasympathetic, sympathetic) and somatic nervous systems (see box). The parasympathetic pelvic nerves arise from the sacral segments S2-S4 and join branches of the hypogastric nerve (sympathetic innervation) in the presacral area to form the inferior hypogastric plexus (mixed, meaning sympathetic and parasympathetic fibers). This plexus is then oriented parasagittally on either side of the rectum, uterine cervix, vaginal fornix, and posterior aspect of the bladder and extends into the base of the broad ligament of the uterus. Injury to the inferior hypogastric plexus, by transection, traction (neurapraxia), tumor infiltration, or inflammation or infection results in various degrees of nerve injury and voiding dysfunction.[8]

The sympathetic innervation of the lower urinary tract is from the thoracolumbar outflow at T10-L2, which forms the superior hypogastric plexus at the level of the pelvic brim and sacral promontory. This plexus is at risk during (1) dissection of the middle rectal arteries at the time of anteroposterior resec-

Lower Genitourinary Tract Innervation

AUTONOMIC PARASYMPATHETIC (S2-S4)
Motor function
Pelvic plexus
Emptying function
AUTONOMIC SYMPATHETIC (T10-L2)
Outlet resistance
Hypogastric plexus
Storage function
SOMATIC (S2-S4)
External striated sphincter
Pudendal nerve
Continence

tion, and (2) retroperitoneal, periaortic lymphadenectomy for pelvic and gynecologic malignancies. Damage to the sympathetic autonomic nervous system reduces the tone and pressures in the bladder neck and the proximal portion of the urethra leading to urgency, frequency, and incontinence. In contrast, parasympathetic denervation results in reduced bladder muscle contractility (hyporeflexia or areflexia) because of lack of cholinergic stimulation. Not infrequently, both the sympathetic and parasympathetic innervation are damaged during pelvic surgery resulting in variable and sometimes unpredictable postoperative voiding symptoms.[2]

Furthermore, in anteroposterior resection the somatic pudendal nerve may be injured during the perineal mobilization of the anus.[9] The pudendal nerve innervates the external striated (voluntary) sphincter in the membranous urethra, and pudendal nerve damage can lead to sphincter compromise and urinary incontinence. The nature of any neurologic lesion to the bladder, urethra, or external sphincter is difficult to predict and is a result of a complex assortment of partial or complete parasympathetic, sympathetic, or somatic denervations. Locally aggressive pelvic visceral tumors may infiltrate the pelvic and hypogastric plexuses and cause preoperative vesicourethral functional derangement.[10]

COLORECTAL SURGERY

The reported incidence of bladder dysfunction after anteroposterior resection for rectal cancer is extremely variable. This variability is attributable to inconsistency of study designs (prospective versus retrospective, selective versus nonselective patients, early versus late timing, the type of study performed, such as urodynamic or questionnaire, and so forth). Earlier studies reported high rates of motor (parasympathetic) denervation approximating 60%,[11,12] but over the first 6-month postoperative period many patients (about 25%) improve spontaneously.[8,9] Obstructive voiding symptoms (slow stream, intermittency, and so forth) and urinary retention occur more commonly than irritative voiding symptoms (urgency, frequency, urge incontinence) and urinary incontinence. In the aggregate, urinary symptoms are most pronounced in the early postoperative period but tend to subside over time.

Postoperative bladder emptying can be impaired by bladder outlet obstruction secondary to benign prostatic hyperplasia (BPH) in men, and a sizable number of men (20% to 30%) with voiding dysfunction after anteroposterior resection require definitive treatment for BPH, such as transurethral resection or pharmacologic therapy with 5-alpha-reductase inhibitors, such as finasteride (Proscar) or alpha-adrenergic sympathetic blockers such as terazosin HCl (Hytrin) or doxazosin mesylate (Cardura). The likelihood of parasympathetic motor compromise of the bladder is increased with tumor extent; that is, it is greater with circumferential, posterior tumors and the radicality of surgery (difficult dissection plane presacrally because of edema, tumor infiltration, infection, and so forth), and it varies according to the experience and expertise of the surgeon.

Recent prospective studies of voiding dysfunction after anteroposterior resection indicate that motor (parasympathetic) denervation of the bladder occurs less frequently than previously reported.[6,13] At 6 months, the incidence approximates 30%, falling to 7.5% to 12% at 1 year. The return of bladder function with time may be attributable to incomplete nerve damage at the time of surgery or nerve regeneration. Motor denervation leads to increased postvoid residuals, frequency, reduced urinary streams, urinary tract infections, and even retention with overflow ("overflow incontinence"). The incidence of motor bladder dysfunction occurring after low anterior resection is less than that after anteroposterior resection.[8,14]

Although the commonest bladder dysfunction after anteroposterior resection is retention with obstructive voiding symptoms, some patients complain of frequency, urgency, and incontinence. Approximately 9% to 17% of patients develop incontinence after anteroposterior or low anterior resection.[10] The risk of incontinence is higher in women than in men (about 3:1) because of the ameliorating effects of the prostate in men. Correspondingly, retention and impaired voiding is more common in men.

Sympathetic nerve compromise to the bladder neck and the proximal part of the urethra results in reduced urethral pressures, bladder neck incompetence, and urinary incontinence. Videourodynamic assessment of the urethral pressure profile (UPP) after anteroposterior resection demonstrated universal evidence of sympathetic denervation (that is, open bladder neck during bladder filling, isobaric pressures in the proximal 1 to 2 cm of the urethra) in a small, selected group of patients referred for postoperative urodynamic studies.[9] Sympathetic denervation may also occur after radical hysterectomy, depending on the extent of the surgical dissection in the vicinity of the cardinal ligaments. Damage to the external striated somatic sphincter also contributes to the likelihood of urinary incontinence. Such damage, usually occurring after anteroposterior resection, results in denervation of the sphincter with loss of urethral closure pressures and incontinence. Somatic nerve damage (pudendal nerve) is nearly always incomplete, and restoration of somatic sphincter muscle activity with time is responsible for the return of active and passive continence in the majority of patients.[2,9]Although incontinence is nearly always secondary to urethral and bladder neck incompetence (damage to the sympathetic and somatic nerves), it occasionally is attributable to parasympathetic nerve damage. Motor denervation, if severe and compounded by outlet obstruction caused by prostatic enlargement, can lead to urinary retention and "overflow" incontinence.[12,15] Motor denervation incontinence (parasympathetic injury) can be distinguished from sympathetic or somatic induced incontinence by the results of measuring the postvoid residual urine volumes.

Another cause of urgency, frequency, and urge incontinence after pelvic visceral surgery is detrusor instability (DI). This is characterized by an overactive bladder detrusor muscle that contracts at low bladder volumes leading to sudden urges to urinate, with urgency and urge incontinence. Some men with BPH have associated detrusor instability (10% to 20%), which can lead to postoperative (as in anteroposterior resection) incontinence, especially if the urethral pressures are low as a result of sympathetic or somatic nerve compromise. The development of de novo detrusor instability is another possibility, especially after gynecologic pelvic surgery, as with Burch and Stamey bladder neck suspensions. A recent careful literature review of patients undergoing careful preoperative and postoperative urodynamic evaluation demonstrated a prevalence of de novo detrusor instability of 17% (range 5% to 27%) after antiincontinence surgery.[16] The exact pathophysiologic mechanism for the development of detrusor instability is unknown, though obstruction, nerve damage during the surgical dissection, prior pelvic surgery, and so forth have all been implicated.[2,16] Therefore prediction of the development of DI in an individual patient is difficult. A sizable proportion of patients with stress incontinence have associated DI ("mixed") incontinence, and precolposuspension DI may be worsened postoperatively.

Radical Hysterectomy

Radical hysterectomy for the treatment of cervical cancer is associated with postoperative voiding dysfunction, including incontinence. Lower urinary tract function is affected by direct surgical trauma to the bladder wall and surrounding vascular and lymphatic structures as well as disruption of the autonomic innervation to the bladder and urethra. If prolonged urinary drainage is not provided to address postoperative bladder hypotonia, the additional problems of bladder overdistension and urinary infection may lead to loss of bladder wall compliance and overflow incontinence.

The degree of dysfunction is directly related to the extent of the dissection and excision of the posterolateral aspects of the cardinal-uterosacral ligament complex.[5] The pelvic plexus of sympathetic and parasympathetic nerves courses through these tissues to pass laterally and anteriorly to the upper third of the vagina as it innervates the bladder and urethra. As surgical radicality increases to include pararectal tissue, the risk of parasympathetic nerve damage increases.[8] Illustrating that preservation of the posterolateral tissues preserves function, Manzl et al. found a 1-year postoperative incontinence rate after Wertheim radical hysterectomy of 4% compared with a rate of 27% with the more radical Latsko radical hysterectomy.[17] Prolonged bladder drainage with a suprapubic catheter provides the best chance for optimizing recovery of bladder function after radical hysterectomy.

Posterior exenteration, with removal of the anorectum and excision of the uterus with wide margins of the cardinal-uterosacral ligaments, is often complicated by urinary incontinence. Additionally, removal of the posterior pelvic structures from behind the bladder, and possible damage to the pudendal innervation of the pelvic floor musculature may lead to pelvic floor prolapse and incontinence. Radical vulvectomy can contribute to pelvic floor prolapse and incontinence through excision of perineal musculature as well as damage to the nerve and blood supply to the area.[18] Additionally, if because of tumor location it is necessary to remove the distal portion of the urethra, overall intrinsic urethral function may be adversely affected.

Hysterectomy for Benign Disease

Abdominal and vaginal hysterectomy for benign disease has been associated with postoperative urinary symptoms including incontinence.[1] However, this relationship is far from clear. Postoperative urinary incontinence is highly dependent on its preoperative presence. There is a statistically significant increase in the prevalence of dysfunctional urinary symptoms, including incontinence, in patients scheduled for benign hysterectomy as compared to the general population.[19,20] Although some patients will have their incontinence resolve postoperatively and others will develop it, the continence status of the majority of patients remains unchanged.[3] Most patients with significant preoperative urinary incontinence will remain incontinent after benign hysterectomy unless a specific procedure, such as bladder neck suspension, is added to address their incontinence. This has also been shown with radical hysterectomy.[21] In summary, the removal of the uterus for benign disease does not in itself cause postoperative urinary incontinence.[22]

Whereas disruption of innervation to the bladder and urethra is a feature of radical hysterectomy that contributes to incontinence, no such alteration has been demonstrated with benign hysterectomy.[23,24] Both abdominal and vaginal hysterectomy avoid dissection of the pelvic plexus as it travels around and over the upper third of the vagina on its way to the bladder and urethra. In radical hysterectomy this area is disrupted, and the upper third of the vagina and much of the parametrial tissue are excised. In benign hysterectomy (transabdominal or transvaginal), direct surgical trauma to the bladder is minimal and the vascularity and lymphatic drainage of the bladder neck area are essentially left intact.

Urodynamic studies after radical hysterectomy have demonstrated bladder denervation reflected in an altered sense (or unawareness) of filling and emptying, elevated postvoid residual volumes, decreased flow rates, and decreased urethral pressures.[25] Similar studies after benign hysterectomy revealed only a transient decrease in bladder capacity with no change in sensory or motor function.[26,27] When an intrafascial transabdominal technique was used, there was no decrease in bladder capacity, implying that the minimal direct surgical trauma involved in the extrafascial technique is responsible for a transient decrease in postoperative capacity.[28]

Denervation of the urogenital tract and pelvic floor musculature may play a larger role in incontinence and pelvic floor prolapse than previously thought.[29] Urodynamic differences may not be apparent in patients undergoing nonradical hysterectomy because nerve routes are not disrupted, or the denervation injury may be subtle and missed when one is measuring end-organ bladder function. Recently, direct neurologic measurement of sacral reflex latencies demonstrated motor and sensory denervation in 31% of previously normal patients after benign hysterectomy.[30] Benson and McClellan noted statistically significant increases in pudendal or perineal nerve terminal motor latencies in 74% of women operated on vaginally for prolapse and 33% of those operated on abdominally for the same problem.[31] An intact innervation of the female urogenital tract and pelvic floor musculature is essential for pelvic organ support as well as urinary and fecal continence.[32] Nerve damage, whether by parturition or through pelvic surgery, is a topic of increasing concern and research study.

INCONTINENCE AND PROLAPSE SURGERY

Urinary incontinence can persist, recur, or arise de novo after surgical procedures intended to treat stress urinary incontinence. Patients perceive their operations as failures if they continue to leak urine, regardless of the cause. A common cause of operative "failure" is an incorrect diagnosis of the type of incontinence the patient has. The patient with detrusor instability will not be cured and may be made worse by an operation for stress urinary incontinence. Patients with "mixed" urinary incontinence (stress urinary incontinence and detrusor instability) will have a 40% to 45% rate of persistence of their detrusor instability after surgical cure of their stress incontinence.[33] Even patients with pure stress urinary incontinence have a 6% to 20% rate of de novo development of detrusor instability after successful stress incontinence surgery.[34,35] Overcorrection of bladder neck descent with a suspension operation can cause detrusor instability or, in the worst case, iatrogenic obstruction with urinary retention, overflow incontinence, and possible injury secondary to bladder overdistension.[36]

Accurate preoperative diagnosis of the cause of a patient's urinary leakage is essential before treatment, be it surgical or otherwise. The patient undergoing surgery for stress incontinence needs to be informed not only of the failure rate of the proposed operation, but also of the possibility of persistent or de novo detrusor instability. Over 200 operations have been described for the surgical treatment of stress urinary incontinence, indicating that there is no one best operation. The main surgical objective is resuspension and stabilization of the patient's usually hypermobile bladder neck to a retropubic, intra-abdominal position. Reported surgical success rates vary and depend on the long-term accomplishment of this objective.[37] True operative failures are those in which stress urinary incontinence persists or recurs shortly after surgery. One group of patients are at particular risk for failure after standard incontinence procedures. These patients have a urethra that can no longer generate its own inherent pressure—a low-pressure urethra, or intrinsic sphincter deficiency. Patients with intrinsic sphincter deficiency have an objective cure rate after Burch colposuspension of only 46%, compared to 82% in patients with normal urethral pressures.[38] Failed previous incontinence surgery, especially anterior colporrhaphy, predisposes patients to sphincter deficiency. Accurate preoperative urodynamic identification of these patients by urethral pressure profilometry and leak point pressure determination allows treatment with a high degree of success utilizing retropubic sling procedures if bladder neck hypermobility coexists, or periurethral bulk collagen injections if the bladder neck is nonmobile.

Patients with pronounced degrees of urogenital prolapse may or may not have coexistent stress urinary incontinence. Those who are continent may have "potential," or "occult," incontinence. Prolapse of the bladder may cause kinking, which increases the urethral pressures to keep the patient continent.[39] If the prolapse is reduced manually by pessary or surgically, the extra boost to urethral pressures is lost, and stress urinary incontinence may be unmasked.[40] Preoperatively it is important to evaluate patients with prolapse for occult incontinence so that a bladder neck suspension can be added, if needed.

UROGENITAL FISTULA

Not all urinary incontinence occurring after gynecologic surgery occurs through the urethra. Intraoperative injury to the ureters, bladder, or urethra can result in extraurethral incontinence because of fistulas. Ureteral injury occurs in approximately 0.5% of major gynecologic procedures.[41] Bladder injuries are more common occurring in 1.8% of abdominal hysterectomies and 0.4% of vaginal hysterectomies.[42] If these injuries are recognized intraoperatively and repaired, a good surgical outcome is almost universal. When an injury goes unnoticed, or a repair breaks down, a urogenital fistula can result.

Vesicovaginal fistula is the most common urogenital fistula in women. Although the incidence has been reported as low as 0.02% after major pelvic operations, it has been noted that 80% of vesicovaginal fistulas in the Western world result from gynecologic surgery for benign conditions such as menorrhagia, fibroids, and uterovaginal prolapse.[43] The remainder result after obstetric procedures, or surgical or radiation treatment of pelvic malignancies. In developing countries, most vesicovaginal fistulas are of obstetric origin and are much more severe. Approximately 20% of small, early, postoperative fistulas heal spontaneously with prolonged bladder drainage. The remainder require surgical correction. Most vesicovaginal fistulas can be repaired transvaginally with success rates approaching 95%.[44]

Other urogenital fistulas occur less commonly. Ureterovaginal fistulas can result from overzealous skeletonizing of the ureters during radical hysterectomy, though most ureterovaginal fistulas develop after surgery for benign gynecologic conditions. Urethrovaginal fistulas occur after urethral diverticulum repair, breakdown of anterior vaginal repair, or obstetric procedures. Lastly, vesicouterine fistula can occur after bladder injury at the time of cesarean section. All these extraurethral causes of urinary incontinence require surgical correction.

Voiding dysfunction is therefore a recognized complication of pelvic visceral surgery, such as anteroposterior resection, low anterior resection, and radical hysterectomy.[8,9,25] Overall, parasympathetic nerve damage appears to be the most common neurourologic lesion, though some studies suggest a high incidence of sympathetic nervous system involvement. Damage to the somatic pudendal nerve may occur after anteroposterior resection or posterior pelvic exenteration, and its incidence is directly related to the extent of the surgical dissection of the anus in the perineum. Motor (parasympathetic) denervation occurs more frequently after anteroposterior resection and radical hysterectomy than after simple hysterectomy, proctocolectomy, or low anterior resection of the rectum.[45] Earlier reports in the literature of a high incidence of postoperative bladder dysfunction after anteroposterior resection have not been corroborated by recent, prospective studies.[6,13]

The risk of nerve damage to the bladder, proximal portion of the urethra, and external striated urethral sphincter is increased in high-stage infiltrative tumors, tumors close to the anal verge, and circumferential tumors involving the posterior rectal wall. A significant percentage of men with bladder dysfunction—obstructive voiding symptoms and urinary retention—after anteroposterior resection and so forth will require definitive treatment for (BPH) in the postoperative period. Some of these men would have had symptoms of "prostatism" (frequency, nocturia, altered stream, hesitancy, and so forth) before their surgery, and these patients should be carefully counseled preoperatively regarding the likelihood of postoperative retention, need for prostate surgery, and so forth. Locally extensive tumors may cause voiding symptoms as a result of the mechanical effect of the tumor or involvement of the pelvic sympathetic and parasympathetic nerves supplying the bladder and urethra. Timely preoperative urologic evaluation and urodynamic assessment will identify such patients and alert the colorectal surgeon to the possibility of local tumor extension and the risk of postoperative voiding problems.

Urinary incontinence complicating gynecologic surgery is not uncommon. Total abdominal or vaginal hysterectomy done for benign indications do not usually cause incontinence. However, radical hysterectomy, with its wider field of dissection and excision, can lead to a denervated bladder and overflow incontinence.[5] Procedures for stress urinary incontinence can fail leaving persistent or recurrent stress incontinence, or they can appear to fail secondary to persistent, recurrent, or de novo detrusor instability.[16,46] Overcorrection of a bladder neck support defect can constitute a functional outlet obstruction and may lead to detrusor instability, urinary retention, and overflow incontinence. Intraoperative urinary tract injury can result in urogenital fistula formation. Patients should be informed of these possible complications before their gynecologic surgical procedures.

The pathogenesis of voiding dysfunction after pelvic surgery is clearly multifactorial (see box). Local tissue effects such as edema, inflammation, tumor involvement, mechanical factors caused by alterations in bladder supports and angulations, and neurologic compromise (autonomic, somatic), contribute to the development of retention, poor voiding, urgency, and incontinence in the postoperative period. Fortunately, many of these symptoms resolve within the first 6 months of surgery, possibly because of nerve regeneration,[47] and treatment decisions should take this into consideration. Thus irreversible therapeutic interventions should be delayed until the vesicourethral dysfunction stabilizes.[9]

Evaluation of Incontinence after Pelvic Surgery

Urinary incontinence after major pelvic surgery (gynecologic or colorectal) occurs less frequently than (approximately half as often as) urinary retention, poor urinary flow, and so on. However, some patients, especially men with coexisting BPH, develop paradoxical incontinence ("overflow incontinence") as a result of bladder muscle motor (parasympathetic) denervation. Patients with overflow incontinence are easily identified when their postvoid residual urine volumes and urinary flow rates are measured (see box).

The presence of urinary tract infection needs to be assessed and, if present, treated. Coexistent drug therapy also needs to be considered because some drugs, such as calcium-channel blocking agents, narcotic analgesics, and epidural anesthesia agents, reduce bladder detrusor contractility and may aggravate bladder hypotonia from surgery or autonomic denervation.[48] Furthermore, alpha-adrenergic agonists (such as ephedrine and phenylpropanolamine) used for treatment of sinusitis and allergies may increase the proximal urethral and bladder neck smooth muscle tone and put a patient into retention. Urgency, urge, and stress incontinence can be pharmacologically mediated by means of the alpha-adrenergic antagonist group of drugs such as antihypertensives, such as prazosin HCl, terazosin HCl (Hytrin), and doxazosin mesylate (Cardura). Thus a careful drug history is an important part of the assessment of patients with postoperative (colorectal and gynecologic) retention or incontinence.[48]

Urodynamic evaluation is not usually indicated in the early postoperative period[2,9] because of the multifactorial causes of the voiding dysfunction—edema, mechanical realignment of the

Pathogenesis of Voiding Dysfunction After Pelvic Surgery

LOCAL TISSUE EFFECTS
Edema
Inflammation
TUMOR EXTENT
MECHANICAL FACTORS
Bladder support
Angulation
NEUROLOGIC DAMAGE
Autonomic
Somatic
SURGICAL EXPERTISE
Antecedent pathologic conditions
Benign prostatic hyperplasia
Incontinence

Clinical Evaluation of Incontinence After Pelvic Surgery

ASSESS PREOPERATIVE SYMPTOMS
Detrusor instability
"Prostatism"
Incontinence
DIAGNOSE AND TREAT URINARY INFECTION
EXCLUDE URINARY RETENTION
Urinary flow rate (UFR)
Postvoid residual volume (PVR)
CONSIDER COEXISTENT PHARMACOLOGIC THERAPY
Calcium-channel blockers
Narcotics
Alpha-adrenergic agonists
Anticholinergics
Alpha-adrenergic blockers

pelvic structures, surgical trauma, temporary nerve compromise, and so forth.[12,49] With time, many of these factors resolve spontaneously, and bladder function returns to normal. Urodynamic studies, particularly the cystometrogram (CMG), may be indicated in instances of mixed voiding dysfunction (obstructive and irritative symptoms), pure irritative voiding dysfunction (frequency, urgency), and incontinence. Simple urodynamic evaluation, comprising a CMG, urinary flow rates, and a postvoid residual urine volume, suffices in the majority of patients (see box). Patients with retention usually can be diagnosed by measurement of the postvoid residual urine volume.

More complex videourodynamic evaluation involving external striated sphincter electromyography (EMG), urethral pressure profile, and other means is required only in patients with prolonged postoperative voiding dysfunction that has stabilized (usually months postoperatively) after major extirpative pelvic surgery such as abdominoperineal resection and radical hysterectomy.[2]

Treatment

The treatment of urinary incontinence after pelvic or colorectal surgical procedures is dependent on its causation. As a general rule, symptoms tend to subside with time, and therefore irreversible surgical procedures should be held in abeyance in the early postoperative period. Urinary retention with "overflow" incontinence is treated with clean intermittent catheterization (CIC), with or without adjunctive pharmacotherapy, such as parasympathomimetic agents, such as bethanechol chloride. Patients with significant BPH, who in the past required prostatectomy, are now treated pharmacologically, as with alpha-adrenergic blockers or 5-alpha-reductase inhibitors. An occasional patient with retention and a history of severe antecedent preoperative prostatism may require transurethral prostatic resection, ablation, or vaporization.

Most patients with postoperative incontinence have either detrusor instability (DI) (persistent or de novo) or urethral or bladder neck incompetence secondary to sympathetic or somatic denervation. DI can be treated with oral anticholinergics, such as propantheline bromide (Probanthine) and oxybutynin. Urethral incompetence can also be managed pharmacologically utilizing alpha-adrenergic agonists such as ephedrine and phenylpropylolamine. If urethral incompetence is severe and persistent, urethral sling procedures or periurethral collagen bulk injection may be needed.

Thus the majority of patients who develop urinary incontinence after pelvic surgery can be managed successfully using clean intermittent catheterization and drug therapy (parasympathomimetic alpha-agonists and anticholinergics) either singly or in combination. Surgical measures, such as slings, periurethral collagen, and prostatic resection, are required only in a small percentage of patients with prolonged (usually months) postoperative voiding dysfunction.

Urodynamic Evaluation of Incontinence After Pelvic Surgery

MAJORITY OF PATIENTS REQUIRE "SIMPLE" URODYNAMICS
Urinary flow rate (UFR)
Postvoid residuals (PVR)
Cystometrogram (CMG)
MINORITY OF PATIENTS REQUIRE "COMPLEX" URODYNAMICS
Sphincter electromyogram (EMG)
Urethral pressure profile (UPP)
Leak point pressure (LPP)

References

1. Hanley HG: The late urological complications of total hysterectomy, *Br J Urol* 41:682, 1969.
2. Yalla SV, Andriole GL: Vesicourethral dysfunction following pelvic visceral ablative surgery, *J Urol* 132:503-509, 1984.
3. Veverst HAM: Changes in the function of the lower urinary tract after hysterectomy, *Int Urogynecol J* 4:350, 1993.
4. Cunsolo A, Bragaglia RB, Manara G, et al: Urogenital dysfunction after abdominoperineal resection for carcinoma of the rectum, *Dis Colon Rectum* 33:918-922, 1990.
5. Debus-Thiede G, Maassen V, Dimpfl T, et al: [Late disorders of bladder function after Wertheim operation—an analysis of urodynamic parameters with reference to surgical radicality], *Geburtshilfe Frauenheilkd* 53(8):424, 1993.
6. Kinn AC, Ohman U: Bladder and sexual function after surgery for rectal cancer, *Dis Colon Rectum* 29:43-48, 1986.
7. Varma JS: Autonomic influences on colorectal motility and pelvic surgery, *World J Surg* 16:811-819, 1992.
8. Mundy AR: An anatomical explanation for bladder dysfunction following rectal and uterine surgery, *Br J Urol* 54:501-504, 1982.
9. Blaivas JG, Barbalias GA: Characteristics of neural injury after abdominoperineal resection, *J Urol* 129:84-87, 1983.
10. Petrelli NJ, Nagel S, Rodríguez-Bigas M, et al: Morbidity and mortality following abdominoperineal resection for rectal adenocarcinoma, *Am Surg* 59:400-404, 1993.
11. Tank ES, Ernst CB, Woolson ST, et al: Urinary tract complications of anorectal surgery, *Am J Surg* 123:118-122, 1972.
12. Fowler JW, Bremmer DN, Moffat LE: The incidence and consequences of damage to the parasympathetic nerve supply to the bladder after abdominoperineal resection of the rectum for carcinoma, *Br J Urol* 50:95-98, 1978.
13. Chang PL, Fan HA: Urodynamic abnormalities before and/or after abdominoperineal resection of the rectum for carcinoma, *J Urol* 130:948-951, 1983.
14. Neal DE, Parker AJ, Williams NS, Johnston D, et al: The long-term effects of proctectomy on bladder function in patients with inflammatory bowel disease, *Br J Surg* 69:349-352, 1982.
15. Eickenberg HU, Amin M, Klompus W, et al: Urologic complications following abdominoperineal resection, *J Urol* 115:180-182, 1976.
16. Vierhout ME, Mulder AFP: De-novo detrusor instability after Burch colposuspension, *Acta Obstet Gynecol Scand* 71:414-416, 1992.
17. Manzl J, Marberger F, Hetzel H, et al: Funktionelle Störungen des unteren Harntraktes nach Radikaloperationen des Kollumkarzinoms, *Geburtshilfe Frauenheilkd* 41:145, 1981.
18. Reid GC, DeLancy JO, Hopkins MP, et al: Urinary incontinence following radical vulvectomy, *Obstet Gynecol* 75:852, 1990.
19. Thomas TM, Plymat KR, Blannin J, Meade TW: Prevalence of urinary incontinence, *Br Med J* 281:1243, 1980.
20. Veverst HAM, et al: Micturition symptoms and urinary incontinence after non-radical hysterectomy, *Acta Obstet Gynecol Scand* 67:141, 1988.
21. Ralph G, Tamussino K, Lichtenegger W: Urodynamic following radical abdominal hysterectomy for cervical cancer, *Arch Gynecol Obstet* 243:215, 1988.
22. Griffith-Jones MD, Tuffnell D: Urinary symptoms after total abdominal hysterectomy: a review, *Int Urogynecol J* 3:61, 1992.
23. Hansen BM, Bonnesen T, Hvidberg JE, et al: Changes in symptoms and colpo-cystourethrography in 35 patients before and after total abdominal hysterectomy: a prospective study, *Urol Int* 40:224-226, 1985.

24. Veverst HAM, et al: Non-radical hysterectomy and the function of the lower urinary tract, Part II: Urodynamic quantification of changes in evacuation function, *Acta Obstet Gynecol Scand* 68:231, 1989.
25. Veverst HAM, et al: Radical hysterectomy and the function of the lower urinary tract: urodynamic quantification of changes in storage and evacuation function, *Acta Obstet Gynecol Scand* 68:331, 1989.
26. Wake CR: The immediate effect of abdominal hysterectomy on intravesical pressure and detrusor activity, *Br J Obstet Gynaecol* 87:901, 1980.
27. Stanton SL, Hilton P, Norton C, Cardozo L: Clinical and urodynamic effects of anterior colporrhaphy and vaginal hysterectomy for prolapse with and without incontinence, *Br J Obstet Gynaecol* 89:459, 1982.
28. Veverst HAM, et al: Non-radical hysterectomy and the function of the lower urinary tract, Part I: Urodynamic quantification of changes in storage function, *Acta Obstet Gynecol Scand* 68:221, 1989.
29. Smith ARB, Hosker GL, Warrell D: The role of partial denervation of the pelvic floor and the aetiology of genitourinary prolapse and stress incontinence of urine: a neurophysiological study. *Br J Obstet Gynaecol* 96:24, 1989.
30. Parys BT, Haylen BT, Hutton JL, Parson KF: The effects of simple hysterectomy on vesicourethral function, *Br J Urol* 64:594-599, 1989.
31. Benson JT, McClellan E: The effect of vaginal dissection on the pudendal nerve, *Obstet Gynecol* 82:387, 1993.
32. Swash M, Snooks SJ, Henry MM: Unifying concept of pelvic floor disorders and incontinence, *J R Soc Med* 78:906, 1985.
33. Sand PK, Bowen LW, Ostergaard DR, et al: The effect of retropubic urethropexy on detrusor instability, *Obstet Gynecol* 71:818, 1988.
34. Cardozo LD, Stanton SL, Williams JE: Detrusor instability following surgery for genuine stress incontinence, *Br J Urol* 51:204, 1979.
35. van Geelin JM, Theeuwes AG, Eskes TK, Martin CB Jr: The clinical and urodynamic effects of anterior vaginal repair and Burch colposuspension, *Am J Obstet Gynecol* 159:137, 1988.
36. Bump RC, Fantl JA, Hurt WG: Dynamic urethral pressure profilometry pressure transmission ratio determinations after continence surgery: understanding the mechanisms of success, failure and complications, *Obstet Gynecol* 72:870, 1988.
37. Bergman A, Elia G: Three surgical procedures for genuine stress incontinence: five-year follow-up of a prospective randomized study, *Am J Obstet Gynecol* 173:66, 1995.
38. Sand PK, Bowen LW, Panganiban R, Ostergard DR: The low pressure urethra as a factor in failed retropubic urethropexy, *Obstet Gynecol* 69:399, 1987.
39. Richardson DA, Bent AE, Ostergard DR: The effect of uterovaginal prolapse on urethrovesical pressure dynamics, *Am J Obstet Gynecol* 146:901, 1983.
40. Virtanen H, Hirvonen T, Mäkinen J, Kiiholma P: Outcome of thirty patients who underwent repair of posthysterectomy prolapse of the vaginal vault with abdominal sacral colpopexy, *J Am Col Surg* 178(3):283, 1994.
41. Mann WJ, Arato M, Patsner B, Stone ML: Ureteral injuries in an obstetrics and gynecology training program: etiology and management, *Obstet Gynecol* 72:82, 1988.
42. Wheelock JB, Krebs HB, Hurt WG: Sparing and repairing the bladder during gynecological surgery, *Contemp Obstet Gynecol* (6):163, 1984.
43. Lee RA, Symmonds RE, Williams TJ: Current status of genitourinary fistula, *Obstet Gynecol* 72:313, 1988.
44. Tancer ML: The post-hysterectomy (vault) vesicovaginal fistula, *J Urol* 123:839, 1980.
45. Kirkegaard P, Hjortrup A, Sanders S: Bladder dysfunction after low anterior resection for mid-rectal cancer, *Am J Surg* 141:266-268, 1981.
46. McGuire EJ: Bladder instability and stress incontinence, *Neurourol Urodyn* 7:563-567, 1988.
47. Neal DE, Bogue PR, Williams RE: Histological appearances of the nerves to the bladder in patients with denervation of the bladder after excision of the rectum, *Br J Urol* 54:658-666, 1982.
48. O'Connell HE, MacGregor RJ, Russell JM: Female urinary incontinence: management in primary care, *Med J Aust* 157:537-544, 1992.
49. Barbaric ZL, Wolfe DE, Segal AS: Urinary tract after abdominoperineal resection, *Radiology* 128:345-348, 1978.

Chapter 46

Spinal Cord Injuries

Delbert C. Rudy

The estimated annual incidence of spinal cord injury (SCI) in the Unites States is over 10,000.[1] The prevalence is estimated at over 200,000.[2] These figures highlight the clinical significance of SCI. More than half of those involved are between 16 and 35 years of age at the time of injury,[3] and more than 80% of those involved are male.[2] Thus the typical SCI patient is a young adult male.

In SCI patients, upper urinary tract disorder as the primary cause of death has been reported in 43% to 75% of such patients.[4] Such upper tract disorder is commonly a direct result of vesicourethral dysfunction secondary to the spinal cord injury. A dramatic improvement in the percentage of renal deaths in Vietnam War veterans compared to World War II and Korean War veterans is largely a result of a better understanding of the pathophysiology of bladder and urethral dysfunction after SCI.[5] This has led to therapeutic improvements that enable patients to be safely managed free of an indwelling catheter.

The key to optimum therapy of voiding dysfunction after SCI is a practical understanding of this dysfunction. The anatomic location of the injury usually gives significant clues about what to expect regarding voiding dysfunction, but urodynamic evaluation to diagnose the specific dysfunction is essential. For the SCI patient, multichannel studies that include electromyography and fluoroscopy are usually necessary. Properly performed, these studies will provide the information necessary to manage the lower urinary tract of the SCI patient regardless of the mechanism of SCI (such as trauma, tumor, vascular disease, disk disease, iatrogenic, diseases, or multiple level involvement). Unlike some common forms of urinary incontinence, the incontinence associated with SCI is more than a social problem. It often indicates inadequate lower urinary tract management, which can result in significant morbidity and mortality.

The goals of urologic management of the SCI patient are preservation of upper urinary tract function and successful management of associated urinary incontinence. A corollary to this is that the least invasive, appropriate therapeutic approach for a given SCI patient should be undertaken. The practicality and high success rate of such an approach have been documented.[6]

Acute Spinal Cord Injury

During the acute phase of spinal cord injury, lower urinary tract management usually consists of the use of an indwelling Foley catheter. Proper fluid management of these patients generally requires continuous monitoring. Typically, during the acute phase of injury, so-called spinal shock is present. This is manifested by absent or suppressed somatic and visceral reflexes mediated by spinal cord segments distal to the level of injury. The bladder is areflexic during this phase.[7] As soon as the fluid status of the patient is stabilized, the indwelling catheter should be converted to intermittent catheterization every 4 hours. Generally, residuals should be kept below 500 ml in an adult. Large fluid intakes and requirements or inadequate frequency of catheterization can lead to overflow incontinence in the spinal shock phase. Typical clinical parameters defined acutely are the level of SCI and the degree of completeness of the injury.

After a variable period of a few days to several months, reflex detrusor activity typically recovers.[8] This recovery usually occurs after return of distal somatic reflexes and onset of lower extremity spasticity with suprasacral SCI. Notable exceptions include complete sacral cord (S2-S4) injuries where reflex bladder contractions may never recover. With supraspinal SCI, resolution of spinal shock frequently coincides with the onset of incontinence. At this point, the incontinence is usually a result of detrusor hyperreflexia. Depending on the level and completeness of SCI, the patient may have definite or only vaguely associated symptoms of urgency or bladder distension. It is appropriate to carry out the initial urodynamic evaluation at this point in the evolution of SCI.

Some patients may continue in apparent spinal shock. If incontinence does not occur by 6 to 12 weeks after injury in patients with SCI, the patient should then undergo urodynamic study. Despite an apparent suprasacral cord injury, incontinence/voiding may not occur for several reasons. The frequent discoordination or dyssynergia of the external urethral sphincter during the bladder contraction may be sufficient to prevent voiding despite even a good-quality bladder contraction at small bladder volumes on an intermittent catheterization regimen. Alternatively, despite an apparent suprasacral cord injury, spinal cord infarction below the level of injury can result in an acontractile (areflexic) bladder.[9] Finally, a sacral cord injury may result in a permanently areflexic or hyporeflexic bladder.

Evolution of bladder and urethral function continues for an extended period of time after SCI. Consequently, during the first year, repetitive urodynamic studies are required to appropriately modify bladder management. This requirement is important both for complete and incomplete SCI. Although exceptions may be made for complete SCI documented by cortical evoked response testing, at least 12 to 18 months must elapse after the final spinal cord injury before permanent and stable lower urinary tract dysfunction can be assumed. However, a clear pattern of vesicourethral dysfunction is usually apparent urodynamically much earlier. Periodic monitoring of upper tract status (by upper tract imaging and the use of serum creatinine) is necessary beginning in the acute phase to help monitor the efficacy of the selected bladder management program.

Chronic Spinal Cord Injury

Established patterns of vesicourethral dysfunction usually correlate with the level of spinal cord injury. There are exceptions. Multiple cord levels may be involved. Cord infarction may result from cord injury extending the involved segment distally.[9] More than one SCI may occur over time. However, even in these complex situations, multichannel urodynamic evaluation with fluoroscopy can sort out the various components of bladder and urethral function and permit rational, optimal patient management.

SCI Above T11

A complete spinal cord injury above T11 and at or below the upper pons in the midbrain will usually result in detrusor hyperreflexia (DH) and detrusor—external sphincter dyssynergia (DESD).[10] DH is defined as bladder overactivity, or involuntary bladder contraction, as a result of a neurologic lesion.[11] DESD is defined as the involuntary contraction of the external urethral sphincter, instead of a normal relaxation, concurrent with a bladder contraction as a result of a neurologic lesion.[11] The characteristic urodynamic findings are depicted in Fig. 46-1. The typical net result is a small-capacity bladder with functional bladder outlet obstruction at the level of the membranous and bulbous urethra in the male and the distal half to third of the urethra in the female. These patients usually have intermittent incontinence with or without defined or vague symptoms of urgency or bladder distension. Initially, postvoid residuals may be small.[8] With gradual detrusor decompensation as a result of outlet obstruction, the residual increases. When the detrusor pressure at which incontinence occurs exceeds 40 cm H_2O, the risk of upper tract compromise becomes significant because ureteral peristalsis and upper urinary tract emptying becomes ineffective in the face of such detrusor pressure.[12,13] Since voiding pressures in SCI patients with DESD usually exceed 40 cm H_2O, incontinence can be used as a significant indicator that further intervention is required. Although significant upper tract damage can occur within a few months, it usually requires years.[14]

It must be noted that not all patients with DESD are certain to damage their upper tracts. A few patients, generally noncompliant or inappropriately managed, appear to defy the odds and maintain normal upper tracts without detrusor decompensation over a long period. The concept that it is the percentage of time that a patient's detrusor pressure exceeds 40 cm H_2O that significantly affects the risk for upper tract compromise has been described and is probably valid.[15] However, the concept is inadequately defined for routine clinical application. In addition, it may take 10 or more years after injury for DESD-induced upper tract compromise to become apparent radiologically. Consequently, at this point in time, DESD with voiding pressures greater than 40 cm H_2O must be assumed to place the patient at high risk for significant morbidity and mortality.

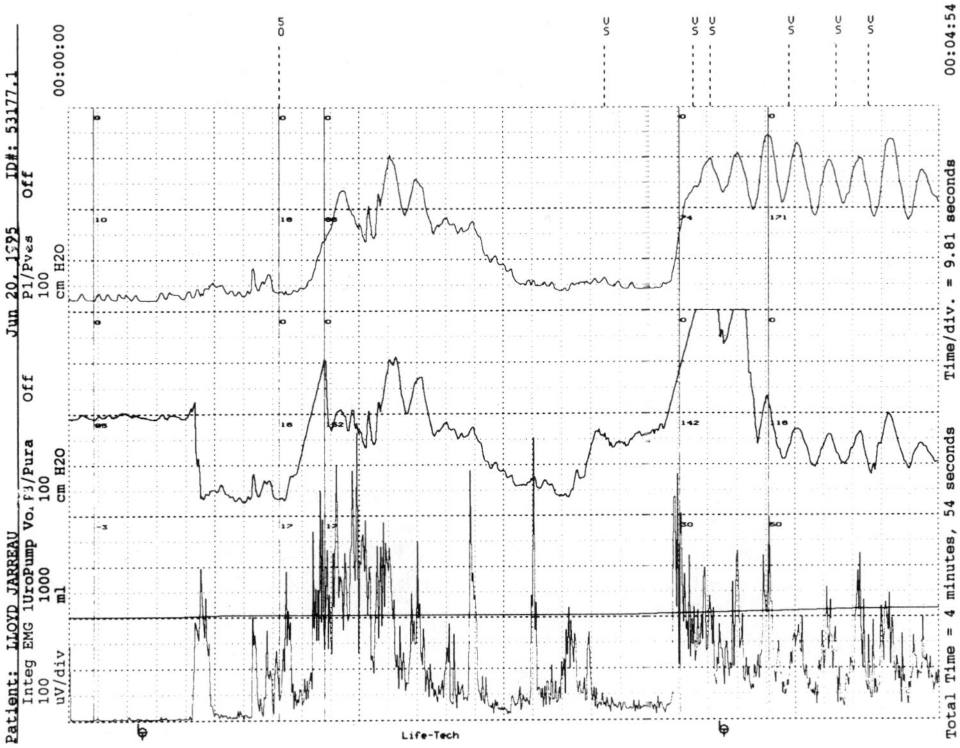

FIG. 46-1 *Multichannel urodynamic study of a 39-year-old man with C5 incomplete spinal cord injury secondary to an assault 7 years earlier.* Top tracing, *Detrusor hyperreflexia on two successive bladder fillings.* Second tracing, *Urethral pressure measurement at the membranous urethra.* Bottom tracing, *Integrated electromyographic activity from the external sphincter. Notice that as bladder pressure increases urethral pressure and EMG activity increase. This is diagnostic for detrusor–external sphincter dyssynergia.* Integ EMG, *Integrated external-sphincter electromyographic activity;* P_{ura}, *urethral pressure;* P_{ves}, *bladder pressure;* Uropump, *bladder volume.*

Optimally, therapy for SCI patients with DH and DESD is directed at the bladder (that is, the hyperreflexia). Anticholinergic therapy is administered to increase the volume threshold of the bladder at which the involuntary contraction is initiated, and clean intermittent catheterization is utilized to empty the bladder, usually every 4 hours, before DH occurs.[6] With DESD, all incontinence and voiding should be prevented. Oxybutynin is the usual drug of choice. Dosages typically start at 5 mg PO bid-tid and can be pushed as high as 40 mg/day. Side effects can limit the tolerated dosage, particularly in the older adult. Alternative anticholinergic agents that can be used alone or in combination include hyoscyamine and propantheline. The tricyclic antidepressant imipramine and the alpha$_1$-adrenergic blockers prazosin, terazosin, and doxazosin can also be useful alone or in combination with the anticholinergic agents. A variety of drugs have been utilized for intravesical instillation in patients with refractory DH. However, their use is laborious and often poorly tolerated by patient or caregivers when used on a chronic basis.

When there is failure of attempted pharmacologic control of DH, the next most practical consideration is augmentation cystoplasty. The goal of this procedure in these patients is to create a large-capacity, low-pressure reservoir for urine storage. This procedure involves isolating a bowel segment, fashioning a patch out of it, and suturing it to a generous incision in the bladder to enlarge the bladder. Although it is a major surgical procedure, success rates of 90% or better, optimally using detubularized ileum, have been reported.[16,17] This is used with clean intermittent catheterization. In obese patients and in patients with severe lower extremity spasticity, severe flexion contractures, or impaired hand function, it may not be possible to catheterize through the urethra, particularly in women. An augmentation cystoplasty with continent abdominal wall stoma, with or without bladder neck or urethral closure, may still permit intermittent catheterization by the patient or caregivers. Obviously this is a more complicated procedure. In addition, stomal problems result in a significant reoperation rate (6%).[17] Complications of augmentation cystoplasty include fistula, bladder stones, bladder rupture, intestinal obstruction, persisting augmented bladder contractions, and metabolic hyperchloremic acidosis.[17,18]

The metabolic acidosis, although a potentially significant clinical problem in patients with impaired renal function, is of unknown long-term clinical significance in patients with normal renal function. Another, largely theoretical, concern with augmentation cystoplasty exists over the long-term risk of malignancy in the augmented bladder.

For quadriplegics with insufficient hand function and inadequate attendant coverage for clean intermittent catheterization, two other reasonable options exist for management of DH and DESD. External urethral sphincterotomy, performed transurethrally, can eliminate the functional urethral obstruction. The resulting low-pressure incontinence, if successful, is managed with an external catheter. This option is obviously not appropriate for females. Although an excellent option in theory, in practice the results are less than desirable. Failure to successfully ablate the external sphincter can be expected in at least 30% of patients.[19] Subsequent failure of the detrusor to contract adequately is also seen. Successful retention of the external catheter may, besides circumcision, require penile prosthesis implantation. Long-term success of external urethral sphincterotomy must be repetitively demonstrated urodynamically.

Another alternative for bladder management in quadriplegics when intermittent catheterization is not feasible is ileovesicostomy.[7,20] This procedure involves isolating a short segment of ileum and anastomosing the proximal end to the fundus of the bladder while the distal end is brought out as a stoma in the right lower quadrant. This procedure "bypasses" the functional urethral obstruction, maintains a low "voiding pressure," and doesn't interfere with the normal vesicoureteral antireflux mechanism. It does require an ostomy appliance and occasionally the urethra must be ligated because of persisting urethral incontinence. Long-term results of the procedure are not currently available.

Other reported therapies for DH and DESD including sacral dorsal root rhizotomy, selective nerve blocks or neurectomies, cystolysis, nerve stimulation, and drug therapy aimed at the dyssynergic external urethral sphincter (with use of baclofen, dantrolene, prazosin, or botulinum toxin) have not achieved routine clinical application.[21]

In patients with incomplete SCI, DH without DESD can occur. The initial management consideration, since voiding is typically not obstructed, should be control of incontinence. Pharmacologic intervention as described previously, but perhaps more limited in dosages employed, in association with timed voiding (that is, voiding every 2 to 4 hours by the clock) may permit spontaneous voiding. For this to work, the SCI must be incomplete to the extent that the patient can initiate a bladder contraction or inhibit voiding long enough to allow voiding in a controlled situation (such as a urinal, bedside commode, or bathroom). Alternatively, males may simply be allowed to void into an external catheter. If an external catheter is used, self-adhesive catheters are preferred. Such catheters are associated with a low incidence of penile injury compared to taped-on external catheters. Unfortunately, such an option does not exist for females. If these attempts at therapy fail, the sequence of management steps described for DH and DESD can be followed.

SCI above T4 to T6, with intact cord segments below, can result in additional vesicourethral and cardiovascular dysfunction. Such an injury can impair or inhibit supraspinal modulation of various sympathetic reflexes. One possibility is urethral and bladder neck smooth muscle (intrinsic or internal sphincter) dyssynergia. Conceptually the result would be similar to DESD, a functional bladder outlet obstruction. Pharmacologic intervention with $alpha_1$-adrenergic blockers or surgical intervention with transurethral incision of the bladder neck would be appropriate. From a practical standpoint, this type of voiding dysfunction is rarely associated with SCI. Multichannel urodynamic evaluation with fluoroscopy is necessary to make this diagnosis.

Patients with C1-C2 SCI, brainstem impairment, and ventilator dependence have been described to have synergic voiding (that is, no DESD) with only DH.[24] This must be quite rare. Instead, such patients will almost invariably show DH and DESD on urodynamic evaluation.

Much more commonly, SCI at levels above T4-T6, with a viable spinal cord distally, is associated with autonomic dysreflexia. Autonomic dysreflexia is defined as an acute syndrome of massive disordered autonomic response to various stimuli below the level of injury in such patients. The reported incidence of autonomic dysreflexia in high thoracic and cervical SCI ranges from 30% to 85%.[25] Time to onset after SCI is variable, appearing as late as 15 years after injury.[25] Autonomic dysreflexia can be acutely life threatening because of systolic blood pressures exceeding 200 mm Hg and diastolic blood pressures exceeding 120 mm Hg. Symptoms include sweating, facial flushing, nasal passage congestion, headache, and tachycardia. Ominously, the patient can also be asymptomatic in the face of dramatic hypertension. This is a particularly dangerous clinical condition. Bladder distension, fecal impaction, and infected decubitus are common promoters of prolonged bouts of autonomic dysreflexia. As a result, blood pressure monitoring of SCI patients during urodynamic testing should be routine. An acute crisis can be managed with calcium-channel blockers, $alpha_1$-adrenergic blockers, chlorpromazine (Thorazine), ganglionic blockers, sodium nitroprusside, diazoxide, or hydralazine. From a urologic standpoint, chronic prophylaxis is often achieved with measures described previously that adequately control DH. When dysreflexia episodes persist despite such control, $alpha_1$-adrenergic blockade (as with terazosin or doxazosin) or calcium-channel blockers (such as nifedipine) are usually effective when administered on an ongoing basis.

SCI from T11 to L2

When SCI is limited to cord segments T11 to L2, complete injuries will also typically result in DH and DESD after resolution of spinal shock. The unique potential feature of SCI at these levels is incompetence of the smooth muscle of the bladder neck and proximal urethra. This is called "intrinsic sphincter deficiency." Thoracolumbar symptomatic nuclei at T11 to L2 innervate the bladder and urethra. Injury to these nuclei will impair the urethral smooth muscle closing function.[26] On voiding cystourethrogram, the SCI patient with this injury will characteristically have an open bladder neck in the absence of a bladder contraction (Fig. 46-2). Clinically patients may complain of typical stress urinary incontinence (that is, incontinence with coughing, straining, transfers, standing, and bowel movements. However, associated DESD may minimize this clinically because any maneuver that increases intra-abdominal pressure, the typical trigger for stress urinary incontinence, will also trigger a dyssynergic external urethral response. Practically speaking, stress incontinence after T11-L2 cord injury with intact sacral cord is more of a problem clinically in women than in men.

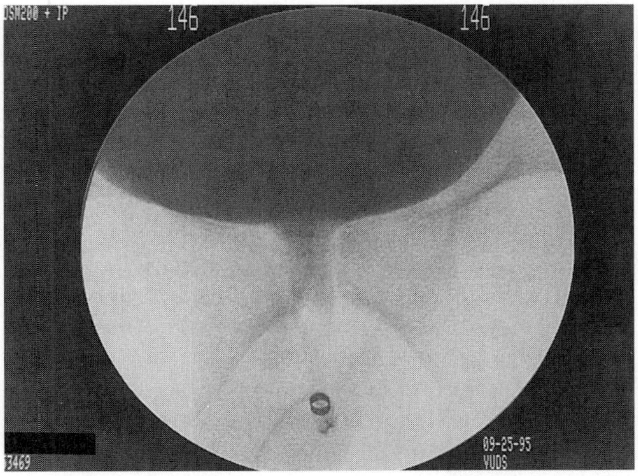

FIG. 46-2 *Forty-three-year-old man with L1 incomplete spinal cord injury secondary to a fall 3 months previously. Typical symptoms of stress urinary incontinence are present. Cystogram phase of videourodynamic study demonstrates an open bladder neck at low intravesical pressure in the absence of a bladder contraction (cystometrogram curve not shown). Notice radiopaque marker on urodynamic catheter at level of membranous urethra.*

It is not uncommon for T11-L2 SCI to be associated with sacral cord injury as well. In this mixed injury, loss of external urethral sphincter function will greatly exacerbate the clinical degree of stress incontinence.

Fluoroscopy at the time of urodynamic study, or videourodynamics, using a radiographic contrast solution to fill the bladder is necessary to make the diagnosis of intrinsic sphincter deficiency. Pressure measurement at the bladder neck and the proximal portion of the urethra will be low or isobaric with the bladder, the bladder neck will open during bladder filling, and Valsalva maneuvers (such as coughing) will generate loss of urine in the absence of a bladder contraction (and often without significant vesicourethral descent in women).

Management of clinically significant stress urinary incontinence associated with T11 to L2 SCI is surgical. The least invasive option is periurethral injection of a bulking agent (that is, autologous fat or collagen), usually an office procedure. Data indicate that this may be particularly well-suited for women with intrinsic sphincter deficiency on a neurogenic basis.[27] Other treatment options include pelvic sling procedure in women[28] and artificial urinary sphincter in men.[29] In properly selected patients, the pelvic sling procedure has a success rate as high as 98%.[30]

A special subset of women with incontinence secondary to intrinsic sphincter deficiency unrelated to neurologic injury consists of female SCI patients treated chronically with an indwelling urethral Foley catheter. Such patients, particularly those with suprasacral SCI, are often incontinent around the catheter or "void" the catheter out. This leads to the use of larger and larger catheters with larger and larger balloons. The result is a huge, patulous, perhaps rigid, incompetent urethra and bladder neck. Optimally, management includes a pelvic sling procedure, but this may fail because of urethral and bladder neck fibrosis and rigidity or complete loss by erosion. In such instances bladder neck and urethral closure may be necessary.[31]

A critically important warning exists when one is managing intrinsic sphincter deficiency in SCI patients. Before one addresses the urethral dysfunction, any bladder dysfunction affecting low-pressure storage and voiding, if appropriate, must be definitively addressed. For example, correcting only the intrinsic sphincter deficiency and associated stress incontinence in the face of a poorly compliant bladder will almost certainly lead, with time, to upper tract compromise and significant morbidity and even mortality.

SCI from S2 to S4 (Sacral Cord)

The detrusor motor nuclei, which provide the preganglionic parasympathetic detrusor innervation that effect a reflex bladder contraction, and the pudendal motor nuclei (Onuf's nucleus) that directly innervate the external urethral sphincter are located in the intermediolateral portions of cord segments S2-S4. Therefore a complete lesion of the sacral cord at these levels will result in loss of reflex bladder contraction, or detrusor areflexia, and a flaccid external urethral sphincter. An incomplete lesion can result in lesser degrees of impairment of contractile bladder or external urethral sphincter contractility. Patients usually develop urinary relation with overflow incontinence. A cystometrogram typically displays a low-pressure filling curve with large bladder capacity and absent reflex detrusor activity after injury (Fig. 46-3). This is indistinguishable from what would be seen urodynamically during the spinal shock phase of a suprasacral SCI. However, suprasacral cord injury is associated with the presence of a positive bulbocavernosus reflex and increasing external urethral sphincter EMG activity during bladder filling (continence reflex).[8] After complete sacral SCI, classically the bulbocavernosus reflex is absent, and the EMG remains quiet during filling. With a normal safe bladder capacity, normal bladder compliance, and intact hand function, patients with sacral SCI are easily managed, at least initially, with self-performed clean intermittent catheterization alone. Loss of external urethral sphincter function, in and of itself, causes no clinically significant voiding dysfunction for males or females, despite commonly held misconceptions.

The significant neurourologic complication that can occur after sacral SCI is a reduction in bladder compliance with time from the injury.[32] This is easily demonstrated on cystometrogram (Fig. 46-4). Although this is more commonly seen with postganglionic pelvic nerve (peripheral nerve) injury, it is seen with conus medullaris and cauda equina (S2-S4 SCI) injuries as well. One proposed mechanism is the occurrence of adrenergic nerve sprouting in the detrusor as a response to parasympathetic denervation of the bladder.[32] Consistent with this hypothesis, alpha-adrenergic blockade can improve bladder compliance in some patients.[32,33] Unfortunately, many such patients fail to respond to at least clinically tolerated levels of alpha-adrenergic blockade. With clean intermittent catheterization, anticholinergics (such as oxybutynin) are more commonly employed to manage the poor bladder compliance, or detrusor hypertonia, pharmacologically.[34] When medication fails, surgical options are the same as those for pharmacologically refrac-

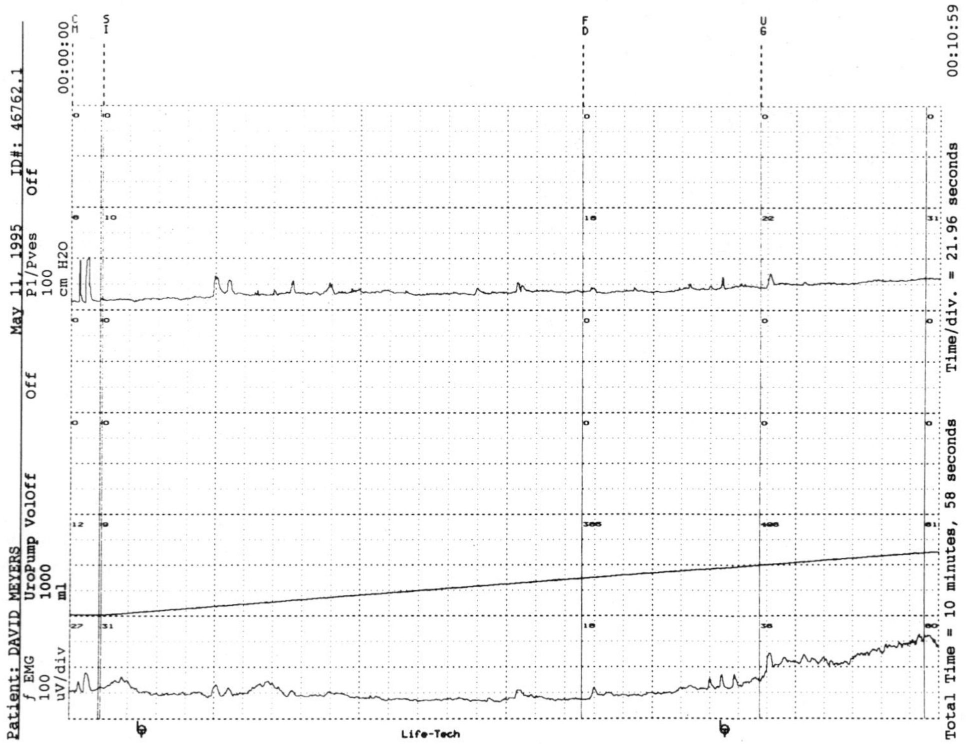

FIG. 46-3 *Multichannel urodynamic study of a 35-year-old man with cauda equina spinal cord injury secondary to a fall 9 months earlier. The patient is in complete urinary retention clinically.* Top tracing, *Areflexic bladder with normal compliance (low bladder filling pressures).* Middle tracing, *Bladder volume.* EMG, *Integrated external sphincter electromyographic activity;* P_{ves}, *bladder pressure;* Uropump Vol, *bladder volume.*

tory DH. Clearly the best current surgical option is augmentation cystoplasty and intermittent catheterization. Credé voiding and voiding by Valsalva maneuver in conjunction with medication are ill advised, since typically the bladder neck fails to relax and voiding pressures are thus elevated. The incidence of detrusor hypertonia in sacral SCI is unknown. It generally takes time, from months to even a few years, for reduced bladder compliance to become evident urodynamically. Thus serial testing with cystometrogram is necessary. Any new onset of persistent overflow incontinence in the sacral SCI patient who is otherwise being appropriately managed should lead to suspected deterioration in bladder compliance. A cystometrogram should then be performed.

It is not uncommon to find a chronically areflexic bladder in patients with low thoracic or lumbar SCI. In such instances, the apparent cause is cord infarction below the level of injury.[9] In this circumstance the apparent cord level of injury may be T11, but the patient will classically have a flaccid lower extremity paralysis, flaccid anal sphincter, and absent bulbocavernosus reflex on a chronic basis. Urodynamically the bladder will be areflexic with intrinsic sphincter deficiency and incontinence at low pressure and volume. To rule out a poorly compliant bladder as a result of sacral cord infarction, one must occlude the bladder neck and make a cystometrogram with filling to at least a normal bladder capacity.[35] Reduced bladder compliance must be successfully managed before one addresses the intrinsic sphincter deficiency, or the patient's upper tracts will be exposed to deleterious intravesical pressures.

Patient Surveillance

During the first 12 to 18 months after SCI, patients should be assessed and reassessed clinically and urodynamically with at least annual upper tract imaging. Any surgical intervention should be delayed until the evolution of the neurologic injury can be assumed complete. Once a definitive long-term lower urinary tract management plan has been successfully instituted, annual follow-up study with upper tract imaging (to evaluate for hydroureteronephrosis, stones, and renal parenchymal loss or scarring), serum creatinine (to follow renal function), and simple urodynamic assessment (cystometrogram ± EMG ± blood pressure monitoring to follow lower urinary tract function) is adequate. Clinical urologic complications (such as pyelonephritis, stone disease, and incontinence) or significant

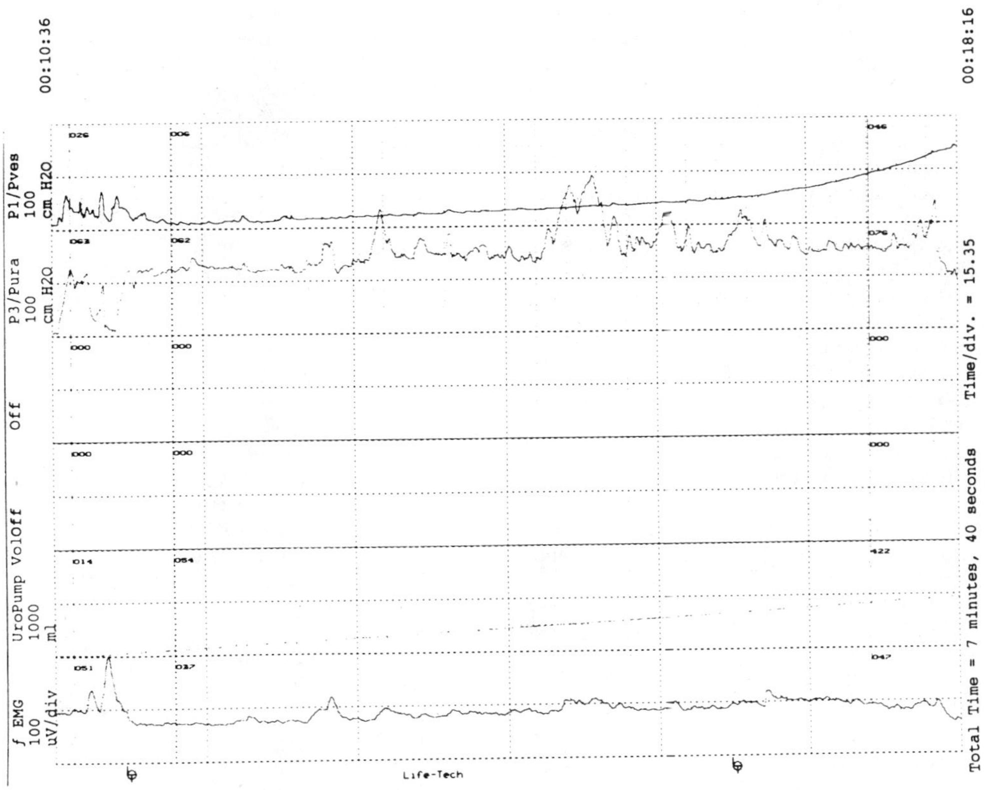

FIG. 46-4 *Multichannel urodynamic study of a 22-year-old man with cauda equina injury status after L5-S1 diskectomy 9 months previously. The patient is in complete urinary retention with occasional overflow and stress urinary incontinence. Top tracing, Areflexic bladder with reduced bladder compliance. Notice pronounced increase of the slope toward the end of filling. Compare to the curve in the top tracing of Fig. 46-3.* Middle tracing, *Bladder volume.* EMG, *Integrated external sphincter electromyographic activity;* P_{ves}, *bladder pressure;* Uropump Vol, *bladder volume.*

changes in neurologic status generally necessitate immediate reevaluation including, perhaps, more sophisticated urodynamic testing.

A variety of clinical situations may occur with time, complicating the urologic management of the SCI patient. Various types of cord myelopathy may occur at the site of SCI with time. Urethral stricture disease from urethral instrumentation (such as intermittent catheterization) can develop. When male SCI patients exceed a range of 45 to 50 years of age, clinically significant benign prostatic hyperplasia may occur with resulting new-onset bladder outlet obstruction. For patients receiving intermittent catheterization or with urinary diversion, this would be irrelevant. For patients managed with external catheter or other forms of spontaneous voiding, significantly obstructive benign prostatic hyperplasia would require therapy. Recurrent SCI can also obviously dramatically affect existing vesicourethral function and thus optimal management.

After the SCI and resulting vesicourethral dysfunction, unless documented recovery of normal bladder and urethral function occurs, patients will require life-long urologic management and surveillance. Using currently available diagnostic and management techniques, an appropriately compliant and managed patient can expect a normal life expectancy from a urologic standpoint with a low incidence of significant associated urologic complications.[6]

References

1. Guttman L: *Spinal cord injuries: comprehensive management and research,* Oxford, 1973, Blackwell Scientific, p 628.
2. Ditunno JF Jr, Formal CS: Chronic spinal cord injury, *N Engl J Med* 330(8):550-556, 1994.
3. Le CT, Price M: Survival from spinal cord injury, *J Chron Dis* 35:487-492, 1982.
4. Hackler RH: A 25-year prospective mortality study in the spinal cord injured patient: comparison with the long-term living paraplegic, *J Urol* 117:486-488, 1977.
5. Borges PM, Hacker RH: The urologic status of the Vietnam War paraplegic: a 15-year prospective follow-up, *J Urol* 127:710-711, 1982.
6. McGuire EJ, et al: A pressure management system for the neurogenic bladder after spinal cord injury, *Neurol Urodyn* 10:223-230, 1991.
7. Awad SA, Bryniak SR, Downie JW, et al,: Urethral pressure profile during the spinal shock stage in man: a preliminary report, *J Urol* 117:91-93, 1977.
8. Rudy DC, Awad SA, Downie JW: External sphincter dyssynergia: an abnormal continence reflex, *J Urol* 140:105-110, 1988.

9. Beric A, Dimitrijevic MR, Light JK: A clinical syndrome of rostral and caudal spinal injury: neurological, neurophysiological and urodynamic evidence for occult sacral lesion, *J Neurol Neurosurg Psychiatry* 50:600-606, 1987.
10. Blaivas JG: The neurophysiology of micturition: a clinical study of 550 patients, *J Urol* 127:958-963, 1982.
11. Abrams P, Blaivas JG, Stanton SL, Andersen JT: The standardisation of terminology of lower urinary tract dysfunction, *World J Urol* 6:233-245, 1989.
12. McGuire EJ, Woodside JR, Borden TA, Weiss RM: Prognostic value of urodynamic testing in myelodysplasia, *J Urol* 126:205, 1981.
13. Coolsaet BLRA, et al: Detrusor pressure versus wall stress in relation to ureterovesical resistance, *Neurourol Urodyn* 1:105-112, 1982.
14. Donnelly J, Hackler RH, Bunts RC: Present urologic status of the World War II paraplegic: 25-year follow-up comparison with status of the 20-year Korean War paraplegic and 5-year Vietnam paraplegic, *J Urol* 108:558-562, 1972.
15. Staskin DR: Hydroureteronephrosis after spinal cord injury: effects of lower urinary tract dysfunction on upper tract anatomy, *Urol Clin N Am* 18:309-316, 1991.
16. Decter RM, Bauer SB, Mandell J, et al: Small bowl augmentation in children with neurogenic bladder: an initial report of urodynamic findings, *J Urol* 138:1014-1016, 1987.
17. Flood HD, Malhotra SJ, O'Connell HE, et al: Long-term results and complications using augmentation cystoplasty in reconstructive urology, *Neurourol Urodyn* 14:297-309, 1995.
18. Nurse DE, Mundy AR: Metabolic complications of cystoplasty, *Br J Urol* 63:165-170, 1989.
19. Noll F, Sauerwein D, Stöhrer M: Transurethral sphincterotomy in quadriplegic patients: long-term follow-up, *Neurourol Urodyn* 14:351-358, 1995.
20. Schwartz SC, et al: Incontinent ileovesicostomy urinary diversion in the treatment of lower urinary tract dysfunction, *J Urol* 152:99-102, 1994.
21. Rudy DC: Detrusor-external sphincter dyssynergia, *Prob Urol* 7:68-93, 1993.
22. Krane RJ, Olsson CA: Phenoxybenzamine in neurogenic bladder dysfunction. I. A theory of micturition, *J Urol* 110:650-652, 1973.
23. Awad SA, Downie JW: Sympathetic dyssynergia in the region of the external sphincter: a possible source of lower urinary tract obstruction, *J Urol* 118:636-640, 1977.
24. McGuire EJ: *Clinical evaluation and treatment of neurogenic vesical dysfunction,* Baltimore, 1984, Williams & Wilkins, p 75.
25. Trop CS, Bennett CJ: Autonomic dysreflexia and its urological implications: a review, *J Urol* 146:1461-1469, 1991.
26. Woodside JR, McGuire EJ: Urethral hypotonicity after supra sacral spinal cord injury, *J Urol* 121:783-785, 1979.
27. McGuire EJ, Appell RA: Transurethral collagen injection for urinary incontinence, *Urology* 43:413-415, 1994.
28. McGuire EJ, O'Connell HE: Surgical treatment of intrinsic urethral dysfunction: slings, *Urol Clin North Am* 22:657-664, 1995.
29. Kreder KJ, Webster GD: Evaluation and management of incontinence after implantation of the artificial urinary sphincter, *Urol Clin North Am* 18:375-381, 1991.
30. McGuire EJ, Bennett CJ, Konnak JA, et al: Experience with pubovaginal slings for urinary incontinence at the University of Michigan, *J Urol* 138:525-526, 1987.
31. Zimmern PE, Hadley HR, Leach GE, Raz S: Transvaginal closure of the bladder neck and placement of a suprapubic catheter for destroyed urethra after long-term indwelling catheterization, *J Urol* 134:554-557, 1985.
32. Sundin T, Dahlström A, Norlén L, et al: The sympathetic innervation and adrenoceptor function of the human lower urinary tract in the normal state and after parasympathetic denervation, *Invest Urol* 14:322-328, 1977.
33. McGuire EJ, et al: Effect of alpha-adrenergic blockade and anticholinergic agents on the decentralized primate bladder, *Neurourol Urodyn* 4:139-142, 1985.
34. Woodside JR, McGuire EJ: Detrusor hypertonicity as a late complication of a Wertheim hysterectomy, *J Urol* 127:1143-1145, 1982.
35. Woodside JR, McGuire EJ: Technique for detection of detrusor hypertonia in the presence of urethral sphincteric incompetence, *J Urol* 127:740-743, 1982.

Chapter 47 Incontinence Caused by Neurologic Disease

Michael J. Kennelly, Delbert C. Rudy

Patients who have changes in bladder function because of an underlying neurologic disease often present clinically with urinary incontinence. Urinary incontinence is a common component of a variety of neurologic diseases. Therefore primary care physicians as well as urologists will frequently encounter patients with neurogenically mediated incontinence, with and without a known neurologic diagnosis. A clinical understanding of how common neurologic diseases cause incontinence is extremely important in both the diagnosis and the management of the urologic component of such diseases.

When evaluating and treating patients with known or suspected neurologic disease and incontinence, a complete evaluation is extremely important. Known neurologic disease and incontinence are not necessarily causally related. Good examples include the multiparous overweight woman with adult-onset diabetes mellitus and stress urinary incontinence secondary to pelvic floor relaxation, which may be unrelated to neurologic disorders of diabetes. Also, urinary urge incontinence in an elderly man with Parkinson's disease and high-grade bladder outlet obstruction secondary to benign prostatic hyperplasia (BPH) may be unrelated to the Parkinson's disease.

Management of patients with neurologic disease should consider all aspects of vesicourethral dysfunction, not just the symptom of urinary incontinence. In a patient with severe lumbar stenosis from disk disease and overflow incontinence, managing the bladder areflexia by intermittent catheterization alone may not address the accompanying poor bladder compliance, which results in a high risk of serious renal complications. Finally, neurologic diseases and the vesicourethral dysfunction resulting in incontinence can change over time. Consequently evaluation and management must also change over time as the neurologic disease changes. A common clinical example of this is multiple sclerosis.

In this chapter we have concentrated on common neurologic disorders associated with urinary incontinence. Emphasis will be placed on the pathophysiologic characteristics of the incontinence from the standpoint of currently available effective therapies. To facilitate the presentation, neurologic diseases are categorized as supraspinal, spinal, peripheral, or mixed (Fig. 47-1).

NEUROUROLOGIC EVALUATION

All patients with neurourologic disease affecting vesicourethral dysfunction require a neurourologic evaluation (see first box on p. 340). Apart from the sensory and motor dermatome examination, the neurologic examination should focus upon reflex activity within the S2 to S4 spinal cord segments (that is, perianal sensation, anal tone, voluntary anal control, and bulbocavernosus reflex). Urodynamic testing is essential in evaluating neurogenic

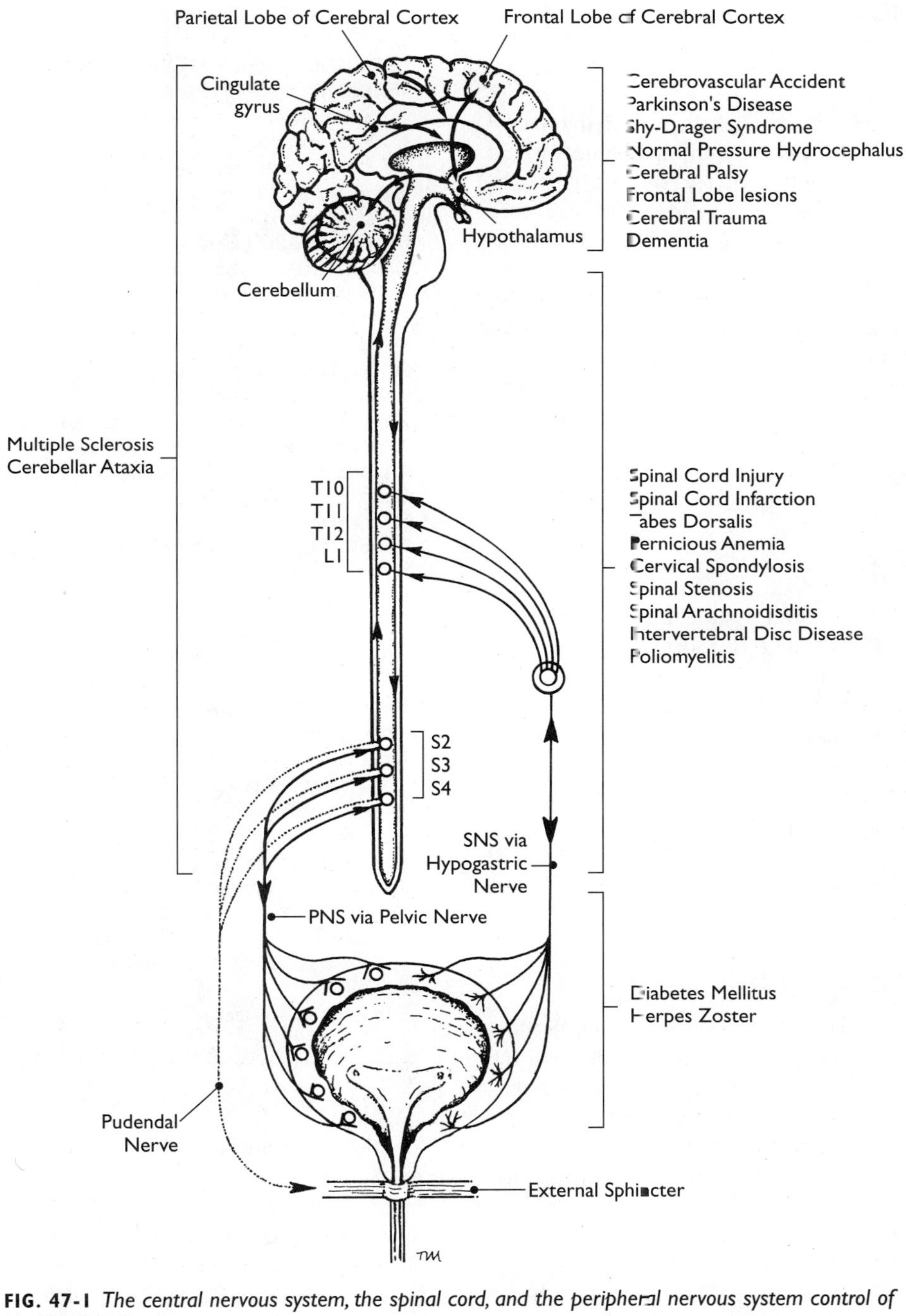

FIG. 47-1 *The central nervous system, the spinal cord, and the peripheral nervous system control of bladder function.*

Evaluation of Incontinence in Patients with Neurologic Disease

History and physical examination
Neurologic examination
Urinalysis with or without urine culture
Renal function study (serum creatinine)
Intravenous pyelogram or renal ultrasound
Endoscopic examination (as indicated)
Urodynamic testing
- Uroflow
- Postvoid residual
- Cystometrogram with or without electromyogram
- Pressure-flow (micturition) study
- Videourodynamic study (multichannel with fluoroscopy)

incontinence because it often determines the underlying neurologic abnormality, categorizes the vesicourethral dysfunction, and provides a basis for appropriate therapy (see box at right). The choice of therapy is based on many factors and should be tailored to each individual patient (see box at lower right). A prudent management scheme begins with simple reversible (medical) therapy before one considers irreversible (surgical) therapy. No uniform treatment exist for all patients with a particular neurologic disease. Rather therapy is individualized and often requires changes until the desired goal is achieved. Although many goals exist in managing neurovesical dysfunction, the main management goal is preservation of upper tract function along with improving the patient's troubling urinary symptoms that impair the quality of life of the individual (see box on p. 341).

SUPRASPINAL DISEASES

The characteristic of vesicourethral dysfunction of supraspinal disorders, if present, is the hyperreflexic bladder.[1,2] Bladder hyperreflexia is defined as an uninhibited bladder contraction with a neurologic cause. Typically this results in urge or indeterminate incontinence, small bladder capacity, small postvoid residual, and no deleterious effects on the upper urinary tract because voiding is unobstructed. A warning here is that supraspinal disease (such as stroke) involving the brainstem (specifically the upper pons) may cause external sphincter dyssynergia (discoordination of bladder and external sphincter) with resulting functional obstruction to voiding and significant risk of renal compromise.[1,3]

CEREBROVASCULAR DISEASE

In the United States, cerebrovascular disease is the third leading cause of death and disability and has an estimated incidence of 160 out of 100,000 people annually.[4,5] Arterial occlusion (primarily atherosclerotic disease with associated diabetes mellitus and hypertension), hemorrhage of congenital malformations, traumatic hemorrhage, and embolus are common mechanisms of cerebrovascular disease. Nearly all stroke survivors (90%) will have some sort of residual functional deficit including urinary incontinence.[6]

The cerebral regulation of the pontine micturition center is primarily inhibitory.[7] Consequently, patients who have had a stroke or CVA (cerebrovascular accident, stroke syndrome) often lose the suprapontine inhibitory control over the spinal reflexes. As the bladder gradually becomes distended, the micturition reflex is automatically activated without the patient's awareness or control, and detrusor hyperreflexia and incontinence can ensue.[8] Incontinence rates in the early recovery period of CVA have ranged from 51% to 83%.[9-13] With time, the prevalence of urinary incontinence decreases. Borrie et al. noted a 60% preva-

Incontinence Management in Neurologic Diseases

DETRUSOR HYPERREFLEXIA
1. Intermittent catheterization
2. Anticholinergics
3. Behavioral therapy and biofeedback
4. Electrical stimulation (TENS)
5. Augmentation cystoplasty
6. Bladder denervation procedure
   a. Ingelman-Sundberg procedure
   b. Subtrigonal phenolization
   c. Cystolysis and bladder transection
   d. Selective sacral rhizotomy
7. External catheter (men)
8. Indwelling Foley catheter
9. Relieve bladder outlet obstruction if present

DETRUSOR HYPERREFLEXIA WITH DETRUSOR EXTERNAL SPHINCTER DYSSYNERGIA
1. Treatment of hyperreflexia (2 to 6 above) and intermittent catheterization
2. External sphincterotomy (men)
3. Urinary diversion
4. Indwelling Foley catheter

DETRUSOR AREFLEXIA
1. Intermittent catheterization
2. Urinary diversion
3. Credé void (women)
4. Indwelling Foley catheter

SPHINCTERIC INCONTINENCE
1. Alpha-sympathetic agents
2. Endoscopic bulking agents (collagen, fat)
3. Pubovaginal sling
4. Bladder neck reconstruction
5. External catheter (men)
6. Urinary diversion
7. Indwelling Foley catheter

Patient Factors to Consider in Choosing Therapy

Prognosis of underlying disease, especially if progressive or malignant disease
Limiting factors: inability to perform certain tasks (hand dexterity, ability to transfer)
Mental status
Motivation
Desire to remain appliance free
Sexual activity status
Reliability
Educability
Psychosocial environment: interest, reliability, and cooperation of family
Economic resources
Age

Goals of Incontinence Management

- Preservation of upper urinary tract
- Maintain adequate bladder capacity with good compliance
- Promote low-pressure micturition
- Avoid bladder overdistension
- Prevent urinary tract infection
- Minimize use of Foley catheter
- Choose therapy that minimizes patient's risks while maximizing his or her social, emotional, and vocational acceptability

lence of incontinence at 1 week that decreased to 42% at 1 month and 29% at 3 months.[13] With rehabilitation, cognitive abilities, motor skills, or detrusor hyperreflexia may improve, resulting in improved continence. Long-term studies report persistent incontinence in approximately 15% of stroke patients.[14]

In addition to neurovesical dysfunction, various other factors play an integral part in development of urinary incontinence in the CVA patient. Cognitive impairments such as dementia, altered sensorium, and loss of communicative skills are associated with the development of incontinence.[15-17] Physical impairments such as immobility and motor deficits that inhibit one's ability to get to the commode or use the urinal contribute significantly to incontinence.[13]

Stroke patients bothered by voiding symptoms will usually complain about urinary urgency, frequency, and urge incontinence. Dysuria, slow stream, and urinary retention are less often reported.[18] Most patients retain sensory awareness after a CVA and exhibit only urgency. The bladder hyperreflexia prompts patients to voluntarily contract their external sphincter, which may inhibit to some degree the detrusor contraction by means of a sacral reflex. Such inhibition fails when the external sphincter fatigues without abating the bladder contraction. In patients with total cortical sensory loss of neurovesical function attributable to CVA, such inhibition is never even attempted.

Proper neurourologic evaluation of voiding dysfunction, including urodynamics, is important in stroke patients.[19,20] The majority of stroke patients studied by means of urodynamics reveal detrusor hyperreflexia with synergic voiding in up to 78% of cases.[18-21] Detrusor areflexia and urinary retention is not uncommon in the acute stages of CVA.[7] Although the exact neurophysiologic explanation remains unknown, lesions in the hypothalamic nuclei and basal ganglia have been implicated.[22] In addition, protracted urinary retention may lead to an overdistension injury and detrusor decompensation, prolonging detrusor areflexia in a cyclic fashion. Electromyography studies reveal that true detrusor–external sphincter dyssynergia rarely occurs (that is, as intrapontine lesions) though patients may have pseudodyssynergia.[1] Wein and Barrett coined the term "pseudodyssynergia" to describe the voluntary contraction of the external sphincter during an involuntary detrusor contraction.[23] Careful analysis of the electromyography tracing will assist in distinguishing pseudodyssynergia from detrusor external sphincter dyssynergia.[24]

Therapeutic management of voiding dysfunction in the stroke patient must be individualized with emphasis placed on the patient's cognitive abilities, motor skills, and rehabilitation potential. Neurologic recovery can be delayed 1 year or more after the initial insult. Therefore initial management should be conservative and reversible whenever possible. A variety of modalities has been reported useful in the management of bladder hyperreflexia.[25] The majority of patients with bladder hyperreflexia can be managed successfully with timed voids alone or supplemented with anticholinergic agents or tricyclic antidepressants. Such pharmacotherapy increases the bladder capacity at first sensation but does not alter the bladder automaticity. Hence it is imperative that patients treated with anticholinergic agents also begin a timed-voiding regimen. Alpha-adrenergic blockade may be useful in some instances. Other pharmacotherapies such as antispasmodics and calcium-channel blockers are of minimal, if any, clinical utility. Side effects of pharmacotherapy for bladder hyperreflexia are particularly significant in the elderly and often prevent the use of optimum drug regimens. Various forms of electrical stimulation have been utilized for bladder hyperreflexia but generally are poorly tolerated by patients. Management of refractory hyperreflexia often includes diapers or condom catheters in males. An indwelling catheter should be the management of last resort because of associated long-term complications.

Appropriately aged male patients with some degree of incontinence after CVA and potential coexisting obstructive benign prostatic hyperplasia (BPH) pose an interesting therapeutic dilemma. In the typical neurologically normal male with BPH-mediated bladder outlet obstruction, transurethral resection of the prostate will alleviate 70% of the associated urge incontinence symptoms. When a prostatectomy follows a stroke, patients often report persistence of voiding symptoms and incontinence.[26,27] To improve the success of prostatectomy in CVA patients, one must demonstrate the coexistence of significant bladder outlet obstruction. Simultaneous measurement of detrusor pressure and uroflow (pressure-flow study) or measurement of the micturitional urethral pressure profile[28] are the most reliable objective modalities to diagnose and quantitate bladder outlet obstruction. If detrusor hyperreflexia and urge incontinence persist after prostatectomy, anticholinergic agents are then often instituted. A preprostatectomy trial of anticholinergic therapy might seem prudent. However, with significant bladder outlet obstruction the risk of resulting urinary retention is very real. Alternative prostatism therapies, primarily medical management, may be better suited for these patients.

Stroke patients with overflow incontinence secondary to detrusor areflexia are ideally managed via clean intermittent catheterization.[29,30] When the social situation or manual dexterity prohibit clean intermittent catheterization, condom catheter drainage with or without diapers are acceptable alternatives. Again, because of the associated long-term complications, indwelling catheter should be the last-resort option.

Parkinson's Disease

Parkinson's disease is characterized by tremor, rigidity, and bradykinesia. In the United States the estimated annual incidence of Parkinson's disease is 0.1 to 0.15%.[31] The disease typically afflicts the 45- to 65-year age group without sex predilection.[14,31]

The exact cause of Parkinson's disease remains unknown. The fundamental defect is a degeneration of dopamine-producing cells in the substantia nigra and locus ceruleus. This causes a net cholinergic effect on the corpus striatum and the classic Parkinson's symptom complex. The extrapyramidal system including the substantia nigra and basal ganglia have an inhibitory effect on the pontine micturition center.[32-35] Therefore Parkinson's disease typically results in a detrusor hyperreflexia caused by lost inhibition on the pontine micturition center.

Various studies document voiding dysfunction in 40% to 70% of patients with Parkinson's disease.[36,37] The majority of patients complain of irritative voiding symptoms (that is, frequency, urgency, and nocturia). In a study of 30 patients by Pavlakis et al., 57% had irritative voiding symptoms, 23% had obstructive voiding symptoms, and 20% had mixed voiding symptoms on presentation.[38] Consistant with the varied voiding symptoms reported, notable urodynamic findings in Parkinson's patients include detrusor hyperreflexia, impaired detrusor contractility, and pseudodyssynergia (bradykinesia) of the external sphincter. Berger et al. evaluated 29 parkinsonian patients and diagnosed detrusor hyperreflexia in 90%.[39] Although two thirds of men will have diminished uroflows suggestive of bladder outlet obstruction, pressure-flow micturition studies frequently reveal impaired bladder contractility as the cause of decreased uroflow.[38] Perineal electromyography often reveals a delayed relaxation of the external sphincter during bladder contraction (bradykinesia or pseudodyssynergia) in 25% to 60% of parkinsonian patients.[38,39] This should not be misinterpreted as detrusor–external sphincter dyssynergia (DESD), which does not occur as a result of Parkinson's disease.

Although standard management of bladder hyperreflexia has been discussed previously, successful evaluation and management of male parkinsonian patients with voiding dysfunction requires an astute urologist. Because obstructive BPH is prevalent in this age group, urodynamic testing is essential. Proper urodynamic testing (cystometry, electromyography, pressure-flow micturition tests, and micturitional urethral pressure profile) can permit one to diagnose and quantitate bladder hyperreflexia, impaired bladder contractility, and coexistent bladder outlet obstruction. Detrusor hyperreflexia with coexisting impaired contractility requires different management from detrusor hyperreflexia with coexisting BPH-mediated obstruction.[40] Even with objectively documented obstruction, prostatectomy is not without increased morbidity in parkinsonian patients. The risk of de novo incontinence after a transurethral prostatectomy (TURP) in parkinsonian men is 20%, compared to 1% after TURP in the neurologically normal men.[41,42] Staskin et al. evaluated 36 post-TURP parkinsonian patients and noted urge incontinence in 83% of patients with poor voluntary external urethral sphincter control versus 4% in patients with good voluntary control.[41] Consequently, patients who lack voluntary control of sphincter function on preoperative EMG are believed to be at high risk for post-TURP incontinence. A subset of males with Parkinson's disease that do well after TURP are those with obstructive voiding symptoms, acute urinary retention, postvoid residuals greater than 200 ml, bladder capacity greater than 200 ml, and voluntary control of the external urethral sphincter.[43] Despite these reports, most urologists are reluctant to perform prostatectomy on parkinsonian patients because these patients often have refractory urgency, frequency, and urge incontinence after TURP. Consequently, in urodynamically obstructed patients, when tolerated, a trial of alpha-adrenergic blockade before TURP would seem prudent. In selected patients with large postvoid residuals, intermittent catheterization with or without anticholinergic therapy for urgency or urge incontinence may be reasonable.

Normal Pressure Hydrocephalus

Normal pressure hydrocephalus is one of the few neurologic diseases associated with urinary incontinence that can be cured if diagnosed and treated appropriately. This syndrome manifests as dementia, dyspraxia of gait, and urinary incontinence associated with cerebral ventricular dilatation with normal lumbar cerebrospinal fluid pressure. Normal pressure hydrocephalus commonly occurs in the elderly after episodes of cerebral inflammation that cause scarring of the arachnoid villi where spinal fluid absorption occurs. Although the exact cause of incontinence in these patients is unknown, urodynamic studies reveal that the majority of these patients have detrusor hyperreflexia and synergic voiding.[44] Successful shunting of the cerebrospinal fluid often resolves all the associated symptoms.

Cerebral Palsy

Cerebral palsy is a general term that describes a nonprogressive motor disorder caused by perinatal or gestational central nervous system damage. Various syndromes of cerebral palsy exist (that is, spastic, athetoid, ataxic, and mixed forms) that describe the motor disability, mental disability, and incoordination of cerebral palsy.[45] An estimated 0.15% of children have cerebral palsy syndromes.[45] The exact cause remains unknown. Neonatal infection, asphyxia, and jaundice have been implicated.

Voiding dysfunction uncommonly develops in patients with cerebral palsy. Most children have normal micturition and achieve continence, though at an older age than expected. Because of the delayed motor development, urodynamic evaluation is usually reserved for teenaged incontinent children. The majority (75%) of incontinent patients exhibit detrusor hyperreflexia when studied urodynamically.[46] Supraspinal and spinal lesions causing detrusor areflexia or detrusor–external sphincter dyssynergia, or both, occur infrequently. Clinical management is based on the urodynamic findings and the patient's overall physical, mental, and social support status.

Miscellaneous Suprasacral Neurologic Disorders

Various frontal lobe lesions caused by metastatic or primary tumors, cerebral trauma, or aneurysms of the anterior communicating artery may result in voiding dysfunction. Cortical awareness of the micturition reflex is centered in the anterior medial superior region of the frontal lobe.[47] Patients with frontal lobe lesions have diminished or absent sensation of the micturition reflex. Urge incontinence develops because they have either partially or totally lost the ability to suppress or inhibit the micturition reflex once it has begun. Urodynamic evaluation in patients with frontal lobe lesions characteristically reveals detrusor hyperreflexia.

Occasionally cerebral trauma resulting in concussion causes temporary voiding dysfunction. Patients may experience initial detrusor areflexia from "spinal shock" with eventual development of detrusor hyperreflexia.[48] The exact neuropathologic reason for temporary detrusor areflexia after concussion remains unknown.

Incontinence coexisting with dementia poses diagnostic and therapeutic challenges for the urologist. There is no simple method of determining if the associated incontinence is secondary to true detrusor hyperreflexia versus voluntary failure to appropriately inhibit the micturition reflex. The incidence of incontinence in dementia has been estimated at up to 40%.[8] Most patients with irritative symptoms respond to anticholinergic agents and timed voids. Incontinent patients who do not complain of irritative symptoms and who urinate in inappropriate settings are usually not curable. Management in these patients usually is with use of diapers in women and external condom catheter or diapers in men.

SPINAL CORD DISEASES

Spinal cord injuries associated with urinary incontinence are discussed in the following chapter. Herein, this review is a brief comment on the more common spinal cord disorders that may cause urinary incontinence.

Spinal Cord Compression Diseases (Intervertebral Disk Disease, Spinal Stenosis, and Cervical Spondylosis)

Spinal cord compression diseases such as intervertebral disk disease, lumbar spinal stenosis, and cervical spondylosis may be associated with voiding dysfunction. Usually spinal cord trauma or aging results in degenerative changes of the intervertebral disk space. Disk degeneration is followed by alterations in vertebral alignment that can cause cord compression. Direct cord compression by a herniated or prolapsed intervertebral disk can also occur as a result of trauma, infection, or aging. The site of cord compression determines the type of voiding dysfunction. For example, patients with voiding dysfunction secondary to cervical spondylosis typically complain of irritative voiding symptoms (urgency, frequency, and urge incontinence) caused by the suprasacral impairment of the reticulospinal tracts.[8] Patients with voiding dysfunction secondary to lumbar spinal stenosis often complain of obstructive symptoms (hesitancy, weak stream, and urine retention) caused by sacral parasympathetic (S2-S4 nerve root) impairment.[49]

Herniated or prolapsed interverterbral disk disease most commonly affects the lumbosacral disk interspaces.[50] Patients typically complain of low back pain in a girdle-like fashion because of inflammation and compression of associated lumbosacral nerve roots. Voiding dysfunction commonly occurs with lesions at the T12-L1, L4-5, or L5-S1 interspaces.[51] Conus medullaris injuries (T12-L1) impair the thoracolumbar sympathetic nuclei and associated sympathetic pathways subserving vesicourethral function. In particular, lesions at this level can impair smooth muscle function at the bladder neck and proximal portion of the urethra (intrinsic urethral sphincter), resulting in stress urinary incontinence.[52] Lesions at the L4-L5 and L5-S1 interspaces impair not only the parasympathetic pelvic nerve, but also the pudendal nerve because of their similar S2-S4 spinal cord distribution.[53,54] Consequently, damage to the conus medullaris or sacral roots causes not only bladder and urethral denervation, but also pelvic floor denervation. Patients with these lesions characteristically present with obstructive voiding symptoms (hesitancy, weak stream, and urine retention) caused by detrusor denervation and incontinence caused by overflow and intrinsic sphincter deficiency.[53,55] Classically neurourologic examination reveals perineal and circumanal sensory loss (S2-S4 dermatome), diminished sensation on the lateral foot (S1-S2 dermatome), decreased external anal sphincter tone (S2-S4 dermatome), and absent bulbocavernosus reflex (pudendal nerve function S2-S4). Urodynamic testing (cystometry with simultaneous electromyography) typically reveals a hyporeflexic or areflexic bladder with evidence of a denervated external urethral sphincter.[53] Bladder compliance may be normal or reduced.[54]

Intermittent catheterization adequately treats the urinary retention and overflow incontinence. Stress incontinence (intrinsic sphincter deficiency) that occurs in conus medullaris lesions may be treated by pubovaginal sling (women only), injectable bulking agents, or artificial sphincters. Decreased bladder compliance should be managed, at least initially, with pharmacologic agents (such as anticholinergics or alpha-adrenergic blockers).

The decision to intervene surgically for the disk disease is usually made by the managing orthopedic surgeon or neurosurgeon. Such a decision is usually made on the basis of somatic function status, which often improves postoperatively. However, resolution of significant associated vesicourethral dysfunction is unfortunately uncommon. This low resolution rate indicates that "early" definitive evidence of vesicourethral dysfunction attributable to cord compression should lead to aggressive clinical management.

Spinal Arachnoiditis

Spinal arachnoiditis is a rare condition that results in adhesions between the leptomeninges. Various factors such as lumbar disk disease, infection, blood in the cerebrospinal fluid, and myelography promote inflammation contributing to spinal arachnoiditis. Scar tissue forms and promotes nerve root compression. Typically spinal arachnoiditis affects the lumbar region; however, any cord segment can be involved. Lumbosacral spinal arachnoiditis with nerve root compression at S2-S4 has been reported to cause detrusor areflexia.[56]

Tabes Dorsalis

Tabes dorsalis, a rare parenchymatous neurosyphilis syndrome, affects the dorsal columns of the spinal cord and posterior sacral roots. Patients typically present with pain, ataxia, and sensory changes. Serologic venereal testing and cerebrospinal fluid analysis are diagnostic. Because the posterior spinal columns mediate bladder sensation, sacral tabes dorsalis often results in voiding dysfunction. Patients typically have partial or complete loss of bladder sensation, large bladder capacity, and elevated postvoid residual urine.[57] Long-standing disease leads to detrusor decompensation and eventual detrusor areflexia. In this setting, patients present with urinary retention and overflow incontinence. Because tabes dorsalis tends to progress despite penicillin therapy, the majority of patients eventually require intermittent catheterization in managing their voiding dysfunction.

Pernicious Anemia

Although pernicious anemia is quite rare, its neurologic manifestations may result in bladder dysfunction. Prolonged vitamin B_{12} deficiency causes degenerative changes in the peripheral nerves and posterior spinal columns. Similar to tabes dorsalis, the voiding dysfunction is secondary to degenerative lesions in the dorsal spinal cord. Patients lack sensory awareness of bladder fullness leading to detrusor areflexia, urinary retention, and overflow incontinence. Despite vitamin B_{12} therapy, these patients often require life-long intermittent catheterization.

Peripheral Nerve Diseases

Diabetes Mellitus

Diabetes mellitus commonly results in peripheral and autonomic neuropathy. Although the exact incidence remains unknown, diabetic neuropathy often occurs with long-standing disease or poorly controlled diabetes. Pathophysiologically, the Schwann cell undergoes metabolic impairment promoting segmental demyelination, axonal degeneration, and impaired nerve conduction.[44,58-60] Afferent sensory nerve pathways usually are impaired before efferent motor nerve pathways.

The bladder dysfunction associated with diabetes mellitus was coined "diabetic cystopathy" by Frimodt-Møller in 1976.[61] Although conflicting reports exist, diabetic cystopathy does not generally begin until after the onset of peripheral autonomic neuropathy.[62-65] Most patients with diabetes mellitus do not complain of symptoms of diabetic cystopathy.[66,67] However, in patients with diabetic neuropathy, up to 85% of patients will have diabetic cystopathy.[58,68,69]

Diabetic cystopathy has an insidious onset and progression with minimal clinical symptoms. Initially patients lose bladder sensation.[61,62,70] With time, the impaired sensation leads to increased bladder volume with overdistension. The patient's awareness of a full bladder is impaired, and infrequent voiding ensues. Ultimately, detrusor decompensation develops, causing an increased postvoid residual, urinary retention, and overflow incontinence.

Although asymptomatic diabetic patients exhibit various urodynamic findings,[71] diabetic cystopathy patients have characteristic findings. Delayed first sensation, increased bladder capacity, decreased bladder contractility, decreased voided flow rate, and elevated postvoid residual commonly occur in diabetic cystopathy.[65] Occasionally detrusor hyperreflexia will coexist.[71] Various pathophysiologic processes such as diabetic microvascular disease of the spinal cord, coexisting obstructing BPH, and aging may contribute to and complicate the voiding dysfunction.[72]

Few effective treatment regimens exist for diabetic cystopathy. Overflow incontinence, urinary retention, and elevated postvoid residual respond to intermittent catheterization or timed voids. Bethanechol chloride,[73-77] alpha-adrenergic blockers,[78] transurethral resection of the bladder neck,[79] and the Credé are not effective. TURP should be considered only when bladder outlet obstruction has been documented (that is, pressure-flow studies demonstrating high pressure with low flow). Control of hyperglycemia prevents not only polydipsia and polyuria, which exacerbate overflow incontinence, but also the glycosuria that potentiates bacteruria and urinary tract infection.

Herpes Zoster

Herpes zoster infection involves reactivation of varicella-zoster virus in the dorsal root ganglia. Patients develop a 3- to 5-day prodrome of fever and malaise before characteristic vesicle eruption and pain within the dermatome distribution of the affected dorsal root ganglia. Herpes zoster involvement of the sacral dorsal root ganglia may result in transient voiding dysfunction. During the prodrome, irritative voiding symptoms (urgency, frequency, and urge incontinence) arise followed by urinary retention lasting up to 6 to 8 weeks.[80] Although rarely seen, herpetic vesicle eruption can occur on the bladder mucosa.[81] Because the disease is self-limiting, the urinary retention is ideally managed by intermittent catheterization.

Neurologic Diseases Affecting Other Locations in the Nervous System

Multiple Sclerosis

Multiple sclerosis is a slowly progressive central nervous system disease characterized by focal neural demyelination (plaques) in the central nervous system white matter. Although the exact cause remains unknown, ongoing research focuses on an autoimmune, viral, or cell mediated immunodeficiency theory.[82,83] This debilitating disease affects young and middle-aged adults with an increased incidence in women, urban dwellers, and inhabitants of temperate climates.[84,85] The multiple focal areas of myelin sheath destruction with perivascular inflammation cause impaired nerve conduction and neurologic deficits.[86] As the perineural edema subsides, nerve conduction at the site of demyelination improves secondary to increased sodium channels along the demyelinated axon.[87] Although the course of disease is variable and unpredictable, most patients have mild temporary neurologic deficits that exacerbate and remit over time. In progressive multiple sclerosis, fibrous gliosis and perineural scarring may cause permanent neurologic deficits. The demyelinating process most commonly involves the posterior and lateral columns of the cervical spinal cord.[88,89] The lumbar and sacral spinal cords have fewer demyelinating plaques compared to the cervical region presumably because of the decreased white matter in those areas.[88]

Since the posterior and lateral columns of the spinal cord subserve bladder and urethral function,[90,91] vesicourethral dysfunction commonly occurs in multiple sclerosis patients.[92-95] Fifty percent to 80% of patients with multiple sclerosis complain of voiding dysfunction during the course of disease, and 10% of patients describe voiding symptoms during initial evaluation.[85,94] Multiple sclerosis patients with voiding dysfunction complain of irritative symptoms (65%), obstructive symptoms, (25%), and mixed symptoms (10%).[84,94]

Because patients with multiple sclerosis have variable presentations and unpredictable clinical courses, a thorough neurourologic evaluation is critical for proper diagnosis and treatment. Although the voiding dysfunction often parallels the exacerbations and remissions of the underlying neurologic deficit,[96] various reports have documented a poor correlation of voiding symptoms and urodynamic findings.[84,94,97] Consequently, urodynamics is an essential component of the neurourologic evaluation.

Detrusor hyperreflexia is the most common urodynamic abnormality detected and occurs in 50% to 90% of cases.[84,94,95] A poorly sustained bladder contraction, variable bladder sensation, and small-capacity bladder often coexist with the detrusor hyperreflexia.[98] About half the patients with detrusor hyperreflexia also have detrusor–external sphincter dyssynergia.[84,94,95] Patients who develop detrusor–external sphincter dyssynergia generally are more neurologically impaired because of progressive disease.[98] Detrusor areflexia or hypocontractility occurs in 20% to 30% of patients, with a substantial proportion progressing to detrusor hyperreflexia.[97,99] Because of the widespread lesions throughout the spinal cord, mixed lesions can occur.

Because of the variable pattern of disease (that is, exacerbations and remissions), optimal management should be conservative, flexible, and minimally invasive. The majority of patients can be successfully managed with a combination of timed voids, anticholinergic agents, and intermittent catheterization. Less than 10% of incontinent patients with multiple sclerosis require surgical intervention.[97] Surgery is reserved for patients with stable disease who have not responded to conservative therapy or for patients with progressive multiple sclerosis with minimal chance of recovery.

Risk factors for upper urinary tract deterioration in patients with multiple sclerosis include indwelling Foley catheter, detrusor–external sphincter dyssynergia in men, and poor bladder compliance.[100,101] In patients with voiding dysfunction, the incidence of urinary tract complication varies between 15% to 25%.[95,102,103] Most complications occur in men with detrusor–external sphincter dyssynergia and women managed with Foley catheter.[100] The use of an indwelling catheter to manage the vesicourethral dysfunction of patients with multiple sclerosis should be avoided. Urosepsis, vesicoureteral reflux, hydronephrosis, recurrent calculi, urethral erosion, nonfunctional urethras, and continued leakage have been well-documented complications of long-term Foley drainage.[104,105] Particularly, Foley drainage in patients with detrusor hyperreflexia and detrusor external sphincter dyssynergia may impair vesicourethral function by chronic erosion, making subsequent conservative therapy (anticholinergic agents and intermittent catheterization) difficult or impossible.

Cerebellar Ataxia

Cerebellar ataxia syndromes are characterized by abnormal motor function (dysmetria, dysarthria, and choreiform movements), poor coordination, and cerebellar deficiency. Diffuse demyelination and neuronal loss occurs not only in the cerebellum, but also at various other sites such as the brainstem, spinal cord (dorsal columns, spinocerebellar tracts, and pyramidal tracts), and dorsal nerve roots. Consequently, voiding dysfunction commonly occurs in patients with cerebellar ataxia. Usually patients with incontinence demonstrate detrusor hyperreflexia with synergic voiding attributable to a supraspinal cerebellar lesion. However, since the ataxia syndrome affects various sites in the nervous system, other voiding dysfunctions such as detrusor hyperreflexia with dyssynergia, detrusor–external sphincter dyssynergia, and detrusor areflexia can occur.[106] As with many of the other neurologic diseases, the management of voiding dysfunction in ataxia syndromes is based on the urodynamic findings. Most patients complaining of urge incontinence respond to anticholinergic agents and timed voids.

Shy-Drager Syndrome

Shy-Drager syndrome was first described in 1960 as a variant of Parkinson's disease.[107] Affected patients exhibit clinical features of Parkinson's disease (tremor, rigidity, and bradykinesia) with associated orthostatic hypotension and anhidrosis. This rare syndrome predominantly affects men and usually occurs in the sixth decade of life.[108] Because of progressive disease and often fatal orthostatic hypotension, the prognosis remains poor with limited (<10-year) life expectancy.[108] Neuronal atrophy and degeneration occur in the substantia nigra, cerebellum, midbrain, peripheral autonomic ganglia, and intermediolateral columns of the thoracolumbar and sacral spinal cord.[107,109]

Nearly all Shy-Drager patients experience some type of voiding dysfunction. Patients complain of irritative symptoms (urgency, frequency, and urge incontinence), obstructive symptoms (hesitancy, straining to void, and urine retention), or mixed symptoms because of the various affected areas of the nervous system. Kirby et al.[110] showed that most patients experienced incontinence caused by detrusor hyperreflexia with associated nonfunctional intrinsic and extrinsic urethral sphincter. A minority of patients in their study had detrusor hyperreflexia with impaired contractility or detrusor areflexia.

Amidst the symptoms and urodynamic findings, continence in patients with Shy-Drager syndrome is usually achieved with anticholinergic agents and timed voids or intermittent catheterization. Patients with documented bladder outlet obstruction should not undergo TURP. With coexisting nonfunctional internal and external urethral sphincters, prostatectomy carries a substantial risk of total urinary incontinence.[111,112] When progressive motor skill deterioration prohibits catheterization, alternative therapies such as condom catheter, diapers, indwelling catheter, or urinary diversion are considered.

References

1. Blaivas JG The neurophysiology of micturition: a clinical study of 550 patients, *J Urol* 127:958, 1982.
2. Khan Z, Hertanu J, Yang WC, et al: Predictive correlation of urodynamic dysfunction and brain injury after cerebrovascular accident, *J Urol* 126:86, 1981.
3. deGroat WC, et al: Neural control of the urinary bladder and large intestine. In Brooks CM, Koizumi K, Sato, editors: *Integrative functions of the autonomic nervous system,* Amsterdam, 1979, Elsevier.
4. Kurtzke JF: Epidemiology of cerebrovascular disease. In McDonawell FM, Caplan LR, editors: *Cerebrovascular survey report for the National Institute of Neurological and Communicatative Disorders and Stroke,* Bethesda, 1985, the Institute.
5. Rose JE: Vascular occlusive disease. In Rosenberg RN, Grossman RG, Schochet SS Jr, et al., editors: *The clinical neuroscience,* vol 2, New York, 1983, Churchill Livingston.

6. Toole JF, et al: Ischaemic cerebrovascular disease. In Toole JF, Cole M, editors: *Clinical neurology,* vol 2, Philadelphia, 1987, Lippincott.
7. Staskin DR: Classification of voiding dysfunction. In *Clinical neuro-urology*, ed 2, Boston, 1991, Little, Brown.
8. Raz S, et al: Neuromuscular dysfunction of the lower urinary tract. In Harrison JH, Gittes RF, Perlmutter AD, et al.: *Campbell's urology*, Philadelphia, 1979, Saunders.
9. Brocklehurst JC, Andrews K, Richards B, Laycock PJ: Incidence and correlates of incontinence in stroke patients, *J Am Geriatr Soc* 33:540, 1985.
10. Rottkamp BC: A holistic approach to identify factors associated with an altered pattern of urinary elimination for stroke patients, *J Neurosurg Nurs* 17:37, 1985.
11. Adams M, Baron M, Caston M: Urinary incontinence in the acute phase of cerebral vascular accident, *Nurs Res* 15:100, 1966.
12. Hingorani K: A study of the hemiplegia bladder, *Br J Clin Pract* 17:515, 1963.
13. Borrie MJ, Campbell AJ, Caradoc-Davies TH, Spears GF: Urinary incontinence after stroke: a prospective study, *Age Ageing* 15:177-181, 1986.
14. Mundy AR, et al: Non-traumatic neurological disorders. In Mundy AR, Stephenson TP, Wein AJ, editors: *Urodynamics: principles, practice and applications* New York, 1984, Churchill-Livingstone.
15. Andrew J, Nathan PW, Spanos NC: Disturbance of micturition and defaecation due to aneurysms of anterior communicating or anterior cerebral arteries, *J Neurosurg* 24:1, 1966.
16. Bradley WE, Timm GW, Scott FB, et al: Inneration of the detrusor muscle and urethral, *Urol Clin North Am* 1:3, 1974.
17. Andrew J, Nathan PW: Lesions of the anterior frontal lobes and disturbances of micturition and defaecation, *Brain* 87:233, 1964.
18. Tsuchida S, Noto H, Yamaguchi O, Itoh M: Urodynamics studies on hemiplegic patients after cerebrovascular accidents, *Urology* 21:315-318, 1983.
19. Motola JA, et al: Cerebrovascular accidents: urodynamic and neuroanatomical findings (abstract), *J Urol* 139:512A, 1988.
20. Badlani GH, et al: Detrusor behavior in patients with dominant hemispheric studies, *Neurourol Urodyn* 10:119, 1991.
21. Arunabh, et al: Urologic problems in cerebrovascular accidents, *Prob Urol* 7(F):41-53, 1993.
22. Uvnas B: Effect of frequency of hypothalamic stimulation upon bladder responses, *Proc Soc Exp Biol Med* 64:181, 1947.
23. Wein A, et al: Etiologic possibilities of increased pelvic floor electromyography activity during cystometry, *J Urol* 127:949, 1982.
24. Rudy DC: Detrusor–external sphincter dyssynergia, *Prob Urol* 7(F):68-93, 1993.
25. Wein AJ: Clinical neuropharmacology of the lower urinary tract. In Yalla SV, editor: *Neurourology and urodynamics: principles and practice,* Macmillian, 1988, New York.
26. Lum SK, Marshall VR: Results of prostatectomy in patients following a cerebrovascular accident, *Br J Urol* 54:186, 1982.
27. Moisey CU, Rees RW: Results of transurethral section of prostate in patients with cerebrovascular disease, *Br J Urol* 50:539, 1978.
28. Yalla SV, Blute R, Waters WB, et al: Urodynamic evaluation of prostatic enlargements with micturitional vesicourethral static pressure profile, *J Urol* 125:677, 1981.
29. Garrett VE, Scott JA, Costich J, et al: Bladder emptying assessment in stroke patients, *Arch Phys Med Rehab* 70:41, 1989.
30. Marks R, et al: How to manage neurologic bladder after stroke, *Geriatrics* 32:50, 1977.
31. Yahr MD: Parkinson's disease: overview of its current status, *Mt Sinai J Med* 44:183, 1977.
32. Yalla SV, DiBenedetto M, Fam BA, et al: Striated urethral sphincter participation in passive distal urinary continence mechanisms: studies in male subjects deprived of proximal sphincter mechanisms, *J Urol* 122:655, 1979.
33. Kurland LT: Epidemiology, incidence, geographic distribution and genetic considerations. In Fields WS, editor: *Pathogenesis and treatment of parkinsonism,* Springfield, Ill., 1958, Charles C. Thomas.
34. Bradley WE: Neurologic disorders affecting the urinary bladder. In Krane RJ, Siroky MB, editors: *Clinical neurourology,* ed 1, Boston, 1978, Little, Brown.
35. Lewin RJ, Dillard GV, Porter RW: Extrapyramidal inhibition of the urinary bladder, *Brain Res* 4:301, 1967.
36. Murnaghan GF: Neurogenic disorders of the bladder in Parkinsonism, *Br J Urol* 33:403, 1961.
37. Porter RW, Bors E: Neurogenic bladder in parkinsonism: effect of thalamotomy, *J Neurosurg* 34:27, 1971.
38. Pavlakis AJ, Siroky MB, Goldstein I, Krane RJ: Neurourologic findings in Parkinson's disease, *J Urol* 129:80, 1983.
39. Berger Y, Blaivas JG, De La Rocha ER, Salinas JM: Urodynamic findings in Parkinson's disease, *J Urol* 138:836, 1987.
40. Resnick NM, Yalla SV, Laurino E: The pathophysiology of urinary incontinence among institutionalized elderly persons, *N Engl J Med* 320:1, 1989.
41. Staskin DS, Vardi Y, Siroky MB: Post-prostatectomy continence in the parkinsonian patient: the significance of poor voluntary sphincter control, *J Urol* 140:117, 1988.
42. Mayo ME, Ansell JS: Urodynamic assessment of incontinence after prostatectomy, *J Urol* 122:60, 1979.
43. Berger Y: When Parkinson's disease disrupts bladder function, *Contemp Urol,* p 37, Aug/Sept 1989.
44. Blaivas JG: Pathophysiology of lower urinary tract dysfunction, *Urol Clin North Am* 12:215, 1985.
45. Bauer SB: Urodynamic evaluation and neuromuscular dyfunction. In Kelalis PP, King LR, Belman AB, editors: *Clinical pediatric urology,* Philadelphia, 1985, Saunders.
46. Khoshbin S, et al: Lower urinary tract function in children with cerebral palsy. (in press).
47. Andrew J, Nathan PW: The cerebral control of micturition, *Proc R Soc Med* 58:553, 1965.
48. McGuire EJ: Neuromuscular dysfunction of the lower urinary tract. In Walsh P, Gittes R, Perlmutter A, Stamey T, editors: *Campbell's urology,* Philadelphia, 1986, Saunders.
49. Smith AY, Woodside JR: Urodynamic evaluation of patients with spinal stenosis, *Urology* 32:474, 1988.
50. Jones RA, Thomson JL: The narrow lumbar canal: a clinical and radiological review, *J Bone Joint Surg* 503:595, 1968.
51. Rosomoff HL, Johnston JD, Gallo AE, et al: Cystometry in the evaluation of nerve compression in lumbar spine disorders, *Surg Gynecol Obstet* 117:263, 1963.
52. McGuire EJ: Urodynamic evaluation after abdominal perineal resection and lumbar intervertebral disk herniation, *Urology* 6:63-70, 1975.
53. Appell RA, et al: Assessment of vesico-urethral dysfunction in lumbar spine disorders. In Sundin T, Mattiasson A, editors: *Proc Eleventh Annual Meeting of the International Incontinence Society,* Trelleborg, Sweden, 1981, Skogs.
54. Appell RA: Voiding dysfunction and lumbar disc disorders, *Probl Urol* 7:135-40, 1993.
55. Andersen JT, Bradley WE: Neurogenic bladder dysfunction in protruded lumbar disc and after laminectomy, *Urology* 8:94, 1976.
56. Shaw MDM, Russell JA, Grossart KW: The changing pattern of spinal arachnoiditis, *J Neuro Neurosurg Psych* 41:97, 1978.
57. Wheeler JS, Culkin DJ, O'Hara RJ, Canning JR: Bladder dysfunction and neurosyphllis, *J Urol* 136:903, 1986.
58. Ellenberg M: Neurologic changes in early diabetes, *Adv Metab Disord* 2(2):459, 1973.
59. Faerman I, Glocer L, Celener D, et al: Autonomic nervous system and diabetes: histological and histochemical study of the autonomic nerve fibers of the urinary bladder in diabetic patients, *Diabetes* 22:225-237, 1973.
60. Frimodt-Moller C: A new method for quantitative evaluation of bladder sensibility, *Scand J Urol Nephrol* 6(15):135, 1972.
61. Frimodt-Moller C: Diabetic cystopathy. I: A clinical study of frequency of bladder dysfunction in diabetics, *Dan Med Bull* 23:267-278, 1976.

62. Watkins PJ: The bladder in diabetes, *Practitioner* 214:56-59, 1975.
63. Buck AC, McRae CU, Chisholm GD: The diabetic bladder, *Proc R Soc Med* 67:81-83, 1974.
64. Fagerberg S-E, Kock NG, Peterén I, et al: Urinary bladder disturbances in diabetics. I. A comparative study of male diabetics and controls aged between 20 and 50 years, *Scand J Urol Nephrol* 1:19-27, 1967.
65. Frimodt-Moller C: Diabetic cystopathy. II. Relationship to some late-diabetic manifestations, *Dan Med Bull* 23:279-287, 1976.
66. Martin MM: Diabetic neuropathy: a clinical study of 150 cases, *Brain* 76:594, 1953.
67. Spring M, et al: Neurogenic bladder dysfunction as a complication of diabetes, *Diabetes* 2:199, 1966.
68. Bartley O, Brolin I, Fagerberg S-E, et al: Neurogenic disorders of the bladder in diabetes mellitus, *Acta Med Scand* 108:187, 1966.
69. Ellenberg M, Weber H: The incipient asymptomatic diabetic bladder, *Diabetes* 16:331, 1967.
70. Schiff HI: The neurogenic bladder in diabetes, *NY State J Med* 82:922-926, 1982.
71. Kaplan SA, Te AE, Blaivas JG: Urodynamic findings in patients with diabetic cystopathy, *J Urol* 153:342-344, 1995.
72. Bradley WE: Diagnosis of urinary bladder dysfunction in diabetes mellitus, *Ann Intern Med* 92(pt 2):323-326, 1980.
73. Barrett DM: The effect of oral bethanechol chloride on voiding in female patients with excesive residual urine: a randomized double blind study, *J Urol* 126:640, 1981.
74. Light KJ, Scott FB: Bethanechol choride and the traumatic cord bladder, *J Urol* 128:85, 1982.
75. Wein AJ, Malloy TR, Shofer F, Raezer DM: The effects of bethanechol chloride on urodynamic parameters in normal women and women with significant residual urine volumes, *J Urol* 124:397, 1980.
76. Wein AJ, et al: The effect of oral bethanechol chloride on the cystometrogram of the normal male adult, *J Urol* 120:330, 1978.
77. Yalla SV, Rossier AB, Fam B: Dyssynergic vesicourethral responses during bladder rehabilitation in spinal cord injury patients: effect of suprapubic percussion, Credé method and bethanechol chloride, *J Urol* 115:575, 1976.
78. Caine M, Pfass A, Perlberg S: The use of alpha adrenergic blockers in benign prostatic obstruction, *Br J Urol* 48:255, 1976.
79. Kahan M, Goldberg PD, Mandel EE: Neurogenic vesical dysfunction and diabetes mellitus, *NY State J Med* 2:2448-2455, 1970.
80. Hald T, Bradley WE: The urinary bladder. In *Neurology and dynamics,* Baltimore, 1982, Williams & Wilkins.
81. Gibbon NOK: A case of herpes zoster with involvement of urinary bladder, *Br J Urol* 129:412, 1956.
82. McFarlin DE, McFarlin HF: Multiple sclerosis, *N Engl J Med* 307:1183, 1982.
83. Poser CM: Exacerbations, activity, and progression in multiple sclerosis, *Arch Neurol* 37:471, 1980.
84. Goldstein I, Siroky MB, Saz DS, Krane RJ: Neurourologic abnormalities in multiple sclerosis, *J Urol* 128:541, 1982.
85. Miller H, Simpson CA, Yeates WK: Bladder dysfunction in multiple sclerosis, *Br Med J* 1:1265, 1965.
86. McDonald WI: Pathophysiology in multiple sclerosis, *Brain* 97:179, 1974.
87. Waxman SG: Membranes, myelin and the pathophysiology of multiple sclerosis, *N Engl J Med* 306:1529, 1982.
88. Fog T: Topographic distribution of plaques in the spinal cord in multiple sclerosis, *Arch Neurol Psychiatry* 63:382-414, 1950.
89. Oppenheimer DP: The cervical cord in multiple sclerosis, *Neuropathol Appl Neurobiol* 4:151, 1978.
90. Barrington FJF: The localization of the paths serving micturition in the spinal cord of the cat, *Brain* 56:126, 1993.
91. Nathan PW, Smith MC: The centrifugal pathway from the bladder and urethra within the spinal cord, *J Neuro Neurosurg Psychiatry* 14:262, 1951.
92. Andersen JT, Bradley WE: Abnormalities of detrusor and sphincter function in multiple sclerosis, *Br J Urol* 48:193, 1976.
93. Awad SA, Gajewski JB, Sogbein SK, et al: Relationship between neurological and urological status in patients with multiple sclerosis, *J Urol* 132:499, 1984.
94. Blaivas JG, Bhimani G, Labib KB: Vesicourethral dysfunction in multiple sclerosis, *J Urol* 122:342, 1979.
95. Blaivas JG: Management of bladder dysfunction in multiple sclerosis, *Neurology* 30(2):12-18, 1980.
96. Wheeler JS Jr, Siroky MB, Pavlakis AJ, et al: The changing neurourologic pattern of multiple sclerosis, *J Urol* 130:1123, 1983.
97. Philip T, et al: The urodynamic characteristics of multiple sclerosis, *Br J Urol* 53:672, 1981.
98. Wheeler JS: Multiple sclerosis. In Krane RJ, Siroky MB, editors: *Neurourology and urodynamics,* Boston, 1991, Little, Brown.
99. Sirls LT, Zimmern PE, Leach GE: Role of limited evaluation and aggressive medical management in multiple sclerosis: a review of 113 patients, *J Urol* 151:946, 1994.
100. Blaivas JG, Barbalias GA: Detrusor-external sphincter dyssynergia in men with multiple sclerosis: an ominous urologic condition, *J Urol* 131:94, 1984.
101. McGuire EJ, Savastano JA: Urodynamic findings and long-term outcome managment of patients with multiple sclerosis–induced lower urinary tract dysfunction, *J Urol* 132:713, 1984.
102. Jameson RM: Management of the bladder in non-traumatic paraplegia, *Paraplegia* 12:92, 1974.
103. Damanski M, et al: Paraplegia of non-traumatic origin and disseminated (multiple) sclerosis: urinary complications, their nature and treatment, *Acta Neurol Psychiatr Belg* 64:495-502, 1964.
104. McGuire EJ, et al: Comparative urological outcome in women with spinal cord injury, *J Urol* 135:730, 1966.
105. Bennett CJ, et al: Comparison of bladder management complications outcomes in female spinal cord injury patients, *J Urol* 153:1458-1460, 1995.
106. Leach GE, Farsaii A, Kark P, Raz S: Urodynamic manifestations of cerebellar ataxia, *J Urol* 128:348, 1982.
107. Shy M, Drager GA: A neurologic syndrome association with orthostatic hypotension, *Arch Neurol* 2:511, 1960.
108. Sotolongo JR Jr, et al: Parkinson's disease, *Prob Urol* 7(1):54-67, 1993.
109. Salinas JM, Berger Y, De La Rocha RE, Blaivas JG: Urological evaluation in the Shy Drager syndrome, *J Urol* 135:741, 1985.
110. Kirby RS, et al: Urethro-vesical dysfunction in the Shy-Drager syndrome, *Proc Second Joint Meeting of the Intenational Continence Society and the Urodynamics Society,* Aachen, pp 303-305, 1983.
111. Sakuta M, Nakanishi T, Toyokura Y: Anal muscle electromyograms differ in amyotrophic lateral sclerosis and Shy-Drager syndrome, *Neurology* 28:1289, 1978.
112. Singh N, et al: Electrophysiologic studies in the Shy-Drager syndrome, *Neurology* 30:394, 1980.

Chapter 48 Bladder Noncompliance

David S. Breslin, David R. Staskin

When the bladder has a change in its normal stretch properties, the usual bladder filling that results in an increase in volume of urine in the bladder can also result in an abnormal increase in pressure within the bladder, and the bladder no longer has normal compliance. Disorders of bladder compliance often result in severe bladder symptoms as well as risk for deterioration of kidney function. Noncompliance is among the most serious problems of the bladder and sometimes is clinically unrecognized until late in the course of the disease. Compliance problems affect primarily the storage function of the urinary bladder.

The basic function of the lower urinary tract (bladder and bladder outlet) is to store and to empty urine while protecting the integrity of the upper urinary tract (kidneys and ureters). To accomplish this purpose, during urinary storage the bladder acts as a compliant low-pressure reservoir, relaxing to accommodate an increasing volume of urine with minimal change in intravesical pressure. This low intravesical pressure permits unimpeded drainage of urine from the upper tracts and facilitates urinary continence. Conversely, during voiding, the bladder performs as a pump while the ureterovesical junctions prevent vesicoureteral reflux and protect the upper tracts from the acute exposure to increased intravesical pressure.

A decrease in bladder compliance is the result of an alteration in the muscular or connective tissue elements of the bladder, or in the intrinsic smooth muscle tone, which is under neurologic control. The clinical conditions that are reviewed in this chapter precipitate a change in the ability of the bladder to store urine at low pressure and may manifest themselves with the classical symptoms of decreased bladder capacity, with an alteration in continence status, or with an effect on upper tract anatomy and function.

Definition

Bladder compliance is defined by the change in intravesical volume divided by the change in intravesical pressure during a volume increment, or $\Delta V/\Delta P$, in units of milliliters per centimeter of water. Normal adult bladder capacity is approximately 300 to 500 ml,[1] and bladder pressure usually increases only 10 to 15 cm H_2O throughout the course of physiologic filling or a diagnostic filling cystometrogram (CMG). Therefore normal bladder compliance usually ranges from 30 to 50 ml/cm H_2O. A study by Andersen[2] assigned the values of 150, 50, and 5 ml/cm H_2O to bladders of high, normal, and low compliance respectively. Gilmour et al. suggest a value of 10 ml/cm H_2O as the lower limit of normal compliance in a series of 69 normal children undergoing filling cystometry.[3]

Bladder compliance can be calculated during filling cystometry. There is ongoing debate among urodynamicists regarding the accuracy of the specific methods of the cystometric examination, such as the filling medium (carbon dioxide versus saline solution), the rate of bladder filling, and the temperature of the liquid medium (room versus body versus cold). Filling rates greater than 100 ml/min are considered *rapid fill,* rates between 10 and 100 ml/min are *medium fill,* and rates less than 10 ml/min are known as *slow fill.*[4] The last rate most closely approximates the physiologic filling rate. A thorough discussion of the debate is outside the scope of this chapter, but in general the nature, the rate, or the temperature of the medium does not significantly alter the results in most normal patients. Undoubtedly performance of cystometry approximating the physiologic state provides the most accurate results but is time consuming. Admittedly, a provocative filling rate may unmask compliance changes, which may or may not be functionally important in the clinical situation. When nonphysiologic filling rates are used, the bladder pressure should be monitored after filling has been completed until a plateau pressure is maintained to more realistically approximate physiologic filling pressures. Additionally, compliance changes at provocative rates may be utilized as a screening tool for a more physiologic test in those found to be abnormal depending on the purpose of the study. A review of 10 reports comparing gas and water cystometry demonstrated unequivocally no qualitative difference between the two filling media.[5]

Relevant Histopathology

The ability of the normal bladder to accommodate near-capacity urine volumes (300 to 500 ml) at pressures as low as 10 cm H_2O is attributable to the passive constituents of the bladder wall, namely collagen, elastin, and smooth muscle fibers. Collagen fibers consist of three polypeptide chains, known as alpha chains, each encoded by its own separate gene, wound in a triple helix as they are secreted into the extracellular matrix. Various combinations of the approximately 20 different alpha chains give rise to only 15 different collagen types described up to now.[6] Types I, II, and III are known as the fibrillar collagens and are responsible for maintaining tensile strength. Type II is usually found in cartilaginous tissue and is rarely found in the urinary bladder. Type I forms large fibers and is usually found in dense connective tissues, such as tendon and bone, and provides tensile strength. In tissues requiring higher levels of compliance, namely, detrusor, lung, and intestine, type III predominates. However, both these fibers may coexist in the various organs, and their interactions may govern the overall structural and dynamic properties of that site.

Elastic fibers consist primarily of the polypeptide elastin, which forms multiple filaments with extensive cross-linking.

These molecules exist in the extracellular matrix as random coils that passively stretch and recoil in a fashion not dissimilar to the action of a rubber band. Elastic fibers provide minimal tensile strength and maximal elasticity, which is in direct contrast to the properties of collagen fibers.[7-9]

Ewalt et al.,[10] using antibodies to collagen types I, III, and IV and elastin, have demonstrated that the lamina propria, by virtue of the localization of these various structural proteins is the primary capacitance layer in normal bladders. They hypothesize that the fascicles of collagen gradually unfold, and only when the unfolding is complete will the pressure increase within the bladder. Elastin is believed to play a part in the refolding of the collagen as the bladder empties. The work of Susset and Regnier support this view because they found that the viscoelastic properties of mucosal strips (and the invariably attached lamina propria) are many times greater than those of muscular strips, in a study of human cadaveric bladder tissue.[11]

Ewalt et al. also performed similar immunohistochemical staining on urodynamically documented noncompliant bladders. There is minimal difference in the appearance of the lamina propria between the normal and abnormal groups; however, the muscularis propria, or detrusor layer, is greatly altered in the pathologic bladder. The interfascicular space has accumulated collagen types I and III and elastin, whereas the pericellular infiltration is mainly type III and elastin. These findings were present and consistent in bladders with neurogenic or obstructed pathologic conditions.[10] Landau et al. determined the percentage of connective tissue and the ratio of connective tissue to smooth muscle in the bladders of 29 patients undergoing bladder augmentation. The percentage of connective tissue was 35.19% ± 2.84% (normal = 10.6% ± 0.020%) and the ratio of connective tissue to smooth muscle was 0.60% ± 0.08% (normal = 0.131% ± 0.021%.[12] Gilpin et al.[13] found that 12 out of 14 obstructed, trabeculated bladders demonstrated circumcellular connective tissue infiltration, whereas no infiltration was seen in normal bladders. It is believed that the smooth muscle cell is responsible for triggering the process of pericellular infiltration. Trabeculation arises from a combination of smooth muscle hypertrophy and connective tissue infiltration, and it is these abnormal muscle layers that no longer allow the bladder to expand and distend with increasing urine volumes.[10]

The forces that govern the bladder's response to filling are the passive component, related to the viscoelastic properties of the structural proteins, namely, collagen and elastin, and the active myoneural component, which in the normal state is dampened by neural reflex mechanisms.[14,15] Elbadawi demonstrated the requirement of "electronic cell-to-cell coupling" in normal, coordinated detrusor function,[16] whereas Shapiro et al. infer that the same mechanism is required for neurologically mediated detrusor relaxation and that abnormal pericellular and interfascicular connective tissue must interfere with the entire process. It has also been noted that the pathologic process described above begins initially in the superficial aspect of the detrusor layer and progresses centrifugally over time. Perhaps the superficial muscle fibers are responding to various inflammatory cell products, as in chronic or recurrent cystitis, elaborated from the lamina propria.[17]

Clinical Significance of Decreased Bladder Compliance

Despite varying causes, the final pathway of all the disease entities mentioned in this chapter is the poorly functional, low-capacity, poorly compliant bladder. (The terms *low* and *decreased compliance* and *noncompliant, hypocompliant,* and *poorly compliant* are used interchangeably within this chapter). Initially the patient may complain of mild irritative symptoms, such as frequency greater than every 2 hours and nocturia greater than two times per night. As the disease progresses, patients may complain of urgency and urge incontinence. Finally, bladder capacity is diminished to the point where voiding occurs more than once per hour, and sleep is severely disrupted.

Patients with the so-called neurogenic bladder, secondary to myelomeningocele, for example, may not complain of the severe irritative symptoms common to the inflammatory or infectious disorders but instead report severe total incontinence secondary to a rigid bladder and a nonfunctional, denervated sphincter mechanism. On the other end of the range, the sphincter may function all too well in these patients with poorly compliant bladders, allowing dangerously high pressures (>40 cm H_2O) to exist for a majority of the bladder-filling cycle, thereby retarding upper tract drainage and causing hydronephrosis and renal insufficiency.

Dilatation of the upper tracts associated with a low-compliance bladder is usually secondary to the development of vesicoureteral reflux or to functional obstruction at the ureterovesical junction (UVJ). True anatomic obstruction of the UVJ in these bladders is rare, unless it is a direct consequence of the overall pathologic process such as tuberculous cystitis. Functional distal ureteral obstruction occurs in normal bladders because of compression of the intramural ureter during bladder contractions, or as a consequence of increased wall tension during bladder filling (increased radius), according to the law of Laplace. In the poorly compliant bladder, however, small increases in volume are associated with large increases in intravesical pressure, thereby exaggerating the risk of ureteral obstruction. An intravesical pressure exceeding 38 to 40 cm H_2O is the value thought to cause functional upper tract obstruction.[18,19]

It is necessary to appreciate the bladder outlet's role in the maintenance of elevated intravesical pressure. Fig. 48-1 illustrates how an incompetent sphincter will allow urinary incontinence yet will protect against hydronephrosis. On the other hand, an overactive sphincter or bladder outlet, in the presence of elevated intravesical pressure, will result in rare incontinence and significant hydronephrosis. Treatment is directed at either reducing bladder outlet resistance (such as sphincterotomy or alpha-adrenergic blockade) or decreasing intravesical pressure (intermittent catheterization with or without anticholinergics or bladder augmentation).

Congenital Disorders

Neurospinal Dysraphism

Myelomeningocele, although decreasing in incidence, is the most common cause of neurogenic bladder dysfunction in the United States and occurs in approximately 1 in 1000 live births.[20] Upper tract deterioration, manifested by pyelonephritis or

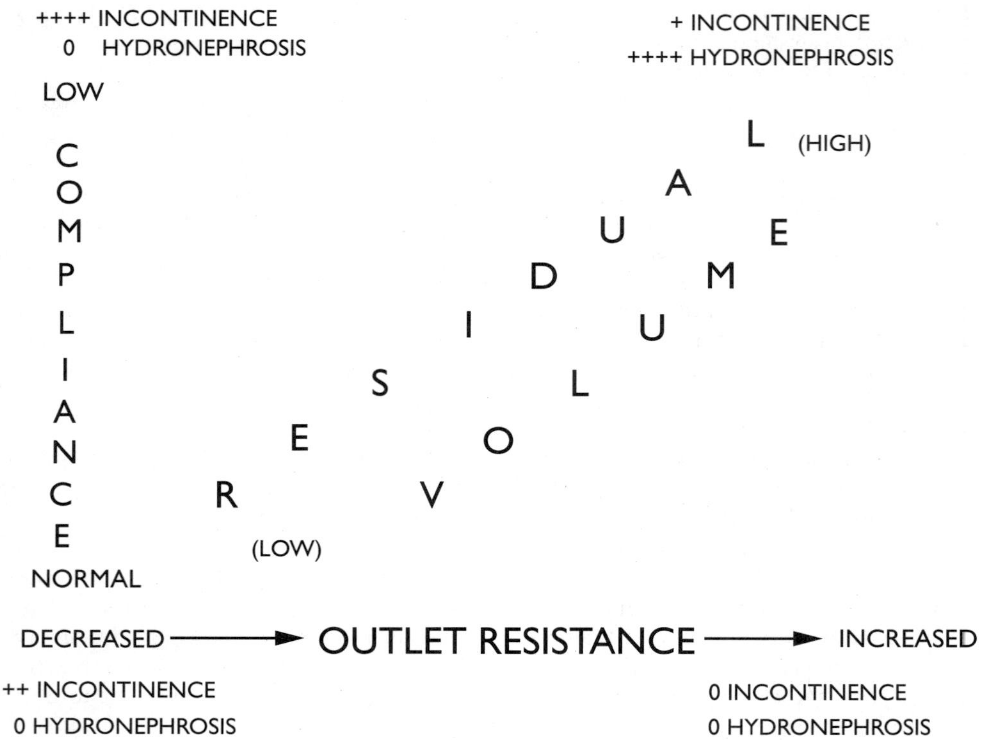

FIG. 48-1 *Relationship between bladder compliance, resting outlet resistance ("leak point pressure"), residual urine volume, and the potential for hydroureteronephrosis versus incontinence.* (From Staskin DR: *Urol Clin North Am* 18:309, 1991.)

hydronephrosis caused by the abnormal bladder, has up to now been the leading cause of illness and death in these young patients. The urologic manifestation of the neurologic lesion is highly unpredictable and may include one or more of the following: detrusor areflexia, detrusor hyperreflexia, hypocompliance, and detrusor–external sphincter dyssynergia.

As discussed above, histopathologic analysis of the bladders of these patients and the comparison to normal controls has documented a pathologic increase in the amount of connective tissue in the smooth muscle layer. Shapiro et al. performed quantitative morphometric analysis on bladder tissue from stillborn fetuses with and without myelomeningocele. Grossly, all the affected bladders were severely trabeculated with cellule formation, and the overall transmural thickness was increased in comparison to controls. Histologic analysis of the normal controls showed a discrete, well-organized layer of smooth muscle embedded in primitive mesenchyme, while four of the five abnormal bladders revealed a diminished size and amount of smooth muscle associated with a threefold increase in the amount of interfascicular and pericellular dense connective tissue.[17]

The manifestation of the above of course is a poorly compliant bladder, as demonstrated cystometrically, with the resultant sequelae of incontinence and renal insufficiency. Ghonheim et al.[21] analyzed the initial and terminal compliance characteristics from carbon dioxide cystometrograms in 32 patients with dysraphism and 15 controls without spinal dysraphism. He then divided the myelodysplastics into two groups with high (mean = 29.7 ml/cm H_2O) and low (mean = 7.3 ml/cm H_2O) initial compliance values. Low initial compliance was associated with vesicoureteral reflux, hydronephrosis, and renal insufficiency. McGuire et al.[19] reported on six myelodysplastic patients with detrusor hypertonia who experienced vesicoureteral reflux or hydronephrosis after initial evaluation. Significant radiographic improvement occurred after the inception of intermittent catheterization with anticholinergic pharmacotherapy. Similar studies have been performed by Weston[22] and Geraniotis.[23]

Treatment options must be geared to the individual situation, but all are directed to reducing bladder-filling pressures and increasing capacity and compliance. Anticholinergic therapy with clean intermittent catheterization is the cornerstone of conservative therapy. Surgical options in patients with upper tract deterioration despite noninvasive management include cutaneous vesicostomy in infants and young children and bladder augmentation in the older population.

Exstrophy

Bladder exstrophy has been estimated to occur between 1 in 10,000 and 1 in 50,000 live births.[24] Muecke[25] attributed the presence of this anomaly to the failure of the cloacal membrane to be reinforced by the medial migration of mesodermal tissue in between layers of endoderm and ectoderm in the infraumbilical abdominal wall. The mesoderm, in normal embryologic development, is destined to become the muscles of the lower abdominal wall and the skeletal structures of the pelvis. Without the support of these various structures, the cloacal membrane prematurely ruptures; the stage of embryologic development at which the rupture occurs will determine the extent of the anatomic defect.

The ultimate fundamental goals of reconstruction of the lower urinary tract are closure of the abdominal wall defect, maintenance of urinary continence, and protection of upper tract renal function. The surgical approach is usually staged over the child's first 3 to 5 years, as described by Jeffs.[26] The success of this complex reconstruction is directly correlated to the histologic condition of the exstrophied bladder. Culp[27] performed histologic analysis of 23 bladders removed from patients with exstrophy at an age of 1 month to 52 years and compared them to normal, postmortem controls. Not one of the study bladders was entirely normal. The most frequent finding was acute and chronic follicular inflammation, with edema of the lamina propria. Areas of acute ulceration and chronic granulation were also commonly noted. Nineteen of the 23 cases demonstrated patchy areas of squamous metaplasia, eight of which showed keratinizing features. Seven of the group displayed pronounced fibrosis of the muscularis layer, whereas 12 were normal.

Despite apparently successful primary bladder closure and subsequent vesical neck reconstruction, a percentage of children will still have persistent urinary incontinence because of small bladder capacity and decreased bladder compliance. Gearhart and Jeffs[28] reported on 12 patients who needed bladder augmentation out of a total of 148 with exstrophy. The indications for the augmentation were poor bladder capacity, hydronephrosis, or incontinence. In a similar series from the Mayo Clinic, Kramer[29] identified 11 patients (mean age, 8 years) requiring enterocystoplasty for decreased capacity (mean = 73 ml) or compliance, or persistent incontinence, out of a total of 201 patients. Other procedures that can be performed at the time of cystoplasty are a Young-Dees-Leadbetter vesical neck plasty, insertion of an artificial urinary sphincter, or a cutaneous continent stoma such as a Mitrofanoff procedure with concomitant closure of the bladder neck.

INFLAMMATORY CONDITIONS

Chemical Cystitis

Various chemotherapeutic agents administered either intravesically for the management of superficial transitional cell carcinoma or intravenously for the treatment of numerous neoplastic and nonneoplastic systemic diseases have been implicated as a cause of bladder contracture. Intravesical immunotherapy in the form of BCG (bacille Calmette-Guérin) is the most prevalent treatment modality, yet some cases require chemotherapeutic alternatives, of which doxorubicin and mitomycin are among the most popular. Cyclophosphamide has been infused intravenously for a variety of autoimmune conditions, such as systemic lupus erythematosus, and for certain hematologic or lymphatic cancers.

Doxorubicin and mitomycin exert their oncolytic influence by intercalation of alkylated compounds into strands of deoxyribonucleic acid, thereby inhibiting its synthesis. The drugs are released and potentially rereleased by cells as they die, as the toxic effects are perpetuated.[30] Uptake by normal cells has been documented.[31] A review of multiple studies[32] has documented a 5% to 100% incidence of chemical cystitis, usually associated with irritative voiding symptoms. In rare cases there was progression to severe bladder contracture with intolerable voiding frequency up to four times per hour, requiring palliative cystectomy and urinary diversion. The histopathologic specimen may demonstrate mucosal edema and superficial hemorrhage, as well as extensive inflammation, ulceration, and necrosis. Fibrosis may extend from its origin in the submucosa, through the muscularis, and into the circumvesical adipose layer.[32,33]

Cystitis has been reported in 4% to 36% of patients receiving cyclophosphamide therapy, usually after high-dose, intermittent, intravenous administration; its symptomatic onset may occur just after initial dosing or years later (especially if cyclophosphamide was administered orally).[34] Gross hematuria may occur years later and require blood transfusion. The offending agent is not the parent drug itself but an active metabolite, acrolein, liberated by hepatic microsomes and excreted in high concentrations in bile and urine.[35] The pathologic changes noted are similar to those described above for doxorubicin and mitomycin.

Cyclophosphamide cystitis may be avoided when the urothelium is protected from the effects of the active metabolite. Methods to accomplish this have included bilateral ureteral and urethral catheterization during the circuminfusion period. Others have simply hydrated patients sufficiently to cause a protective, dilutional diuresis during the period that the metabolite is being excreted into the urine. In severe cases surgical palliation is required, usually in the form of bladder augmentation with or without partial or supratrigonal cystectomy, or total urinary diversion with cystectomy.

Pelvic Irradiation

Pelvic malignancies account for 19% and 28% of all malignancies in the female and male respectively and include neoplasms of the gynecologogic, urologic, and alimentary systems. The majority of these tumors may be treated with radiation or surgery, or both, for definitive or palliative therapy.[36,37] Radiation is usually administered either by interstitially applied radioactive seeds (brachytherapy) or by external-beam linear accelerators (teletherapy). Advanced carcinomas of the cervix may require dual therapy.[38] Complications associated with radiation therapy are associated with the specific organ treated, the method of delivery, the isotope utilized, and, above all, the total dosage administered. The incidence of severe bladder symptoms after radiation for cervical carcinoma has been demonstrated to be dose related in multiple studies; 70% of the patients with such symptoms received greater than 6000 rad.[39]

The clinical presentation of radiation cystitis may closely mimic the irritative symptoms of bacterial cystitis and can feature frequency, urgency, nocturia, dysuria, and hematuria. In landmark studies, Dean and Lytton[40] and Kottmeier and Gray[41] showed that acute radiation cystitis occurs in less than 5% of patients, at cumulative doses exceeding 3000 rad. Dean and Lytton also showed in their study of 964 patients that only 2.5% of the complications (cystitis, hematuria, ureteral obstruction, fistula) associated with pelvic irradiation for malignancy were attributable to the effects of the radiation alone, whereas the majority of the complications were secondary to persistent or recurrent tumor. Bladder contracture is rare and usually occurs when an associated operation has been performed.[42,43]

Cystoscopy characteristically demonstrates mucosal edema and diffuse erythema, with increased vascular injection in the acute stages. The appearance of the mucosa in the chronic phase is notable for areas of extreme pallor, with diffuse atrophy and areas of telangiectasia. Histologically there is interstitial fibrosis and endarteritis obliterans. In severe cases, fibrotic scarring spreads to the muscularis, with an associated decrease in compliance.[42,43]

The majority of bladder symptoms are managed medically. Anticholinergics may be helpful to increase bladder capacity and decrease the incidence of debilitating urinary frequency. Hemorrhagic cystitis may be managed by a variety of instillational agents such as dimethyl sulfoxide (DMSO) or formalin. Severe hemorrhage or bladder contracture may require diversion or cystectomy.

Interstitial Cystitis

Since first being described by Nitze[44] in 1907, this condition has eluded complete characterization because an exact cause has yet to be discovered. Patients are usually middle-aged women, presenting with often debilitating irritative voiding symptoms and severe suprapubic pain usually diminished or relieved by voiding. Urine cultures and cytologic tests are negative, and urinalysis may show microhematuria.[45] Cystoscopy demonstrates multiple petechial hemorrhages, known as glomerulations, on the second fill, after initial distension of the bladder to obtain a pressure greater than 70 cm H_2O.[46] The presence of single or multiple radiating ulcers as described by Hunner has proved to be extremely rare.[47]

Early histopathologic descriptions reported a transmural pancystitis with inflammation and fibrosis extending into the muscularis.[48,49] These initial studies included only patients with small-capacity bladders. Later studies with the more current, broader inclusion criteria reported that the principle microscopic findings are a normal-appearing epithelium and muscularis, with vasodilatation and edema occurring in the submucosa. Mast cells and edema are noted in the muscularis only in cases of excessive mastocytosis.[50] Fibrosis of either the submucosa or muscularis layers is a rare finding.[45] Messing and Stamey identified patients with two forms of the disease: the group with a small capacity bladder and a Hunner's ulcer were placed in the "classic" category, whereas the remainder with a normal capacity and no ulcer were placed in the "early" group. Interestingly, fibrosis was seen in only 4 of 15 patients in the early group (muscle was not demonstrated in the remaining 4), and in 4 of 19 in the classic group.[45] Most patients currently diagnosed with this condition demonstrate normal bladder capacities while under general anesthesia; severe sensory urgency while the patient is awake prevents filling volumes to even one half the capacity seen under anesthesia.

INFECTIOUS DISEASES

Schistosomiasis

The urologic manifestations characteristic of infection with the parasite *Schistosoma haematobium,* that is, gross hematuria and terminal dysuria, have been known for 4000 years, since the Twelfth Dynasty of ancient Egypt. This entity is still a major health concern in the fertile farming lands of the Middle East because 80 to 90 million people are believed to be infected by *S. haematobium.*[51]

Adults of the species *S. haematobium* lodge in the veins of the perivesical plexus and may deposit 200 to 500 eggs per day for an average life span of 3.4 years.[52] The majority of eggs remain in the walls of the hollow viscera in which they are laid and where they stimulate in the host the characteristic granulomatous reaction.[53] A mild inflammatory reaction occurs as the eggs leave terminal venules and enter the bladder wall. Although only 20% of the eggs successfully migrate to the lumen for subsequent excretion, the remainder become trapped in the submucosa and epithelium by the developing fibrosis and scar tissue.[54] An intense foreign-body reaction and eosinophilic cellular infiltration occurs and may form the characteristic tubercle, known as a bilharzioma. Calcification of the ovum may occur. Small ulcers form as the ova penetrate the epithelial layer to enter the lumen; these ulcers may coalesce to form larger ulcers associated with gross hematuria. As the process continues, the blood supply to the mucosa diminishes; further ulceration and hemorrhage occur. Progressive involvement of the deeper layers causes the entire muscularis to be replaced by fibrotic, sclerotic, disorganized tissue; in 1% of patients the capacity is less than 60 ml. The resultant fibrosis may obstruct the ureteral orifices with resultant renal failure. Squamous cell carcinoma is found in 60% to 90% of bilharzial cancers, and adenocarcinoma of the bladder in 5% to 15%.[55,56] Early cases of schistosomiasis caused by *S. haematobium* are effectively treated with various parasiticidal compounds. Chronically contracted bladders have been managed in the past by denervation, hydrodistension, and augmentation cystoplasty.

Tuberculosis

Bladder involvement is secondary to antegrade flow of the tubercle bacillus from the involved kidney and occurs in about 1% of cases with genitourinary tuberculosis. The classic cystographic picture of tuberculous cystitis characteristically shows a small, irregularly shaped bladder with bilateral vesicoureteral reflux and varying degrees of pelvicalicectasis and ureterectasis.[57] The orifice is initially obscured by mucosal edema. Inflammation and the resultant fibrosis usually starts from the ureteral orifice on the affected side and then progresses to the entire bladder transmurally, involving the muscularis propria. The periureteral fibrosis causes contraction of the orifice, which then becomes rigid and often dilated, described previously as a "golf-hole." Vesicoureteral reflux may result from the scarring in the ureter's lower third because the normally coapted flap-valve mechanism no longer functions effectively[58]; or the disease in the distal portion of the ureter may cause ureteral stricture, obstruction, and autonephrectomy.[59] Ulcers, although rare, usually occur initially near the orifice but may be found throughout as the disease spreads. The appearance of discrete tubercles, also seen in proximity to the ureteral orifice, is a very infrequent finding.[58]

In severe and advanced cases the entire mucosal lining is replaced by ulceration and granulation tissue. The bladder in the end stage is small, spherical, and contracted with severely diminished capacity.[58,59] Treatment is obviously directed to the anatomic site and the severity of the disease at the time of diagnosis. Early treatment with multidrug regimens including rifampin, pyrazinamide, isoniazid, and ethambutol is usually effective. In advanced cases, surgery usually follows the pharmacologic intervention and may require the use of intestinal segments to replace a strictured ureter or a contracted bladder. Augmentation cystoplasty should be performed in patients with bladder capacities less than 100 ml.

TRAUMA

Spinal Cord and Neural Injury

Classification schemas that describe residual bladder function after neurologic insult have relied primarily upon the specific anatomic location and spinal cord level of the injury. Classically a suprasacral (upper motor neuron) disorder, including intracerebral lesions, causes detrusor hyperreflexia, whereas lesions of the conus medullaris (lower motor neuron), which contain the S1 to S5 spinal segments, cause detrusor areflexia. The conus is approximately 1.5 cm long and is located at vertebral level T12 to L1. It should be noted that many lesions may not conform to a convenient anatomically based classification system, and hence the clinical appearance may reflect a combination of upper and lower motor neuron features.

Low bladder compliance may result from injuries to the sacral segments of the conus medullaris or to the parasympathetic nerves of the pelvic plexus. Gunasekera et al.[60] found, in a study of 70 patients with localized, surgically treatable spinal cord lesions, that all 34 patients with an upper motor neuron lesion displayed normal bladder compliance; reduced compliance was seen only in patients with lower motor neuron lesions. Hackler et al[61] identified low compliance (20 ml/cm H_2O) in 50% of patients with lower motor neuron lesions, compared to only 10% of patients with suprasacral lesions. Parasympathetic denervation may also occur during extirpative pelvic surgery, as with a radical hysterectomy or an abdominoperineal resection. Sislow and Mayo[62] compared the bladder compliance of patients with injuries to the conus or cauda equina to that of patients who underwent extensive pelvic surgery. Interestingly, of the 31 patients in the pelvic surgery group, 18 had abnormal compliance compared to only 4 of the 33 patients in the conal–cauda equina group. The median bladder capacity was higher in the conal–cauda equina group (450 ml) than in the pelvic surgery group (305 ml).

The exact mechanism by which parasympathetic decentralization causes detrusor hypocompliance has up to now not been fully clarified, though most theories indicate a possibly exaggerated alpha-adrenergic mediated smooth muscle tonus rather than the normally present beta-adrenergic mediated smooth muscle relaxation, which facilitates accommodation of increasing bladder volumes.[63] In a feline model, Hanno et al[64] confirmed that parasympathetic denervation resulted in adrenergic hyperinnervation of the detrusor. In contrast, Neal et al.[65] demonstrated no change in adrenergic innervation but an increase in cholinergic innervation associated with decreased compliance.

Ghoniem and colleagues[15] performed complete parasympathetic decentralization by means of a lumbosacral laminectomy in five dogs; a full-thickness bladder biopsy specimen was taken before the procedure and again 12 weeks postoperatively. Bladder capacity was decreased after denervation compared to normals (119 versus 198 ml) but was not statistically significant. Bladder compliance, however was greatly diminished after denervation (1.29 versus 4.2 ml/cm H_2O, $p < 0.05$). Histologic analysis of the denervated bladders demonstrated a lymphocytic infiltrate and fibrosis in the submucosal layer and a similar fibrosis and collagenosis in the muscularis layer. The muscularis layer demonstrated increased thickening and a higher density of cell nuclei (275 vs 166 per mm^2). This is strong evidence that histologic changes and the resultant hypocompliance are neurally mediated.

As above, treatment is geared to maintaining low detrusor pressures and preventing upper tract deterioration. Anticholinergics with or without intermittent catheterization is the initial treatment of choice.

OBSTRUCTIVE PHENOMENA

Fetal and Neonatal Bladder Outlet Obstruction

The most common cause of congenital bladder outlet obstruction is posterior urethral valves, found only in males, and located at the distal part of the prostatic urethra. The valve leaflets are mucosal folds that cause varying degrees of obstruction. The infants may present with a poor urinary flow, sepsis, or a palpable lower abdominal mass, resulting from a distended bladder. Failure to thrive is usually associated with azotemia and anemia. Abdominal ultrasound survey will usually demonstrate hydronephrosis and a distended bladder in both the pediatric and the fetal populations.

These "valve" bladders are grossly thickened and trabeculated. In many cases, the bladder dysfunction and resultant hydroureteronephrosis persists even after the outlet obstruction is relieved.[66] Three distinct urodynamic findings have been identified in these patients: myogenic failure, detrusor hyperreflexia, and detrusor hypertonia.[67] The last group, with a poorly compliant bladder, is at the highest risk for upper tract deterioration.

Various studies have attempted to dispel the previously held notion that bladder hypocontractility and hypocompliance are the result of obstruction-related collagen deposition. Workman and Kogan[68] studied the bladders of stillborn or aborted fetuses with posterior valves and compared them to that of controls. The affected bladders had increased bladder thickness (1.7 ±0.3 versus 0.9 ±0.2 mm) and a slightly increased ratio of connective tissue (38% ±6% versus 31% ±7 %). They concluded, based on the minimal degree of collagen deposition, that the deposition itself was not the cause of bladder dysfunction and suggested that an alteration in the collagen subtypes might be responsible. Kim et al.[67] indeed studied the effects of obstruction on collagen subtypes in fetal bladders against age-matched controls and found a sharp increase in the ratio of thick-to-thin collagen fibers in the obstructed bladders. In severe cases, thick collagen infiltrated between individual muscle fibers. This phenomenon indicates that pathologic collagen deposition may not only affect compliance, but contractility as well. Interestingly, Peters et al.[69] demonstrated only smooth muscle hypertrophy and hyperplasia and not connective tissue infiltration, in an in utero sheep model. They demonstrated a sixfold increase in smooth muscle mass and cystometric evidence of reduced compliance.

Adult Bladder Outlet Obstruction

The overwhelming number of adults with abnormal bladder compliance are men greater than 50 years of age with prostate-related voiding dysfunction. Benign prostatic hypertrophy (BPH) of some degree is nearly ubiquitous in men in this age group, yet the clinical presentation with respect to irritative versus obstructive symptoms is highly variable Various studies have examined the structural morphology responsible for the detrusor dysfunction.

Elbadawi et al.[70] investigated obstructive and nonobstructive bladder dysfunction in a prospective ultrastructural and urodynamic study with blinded clinical and urodynamic information. Patients with urodynamically confirmed obstruction demonstrated a myohypertrophy pattern that is characterized by (1) widening of spaces between smooth muscle cells, (2) massive deposits of collagen and elastin between the abnormally separated muscle cells, (3) smooth muscle hypertrophy, and (4) nonuniform distribution of the three previous attributes in the muscle fascicles. The relative amounts of collagen versus elastin is believed to govern the distensibility of the bladder wall in each individual patient, just as in the fetal population, discussed above. Gilpin et al.[13] demonstrated collagen infiltration among muscle bundles in 12 out of 14 urodynamically obstructed men and an absence of infiltration in all patients without obstruction.

CONCLUSION

The conditions discussed above are not an all-inclusive list of the entities that are known to produce poorly compliant bladders but are simply among the most well characterized. Each can cause varying degrees of abnormal compliance and hence can produce a broad spectrum of clinical presentations, ranging from annoying irritative voiding symptoms to life-threatening renal failure. Therapy is therefore directed appropriately. The overriding goal when severe bladder disorder is present is preservation of renal function; this is usually accomplished by medical or surgical means designed to decrease resting storage pressure, thereby allowing unimpeded drainage of upper tract urine. The mainstay of medical therapy remains anticholinergic pharmacotherapy with or without clean intermittent catheterization. Bladder augmentation, reserved for cases refractory to more conservative therapies, has produced excellent results.

REFERENCES

1. Stephenson TP: The interpretation of conventional urodynamics. In Mundy AR, Stephenson TP, Wein AJ, editors: *Urodynamics: principles, practice and application,* ed 2, Edinburgh, 1994, Churchill Livingstone.
2. Andersen JT: Detrusor hyperreflexia in benign intravesical obstruction, a cystometric study, *J Urol* 115:532, 1976.
3. Gilmour RF, Churchill BM, Steckler RE, et al: A new technique for dynamic analysis of bladder compliance, *J Urol* 150:1200, 1993.
4. McInerney PD: The practice of urodynamics. In Mundy AR, Stephenson TP, Wein AJ, editors: *Urodynamics: principles, practice and application,* ed 2, Edinburgh, 1994, Churchill Livingstone.
5. Churchill BM, Gilmour RF, Williot P: Urodynamics, *Pediatr Clin North Am* 34:1133, 1987.
6. Vuorio E, de Crombugge B: The family of collagen genes, *Ann Rev Biochem* 59:837, 1990.
7. Bornstein P, Sage H: Structurally distinct collagen types, *Ann Rev Biochem* 49:957, 1980.
8. Gathercole LJ, Keller A: Crimp morphology in the fiber-forming collagens, *Matrix* 11:214, 1991.
9. Burgeson RE: New collagens, new concepts, *Ann Rev Cell Biol* 4:551, 1988.
10. Ewalt DH, Howard PS, Blyth B, et al: Is lamina propria matrix responsible for normal bladder compliance? *J Urol* 148:544, 1992.
11. Susset JG, Regnier JG: Viscolelastic properties of bladder strips: standardization of a technique, *Invest Urol* 18:445, 1981.
12. Landau EH, Jayanthi VR, Churchill BM, et al: Loss of elasticity in dysfunctional bladders: urodynamic and histochemical correlation, *J Urol* 152:702, 1994.
13. Gilpin SA, Gosling JA, Barnard RJ: Morphological and morphometric studies of the human obstructed, trabeculated urinary bladder, *Br J Urol* 57:525, 1985.
14. McGuire EJ, Savastano JA: Effect of alpha-adrenergic blockade and anticholinergic agents on decentralized primate bladder, *Neurourol Urodyn* 4:139, 1985.
15. Ghonhiem GM et al: Effect of bilateral sacral decentralization on detrusor contractility and passive properties in dog, *Neurourol Urodyn* 3:23, 1984.
16. Elbadawi A: Ultrastructure of vesicourethral innervation. I. Neuroeffector and cell junctions in the male internal sphincter, *J Urol* 128:180, 1982.
17. Shapiro E, Becich MJ, Perlman E, Lepor H: Bladder wall abnormalities in myelodysplastic bladders: a computer assisted morphometric analysis, *J Urol* 145:1024, 1991.
18. Staskin DR: Hydroureteronephrosis after spinal cord injury: effects of lower urinary tract dysfunction on upper tract anatomy, *Urol Clin North Am* 18:309, 1991.
19. McGuire EJ, Woodside JR, Borden T: Upper urinary tract deterioration in patients with myelodysplasia and detrusor hypertonia: a followup study, *J Urol* 1 29:823, 1983.
20. Kroovand RL: Myelomeningocele. In Walsh PC, Gittes R, Perlmutter A, Stamey T, editors: *Campbell's urology,* ed 5, Philadelphia, 1986, Saunders.
21. Ghonhiem GM, Bloom DA, McGuire EJ, Stewart KL: Bladder compliance in meningomyelocele children, *J Urol* 141:1404, 1989.
22. Weston PMT, Robinson LQ, Williams S, et al: Poor compliance early in filling in the neuropathic bladder, *Br J Urol* 63:28, 1989.
23. Geraniotis E, Koff SA, Enrile B: The prophylactic use of clean intermittent catheterization in the treatment of infants and young children with myelomeningocele and neurogenic bladder dysfunction, *J Urol* 139:85, 1988.
24. Lattimer JK, Smith MJK: Exstrophy closure: a followup on 70 cases, *J Urol* 95:356, 1966.
25. Muecke EC: The role of the cloacal membrane in exstrophy: the first successful experimental study, *J Urol* 92:659, 1964.
26. Jeffs RD: Exstrophy and cloacal exstrophy, *Urol Clin North Am* 5:127, 1978.
27. Culp DA: The histology of the exstrophied bladder, *J Urol* 91:539, 1964.
28. Gearhart JP, Jeffs RD: Augmentation cystoplasty in the failed exstrophy reconstruction, *J Urol* 139:790, 1988.
29. Kramer SA: Augmentation cystoplasty in patients with exstrophy-epispadias, *J Pediatr Surg* 24:1293, 1989.
30. Baker WC, Russo MA, deVere White RW: Severe bladder contracture in patient receiving intravesical mitomycin C for superficial bladder cancer, *Urology* 30:357, 1987.
31. Rudolph R, Stein RS, Patillo RA: Skin ulcers due to adriamycin, *Cancer* 38:1087, 1976.
32. Dmochowski R, Rudy DC: Bladder contracture following intravesical doxorubicin therapy: case report and review of the literature, *J Urol* 143:816, 1990.
33. Wajsman Z, McGill W, Emglander L, et al: Severely contracted bladder following intravesical mitomycin C therapy, *J Urol* 130:340, 1983.
34. Marsh FP, Vince FP, Pollock DJ, et al: Cyclophosphamide necrosis of bladder causing calcification contracture and reflux; treated by colocystoplasty, *Br J Urol* 43:324, 1971.

35. Brock N, Hohorst HJ: Metabolism of cyclophosphamide, *Cancer* 20:900, 1967.
36. Brady LW, Markoe AM, Sheline GE, et al: Radiation oncology: programs for the present and future, *Cancer* 55:2037, 1985.
37. *1985 Cancer facts and figures,* New York, 1985, American Cancer Society.
38. *1980 Cancer facts and figures,* New York, 1979, American Cancer Society.
39. Kottmeier HL, Gray MJ: Rectal and bladder injuries in relation to radiation dosage in carcinoma of the cervix: a 5 year follow up, *Am J Obstet Gynecol* 82:74, 1961.
40. Dean RJ, Lytton B: Urologic complications of pelvic irradiation, *J Urol* 119:64, 1978.
41. Gray MJ, Kottmeier HL: Rectal and bladder injuries following radium therapy for carcinoma of the cervix at the Radiumhemmet, *Am J Obstet Gynecol* 74:1294, 1957.
42. Galleher EP Jr, Young JD Jr, Mowad JJ, et al: A followup study of supervoltage irradiation followed by cystectomy for bladder cancer, *J Urol* 99:59, 1968.
43. Liegner LM, Taylor JA, Michaud NJ: Supervoltage cobalt-60 treatment of bladder cancer: palliation or cure? *J Urol* 87:373, 1962.
44. Messing EM: Interstitial cystitis and related syndromes. In Walsh PC, Retik Ab, Stamey TA, Vaughan ED Jr, editors: *Campbell's urology,* ed 6, Philadelphia, 1992, Saunders.
45. Messing EM, Stamey TA: Interstitial cystitis: early diagnosis, pathology and treatment, *Urology* 12:381, 1978.
46. Walsh A: Interstitial cystitis. In Harrison JH et al, editors: *Campbell's urology,* ed 4, Philadelphia, 1978, Saunders.
47. Hanno PM, Levin RM, Monson FC, et al: Diagnosis of interstitial cystitis, *J Urol* 141:846, 1989.
48. Hand JR: Interstitial cystitis, *J Urol* 61:291, 1949.
49. Smith BH, Dehner LP: Chronic ulcerating cystitis (Hunner's ulcer): a study of 28 cases, *Arch Pathol* 93:76, 1972.
50. Johansson SL: Light microscopic findings in bladders of patients with interstitial cystitis. In Hanno PM, et al, editors: *Interstitital cystitis,* New York, 1990, Springer-Verlag.
51. Dittrich M, Doehring E: Ultrasonographical aspects of urinary schistosomiasis: assessment of morphological lesions in the upper and lower urinary tract, *Pediatr Radiol* 16:225, 1986.
52. Butterworth AE, et al: Longitudinal studies on human schistosomiasis, *Philos Trans R Soc Lond (Biol)* 321:495, 1988.
53. Cheever AW, Byram JE, Hieny S, et al: Immunopathology of *Schistosoma japonicum* and *S. mansoni* infection in B-cell depleted mice, *Parasite Immunol* 7:399, 1985.
54. Cheever AW, Anderson LA: Rate of destruction of *Schistosoma mansoni* eggs in the tissues of mice, *Am J Trop Med Hyg* 20:62, 1971.
55. Dimmette RM, Sayegh ES, Sproat HF: Chronic ulcer of the bladder associated with schistosomiasis, *Surg Gynecol Obstet* 101:721, 1955.
56. Sayegh ES: Late complications of urinary bilharziasis, *J Urol* 63:353, 1950.
57. Sculley RE, et al: Weekly clinicopathological exercises, Case 11-1987, *N Engl J Med* 316:676, 1987.
58. Barrie HJ, Kerr WK, Gale GL: The incidence and pathogenesis of tuberculous strictures of the renal pelvis, *J Urol* 98:584, 1967.
59. Gunasekera WSL, Richardson AE, Seneviratne KN, et al: Detrusor hyperreflexia in neurogenic bladder disorders caused by localized partial lesions of the spinal cord and cauda equina, *Surg Neurol* 20:63, 1983.
60. Hackler RH Hall MK, Zampieri TA: Bladder hypocompliance in the spinal cord injury population, *J Urol* 141:1390, 1989.
61. Sislow JG, Mayo ME: Reduction in human bladder compliance following decentralization, *J Urol* 144:945, 1990.
62. Sundin T, Dahlström A: The sympathetic innervation of the urinary bladder and urethra in the normal state and after parasympathetic denervation at the spinal root level: an experimental study in cats, *Scand J Urol Nephrol* 7:131, 1973.
63. Hanno AGE, Atta MA, Elbadawi A: Intrinsic neuromuscular defects in the neurogenic bladder: IX. Effects of combined parasympathetic decentralization and hypogastric neurectomy on neuromuscular ultrtastructure of the feline bladder base, *Neurourol Urodyn* 7:93:1988.
64. Neal DE, Bogue PR, Williams RE: Histological appearances of the nerves of the bladder in patients with denervation of the bladder after excision of the rectum, *Br J Urol* 54:658, 1982.
65. Parkhouse HF, et al: Long-term outcome of boys with posterior urethral valves, *Br J Urol* 62:59, 1988.
66. Kim KM, Kogan BA, Massad CA, Huang YC: Collagen and elastin in the obstructed fetal bladder, *J Urol* 146:528, 1991.
67. Workman SJ Kogan BA: Fetal bladder histology in posterior urethral valves, *J Urol* 144:337, 1990.
68. Peters CA, Vasavada S, Dator D, et al: The effect of obstruction on the developing bladder, *J Urol* 148:491, 1992.
69. Elbadawi A, Yalla SV, Resnick NM: Structural basis of geriatric voiding dysfunction. IV. Bladder outlet obstruction, *J Urol* 150:1681, 1993.

Chapter 49 Continent Diversion

Randall G. Rowland

When urinary diversion is required for the management of any problem that involves the lower urinary tract, a very important issue in the quality of life of the patient is continence. Noncontinent diversions such as ileal or colon conduits have been used in the past. In recent years, procedures have evolved that make the use of continent cutaneous urinary reservoirs practical. These continent cutaneous procedures offer the patient the ability to avoid having to use ostomy appliances and enjoy a better quality of life. Although neobladder procedures have been developed for urinary reconstruction, these procedures are generally not applicable in patients whose indications for surgery is incontinence. As a result, only selected continent cutaneous urinary reservoirs are presented in this chapter. The Indiana, Kock, and Mainz pouches are described along with a transverse colon–gastric tube pouch that is suitable for heavily radiated patients.

Patients along with their families and primary care physicians who help in the management of the patient over the long term often have many questions about continent diversion. Illustrations of the surgical procedures are invaluable in helping the patient and those individuals involved in the long-term postoperative management of the patient to understand the operative procedure and the concepts upon which the operative procedure is based. For this reason, step-by-step illustrations are provided for physicians to review and present to patients to help them conceptualize the operative procedures involved in continent diversion.

Regardless of the type of reservoir that is constructed, several general considerations need to be made. An ideal continent cutaneous reservoir should be a low-pressure, compliant vessel that uses the minimum amount of bowel possible to achieve a capacity sufficient to allow the patient to go 4 to 6 hours between catheterizations. Since the reservoir is being emptied by clean intermittent catheterization and will normally be colonized with bacteria, an effective antireflux mechanism is needed. If the patient's quality of life is to be improved, a reliable continence mechanism is necessary. The procedures should also offer low complication and reoperation rates.

Detubularization of the bowel segment or segments to be used for the reservoir is an important concept that offers two major advantages. First, detubularization changes a cylindrical segment of bowel to a shape approximating a sphere. This increases the volume of the reservoir relative to the amount of bowel used.[1] A sphere gives the maximum volume for a given surface area. Even though a perfect sphere is not obtained, an ellipsoid with its length no more than twice its width will hold over 90% of the maximum volume of a perfect sphere. This 2:1 ellipsoid can be achieved by a single folding over of a colonic segment. The other advantage of detubularization is a reduction in the pressure within the reservoir. According to Laplace's law, the pressure within a vessel is proportional to the tension in the wall of the vessel and inversely proportional to the radius of the vessel. Since detubularization increases the radius of the reservoir, the intrareservoir pressure decreases.

SELECTED CURRENT PROCEDURES

The Indiana Pouch

The Indiana pouch was first described in 1985 as a modification of the Gilchrist procedure.[2] Over the last 10 years, modifications that have improved the reliability of the procedure, decreased operative time, and decreased the need for revisions have been made. The current technique uses 8 to 10 cm of terminal ileum and 25 to 30 cm of cecum and ascending colon.[3] The colonic segment that is used for the reservoir is completely detubularized. One can accomplish this by splitting the segment along the antimesenteric surface as shown in Fig. 49-1. The cephalad end is folded down to the apex of the antimesenteric incision, and the reservoir is closed transversely. This creates an ellipsoid with approximately a 2:1 length-width ratio. Recently the hand-sewn detubularization technique has been modified by using absorbable GIA and TA_{55} staplers to detubularize and close the reservoir,[4] as shown in Fig. 49-2. This technique saves about 1 hour of operative time.

Before reconfiguration and closure of the reservoir, one creates the continence mechanism and efferent limb by tapering the terminal ileal segment with metal staples and plicating the ileocecal valve, as shown in Fig. 49-3. After the efferent limb and continence mechanism have been completed, the reservoir is detubularized and closed. The locations of the reservoir and stoma site (usually in the right lower quadrant or the umbilicus) are selected. The ureters are implanted using tunneled tenial implantations to prevent reflux. A 2:1 or 3:1 tunnel length–ureteral diameter ratio is created as shown in Fig. 49-4. Ureteral stents and a cecostomy tube are left in place in the initial postoperative period.

The Kock Pouch

The Kock pouch urinary diversion is a modification of the Kock continent ileostomy procedure developed for patients who have had a total colectomy.[5] The procedure has undergone several modifications to achieve the current form.[6] The pouch is made from a 78 cm segment of ileum. The central 44 cm is split along the antimesenteric border to detubularize this portion. This portion is configured into a U shape, and the medial edges are sewn together, as shown in Fig. 49-5. Intussuscepted ileal valves are formed in the remaining afferent and efferent limbs to create the antireflux and continence mechanisms (Fig. 49-6). After the intussuscepted valves are completed, the bottom of the detubularized central portion of the segment is folded over to complete the reservoir (Fig. 49-7). The ureters are anastomosed to the afferent limb in an end-to-side manner as in a Bricker procedure. A flush stoma is usually created in the right lower quadrant. It is important to make the efferent limb as straight and as short as possible to facilitate catheterization. Ureteral stents and a large Medina tube in the efferent limb are left in place at the end of the procedure.

The Mainz Pouch

The Mainz pouch is a composite ileocecal reservoir. Initially the continence mechanism was based on an intussuscepted ileal segment. Several modifications were made on this portion of the technique, which evolved into placing the intussuscepted ileal segment through the ileocecal valve to reinforce it.[7] The technique of forming the composite reservoir is shown in Fig. 49-8. The efferent limb and continence mechanism techniques are shown in Fig. 49-9. More recently, a continent appendix stoma has been used when a good appendix is available. The appendix is tunneled in a tenia to create the continence mechanism as shown in Fig. 49-10. Care must be taken to keep the appendiceal blood supply intact. The ureters are brought into the reservoir through the colonic segment using a tunneled submucosal technique.

The Transverse Colon–Gastric Tube Pouch

Although all three of the previously described pouches have been used in radiated patients, Bihrle and his associates developed a pouch made from bowel segments that are normally out of the field of radiation for pelvic malignancies.[8]

The reservoir is made from a detubularized segment of transverse colon as shown in Fig. 49-11. A gastric tube is harvested from the greater curvature of the stomach and is supported by one of the gastroepiploic vessels (Fig. 49-12). The tube is implanted into the reservoir by a tunneled tenial technique as shown in Fig. 49-13.

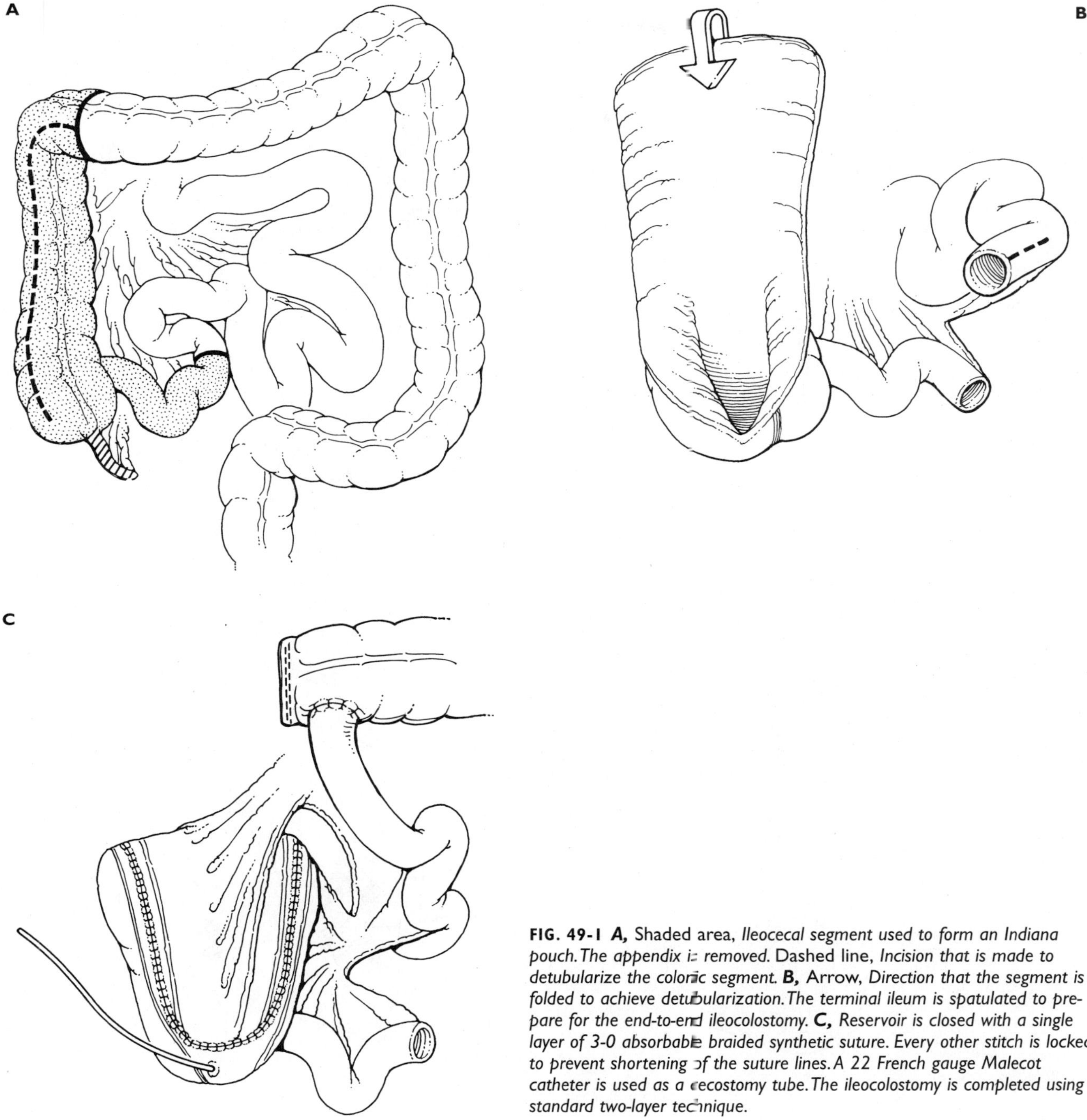

FIG. 49-1 ***A,*** Shaded area, *Ileocecal segment used to form an Indiana pouch. The appendix is removed.* Dashed line, *Incision that is made to detubularize the colonic segment.* ***B,*** Arrow, *Direction that the segment is folded to achieve detubularization. The terminal ileum is spatulated to prepare for the end-to-end ileocolostomy.* ***C,*** *Reservoir is closed with a single layer of 3-0 absorbable braided synthetic suture. Every other stitch is locked to prevent shortening of the suture lines. A 22 French gauge Malecot catheter is used as a cecostomy tube. The ileocolostomy is completed using a standard two-layer technique.*

The ureters are also implanted into the reservoir using the antirefluxing tunneled tenial technique (Fig. 49-14). The stoma is usually created in the upper portion of the abdomen.

Postoperative Management and Follow-Up Study

Regardless of which technique is used for continent cutaneous urinary diversion, the ureterointestinal anastomosis has to be evaluated before stent removal. Usually x-ray contrast material is injected through the stents. If the contrast runs around the stents into the reservoir, the stents are removed at about 1 week.

The reservoir is kept at rest with a cecostomy tube or a tube through the efferent limb for 2 to 3 weeks. The reservoir is checked with a pouchogram. If no leaks are present, the patient is started on intermittent catheterization. The upper tracts are checked for any evidence of obstruction with an intravenous pyelogram.

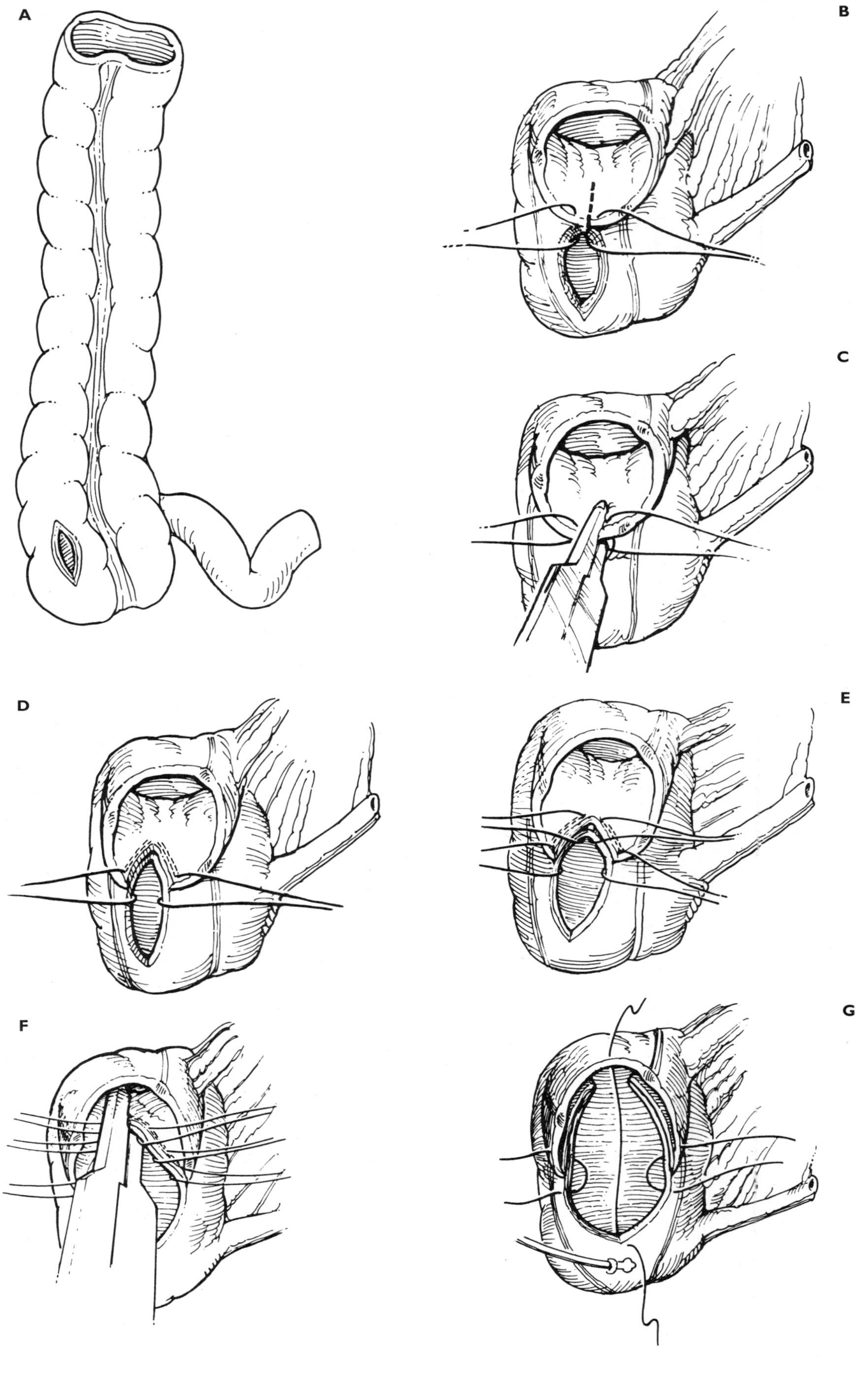
A
B
C
D
E
F
G

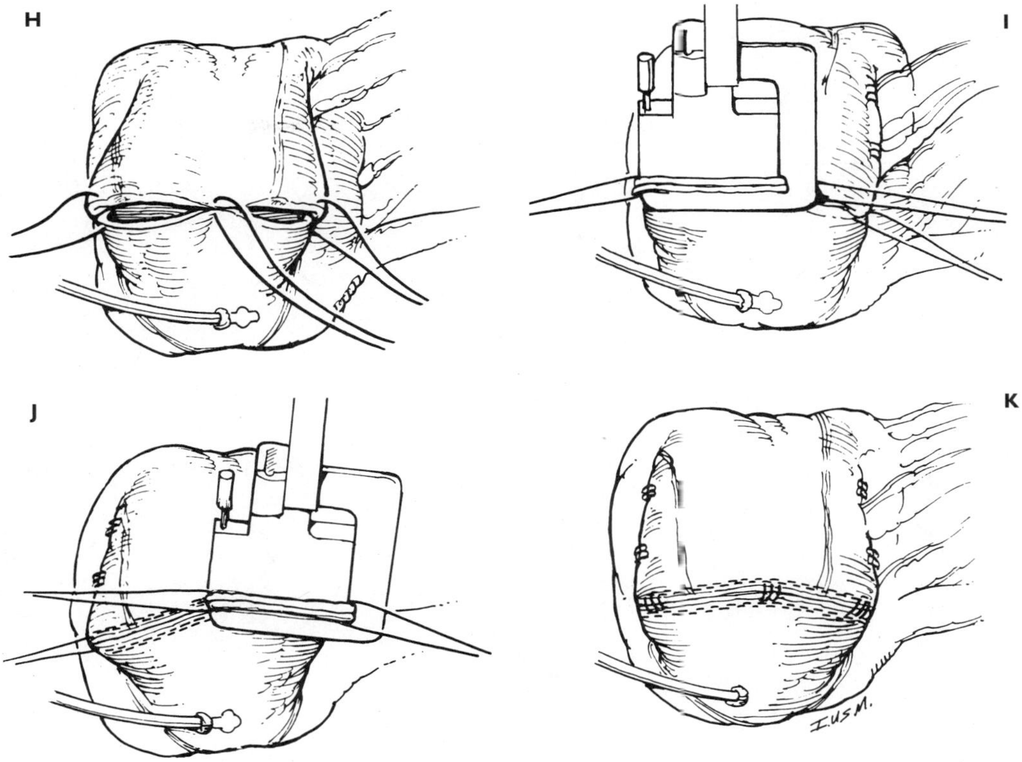

FIG. 49-2 ***A,*** *When absorbable staples are used to detubularize and close the reservoir, the same ileocecal segment is isolated as with the hand-sewn technique. A 2 to 3 cm cecotomy is made on the antimesenteric surface across from the ileocecal valve. This gives good access to the ileocecal valve for tapering of the efferent limb and creation of the continence mechanism at the ileocecal valve.* ***B,*** *After the efferent limb and continence mechanism have been completed, holding sutures are placed to align the antimesenteric portion of the cephalad end of the segment with cecotomy.* Dashed line, *Where the absorbable GIA stapler will be applied.* ***C,*** *The 75 mm GIA absorbable stapler is fired.* ***D,*** *After firing the stapler, partial detubularization is achieved.* ***E,*** *The incision between the two staple lines must be extended 5 mm beyond the end of the staples. New holding sutures are placed to help with positioning the bowel for application of a second stapler.* ***F,*** *Usually a third stapler application is required to complete the detubularization. The holding sutures are used to close the small gaps between staple lines, since absorbable staples cannot be overlapped.* ***G,*** *Holding sutures are placed in preparation for closure of the reservoir.* ***H,*** *Before closure, a cecostomy tube is placed.* ***I,*** *A TA_{55} low-profile absorbable staple cartridge is applied to partially close the reservoir.* ***J,*** *A second TA_{55} application is used to complete the closure.* ***K,*** *The holding sutures are used to close the gaps between staple lines.*

Mucus is produced by the bowel segments. This must be irrigated from the reservoir starting immediately postoperatively four times per day. Reservoir irrigations must be continued after the patient begins intermittent catheterization. The frequency of irrigation can be decreased as mucus production slows down. This author advises at least daily irrigation long term. Occasionally pouch stones occur in patients who have stopped irrigating their reservoir.

Renal function, electrolytes, and hemoglobin should be followed on a long-term basis. Patients who have had larger segments of terminal ileum resected (Kock pouch) can experience B_{12} deficiency and anemia after several years.

Radiographic visualization of the pouch and upper tracts using pouchograms and intravenous pyelograms should be performed every 6 to 12 months initially to monitor patients for reflux or upper tract filling defects or obstruction. If no abnormalities are demonstrated with the first two or three sets of studies, follow-up exams can be less frequent.

Although there have been no reports of transitional cell carcinoma or adenocarcinoma in reservoirs that I am aware of at this time, the potential for tumor exists. Despite the low likelihood of tumor development, the patients should be monitored for pouch tumors starting 5 to 10 years after the procedure or sooner if unexplained bleeding occurs or if a mass is seen on x-ray studies.

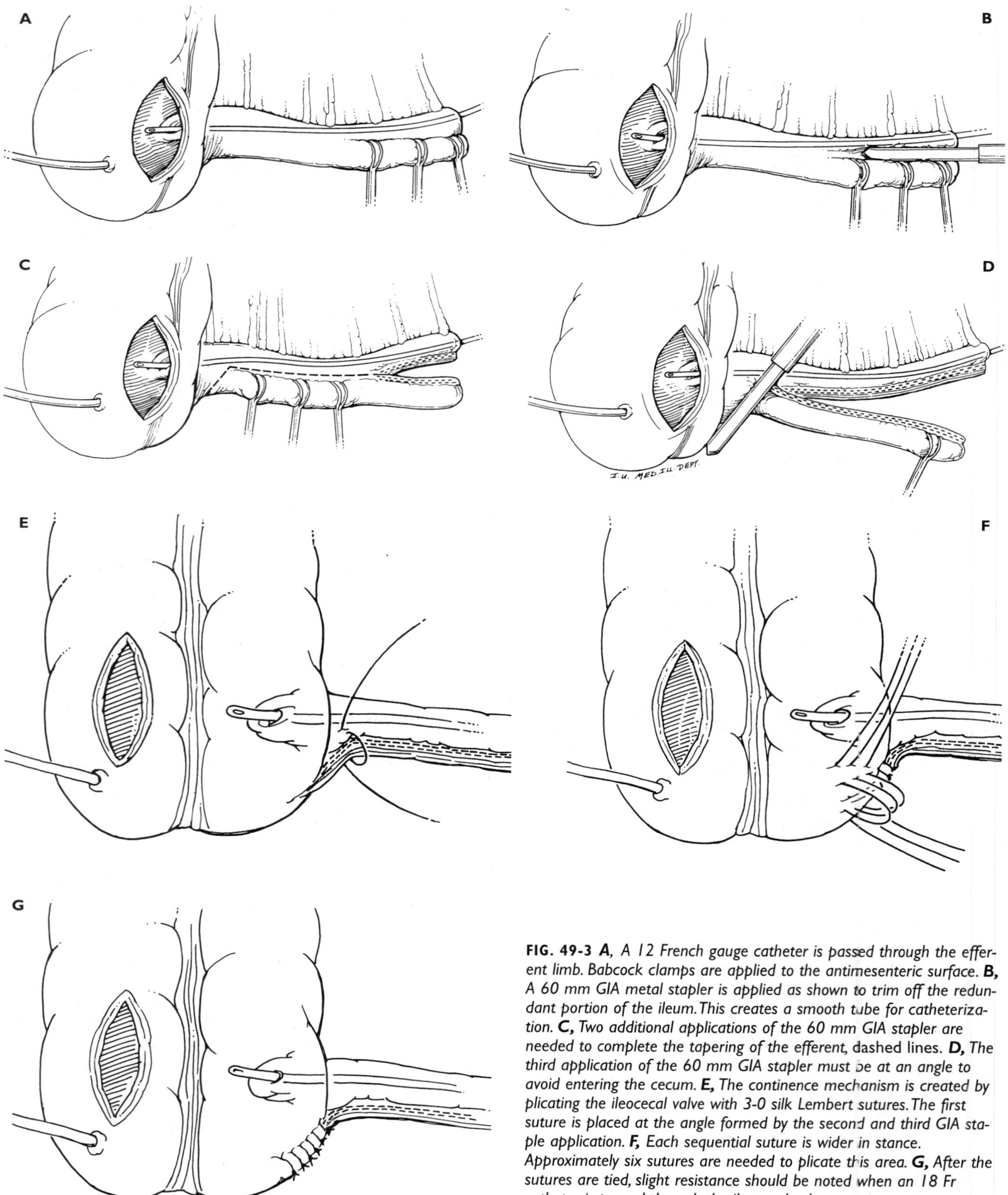

FIG. 49-3 ***A***, *A 12 French gauge catheter is passed through the efferent limb. Babcock clamps are applied to the antimesenteric surface.* ***B,*** *A 60 mm GIA metal stapler is applied as shown to trim off the redundant portion of the ileum. This creates a smooth tube for catheterization.* ***C,*** *Two additional applications of the 60 mm GIA stapler are needed to complete the tapering of the efferent, dashed lines.* ***D,*** *The third application of the 60 mm GIA stapler must be at an angle to avoid entering the cecum.* ***E,*** *The continence mechanism is created by plicating the ileocecal valve with 3-0 silk Lembert sutures. The first suture is placed at the angle formed by the second and third GIA staple application.* ***F,*** *Each sequential suture is wider in stance. Approximately six sutures are needed to plicate this area.* ***G,*** *After the sutures are tied, slight resistance should be noted when an 18 Fr catheter is passed through the ileocecal valve area.*

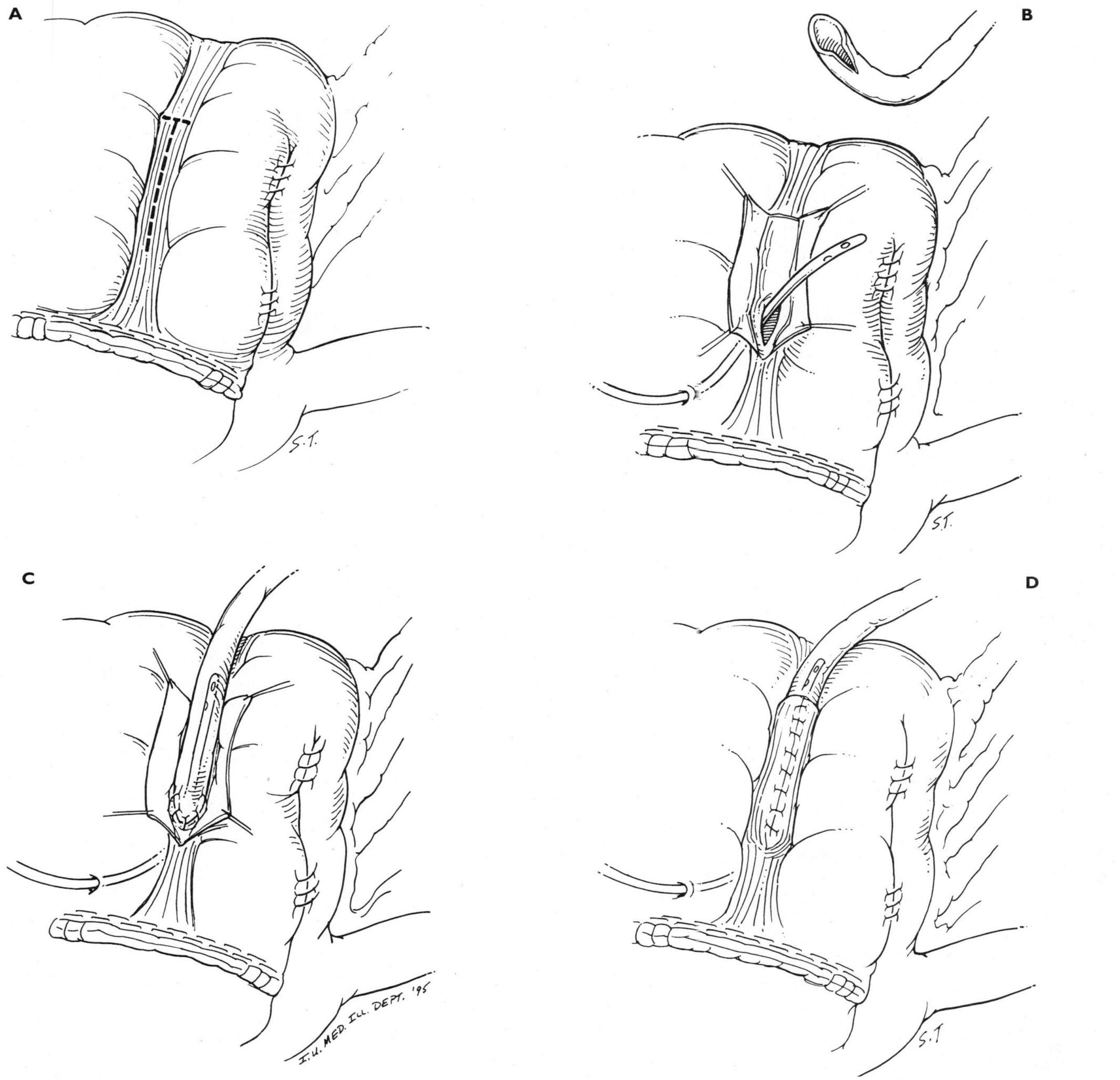

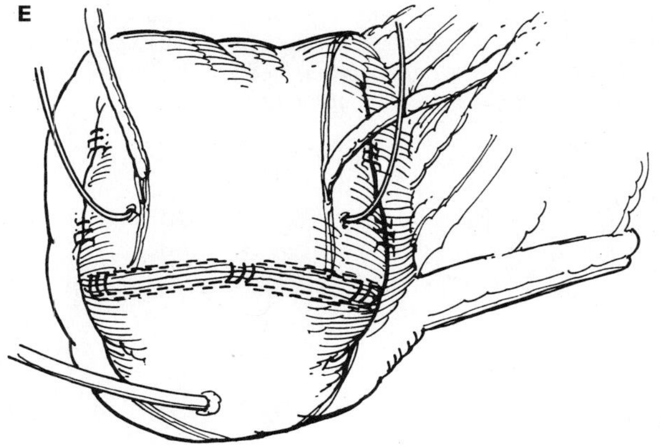

FIG. 49-4 ***A,*** *Ureteral implantation sites are selected along teniae that allow good alignment with the ureters. The dashed T indicates where the tenial incision will be made. The crossbar of the T completely transects the tenia to prevent compression of the ureter at the hiatus.* ***B,*** *After the tenial flaps are raised, one makes a mucosal incision that will become the anastomotic site for the ureteral orifice. A stent is passed through a separate stab wound and is brought through the orifice site. The ureter is cut obliquely or spatulated to increase the size of the anastomosis.* ***C,*** *The ureteral orifice is created using 5-0 monofilament absorbable interrupted sutures. The stent is passed up the ureter and secured to the wall of the reservoir with an absorbable suture.* ***D,*** *The tenial flaps are closed over the ureter using a running locked 5-0 braided synthetic nonabsorbable suture. The adventitia of the ureter is caught with several of the sutures to prevent telescoping of the ureter out of the tunnel.* ***E,*** *A completed Indiana pouch. The left ureter is often led through the mesentery to the reservoir to achieve good alignment with a tenia.*

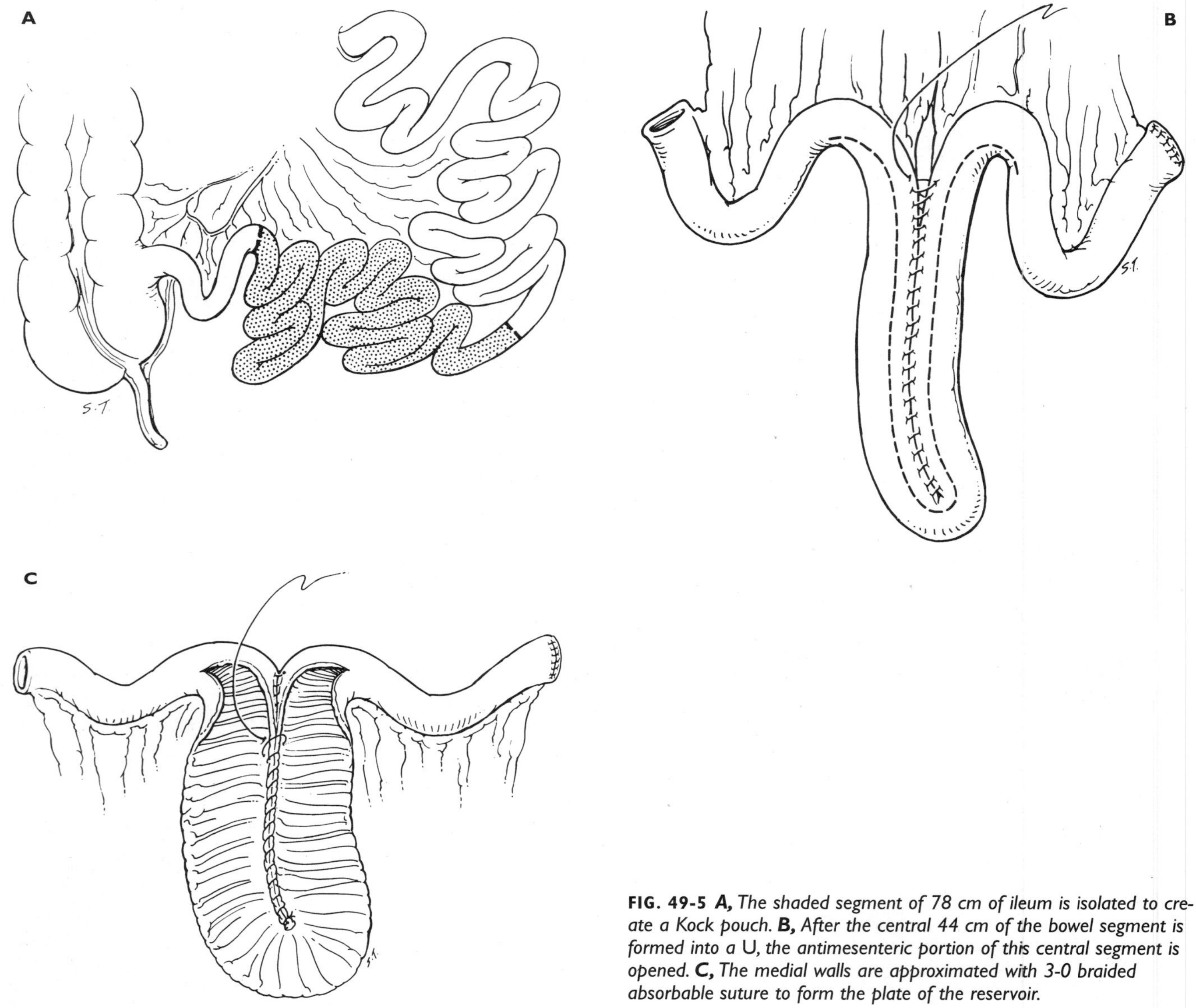

FIG. 49-5 ***A,*** *The shaded segment of 78 cm of ileum is isolated to create a Kock pouch.* ***B,*** *After the central 44 cm of the bowel segment is formed into a U, the antimesenteric portion of this central segment is opened.* ***C,*** *The medial walls are approximated with 3-0 braided absorbable suture to form the plate of the reservoir.*

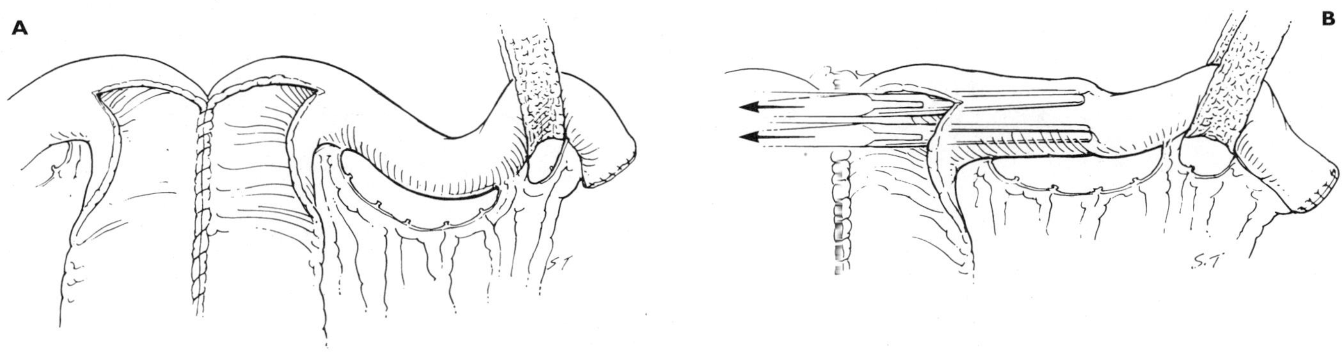

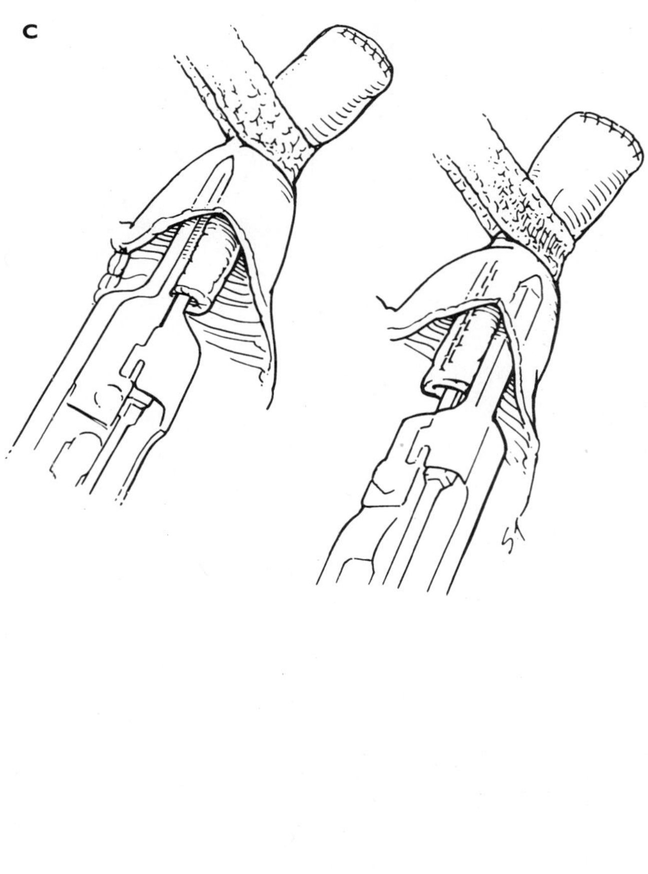

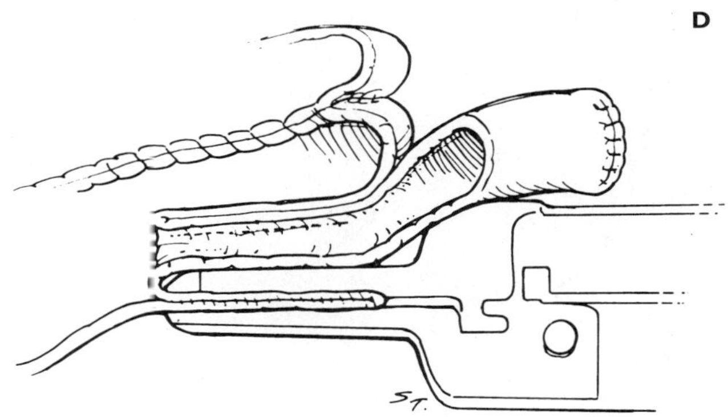

FIG. 49-6 ***A,*** *Eight centimeters of mesentery is taken down at the midportion of the afferent and efferent segments to facilitate creation of intussuscepted nipple valves. A polyglycolic acid mesh strip is passed through a mesenteric window. This strip will be used to secure the intussusception.* ***B,*** *Allis clamps are used to intussuscept the bowel segments.* ***C,*** *The intussuscepted segments are secured with TA_{55} or modified GIA staplers without knives. Two or three applications are made through the nipple.* ***D,*** *A final staple row is placed from outside the reservoir to fix each nipple to the reservoir wall.*

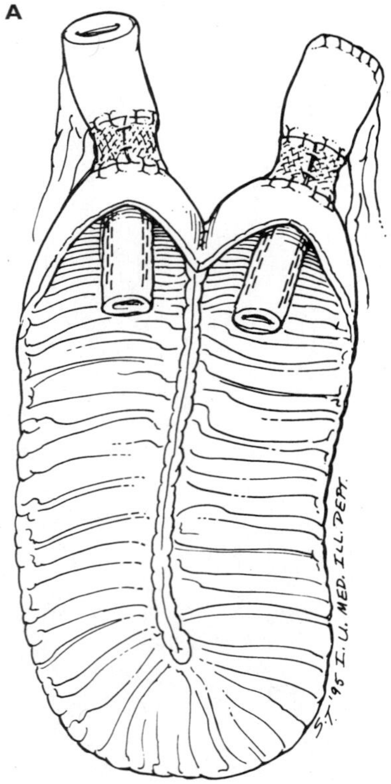

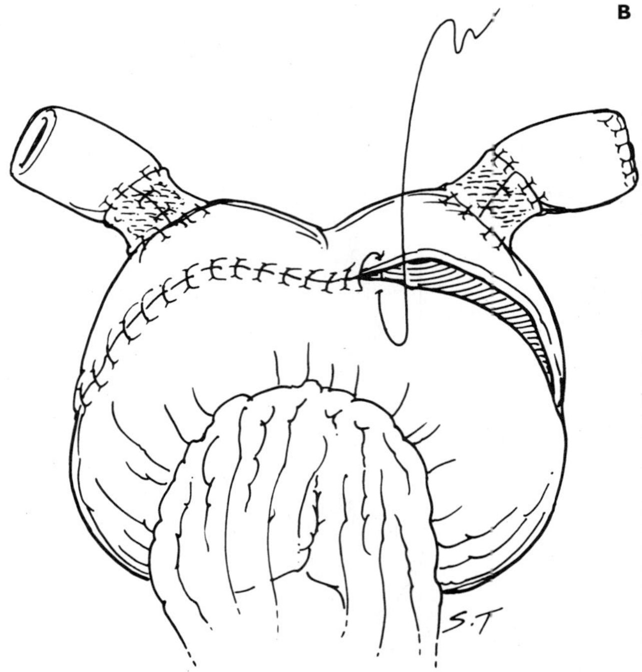

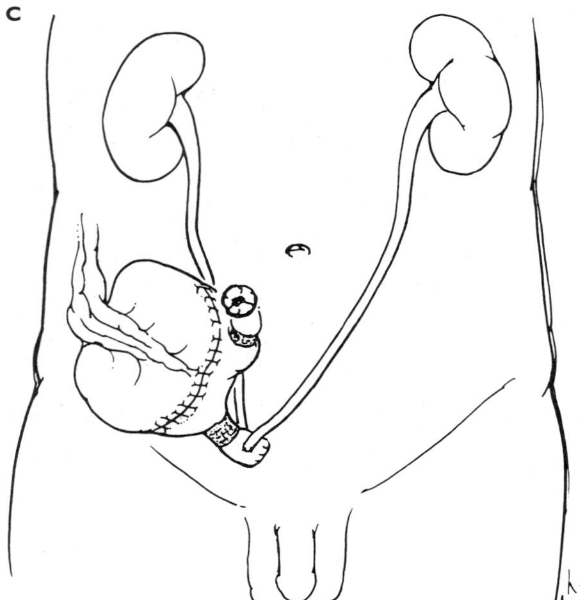

FIG. 49-7 ***A,*** *Completed afferent and efferent limbs and nipple valves.* ***B,*** *The bottom of the U is folded upwards to close the pouch.* ***C,*** *The ureters are sewn to the afferent limb in a Bricker fashion. The efferent limb is brought up to create a short straight segment with a flush stoma. A polyglycolic acid strut is used to secure the mesentery of the efferent limb to the abdominal wall. Stents and a 30 Fr Medina tube are brought out the efferent limb.*

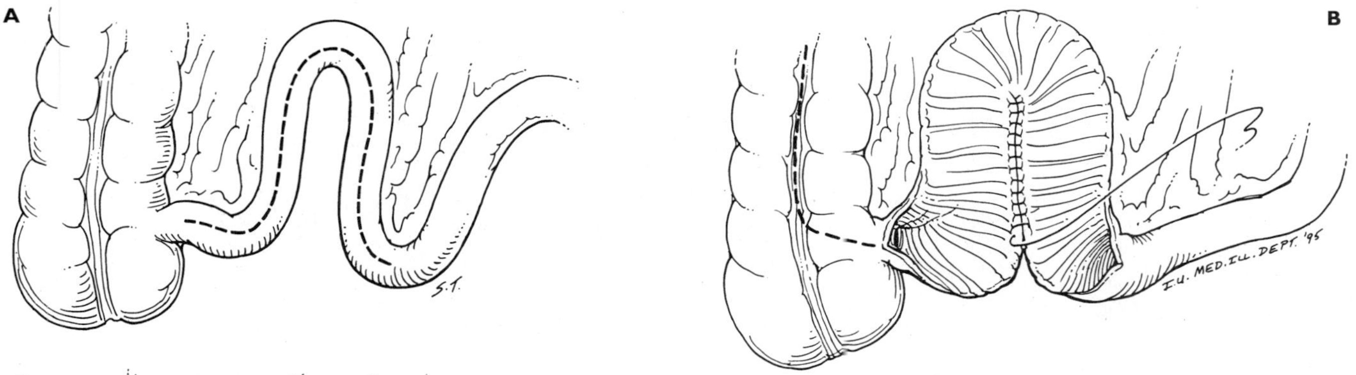

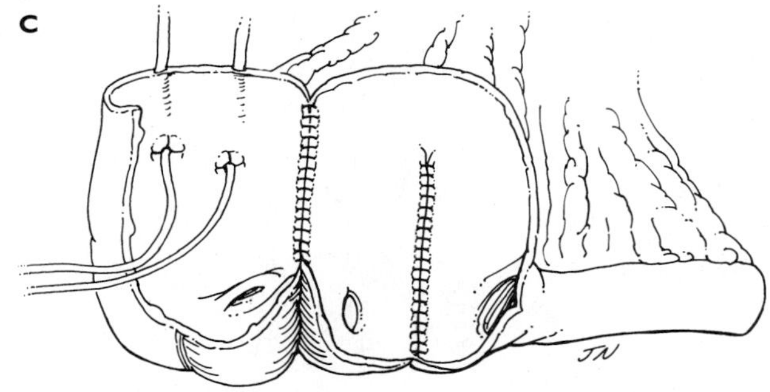

FIG. 49-8 ***A,*** *Bowel segment that is isolated to create a Mainz pouch.* Dashed line, *Incision to be made along the antimesenteric portion of the most distal 24 cm of ileum to create the anterior wall of the reservoir.* ***B,*** *The anterior wall is prepared.* Dashed line, *Cecal incision that will be made to create the posterior wall of the reservoir.* ***C,*** *The ureters are implanted using a submucosal technique. Stents are placed.*

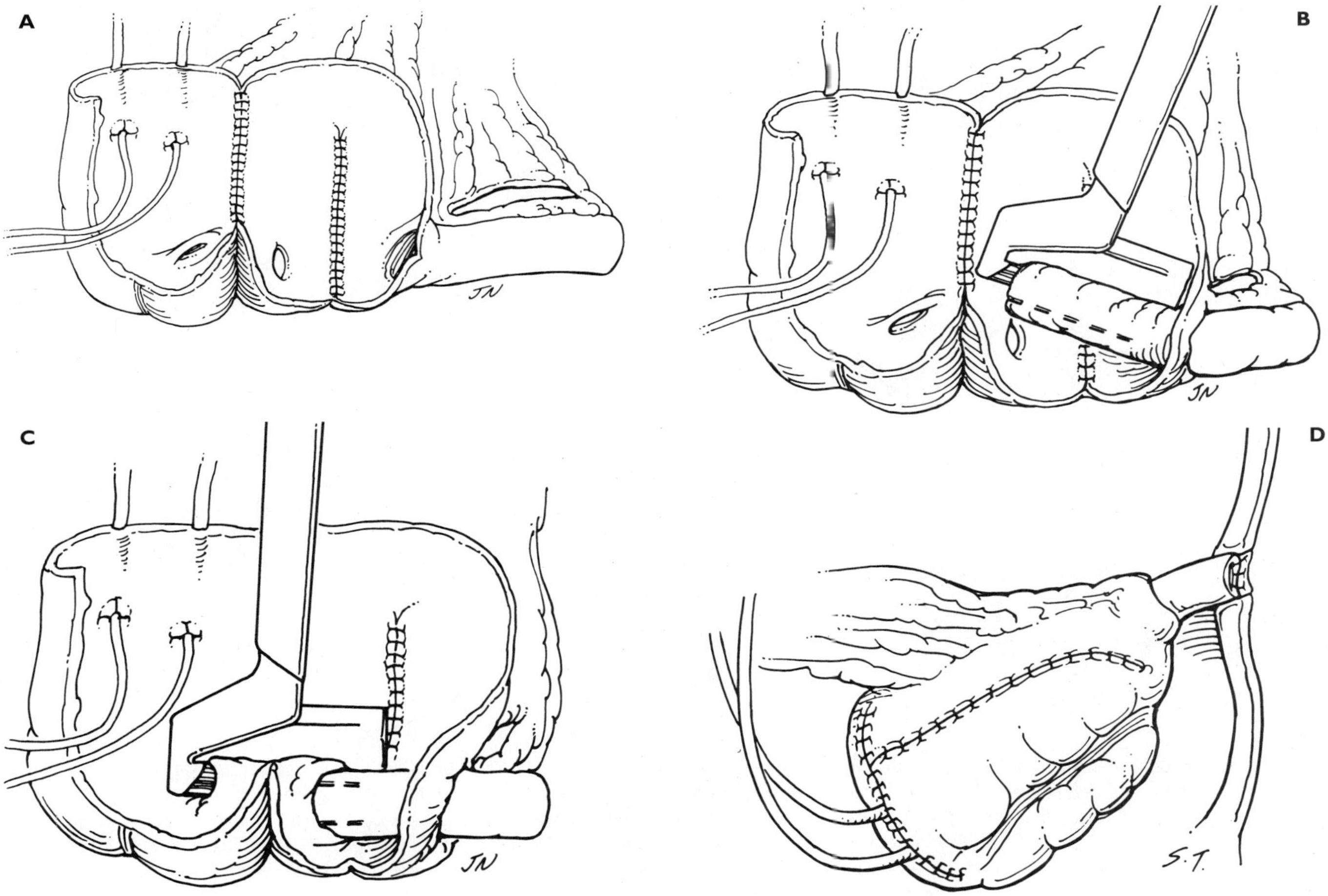

FIG. 49-9 ***A,*** *The mesentery is taken down for 6 cm to prepare for intussusception.* ***B,*** *Two staple rows are applied through the nipple for fixation of the intussusception with* TA_{55} *or knifeless GIA staplers.* ***C,*** *The intussuscepted ileum is passed through the ileocecal valve and fixed with an additional staple cartridge.* ***D,*** *The efferent limb of the completed reservoir is used to create a stoma. The umbilicus is frequently used.*

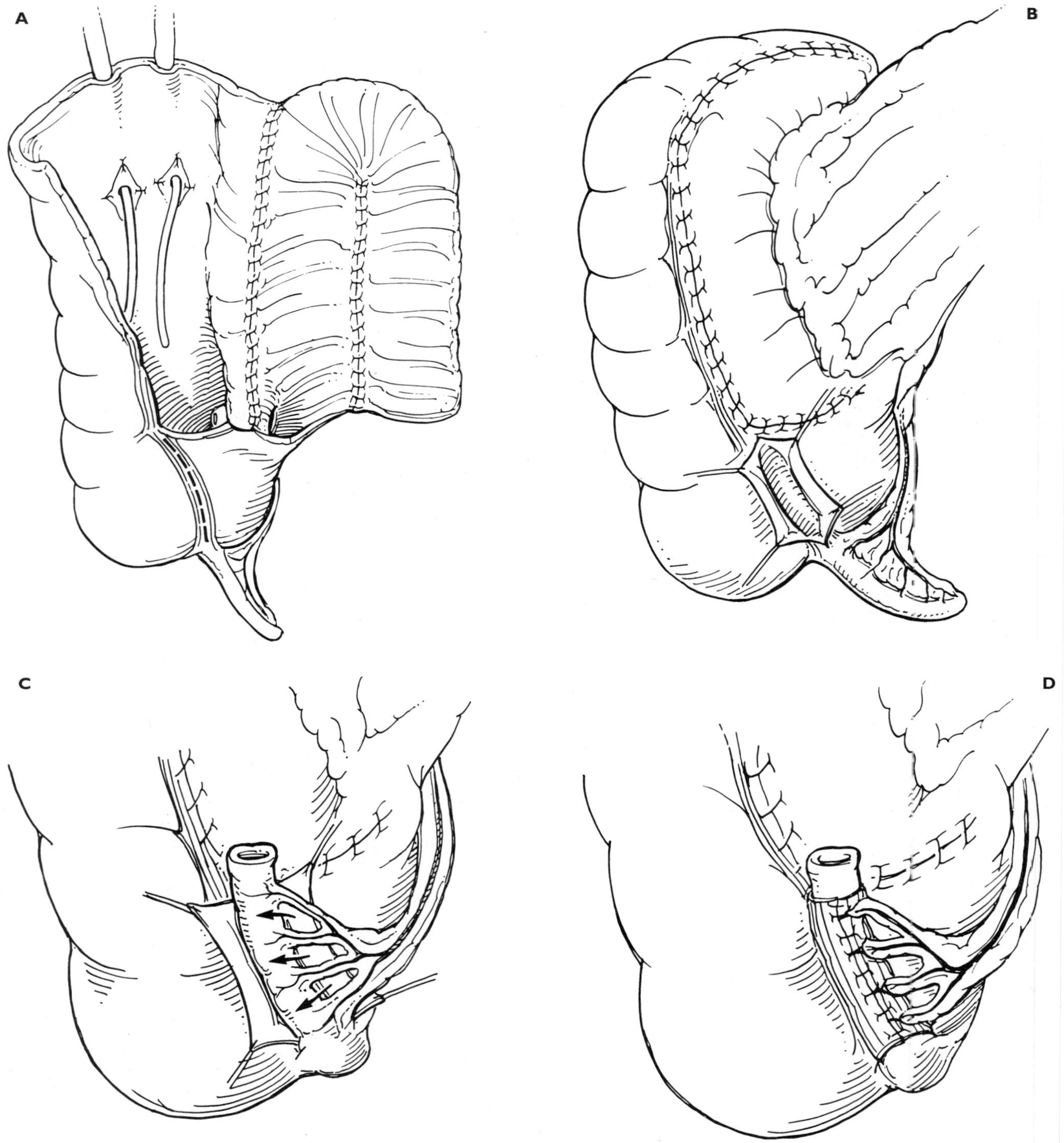

FIG. 49-10 ***A,*** *In a variation of the procedure, the appendix can be used to form the efferent limb and continence mechanism. The detubularization of the cecum is modified to preserve the cap of the cecum for implantation of the appendix.* Dashed line, *Where the appendix will be embedded to create the continence mechanism.* ***B,*** *A tenial tunnel is prepared to accept the appendix.* ***C,*** *The mesenteric vessels of the appendix are skeletonized. Interrupted sutures are placed to close the tenia and preserve the appendiceal blood supply. The arrows show the locations where sutures will be placed.* ***D,*** *The tunneled appendix will be anastomosed to the stump of the umbilicus.*

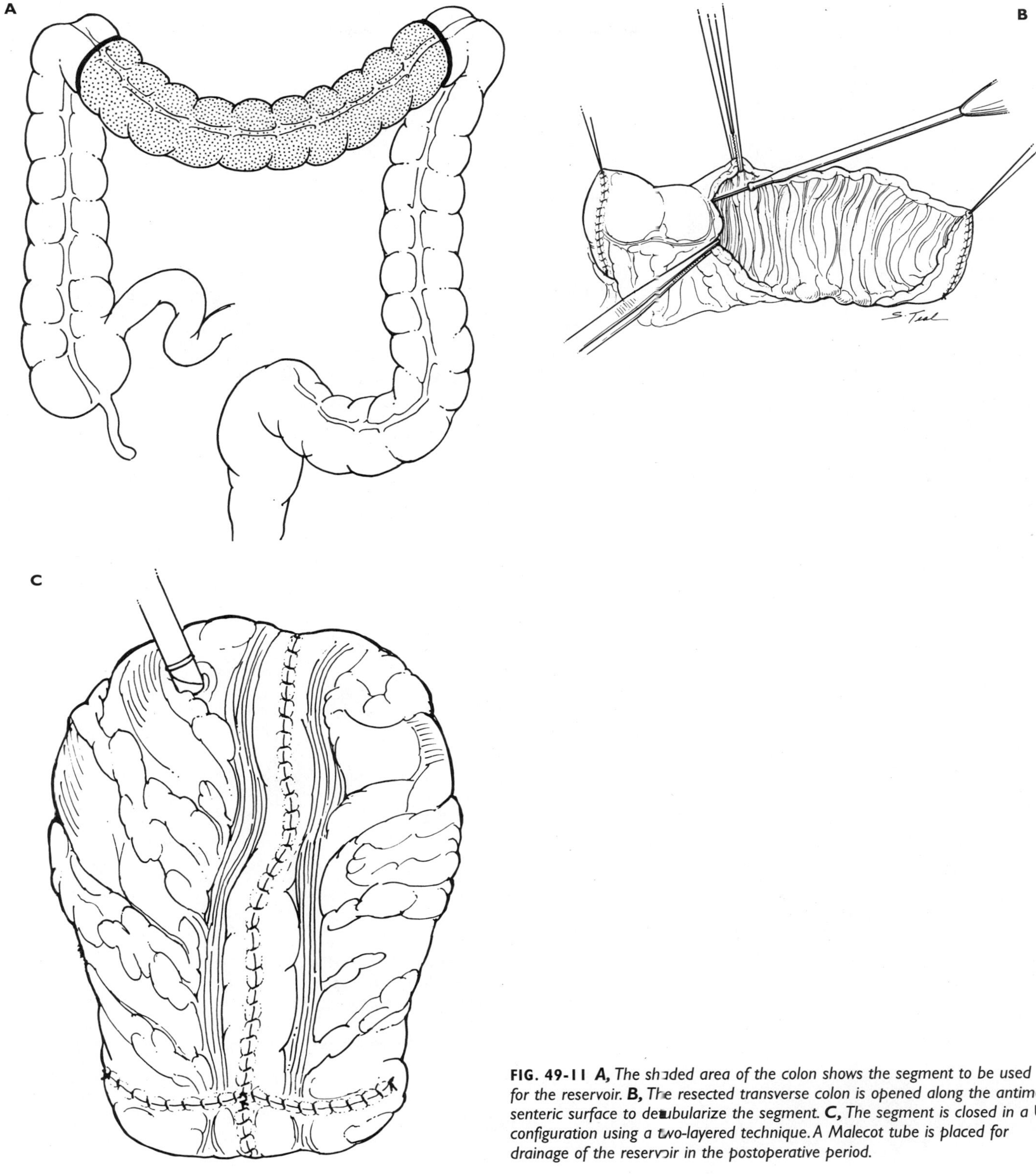

FIG. 49-11 ***A,*** *The shaded area of the colon shows the segment to be used for the reservoir.* ***B,*** *The resected transverse colon is opened along the antimesenteric surface to detubularize the segment.* ***C,*** *The segment is closed in a U configuration using a two-layered technique. A Malecot tube is placed for drainage of the reservoir in the postoperative period.*

A

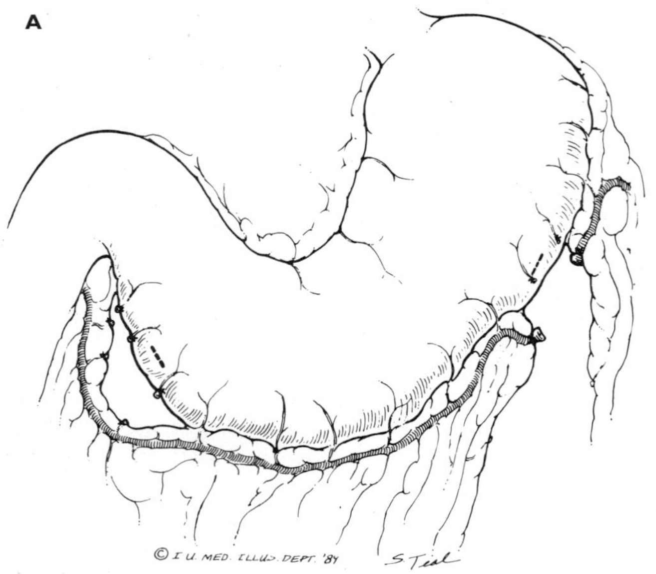

B

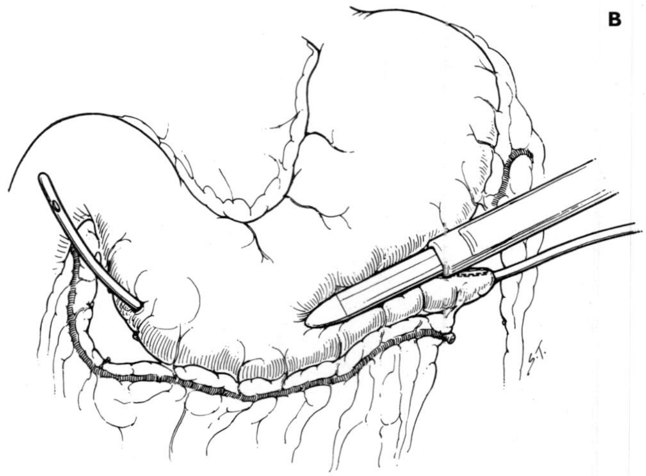

C

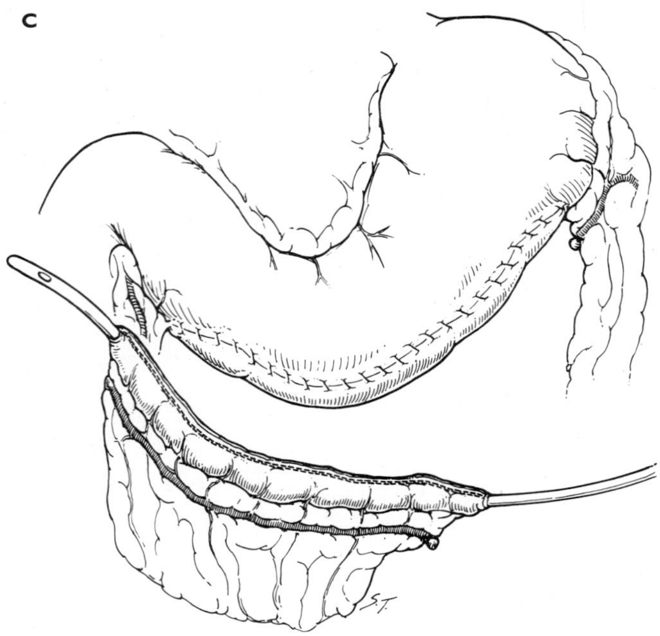

FIG. 49-12 ***A,*** *The stomach is prepared for the harvesting of a greater curvature tube that is supported by the right gastroepiploic vessels.* ***B,*** *A series of GIA metal staple cartridges is used to harvest a tube over a 12 Fr catheter. Usually a 12 to 15 cm tube is created.* ***C,*** *This illustration shows the isolated gastric tube that will be used as the efferent limb.*

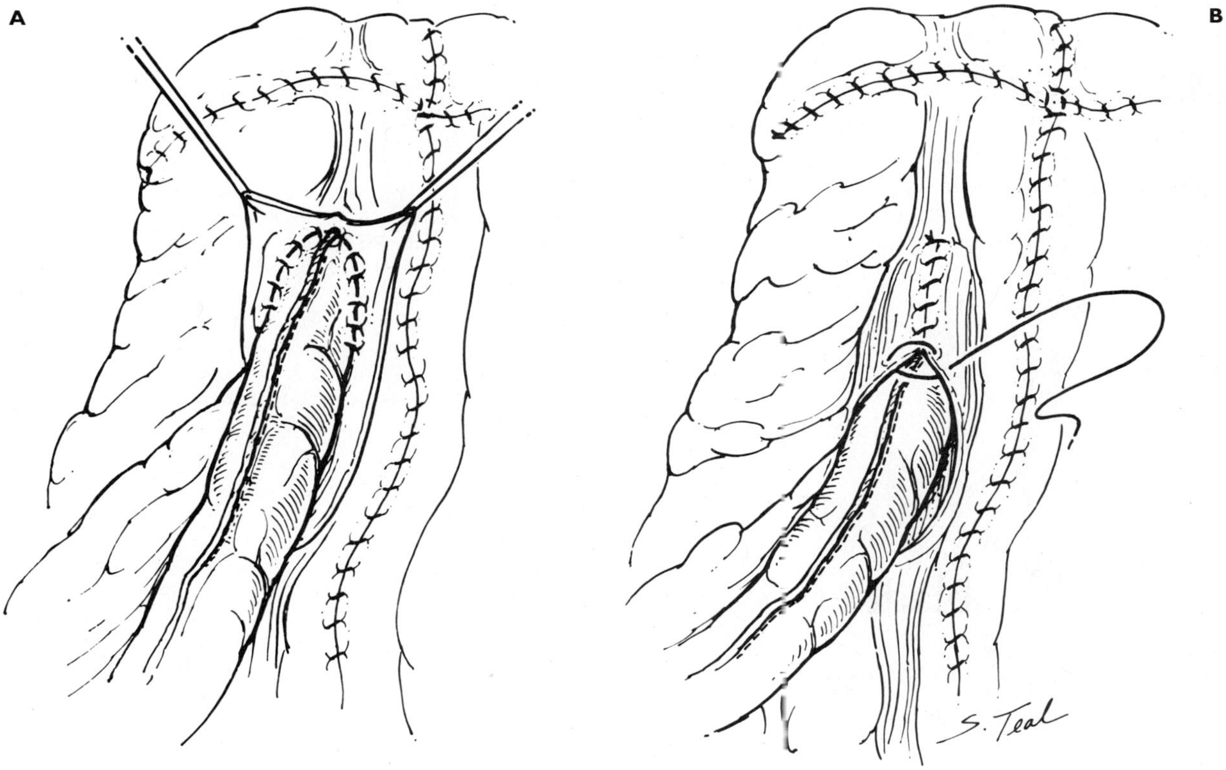

FIG. 49-13 ***A,*** *A tenial tunnel is prepared for implantation of the gastric tube on the anterior wall of the reservoir.* ***B,*** *The tenia is closed over the gastric tube to create the continence mechanism.*

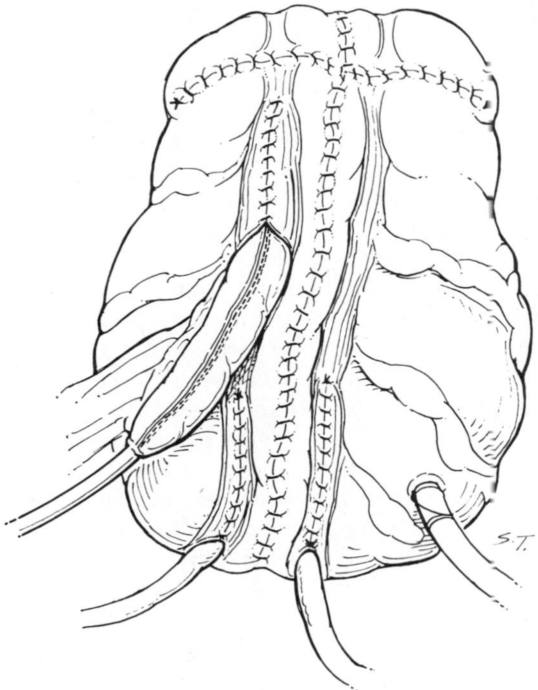

FIG. 49-14 *The ureters are tunneled into other tenial sites in an antirefluxing manner.*

SUMMARY

Several different continent cutaneous reservoirs can be used successfully in patients who require urinary diversion for any reason, including intractable incontinence. The choice of the procedure should be tailored to the specific needs and circumstances of each patient. Patients require a support system to help them in the first few months after surgery. Depending on local conditions, this support comes from the urologist, the hospital and office nursing staffs, and enterostomal therapists. Long-term, compulsive follow-up study is needed to be certain that the patient is being well served by his or her continent cutaneous reservoir.

REFERENCES

1. Hinman F: Selection of intestinal segments for bladder substitution: physical and physiological characteristics, *J Urol* 139:519, 1988.
2. Rowland RG, Mitchell ME, Bihrle R: The cecoileal continent urinary reservoir, *World J Urol* 3:185, 1985.
3. Rowland RG, Kropp BP: Evolution of the Indiana continent urinary reservoir, *J Urol* 152:2274, 1994.
4. Rowland RG: Present experience with the Indiana pouch, *World J Urol* In press 9-95.
5. Kock NG: Continent ileostomy, *Prog Surg* 12: 180, 1973.
6. Lieskovsky G, Boyd SD, Skinner DG: Cutaneous Kock pouch urinary diversion, *Probl Urol* 5:256, 1991.
7. Riedmiller H, Thüroff J, Hohenfellner R: Continent urinary diversion: the Mainz-pouch procedure, *Probl Urol* 5:283, 1991.
8. Bihrle R, Klee LW, Adams MC, et al: Early clinical experience with the transverse colon–gastric tube continent urinary reservoir, *J Urol* 146:751, 1991.

Chapter 50 Neobladder

George D. Webster

The term "neobladder" describes the replacement of the native bladder by an intestinal reservoir anastomosed to the urethra. Such orthotopic bladder replacement procedures were first described at the turn of the century; however, in the modern surgical era they were popularized by Camey of Paris.[1] These procedures were performed primarily in patients requiring radical cystectomy for carcinoma of the bladder and until very recently had been recommended only in males. The impetus for their recently popularity has been disillusionment with the long-term medical results and the social implications of the alternative, the appliance-dependent urostomy. Their performance ideally requires that the native urethra can be preserved and that the distal sphincter mechanism remains intact. In cases where this is not assured the preferable alternative would be to construct a continent urinary reservoir with catheterizable abdominal stoma.

The ideal neobladder should mimic bladder function as closely as possible. It should provide a low-pressure capacious reservoir, achieve continence, and allow for complete emptying either by voluntary explusion or by easy catheterization. In addition, it should protect the upper tracts from reflux or obstruction and avoid metabolic disturbances and subsequent malignant change. It is doubtful that any current urinary diversion can consistently achieve all these goals; however, when compared to the standard ileal conduit, the procedure certainly promotes an improved quality of life and body image, and it fosters psychologic well-being because it more closely mirrors normal bladder function.

PATIENT SELECTION

As noted earlier, the leading indication for orthotopic bladder replacement is after radical cystectomy for bladder cancer. Other diagnoses that may lead to urinary diversion include patients with neurogenic bladder dysfunction, intractable urinary incontinence, and those with devastated outlets. These patients are not candidates for neobladder construction that relies on the functional integrity of the urethra, and this patient group is more appropriately treated by continent urinary diversion to an abdominal stoma.

Patients with bladder cancer considered for neobladder construction should fulfill several selection criteria. Most important is the tumor prognosis and the risk of urethral recurrence. Potentially curative measures should not be limited in the interests of pursuing orthotopic bladder replacement, nor should the neobladder be endangered by a high likelihood of local recurrent disease. Additionally management of any recurrent disease, perhaps by radiation therapy, should not be limited by the presence of the diversion. Some have expressed a reservation about performing orthotopic bladder replacement in patients with pT3/pT4 or N+ bladder cancer because of the risk of pelvic recurrence, which could complicate the neobladder. However, reports indicate that tumor recurrence in the pelvis appears uncommon, even in patients with node-positive disease.[2] Nonetheless, the fact that 50% of patients with such advanced tumor stage or lymph node involvement finally die from widespread metastases and have a mean survival time of less than 1.5 years demands consideration, and hence in this group the decision must be individualized. Skinner has a considerable experience with orthotopic bladder replacement and does not consider nodal disease or involvement of the perivesical fat necessarily to be a contraindication. In a series of 119 patients, 5 suffered pelvic recurrence 4 to 8 months postoperatively, and their attendant voiding problems necessitated intermittent catheterization.[3]

Urethral recurrence is reported to occur in 4% to 15% of patients undergoing cystoprostatectomy without simultaneous urethrectomy.[2] In compiling these data Seeman reviewed 3000 patients but comments on the considerable differences between the evaluated populations and questions this incidence. In the past the indications for simultaneous urethrectomy with radical cystectomy included patients with diffuse carcinoma in situ, patients with multifocal bladder tumors, patients with tumors in proximity to the bladder neck, and those with prostatic urethral involvement. There is now an ongoing attempt to redefine which factors have significant prognostic value in identifying a risk of urethral recurrence and therefore would preclude orthotopic bladder replacement, and currently I exclude patients who have prostatic urethral involvement with stromal or ductal involvement, those who have a positive urethral margin, and patients with locally extensive disease, which would be predictive of a high risk of local recurrence.

Several nononcologic factors may deter one from orthotopic replacement, and they include those in whom the pelvic floor dissection was "nonanatomic," in whom preservation of the distal sphincter mechanism is questionable. Prior radiation therapy does not necessarily contraindicate this surgery, provided that the intestinal segment used does not have pronounced radiation change. Skinner reported no high complication rate in this group.[4] There are also rare anatomic factors that preclude approximation of the bowel segment to the pelvic floor. It may also be inadvisable in the aged, the poorly motivated patient, the infirm individual, or the patient unprepared to accept the possibility of continence problems, enuresis, and voiding dysfunction, which may require self-catheterization.

Obesity is not a contraindication to orthotopic bladder replacement but certainly renders the procedure more difficult. The fat-laden mesentery is difficult to fold and complicates the construction of the reservoir. Patients who have previously undergone bowel resection and those with preexisting bowel dysfunction are at risk for protracted bowel dysfunction after further extensive bowel resection for reservoir construction. If reservoir construction is still to be considered, contrast study of the bowel should be performed in this group, though it is not routinely performed preoperatively in the absence of such factors.

Impaired renal function with serum creatinine in excess of 1.5 mg% raises concern, and 3.5 mg% is a contraindication to the formation of a urinary reservoir. Although many patients develop mild metabolic acidosis, this is rarely clinically manifested nor does it require therapy. The ileal mucosa may adapt with time, loosing much of its absorptive surface because of the chronic exposure to urine, reducing the significance of electrolyte abnormalities.

Historically women were not considered candidates for orthotopic bladder replacement; however, this posture has recently been challenged, and reports are now emerging of its successful use.[5]

Suffice it to say that once the patient has been selected for radical cystectomy the decision regarding type of diversion is going to be based on a careful evaluation that will include endoscopic, histopathologic, and radiographic study to determine the extent of the disease. The final decision will generally be made at the time of surgery, and hence it is essential that patients be carefully preoperatively counseled about the factors that will determine this decision.

Preoperative Preparation and Counseling

Thorough preoperative counseling will ensure that the patient has realistic expectations of outcome and is not surprised by any subsequent untoward events. A simple diagram explaining the differences between the various diversion techniques is useful, and patients find it extremely helpful to speak with a patient who has previously undergone a similar procedure. The patient is informed of the more common early and late complications of the surgery and how his or her lifestyle will change, especially with the need for regular bathrooming or, in some cases, for intermittent catheterization. It is my experience that a small number of patients will decline a continent urinary diversion in lieu of a simple urinary ileostomy based on an honest reporting to them of the duration of surgery and hospitalization together with the incidence of early and late complications. This dropout rate is certainly better than dealing with an unhappy, poorly informed patient who has subsequently encountered problems!

Preoperative studies will to some degree be determined by the cause of the disease leading to the continent urinary diversion. Assessment of renal function should include a serum creatinine and imaging of the upper urinary tracts preferably by urography. If abnormalities are found, renal function can be better evaluated by a DPTA (diethylenetriaminepentacetic acid) renogram. Bowel contrast study should be performed in patients in whom a bowel disorder is suspected, or in those in whom prior intestinal surgery may influence one's choice of the bowel segment to be used.

Preoperatively the enterostomal therapist should mark the patient for an appropriate stoma site for an appliance-dependent ostomy, lest intraoperative findings dictate that this must be done. The continent stoma, on the other hand, has few rigid siting criteria, though bringing it through the rectus muscle may reduce the incidence of peristomal hernia. Most patients prefer an unobtrusive site low on the abdominal wall, even in a skin crease, to improve concealability. Some surgeons advise an umbilical stoma.

Before surgery the intestines are prepared by lavage or mechanical preparation and antibiotics according to the surgeon's preference. I prefer to start clear fluids only by mouth 2 days before surgery and the use of Go-Litely (TM Braintree Laboratories, Inc., Braintree, Mass.), a polyethylene glycol electrolyte gastrointestinal lavage solution, the day before surgery. For adults, a volume of up to 4000 ml may be required to lavage the bowel until the rectal efflux is clear. One should avoid dehydration by starting intravenous fluids the day before surgery. Those with poor nutrition may benefit from a period of preoperative hyperalimentation.

Surgical Techniques

The ileum, right colon, and sigmoid colon have all been used for orthotopic bladder replacement, and as yet no specific bowel segment appears to be superior to another. The ileum has been used in procedures described by Camey, Hautmann, and Studer, with these procedures differing in the mode of detubularization and bowel reconfiguration and the technique used to protect against reflux.[6-8] Reservoirs using the ileocolonic region include the Mainz pouch and LeBag, among others.[9,10] Use of the sigmoid colon has been popularized by Reddy.[11]

Hemi-Kock Technique

My major experience is with the hemi-Kock technique using detubularized ileum, which is to be described.

Regardless of technique, the radical cystoprostatectomy will have been completed, frozen-section biopsy specimen of the urethral margin will be normal, and there will be no other findings contraindicating orthotopic bladder replacement. The pelvic floor dissection should have been with care to avoid injury to the distal sphincter mechanism, in the same fashion as one would dissect the prostatic apex performing radical prostatectomy for prostate cancer. The left ureter is transposed beneath the sigmoid mesocolon to approximate the right, and the ureters are clipped to dilate so as to facilitate anastomosis. Approximately 60 cm of ileum is then isolated on its mesentery, with use of the same anatomic landmarks as previously described, the most important being that the distal margin of bowel be at the watershed between the distal branches of the superior mesenteric artery and the ileocolic artery. Ileoileal reanastomosis cephalad to the isolated segment is performed by use of the staple or suture technique and the isolated segment of bowel is irrigated clean. The isolated bowel segment is marked into three separate segments measuring 22 cm, 22 cm, and 16 cm (Fig. 50-1). The proximal 16 cm segment is used for construction of the afferent nipple, which prevents reflux.

Initially an 8 cm mesenteric window is created in the afferent limb of the pouch by individual cauterizing and sectioning of the mesenteric vessels close to the bowel wall. One should avoid electrocautery injury to the bowel, and the amount of fat remaining on the bowel wall should be limited. Two vascular arcades are spared, and then a second small window is made in the mesentery through which a 2 cm wide folded strip of tetracycline-soaked polyglycolic acid (PGA) mesh may be passed (optional). This mesh strip will ultimately form a collar around the entering and exiting limbs to the reservoir, stabilizing the nipple. One now creates the nipple by intussuscepting the section of bowel that has been stripped of its mesentery over the ileal plate using Babcock clamps that have been passed up the intestinal lumen for traction. In this fashion a 5 to 6 cm intussusception is created proximally and distally. The nipple is secured by the placement of three parallel rows of TA_{55} intestinal staples. Staples are of a 4.8 mm size and are nonhemostatic, and two staple cartridges for each nipple are modified with removal of the terminal six staples from the base of the cartridge, before being fired. These may either be removed by the surgeon, though a cartridge modified in this fashion is available. The absence of the terminal staples ensures that there are no staples at the tip of the nipple where exposure to urine because of nipple ischemia is more likely, and their slough into the reservoir might predispose to stone formation. The two modified staple cartridges fix the intussusception at the 10 o'clock and 2 o'clock positions, the TA_{55} stabilization-pin hole being oversewn with a 3-0 Vicryl (polyglactin 910) suture. The third staple line fixes the nipple to the back wall of the ileal plate, and it need not be of a modified variety. Two techniques are available for placement of this staple line, with the preferable technique encompassing only the outer wall of the intussusception and the back wall of the ileal plate, as shown in Fig. 50-1. The tip of the nipple is additionally secured to the back wall of the ileal plate by two 3-0 PGA sutures fixing the posterior wall of the tip of the nipple to the wall of the ileal plate. The PGA meshed strip is now secured as a collar around the entering ileal segment using interrupted 3-0 PGA sutures.

The two distal 22 cm segments are then laid out in a U-shape and once again anastomosed side to side, the bowel opened to create an ileal plate, and the reservoir is formed by folding the ileal plate upon itself. However, the most dependent portion of the reservoir is left open for anastomosis to the urethra, and, in addition, a small working hiatus is left open on the anterior portion of the reservoir closure, through which subsequent stent and drainage catheter attachment can be accomplished. The dependent portion of the reservoir reaches the pelvic floor in the majority of cases with little difficulty. In the event tension appears excessive, the abdominal wall retraction should be relaxed, the abdominal packs that are used to displace other visceral contents cephalad should be released, and a break in the operating table should be flattened. The urethral anastomosis is performed with interrupted 3-0 PGA suture. The posterior sutures (4, 6, and 8 o'clock positions) are initially placed through the urethral wall and its corresponding location on the reservoir opening, and the knots to be tied inside the lumen are tagged to be tied later. The lateral and anterior anastomotic sutures are placed such that the knots are tied externally. The sutures are tied after the pouch has been approximated to the pelvic floor, reducing tension. Posterior sutures are tied within the lumen first, and attention is then directed to the ureteral anastomoses, which are performed using the Wallace technique, stented with 8 Fr single-J stents. The tips of the stents are passed through the afferent limb and nipple and out through the working hiatus on the anterior pouch closure. A 22 Fr urethral Foley catheter is inserted to stent the urethral anastomosis, and its tip is similarly delivered through the hiatus. The stents are trimmed in length and fixed to the tip of the urethral catheter with a single 3-0 Prolene (polypropylene) suture and then internalized into the reservoir, and the working hiatus is closed (Fig. 50-2). An alternative is for the stents to be brought through the anterior pouch and abdominal wall and the urine drainage to be exteriorized, and some also prefer to place a suprapubic tube. I routinely use an internalized drainage system with no suprapubic catheter unless adverse intraoperative events, such as urethral anastomotic tension, are identified. Drainage is once again using suction drains to drain the pelvic floor and reservoir, and a gastrostomy tube is routinely placed.[12]

POSTOPERATIVE MANAGEMENT

A 24-hour period of postoperative intensive care nursing is advised. Broad-spectrum antibiotics are continued for 3 days postoperatively, and nasogastric or gastrostomy tube drainage is continued for 4 to 7 days until intestinal motility returns, and graduated oral feeding is then begun. Catheter and stent irrigation is performed each 4 hours depending on the catheter drainage technique used. The suction drains are removed

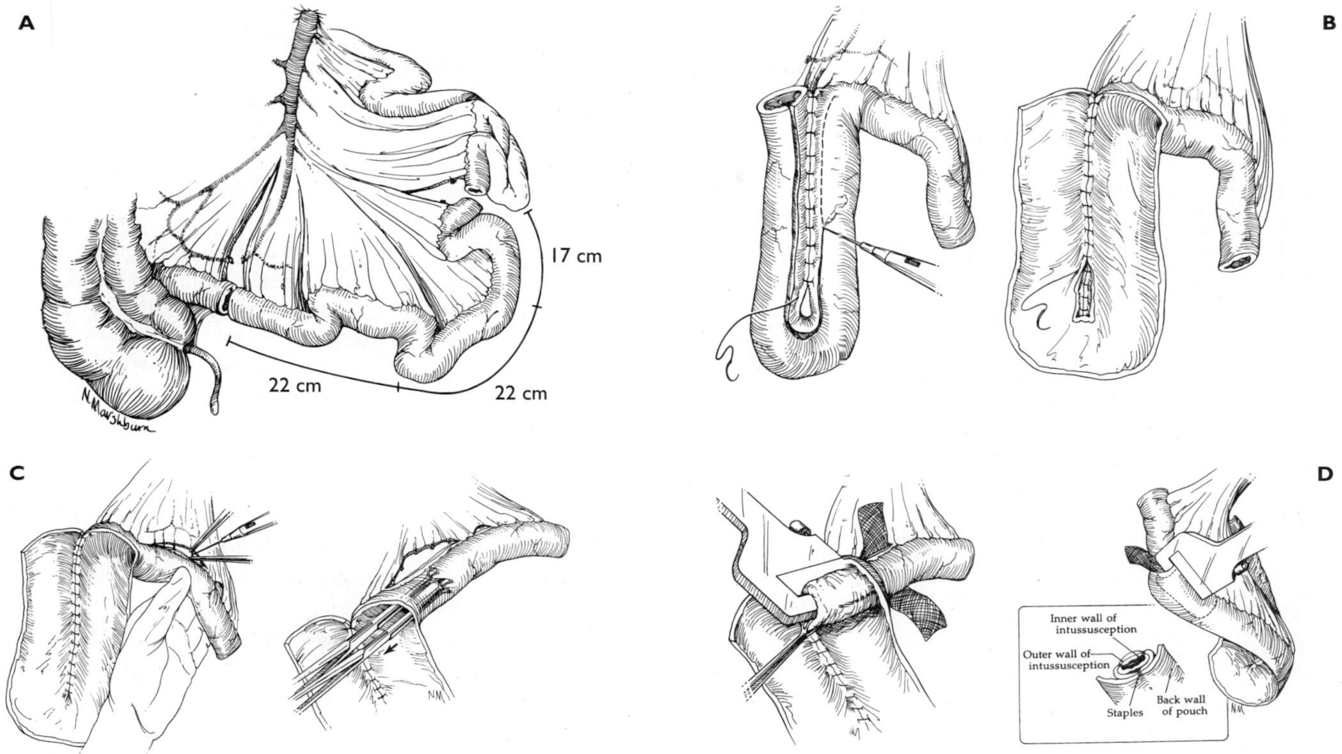

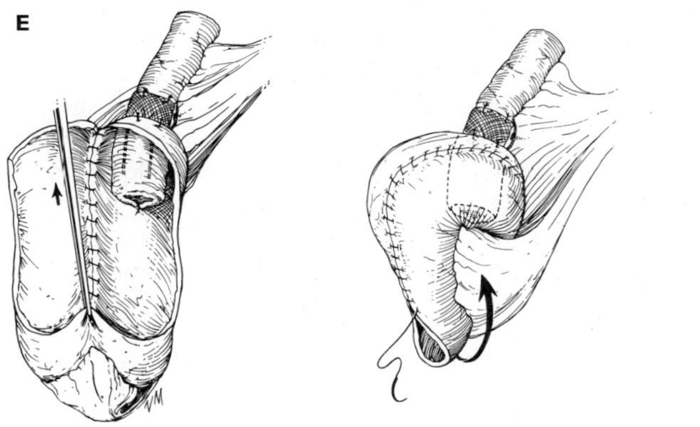

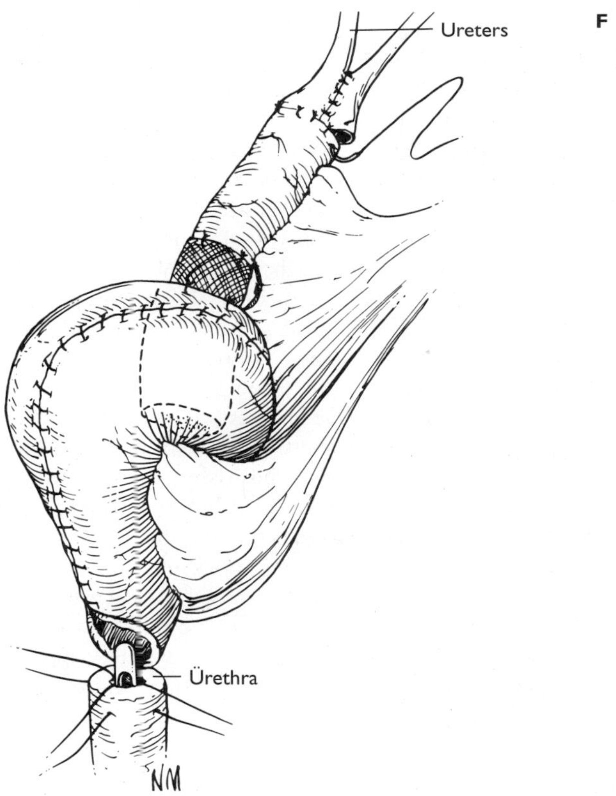

FIG. 50-1 *Hemi-Kock technique.* ***A,*** *The hemi-Kock orthotopic bladder is constructed from 60 cm of ileum. The inlet and nonrefluxing intussusception derive from a proximal 17 cm section, and the two distal 22 cm sections are used to construct the reservoir.* ***B,*** *The two distal 22 cm sections are laid side by side and joined with a continuous seromuscular suture. The bowel is then opened with electrocautery, and the suture line is reinforced with a continuous through and through suture.* ***C,*** *The mesentery is stripped from an 8 cm length of the proximal portion of the intact ileum just next to the reservoir, and a second 1 cm window is created one vascular arcade proximally to accommodate a mesh collar. The bowel is intussuscepted with two Babcock clamps to create a nipple approximately 5 cm in length.* ***D,*** *The intussusception is stabilized with two or three rows of staples that encompass the two walls of the intussusception. Another row of staples anchors the outer wall of the intussusception to the back wall of the reservoir.* ***E,*** *The mesh collar is wrapped around the inlet and anchored with seromuscular sutures, and the sheet of ileum is folded upward and closed in two layers with continuous sutures.* ***F,*** *The reservoir inlet is trimmed as needed to avoid redundancy and anastomosed with the ureters in an end-to-end manner. Six to eight through-and-through sutures are used to anastomose the reservoir and the urethra.* (From Webster GD, Kreder KJ: Orthotopic bladder replacement in men. In Fowler JE, editor: *Mastery of surgery: urologic surgery,* Boston, 1992, Little, Brown.)

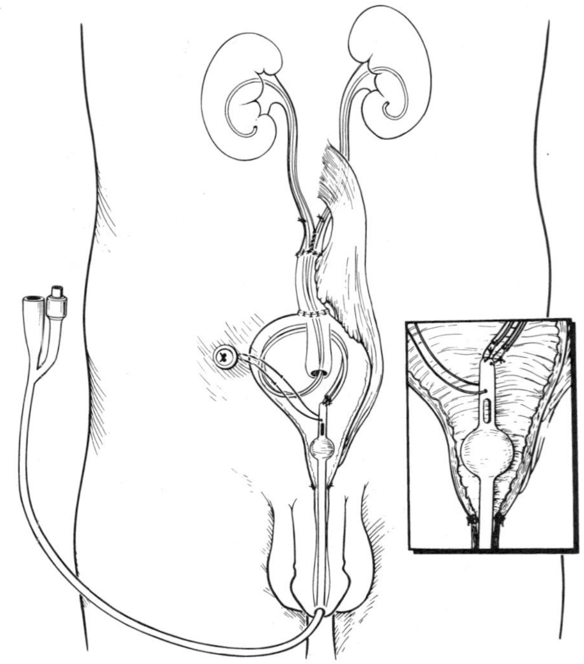

FIG. 50-2 *Schema of urinary drainage system.* (From Mark SD, Webster GD: *J Urol* 153:334-335, 1995.)

sequentially, the first on postoperative day 7 or 8 and the second on postoperative day 9 or 10. The patient is usually discharged between day 9 and day 11 with the orthotopic reservoir drained by the urethral catheter.

The patient is readmitted 3 weeks after surgery, an excretory urogram and pouchogram are obtained, and the system is activated by removal of the catheter and the attached stents, if no extravasation was seen. Initially continence is poor, but the patient is urged to void every 2 hours, and a postvoid residual urine is checked. The latter is customarily low initially. A few patients achieved daytime social continence within the first 3 weeks, and by 3 months the majority have done so, and the interval between voids may be 2 to 4 hours. Emptying efficiency is moderate, but a residual urine in excess of 100 ml is fairly common and is acceptable. Unlike using continent urinary diversion with a catheterizable stoma that is invariably colonized with bacteria, one can attempt to sterilize the orthotopic system provided that intermittent catheterization is not required.

Follow-up studies include an excretory urogram and pouchogram (cystogram) 3 months after surgery, and customarily a urodynamic study of the system is also obtained. Oncologic surveillance of the urethra is needed, urine cytologic specimens are obtained at each cancer follow-up exam, and endoscopy may be indicated.

Results

Early complications are no different from those that may follow any major intra-abdominal procedure, and the complications specific to this procedure include a higher risk of intestinal ileus, reservoir leak with resultant significant drainage, or intraperitoneal abscess (see box). The later problems include daytime urinary incontinence and enuresis, voiding problems and urethral anastomotic contracture, urethral tumor recurrence, and problems related to the reservoir itself such as small capacity, electrolyte and metabolic disturbance, and urinary infection. Upper tract problems are uncommon and include ureteroileal stenosis and reflux.

Skinner has reported a series of 126 male patients undergoing this procedure.[3] They reported the average operating time to be 4 hours and 20 minutes (a range of 3.5 to 5.5 hours), and they had an early complication rate of 11% and two perioperative deaths (1.6%). The early complication required surgical intervention in three cases, one because of a rectoreservoir fistula, one urinoma requiring drainage, and one wound dehiscence. Late complications were uncommon, with one patient having a nipple prolapse causing reflux and one developing a reservoir calculus requiring endoscopic removal. There were no cases of ureteroileal stenosis, and reflux has been seen in only two. Of 121 patients available for continence evaluation, 114 patients (94%) were dry by day, four (3.3%) required protective pads, and only three had severe daytime incontinence. They had nine patients (7.4%) who needed intermittent catheterization because of voiding problems, and in four of these patients this catheterization was attributable to pelvic tumor recurrence. Nighttime continence was achieved in 35 patients (29%), 67 (55.3%) being dry by night provided that they awakened two or three times to void. Nineteen patients (15.7%) had nighttime incontinence, though it is important to note that this leakage is often merely a small-volume seepage rather than total incontinence.

Ghoniem has also reported a large series, and his results are not dissimilar from Skinner's other than a higher late complication rate.[13] He reports eight patients with ureteral stricture, requiring open surgical correction in five and endoscopic management in three. He also had six patients with urethral anastomotic contracture, requiring endoscopic incision, and 21 patients developed stones on the antireflux mechanism.

Potential Complications of Continent Urinary Diversion

EARLY
General
Procedure specific
- Prolonged ileus
- Bowel anastomotic leak
- Reservoir leak
- Temporary upper tract obstruction

LATE
Procedure specific
- Ureteral
- Stenosis
- Reflux

Reservoir
High pressure
- Calculi
- Mucus obstruction
- Outlet Incontinence
- Stenosis
- Other infection
- Gastrointestinal disturbance
- Metabolic disturbance
- Recurrent malignancy

Conclusions

Continent urinary diversion and orthotopic bladder replacement has greatly improved the quality of life of the patient undergoing bladder removal for cancer. The closer one can approximate normal bladder function, the more accepting the patient will be, and the less devastated each will feel about the prospect of bladder removal, and hence orthotopic replacement would seem the optimal approach. In men, the primary needs are that we better identify those patients in whom this is an acceptable alternative, that is, those who do not require urethrectomy. The role of the procedure in the management of women undergoing cystectomy needs continued elaboration but is certainly going to become a more popular choice.

References

1. Camey M, Le Duc A: L'entérocystoplastie avec cysto-prostatectomie totale pour cancer de la vessie, *Ann d'Urol* 13:114-123, 1979.
2. Seeman O, Junemann KP, Alken P: Patient selection criteria for orthotopic bladder replacement. In Webster GD, Goldwasser B, editors: *Urinary diversion,* Oxford, 1995, Isis Medical Media.
3. Skinner DG, Boyd SD, Lieskovsky G, et al: Lower urinary tract reconstruction following cystectomy: experience and results in 126 patients using the Kock ileal reservoir with bilateral ureteroileal urethrostomy, *J Urol* 146:756-760, 1991.
4. Ahlering TE, Kanellos A, Boyd SD, et al: A comparative study of perioperative complications with Kock pouch urinary diversion in highly irradiated versus nonirradiated patients, *J Urol* 139:1202-1204, 1988.
5. Montie JE: Orthotopic bladder replacement in women. In Webster GD, Goldwasser B, editors: *Urinary diversion,* Oxford, 1995, Isis Medical Media.
6. Mark SD, Webster GD: Ileal reservoirs (Camey II, Hautmann, Kock, Studer). In Webster GD, Goldwasser B, editors: *Urinary diversion,* Oxford, 1995, Isis Medical Media.
7. Hautmann RE, Miller K, Steiner U, Wenderoth U: The ileal neobladder: six years of experience with more than 200 patients, *J Urol* 150:40-45, 1993.
8. Studer UE, Gerber E, Springer J, Zingg EJ: Bladder reconstruction with bowel after radical cystectomy, *World J Urol* 10:11-19, 1992.
9. Thüroff JW, Alken P, Engelmann U, et al: The Mainz pouch (mixed augmentation ileum and zoecum) for bladder augmentation and continent urinary diversion, *Eur Urol* 11:152-160, 1985.
10. Light JK, Marks JL: Total bladder replacement in the male and female using the ileocolonic segment (Le Bag), *Br J Urol* 65:467-472, 1990.
11. Reddy PK, Lange PH, Fraley EE: Total bladder replacement using detubularized sigmoid colon: technique and results, *J Urol* 145:51-55, 1991.
12. Mark SD, Webster GD: Simplified urinary drainage following orthotopic or continent bladder replacement, *J Urol* 153:334-335, 1995.
13. Ghoniem MA, Shaban AA, Mahran MR, Kock NG: Further experience with the urethral Kock pouch, *J Urol* 147:361-365, 1992.

Chapter 51

Augmentation Cystoplasty

Anthony R. Stone, Michael Rentzepis

For patients whose quality of life is significantly compromised by voiding symptoms caused by low bladder capacity, low compliance, or bladder hyperactivity, an augmentation cystoplasty provides a treatment option that can rehabilitate the patient to an acceptable quality of life as well as protect the kidneys from subsequent deterioration of function. Voiding dysfunction can be manifested by the inability to store urine properly, the inability to empty effectively, or a combination of both. Depending on the nature of the storage failure, medical or surgical options are available for the management of these patients. In those patients with functionally or anatomically contracted bladders with low compliance, poor capacity, or, in those with hyperreflexic detrusors, adequate accommodation and storage may not always be achieved by conservative measures. In this group of patients, an augmentation cystoplasty may be the procedure of choice to reestablish the bladder's ability to store urine.

Historical Perspective

In 1888 Tizzoni and Foggi described ileal augmentation cystoplasty in dogs,[1] but in 1898 Mikulicz performed the first human operation in 1898.[2] In 1917, Neuhof used free fascial grafts to repair defects and reconstruct partially resected bladders in animals.[3] He noted that transitional epithelium overgrew onto the graft. He noted ossification of his grafts as well as graft shrinkage. Interestingly, Lay[4] used preserved gallbladder as a bladder substitute; however, the patient died of postoperative uremia. Other investigators used the sigmoid colon, an ileocecal segment, or the cecum and ascending colon for augmentation or bladder substitutions.[5-7] Augmentation cystoplasty gained greater popularity with the work by Goodwin[8] and Turner-Warwick[9] in the 1950s and 1960s, and it appears that the time was right for this work to act as a catalyst for a significant increase in lower urinary tract reconstruction. Emptying of the bladder remained of great concern in these patients, and with the advent and acceptance of clean intermittent catheterization a significant hurdle was overcome. Our current techniques have built upon these foundations to include not only the work done in augmenting bladders, but also the advances in preventing vesicoureteral reflux and continent reconstruction with abdominal stomas. In addition, the use of pubovaginal slings and artificial urinary sphincters have helped improve the continence rates of those patients with associated intrinsic urethral deficiency.

Definitions

In the past, the term "augmentation cystoplasty" has been used generically to refer to any procedure where bowel is used to enlarge or substitute for bladder tissue. Recently a subcommittee of the International Continence Society has attempted to standardize the terms used for these procedures. Thus augmentation cystoplasty should refer to a surgical procedure for increasing bladder capacity. They go on to state that this may be accomplished without other tissues (such as autoaugmentation) or with incorporation of other tissues such as intestine (enterocystoplasty, intestinocystoplasty), with or without changing the shape of such intestine (that is, detubularization and reconfiguration), and with or without resection of a portion of the original bladder. This distinguishes augmentation cystoplasty from bladder substitution, which refers to a surgical procedure for in situ (orthotopic) total substitution or replacement of the bladder by other tissue such as isolated intestine. After subtotal excision of the original bladder (as in interstitial cystitis) the intestinal urinary reservoir may be connected to the bladder neck (bladder substitution to the bladder neck) and after complete excision of the original bladder (radical cystoprostatectomy), the reservoir may be connected to the urethra as a continent outlet (bladder substitution to urethra). This chapter is concentrated on the discussion of bladder augmentation as defined above.

INDICATIONS

Augmentation of the bladder facilitates improved storage of urine without significant increases in detrusor pressure and therefore has most often been used in those conditions that lead to a contracted bladder. Radiation cystitis, tuberculosis, or schistosomiasis[10] represent exogenous sources for "anatomic" contraction of the bladder, whereas neurologic entities such as spina bifida or spinal cord injury lead to "functional" or neuropathic contraction. A variety of alternative therapies has also been tried to convert the functionally contracted bladder to low-pressure, lower-motor-neuron type of behavior, including subarachnoid blocks, sacral rhizotomy, presacral denervation, and subtrigonal injection of phenol or alcohol. In general, these therapies have not succeeded in altering detrusor characteristics significantly or have inappropriate complications.

EVALUATION

In the patient with urine storage failure, a complete history and physical exam is an essential part of the evaluation to determine the cause of the dysfunction and therefore facilitate determination of a logical treatment regimen. A medication history and surgical history are of importance to narrow options. Because conservative measures have been discussed in other chapters, it is assumed that at this point the patient has failed these measures, and now a surgical approach is being considered.

For children, age may be a limiting factor from a technical standpoint. Children under 7 years of age often have a urethra that is not of sufficient caliber to accept an "appropriate" catheter to evacuate secreted mucus. The use of gastric segments or autoaugmentation procedures with or without deepithelialized intestine may theoretically obviate this concern, and these procedures are discussed later in this chapter. In addition, these evacuation problems may be helped by the construction of a continent abdominal stoma at the time of cystoplasty, again to facilitate bladder emptying.

In the past, impaired renal function (creatine greater than 2, creatinine clearance less than 35) was considered to be a contraindication to enterocystoplasty because of the reabsorption phenomena found with augmented segments (see below). The source of renal failure is important in these situations; however, because those patients who are in failure caused by elevated bladder pressures may stabilize or improve after augmentation. Even if renal function continues to deteriorate, the lower urinary tract will be better suited to receive a transplant.[11] In other patients with renal failure, particularly children, the use of gastric segments may help to prevent or improve the metabolic acidosis associated with this procedure.

Urodynamic Evaluation

Urodynamic evaluation allows for a formal objective assessment of bladder function before the initiation of therapy. Videourodynamic testing provides a means to assess visually the bladder for evidence of reflux and provide an opportunity to check for intrinsic sphincter deficiency at one sitting. A Valsalva leak point pressure can be used in lieu of video confirmation, particularly in those patients in whom intrinsic sphincter deficiency is likely, that is, patients with myelomeningocele or the exstrophy-epispadias complex.

Radiologic Evaluation

If a videourodynamic study is not performed, a cystogram is necessary to rule out reflux. An intravenous pyelogram should be done for assessment of the upper tracts and to assist in planning possible ureteral reconstruction. Most patients with storage failure have been followed with serial renal ultrasonograms during their course and should have a recent one available before surgery to act as a baseline reference. If renal function is marginal, a nuclear renogram will provide differential function, which can also determine if ureteral obstruction is present. Imaging of the bowel is usually not necessary unless an underlying disorder is suggested, such as diverticular disease, inflammatory bowel disease, or previous intestinal surgery.

Laboratory Studies

In addition to a complete blood count to help in the assessment for anemia associated with chronic disease, a chemistry panel is essential to evaluate renal function and acid-base status. A creatinine clearance is an excellent, easily obtainable measure of true renal function, particularly in those patients with evidence of chronic renal insufficiency. It also serves as a baseline reference for follow-up. In addition, a preoperative urine culture is necessary for one to treat any specific organism before surgery.

Endoscopy

Cystourethroscopy is often the least important aspect of the preoperative evaluation; however, in those patients who previously have had outlet procedures performed, as in the exstrophy and epispadias population, it takes on significant importance, in that it can determine how appropriate the urethra will be for catheterization. In addition, it is used to verify an absence of diverticula and to identify small calculi within the bladder that may be missed by routine x-ray examination.

General Preoperative Considerations

As the patient undergoes evaluation for augmentation cystoplasty, a plan for reconstruction must develop based on the patient's history and physical exam, metabolic status, urodynamic evaluation, and radiologic appearance. Those patients with a metabolic acidosis may benefit most from use of a gastric segment, and this may also be a consideration in the irradiated patient. Those patients with intrinsic sphincter deficiency should undergo a procedure to enhance the outlet at the same sitting. Vesicoureteral reflux will generally necessitate reimplantation of the ureters at the time of surgery.

In patients who are wheelchair bound, particularly females, a discussion of the creation of a continent, catheterizable, abdominal stoma at the time of surgery, with or without an associated bladder neck procedure, should occur. This should also be considered in the younger child undergoing reconstruction when catheter size is a consideration.

Finally, during the multiple meetings with the patient who may ultimately undergo an augmentation cystoplasty, it is of utmost importance to reinforce in the patient the need to remain motivated after surgery because intermittent catheterization will most likely be necessary. In addition, the patient must understand the risks and limitations of the procedure as well as the possible need for subsequent procedures.

By fully evaluating the patient with inadequate storage ability, a rational approach to surgical treatment can be planned with a minimum of additional procedures. The informed patient who understands the expectations of the procedure and understands the subsequent responsibilities of managing an augmented bladder is best capable of taking full advantage of his or her new potential freedom.

SURGICAL TECHNIQUES

Bowel preparation is essential unless a gastric segment will without a doubt be used. All other cases require a bowel preparation, which is particularly of importance in patients with spina bifida or those affected by a neuropathic bowel. For this reason, we encourage a bowel-cleansing regimen in this population, beginning a week in advance, consisting of the use of daily enemas and moving toward a more liquid diet if possible. We then have the patients undergo a mechanical bowel prep with GoLYTELY (polyethylene glycol 3350 and electrolytes) or magnesium citrate the day before surgery, in addition to an antibiotic bowel prep with neomycin and erythromycin. The patients are also instructed in incentive spirometry before surgery.

In those patients with spina bifida, strict latex precautions are enforced even if the patient has had no previous latex reactions. Anaphylactic reactions to latex can occur after repeated exposures and may occur intraoperatively, as has happened at our institution. For this reason, our nursing and operating room staff have been fully educated in this latex-free protocol, and it is written clearly in the chart.

Patients are positioned in the low lithotomy position for females and supine position for males. The incision is most often made in the lower midline; however, we have used a Pfannenstiel incision in women who have an existing scar. If a gastric segment is to be used, the lower midline incision can be extended cephalad to facilitate resection of the stomach after the bladder dissection.

With the patient in the Trendelenburg position, the bowel falls into the upper abdomen and a self-retaining retractor can be used to provide excellent pelvic exposure. The bladder is grasped between Allis clamps, and the lateral peritoneal attachments are taken down with the Bovie knife to the vas deferens in the male and to the superior pedicles in the female. Blunt dissection then allows for anterior and lateral mobilization of the bladder.

The bladder is then opened at the dome transversely down to the trigone on each side. The incision is extended in front of the ureters on either side to prevent an hourglass deformity after reconstruction (Fig. 51-1). With the bladder bivalved in this way, the greatest volume of augmentation can be achieved with the least amount of material, retaining the spherical orientation of the bladder. Criticism of this coronal dissection has been voiced because of the potential hazards of interference with the native ureterovesical junctions. This has not been a problem in our hands. However, the bladder may be bivalved in the sagittal plane if this is a concern. Whichever dissection technique is used, it is essential to extend the incision down to the trigone as previously described.

If an artificial urinary sphincter (AUS) or fascial sling is to be used, these procedures may be appropriately performed at this point in the operation. The open bladder allows for correct positioning of the cuff or the fascia at the bladder neck at this time.

If the ureters need to be reimplanted, they may be dissected from the bladder at this time. It is not necessary to extend the dissection into the bladder unless significant lower ureteric dilatation is present.

In the majority of patients, bladder tissue does not have to be excised. Supratrigonal cystectomy may be carried out in patients with interstitial cystitis or with severe detrusor hyperreflexia, where it is deemed appropriate to remove most of the diseased bladder. In this case, if supratrigonal cystectomy is required, the

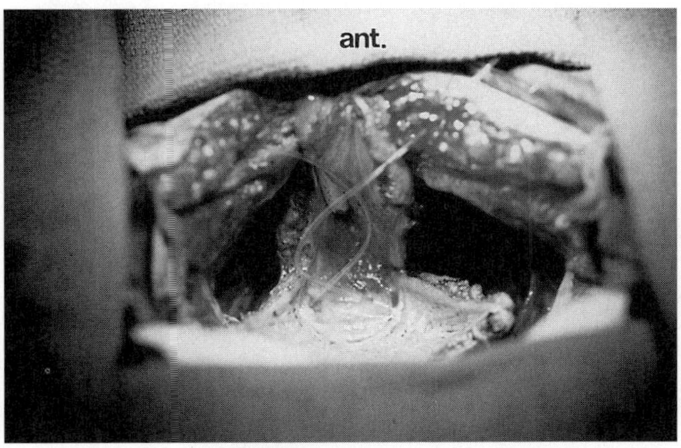

FIG. 51-1 *The bladder is opened in the coronal plane with incision extended into trigone in front of ureteral orifices.* ant., *Anterior.*

bladder is initially opened sagittally. The mucosa is then scored with the Bovie knife just above the ureters posteriorly and laterally. Each half of the bladder is then carefully dissected off the ureters on each side, with vessels being fulgurated as they are identified. A small fringe of bladder is left anteriorly, and just enough bladder is left above the ureters and across the trigone to allow an adequate enterovesical anastomosis to be carried out (Fig. 51-2).

Infratrigonal cystoplasty may be accomplished in a similar way. In this case, the ureters should be detached from the bladder. It may help to identify the superior pedicles on either side and to incise and ligate them. The two halves of the bladder are removed as before, leaving a small fringe of bladder above the internal meatus.

CHOICE OF BOWEL SEGMENT

Ileum

Ileum is commonly used for augmentation because of its availability, mobility, and reasonable management of electrolyte disturbances. Indeed, most urologists are comfortable with the use of ileum because it has been used for ileal conduit diversion for many years. A segment of ileum approximately 25 to 40 cm in length is isolated on its mesentery, commencing approximately 15 cm from the ileocecal valve. The length of segment is dependent on the incision made in the bladder. Careful measurement of the bladder incision is not necessary because the detubularized ileum is an extremely compliant material. Detubularization interrupts the circular muscle fibers of the bowel segment, helping to prevent any residual high-pressure contractions. The terminal portion of the ileum should not be contained within the mobilized segment to prevent the possibility of later onset of vitamin B_{12} deficiency. A side-to-side stapled or sewn anastomosis is performed to reconstitute bowel continuity. The isolated segment is placed caudally to this anastomosis in a U-shaped configuration, with the curve of the U directed inferiorly. The contiguous borders of this bowel segment are sutured together with a running seromuscular 3-0 polyglycolic acid (PGA) suture (Fig. 51-3). The bowel is then opened along this suture line to completely detubularize it. This suture line is then reinforced with another running 3-0 PGA suture through all layers. Recently, this maneuver has been achieved using absorbable staples (Polysorb GIA 75 stapler). This stapling device provides an excellent, quickly performed, two-layer, water-tight closure (Fig. 51-4).

The dependent portion of the opened bowel is sutured to the apex of the posterior aspect of the "clammed" bladder. This anastomosis is continued down both sides of the posterior wing of the "clam," with the bowel being sutured down into the open corners of the bladder. Infant feeding tubes, 5 or 8 Fr, may be placed in the ureters during this portion of the anastomosis to ensure that the ureters are not damaged in any way. Once the suture lines reach the anterior aspect of the opened bladder, the upper aspect of the bowel segment is then folded over and anastomosed to the anterior wing of the "clam." This suture line is then continued until the ileovesical closure is completed. Any redundant bowel may be sutured to itself. We prefer to suture the open bowel segment into the "clammed" bladder in this way rather than reconfiguring the segment into a "cap" first because this allows the bowel to be easily tailored to any size of opened bladder without complicated measuring techniques being required (Fig. 51-5).

Before closure of the vesicointestinal anastomosis, a Malecot catheter is placed through a stab incision in the bowel portion of

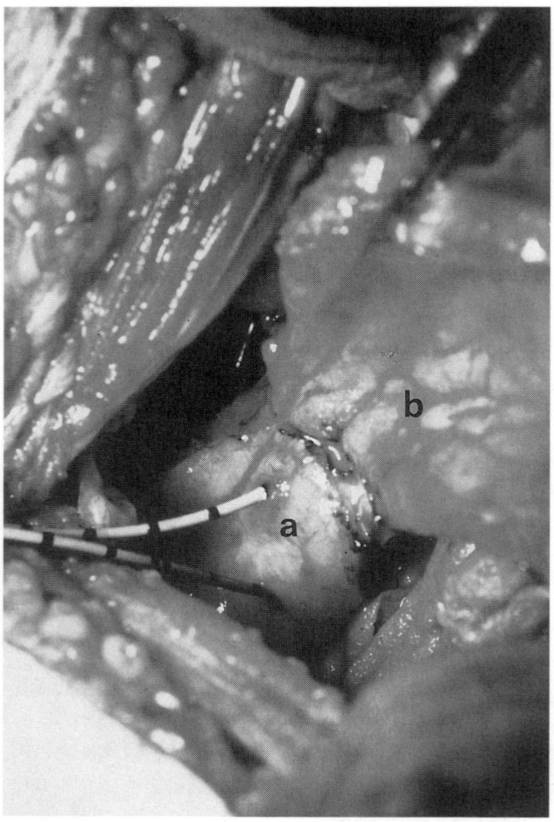

FIG. 51-2 *Supratrigonal cystectomy. a, Small fringe of bladder retained above ureteral orifices; b, Bowel segment being anastomosed to bladder remnant.*

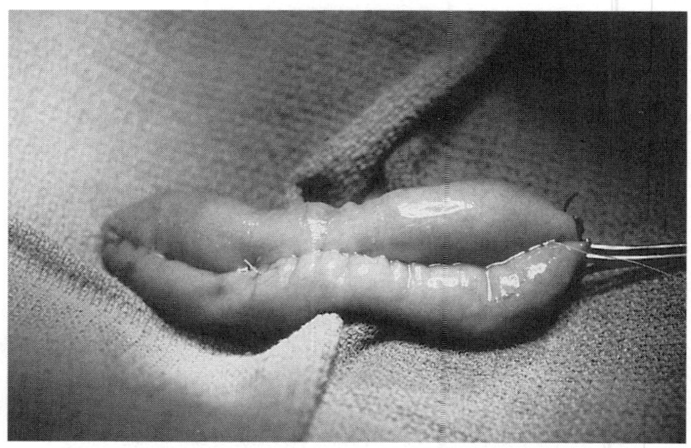

FIG. 51-3 *Contiguous borders of bowel segment sutured together before detubularization.*

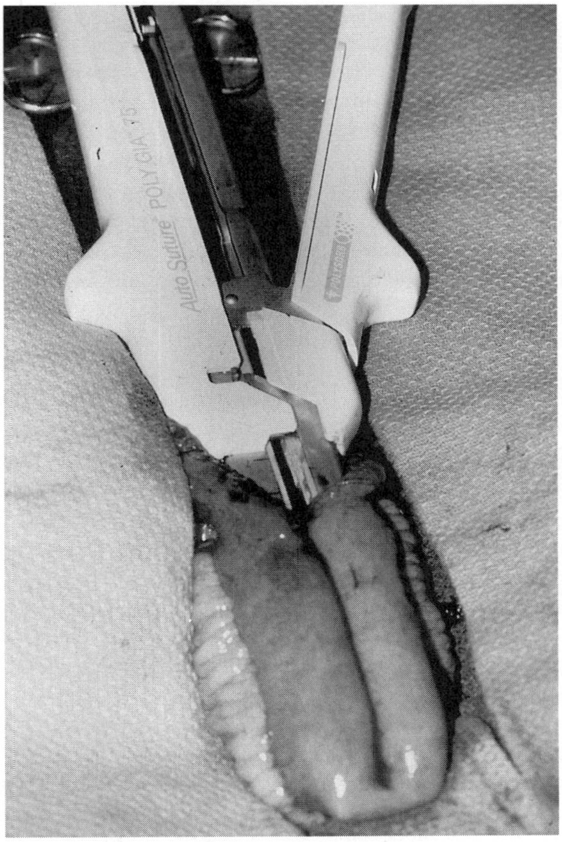

FIG. 51-4 *Absorbable staples may be used to detubularize and reconfigure bowel segment.*

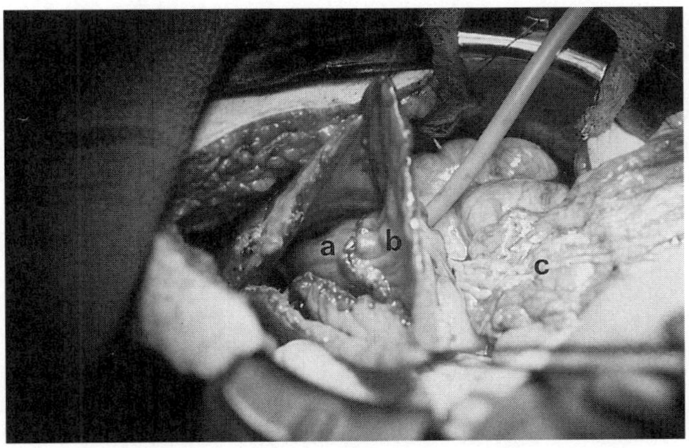

FIG. 51-5 a, *Posterior "wing" of clammed bladder;* b, *detubularized, reconfigured bowel segment before completion of ileovesical anastomosis;* c, *omentum.*

the cystoplasty. A purse-string suture is placed around this exiting tube to prevent leakage at this point. Suprapubic drainage with a wide-bore catheter such as a Malecot is essential to efficiently remove mucus and clots postoperatively.

At this time the ileocecal anastomosis is tested by filling the cystoplasty with saline solution and closing any obvious leakage points with interrupted absorbable sutures. We do not attempt to place a complete invaginating second layer of suture because this has been found to be unnecessary.

This technique provides a reliable, low-pressure, spherical reservoir. It should be noted, however, that some authors do not believe it necessary to reconfigure the bowel segment but merely detubularize and suture this open segment into the bladder.[11]

If possible, the omentum is mobilized from the transverse colon and pedicled down either of the pericolic gutters. The omentum is then wrapped around the cystoplasty and sutured in place with two or three interrupted absorbable sutures. The omentum is specifically attached to the cystoplasty adherent to the exiting catheter, and this is then sutured to the anterior abdominal wall adjacent to the exiting catheter to seal any potential leaks that might occur when this tube is removed.

Sigmoid Colon[12]

On occasion, the ileum may be matted within adhesions, or the mesentery may be too short to allow adequate mobilization. In these cases, the use of a sigmoid segment is reasonable. A segment of approximately 15 cm is usually appropriate. In this case it need not be reconfigured into a U-shape but is detubularized and sutured into the opened bladder. A Malecot catheter for drainage and omental wrap are employed as previously described. Sigmoid continuity may be restored with either an end-to-end sutured or side-to-side stapled or sewn anastomosis.

Cecum and Right Colon

The cecum and right colon may also be used, though this segment is more often used for bladder substitution or orthotopic bladder replacement because it provides a larger reservoir. It is mobilized on an ileocolic vascular pedicle and should include the hepatic flexure and transverse colon up to the middle colic artery. The segment is opened through the anterior tenia and then folded over on itself. The sides of the segment are sewn to each other to form a pouch. The inferior open portion of the pouch is then sewn into the opened bladder to form the cystoplasty.

Transverse Colon

In the irradiated patient the transverse colon may be the most appropriate segment for use in the augmentation. The segment is isolated on a middle colic pedicle, which will usually allow it to reach down to the bladder easily. As with the sigmoid colon, this segment needs only to be detubularized.

Stomach[13]

Gastrocystoplasty has recently gained acceptance by the urologic community, especially in children with renal insufficiency or in adults in whom irradiated bowel precludes the use of other segments. The gastric segment has the specific advantage of not absorbing electrolytes from the urine, thus eliminating the development of a hyperchloremic metabolic acidosis with its attendant effects on calcium and bone metabolism. The mucus produced by the stomach is thin and watery, thus allowing for easier irrigation in the younger patient with a smaller-caliber urethra. In addition, the urine is more often sterile because of its acidic pH.

Antral gastrocystoplasty was originally introduced in Hong Kong.[14] However, its long-term results are not impressive. The "wedge" gastrocystoplasty popularized by Mitchell using a stomach patch from the greater curvature on a right or left gastroepiploic pedicle has had greater success.[13]

In this procedure, one mobilizes the greater curvature of the stomach by dissecting the omentum off the transverse colon to enter the lesser sac. One then develops a right gastroepiploic pedicle by ligating and dividing the short gastric vessels between the greater curvature to the medial aspect of the gastric wedge. Bissada has recommended testing the patency of the left and right gastroepiploic vessels before harvesting the vascular pedicle to detect possible poor flow from one side.[15] The omentum may be left attached to the pedicle or separated. One then isolates the gastric wedge from the stomach using two rows of GIA staples (GIA 90 instrument, Fig. 51-6). Initially the technique necessitated removal of the staples from the stomach side of the incision and reanastomosing of the edges of the stomach to restore gastric anatomy. The technique has now been modified such that a shallow wedge is excised, leaving sufficient gastric continuity at the lesser curvature, obviating the need for reanastomosis of the stomach. This maneuver cuts down considerably on blood loss and operative time.

The gastric wedge on its right gastroepiploic pedicle with or without attached omentum is then led behind the transverse mesocolon and root of the small bowel mesentery to lie easily within the pelvis. The staples along the edges of the wedge are then removed and gastrovesical anastomosis is carried out with a running 3-0 PGA suture. The omentum is conveniently placed to wrap around the gastrocystoplasty once the anastomosis is complete.

Whichever segment of bowel is used to accomplish the augmentation, it is imperative to leave a peritoneal drain in place. We prefer a round suction drain (10 Fr Jackson-Pratt). Persistent drainage can be sent for a sufficient creatinine level to be checked to determine the source of leakage during the postoperative period.

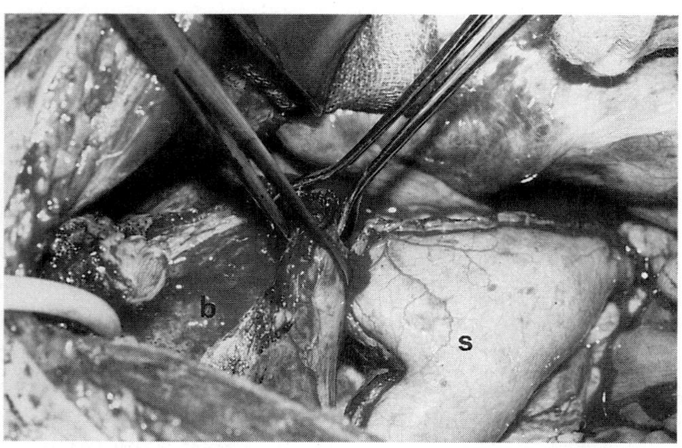

FIG. 51-6 b, *Opened bladder;* s, *gastric segment (stapled), lead underneath the mesentery before gastrovesical anastomosis.*

Postoperative Care

In the early postoperative period, the cystoplasty is irrigated with 30 to 40 ml of normal saline every 8 hours to ensure good drainage and to prevent mucus accumulation and plugging. The patient continues to receive fluids intravenously and nasogastric aspiration until bowel function returns, and the peritoneal drain is left in place until drainage is minimal. The patient is discharged to home after a regular diet can be tolerated and after instruction in catheter care has been given. The suprapubic catheter is irrigated by the patient twice per day while at home.

A cystogram is performed 2½ to 3 weeks postoperatively through the suprapubic tube. If no extravasation is seen, the tube is removed, and the patient may begin clean intermittent catheterization. If the ureters had been reimplanted at the time of surgery, the ureteral stents are removed at this time as well. A minority of patients may be able to empty their bladders volitionally, but even in this group we recommend intermittent catheterization at least initially to ensure complete emptying. The catheterization schedule consists of 2-hourly catheterizations during the day and at least once at night. Over the next 4 to 6 weeks this regimen can be extended so that the patient is catheterizing approximately 4-hourly during the day and sleeps through the night.

Subsequent follow-up includes following renal and metabolic status with regular serum creatinine and electrolyte checks. If the renal status appears to be impaired, creatinine clearance can be measured to obtain a more precise evaluation of renal function. In routine cases we check labs every 3 months for the first year and then yearly. In addition, a urine culture should be checked at each follow-up visit. We routinely treat bacteriuria caused by urease-producing organisms but reserve treatment for other bacteria based on the clinical setting. There is no evidence that prophylactic antibiotics are advantageous after augmentation cystoplasty, even in those patients on clean intermittent catheterization.

Upper tracts are evaluated at 3, 6, and 12 months postoperatively to evaluate for hydronephrosis, thinning of parenchyma, and stones. If the cystoplasty was performed in part to maintain or improve renal function, a nuclear renogram or repeat creatinine clearance may be obtained.

Cystourethroscopy is performed yearly to evaluate for small stones and also to exclude carcinomatous changes.

Complications

Early complications include the leakage of urine, which most often can be managed conservatively or by percutaneous nephrostomy tube drainage.

Despite detubularization and reconfiguration of the bowel segment, continued peristaltic activity and hyperactivity may occur (Fig. 51-7). The principal side effect of this may be incontinence; however, this is usually attributable to insufficient outlet resistance. Continued overactivity of the bladder segment may produce associated bladder neck opening with subsequent leakage. Hyperactivity may be managed with anticholinergic medication as with the intact bladder. Occasionally an additional patch of bowel needs to be inserted into the cystoplasty to resolve this problem.

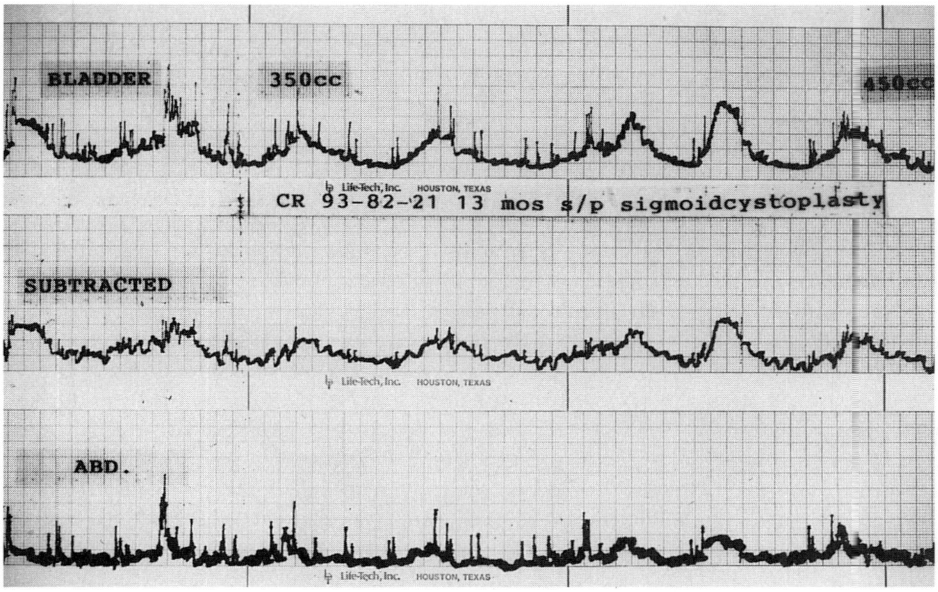

FIG. 51-7 *Persistent contractions in a sigmoid cystoplasty, potential cause of recurrent incontinence after cystoplasty.*

Metabolic and renal problems can occur because of the reabsorption of electrolytes from the urine. Chloride ions are absorbed along with hydrogen ions with subsequent loss of bicarbonate and potassium into the urine, giving rise to a hyperchloremic acidosis. Adequate renal function will normally compensate for this problem. Patients with impaired renal function should be monitored carefully after cystoplasty for this phenomenon. Oral bicarbonate therapy will correct this in most cases. Exacerbation may occur in relation to urinary tract infection. If the acidosis is not corrected, this may interfere with calcium metabolism, which may have significant consequences in children in terms of growth.

With gastrocystoplasty, metabolic problems may arise from the secretion of hydrogen ions into the urine. Some children may develop a metabolic alkalosis and require treatment with histamine (H_2-receptor) blockers. In addition, the secretion of gastric acid in the sensate patient may lead to the "hematuria-dysuria" syndrome.[16] In this syndrome, patients will have episodic hematuria associated with bladder discomfort. Often these patients respond to H_2 blockers. It is our practice to maintain patients who have undergone a gastrocystoplasty on H_2 blockers for 3 months postoperatively and then wean them off. Omeprazole (a protein pump inhibitor) has been used successfully in cases of refractory metabolic alkalosis and severe aciduria.[17]

The bowel segment will continue to produce mucus. Occasionally this will accumulate in the cystoplasty, causing catheterizing difficulties. In general, this may be presented by adequate catheter drainage. Daily saline irrigation in the early postoperative period may prevent this problem. Mucus production, though never ceasing completely, will decrease with time.

Spontaneous perforation of the augmentation cystoplasty has been reported.[18-21] It occurs most commonly in those patients who have undergone artificial urinary sphincter placement and who are receiving intermittent catheterization. Perforation usually occurs in the cystoplasty bowel segment and not at the anastomosis. Ischemia of the bowel caused by overdistension is generally the implicated underlying disorder. The consequences of perforation may be grave, especially in the nonsensate patient, who often will present in the later stages of peritonitis. Patients and their families must thus be adequately counseled as to the dangers of failure to appropriately empty the cystoplasty on a regular basis.

The development of stones, believed to be caused by chronic bacteriuria and urinary stasis or the presence of staples from the anastomosis, has increasingly been reported, with an incidence of 30% to 50%.[22,23] Stones have been found to be made of apatite, struvite, and ammonium urate among others.[24] Both open and endourologic treatments have been used successfully.

The risks of carcinoma formation in the ureterosigmoidostomy are well documented.[25] Despite removal of the anastomosis away from the fecal stream, a growing number of tumors in cystoplasties (usually adenocarcinoma) have been reported,[26] with a mean latency of 18 years. Both small and large bowel segments appear to be involved equally,[27,28] and as yet no human cases have been found with gastrocystoplasty. Chronic bacterial colonization seems to be the common oncogenic etiologic factor. Experimental studies have implicated the high concentration of nitrosamines produced by these bacteria as a possible cause of the tumors. The reactivity of cellular elements is believed to be important in this process, and there is some evidence that this may be reversed by nonsteroidal antiinflammatory drugs (NSAIDs).

The risk of pregnancy in cystoplasty patients has been examined.[29] Sixty percent of the women in the group developed urinary tract infections while pregnant. The principal concern was that of preventing the development of incontinence after delivery; one of 10 patients with a normal outlet before delivery was incontinent afterwards. Two women with normal outlets had cesarean sections unrelated to their urologic condition. Cesarean sections were performed in the three women who had had continence procedures; all three women remained continent. It was recommended that women undergoing cesarean section should have a urologist as part of the operative team to help identify the unusual anatomy and assist in the dissection of the cystoplasty off the uterus.

Future Directions and Novel Approaches

To prevent the associated problems inherent in using bowel or gastric segments, a variety of synthetic tissues, including silicon rubber, Teflon, and gelatin sponge, have been tried with limited success. Lyophilized human dura, bovine pericardium, fascial free grafts, peritoneum, and omentum have also been tried.[30-34] None of these materials has succeeded in supplanting the use of bowel or stomach for a variety of reasons. Attempts to grow transitional epithelium on collagen matrices continue to be carried out in vitro and in the animal model[35] and may eventually lead to an alternative approach.

Deepithelialized sigmoid colon has been used to augment the bladder with the hope that the transitional epithelium will regenerate over its surface and thus prevent the absorptive sequelae associated with intestinal segments. Motely et al. noted that 10 of 11 calves had complete coverage of the deepithelialized grafts, but all had residual colonic mucosa or developed mucoceles.[36] In several animals, however, significant fibrosis and contraction occurred. It was believed that removal of the colonic mucosa was a tedious procedure and that early distension of the graft may be essential in avoiding graft fibrosis. It has also been postulated that the act of stripping the mucosa may set up the inflammatory reaction that is aggravated by the contact with urine.

Reversed seromuscular grafts have been used[37] to augment the bladder. Again, moderate to severe fibrosis and contraction of the flap developed in many cases. Mucosal stripping would be necessary to prevent the secretion of mucus into the abdomen.

Autoaugmentation is a novel approach to increasing the capacity of the bladder without the use of bowel or stomach segments, with the hope of avoiding the associated complications found with their use. In this procedure, the detrusor is removed from the dome of the bladder, leaving the mucosa intact.[38] This maneuver creates a large bladder diverticulum, thus theoretically reducing abnormal contractility and improving functional capacity. The long-term results, however, have suggested that significant mucosal contraction can occur. Clinical results in terms of improved continence and stabilization of upper tracts have been favorable; however, objective results, gained by urodynamics, have shown little improvement.[39] Concern has also been raised on the incidence of late contracture of the exposed bladder mucosal segment. Further long-term studies are needed to determine the merits and limitations of this technique.

Autoaugmentation associated with enterocystoplasty[40] or gastrocystoplasty[41] is another novel approach to augmentation. Detrusorectomy is carried out as described above, and the missing area is covered with a gastric or bowel segment from which the mucosa has been removed. It is hoped that an approach such as this might combine the advantages of autoaugmentation and prevent contractures of the transitional epithelium. Nonsecretory sigmoid cystoplasty has been performed experimentally in dogs and followed up with human patients.[42] The deepithelialized colon was sutured over the bladder dome with 5-0 chromic catgut. The investigators found that compliance increased in all animals in the combined group. In the patient cohort, bladder capacity increased significantly. Although still experimental, this approach may combine the advantages of retaining transitional epithelium without the additional concerns of mucosal fibrosis and greater susceptibility to trauma, that is, catheterization as may happen with simple autoaugmentation.

Ureterocystoplasty is an approach that can be utilized when one kidney has become nonfunctional because of severe reflux or obstruction. In these cases the nonfunctioning kidney is removed and the ureter can be split longitudinally on its anterior aspect and mobilized along its upper two-thirds extent. Care is taken to preserve the blood supply to the intact lower third. The ureter is then folded over or reconfigured and sutured into the "clammed" bladder (Fig. 51-8). The small series reported on this technique has generally shown good results.[43-44] One significant advantage is that there should be no need to irrigate the augmented bladder, which makes this procedure ideal for the young patient. Although the long-term sequelae are unknown, it may prove of use in buying time for the patient until he or she is old enough to successfully undergo formal enterocystoplasty.

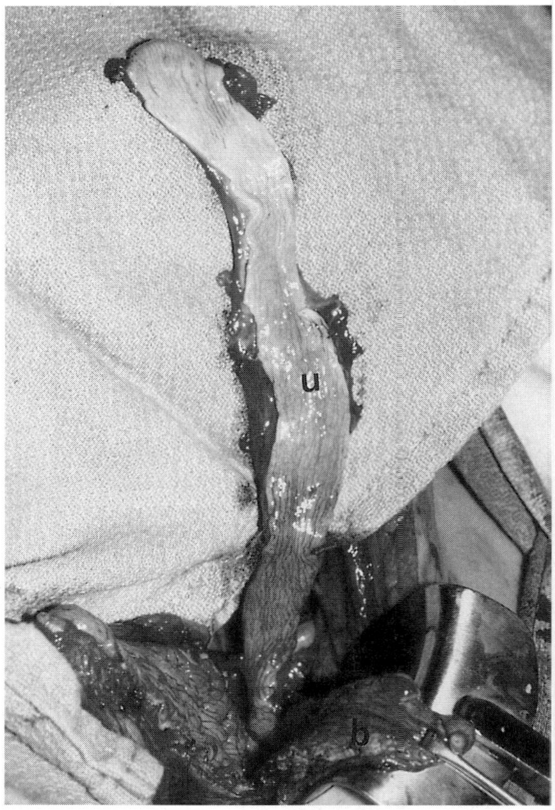

FIG. 51-8 *Ureterocystoplasty.* b, *Clammed bladder;* u, *opened ureter, ready to be anastomosed for cystoplasty.*

Summary

Despite the limitations of enterocystoplasty, augmentation of the bladder remains a feasible and useful alternative for those patients with a functionally or anatomically contracted bladder. Stabilization of renal function and improved continence may allow the patient to have a more socially acceptable life and provide him with a sense of independence. Careful patient selection, meticulous technique, and scrupulous commitment to follow-up study are essential in the success of augmentation cystoplasty.

References

1. Tizzoni F: Die weiderherstellung de harnblase, *Zentralbl Chir* 15:921-924, 1888.
2. Mikulicz J: Zur operation der angerborener blasensplate, *Zentralbl Chir* 26:641, 1899.
3. Neuhof H: Fascia transplantation into visceral defects: an experimental and clinical study, *Surg Gynecol Obstet* 24:383, 1917.
4. Lay EB: Bladder made from gallbladder, *Arch Ital di Chir* 11:333, 1925.
5. Bisgard J: Substitution of the urinary bladder with a segment of sigmoid, *Ann Surg* 117:106, 1943.
6. Bricker E, Eiseman B: Bladder reconstruction from cecum and ascending colonfollowing resection of pelvic viscera, *Ann Surg* 132:77, 1950.
7. Gilchrist R, Merricks J, Hamlin H, Reiger I: Construction of a substitute bladder and urethra, *Surg Gynecol Obstet* 90:752, 1950.
8. Goodwin WE, Winter CC, Barker WF: "Cup-patch" technique of ileocystoplasty for bladder enlargement or partial substitution, *Surg Gynecol Obstet* 108:317, 1959.
9. Turner-Warwick RT, Ashkin MA: The functional results of partial, subtotal, and total cystoplasty with special reference to ureterocecoplasty, selective sphincterotomy, and cystocystoplasty, *Br J Urol* 39:3-12, 1967.
10. Couvelaire R: La "petite vessie" des tuberculeux génito-urinaires: essai de classification, place et variantes des cysto-intestino-plasties, *J Urol* (Paris) 56:381, 1950.
11. Mundy AR: Detrusor instability. In Mundy AR, editor: *Urodynamic and reconstructive surgery of the lower urinary tract*, Edinburgh, 1993, Churchill Livingstone.
12. Webster GD, Kreder KJ, Ramon J: Right colocystoplasty and sigmoidocystoplasty. In Whitehead EW, editor: *Atlas of surgical techniques*, in press.
13. Mitchell ME: Stomach for bladder augmentation and replacement. In King LR, Stone AR, Webster GD, editors: *Bladder reconstruction and continent urinary diversion*, ed 2, St Louis, 1991, Mosby.
14. Leong CH: Use of the stomach for bladder replacement and urinary diversion, *Ann R Coll Surg Engl* 60:283, 1978.
15. Bissada SA, Bissasa NK: Choice of gastroepiploic vessels for gastrocystoplasty, *J Urol* 148:101, 1992.
16. Nguyen DH, Bain MA, Salmonson KL, et al: The syndrome of dysuria and hematuria in pediatric urinary reconstruction with stomach, *J Urol* 150:707-709, 1993.
17. Kinahan TJ, Khoury AE, McLorie GA, Churchill BM: Omeprazole in post-gastrocystoplasty metabolic alkalosis and aciduria, *J Urol* 147:435, 1992.
18. Slataon JW, Kropp KA: Conservative management of suspected bladder rupture after augmentation enterocystoplasty, *J Urol* 152:713, 1994.
19. Rushton HG, Woodward JR, Parrot TS, et al: Delayed bladder rupture after augmentation enterocystoplasty, *J Urol* 140:344, 1988.
20. Elder JS, Snyder HM, Hulbert WC, Duckett JW: Perforation of the augmented bladder in patients undergoing clean intermittent catheterization, *J Urol* 140:1159, 1981.
21. Couillard DR, Vapnek JM, Rentzepis MJ, Stone AR: Fatal perforation of an augmentation cystoplasty in an adult, *Urology* 42:5, 1993.
22. Hendren WH, Hendren RB: Bladder augmentation: experience with 129 children and young adults, *J Urol* 144:445, 1990.
23. Palmer LS, Franco I, Reda EF, et al: Endoscopic management of bladder calculi following augmentation cystoplasty, *Urology* 44:902, 1994.
24. Palmer LS, Franco I, Kogan SJ, et al: Urolithiasis in children following augmentation cystoplasty, *J Urol* 150:726, 1993.
25. Spence HM, Hoffman WW, Fosmire GP: Tumor of the colon as a late complication of ureterosigmoidostomy for exstrophyof the bladder, *Br J Urol* 51:466, 1979.
26. Stone AR: Tumors associated with lower tract reconstruction using isolated bowel segments. In King LR, Stone AR, Webster GD, editors: *Bladder reconstruction and continent urinary diversion,* ed 2, St Louis, 1991, Mosby.
27. Kirby RS, Lloyd-Davies RW: Adenocarcinoma occurring with a caecocystoplasty, *Br J Urol* 57:357, 1985.
28. Golomb J, Klutke CG, Lewis KJ, et al: Bladder neoplasms associated with augmentation cystoplasty: report of 2 cases and literature review, *J Urol* 142:377, 1989.
29. Hill DE, Kramer SA: Management of pregnancy after augmentation cystoplasty, *J Urol* 144:457, 1990.
30. Stone AR, Radomski SB, Roach MB, Gandour-Edwards R: Human dehydrated dura cystoplasty: a suitable alternative to bowel? *Scand J Urol Nephrol* 142:146-147, 1992.
31. Novick AC, Straffon RA, Banowsky LH, et al: Experimental bladder substitution using biodegradable graft or natural tissue, *Urology* 10:118, 1977.
32. Kudish HG: The use of polyvinyl sponge for experimental cystoplasty, *J Urol* 78:232, 1957.
33. Orkasa S, Tsuji I: Enlargement of contracted bladder by use of gelatin sponge bladder, *J Urol* 104:107, 1970.
34. Kelami A: Duraplasty of the urinary bladder: results after two to six years, *Eur Urol* 1:178, 1975.
35. Tsuji I, Ishida H, Fujieda J: Experimental cystoplasty using preserved bladder graft, *J Urol* 85:42, 1961.
36. Motley RC, Montgomery BT, Zollman PE, et al: Augmentation cystoplasty utilizing de-epithelialized sigmoid colon: a preliminary study, *J Urol* 143:1257, 1990.
37. Grotzinger P, Shoemaker W, Marucci H, et al: The use of inverted seromuscular grafts from the ileum for reconstruction of the urinary bladder, *Ann Surg* 140:834, 1954.
38. Snow BW, Cartwright PC: Bladder autoaugmentation. In King LR, Stone AR, Webster GD, editors: *Bladder reconstruction and continent urinary diversion,* ed 2, St Louis, 1991, Mosby.
39. Rudy DC, Kenelly MJ, Mcguire EJ: Detrusor myomectomy (bladder autoaugmentation): experience in myelodysplastic patients, *Proc Second International Meeting on Continent Urinary Reconstruction,* Mainz, 1995.
40. Dewan PA, Stefanek W: Autoaugmentation colocystoplasty: a case report, *Pediatr Surg Int* 1994: in press.
41. Dewan PA, Stefanek W: Autoaugmentation gastrocystoplasty: early clinical results, *Br J Urol* 74:460-464, 1994.
42. Lima SVC, Araujo LAP, Vilar FO, et al: Nonsecretory sigmoid cystoplasty: experimental and clinical results, *J Urol* 153:1641, 1995.
43. Churchill BM, Aliabadi H, Landau EH, et al: Ureteral bladder augmentation, *J Urol* 150:716, 1993.
44. Bellinger MF: Ureterocystoplasty: a unique method for vesical augmentation in children, *J Urol* 149:811, 1993.
46. Landau EH, Jayanthi VR, Khoury AE, et al: Bladder augmentation: ureterocystoplasty versus ileocystoplasty, *J Urol* 152:716, 1994.

Chapter 52

Management of Complicated Incontinence in Women

Victor W. Nitti, Mark W. Plawker

Urinary incontinence may be considered "complicated" when multiple causes are involved in producing the symptoms experienced by the patient. In most of these patients, multiple previous therapies have been used without success. Because the cause of incontinence in these patients is complex, the initial evaluation with the incontinence history and physical examination may not provide a clear indication of the problem. In these patients, the endoscopic, radiographic, and urodynamic studies are extremely important to validate the findings on history and physical exam as well as to further delineate the cause of the patient's symptoms. When the initial history and physical are complete and the diagnosis appears to be complicated, the clinician must rely on the other studies to further evaluate the patient to establish the diagnosis rather than to confirm the initial clinical impression as in uncomplicated patients.

As each step in the evaluation of incontinence is completed in most patients, the physician can be comfortable with the diagnosis when the previous findings are confirmed by each additional study. However, in the complicated patient, a carefully performed complete evaluation can not only confirm the initial clinical impression but also demonstrate other underlying causes for the symptoms experienced by the patient. Also, the cause of incontinence in these patients may be uncommon and unrecognized during previous evaluations.

The physician should be cautious in the management of any patient in whom multiple pharmacologic regimens or previous surgery has failed. These individuals warrant a complete evaluation including a meticulous history and physical examination as well as an attentive, compassionate approach to their symptoms, since they are often doubtful, hopeless, and frustrated.

In patients with "complicated incontinence" all contributing factors must be carefully considered before the institution of any treatment. For example, increasing age is associated with greater intrinsic sphincter deficiency, more pronounced anatomic changes secondary to pelvic floor laxity, and the development of varying degrees of detrusor hyperactivity and instability. One may assume then that the elderly patient may suffer a more refractory course. In addition, the physician must consider the patient's attitude, dexterity, and access to assistance. In cases of complicated incontinence, the patient might be expected to comply with indefinite pharmacologic regimens or self-catheterization. When surgery is a consideration, the patient should be aware that the postoperative course might be marked by the need for a secondary or adjunct procedure, temporary or permanent outflow obstruction, or transient exacerbated urge incontinence.

CLINICAL EVALUATION

When one is evaluating voiding dysfunction, and specifically incontinence, it is helpful to consider both the anatomic and functional aspects of the underlying problem. From a functional or physiologic standpoint, voiding dysfunction can be divided into two broad categories: a failure to empty or a failure to store urine.[1] Anatomically the bladder or the urethra may be abnormal or dysfunctional. These problems are not mutually exclusive because one may have a concurrent failure to store and empty as a result of bladder or urethral dysfunction. By using these very simple classifications, we have been able to simplify the diagnosis and treatment of complicated incontinence. If each element is evaluated separately, a complete diagnosis can be made and treatment subsequently directed at each cause of the incontinence.

History and physical examination as well as urodynamics, radiologic, and endoscopic assessment may all be employed to completely evaluate the complex patient. Regardless of its cause, a properly performed incontinence evaluation will discern a failure to store versus a failure to empty and further delineate bladder or urethral dysfunction.

Fig. 52-1 summarizes the concepts presented above and incorporates the four types of incontinence that are classically described. Stress urinary incontinence is the involuntary loss of urine with increases in intra-abdominal pressure in the absence of an increase in detrusor pressure. It is caused by functional or anatomic abnormalities of the urethra. Some degree of stress incontinence is usually a component of complicated incontinence. Urge incontinence is generally thought of as a loss of urine preceded by an urge to void. We would like to broaden this to include any involuntary loss of urine attributable to uninhibited bladder contractions, high urine storage pressures, poor compliance, or small functional capacity. Urge incontinence therefore is also almost always a component of complicated incontinence. Overflow incontinence is the loss of urine associated with urinary retention and can result in associated symptoms of urgency. Mixed incontinence is a relatively common problem where stress and urge incontinence coexist and probably, to varying degrees, comprises the majority of the patients described in this chapter. It is well known that in patients who have mixed incontinence, correcting the sphincteric incompetence component will usually result in significant improvement in the subsequent urge incontinence. However, in patients who have a significant component of urge incontinence with coexisting severe intrinsic sphincteric deficiency (ISD), any procedure that results in obstruction of the urethra will greatly aggravate the urge component of the incontinence problem during the first few weeks or months after the operative procedure.

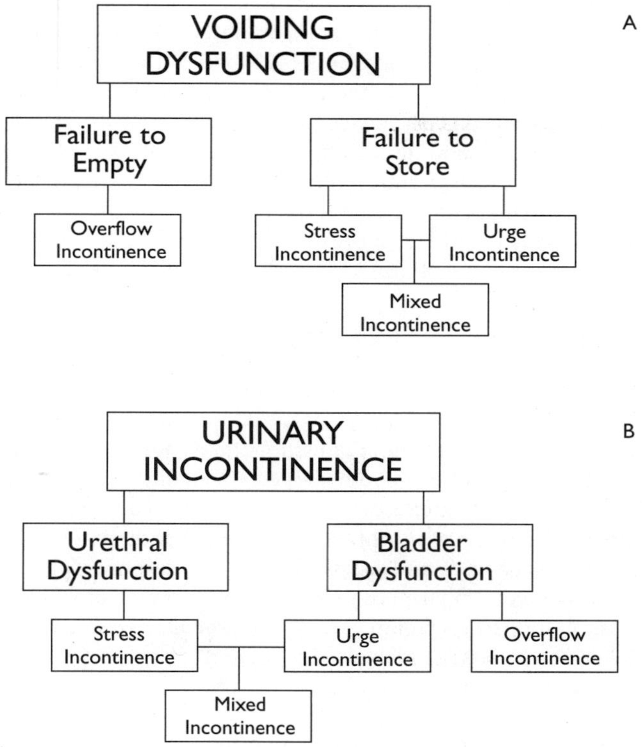

FIG. 52-1 *Classification of voiding dysfunction and incontinence according to functional,* ***A,*** *and anatomic,* ***B,*** *characteristics.*

MULTIPLE CAUSES

Multiple-cause incontinence occurs when there is more than one underlying voiding dysfunction causing incontinence. This may happen from a single disease process that affects more than one part of the lower urinary tract (such as a radiation or spinal cord injury) or when two separate diseases coexist (such as cerebrovascular accident and anatomic stress urinary incontinence). Many neurologic conditions can simultaneously affect urine storage and emptying. For example, a suprasacral spinal cord injury can result in frequent uninhibited detrusor contractions with associated urge incontinence (failure to store) as well as in detrusor–external sphincter dyssynergia (failure to empty). Demyelinating diseases, such as multiple sclerosis, may do the same. Damage to the cauda equina may result in an acontractile bladder secondary to lower motor neuron damage (failure to empty with overflow incontinence) or a denervated sphincter (failure to store). In addition, neurologic disease may be associated with nonneurogenic causes of incontinence. Multiple sclerosis or cerebrovascular accident with stress incontinence could present with neurologically mediated detrusor hyperreflexia (failure to store secondary to bladder dysfunction) and nonneurologically mediated anatomic stress incontinence (failure to store secondary to urethral dysfunction). By evaluating and treating each potential cause of incontinence, the clinician will have the greatest chance for successful treatment.

RADIATION

Radiation therapy is commonly used to treat gynecologic and rectal malignancies. Unfortunately it is not without complications, especially on the urinary tract. Urinary incontinence may result from injury to the bladder, urethra, or both. As early as the 1920s and reported in many subsequent papers, radiation-induced damage to the bladder has been recognized as a real source of morbidity with respect to urinary dysfunction.[2,3] Although the overall incidence of clinically significant changes in the bladder is unknown, it is reported to be 2% to 20%. This disparity undoubtedly represents a range of dose exposure, technique, and variations in patient characteristics. A recent paper has accepted a rate of 2% to 4% for early disease and 10% to 15% for advanced disease.[4] It has been demonstrated that there is a direct correlation between the success of treatment and the rate of complications,[5] and those with a lower complication rate have a higher rate of pelvic recurrence. Despite the bladder's relative radioresistant properties, an overall morbidity as high as 25% can be expected after a combined dose of 7500 rad.

Clinical sequelae may be categorized as either acute or chronic and manifested in a distinct or overlapping fashion accordingly.[5] As expected, the varying grades of radiation-induced cystitis correlate with a degree of irritability and may manifest as frequency, urgency, dysuria, and microscopic to gross hematuria. Early bladder reaction may be predictive of late, permanent changes, especially fistulas.[7] Perhaps a more significant dilemma to the physician is the patient whose extended survival subjects them to the late-phase consequences. These changes can be anticipated at a range of 22 to 48 months with a minimum latent period of about 6 months for symptoms to ensue.[5,6] We have seen incontinence as a result of radiation-induced changes initially present 20 years after radiation.

On a cellular level there is pronounced fibrosis in the lamina propria and muscular layers with eventual muscle cell death.[8] Enlarged intercellular gaps in both the circular and longitudinally arranged muscle fibers result in spasms and poorly coordinated detrusor contractions.[9] If allowed to progress, long-term radiation injury is manifested as a hypocontractile or areflexive, small-capacity, poorly compliant bladder.[10] Thus the effects on the bladder alone may cause a multitude of problems. The small-capacity, poorly compliant bladder is unable to store urine at low pressures, and urge incontinence may result. In addition, the absence of normal contractility may prevent emptying. Although less well documented, radiation may also result in fibrosis of the external urethral sphincter in males that subsequently becomes poorly compliant and paretic.[11] Urethral incompetence has also been demonstrated in the female after cervical radiation.[10] This intrinsic sphincter dysfunction results in a failure to store, which presents as stress incontinence. Thus, in the most complicated cases, both the bladder and urethra may be affected with subsequent failure to empty secondary to decreased bladder contractility and failure to store caused by a poorly compliant bladder (urge incontinence) and a dysfunctional urethra (stress incontinence). The clinical picture may mimic that of urge incontinence or stress incontinence and may therefore only be discernible after videourodynamic and cystoscopic evaluation. Individual evaluation of each potential effect of radiation is mandatory for a complete diagnosis and subsequent proper therapy.

Anticholinergic or antispasmodic therapy may ameliorate minor symptoms. Patients with more pronounced incontinence, upper tract deterioration, or development of a fistula may ultimately require bladder augmentation or substitution. In our experience medical therapy has not been successful in most severe cases of radiation cystitis. Although patients with an accompanying incompetent urethra may have lower leak point pressures (thus preserving renal function), those who desire to be dry may need an additional procedure. Pubovaginal slings or periurethral collagen injections may be used to treat the intrinsic sphincter deficiency caused by radiation. In cases of severe damage to the urethra where these procedures have failed, we have resorted to closure of the bladder neck and urethra with augmentation cystoplasty and creation of a continent, catheterizable abdominal stoma (see below). Indwelling catheters, though less desirable, may be the only option in select debilitated patients or those not amenable to alternative treatment modalities. This should be considered only as a last resort.

DETRUSOR HYPERACTIVITY

With a rapidly expanding elderly population, geriatric incontinence has become an increasing problem. Because this cohort is subject to multiple medications, limited mobility, mental status changes, and fecal impaction among other unfavorable conditions, the cause of their incontinence becomes more complex. In women, previous pelvic surgery, radiation, or anatomic changes (such as pelvic prolapse or atrophic vaginitis) may further complicate the scenario. Regardless of sexual type, however, detrusor hyperactivity is the most common independent factor resulting in incontinence in the elderly.[12] This is essentially urge incontinence and is characterized by an unexpected detrusor contraction, an inability to inhibit flow, and a subsequent loss of urine. In the elderly, this may occur with greater frequency secondary to diminished bladder capacity.

More recently, Resnick and Yalla described the entity of "detrusor hyperactivity with impaired contractility"[13,14] (DHIC). It was proposed while they were studying a group of elderly, institutionalized, incontinent patients. The authors noted that 30% of these patients had an alteration in bladder reflex and contractile function in an opposite fashion such that uninhibited contractions emptied less than half the volume of the bladder despite the absence of obstruction. This phenomena, though clinically mimicking simple detrusor hyperactivity, is actually a failure to empty resulting from a decreased speed of detrusor contraction. The peak and duration of detrusor pressures as well as the voided volumes are unchanged. Although augmentation of voiding with abdominal straining and decreased flow rate are present in the majority of these patients, there is no anatomic or neurologic basis of obstruction. The result of DHIC is a combined failure to empty and failure to store, both based on detrusor dysfunction. In the group studied, DHIC was found to be the second most common cause of incontinence after simple detrusor hyperactivity.[13,14]

Although the pathophysiologic characteristics underlying DHIC are unknown, it may be associated with long-standing detrusor hyperactivity. This becomes an important consideration in institutionalized settings where therapies might need to be altered as the underlying bladder function changes. Although none of the studied patients in the original study were found to be in urinary retention, large postvoid residual urine volumes can be a significant concern. In these patients, any one or more of the above-mentioned coexisting conditions would potentially result in retention. In addition, traditional treatments for detrusor hyperactivity, such as anticholinergics, might exacerbate incomplete emptying, and incontinence could become "overflow" in nature. This could further lead to myogenic bladder failure, increased incidence of urinary infection, and renal deterioration.

REFRACTORY INCONTINENCE

Refractory incontinence is incontinence that has failed to respond to seemingly appropriate therapy. Incontinence may persist for several reasons: (1) failure of appropriate treatment, (2) effects of treatment on other aspects of voiding function, and (3) incomplete diagnosis before treatment. Two commonly seen causes of refractory incontinence are failed surgery for stress incontinence and inadequate therapeutic response of urge incontinence to pharmacologic treatment. These complicated cases almost always require a complete urologic investigation to delineate the reasons for failure because the next step in treatment often requires invasive therapy.

INCONTINENCE AFTER FAILED INCONTINENCE SURGERY

Recurrent or persistent stress incontinence after incontinence surgery (that is, bladder neck suspension) may be attributable to an initially complex problem in which the patient almost seems destined for recurrence. However, the physician must consider inadequate correction of the anatomic abnormality or a missed diagnosis of intrinsic sphincteric deficiency. Although the former may represent recurrent anatomic abnormalities, the latter involves a poorly functioning urethra that was overshadowed by the more obvious anatomic abnormality. In each of these cases, the patient with persistent incontinence continues to suffer from a failure to store secondary to urethral dysfunction, whether anatomic or intrinsic. In a series of 206 bladder neck suspensions, an overall 90% short-term success rate (mean follow-up time 17 months) for cure of stress incontinence was described.[15] Of the 20 failures, only two were attributable to recurrent anatomic incontinence, and the remainder were secondary to intrinsic sphincteric damage. It was concluded that short-term failures are more likely secondary to intrinsic sphincter deficiency. Other studies have shown much higher long-term failure rates, but these fail to distinguish between anatomic and intrinsic causes.[16]

Another cause of "failed" stress incontinence surgery is postoperative urge incontinence. This can be a major problem because patients still require pads or diapers despite the fact that their stress incontinence has been cured. Incontinence has been "converted" from a failure to store secondary to urethral dysfunction to a failure to store secondary to bladder dysfunction. Preexisting urge incontinence will resolve in about 65% of patients after stress incontinence surgery but will persist in 35%.[15,17] In that series, de novo urge incontinence occurred in 7.5% of patients after bladder neck suspension.[15] Fortunately, then, the severity of symptoms of urgency and urge incontinence almost always improve over time after incontinence surgery.

Patients who have failed incontinence procedures should be carefully evaluated before embarking on further treatment. It is essential to be absolutely certain about the reason for failure or persistent symptoms. Therefore we recommend a complete videourodynamic evaluation and cystoscopy in addition to a meticulous history and physical. Special attention is given to differentiating between recurrent stress incontinence and persistent or de novo urge incontinence. Obstruction caused by the failed procedure must also be considered (see below). In cases where stress incontinence is established, recurrent hypermobility must be distinguished from intrinsic sphincter dysfunction. Once the correct diagnosis is established treatment can be instituted irrespective of prior surgical attempts. Ramon et al. have shown an excellent success rate for transvaginal needle suspension for recurrent stress incontinence when bladder neck hypermobility was demonstrated,[18] and others have reported similar results.[15] When persistent or recurrent incontinence is due to intrinsic sphincter deficiency without urethral hypermobility, a sling procedure or periurethral injection would be a better choice.

Obstruction and Incontinence After Incontinence Procedures

Most surgical procedures performed to treat anatomic stress incontinence (such as bladder neck suspension, urethropexy, colposuspension) alter anatomic features. A potential complication of any such procedure is iatrogenic bladder outlet obstruction. This may result in obstructive symptoms with partial or total urinary retention, recurrent urinary tract infections, or severe irritative symptoms such as frequency, urgency, and urge incontinence. The true incidence of iatrogenic obstruction and voiding dysfunction after incontinence procedures is not known, but it has been estimated at 2.5% to 24% for different procedures.[19-23] The presence of iatrogenically induced obstruction does not preclude the persistence of stress incontinence. Thus incontinence may occur as a result of persistent "outlet failure" (stress incontinence) or detrusor activity from the obstruction itself (urge incontinence).

In the three major series reported on this subject, 39% to 67% of obstructed patients experienced urge incontinence, whereas none to 46% had persistent stress incontinence.[24-26] Stress incontinence in these cases is best explained by technical considerations. Irrespective of the selected procedure, proper suture placement is crucial. For example, sutures placed too distally can kink the urethra and result in obstruction and continued stress incontinence. In this instance, the bladder neck and the proximal portion of the urethra have not been adequately supported. Also the intrinsic properties of the urethra and periurethral scarring after surgery can lead to recurrent stress incontinence with obstruction. In these cases obstruction is not always an easy diagnosis. Urodynamic criteria alone may not be accurate because these patients do not necessarily manifest the high-pressure, low-flow voiding dynamics characteristic of bladder outlet obstruction.[26] Careful evaluation of the patient with obstruction and persistent stress incontinence after incontinence surgery will uncover the failure to empty secondary to obstruction (bladder outlet dysfunction) and the failure to store secondary to persistent urethral hypermobility (also bladder outlet dysfunction). Endoscopy and videourodynamics (with simultaneous fluoroscopic imaging of the bladder outlet during voiding) are important tools in making the diagnosis of iatrogenic obstruction.

The treatment for obstruction and recurrent stress incontinence is complete urethrolysis, taking down the prior surgery, followed by resuspension of the bladder neck. This can be accomplished by the transvaginal or retropubic route.[24-26] The presence of obstruction does not affect the outcome of the stress incontinence surgery because 95% success rates have been achieved with a 21-month follow-up time.[26] Successful treatment of obstruction ranges from 65% to 93%.[24-26]

Refractory Urge Incontinence

The most common bladder problem associated with complicated incontinence is detrusor hyperactivity. Pharmacotherapy, specifically by anticholinergics and antispasmodics, has been the traditional first-line treatment for urge incontinence (failure to store) caused by "bladder hyperactivity" as a result of detrusor instability or hyperreflexia, poor compliance, or a bladder with small functional capacity. Some patients are refractory to medical therapy or cannot tolerate the side effects and consequently suffer intractable incontinence. Behavior modification, biofeedback, and electrical stimulation provide alternative options. These modalities require ultimate patient cooperation but offer the distinct advantage of being minimally invasive and inexpensive. In cases where this too has failed, patients may be left only with the option of bladder augmentation. In situations where the symptom of incontinence is the reason for treatment, the prospect of major reconstructive surgery must be carefully weighed by the patient. However, in many cases this will offer a realistic option for achieving dryness. In cases of poor compliance and high storage pressures, bladder augmentation may be "less elective" because renal function must be preserved.

Although urinary diversion was once the mainstay of treatment for these refractory patients, improvement in urodynamics as well as in the evaluation and treatment of outlet dysfunction has made bladder augmentation a more practical solution. And whereas renal insufficiency was considered a contraindication in the past,[27] augmentation cystoplasty has been demonstrated to improve or not affect renal function.[28,29] The goal of bladder augmentation is to increase functional capacity, lower storage pressures, and eliminate uninhibited detrusor contractions or at least increase the volume at which they occur. Care must be taken to ensure that the patient is able and willing to perform intermittent self-catheterization in the event that spontaneous bladder emptying cannot be achieved postoperatively. Equally important is that the true cause of the incontinence is firmly established and that all less-invasive modalities have been exhausted before one embarks on major urinary tract reconstruction.

From a technical standpoint, a detubularized portion of the cecum, the ileum, or a combination, has been employed with good reported success.[28-31] Some authors have cautioned against augmentation for a postradiation bladder (as in the treatment of cervical cancer)[33]; however, we have not encountered significantly increased intraoperative or postoperative problems.

Bladder augmentation may also be combined with procedures to treat bladder outlet dysfunction and coexisting stress incontinence (bladder neck suspension, colposuspension or sling, collagen injections, or an artificial sphincter).

Bladder Neck Closure for Intractable Incontinence

Although not commonly performed, bladder neck closure in the female is a feasible option for the treatment of refractory bladder outlet dysfunction. However, it is irreversible and should not be done hastily. We have found it particularly useful in three situations. The first is for extensive urethral damage as a sequela of long-term indwelling urethral catheters. This is often seen particularly in women with neurogenic bladders who are unable to catheterize the urethra (as in severe multiple sclerosis).[34] Typically these patients eventually begin to leak around the catheter. With successive catheter upsizing the urethra looses any ability to coapt around the catheter, resulting in further leakage. Bladder neck closure may be combined with the placement of a permanent suprapubic tube or with augmentation cystoplasty and creation of a continent catheterizable stoma. A second indication for bladder neck closure is in the patient (that is, a female paraplegic) who would never be able to manage permanent urethral self-catheterization after correction of intrinsic urethral dysfunction (with or without vesical dysfunction). In this case the closure is combined with a continent catheterizable abdominal stoma with or without bladder augmentation. The third indication is in female intrinsic urethral dysfunction that has failed all reasonable attempts at correction. We have recently found this useful in cases of severe radiation fibrosis that failed pubovaginal sling and multiple periurethral injections. Bladder neck closure may be accomplished by the transvaginal, transvesical, or combined approach.[35,36] We prefer the transvaginal route whenever possible because it has been effective with few complications.

Urologic Conditions Associated with Incontinence

Urinary incontinence may be associated with other urologic conditions that might independently require surgical correction. When the incontinence is surgically correctable, alternative plans may be warranted to accommodate both problems. In these cases it is important to fully evaluate the incontinence before initiating treatment. Two such conditions where this is applicable are urethral diverticulum and vesicovaginal fistula.

Urethral Diverticulum

A diverticulum of the female urethra arises from the urethral wall and consists of an epithelium-lined fibrous sac. It is believed to occur as a result of obstruction to the periurethral glands with subsequent retention of secretions, infection, and abscess formation.[37,38] Rupture of the abscess into the urethra forms the diverticulum. Typically, women present with recurrent urinary tract infections, dyspareunia, urethral pain, and irritative voiding symptoms.[39,40] The definitive treatment is surgical with complete excision of the diverticulum.[41]

Incontinence has been reported to be present in about 70% of patients with a urethral diverticulum.[42,43] Therefore it is important to diagnose the cause of the incontinence preoperatively so that if surgery is necessary it can be performed at the same time as the diverticulectomy. Incontinence associated with urethral diverticulum may be either stress incontinence, urge incontinence secondary to detrusor instability, or paradoxical incontinence. Paradoxical incontinence, sometimes confused with stress incontinence, is not actually related to the loss of urine across the bladder neck but rather to a loss from urine pooled in the diverticulum.[44] Ganabathi et al. recently reported on a series of 63 women who underwent treatment of urethral diverticulum.[43] They used the previously established guidelines for preoperative urodynamic evaluation, which include a history of stress or urge incontinence, symptoms of bladder dysfunction, or urethral hypermobility.[40] Fifty-eight women (92%) had at least one of these and underwent urodynamic evaluation. Sixty-two percent had abnormal findings (Table 52-1).

A complete evaluation is helpful in cases where incontinence coexists with a urethral diverticulum. If stress incontinence is discovered, surgical correction can be combined with urethral diverticulectomy. If detrusor instability is found, this may influence the use of postoperative anticholinergic therapy. In the past, simultaneous incontinence surgery and urethral diverticulectomy was avoided for fear of infection in the retropubic space. However, in 1987, Leach and Bavendam reported no increased risk when needle suspension was performed with urethral diverticulectomy.[40] They recommended that the transvaginal needle suspension sutures be placed and transferred before manipulation of the diverticulum. In fact, they further recommended that a simultaneous bladder neck suspension be performed if there was stress urinary incontinence, severe urethral hypermobility only, or a large diverticulum extending beneath the proximal urethra and bladder neck. Subsequent studies by the same authors reported success rates of about 72% for stress incontinence treatment.[43,44] In 1993, Swierzewski and McGuire described the use of a pubovaginal sling in conjunction with urethral diverticulectomy.[42] With short-term follow-up all were continent. The pubovaginal sling has the advantage of simultaneously treating intrinsic sphincter deficiency. When choosing an incontinence procedure to perform with urethral diverticulectomy, we prefer a needle suspension (Raz procedure) for patients with pure anatomic incontinence. Pubovaginal sling may be better for patients with intrinsic sphincter deficiency (no

Table 52-1 Urodynamic Findings in 58 Women with Urethral Diverticulum

Findings	Percentage
Normal urodynamics	38
Stress urinary incontinence only	34
Stress urinary incontinence and detrusor instability	14
Detrusor instability only	10
Myogenic decompensation	2
Sensory urgency	2

From Ganabathi K, Leach GE, et al: *J Urol* 152:1445, 1994.

A

B

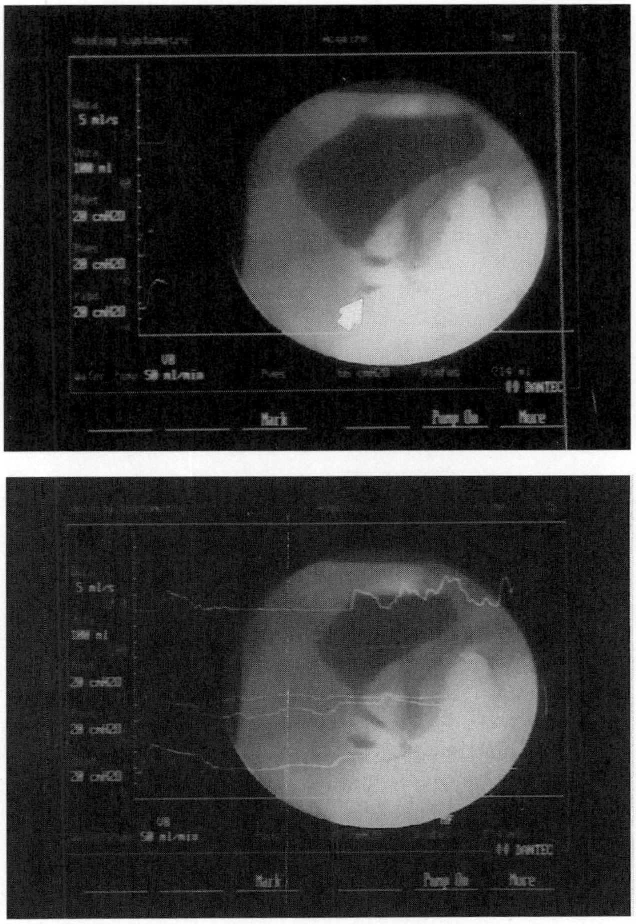

FIG. 52-2 *Stress incontinence and urethral diverticulum. This 41-year-old woman complained of severe urethral and postvoiding pain as well as progressive stress incontinence. Physical examination revealed a tender cystic urethral mass and stress incontinence in the lithotomy position. The above videourodynamic evaluation was performed.* ***A,*** *Patient performing the Valsalva maneuver, which demonstrates urethral hypermobility and stress incontinence at a Valsalva leak point pressure (vesical pressure attained when stress incontinence is demonstrated) of 66 cm H_2O. The diverticulum also fills slightly, arrow.* ***B,*** *Voiding study shows more pronounced filling of the diverticulum. Because of the stress incontinence associated with a low Valsalva leak-point pressure, a simultaneous pubovaginal sling and urethral diverticulectomy were recommended.*

hypermobility or hypermobility with a Valsalva leak-point pressure of 90 cm H_2O or less). Fig. 52-2 shows the videourodynamic evaluation and suggested treatment in a patient with urinary incontinence and a urethral diverticulum.

Vesicovaginal Fistula

A vesicovaginal fistula causes incontinence for obvious reasons. However, in addition to the urine lost through the fistula, patients may suffer from involuntary loss of urine through the urethra secondary to urethral or bladder dysfunction. Often the fistula and the bladder-urethral dysfunction are of the same cause (such as radiation), whereas at other times they may be independent processes (such as posthysterectomy vesicovaginal fistula with concomitant anatomic stress incontinence). Common causes of vesicovaginal fistula include gynecologic and urologic surgery, radiation, and obstetric trauma.[45,46] A history of radiation or incontinence before development of the fistula should prompt an investigation of another cause of the incontinence. Evaluation of urine loss through the urethra can be challenging in a patient with a large vesicovaginal fistula because it is often difficult to fill the bladder. It may be necessary to pack the vagina to limit the leakage from the fistula. In cases of radiation-induced fistula, we have performed a cystometrogram with the patient under anesthesia and the vagina tightly packed to assess bladder capacity and compliance and to further determine whether simultaneous bladder augmentation was necessary. If the cause of incontinence through the urethra is found to be surgically treatable, it can often be fixed at the time of fistula repair.

References

1. Wein AJ, Barrett DM: *Voiding function and dysfunction,* St Louis, 1988, Mosby.
2. Watson EM, Herger CC, Sauer HR: Irradiation reaction in the bladder: their occurrence and clinical course following the use of X-ray and radium in the treatment of female pelvic disease, *J Urol* 57:1038-1053, 1947.
3. Herger CC, Sauer HR: Treatment of alkaline incrustations of urinary tract with solution, *J Urol* 53:696, 1945.
4. Kagan AR: Bladder, testicle, and prostate irradiation injury, *Front Radiat Ther Oncol* 23:323-337, 1989.
5. Orton CG, Wolf-Rosenblum S: Dose dependence of complication rates in cervix cancer radiotherapy, *Int J Radiat Oncol Biol Phys* 12:37-44, 1985.
6. Perez C, Breaux S, Bedwinek J, et al: Radiation therapy alone in the treatment of carcinoma of the uterine cervix, *Cancer* 54:235-246, 1984 .
7. van Nagell JR Jr, Parker JC Jr, Maruyama Y, et al: Bladder or rectal injury following radiation therapy for cervical cancer, *Am J Obstet Gynecol* 119:727-732, 1974.
8. Antonakopoulous GN, Hicks RM, Berry RJ: The subcellular basis of damage to the human urinary bladder induced by radiation, *J Path* 143:103-116, 1984.
9. Michailov MCH, Elsässer E, Welscher UE: Immediate mechanical reactions of isolated human detrusor muscle on x-irradiation, *Strahlentherapie* 155:284-286, 1979.
10. Zoubek J, McGuire EJ, Noll F, DeLancey JOL: The late occurrence of urinary tract damage in patients successfully treated by radiotherapy for cervical carcinoma, *J Urol* 141:1347-1349, 1989.
11. Kaufman JJ, Smith RB, Raz S: Radiation therapy in carcinoma of the prostate: a contributing cause of urinary incontinence, *J Urol* 132:998-999, 1984.
12. Castleden CM, Duffin HM, Asher MJ: Clinical and urodynamic studies in 100 elderly incontinent patients, *Br J Med* 282:1103-1105, 1981.
13. Resnick NM, Yalla SV: Detrusor hyperactivity with impaired contractile function: an unrecognized but common cause of incontinence in elderly patients, *JAMA* 257:3076-3081, 1987.
14. Resnick NM, Yalla SV, Laurino E: The pathophysiology of urinary incontinence among institutional elderly persons, *N Engl J Med* 320:1-7, 1989.
15. Raz S, Sussman EM, Erikson DE, et al: The Raz bladder neck suspension: results in 206 patients, *J Urol* 148:845, 1992.
16. Korman HJ, Sirls LT, Kirkemo AK: Success rate of modified Pereyra bladder neck suspension determined by outcomes analysis, *J Urol* 152:1453, 1994.
17. McGuire EJ, Savastano JA : Stress incontinence and detrusor instability/urge incontinence, *Neurourol Urodyn* 4:313, 1985.

18. Ramon J, Mekas J, Webster GD: Transvaginal needle suspension procedures for recurrent stress incontinence, *Urology* 38:519, 1991.
19. Juma S, Sdrales L: Etiology of urinary retention after bladder neck suspension, *J Urol* 149:400A, (abstract), 1993.
20. Spencer JR, O'Conor VJ Jr, Schaeffer AJ: Comparison of endoscopic suspension of the vesical neck with suprapubic vesicourethropexy for treatment of stress urinary incontinence, *J Urol* 137:411, 1987.
21. Rost A, Fiedler U, Fester C: Comparative analysis of the results of suspension-urethroplasty according to Marshall-Marchetti-Krantz and of urethrovesicopexy with adhesive, *Urol Int* 34:167, 1979.
22. Mundy AR: A trial comparing the Stamey bladder neck suspension with colposuspension for the treatment of stress incontinence, *Br J Urol* 55:687, 1983.
23. Cardoza LD, Stanton SL, Williams JE: Detrusor instability following surgery for genuine stress incontinence, *Br J Urol* 51:204, 1979.
24. Webster GD, Kreder KJ: Voiding dysfunction following cystourethropexy: its evaluation and management, *J Urol* 144:670, 1990.
25. Foster HE, McGuire EJ: Management of urethral obstruction with transvaginal urethrolysis, *J Urol* 150:1448, 1993.
26. Nitti VW, Raz S: Obstruction following anti-incontinence procedures: diagnosis and treatment with transvaginal urethrolysis, *J Urol* 152:93, 1994.
27. Smith RB, VanCangh P, Skinner DG, et al: Augmentation enteroplasty: a critical review, *J Urol* 118:35, 1977.
28. Downis A, Abel BJ, Gow JG: Cecoplasty for bladder augmentation, *J Urol* 123:164-167, 1980.
29. Hanley HG: Ileocystoplasty: a clinical review, *J Urol* 82:317, 1959.
30. Lockhart JL, Bejany D, Politano VA: Augmentation cystoplasty in the management of neurogenic bladder disease and urinary incontinence, *J Urol* 135:969-971, 1986.
31. Luangkhot R, Peng BCH, Blaivas JG: Ileocystoplasty for the management of refractory neurogenic bladder: surgical technique and urodynamic findings, *J Urol* 146:1340-1344, 1991.
32. Couvelaire R: La "petite vessie" des tuberculeux génito-urinaires: essai de classification, place et variantes des cysto-intestino-plasties, *J d'Urol* 56:381, 1950.
33. Goldwasser B, Webster GD: Augmentation and substitution enterocystoplasty, *J Urol* 135:215-224, 1986.
34. Zimmern PE, Hadley HR, Leach GE, Raz S.: Transvaginal closure of the bladder neck and placement of a suprapubic catheter for destroyed urethra after long-term indwelling catheterization, *J Urol* 134:554, 1985.
35. Zimmern PE, Leach GE, Hadley HR, et al: Transvaginal closure of the bladder neck, *Semin Urol* 6:30, 1986.
36. Levy JB, Jacobs JJ, Wein AJ: Combined abdominal and vaginal approach for bladder neck closure and permanent suprapubic tube urinary diversion in the neurologically impaired female, *J Urol* 149:292A, 1993.
37. Routh A: Urethral diverticula, *Br Med J* 1:361, 1890.
38. Huffman JW: The detailed anatomy of paraurethral ducts in the adult female, *Am J Obstet Gynecol* 55:86, 1948.
39. Davis HJ, Telinde RW: Urethral diverticula: an assay of 121 cases, *J Urol* 80:34, 1958.
40. Leach GE, Bavendam TG: Female urethral diverticulum, *Urology* 30:407, 1987.
41. Leach GE, Schmidbauer CP, Hadley HR, et al: Surgical treatment of female urethral diverticulum, *Semin Urol* 4:33,1986.
42. Swierzewski SJ III, McGuire EJ: Pubovaginal sling for the treatment of female stress urinary incontinence complicated by urethral diverticulum, *J Urol* 149:1012, 1993.
43. Ganabathi K, Leach GE, Zimmern PE, Dmochowski R: Experience with management of urethral diverticulum in 63 women, *J Urol* 152:1445, 1994.
44. Bass JL, Leach GE: Surgical treatment of concomitant urethral diverticulum and stress incontinence, *Urol Clin North Am* 18:365, 1991.
45. Everett HS, Mattingly RF: Urinary tract injuries resulting from pelvic surgery, *Am J Obstet Gynecol* 71:502, 1956.
46. Goodwin WE, Scardino PT: Vesicovaginal and ureterovaginal fistulas: a summary of 25 years experience, *J Urol* 123:370, 1980.

Chapter 53

Clean Intermittent Catheterization

Jay B. Hollander, Ananias C. Diokno

Clean intermittent self-catheterization (CIC) was introduced in 1972 by Lapides.[1] Since then, the management of neurogenic voiding dysfunction has changed radically. Ileal conduit supravesical urinary diversion for neurogenic bladder is largely a thing of the past. Bladder substitution procedures for patients requiring cystectomy can now provide for continent (appliance-free) reservoirs fashioned from bowel all because CIC has been proved safe and effective. Chronic urinary retention need no longer be managed by indwelling catheters in most cases.

Today CIC is widely accepted by the medical community and should be available as a treatment option in any medical center that deals with patients who have either bladder-emptying dysfunction or neurogenic incontinence.

HISTORICAL BACKGROUND

The role of CIC in the management of urinary incontinence applies to patients with overflow incontinence or neurogenic incontinence or those who after treatment of incontinence have a component of bladder-emptying dysfunction. It is fitting that the first patient Lapides treated by CIC had neurogenic incontinence. She was a 30-year-old woman with multiple sclerosis and urge incontinence secondary to detrusor hyperreflexia (uninhibited bladder contractions) with incomplete emptying. She was prescribed anticholinergics to control the hyperreflexia and CIC to empty the bladder. Not only did she become continent, but she also remained free from problems with infections. Lapides reported on the success of CIC, showed safety and efficacy with short-term and long-term follow-up study, and eventually witnessed its acceptance and use worldwide.[2,3] Although it might now seem logical that CIC would be well accepted, when Lapides conceived of the idea, the prevailing medical thought would have predicted failure. Self-catheterization by nonmedical personnel was a foreign concept to most medical professionals, let alone their patients. Furthermore and perhaps more importantly was the fear that introducing a nonsterile catheter with "clean" but nongloved hands into the urethra and bladder would introduce bacteria and put the patient at great risk for infection. Indeed these same fears exist for patients today, and medical personnel must be able to explain to patients the logic that allows CIC to be safe and effective.

Lapides initially had fears that CIC might be risky for patients. His first patient was taught to resterilize the catheters initially, but after learning that she was successfully reusing the same catheter without resterilizing he began to study and promote CIC. Lapides's concepts regarding CIC still help in explaining to patients the logic behind CIC. He believed that even though bacteria were being introduced into the bladder with CIC, the bladder's natural resistance to infection was preventing the bacteria from doing any harm. Furthermore, regular bladder emptying with CIC was optimizing the bladder to resist infection. He theorized that high intravesical pressures and overdistension diminished one of the major barriers to infection, good vascularity. When the bladder was allowed to store at low pressures without overdistension, bladder mucosal vascularity was optimized.[4] In addition, regular bladder emptying reduced the time for bacteria to multiply, perhaps further diminishing the risk of infection as had been suggested by others.[5]

The concept of CIC provided for patient independence from indwelling catheters. Clean technique did not require sterile gloved preparation of skin or sophisticated sterile techniques. This made the technique convenient for patients. Since the same catheter could be used for weeks at a time, the technique could be cost effective, a notion that has great implications today. Finally, the disadvantages of an indwelling Foley catheter could be avoided. Urethritis, epididymitis, erosion, and fistulas were not uncommon with chronic indwelling Foley catheters. Freedom from Foley catheter discomfort and collection bags was also desirable. Sexual intercourse could be possible.

Indications for Managing Incontinence with CIC

There are two major indications for managing incontinence with CIC: incontinence that occurs from overflow and incontinence that after medical or surgical management results in retention or high postvoid residuals. In the former case overflow incontinence may be secondary to bladder hypotonia, areflexia, or outlet obstruction. An attempt to manage outlet obstruction either medically or surgically should be made before one commits patients to long-term CIC unless the risks of such therapy are too great to attempt.

Many primary conditions can result in urinary incontinence that might be managed in part by CIC (see first box). Neurologic disorders including spinal cord injury, myelodysplasia, and multiple sclerosis can result in long-term bladder dysfunction with incontinence because of either poor emptying or hyperreflexic bladder contractions that when suppressed with anticholinergic medications result in poor bladder emptying. CIC plays a major role in managing such patients. Any chronic outlet obstruction can result in bladder overdistension and eventually bladder decompensation such that overflow incontinence results. Even if the outlet obstruction is relieved, the bladder may still have trouble emptying. In urinary retention from benign prostatic hyperplasia (BPH), CIC may be a management option as a preoperative maneuver to avoid an indwelling Foley catheter before surgery. CIC can be used as a long-term management alternative to avoid surgery, or postoperatively if retention persists.

Finally, CIC can be used as part of surgical planning when procedures designed to treat incontinence result in retention either as a planned sequela or as an expected possible complication (see second box below). Urinary retention commonly occurs temporarily after bladder suspension procedures, and CIC allows these patients to be free of indwelling catheters until voiding begins. Augmentation cystoplasty may be recommended for patients with incontinence secondary to small-capacity, high-pressure bladder storage. The procedure that uses bowel to enlarge the bladder may result in poor bladder emptying or retention, and CIC may be required to empty the augmented but now continent bladder. Before the use of CIC neurogenic bladder dysfunction was too often managed by supravesical urinary diversion with procedures such as the ileal conduit. With the advent of CIC many of these procedures were reversed or undiverted.[6,7] The success of such procedures was dependent on improved and creative reconstruction technique that developed with the knowledge that CIC could be utilized to empty the newly created storage reservoir or bladder.

The success of urinary diversion procedures paved the way for development of continent urinary diversion procedures and neobladder procedures where the bladder is either removed or no

Conditions that can result in incontinence that may be managed with clean intermittent catheterization

NEUROGENIC VOIDING DYSFUNCTION
Spinal cord injury
Multiple sclerosis
Myelodysplasia
Peripheral neuropathy (that is, diabetes with overflow incontinence)
NONNEUROGENIC RETENTION WITH OVERFLOW
Atonic and decompensated bladder
Outlet obstruction (nonsurgical candidate, refusal, or awaiting surgery)

Surgical procedures for incontinence causing retention that may require clean intermittent catheterization

Bladder suspension
Anterior colporrhaphy
Urethral sling
Augmentation cystoplasty
Continent urinary reservoir

longer available for reconstruction. Bowel fashioned into a urinary reservoir is emptied with CIC via a continent abdominal stoma in the case of continent diversion procedures. Similar reservoirs can be attached to the urethra if the bladder has been removed. This so-called neobladder may empty by patient maneuvers such as that of Valsalva or Credé, but CIC is often required.

Contraindications

CIC is contraindicated whenever the urethra cannot be safely catheterized. False passages or urethral stricture disease must be managed first to subsequently allow safe, trauma-free CIC. The technique is contraindicated if the patient lacks the manual dexterity to perform the procedure or the mental capacity to perform the technique reliably. If the urethra is not accessible because of obesity or flexion contractures, CIC may not be a good option. Using a significant other to perform CIC should be considered thoughtfully because it may create a situation of total dependence. The quality of the relationship and reliability of the significant other should be evaluated thoroughly before one institutes the program, especially if CIC is expected to be lifelong. CIC can be performed in patients with a penile prosthesis or an artificial urinary sphincter.[8] The sphincter must be in the open position when the catheter is passed. CIC can also be considered if there is a need in immunocompromised patients. CIC has been reported to be safe in transplant patients.[9]

Pretreatment Evaluation

When CIC is used to assist in management of urinary incontinence, it should be done so only after a thorough urologic work-up beginning with acquisition of a history and physical examination. It is important to realize that the primary problem resulting in urinary incontinence might also result in recurrent urinary tract infections or deterioration of the upper urinary tract. In the case of neurogenic incontinence, a work-up should include upper urinary tract imaging, cystoscopy, and an appropriately tailored urodynamic work-up. The indications and details of such a work-up are covered elsewhere in this text, but are essential to understand in order to arrive at a safe effective bladder management plan, which may include CIC.

In cases of overflow incontinence, it is also especially important to determine the cause for overflow incontinence and to rule out upper urinary tract deterioration or postrenal insufficiency. Every patient who presents with urinary incontinence should have a postvoid residual checked. If retention is present, it should be obvious because of the large and at times massive retention volume. Patients with overflow incontinence must have their renal function screened with a serum creatinine measurement and hydronephrosis being ruled out with a renal ultrasonogram. Cystoscopy can assist with determining if outlet obstruction is the source for retention, and if there is doubt, a more sophisticated neurourologic work-up may be indicated. The goal of evaluation is to determine the most appropriate management plan for a particular patient. Both patient preference and urinary tract status must be considered to arrive at a plan that will provide for optimal urinary tract preservation while, if possible, improving the quality of life. Many patients with neurogenic incontinence are amazed at how happy they are continent using CIC when initially the concept seemed foreign and undesirable.

CIC Instructions

Individualized instruction is required to learn CIC. Although reading materials and videotapes are valuable adjuncts, these are no substitution for a trained health care professional who can instruct the patient and adapt a program, along with the physician, that best suits the patient.

The preinstruction evaluation should have arrived at recommendations to tailor an individualized program. This may include institution of medications to assist with bladder storage. Behavioral modification may be required to optimize fluid intake. Fluid intake may be temporarily diminished or adjusted to plan for activities that may preclude convenient CIC. Overall, however, total daily fluid intake should remain normal to maintain good hydration. Timed bladder emptying is important to avoid overdistension, which might result in overflow or urge incontinence. The patient must understand the importance of interval bladder emptying to allow for the bladder to be limited to a prescribed maximum volume (usually less than 400 ml). Patients will generally need to catheterize 4 to 6 times per day to avoid overdistending the bladder.

Patients must be instructed on their pelvic anatomy, and a catheter appropriate for the particular patient is selected. A variety of catheters is available for self-catheterization. The most common types are clear plastic 14 or 16 Fr straight catheters designed specifically for CIC. Female catheters are shortened for more convenient use and storage. The catheter that the patient finds easiest to pass and use is generally the one that should be selected. Catheter materials from plastic to rubber to silicone with a variety of tips and flexibility are available. Clear catheters allow for identification of fluid within the lumen, and such identification can assist patients with proper catheter placement and cleansing.

Patients should have a clear understanding of CIC principles. Catheters can be reused after a wash and rinse with soap and water. Even if washing is not possible, catheterization should be performed at regular intervals because doing so will be better for the patient than deferring catheterization and risking overdistension, incontinence, and infection. Although bacteria are present on the hands and catheters, the regular emptying of a bladder with normal host defense mechanisms, which resist bacterial invasion, will provide for a low incidence of infections and means of continent bladder emptying. CIC has even been shown to be a safe and acceptable treatment alternative in transplant patients with bladder-emptying problems. These patients have diminished host defense mechanisms, and yet with regular bladder emptying few serious problems occur.

Females are first shown anatomic landmarks with the assistance of a mirror. The labia, urethral meatus, and vaginal introitus are identified both visually and by touch. Once familiar with her anatomic features the woman or girl can sit on the toilet seat with knees apart or stand with one foot on the toilet seat. The second and fourth digits of the nondominant hand can spread the labia with the middle finger identifying the urethral meatus. The dominant hand guides the catheter (which can be prelubricated with a water-soluble lubricant) into the urethral meatus until it passes into the bladder and the urine is drained. After the bladder is emptied, the catheter is removed slowly so that the small amount of urine below the catheter eyes can then drain for complete emptying. The catheter can then again be washed and rinsed as before catheterization, after which it can be stored in a makeup case, plastic baggy, or towel in the purse.

In males the technique again requires washing the hands and catheter, if possible, before the procedure. A water-soluble lubricant is again placed on the tip of the catheter, and the catheter is passed while the patient sits on the toilet or stands so that when urine begins to drain it will do so into the toilet or appropriate receptacle. Males must learn the sensation as the catheter passes the resistance of the external urethral sphincter and prostate. In patients with no urethral sensation, the tactile sensation of the fingers can perceive the resistance and gentle pressure necessary for atraumatic catheterization. In males, once the urine begins to flow, the catheter is passed another few centimeters to ensure that the eye of the catheter is well into the bladder. When the bladder is emptied, the catheter is slowly removed. Resterilization of catheters or one-time-use catheters are generally not necessary. Catheters can be reused for weeks at a time. This can provide for a safe, convenient, cost-effective program.

When anatomic barriers make CIC difficult, creative devices have been invented to facilitate the procedure in patients with poor hand function, spastic legs, and difficulty transferring.[10,11] Further details on CIC teaching techniques can be found elsewhere.[12-14] We generally begin all patients learning CIC on a low-dose oral antibacterial for the first 2 to 4 weeks of the program, after which no antibiotics are given unless necessary.

Complications and Follow-Up Study

Minor local complications caused by CIC may occur. Occasionally urethral bleeding or gross hematuria can occur and is usually self-limited. Occasionally bladder stones occur. Urethral trauma can occur resulting in false urethral passages or strictures. These problems are all uncommon and are usually easily managed by the urologist.

Urinary tract infection is the most common complication of CIC. Asymptomatic bacteriuria is a frequent finding in patients using CIC. If the patient is otherwise doing well, the finding can be ignored, since long-term observation of bacteriuria in CIC patients has not been found to be deleterious.[15] Clinical infections are those that result in signs or symptoms of a urinary tract infection. Among spinal cord patients with no sensation, signs of urinary tract infection may be increased spasticity, signs of autonomic hyperreflexia, fever, hematuria, or foul-smelling, cloudy urine. Clinical infections should be treated with short-course oral antibiotics. A 10-year follow-up study of patients using CIC showed an incidence of bacteriuria of 74%, most of which was asymptomatic.[3] Febrile or pyelonephritic infections were uncommon. Recurrent clinical infections may occasionally dictate long-term low-dose oral antibacterial prophylaxis in certain individuals.

Vesicoureteral reflux increases the risk of upper urinary tract infection in patients using CIC. In these individuals chronic antibiotic prophylaxis may be considered. In most patients using CIC, vesicoureteral reflux does not occur if it was known not to be present initially. If vesicoureteral reflux is acquired while a patient is using CIC, the program should be reevaluated and improved.

Upper urinary tract deterioration is uncommon in CIC patients unless bladder storage pressures are abnormally high or vesicoureteral reflux is present. Pretreatment evaluation should be able to determine which patients are at risk, and the program should be designed to minimize upper urinary tract deterioration. Regardless, long-term follow-up is required to ensure that the appearance and function of the urinary tract is preserved.

After the patient is following a stable CIC program, we see patients at least yearly to update their history and urologic physical examinations. Patients are asked to obtain a urine specimen with a new catheter for urinalysis and possible culture and sensitivity changes. The frequency of catheterization, catheter volumes, and any problems the patient may have had, such as recurrent incontinence, must be determined to retailor the program if necessary. Medications prescribed long term for bladder management, such as an anticholinergic, must be reviewed with dosage adjusted if needed. A serum creatinine can ensure that the renal function remains stable. A renal ultrasonogram can rule out hydronephrosis if any question of renal-function deterioration exists. Hydronephrosis can occur because of lower urinary tract dysfunction from chronic overdistension of the bladder or chronic high-pressure urinary storage. Periodic cystoscopy may be indicated, especially in patients who show signs of renal deterioration, recurrent clinical infections, or problems with hematuria. As a routine, we generally will perform surveillance cystoscopy every 2 to 3 years to ensure that the bladder appearance remains unchanged without stones or tumors or significant inflammation. Although renal deterioration is uncommon in a patient using CIC, such findings dictate reevaluation of the CIC program to either improve it or find another alternative.

Summary

Clean intermittent catheterization has been established as a fundamental modality for bladder emptying that cannot be accomplished by normal voiding. The use of CIC in the management of urinary incontinence has a wide range of applications from managing overflow incontinence to urinary retention that results from the primary treatment of incontinence either surgical or medical. The technique has been proved safe and effective in long-term follow-up study. CIC can be easily taught in an outpatient setting and followed by primary caregivers who have a basic understanding of the technique and access to urologic referral when needed.

References

1. Silber SJ: Clean intermittent self-catheterization in the treatment of urinary tract disease, *J Urol* 107:458-461, 1972.
2. Lapides J, Diokno AC, Lowe BS: Followup on unsterile, intermittent self catheterization, *J Urol* 111:184-187, 1974.
3. Diokno AC, Sonda LP, Hollander J: Fate of patients started on clean intermittent self-catheterization therapy ten years ago, *J Urol* 129:1120-1122, 1983.
4. Lapides J: Pathophysiology of urinary tract infection, *Univ Mich Med Center J* 39:103-112, 1973.

5. Hinman F, Cox C: The voiding vesical defense mechanism: the mathematical effect of residual urine, voiding interval and volume on bacteriuria, *J Urol* 91:491-498, 1966.
6. Hendren WH: Urinary tract refunctionalization after prior diversion in children, *Ann Surg* 180:494, 1974.
7. Mitchell ME: Urinary tract diversion and undiversion in the pediatric age group, *Surg Clin North Am* 61:1147, 1981.
8. Diokno AC, Sonda LP: Compatibility of genitourinary prostheses and intermittent self-catheterization, *J Urol* 125:659-660, 1981.
9. Barnett M, Bruskewitz R, Glass N, et al: Long-term clean intermittent self-catheterization in renal transplant recipients, *J Urol* 134:654-657, 1985.
10. Hunt GM, Whitaker RH: A new device for self-catheterization in wheelchair bound women, *Br J Urol* 66:162-163, 1990.
11. Rosenbaum TP: The autocath: an assistive device for females on clean intermittent catheterization, *Urologic Nurs* 10:23, 1990.
12. Webber-Jones JE: Performing clean, intermittent self-catheterization appears in nursing, *Nursing* 21:56-59, 1991.
13. Rosen N, Ravalli R: Intermittent self-catheterization, *Clin Ger Med* 6:101, 1990.
14. Duffy L: Teaching clean intermittent self catheterization: a nursing process, *AUAA J* 4:12, 1984.
15. Mohler JL, Cowen DL, Flanigan RC: Suppression and treatment of urinary tract infection in patients with an intermittently catheterized neurogenic bladder, *J Urol* 138:336-340, 1987.

Chapter 54 Clinical Management Decisions

Kevin Pranikoff

The segment of our population over 65 years of age is growing, with a 21% increase seen from 1980 to 1989. Within this group, there is a disproportionate increase in the oldest segment, those 85 years and older. This growth is expected to continue well into the twenty-first century.[1] The prevalence of urinary incontinence in community-dwelling persons greater than 60 years of age was found to be 18.9% in men and 37.7% in women utilizing a survey technique in the MESA Project.[2] Among institutionalized older persons, the generally accepted rate is about 50%.[3] Hu has estimated that the great economic cost of caring for urinary incontinence was about $8.1 billion in 1984. His estimate for the costs of incontinence care in nursing homes is about $2 billion annually, or about 10% of total nursing care costs. He notes that these figures are conservative and quotes other data estimating costs in nursing homes ranging from $0.5 to $8 billion per year.[4]

There is general agreement that urinary incontinence is a cause for embarrassment, social isolation, and depression.[5-7] It is also a source of stress for caregivers and often plays an important role in the decision to institutionalize a family member.[8] There is an association, though not necessarily a cause-and-effect relationship, between incontinence and other geriatric syndromes.[9] Although it may be a physical health hazard by promoting skin breakdown in the face of poor hygiene, incontinence does not appear to be a risk factor for death, at least for community-dwelling individuals.[10]

THE ELDERLY PATIENT

Medical decision making for the elderly with incontinence encompasses the same general principles as for any population. Their care, however, is confounded by the high prevalence of comorbid states causing physical or cognitive impairments that may affect treatment outcomes, complications, or prognosis independent of urinary incontinence. These patients are also more likely to have special considerations in the psychosocial area with inadequate social support systems or financial resources to see them through a hospitalization or prolonged recovery period. An adequate evaluation of all factors may require multidisciplinary input encompassing the principles of a comprehensive geriatric assessment emphasizing functional status and quality-of-life issues. The expertise of a social worker and geriatrician in addition to the primary physician and urologist may be invaluable.[11]

In the event of a planned surgical intervention, the preoperative assessment will alert the caregiver to potential areas in need of special consideration to successfully rehabilitate the geriatric patient. Acute hospitalization in this age group is often complicated by increased disorientation and confusion caused by loss of familiar surroundings and routine and physical deconditioning. Early attention to remobilization efforts is a fundamental principle in the care of the acutely ill elderly patient.[12] If one restores continence in a previously community-dwelling patient who postoperatively requires long-term nursing home management indefinitely, the treatment has failed to improve the patient's quality of life.

Physicians are obligated to educate their patients and make them aware that treatment is available if it is desired. This treatment should be offered to the elderly age group, especially because they are less likely to proactively seek medical information on their own.[5] Burgio et al. found that the majority of older patients with incontinence do not report it to their doctors. Severity of incontinence, physical disability, and a pattern of regular health care utilization appeared to be the strongest predictors of treatment-seeking behavior. Even of those who considered their incontinence to be a problem, only 59% reported it.[13]

Today there is also a myriad of effective pads and barrier products available for the noncurative treatment of urinary incontinence. Many individuals develop effective coping mechanisms and do not see incontinence as affecting their quality of life and are not limited by it. The physician must be careful not to proselytize for further intervention in these patients but just to let them know it is available if and when desired. There is evidence, in fact, that people with more effective coping styles in the face of illness will have better outcomes.[5]

Despite the prevalence of urinary incontinence, it remains underdiagnosed and underreported.[14] When it is reported, it may be ignored. In the elderly, this is often the result of the erroneous belief by the practitioner that incontinence is an inevitability of old age or an untreated secondary complication of dementia. The majority of elderly, however, are continent.[2,15]

One primary difficulty in dealing with the older age group is developing an adequate data set on which to base our clinical decisions. Part of this may be related to the elderly's passive nature in medical situations.[5] Other factors include failing memory and wanting to please the physician rather than complain. This situation is compounded when the medical history is complicated and the medication list is long.

It is very important that patients see the physician with an accompanying family member or caregiver whenever it is possible. They can often aid in filling in the details and providing another view on such matters as how often the patient voids or needs to change his or her clothes because of wetness. It is also important in rapport building to treat the patient with dignity. Speak to the elderly patient, not just to the accompanying person, and give the patient the opportunity at some time to speak with you privately in case he or she has concerns that he or she would feel better not sharing.

It is also important to avoid addressing patients with inappropriate phrases of familiarity. Most older patients will tell you that they resent being addressed as "sweetie" or "honey" by medical professionals they just met who are usually many decades their junior. Most of us would also. It is very important always to address older patients by their surname unless invited by them to do otherwise.

The development of a data set for the patient becomes even more complicated as dementia increases especially if there is no interested accompanying caregiver. One should encourage referral sources to send information when possible, and the physician may wish to telephone children or the caregiver in a nursing home while the patient is still in the office. This often helps to clarify issues. Unfortunately, sometimes the information needed is as basic as determining exactly why the patient was sent or what is the character of his or her incontinence (such as nighttime only or only while restrained in a chair).

When a nursing home has a large enough volume of consultations to justify it, one should consider performing them at the facility. We have had such a program in effect for 13 years at a 600-bed nursing home. The institution is serviced by one half-day session monthly when 12 to 18 consultations are performed. At the time of seeing the patient, their clinical data are maximized by the availability of their medical chart and the nursing staff who care for them daily. Using the chart, we can request specific information or for observations to be done and the data to be present at our next visit. The families are aware of when we will be there and can accompany the patient if they wish.

Previous to this, the patients were sent to the hospital clinic usually with a one-page referral sheet often saying "incontinence." (Read: bed sheets were wet, nurse called the physician who ordered a consultion, the demented patient had no idea why he was there.) The interaction was often unsatisfactory for all parties: the patient, the physician, and the facility. By going to the facility and improving communications by personal contact or use of the chart, one can significantly improve the quality and efficiency of the interaction for all involved. Additionally this organization can facilitate the use of patient care protocols and result in significant cost savings by decreasing transportation costs involved in sending patients out.[16,17]

Cautions to this organization include that the facility must have enough consultation requests to justify a physician's time to travel to it. There is also added burden in that the facility must expend some resources to run the clinic (staff, supplies, space, and so forth). The cost savings are realized by the third-party payors who save transportation costs. Although insurers would readily spend hundreds of dollars to transport to a hospital, there may not be an easy mechanism available to the nursing home for recovering its nominal expenditures to have the patient seen on site.[17]

TREATMENT DECISIONS IN OLDER PEOPLE

The treatment of urinary incontinence in the elderly is a legitimate undertaking in both the community-dwelling and the nursing home populations.* The tools to successfully accomplish this include evaluation and treatment algorithms, behavioral therapies, pharmacotherapy, and surgery.[14,16,18,19,20]

Before one embarks on treatment, the amount of recommended work-up required is controversial, with many authors' minimal recommendation ranging from a clinical evaluation with a postvoid residual urine and urinalysis to a full videourodynamic evaluation.[16,21-24,26.] Most of these authors agree, however, that the assessment should be individualized based on the presence of any transient causes of incontinence, the risk to the patient of an empiric treatment trial, and the degree to which invasive testing would alter treatment decisions.[15,25,26]

The assessment of urinary incontinence as in any medical assessment must include a general medical history. Certainly dementia and decreased mobility may affect continence status.

Although there is a strong association between the severity of incontinence and the degree of dementia, such association does not necessarily imply causation. The reported rate of incontinence in the demented elderly range from 11% to 90%.[26] If the abilities to transfer and dress independently are preserved, however, even patients with severe dementia are likely to be continent.[26-28] The cause of incontinence in this group is often multifactorial. Treatment of one factor may often make the contribution from the other factors manageable. An example of this might be the improvement of mobility in a severely arthritic person with dementia to the point that incontinence could be aided by a prompted voiding program. Abnormalities of fluid balance such as lower extremity edema may contribute to nocturia when this fluid is mobilized. The absence of estrogen replacement in postmenopausal females may be helpful in developing a treatment strategy. There is evidence that exogenous estrogens may improve the mucosal seal as well as synergistically improve the effects of alpha-adrenergic receptor stimulation by increasing receptors in the urethra.[29] A history of narrow-angle glaucoma is a contraindication to the use of anticholinergic agents, and, when in doubt, one should always consult with the patient's ophthalmologist before instituting such therapy.[30]

*References 3,7,8,14,15,26.

The incontinence-specific history must allow one to determine the character of the incontinence and to search for readily reversible causes of transient incontinence.[15,26] Multiple algorithms are available to guide the assessment and treatment.[14,16,21] A minimal physical evaluation will generally include a urinalysis and a postvoid residual urine. One must remember that asymptomatic bacteriuria is a frequent finding in the elderly population.[31,32] Its coexistence with urinary incontinence is not necessarily an indication of its etiologic significance. In our experience its contribution to incontinence is rare.[16] As a practical matter, one should attempt treatment of bacteriuria with specific antibiotics based on cultures after its initial discovery and should ask for careful observation by the patient or caregiver concerning any change in incontinence. If it transiently clears with no improvement in incontinence, it is no longer treated. In the presence of dementia or severe physical limitation, it is an important consideration to examine a catheterized specimen to ensure accuracy of collection. The risk of this minimal invasion is limited to a rare urinary tract infection, and doubt about the collection is removed. Ouslander et al. documented that in a frail elderly female nursing-home population, accurate clean-catch urine collections can be accomplished. Their protocol utilized specially trained research personnel, however, and excluded bedridden and noncommunicative patients. He admits that "similar results might not be obtained by nursing home staff without adequate training and continuous quality improvement strategies."[33]

Postvoid residual urine determination is a universal part of assessment protocols. It is important to remember that these may be variable within a patient and may be affected by technique, patient relaxation, and timing.[22,34] As a rule, one should obtain three measurements in nursing-home patients and in community-dwelling patients and not make a decision based on one residual measurement. In general, one should ask patients to give a urine sample first and only after they have voided explain that a residual urine is being measured. Although this is less time efficient, it does not stress patients and interfere with their ability to relax and void because they are worried about being catheterized.

One must also remember that a large amount of postvoid residual urine may be detrimental to the patient but it is only one factor in the global circumstance. It is well accepted that urine storage pressures and not residual volume is the major factor leading to life-threatening urinary tract decompensation.[35] Certainly a large amount of residual urine may contribute to symptomatic urinary tract infections or incontinence, but it might not. It is difficult to give an exact number to the volume of postvoid residual urine that is considered unacceptable. We know that some patients with detrusor instability and without obstruction are unable to empty to completion.[36] It is also not uncommon to have a patient who clinically responds to anticholinergic therapy increase his or her residual, occasionally to a degree that makes one uncomfortable, that is, 200 to 300 ml. Nevertheless, if it is tolerated and is of low pressure and the patient becomes comfortable and continent, it by itself does not in my mind mitigate against continued use of the medication. It does require careful monitoring.

Once a basic assessment has been accomplished a decision must be made as to whether a definite or probable cause of the incontinence has been identified and whether a specific or empiric treatment trial is indicated. In general, one should consider an initial treatment at this juncture, which will usually require a behavioral or pharmacologic intervention. There is a wide body of literature attesting to the success of behavioral and pharmacologic therapy.[14,16,18-20,29,37] One should usually consider the simplest and least-invasive therapies first, but the specific recommendation must be individualized based on home environment involvement and availability of caregivers, comorbidities, contraindications to pharmacologic agents, and cost. When one is instituting a timed or prompted voiding schedule, it is often useful for the patient to wear a watch with an alarm. This can be easily set for the next scheduled voiding attempt. When it goes off, it may serve as a reminder to the patient to void, or, if not, it will remind the caregiver to prompt.

Occasionally intermittent catheterization may need to be used to allow a large postvoid residual to be tolerated. This must be individualized, however, because many elderly patients cannot perform this on their own and it becomes burdensome to caregivers and staff intensive in nursing homes. For this reason, one should not institute this therapy if it cannot be accomplished independently by the patient. Schnelle and Ouslander have noted that the staff-dependent intervention of prompted voiding is often difficult to maintain when the research team leaves the nursing home and the regular staff assumes the duty.[38,39] Besides staff time constraints, another factor that may be operative is the lack of positive feedback to the staff tasked with the work. In estimating the cost of incontinence care in nursing homes, Hu estimates labor costs at $2 to $5.50 per day, with total costs (labor, supplies, and laundry) at $3.80 to $8.80 per day.[4] Therefore the staff is still tasked with the work and must learn a new skill, but if the prompting intervention is successful, the benefit savings are seen elsewhere in the organization (decreased laundry and supply utilization). Finding a way to motivate staff and allow them positive feedback is a major factor in converting many research protocols into successful patient care.[40,41]

When one is using pharmacotherapy, it is generally accepted that the elderly should be treated with lower doses initially because they may be quite sensitive to various agents. It is often beneficial when bladder relaxants are needed in large doses to combine agents with different mechanisms of action in lower doses than might be required if they were used singularly, thereby avoiding some side effects.

If initial therapy has failed and it is a consideration to try higher doses of pharmacologic agents or surgery for stress incontinence, it is recommended that urodynamics be performed. This can be accomplished in most but not all patients. Those with severe dementia may not be able to cooperate and may became quite scared in the laboratory.[26]

It has been shown that major surgery can be tolerated by the elderly and that age alone should not mitigate against appropriate surgery for stress incontinence when indicated.[42-44] Of course surgery for stress urinary incontinence ranges from injection procedures and needle suspensions requiring no or minimal dissection to retropubic or combined abdominal and vaginal procedures requiring extensive dissection and causing significant incidents of postoperative urinary retention. Detailed work-up and proper patient selection are important when these approaches are required.

SUMMARY

The needs of the elderly will increasingly occupy the attention of physicians. Urinary incontinence is not an inevitable condition of being old and its evaluation deserves our thoughtful attention. Clinical management decisions in this population must take into consideration the pathophysiologic characteristics of the incontinence and the increased comorbidities and psychosocial complexities that our patients face. I feel strongly that with appropriate systems and attitudes this can be accomplished with a maximum of satisfaction for the patient and the physician.

REFERENCES

1. Furner SE, Grant MD, Brody JA: The aging population. In O'Donnell PD, editor: *Geriatric urology,* Boston, 1994, Little, Brown.
2. Diokno AC, Brock BM, Brown MB, Herzog AR: Prevalence of urinary incontinence and other urological symptoms in the noninstitutionalized elderly, *J Urol* 136:1022, 1986.
3. Urinary incontinence in adults: NIH Consensus Conference, *JAMA* 261:2685, 1989.
4. Hu TW: The economic impact of urinary incontinence, *Clin Geriatr Med* 2:673, 1986.
5. Light E, Lebowitz BD: Psychosocial factors in urologic disorders. In O'Donnell PD, editor: *Geriatric urology,* Boston, 1994, Little, Brown.
6. Wyman JF, Harkin SW, Fantl JA: Psychosocial impact of urinary incontinence in the community-dwelling population, *J Am Geriatr Soc* 38:3, 1990
7. Resnick NM, Yalla, SV: Management of urinary incontinence in the elderly, *N Engl J Med* 313:800, 1985.
8. Ouslander JG, Zarit SH, Orr NK, Muira SA: Incontinence among elderly community-dwelling dementia patients: characteristics, management and impact on caregivers, *J Am Geriatr Soc* 38:440,1990.
9. Tinetti ME, Inouye SK, Gil TM, Doucette JT: Shared risk factors for falls, incontinence and functional dependence, unifying the approach to geriatric syndromes, *JAMA* 273:1348, 1995.
10. Herzog AR, Diokno AC, Brown MB, et al: Urinary incontinence as a risk factor for mortality, *J Am Geriatr Soc* 42:264, 1994.
11. Resnick MI, Palmer RM: Surgical decisions. In O'Donnell PD, editor: *Geriatric urology,* Boston, 1994, Little, Brown.
12. Robinson KM, Siebens H: Rehabilitation. In O'Donnell PD, editor: *Geriatric urology,* Boston, 1994, Little, Brown.
13. Burgio KL, Ives DG, Locher JL, et al: Treatment seeking for urinary incontinence in older adults, *J Am Geriatr Soc* 42:208, 1994.
14. Urinary Incontinence Guideline Panel: *Urinary incontinence in adults: clinical practice guideline,* AHCPR Pub No 92-0038 Rockville, Md., 1992, Agency for Health Care Policy and Research, Public Health Service, U.S. Department of Health and Human Services.
15. Resnick NM: Geriatric urinary incontinence, *AUA Update Series* vol 5, lesson 9, Baltimore, Md., 1992, American Urological Society.
16. Constantino G, Pranikoff K: Female urinary incontinence: an algorithmic approach, *Urologic Nurs* 9:7, 1988.
17. Pranikoff K, Bertolino J, Constantino G: On-site nursing home specialty care: a cost-effective model, *J Am Geriatr Soc* 40:SA60, 1992.
18. Burns PA, Pranikoff K, Nochajski TH, et al: A comparison of effectiveness of biofeedback and pelvic muscle exercise treatment of stress incontinence in older community-dwelling women, *J Gerontol* 48:M167, 1993.
19. Schnelle JF: Prompted voiding treatment of urinary incontinence in nursing home patients: a behavioral management approach for nursing home staff, *J Am Geriatr Soc* 37:1051, 1989.
20. O'Donnell PD, editor: *Geriatric urology,* Boston, 1994, Little, Brown.
21. Hilton P, Stanton SL: Algorithmic method for assessing urinary incontinence in elderly women, *Br Med J* 282:940, 1981.
22. Dubeau CE, Resnick NM: Evaluation of the causes and severity of geriatric incontinence: a critical appraisal, *Urol Clin North Am* 18:243, 1991.
23. Ouslander J, Staskin D, Raz S, et al: Clinical versus urodynamic diagnosis in an incontinent geriatric female population, *J Urol* 137:68, 1987.
24. Diokno AJ: Diagnostic categories of incontinence and the role of urodynamic testing, *J Am Geriatr Soc* 38:300, 1990.
25. Wein AJ: Editorial comment to Ouslander J, Staskin D, Raz S, et al: Clinical versus urodynamic diagnosis in an incontinent geriatric female population, *J Urol* 137:68, 1987.
26. Skelly J, Flint AJ: Urinary incontinence associated with dementia, *J Am Geriatr Soc* 43:286, 1995.
27. DuBeau CE, Resnick NM: Urinary incontinence and dementia: the perils of guilt by association, *J Am Geriatr Soc* 43:310, 1995.
28. Resnick NM, et al: Risk factors for incontinence in the nursing home: a multivariate study, *Neurourol Urodyn* 7:274, 1988.
29. Wein AJ: Practical uropharmacology, *Urol Clin North Am* 18:269, 1991.
30. Wall LL, Norton PA, Delancey JOL: *Practical urogynecology,* Baltimore, 1993, William & Wilkins.
31. Nicolle LE, Bjornson J, Hardin GK, MacDonell JA: Bacteriuria in elderly institutionalized men, *N Engl J Med* 309:1420, 1983
32. Abrutyn E, Mossey J, Levison M, et al: Epidemiology of asymptomatic bacteriuria in elderly women, *J Am Geriatr Soc* 39:388, 1991.
33. Ouslander JG, Schapira M, Schnelle JF: Urine specimen collection from incontinent female nursing home residents, *J Am Geriatr Soc* 43:279, 1995.
34. Stoller ML, Millard RJ: The accuracy of a catheterized residual urine, *J Urol* 141:15,1989.
35. McQuire EJ: Interaction of bladder filling behavior and urethral function, *World J Urol* 8:194,1990.
36. Resnick NM, Yalla SV, Laurince E: The pathophysiology of urinary incontinence among institutionalized elderly persons, *N Engl J Med* 320:1, 1989.
37. Fantl JA, Wyman JF, McClish DH, et al: Efficacy of bladder training in older women with urinary incontinence, *JAMA* 265:609, 1991.
38. Ouslander JG, Schnelle FJ, Uman G, et al: Predictors of successful prompted voiding among incontinence nursing home residents, *JAMA* 273:1366, 1995.
39. Schnelle JF: Personal communication
40. Burgio LD, McCormick KA, Scheve AS, et al: The effects of changing prompted voiding schedules in the treatment of incontinence in nursing home residents, *J Am Geriatr Soc* 42:315, 1994.
41. Burgio LD, Engel BT, Hawkins A, et al: A staff management system for maintaining improvements in continence with elderly nursing home residents, *J Appl Behav Anal* 23:111, 1990.
42. Hosking MP, Warner MA, Lobdel CM, et al: Outcome of surgery in patients 90 years of age and older, *JAMA* 261:1909, 1989.
43. Nitti VW, Bregg KJ, Sussman EM, Raz S: The Raz bladder neck suspension in patients 65 years old and older, *J Urol* 149:802, 1993.
44. McGuire EJ: Identifying and managing stress incontinence in the elderly, *Geriatrics* 45:44, 1990.

Chapter 55

Incontinence Assessment

Jean F. Wyman, Joyce Colling, Pat D. O'Donnell

Assessment of Community-Dwelling Women

Urinary incontinence is a significant problem among aging women. Approximately 30% to 38% of women over 60 years of age suffer from incontinence.[1,2] Older women are twice as likely to be incontinent as men in their age group. The prevalence of the different types of incontinence varies based on the study population and diagnostic criteria used.[1,2] In contrast to younger women, a majority of older women report mixed incontinence with both stress and urge symptoms present. Detrusor instability increases with age; however, it can present either with severe urgency or as sudden uncontrollable urine loss without any warning of urgency.

Although the prevalence of incontinence tends to increase with advancing age, age alone is not considered a risk factor for its development. The most consistent risk factors identified across studies are being female and having cognitive or mobility impairments. Other risk factors that have been implicated include medication use (such as diuretics), hypoestrogenism, comorbidity of chronic illness (such as depression, diabetes, stroke, arthritis, pulmonary disease), pelvic muscle weakness, childbirth, and smoking.[3-5] Thus incontinence should not be considered a normal part of the aging process by itself; rather it should be considered a pathophysiologic condition usually multifactorial in cause that warrants careful evaluation and management.

This section is a description of the clinical evaluation of the incontinent older woman, and it can easily be conducted in primary care practice. This assessment follows the same initial evaluation recommended by the Agency for Health Care Policy and Research in their *Clinical Practice Guideline on Urinary Incontinence in Adults.*[6] Indications for referral to an incontinence specialist are provided.

Aging Changes Affecting Continence

Aging is associated with many normal changes in the genitourinary system, and some may predispose women to the development of incontinence. The most significant change is the loss of estrogen that occurs after menopause. The bladder, urethra, and vagina are estrogen-dependent organs. Decreased estrogen can lead to atrophy resulting in tissue friability, inflammation, diminished periurethral blood flow, decreased pelvic muscle strength, pelvic prolapse, and susceptibility to infection, all of which can cause urinary symptoms.

An individual's risk of incontinence increases with superimposed pathophysiologic or pharmacologic factors that can change the delicate balance between normal and abnormal lower urinary tract functioning. For example, a chronic cough may precipitate stress incontinence; arthritis may compromise mobility status making it difficult to reach the toilet in time especially when there is a late signal for the need to void; and diuretic agents needed to manage congestive heart failure may initiate incontinence because of rapid diuresis.

Clinical Evaluation

The clinical evaluation of an incontinent older woman is similar to that of the younger woman. However, the older woman may present with more complex symptoms because of comorbidity of chronic illnesses, greater medication use, previous gynecologic (including anti-incontinence) surgery, and impaired functional status making interpretation of the findings more difficult. The significance of the symptoms must be viewed within a broad context of information collected. All potentially reversible causes of incontinence should be identified and treated. Resnick[7] coined the useful mnemonic "DIAPPERS" to categorize the reversible causes of urinary incontinence that are common in the elderly (see box).

Clinical History

The symptom of urine loss should be elicited through careful questioning on annual examinations. Many older women may underreport their incontinence because they misinterpret the question being asked, they do not perceive incontinence to be a serious problem, they believe that it is a normal consequence of aging or of being female, or there is embarrassment, lack of knowledge of treatment options, fear of surgery, and hopelessness or low expectation of treatment success. Because incontinence is frequently underreported, it may be necessary to use several open-ended questions to detect whether incontinence is

Reversible Causes of Urinary Incontinence

D elirium
I nfection—urinary (symptomatic)
A trophic urethritis and vaginitis
P harmacologic causes
P sychologic causes, especially depression
E xcess fluid excretion (e.g., from heart failure or hyperglycemia)
R estricted mobility
S tool impaction

From Abrams WB, Beers MH, Berkow R, et al, editors: Urinary incontinence. *The Merck manual of geriatrics,* ed 2, Whitehouse Station, N.J., 1995, Merck Research Laboratories.

actually present. An initial statement such as "Many women your age begin to have problems making it to the bathroom in time and have an accident" may help ease a patient's discomfort in discussing an embarrassing subject and help her to realize that she is not alone. This statement can then be followed by questions, such as "Do you have trouble getting to the bathroom in time?" or "Do you have trouble holding your urine (water)?" Additional questions to elicit incontinence even after a negative response to the previous question include "Do you ever lose urine when you don't want to?" and "Do you ever wear a pad or other protective device to collect your urine?"[6] Surprisingly, many women will answer no to all questions until the question regarding pad usage.

Once the symptom of incontinence is identified, a continence history along with a focused medical, neurologic, and genitourinary history and medication review of prescription and over-the-counter drugs should be obtained. The continence history includes a detailed description of the incontinence including its onset, duration, type, frequency, pattern, precipitating circumstances, associated symptoms, and past and current management methods. The patient should be questioned about her most bothersome symptom and the effect of her symptoms on her quality of life (see the discussion of Incontinence Severity Assessment on p. 400). When mixed incontinence is present, often the treatment plan will be developed to manage the most bothersome symptom. The patient should be questioned on her fluid-intake pattern, including caffeine intake, and her motivation, expectations, and goals for treatment. In addition, questions on relevant medical conditions and medication use that can contribute to the development or exacerbation of urinary incontinence should be asked.

A functional assessment focused on the individual's abilities for self-toileting and for complying with treatment regimens should be conducted. This would include the ability to walk at an adequate speed to reach the toilet, the manual dexterity to disrobe for toileting or to perform self-catheterization if required, and the mental abilities to remember to follow a voiding schedule or take medications as prescribed. An environmental assessment, including location of the toilet in relationship to the bedroom and where the majority of time is spent at home, and an evaluation of caregiver burden and support are essential for elderly women with cognitive and mobility impairments.

Physical Examination

The physical examination of the incontinent older woman requires greater attention to general health status, since many chronic conditions such as congestive heart failure, peripheral edema, and arthritis common in the elderly can significantly contribute to incontinence. In addition, pelvic, rectal, and neurologic examinations are conducted.

The pelvic examination includes assessment of perineal skin condition, pelvic floor defects (uterine prolapse, vaginal vault prolapse, cystocele, enterocele, rectocele), atrophic vaginitis, and pelvic muscle tone and function. To assess for pelvic floor defects, separate the blades of the vaginal speculum, insert one blade sequentially at the anterior and posterior vaginal walls, and ask the patient to strain or cough. Bulging of the anterior wall when the posterior wall is held down indicates a cystocele, whereas bulging of the posterior wall when the anterior wall is held down indicates a rectocele or enterocele. Ideally, prolapse should be assessed with the patient in the supine and standing positions because the extent of the prolapse may be underestimated in the supine position only. Women with pelvic prolapse beyond the introitus or those who are symptomatic need referral to a gynecologist who specializes in prolapse treatment. However, the presence of a pelvic floor defect is a nonspecific finding that may have no relationship to the cause of the incontinence or warrant immediate consideration of a surgical repair.[8]

Pelvic muscle tone and function can be assessed through digital palpation of the puborectalis and puboccygeus muscles, which are located approximately 5 cm inside the vaginal introitus at the 5 o'clock and 7 o'clock positions. The patient is asked to contract her pelvic floor muscles against the examiner's finger or fingers as if she were using the muscles to stop her urine stream or to stop the passing of flatus. Simultaneously, the examiner should place a hand on the patient's abdomen to determine whether the patient is straining with her abdominal muscles in her attempt to contract her pelvic floor muscles. In addition, timing the duration of contraction is another measure of muscle strength. The lack of the ability to voluntarily contract the pelvic floor muscles does not necessarily imply that nerve damage has occurred.

The vagina should be inspected for signs of atrophic vaginitis, such as friability, erosions, petechiae, and telangiectasia. The observation of a pale, shiny mucosa with loss of rugal folds is a sign of vaginal atrophy, whereas the observation of an inflammatory process is evidence of atrophic vaginitis.

The rectal examination includes observation for fecal impaction, masses, sphincter tone, and sacral reflexes. A similar digital test as vaginal palpation can be used to assess the anal sphincter tone and contraction. Assessment of sacral innervation is to check for the anal wink reflex. This is done by gentle clitoral stroking with a cotton applicator and observing for the closing of the anus or a lifting of the levator ani. Approximately 25% of older women will not demonstrate this reflex; thus absence of the anal wink reflex is not necessarily pathologic.[9]

A screening neurologic examination should include assessment of mental status and evaluation of neurologic disorders that can affect bladder function. Delirium, dementia, stroke, Parkinson's disease, lumbar and cervical spondylosis, diabetic neuropathy, and normal-pressure hydrocephalus are more common in the elderly.

Incontinence Severity Assessment

A urinary diary is an essential part of the initial clinical evaluation (Appendix I). It helps to document the severity of incontinence, determine if associated irritative symptoms (that is, frequency and nocturia) are present, establish if there is a pattern to the incontinence, identify precipitating events, and determine the treatment goals and plan. The diary is also critical in establishing a baseline measure for assessment of treatment outcome. There is a variety of diaries available depending on what information is of most interest to collect. Ideally a diary should be kept for a 1-week period.

Quality of Life

Assessment of symptom distress and quality of life is becoming increasingly important in evaluating the severity of health conditions. One can assess symptom distress simply by asking the patient to describe the "bothersome" nature of her symptoms using a rating scale of "not at all" to "greatly," or a scale of 0 to 10. Similarly, one can assess quality of life by asking the patient how much her incontinence has affected her daily life. Two self-administered questionnaires for assessing quality of life specific to urinary incontinence, the Urogenital Distress Inventory and the Incontinence Impact Questionnaire,[10,11] have validated shorter versions that can easily be used in office practice (Appendix J). Both instruments are highly responsive to detecting treatment effects and can be used in the evaluation of treatment outcomes.

Laboratory Tests

A midstream urine specimen should be obtained for urinalysis. If warranted, a urine culture should be performed. Generally, blood chemistry determinations are not recommended unless there is suspicion of underlying disease causing the symptoms. Blood glucose and calcium should be tested in patients with suspected polyuria in the absence of excessive fluid intake or use of diuretics. Blood urea nitrogen and serum creatinine levels should be determined if patients are suspected of having obstruction or urinary retention.

Bladder Function Tests

Simple tests of bladder function can be easily performed in office practice. All patients should have a postvoid residual volume determination through straight catheterization or the use of bladder ultrasonography. Patients with postvoid residual volumes of greater than 50 ml should be referred for urologic evaluation. The provocative stress test is used to aid in the diagnosis of stress incontinence. One performs this by asking the patient who has a full bladder to cough forcefully at least three times while in the standing position with a small pad underneath her feet. The presence of urine loss at the height of the cough exertion is considered stress incontinence, whereas leakage that is delayed is suggestive of detrusor overactivity. In patients who report difficulty in emptying their bladders, it is helpful to listen to their voiding. Signs of voiding difficulty such as hesitancy, straining, or intermittent stream may be suggestive of obstruction or detrusor contractility problems.

Simple cystometry can be performed in a clinic setting to help clarify the clinical diagnosis or if neurologic disorders are suspected. Ouslander et al.[12] described a method that can be conducted without the use of special equipment. The procedure involves the use of a 14 French straight catheter attached to a 50 ml syringe without its piston or bulb. The patient's bladder is filled with 25 to 50 ml aliquots of room-temperature sterile water with the syringe held approximately 15 cm above the pubic symphysis (bladder pressure should not normally exceed 15 cm H_2O during filling). The patient is asked to report when she first experiences the need to void and then to report when she has reached maximum capacity and "cannot hold anymore." The presence of involuntary bladder contractions is detected by the continuous upward movement of fluid sometimes accompanied by leaking around or expulsion of the catheter. Involuntary contractions or severe urgency at low bladder volumes less than a range of 250 to 300 ml are suggestive of detrusor instability, especially if consistent with the patient's symptoms.

Indications for Referral

An initial diagnosis and management plan can be determined for most incontinent older women using the clinical evaluation described above. However, the primary care physician may want to refer the patient for further evaluation or treatment for several reasons:

- The diagnosis is unclear and a management plan cannot be determined.[6]
- Failure of a therapeutic trial.[6]
- Hematuria without infection.[6]
- Presence of other comorbid conditions:[6]
  - Recurrent symptomatic urinary tract infections
  - Abnormal postvoid residual volume
  - Severe or symptomatic pelvic prolapse
  - Suspected neurologic cause of incontinence
- Patient desires surgical procedure or collagen injections.
- Patient requires intensive behavioral intervention, such as bladder training, biofeedback-assisted instruction, electrical stimulation.
- Patient has intractable incontinence or severe cognitive or physical impairments and requires assistance with managing skin protection and comfort.

Depending on the reason for referral, the primary care physician may refer to a urologist or gynecologist for additional evaluation and treatment, or to a continence nurse specialist for evaluation and behavioral therapy or supportive interventions.

Assessment of Institutionalized Elderly Women

The population in most nursing homes is about 70% female, and of this group over 50% are incontinent of urine, usually on a daily basis.[6] Often incontinence and cognitive impairment are linked in this population, and virtually all incontinent residents need physical assistance to manage their elimination needs. The approach to assessing incontinent residents who are cognitively or physically impaired contains some variations from those who are intact functionally and cognitively because impaired residents are often unreliable historians and sometimes performing an adequate physical examination is upsetting for them.[12] Further, it is often impractical and fatiguing for residents to carry out bladder function studies so that the physician can arrive at a definitive diagnosis. The following section emphasizes assessments that are appropriate for health professionals to use with those who are cognitively or physically impaired and in whom urinary incontinence (UI) has been detected.

Detection of Urinary Incontinence

In the nursing home, initial UI detection usually occurs through the use of the Minimum Data Set (MDS), which is a standardized, comprehensive screening tool now mandated on residents' admission in all nursing homes.[13] When incontinence is detected using the MDS, a Resident Assessment Profile (RAP), the assessment and treatment decision making part of the MDS, is then used to identify potentially reversible causes of UI and select other management strategies if UI is not resolved by removal of the reversible causes. What is not made explicit in the RAP is how to carry out the various assessments that will provide answers to assessment questions with minimal disruption to the resident and with maximal efficiency for the person charged with performing the evaluation.

Clinical Assessment

Because UI is a symptom and not a specific disease condition in the institutionalized woman, aspects both internal and external to the resident can influence the impaired person's continence status. Five areas should be assessed before one considers a treatment or management program for impaired persons with UI. The five areas are (1) a health history, including medication and fluid intake profile; (2) a history of the UI, including a voiding diary; (3) a focused physical, which includes a cognitive and functional assessment; (4) a urinalysis; and (5) an environmental assessment. This information will screen for transitory causes of UI such as a bladder infection or drug-induced UI, help identify the type of UI, screen for problems that should be evaluated further, and direct the health professional toward specific treatment options for the resident.

Health history and history of incontinence. The health history includes a review of health conditions, particularly a history of neurologic problems such as stroke, multiple sclerosis, or spinal surgery that may interrupt normal innervation to the lower urinary tract. In addition, the presence of diabetes can contribute to UI because of polyuria with hyperglycemia. Congestive heart failure may also be a factor in UI because of impaired circulation and pooling of fluid in dependent extremities during the day, which is then excreted at night when the person is horizontal. A query about frequent urinary tract infections, vaginitis, and fecal impaction is also warranted because these conditions can also cause or exacerbate UI.

A careful examination of the current prescribed and over-the-counter medications is an important aspect of the health history because several medications are known to affect incontinence. Even if drugs cannot be eliminated, the timing of administration may be altered to minimize their effect on UI such as giving diuretics early in the day to decrease nighttime incontinence. It may also be possible to substitute drugs that do not affect incontinence or to switch to nondrug alternatives such as a backrub or warm milk as a sedative for sleep rather than a drug with sedative properties. Sometimes drugs ordered for a purpose other than UI can also improve UI, such as if the person has urge UI symptoms an antihistamine drug may decrease bladder muscle irritability and urgency symptoms.

Another component of the health history is a review of the fluid status. This should include the timing and amount during a 24-hour period and the type of fluids consumed. Beverages containing caffeine should be eliminated or limited because they have a diuretic effect. Some common beverages containing caffeine are coffee, tea, some carbonated drinks, and chocolate.[14] Alcohol intake should also be assessed because alcohol also has strong diuretic properties. Beverages containing artificial sweeteners such as NutraSweet should be used on a limited basis because they can irritate the bladder, making urine control more difficult. Inadequate fluid intake can also irritate the bladder causing urgency. The general rule for determining the adequacy of fluid intake in an older adult is 25 ml of water for every kilogram of body weight. One simple objective measure of the adequacy of fluid volume is to measure the specific gravity of the resident's urine (normal range, 1.003 to 1.030).

Incontinence history. At a minimum, the incontinence history in institutionalized women should include the onset, frequency, timing and volume of UI, what makes it worse or better, whether there is nocturia or enuresis, and the present means of management. This information can be obtained from the resident or caregiver; however, a voiding diary of at least 1 and preferably 2 or 3 days is a valuable tool for obtaining the timing, amount, and factors or activities that seem to make UI occur. Appendix I shows an example of a voiding diary. Much or all of the history may need to be obtained from a careful examination of the resident's records and by interviewing nursing staff or family members.

Focused physical examination. The physical examination should include the following: (1) an abdominal examination to check for bladder distension, tenderness, and masses; (2) a pelvic examination to inspect the perineal skin condition, presence of atrophic vaginitis (mucosa bleeds when touched if severe), presence of urethral inflammation, and presence of vaginal prolapse (prolapse is severe if uterus or vaginal vault is bulging from the vagina after the resident is asked to bear down); and (3) a digital examination of the rectum to determine fecal impaction, masses, and sphincter tone. The physical exam should also include an evaluation of cognitive status and an evaluation for depression. The Folstein Mini-Mental State Examination (MMSE)[15] and the Geriatric Depression Scale are two commonly used standardized measures to test cognitive status and to test for depression respectively. If the person has dementia and is unable to answer questions, the Cornell Scale for Depression is a useful alternative.[16] The physical examination may need to be accomplished in two different time periods if the resident is easily fatigued or upset. It may also be advisable to ask a staff member familiar with the resident to be present to help with the physical examination.

Finally, because impaired mobility is one of the major factors in functional incontinence of institutionalized women, a careful evaluation of the resident's mobility status is important. Evaluation of the resident's ability to ambulate, transfer to the toilet, disrobe, and use assistive devices should be observed as well as the time needed to complete these activities. Again, asking the staff what the resident is capable of doing may assist in determining the person's actual ability because residents sometimes will not cooperate fully for a stranger. Every effort should be made to maximize the resident's existing mobility skills with assistive devices and, if possible, to enhance mobility through a regular mobility and exercise program.

Urinalysis. Obtain a clean-catch or catheterized urine specimen to determine the presence of a urinary tract infection (UTI). Use of a FemCath is a convenient and less traumatic means of obtaining a sterile specimen than the usual catheter, especially in demented patients. A dipstick is a quick and inexpensive way to screen for the presence or absence of urinary abnormalities before sending the urine to a laboratory for further analysis. UTIs are defined as bacteriuria of more than 10^5 CFU/ml of urine. Pain, burning, and fever, the cardinal signs of a UTI, may be absent in older adults, and if they are cognitively impaired, they may not be able to verbalize their symptoms. In addition, greater frequency of voiding, another sign of a UTI, may go undetected if the resident is frequently incontinent. Consequently, a urinalysis may be the only means to determine the presence of a significant UTI. If hematuria, glycosuria, or proteinuria are present, further evaluation is warranted. If the resident is catheterized, a postvoid residual determination can also be done at this time. An alternative method is to use a bladder ultrasound device. Residuals under 200 ml are considered normal in this age group, but this figure should also be compared to the person's bladder capacity. It is not uncommon for older persons to have a bladder capacity of only 250 to 300 ml as compared with 500 to 600 ml in younger persons.

Environmental assessment. An environmental assessment of institutionalized women should include adequacy and accessibility of toileting facilities, presence of toileting aids such as commodes or urinals (a variety of female urinals are available), and the willingness and ability of the nursing staff to assist the patient to the toilet, if necessary. In addition, the nursing aide should be questioned as to her understanding of how to manage the resident's UI.[17,18] This will also provide an evaluation of current management.

If UI does not resolve, once transitory causes or contributing factors to UI have been eliminated or modified as much as possible, then persistent or chronic UI is believed to be present. Four major types of persistent UI have been identified: urge, stress, overflow, and functional. Many older women have combinations of the different types of incontinence, which makes the diagnosis and management especially difficult in this group of patients. Much of the information from the UI assessment can help to identify the probable type or types of incontinence that exist and to determine what combination of strategies for managing the UI would be most successful for a particular resident.

Assessment of Community-Dwelling Elderly Men

The incidence of urinary incontinence in community-dwelling elderly men is approximately 19%.[2] Unlike in elderly women, stress incontinence caused by sphincteric incompetence is extremely rare in men who have had previous prostate or pelvic surgery.[19] Therefore incontinence in elderly men is almost always associated with involuntary detrusor contractions. Elderly community-dwelling men with incontinence usually present with symptoms of urgency and urge incontinence. As in older women, the episodes of incontinence occur without warning, with the first awareness of an impending detrusor contraction usually being the involuntary flow of urine. The assessment of elderly men begins with a history of voiding symptoms and an evaluation of the functional status of the patient using the same evaluation techniques described above for elderly women.

History

Again, it is important to remember that, unlike in elderly women, stress incontinence is extremely rare in older men who have not had previous prostate or pelvic surgery. In patients who have stress incontinence, the onset usually occurs immediately after prostate or pelvic surgery and makes the diagnosis reasonably obvious, based on the time of onset. Stress incontinence in men after prostate or pelvic surgery is almost always attributable to intrinsic sphincteric deficiency (ISD), which is described in Chapter 30. Treatment of ISD in men usually involves intraurethral collagen (Chapter 33) or an artificial urinary sphincter (Chapter 38). It is always important to realize that coexisting detrusor hyperactivity may be a major factor contributing to incontinence in patients with ISD.

Elderly community-dwelling men with urinary incontinence who have not had previous prostate or pelvic surgery usually have a history consistent with urge incontinence. As is seen in elderly women, the character of the urge incontinence is often one of no warning of an impending incontinence episode. The history of episodes of urge incontinence without warning is a distinguishing characteristic that is common among older people and rare among younger people. The elderly community-dwelling man with urinary incontinence also needs to be carefully interviewed for voiding symptoms that are consistent with bladder outlet obstruction. Frequency of urination, urgency, and nocturia are symptoms of bladder outlet obstruction as well as symptoms that frequently occur in elderly men with urinary incontinence without bladder outlet obstruction. Also, hesitancy of voiding is a symptom of bladder outlet obstruction and a symptom often associated with incontinence in older men. A small urinary stream and an intermittent stream is a symptom of bladder outlet obstruction that is not commonly associated with incontinence in older men without bladder outlet obstruction. The voiding history of the older man is often difficult to obtain accurately but can be extremely helpful in developing a clinical impression of the presence of bladder outlet obstruction.

Clinical Assessment

On initial evaluation, the older community-dwelling man with urinary incontinence needs to have a digital rectal examination to evaluate the prostate. The clinical estimation of the size of the prostate does not indicate the presence or absence of bladder outlet obstruction in most patients. A small prostate on physical examination can produce significant bladder outlet obstruction, whereas a large prostate on digital rectal examination may result in no detectable bladder outlet obstruction. The presence of prostate cancer in the prostate gland can produce irritative bladder symptoms which may precipitate urge incontinence in some patients. The office evaluation of a community dwelling man with urinary incontinence should include a urinary flow rate with an ultrasonographic residual urine measurement, a digital rectal examination, and a prostate-specific antigen determination. Elderly community-dwelling men with urinary incontinence and associated prostate cancer may enjoy an improved quality of life related to bladder symptoms with appropriate therapy of the prostate cancer.

The diagnosis of bladder outlet obstruction can best be made with urodynamic studies that include a pressure-flow study as described in Chapter 12. Most elderly community-dwelling men can tolerate urodynamic studies without significant distress. The decision to perform complete urodynamic studies in elderly patients is an extremely important one. The clinician usually cannot manage the patient well over the long term without the information provided by complete urodynamic studies that define the nature of the clinical problem. However, the clinician does not want to subject the elderly patient to extensive testing that does not contribute significantly to the management decisions. Community-dwelling patients usually have a higher functional status and a longer expected survival and tolerate the studies better than chronic care patients do.

In the evaluation of older men with urinary incontinence, a complete neurologic examination is always important. It is common for older men with incontinence to have coexisting deterioration of mental function. Because changes in mental status may occur in this group, diseases such as brain tumors frequently are not diagnosed early in these patients. When one is evaluating older men with urinary incontinence, it is important to be sure that a neurologic cause is not present before establishing a treatment plan for the patient.

The assessment of the severity of incontinence in the community-dwelling man can be done by use of a voiding diary as described previously for elderly women (Appendix I). The clinical evaluation of the functional status of the patient as described previously for women will indicate whether a voiding diary that is prepared by the patient is likely to be useful in the assessment of the severity of incontinence. Usually the level of functional status required to exist in a community-dwelling environment is adequate to maintain an accurate voiding diary. It is always important to evaluate the mental status and activity status of the patient before the incontinence assessment.

Assessment of Chronic-Care Elderly Men

Chronic-care older men tend to perform at a much lower level than community-dwelling elderly men. Therefore the evaluation of the functional status of elderly chronic-care men with urinary incontinence is of critical importance in the approach to both evaluation and management of the patient. Also, the general medical condition of the patient is likely more complicated, and a medical assessment is important in decisions regarding evaluation and treatment of urinary incontinence.

The treatment plan for management of urinary incontinence in older men needs to be based on the incontinence diagnosis determined by the history, physical exam, and urodynamic studies. The decision to perform extensive urodynamic studies in chronic-care older men is even more difficult than in community-dwelling men because the potential benefit from the studies in the long-term management decisions is usually less in chronic-care patients. However, the studies are tolerated reasonably well by most elderly men, and the risk is minimal. The quality of life of the elderly man must be improved over the long term by improved management decisions as a result of the performing of the studies to justify recommending the studies to the patient and the patient's family.

The initial assessment of severity of incontinence in elderly men can be made on the basis of the clinical management of the patient by the caregivers.[20] In a research environment, incontinence-detection devices can be used to determine the occurrence of an incontinence episode.[21-24] In any circumstance where accurate measurement of incontinence is desired, the factor that determines the accuracy of the measurement is the method of detection. In community-dwelling elderly men, the mental status of the patient is usually adequate to use the voiding diary for accurate measurement of incontinence severity. In the chronic-care environment, elderly incontinent men usually have cortical impairment, which precludes the use of a diary for measurement of severity, and the assessment must be done by caregivers.

Summary

The long-term treatment plan for the management of incontinence in elderly people must be based on accurate information from an assessment of the patient. In older people, many issues are of critical importance in the management plan of the patient that not only include the diagnostic characteristics of incontinence, but also include the functional status of the patient as well as the great effect that treatment can have on the quality of life of the individual.

References

1. Herzog A, Fultz NH: Prevalence and incidence of urinary incontinence in community-dwelling populations, *J Am Geriatr Soc* 38:273, 1990.
2. Diokno AC, Brock BM, Brown MB, et al: Prevalence of urinary incontinence and other urological symptoms in the noninstitutionalized elderly, *J Urol* 136:1022, 1986.
3. Diokno AC, Brock BM, Brown HB, et al.: Medical correlates of urinary incontinence in the elderly, *Urology* 36:129, 1990.
4. Wetle T, Scherr P, Branch LG, et al: Difficulty with holding urine among older persons in a geographically defined community: prevalence and correlates, *J Am Geriatr Soc* 43:349, 1995.
5. Burns P, Nochajski T, Pranikoff K: Predictors of incontinence in older women, *Neurourol Urodyn* 12:432, 1993.
6. Urinary Incontinence Guideline Panel: *Urinary incontinence in adults: clinical practice guideline,* AHCPR Pub No 92-0038, Rockville, Md., 1992, Agency for Health Care Policy and Research, Public Health Service, US Department of Health and Human Services.
7. Resnick NM: Urinary incontinence in the elderly, *Med Grand Rounds* 3:281, 1984.
8. Ouslander JG: Geriatric urinary incontinence, *Dis Month* 38(2):71, 1992.
9. Wall LL, Norton PA, DeLancey JOL: Special considerations in the elderly. In *Practical urogynecology,* Baltimore, 1993, Williams and Wilkins.
10. Shumaker SA, Wyman JF, Uebersax JS, et al.: Health-related quality of life measures for women with urinary incontinence: the Incontinence Impact Questionnaire and the Urogenital Distress Inventory, *Qual Life Res* 3:291, 1994.
11. Uebersax JS, Wyman JF, Shumaker SA, et al.: Short forms to assess life quality and symptom distress for urinary incontinence in women: the Incontinence Impact Questionnaire and the Urogenital Distress Inventory, *Neurourol Urodyn* 14:131, 1995.
12. Colling JC, Ouslander JG, Hadley BJ, et al: The effects of patterned urge-response toileting (PURT) on urinary incontinence among nursing home residents, *J Am Geriatr Soc* 40:135-141, 1992.
13. Department of Health and Human Services: rules and regulations, *Fed Reg* 54(21):5333-5334, 5365, Feb 2, 1989.
14. Guthrie H: *Introductory nutrition,* ed 7, St Louis, 1989, Mosby.

15. Folstein MF, Folstein S, McHugh PR: Mini mental state: a practical method for grading the cognitive status of patients for the clinician, *J Psychiatr Res* 12:189-198, 1987.
16. Alexopoulos GS, Abrams RC, Young RC, Shamoian CA: Cornell scale for depression in dementia, *Soc Biol Psychiatry* 23:271-284, 1988.
17. Colling JC, Wagner A. Understanding aides' resistance to change in the nursing home, *J Long-Term Administration* 21:27-30, 1993.
18. Campbell EB, Knight M, Benson M, Colling JC: Effect of an incontinence training program on nursing home staffs' knowledge, attitudes, and behavior, *Gerontologist* 31:788-794, 1991.
19. Woodside JR: Stress urinary incontinence in men, *J Urol* 128:1246, 1982.
20. O'Donnell PD, Calandro V: Incontinence management scale in elderly inpatient men, *Urology* 37(3):220-223, 1991.
21. O'Donnell PD, Sutton LE, Beck CE: Urinary incontinence detection in elderly inpatient men, *Neurourol Urodyn* 6(20):101-108, 1987.
22. O'Donnell PD, Marshall M: Telemetric ambulatory urinary incontinence detection in the elderly, *J Ambul Monit* 1(3):233-240, 1988.
23. O'Donnell PD, Beck CM, Finkbeiner AE: Incontinence volume measurements in elderly inpatient men, *Urology* 35(6):499-503, 1990.
24. O'Donnell PD: A microcomputer based incontinence data management system for elderly inpatients, *J Neurourol Urodyn* 9:145-153, 1990.

Chapter 56 Management of Incontinence in Long-Term Care

John F. Schnelle, Joseph G. Ouslander

There are many extremely important clinical issues involving the management of incontinence in nursing home residents that are unique to this select population. First, one must consider the prevalence and severity of incontinence in this group as well as the most common types of incontinence seen in the nursing home population. Next, it is important to determine the initial evaluations that should be conducted, in particular consideration of the nursing home resident who is often both demented and mobility impaired. Because of these impairments, it is important to emphasize an early assessment of resident responsiveness to a prompted voiding (PV) protocol designed to compensate for a resident's functional and cognitive impairment. Finally, one should evaluate alternative treatment options that can be considered either in combination with or separate from the prompted voiding protocol.

Urinary incontinence affects approximately 50% of all nursing home residents.[1] Typically, this incontinence is severe in frequency, volume, and influence on quality of life. In a recent study in which residents were checked every 2 hours, nursing home residents were found to be wet an average of six times in a 20-hour period (7 A.M. to 5 P.M. and 7 P.M. to 5 A.M.).[2] The average volume per incontinent episode was 115 ml during the daytime and 160 ml during the night. In addition, almost all residents with urinary incontinence also suffer from fecal incontinence. In a recent study, the average frequency of fecal incontinence per day in a sample of 165 nursing home residents who were incontinent of urine was 1.1.[3]

The severity of incontinence in the nursing home is also manifested by its association with a wide range of illnesses. It is related to skin irritation and makes pressure sores more difficult to heal.[4] In consideration of the effects of incontinence on skin health, a primary recommendation of the Agency for Health Care Policy and Research (AHCPR) practice guidelines for pressure-sore prevention is to control moisture.[5]

Mobility problems are also commonly associated with incontinence in nursing home residents. These mobility problems may lead to falls among residents with nocturia and nocturnal incontinence. Immobility and incontinence have also been identified as primary risk factors in the nursing home for the development of infections requiring hospitalizations.[6]

It is difficult to evaluate the psychologic effects of incontinence in nursing home residents, since most incontinent residents are also demented. However, there is evidence that families of nondemented residents place high value on incontinence rehabilitation programs. In a recent preference survey, respondents chose an incontinence rehabilitation program over such highly valued alternatives as moving to a private room and better food.[7]

Basic Causes and Types of Urinary Incontinence

The pathogenesis of urinary incontinence among nursing home residents is often multifactorial, involving urologic and gynecologic conditions, neurologic disorders, behavioral and psychologic factors, and functional impairments. Thus the approach to assessment and treatment must be comprehensive and involve consideration of all of these potential factors. The most important factors to consider are those that are *reversible.* Potentially reversible conditions that can contribute to urinary incontinence in nursing home residents are listed in Table 56-1. Although identification and management of these reversible factors may not cure the urinary incontinence, the severity of the urinary incontinence may be reduced, and, thereby, the incontinence made more manageable by other interventions. In addition, identification and management of these conditions may have important benefits for the residents' overall functioning and quality of life.

Table 56-2 illustrates a classification of the basic types of persistent urinary incontinence. Three important features of this classification should be noted. First, from a neurourologic perspective, this classification is greatly simplified and does not include all the pathophysiologic types of urinary incontinence. For example patients with suprasacral spinal cord lesions such as those that can occur in multiple sclerosis may have detrusor

Table 56-1 Potentially Reversible Conditions that Can Cause or Contribute to Urinary Incontinence in Nursing Home Residents

CONDITIONS	MANAGEMENT
IMPAIRED ABILITY OR WILLINGNESS TO REACH A TOILET	
Delirium	Diagnosis and treatment of underlying cause or causes of acute confusional state
Illness, injury, or restraint that interferes with mobility	Regular toileting assistance Use of toilet substitutes Environmental alterations (such as bedside commode)
Depression	Appropriate pharmacologic or nonpharmacologic treatment
IRRITATION OR INFLAMMATION IN OR AROUND THE LOWER URINARY TRACT	
Urinary tract infection (symptomatic with frequency, urgency, sudden onset or worsening of incontinence, unexplained fever or functional decline)	Antimicrobial therapy*
Atrophic vaginitis or urethritis	Oral or topical estrogen†
Stool impaction	Disimpaction Appropriate use of stool softeners and laxatives if necessary Adequate mobility and fluid intake
INCREASED URINE PRODUCTION	
Metabolic (hyperglycemia, hypercalcemia)	Better control of diabetes mellitus Therapy for hypercalcemia depends on underlying cause
Excess fluid intake	Reduction in intake of diuretic fluids (such as caffeinated beverages)
Volume overload	
Venous insufficiency with edema	Support stockings Leg evaluation Sodium restriction Diuretic therapy
Congestive heart failure	Medical therapy
DRUG SIDE EFFECTS	Discontinuation of the offending medication if possible
Rapid-acting diuretics causing frequency and urgency	Dosage reduction or modification (such as flexible scheduling of rapid-acting diuretics)
Anticholinergics, narcotics, calcium-channel blockers, alpha-adrenergic agonists (in men) causing urinary retention	
Alpha-adrenergic antagonists causing urethral relaxation and stress incontinence	
Psychotropic drugs with sedative or extrapyramidal effects causing sedation and immobility that interfere with toileting	

*For nursing home residents with bacteriuria (with or without pyuria) who have chronic, stable symptoms of incontinence and no other symptoms of urinary tract infection, antimicrobial therapy is not indicated (see text).
†See text for specific recommendations.

Table 56-2 **Basic Types and Causes of Urinary Incontinence**

TYPE	SYMPTOMS	COMMON CAUSES
Stress	Involuntary loss of urine (usually small amounts) simultaneous with increases in intra-abdominal pressure such as those caused by coughing, sneezing, laughing)	Weakness and laxity of pelvic floor musculature resulting in hypermobility of the bladder base and proximal portion of the urethra Bladder outlet or urethral sphincter weakness (intrinsic sphincter deficiency) related to prior surgery or trauma
Urge	Leakage of urine (usually larger but often variable volumes) because of inability to delay voiding after sensation of bladder fullness is perceived	Detrusor hyperactivity isolated or associated with one or more of the following: Local genitourinary condition such as cystitis, urethritis, tumors, stones, diverticula, outflow obstruction, impaired bladder contractility (DHIC) Central nervous system disorders such as stroke, dementia, parkinsonism, spinal cord injury, or disease
Overflow	Leakage of urine (usually small amounts) resulting from mechanical forces on an over-distended bladder	Anatomic obstruction by prostate, large cystocele Acontractile bladder associated with diabetes mellitus or spinal cord injury
Functional*	Urinary leakage associated with inability to toilet because of impairment of cognitive or physical functioning, psychologic unwillingness, or environmental barriers	Severe dementia Immobility Physical restraints Inaccessible toilets Unavailability of regular toileting assistance Depression

*Functional incontinence should be a diagnosis of exclusion. Most nursing home residents have functional factors that may contribute to incontinence but may also have reversible and specifically treatable conditions underlying the incontinence.

hyperreflexia with external sphincter dyssynergy that can result in incontinence and incomplete bladder emptying ("detrusor–external sphincter dyssynergy").

Second, many incontinent nursing home residents suffer from a combination of two or more types of incontinence. However, this classification includes the predominant types of urinary incontinence in a nursing home population. The predominant abnormality of lower urinary tract functioning found among nursing home residents is detrusor hyperactivity (involuntary bladder contractions found by cystometry), also termed "detrusor instability," "unstable bladder," and "detrusor hyperreflexia" (the last in the presence of a neurologic disorder). Although most often associated with the urge type of urinary incontinence, detrusor hyperactivity is commonly seen with sphincter weakness and stress urinary incontinence in women and with obstruction with benign or malignant prostatic enlargement in men. Of important note is that detrusor hyperactivity is also seen in continent elderly people (men more commonly than women), and thus its precise role in the pathogenesis of incontinence in the nursing home population is incompletely understood.[5] Detrusor hyperactivity in nursing home residents is commonly associated with impaired bladder contractility resulting in incomplete bladder emptying (termed "detrusor hyperactivity with impaired contractility," or "DHIC").[6] Nursing home residents with DHIC may have symptoms that mimic stress or overflow incontinence as well as urge incontinence.

Third and most importantly, functional urinary incontinence should be a diagnosis of exclusion because most nursing home residents have impairments of cognitive or physical functioning that may interfere with their ability to toilet. These residents may also have other potentially treatable conditions contributing to their urinary incontinence. Thus a search for reversible factors and other types of urinary incontinence should be completed before one labels a nursing home resident's urinary incontinence as "functional."

Issues in Assessment and Treatment

Most incontinent nursing home residents are extremely frail even when compared to other residents who are not incontinent but nonetheless require nursing home care. Two major aspects of this frailty influence how assessment and treatment of incontinence should progress in a nursing home. First, a mobility assessment must be an early assessment priority. In a recent clinical trial in six nursing homes, only 38% of the residents were capable of independent ambulation even with the use of a walking device.[7]

In addition, among these residents who were capable of independent ambulation, many residents showed severe gait, balance, or endurance problems that adversely affected their ability to use the toilet independently. Thus attempts to correct or at least compensate for these mobility problems must be a primary concern in the treatment of incontinence for the majority of nursing home residents. Incontinence would not be successfully treated by improving bladder functioning if those residents who have impaired mobility are still not able to reach the toilet in time.

Secondly, most incontinent residents have dementia, which is often severe. Dementia not only makes assessment problematic, but also limits treatment options, since it is doubtful that severely demented residents can follow treatment protocols that require active learning and participation. Unfortunately, conventional mental status examinations do not permit prediction of how well incontinent residents will respond to rehabilitative interventions.[8] Therefore, later in this chapter, we recommend a behavioral assessment strategy that is based on an evaluation of the residents' ability to perform tasks actually required in a potential treatment program. Since the cognitive status and mobility of incontinent residents play such important roles in determining what type of treatment is possible, we also recommend a staging approach to assessment that initially emphasizes measurements of a resident's ability and motivation to toilet and to stay dry. The intent is to limit the more invasive assessments and treatments to those residents for whom such procedures may produce beneficial results. Fig. 56-1 illustrates the assessment steps and potential treatment options that emerge from each assessment stage that we recommend. We divide the assessment and treatment into two phases: a basic evaluation, which is recommended for all incontinent residents, and a further evaluation stage that is recommended for only those residents who meet specific criteria in the basic evaluation phase. The steps in Fig. 56-1 are described in the remainder of this chapter.

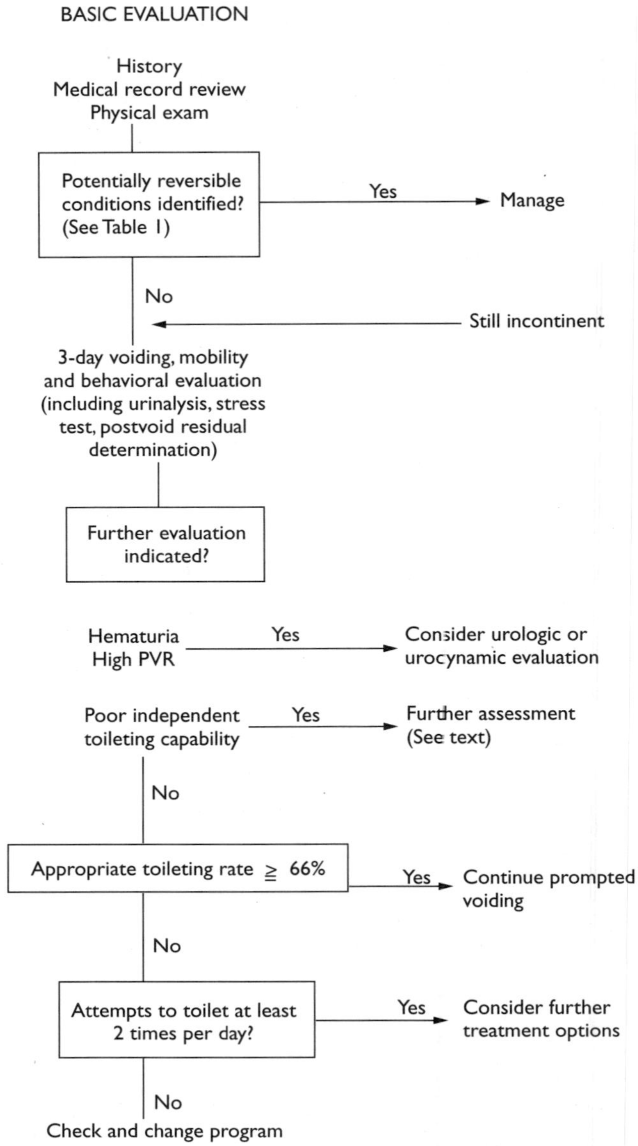

FIG. 56-1 *Assessment and treatment steps for urinary incontinence.*

Basic Evaluation of Incontinent Residents

History

A medical record review should be undertaken to identify medications, medical conditions, and past genitourinary history that may be relevant to the resident's incontinence. A precise history and report of symptoms may be difficult to obtain from many nursing home residents because incontinence is closely associated with dementia in this population. Residents who can reliably report symptoms should be questioned about irritative and other symptoms that are suggestive of urge incontinence (frequency, urgency, nocturia [more than two episodes]), symptoms of stress incontinence (leakage simultaneous with coughing, sneezing, laughing, bending), voiding difficulty (hesitancy, poor or intermittent stream, straining to finish voiding), and other associated symptoms such as dysuria or pain. Pain related to voiding is unusual and should be carefully evaluated.

Physical Examination

The general physical examination should be designed to exclude volume overload (that is, venous insufficiency, congestive heart failure) and previously undiagnosed neurologic conditions that might contribute to the incontinence (such as signs of parkinsonism, spinal cord compression). Rectal examination is done to allow one to assess resting and active sphincter tone, to exclude fecal impaction, and to assess the prostate in men. It should be noted that the size of the prostate on physical examination can neither diagnose nor exclude the presence of urethral obstruction.

The pelvic examination should include assessment of perineal and vulvar skin condition, exclude pelvic masses and pronounced pelvic prolapse (that is, uterine descensus or a cystocele that protrudes through the vaginal introitus), and allow one to evaluate the vaginal epithelium for signs of inflammation (erythema, friability, bleeding) that are suggestive of atrophic vaginitis. Female residents with pronounced pelvic prolapse should be considered for gynecologic evaluation to determine the need for a pessary or for surgery in those who are candidates. A cough test to detect stress incontinence can also be done at the time of the pelvic examination, but it is best performed in the standing position with at least 200 ml in the bladder. Since many incontinent residents cannot easily void after a one-time instruction to do so, the stress test is most easily conducted during the 3-day period in which a voiding and behavioral assessment evaluation is being conducted (see below).

Three-Day Voiding and Behavioral Evaluation

The three-day voiding and behavioral evaluation is designed to address six major questions:

1. Is the resident responsive to a prompted voiding program?
2. Does the resident show cognitive, physical, or motivational problems that will affect treatment of his or her incontinence?
3. Should all further evaluation and treatment be stopped and the resident's incontinence managed with palliative techniques such as diapers with a regular checking and changing program?
4. Does the resident have a high postvoid residual volume or abnormal urinalysis results?
5. Does the resident show signs of stress incontinence?
6. Does the resident show mobility problems that will prevent independent toileting or make independent toileting unsafe?

One can address these questions by modifying a standard prompted voiding protocol. This standard prompted voiding protocol is briefly described here, since it has been described comprehensively in several places.[9-11] The prompting voiding protocol involves four major steps, as listed in the box below.

During the 3-day assessment, residents are exposed to the protocol every 2 hours between 8 A.M. and 4 P.M. (4 prompts per day, or 12 prompts over a 3-day period). After each prompting a recording is made as to each resident's incontinent status when initially checked (wet/dry), the resident's response to the prompt (attempted toilet successfully, attempted to toilet unsuccessfully, did not attempt to toilet), and the resident's behavioral response to the prompts (showed resistance, agitation, or cooperation). These data can be used to address assessment questions 1 to 3 above.

With regard to question 1, if residents respond to the 12 prompts with a 66% appropriate toileting ratio, they are excellent candidates for ongoing management with prompted voiding.[12] The appropriate toileting ratio is calculated when one divides the total number of voids in a toilet by the total number of continent and incontinent voids. Residents who are responsive to prompted voiding very likely showed impaired ability or willingness to use the toilet before that prompted voiding (see Table 56-1). Prompted voiding compensates for these factors.

Data relevant to questions 2 and 3 (motivational and cognitive capacity and should a changing program be considered) are provided when one analyzes the resident's attempts to toilet. If the resident attempts to toilet one time a day or less and continues to be wet two or more times a day, or if he or she shows resistance to being given toileting assistance, the resident is determined to be unsuitable for prompted voiding. Resistance can be objectively rated by a resident's verbal self-statement that he or she does not want to be bothered by the prompting or by demonstrating increased agitation when attempts are made to toilet or change them. In our previous work, approximately 15% to 25% of nursing home residents are found to demonstrate either resistance or a low motivation to toilet. It is unlikely that these residents will have the motivation to cooperate with any further treatment that would require even more active involvement than prompted voiding, and hence we recommend these residents be prescribed a changing program to control the effects of moisture on skin health. Regardless of the resident's response to the prompted voiding protocol, all residents should be assessed for conditions that may justify further evaluation. The following sections describe three modifications to the basic prompted voiding protocol that are designed to identify the presence of these conditions.

Prompted Voiding Protocol

1. Contact the resident every 2 hours from 7 A.M. to 7 P.M.
2. Focus his or her attention on voiding by asking whether he or she is wet or dry.
3. Check for wetness, record on bladder record, and give feedback on whether he or she was correct or incorrect.
4. Whether the resident is wet or dry, ask the resident if he or she would like to use the toilet (or urinal).
   a. If yes:
      (1) Assist the resident.
      (2) Record the results on the bladder record.
      (3) Give him or her positive reinforcement by spending an extra minute or two talking with him or her.
   b. If no:
      (1) In the event the resident has not attempted to void in the last 4 hours, repeat the request to use the toilet once or twice before leaving.
      (2) Inform the resident that you will be back in 2 hours and request him or her to try to delay voiding until then.

Postvoid Residual Determination and Urinalysis

The first modification of the protocol is designed to obtain a clean-catch urinalysis and an estimate of postvoid residual volume. An attempt is made to collect these data the first time the resident toilets during the 3 days of prompted voiding rounds. The urinalysis collection procedure will be discussed first. Clean urine may be difficult to obtain from incontinent, cognitively impaired, immobile nursing home residents. If the resident will be catheterized for a postvoid residual determination, the urine obtained by catheterization can be used for the urinalysis. However, it is also possible to noninvasively obtain, from both men and women, a clean-catch urine specimen that accurately matches culture results from a catheterized specimen. For women, the technique involves careful cleaning of the perineum with a sterile preparation kit and then having them void into a disinfected collection device (toileting insert or "hat," or fracture bedpan).[13] For men, a clean condom catheter can be applied after the penis is cleaned with a sterile preparation such as povidone-iodine complex (betadine).[14]

The primary purpose of the urinalysis is to exclude hematuria unless the resident has symptoms other than incontinence that are suggestive of a urinary tract infection (dysuria, recent onset or worsening of their incontinence, unexplained fever, or functional decline). Bacteriuria should not be treated because eradicating the bacteriuria has no effect on the severity of the incontinence in nursing home residents. The urinalysis can also exclude sterile hematuria, which may be a sign of bladder or upper urinary tract disorder. Glucosuria resulting from poorly controlled diabetes can also be detected. This may cause polyuria and exacerbate the incontinence.

Although rapid urine screening methods are generally thought of as inaccurate in the nursing home population, they can be used to exclude bacteriuria with reasonable accuracy. The combination of negative dipstick tests for both nitrite and leukocyte esterase and a negative enzyme-based screen for bacteriuria (Uriscreen, Ventrex Laboratories, Portland, Maine) has a negative predictive value of over 95% for significant bacteriuria among incontinent nursing home residents.[15] Whether such screening tests are practical depends on the availability of personnel who can reliably collect the urine and perform the tests and the costs relative to sending a specimen to the laboratory for urinalysis.

Significant degrees of urinary retention can occur in the absence of symptoms or signs of obstruction or bladder contractility problems. In addition, physical examination (suprapubic palpation, bimanual examination) is neither sensitive or specific in detecting significant residual volume. Postvoid residual volume is usually determined by catheterization, but there is now available a portable ultrasound device that can noninvasively measure residual urine with reasonably good accuracy.[16] It is important to understand that postvoid residual volume can have substantial intraindividual variability. The timing of the determination in relation to a void, the degree to which the void was natural for the patient, the nature of instructions given to the patient, the amount of straining, and the body position can all influence the postvoid volume obtained. Thus, when moderately elevated volumes are detected (such as 150-300 ml), repeated determinations may be appropriate. In these situations, the use of ultrasound may be especially valuable in avoiding the need for repeated catheterizations. Repeated residual volumes of more than 200 ml should prompt consideration of whether the resident should be referred for further evaluation.

Pad Test for Stress Incontinence

The second modification to the prompted voiding protocol evaluates if the resident has signs of stress incontinence. Because the presence or absence of stress incontinence does not predict responsiveness to prompted voiding, results of the stress test are helpful only for those residents who fail a trial of prompted voiding and who are candidates for specific therapy for stress incontinence (see the discussion of treatment options for stress incontinence). The stress test can be performed during the same toileting episodes in which a clean urine and a postvoid residual volume is being obtained. The stress test is performed by having the resident cough several times in the standing position. The test is positive if there is leakage of urine simultaneous with the cough. If the test is negative and if the total bladder volume (voided volume and residual) is less than 200 ml, the test should be repeated because a low bladder volume can cause a false-negative test. In many cases, it is impossible to obtain an adequate stress test because of either low bladder volumes caused by involuntary bladder contraction or low frequency of toileting or because of difficulty in following the coughing instructions. Because of these difficulties, attempts to obtain a stress test should be terminated if it cannot be successfully completed during the first few attempts to toilet.

Mobility Assessment

The third modification to the prompted voiding protocol evaluates the resident's mobility skills to independently toilet and to do so safely. There are two questions addressed by the mobility assessment protocol: (1) Will a resident require ongoing prompted voiding management because of physical inability to safely use the toilet? (2) Should a resident be prescribed a rehabilitation program to improve skills related to toileting?

The extent to which a resident can safely perform the physical steps involved in toileting can be most effectively evaluated during the prompted voiding rounds when the resident must move for either changing or toileting assistance. These incontinence care activities offer a natural opportunity to evaluate the resident's ability to perform three critical skills for independent toileting: standing, moving (either walking or wheeling) to the toilet, and transferring. We have designed a standardized assessment protocol to assess these skills.[17] The instructions to the resident involved in this protocol are designed to elicit the maximum possible independent effort. A resident can be said to be capable of independent toileting if he or she performs all three of the tasks if either instructed to do so or with instructions and gentle manual guidance. We have found 30% to 40% of nursing home residents in our studies are capable of independently performing all three skills necessary for independent toileting.

Residents who are not capable of toileting independence will have to be maintained on prompted voiding so as to receive toileting assistance even if other treatments for incontinence are attempted and successful. For example, even if a resident is capable of maintaining dryness for several hours at a time because of an intervention such as drug therapy, this resident will be continent only to the extent that the staff offers him or her an opportunity to toilet on a regular basis. In addition, many of the residents who are capable of independently performing all toileting tasks are either very slow or show poor strength and endurance. For example, we have reported that the average time it took an incontinent resident to stand was 6 seconds, and the average time incontinent residents could walk in a standardized endurance test was 2.6 minutes.[17] These mobility problems limit the resident's ability to stay dry, and the muscle weakness associated with the slowness and poor endurance place the residents at risk for falling if they do attempt to toilet. Thus many such residents will also have to be maintained on prompted voiding so that toileting assistance can be provided for the purpose of getting the residents to the bathroom quickly and safely. The issues involved in the maintenance of prompted voiding are complex and require an effective quality assurance system. Descriptions of such a system have been provided in several places.[18,19]

Who Are Candidates for Further Evaluation?

Urologic or urodynamic evaluation should be considered for residents with sterile hematuria or high postvoid residual (residual volumes greater than 200 ml). Only residents who are candidates for specific interventions based on the results of these evaluations should be referred. Further evaluation may also be indicated for those residents who show stress symptoms or high wetness frequency (2+ times per day), despite attempts to toilet two or more times a day. In these cases, either a stress or an urge incontinence diagnosis is suspected, and there are treatment options available for these conditions that have been proved effective with elderly people who do not live in nursing homes. By virtue of their attempts to toilet two or more times a day, these nursing home residents who show signs of stress or urge incontinence have also demonstrated that they have at least the minimal cognitive capacity and motivation to make them candidates for these further types of treatment. They would not have been responsive to the prompts and attempts to toilet if they were not motivated to be dry. Further evaluation by a physical therapist is also recommended for residents who either cannot independently perform all three mobility skills related to toileting or who do so very poorly and who are believed to have some potential for improving these skills. Based on previous work, we estimate that most incontinent residents will be in need of either a physical therapist consultation or a nursing exercise program designed to improve endurance and muscle strength. We review some of the treatment options that are available for those residents who have problems that require further evaluation.

Treatment Options for Stress Incontinence

Behavioral Interventions

All of the behavioral interventions discussed in this section and also the section on behavioral treatment for urge incontinence require that residents follow multistep instructions. Despite a high motivation to be continent, it may be difficult for many nursing home residents to do so because of severe dementia. If the residents are to be considered candidates for the more active behavioral interventions, we suggest that the best way to determine if she or he is capable of adhering to the behavioral protocol is to actually attempt the protocol for a brief two or three trial run-in period. This "run-in" assessment approach is identical to the logic of the 3-day prompted voiding assessment. If the resident shows the ability to follow the instructions involved in the behavioral intervention during this run-in period, further treatment with the behavioral intervention may be possible. If a resident proves incapable of following the instructions required for a behavioral protocol, other treatments that do not require such active resident involvement may be tried. The logic of this "run-in" assessment strategy is discussed in more detail in other places.[8]

Behavioral treatment for stress incontinence generally involves pelvic muscle, or Kegel, exercises. Biofeedback is often used to assist patients to learn pelvic muscle exercises. Biofeedback is the use of electrical or mechanical instrumentation to relay information to patients about their physical activity. In relation to stress incontinence, patients are taught to tighten their sphincter without increasing abdominal pressure. In some cases, vaginal cones are also used to supplement the pelvic muscle exercises.

Biofeedback and pelvic muscle exercises have been shown to reduce incontinence frequency in older women, but these procedures have not been adequately tested with the frail nursing home population.[20]

Drug Therapy

For sphincter weakness with stress urinary incontinence in women, drug treatment involves a combination of estrogen and an alpha-adrenergic agonist. Estrogen can be given by vaginal cream, 1 g at bedtime, or orally as 0.625 mg of conjugated estrogen daily. Data supporting the effectiveness of estrogen, especially when given alone, for the treatment of stress incontinence are sparse.[21,22] Either pseudoephedrine, 30 to 60 mg three times per day, or phenylpropanolamine, 75 mg twice per day, can be used as the alpha-agonist. Phenylpropanolamine has been shown to be as effective as pelvic muscle exercises among noninstitutionalized older women with stress incontinence.[23] Drug treatment for stress urinary incontinence should be combined with a toileting program (to keep the bladder volume as low as possible) and pelvic muscle exercises (for residents who can cooperate). Women who have prominent pelvic prolapse or who fail a 3- to 6-month trial of drug or behavioral therapy, or both, should be considered for surgical intervention.

For women with mixed urge and stress urinary incontinence, a combination of the above approaches can be used. Imipramine, in doses of 10 to 25 mg three times per day, may be tried as a combination anticholinergic and alpha-agonist. Imipramine can worsen cardiac conduction abnormalities and, in addition to its anticholinergic side effects, can cause significant orthostatic hypotension in nursing home residents who are ambulatory. Thus this drug should be used cautiously in the nursing home population.

Surgery

Surgical intervention for urinary incontinence is a consideration for a small but important subgroup of incontinent nursing home residents. Since urinary incontinence is not a life-threatening problem, it must be bothersome enough to a resident who is a candidate for elective surgery to pursue surgical treatment (that is, one who is medically stable, is not terminally ill, and desires further treatment for the incontinence).

Surgery for urinary incontinence is basically of two types. First, women with stress urinary incontinence associated with significant pelvic prolapse and urethral hypermobility may benefit from bladder neck suspension and repair of the pelvic prolapse. Although studies have not been done in the nursing home population, the short-term (1- to 5-year) success of this type of surgery for properly selected older women has been found to be in the range of 75% for significant reduction or elimination of wetness. For commonly dwelling residents with stress incontinence associated with intrinsic urethral deficiency, artificial urinary sphincters have been used. This requires a relatively major surgical procedure and is probably not an appropriate option in the nursing home population. Periurethral injections of collagen have recently been approved for residents with intrinsic urethral deficiency. Although studies have not yet included very frail residents, periurethral injection has been reported to be effective in younger residents.[24]

The other type of surgical intervention for urinary incontinence is the removal of anatomic obstruction, most commonly an enlarged prostate in males or a urethral stricture. Detailed discussion of the evaluation and surgical treatment of lower urinary tract obstruction is beyond the scope of this chapter. Suffice it to say that nursing home residents who are candidates for surgery should be referred for complex urodynamic evaluation. Newer, less invasive techniques are now available for the surgical relief of obstruction in men and may be especially appropriate for consideration in frail, older nursing home residents.

TREATMENT OPTIONS FOR URGE INCONTINENCE

Behavioral Treatment

A bladder retraining program is perhaps the primary behavioral treatment used for urge incontinence. A bladder retraining program requires the participant to resist or inhibit the sensation of urgency to postpone voiding and to urinate according to a timetable rather than according to the urge to void. Initially the time goal is usually set between 2 and 3 hours and is then extended. A recent randomized controlled study reported that 12% of older community-dwelling women who underwent bladder training became continent and 75% improved by at least a 50% reduction in the number of incontinence episodes.[25] The number of incontinent nursing home residents who are capable of responding to bladder training is not known but is probably very small.

Drug Treatment

Drugs with anticholinergic effects, including propantheline (15 to 30 mg three to four times per day), oxybutynin (2.5 to 5 mg two to four times per day), and imipramine (10 to 25 mg three times per day) have been most commonly used as bladder relaxants. Several studies suggest that frail and functionally impaired incontinent residents do not respond well to bladder-relaxant medications.[26-30]A recent placebo-controlled trial in which oxybutynin was added to prompted voiding indicates that a modest subgroup (approximately 25%) of incontinent nursing home residents with detrusor hyperactivity may benefit from this drug when added to a prompted voiding protocol. If a therapeutic trial of one of these medications is undertaken, careful observation is needed for anticholinergic side effects including dry mouth, constipation and fecal impaction, blurry vision, urinary retention, and worsening cognitive function. Imipramine can also cause orthostatic hypotension. Women with urge incontinence associated with atrophic vaginitis should be treated with estrogen as described earlier. New types of bladder-relaxant drugs and long-acting preparations (such as slow-release capsules, skin patches) are being developed but are not currently available.

TREATMENT FOR OVERFLOW INCONTINENCE

As stated earlier, residents with large postvoid residual volumes should be considered for urodynamic evaluation to determine the cause or causes if the problem can be surgically corrected and the resident is a candidate for surgery (that is, is medically stable, is not terminally ill, and desires further treatment). For other residents, there are basically three options. First, if the residual volumes are in an intermediate range (that is, 200 to 400 ml), the resident can be observed without specific intervention. If renal function deteriorates or if symptomatic infections occur, treatment should be initiated. Second is intermittent catheterization. This may be uncomfortable for many nursing home residents and difficult to perform for nurses because of resistance from the resident. In addition, although it may be possible to safely perform clean (as opposed to sterile) catheterizations in a nursing home setting, infection-control concerns will generally necessitate sterile catheterizations in most typical nursing homes. Third is a long-term individual catheter. Although long-term catheterization is known to be associated with substantial morbidity in the nursing home population, careful attention to catheter-care guidelines may help prevent complications in residents who need continuous bladder drainage. There is no evidence that drug therapy is an effective approach to overflow incontinence in the nursing home population.

TREATMENT FOR MOBILITY PROBLEMS THAT LIMIT INDEPENDENT TOILETING

It is unknown how often physical therapy assessment and treatment would be helpful for incontinent residents who are chronically ill or demented and who require maximal assistance to perform the three mobility skills related to independent toileting. These skills are standing, moving to the toilet by use of a wheelchair or walking, and transferring. We have not been successful in significantly improving the independence level of these very dependent residents in two separate exercise rehabilitation trials that have lasted for 9-week periods.[17,31] However, we have been able to improve the endurance, speed, and safety levels in all three mobility skills with those residents who are capable of performing these three skills independently or with minimal physical assistance.

The mobility intervention we have tested is called FIT (functional incidental training) and involves two primary additions to prompted voiding. The two additional FIT steps are done each time prompted voiding occurs when the resident is out of bed. First, the resident is encouraged to perform the toileting-related activities with minimal staff assistance. Because of staff time constraints, aides typically provide maximal assistance to the residents in completing the prompted voiding sequence. For example, walking a slow and unsteady resident to the bathroom takes more time than wheeling the resident to the bathroom. In the absence of functional considerations, it is more efficient to provide such maximal assistance and to minimize the resident's involvement. The FIT intervention promotes functional activity. Second, the resident is given repeated practice in each functional activity (such as standing twice) and works toward an individualized goal. This individualized goal is increased progressively as the resident demonstrates improvement. The application of the FIT protocol three times a day for 9 weeks has been shown to result in significant improvement in walking endurance, standing speed, wheelchair endurance, and safety measures for a group of 38 residents in a controlled trial.[17]

References

1. Ouslander JG, Kane RL, Abrass IB: Urinary incontinence in elderly nursing home patients, *JAMA* 248:1194-1198, 1982.
2. Schnelle JF, et al: The dark side of incontinence: Incontinence at night in nursing homes, *J Am Geriatr Soc* 41:371-376, 1993.
3. Ouslander JG, et al: Effects of prompted voiding on fecal continence among nursing home residents, *J Am Geriatr Soc* (Submitted).
4. Panel for the Prediction and Prevention of Pressure Ulcers in Adults: *Pressure ulcers in adults: prediction and prevention: clinical practice guideline,* No 3,. AHCPR Publication No. 92-0047. Rockville, Md., 1992, Agency for Health Care Policy and Research, Public Health Service, U.S. Department of Health and Human Services.
5. Diokno AC, Brown MB, Brock BM, et al: Clinical and cystometric characteristics of continent and incontinent noninstitutionalized elderly, *J Urol* 140:567-571, 1988.
6. Resnick N, Yalla SV: Detrusor hyperactivity with impaired contractile function: an unrecognized but common cause of incontinence in elderly patients, *JAMA* 257:3076-3081, 1987.
7. Ouslander JG, Schnelle JF, Uman G, et al: Does oxybutynin add to the effectiveness of prompted voiding for urinary incontinence among nursing home residents? *J Am Geriatr Soc* 43:610-617, 1995.
8. Schnelle JF, et al: A subject screening strategy for nursing home residents: run-in versus mental status testing, *Behav Health Aging* 3(1):13-21, 1993.
9. Schnelle JF: *Managing urinary incontinence in the elderly,* New York, 1991, Springer Publishing.
10. Schnelle JF, Ouslander JG, Simmons SF: Predicting nursing home resident responsiveness to a urinary incontinence treatment protocol, *Int Urogynecol J* 4:89-94, 1993.
11. Schnelle JF: Treatment of urinary incontinence in nursing home patients by prompted voiding, *J Am Geriatr Soc* 37:1051-1057, 1989.
12. Ouslander J, et al: Predictors of responsiveness to prompted voiding among incontinent nursing home residents, *J Am Geriatr Soc* 11:SA25, 1994.
13. Ouslander JG, Schapira M, Schnelle JF: Urine specimen collection from incontinent female nursing home residents (Abstract), *J Am Geriatr Soc* 43:279-281, 1995.
14. Ouslander JG, Greengold BA, Silverblatt FJ, Garcia JP: An accurate method to obtain urine for culture in men with external catheters, *Arch Intern Med* 147:286-288, 1987.
15. Schapira M, et al: Accuracy of rapid screening methods for bacteriuria among incontinent nursing home residents, *J Am Geriatr Soc* 11:SA4, 1994.
16. Ouslander J, Simmons S, Turco E, et al: Use of a portable ultrasound device to measure postvoid residual volume among incontinent nursing home residents, *J Am Geriatr Soc* 42:1189-1192, 1994.
17. Schnelle JF, Mackae PG, Ouslander JG, et al: Functional incidental training, mobility performance, and incontinence care with nursing home residents, *J Am Geriatr Soc* 43:1356-1362, 1995; comment in 43:1439-1440, 1995.
18. Schnelle JF, Newman D, White M, et al: Maintaining continence in nursing home residents through the application of industrial quality control, *Gerontologist* 33:114-121, 1992.
19. Schnelle JF, McNees P, Crooks V, Ouslander JG: The use of a computer-based model to implement an incontinence management program, *Gerontologist* 35:656-665, 1995.
20. Burns PA, Pranikoff K, Nochajski T, et al: Treatment of stress incontinence with pelvic floor exercise and biofeedback, *J Am Geriatr Soc* 38:341-344, 1990.
21. Urinary Incontinence Guidelines Panel: *Urinary incontinence in adults: clinical practice guideline,* AHCPR Pub No 92-0038, Rockville, Md., 1992, Agency for Health Care Policy and Research, Public Health Service, U.S. Department of Health and Human Services.
22. Fantl JA, Cardozo L, McClish DK, and The Hormones and Urogenital Therapy Committee: Estrogen therapy in the management of urinary incontinence in postmenopausal women: a meta-analysis. First report of the hormones and urogenital therapy committee, *Obstet Gynecol* 83:12-18, 1994.
23. Wells TJ, Brink CA, Diokno AC, et al: Pelvic muscle exercise for stress urinary incontinence in elderly women, *J Am Geriatr Soc* 39:785-791, 1991.
24. Cole HM: Diagnostic and therapeutic technology assessment (DATTA): use of Teflon preparations for urinary incontinence and vesicoureteral reflux, *JAMA* 269:2975-2980, 1993.
25. Fantl JA, Wyman JF, McClish DK, et al: Efficacy of bladder training in older women with urinary incontinence, *JAMA* 265:609-613, 1991.
26. Castleden CM, Duffin HM, Asher MJ, Yeomanson CW: Factors influencing outcome in elderly patients with urinary incontinence and detrusor instability, *Age Ageing* 14:303-307, 1985.
27. Zorzitto ML, et al: Effectiveness of propantheline bromide in the treatment of geriatric patients with detrusor instability, *Neurourol Urodyn* 5:133-140, 1986.
28. Zorzitto ML, Holliday PJ, Jewett MA, et al: Oxybutynin chloride for geriatric urinary dysfunction: a double-blind placebo-controlled study, *Age Ageing* 18:195-200, 1989.
29. Tobin GW, Brocklehurst JC: The management of urinary incontinence in local authority residential homes for the elderly, *Age Ageing* 15:292-298, 1986.
30. Wiseman PA, Malone-Lee J, Rai GS: Terodiline with bladder retraining for treating detrusor instability in elderly people, *Br Med J* 302:994-996, 1991.
31. Schnelle JF, MacRae PG, Giacobassi K, et al: Exercise with physically restrained nursing home residents: maximizing benefits of restraint reduction, *J Am Geriatr Soc* 44:507-512, 1996.

Chapter 57

Etiology of Urinary Incontinence

Simon Jackson, Paul Abrams

Urinary incontinence is an immense problem among older people, with approximately 38% of the community-dwelling women suffering from incontinence, whereas approximately 19% of older men in the community have incontinence.[1-3] Of older people in chronic care facilities, approximately 55% experience urinary incontinence.[4] Not only does incontinence cause emotional disturbance and social isolation,[5] but it also is a common cause of institutionalization in the elderly. On urodynamic evaluation of older people who have urinary incontinence, involuntary detrusor contractions are commonly observed, and they may be a sign of detrusor instability (DI) or detrusor hyperreflexia. In older women, sphincteric incompetence may be present alone or in combination with detrusor hyperactivity. The effects of aging on the nervous system and lower urinary tract exacerbate any conditions that predispose the patient to urinary incontinence such as bladder outlet obstruction in older men or intrinsic sphincter deficiency in older women. In up to 35% of older subjects the pathophysiologic condition of urinary incontinence may be multifactorial.[6]

It is extremely important to determine the cause of incontinence in older people, since successful therapy must be based on the cause, which may be multiple as stated above. If sphincter weakness or outlet obstruction exists in older patients, it is possible to treat it successfully even in the frail elderly.[7-13] This will often involve urodynamic evaluation, which also can be done with the frail elderly. Cystometry aims to give a pathophysiologic explanation for a clinical problem; treatment can then be targeted appropriately.

Etiology

First we consider in some depth the pathophysiologic processes believed to cause both DI and sphincter weakness, these being the most common causes of urinary incontinence in the elderly. We then consider some of the other pathologic processes that afflict the elderly patient in particular and cause or aggravate urinary incontinence.

Detrusor Instability

Detrusor instability increases with age[14] and has been found to be the underlying etiology in 39% to 68% of elderly incontinent patients.[15,16] Although idiopathic DI still predominates, in the elderly there is an increasing incidence of detrusor hyperreflexia (DHR), defined as DI in the presence of a neurologic disease. Common neurologic disorders associated with DHR include stroke and multiinfarct dementia, and Parkinson's disease is also implicated[17] because of involvement of the micturition reflex at the level of the basal ganglia. Rarer causes of DHR in the elderly include brain tumors, multiple sclerosis,[18] and Shy-Drager syndrome.[19] Even in the absence of obvious neuropathy, urge incontinence can be associated with a reduction in cognitive function, with reduced cortical perfusion demonstrated on single–photon emission computed tomography.[20] This finding indicates that covert cortical neuropathy may account, at least in part, for the increasing incidence of DI in the elderly.

Bladder outlet obstruction secondary to benign prostatic obstruction is said to be the most common cause of obstructive instability, and its incidence rises with age; more than 50% of older men with lower urinary tract symptoms have DI.[21] Relief of prostatic obstruction reverses DI in up to two thirds of patients,[21] though in the elderly population reversal rates for DI after transurethral resection of prostate may be considerably lower than this number.[22] This finding implies that the pathophysiologic features of much DI in the elderly male may not simply be secondary to obstruction.

The cause of detrusor instability and detrusor hyperreflexia is not always clear. Also, bladder outlet obstruction appears to increase the problem of detrusor instability and detrusor hyperreflexia. It is unclear if the pathophysiologic characteristics of detrusor hyperactivity are the same in patients with bladder outlet obstruction compared with patients without obstruction. Detrusor muscle bundles within the bladder wall frequently exchange fibers with adjacent bundles, so that from a structural and mechanical point of view the detrusor comprises a single unit of branching and reuniting smooth muscle bundles. However, detrusor muscle is unusual in that the electrical coupling between cells is poorly developed,[23] preventing ready spread of electrical activity between neighboring cells. This is important functionally if activity in individual detrusor smooth muscle cells during filling is not to cause a coordinated detrusor contraction with a consequent rise in intravesical pressure. Such activity is achieved only through excitatory nerves, which branch extensively throughout the detrusor, activating most cells. An unstable detrusor appears to be better coupled electrically, possibly secondary to denervation. Let us consider the evidence for this statement.

Increased electrical coupling may be involved in detrusor hyperactivity. There is some histologic evidence that intercellular junctions alter with age, with an increase in ultraclose cell abutments correlating with increasing incidence of DI.[24] These cell junctions may result in increased cellular electrical coupling. These histologic studies also demonstrated muscle degeneration, which correlated with impaired detrusor contractility. This correlation could account for the observed association between detrusor hyperreflexia and impaired contractility described by Resnick.[25] In obstructed animal bladders it has been shown that smooth muscle cells appear better coupled electrically when compared with normal bladder.[26] Kinder and Mundy reported increased spontaneous activity and tetanic contractions in smooth muscle from both DI and DHR.[27] Detrusor from DHR taken at the time of cystoplasty demonstrated increased spontaneous activity and supersensitivity to agonists such as carbachol, acetylcholine, and potassium.[28]

Denervation may be involved in detrusor hyperactivity. In addition to improved electrical coupling, DI appears to be associated with denervation. In animal work, using a pig model where DI develops secondary to an induced bladder outlet obstruction, histologic examination has shown a reduction in the density of acetylcholinesterase-positive nerves in an unstable bladder.[29] The findings are similar in the rabbit.[30] There is limited evidence in the human, but these features have also been seen in bladders of men with prostatic hypertrophy,[31,32] and reinnervation after prostatectomy has been observed.[33] Detrusor muscle from patients with DHR taken at the time of cystoplasty has also been shown to be partially denervated.[28]

Although it is easy to postulate why denervation may occur in DHR, explaining denervation in the presence of outlet obstruction is more problematic. The rat model does not suffer from denervation when the bladder outlet is obstructed. In the rat there are no detrusor intramural ganglia, whereas these are seen in all species where obstruction causes denervation. It therefore seems possible that the rat is protected by its ganglia being extravesical. Brading suggests that increased intravesical pressure occurring during voiding causes intramural ischemia, resulting in damage to the ganglia. This is exacerbated by outlet obstruction with its increased duration of the voiding contraction.[34]

Furthermore, it appears that the observed increased electrical coupling may be secondary to denervation; experimental denervation of smooth muscle cells results in supersensitivity to agonists and increased cell excitability.[35,36] Sethia[37] has demonstrated that denervation of pig bladder by full-thickness bladder transection leads to instability.

In conclusion, evidence from both animal models and humans indicate that in DHR or instability associated with bladder outlet obstruction one underlying factor is an alteration in the properties of smooth muscle resulting from denervation of the detrusor. The cause of idiopathic DI remains unknown, though its observed increasing incidence with age may be secondary to altered intercellular junctions. There have been reports of alterations in receptor density in unstable human bladders, including alpha-adrenoreceptors,[38] presynaptic alpha-adrenoreceptor activity,[39] and increased atropine resistance.[40] The situation is clearly complex; a central neurologic element must also play a part as demonstrated by those patients in whom incontinence follows trigger factors such as putting the key in the front door ("latch-key incontinence") and hand washing. At present it would appear that we still have to postulate a variety of mechanisms to explain the observed changes in detrusor excitatory and inhibitory inputs.

Sphincter Weakness

Urethral sphincter incompetence occurs in up to 76% of elderly women,[14] and it has been shown that urethral closure pressure decreases with age in both stress incontinent women and normal controls.[41] Childbirth and the menopause appear to be the two most important contributing factors. It is well established that neuromuscular damage, both to the pelvic floor and to the urethral sphincter, occurring at the time of childbirth, contributes to the onset of female urinary stress incontinence, whereas the menopause appears to be an important additional factor. Rekers et al.[42] looked at the relationship between urinary symptoms and the menopause and demonstrated, using multivariate analysis, that it contributed significantly to their onset. It therefore seems likely that estrogen deficiency is an important implicating factor, though the mechanisms remain unclear.

For a tube to occlude perfectly it is important that the inner walls be soft and compressible.[43] The inner urethral epithelial surface is folded to allow complete apposition of the mucosa. The submucosa consists of collagen fibers, elastic tissue, and a rich vascular network, forming a spongy tissue that is likely to contribute to urethral sealing. It seems probable that these factors play an important role in maintaining urinary continence and may well be implicated in the onset of postmenopausal sphincter incompetence. We consider some of these possible etiologic factors in more detail.

Urethral Blood Flow

One can propose a model whereby the vascular flow within the urethral submucosa contributes pressure and provides occlusive force by means of a hermetic seal. It seems likely that an increased flow through the rich submucosal vascular plexus will increase this occlusive pressure whereas a decreased flow, as may occur in the atrophic postmenopausal genitourinary tract, could predispose to urinary incontinence. A role for the vascular component of the urethra was first described by Berkow,[44] who felt that the venous plexus had a function like a washer in a tap (faucet). Vascular pulsations in the urethral high-pressure zone were described by Enhorning,[45] who also regarded the rich venous network as an auxiliary closure mechanism. Subsequent studies have confirmed these initial findings; animal studies have shown that occlusion of the arterial input to the urethra brings about a significant fall in urethral luminal pressure,[46,47] and a negative correlation has been demonstrated between vascular pulsations seen on urethral pressure profilometry and menopausal age.[48] Tsai,[49] using a thermistor technique, has estimated blood flow in the vagina of postmenopausal women and concluded that the blood flow values were lower than those for premenopausal women reported in the literature. Therefore, although further research is required, it seems likely that blood flow plays a key role in maintaining urethral occlusion, and an apparent reduction in flow after the menopause could explain the observed increased incidence of sphincter incompetence in this age group.

Collagen

The major component in the urethra is collagen, the fibers of which are arranged predominantly longitudinally with some circular fibers and are crucial to optimum functioning during bladder neck closure. Versi[50] reported a correlation between lower resting urethral pressure and reduced skin collagen in postmenopausal women, whereas stress incontinence is associated with reductions in total collagen in skin, ligamentum rotundum,[51] and the vesicovaginal fascia.[52] Furthermore, stress incontinent women synthesize less collagen[53] and not only have a reduction in the total collagen in the tissue but also a mechanically weaker fiber as demonstrated by an alteration in the cross-links that stabilize the collagen fibers.[54] Genitourinary prolapse is often implicated in causing stress incontinence, and this too appears to be secondary to collagen deficiency.[55]

Collagen levels fall after the menopause, but there is a negative correlation between menopausal age and skin collagen content.[56] Hormonal replacement therapy not only prevents this decline but actually replaces collagen content,[57] alters collagen type ratios,[58] and stabilizes cross-links.[59]

Therefore it seems that collagen deficiency is implicated in both stress incontinence and genitourinary prolapse and that the metabolism of collagen is adversely affected by the altered hormonal environment after the menopause. The therapeutic implications of this are worthy of further research.

DENERVATION

An association between urinary stress incontinence and denervation of the urethral sphincter, pelvic floor striated musculature, and anal sphincter has been demonstrated.[60-63] Furthermore, denervation increases with age.[64]

It is well known that there is an association between childbirth and urinary incontinence. The reason is believed to be a combination of mechanical sphincter and muscle damage and denervation injury. Electrophysiologic studies have shown that in most cases there is evidence of denervation of the pelvic floor muscles,[65] there being significantly prolonged pudendal-nerve terminal motor latencies when one is comparing women after vaginal delivery with those delivering by cesarean section and controls. Additionally, prolonged second stage of labor and forceps delivery correlated with neurophysiologic evidence of pudendal neuropathy and partial denervation of the pelvic floor striated sphincter musculature, with this evidence being more pronounced in those women who had developed incontinence at a 5-year follow-up rather than earlier.[66] Concentric needle electromyographic work has confirmed nerve damage after vaginal delivery in 80% of women delivering their first child with a long active second stage, and the birth of heavier babies is associated with the most damage.[67]

MUSCLE DAMAGE

Although little work has been undertaken looking at the anatomy of the lower urinary tract after childbirth, anal endosonography has clearly shown it to be associated with disruption of the pelvic floor, since there has been damage to the anal sphincter and perineal body.[68,69] It seems likely that this results in urinary and fecal incontinence. Histochemical studies of pelvic floor muscle biopsy specimens from women with urinary stress incontinence have supported the neurophysiologic findings by demonstrating evidence of muscle fiber damage.[70]

In summary, the cause of sphincter incompetence appears to be neuromuscular damage associated with childbirth, with this damage persisting into old age. Aging results in further denervation, and the hypoestrogenic postmenopausal state further contributes through observed alterations in pelvic collagen metabolism and a possible reduction in urethral blood flow.

OVERFLOW INCONTINENCE

The most common voiding disorder in the elderly is that secondary to male prostatic obstruction. In addition there is a high incidence of poor detrusor contractility, which can affect either sex and may impair voiding even in the absence of outlet obstruction. This may relate to muscle cell degeneration.[24] These factors make the elderly susceptible to urinary retention, which, if chronic, can be painless and can be complicated by overflow urinary incontinence.

Factors that can precipitate urinary retention in the elderly include constipation, drugs (such as alpha-adrenergic agonists or drugs with anticholinergic properties; see below), and bed confinement. These factors probably unmask a previous subclinical voiding dysfunction. Neurologic disorders likely to cause voiding dysfunction and retention in the elderly include spinal cord compression secondary to vertebral collapse and spinal cord lesions such as tumors. Strokes impair detrusor contractility initially, but this is commonly later replaced by detrusor hyperreflexia, whereas Parkinson's can also cause voiding dysfunction as a result of sphincter dyssynergia[71] or poor detrusor contractility.[72]

Sensory loss may lead to progressive bladder distension, voiding dysfunction, and eventual acontractility and urinary overflow incontinence. Diabetes mellitus is the commonest disorder implicated, with tabes dorsalis being rare now. Up to 70% of diabetics can have impaired bladder sensation, with 15% being acontractile.[73]

URINARY TRACT INFECTIONS

Urinary infections are more common in the elderly, occurring in up to 46% of long-stay geriatric patients over the course of a year.[74] By altering bladder sensation they can cause urinary incontinence, characteristically sensory urge incontinence. Impaired immunologic response, voiding dysfunction and urinary stasis, atrophic genital changes, concurrent fecal incontinence, and poor fluid intake are some of the factors that predispose to the higher incidence of urinary tract infections in the elderly.

CONFUSIONAL STATES

Structural brain damage, poor cerebral circulation, metabolic disorders, infections, or drug toxicity can cause acute or chronic confusional states, often resulting in the loss of social conditioning with micturition at inappropriate times and in inappropriate places. In addition, as discussed above, neurologic pathologic states are frequently associated with DHR, and reduced cerebral perfusion can be the cause of "idiopathic" DI.[20]

IMMOBILITY

If the patient suffers with detrusor instability, immobility that results in delay getting to the toilet or delay undressing once there can result in urinary incontinence rather than the frequency and urgency that may be the less troublesome symptoms in the more mobile and dextrous person.

Drug Therapy

Polypharmacy, or the use of multiple medications concurrently, is common among the elderly. Older Americans consume concurrently an average of over four medications each, and 40% of nursing home residents take inappropriate drugs.[75] Iatrogenic incontinence is common; up to 60% of patients with incontinence are taking between one and four drugs with potentially adverse lower urinary tract effects.[76] Drugs can adversely affect the lower urinary tract in the following ways:

1. *Increased urine production.* Diuretic medication, including alcohol, aggravates any lower urinary tract symptoms (LUTS) by increasing the rate of bladder filling.
2. *Decreased bladder contractility.* Drugs with an anticholinergic action, alpha-adrenergic agonists, and calcium-channel blockers have the potential to decrease bladder contractility. When they are combined with the poor intrinsic detrusor contractility that can occur in the elderly, there is a risk that these preparations can induce urinary retention and subsequent overflow urinary incontinence.
3. *Increased urethral tone.* Alpha-adrenergic receptors may be responsible for exerting a tonic sympathetic stimulation on the smooth musculature around the bladder neck and proximal portion of the urethra. Phenylpropanolamine has been shown to improve urethral sphincteric insufficiency,[77] and there is potential for such drugs to precipitate urinary retention in patients with an underlying predisposition.
4. *Decreased urethral tone.* On the other hand, the use of alpha-adrenergic blockers can often be correlated with a decrease in urethral-profile closure pressures. Beta-adrenergic agonists, particularly those with beta$_2$-adrenergic characteristics, are able to produce relaxation of slow-twitch skeletal muscle, such as that occurring in the outermost urethral wall, which may account for the decrease in urethral-profile parameters seen with terbutaline. The benzodiazepines also have muscle-relaxant effects, probably secondary to central activity on GABA receptor sites on central nervous system membranes. Whether they exert any effect on the urethral pressure profile is unknown, but they have been shown to be effective promoters of spontaneous voiding after colposuspension surgery.[78] The use of all these compounds may therefore reasonably be expected to aggravate urinary stress incontinence.

Conclusions

The approach to urinary incontinence in the elderly population differs little from that in younger patients. False preconceptions that urinary incontinence in most elderly patients is associated with immobility and cerebral disease originate from early reports on geriatric inpatients,[79,80] and it is now accepted that the pathophysiologic characteristics of incontinence, even in the severely disabled elderly with dementia or severe immobility, does not differ greatly from their peers without such an impairment.[6] Before extensive investigation is embarked upon, simple measures should be taken to exclude or rectify constipation, infection, urinary retention, and inappropriate medication and to improve mobility and toilet access. Once this has been done evaluation of the lower urinary tract function is recommended; a urodynamic assessment may avoid prolonged medication with inappropriate and poorly tolerated drugs and allow contemplation of surgery. Patients should not be denied these benefits on the basis of their age alone.

References

1. Diokno AC, Brock BM, Brown MB, et al: Prevalence of urinary incontinence and other urological symptoms in the noninstitutionalized elderly, *J Urol* 136:1022-1025, 1986.
2. Yarnell JWG, St Leger AS: The prevalence, severity and factors associated with urinary incontinence in a random sample of the elderly, *Age Ageing* 8:81-85, 1979.
3. Thomas TM, Plymat KR, Blannin J, et al: Prevalence of urinary incontinence, *Br Med J* 281:1243-1245, 1980.
4. Ehrman JS: Correspondence from Washington, use of biofeedback to treat incontinence, *J Am Geriatr Soc* 31:182-184, 1983.
5. Grimby A, Milson I, Molander U, et al: The influence of urinary incontinence on the quality of lifeof elderly women, *Age Ageing* 22:82-89, 1993.
6. Resnick NM, Yalla SV, Laurino E: The pathophysiology of urinary incontinence among institutionalised elderly persons, *N Engl J Med* 320:1-7, 1989.
7. Stamey TA: Endoscopic suspension of the vesical neck for urinary incontinence in females: report on 203 consecutive patients, *Ann Surg* 192:465-471, 1980.
8. Stanton SL, Cardozo LD: Surgical treatment of incontinence in elderly women, *Surg Gynecol Obstet* 150:555-557, 1980.
9. Gillon G, Stanton SL: Long-term follow-up of surgery for urinary incontinence in elderly women, *Br J Urol* 56:478-481, 1984.
10. Shafik A: Prostatic commissurotomy: a simple techniqe for the treatment of benign prostatic hypertrophy, *Br J Urol* 58:157-160, 1986.
11. Griffiths Jones MD, Abrams PA: The Stamey endoscopic bladder neck suspension in the elderly, *Br J Urol* 65:170-172, 1990.
12. Couillard DR, Deckard-Janatpour KA, Stone AR: The vaginal wall sling: a compressivesuspension procedure for recurrent incontinence in elderly patients, *Urology* 43:203-208, 1994.
13. Golomb J, Goldwasser B, Mashiach S: Raz bladder neck suspension in women younger than sixty-five years compared with elderly women: three years experience, *Urology* 43:40-43, 1994.
14. Keane DP, Eckford SD, Shepherd AM, et al: Referral patterns and diagnoses in women attending a urodynamic unit, *Br Med J* 305:808, 1992.
15. Hilton P, Stanton SL: Algorithmic method of assessing urinary incontinence in elderly women, *Br Med J* 282:940-942, 1981.
16. Castleden CM, Duffin HM, Asher MJ: Clinical and urodynamic studies in 100 elderly incontinent patients, *Br Med J* 282:1103-1105, 1981.
17. Fitzmaurice H, Fowler CJ, Rickards D, et al: Micturition disturbances in Parkinsons disease, *Br J Urol* 57:625-626, 1985.
18. Philp T, Read DJ, Higson RH: The urodynamic characteristics of multiple sclerosis, *Br J Urol* 53:672-675, 1981.
19. Lockhart JL, Webster GD, Sheremata W, et al: Neurogenic bladder dysfunction in the Shy-Drager syndrome, *J Urol* 126:119-121, 1981.
20. Griffiths DJ, MaCracken PN, Harrison GM, et al: Cerebral aetiology of urinary urge incontinence in elderly people, *Age Ageing* 23:246-250, 1994.
21. Abrams PH, Farrar DJ, Turner-Warwick RT, et al. The results of prostatectomy: a symptomatic and urodynamic analysis of 152 patients, *J Urol* 121:640-642, 1979.

22. Gormley EA, Griffiths DJ, McCracken PN, et al: Effect of transurethral resection of the prostate on detrusor instability and urge incontinence in elderly males, *Neurourol Urodyn* 12:445-453, 1993.
23. Brading AF, Parekh AB, Tomita T: Tissue impedance of smooth muscles isolated from guinea-pig, *J Physiol* 417:63, 1989.
24. Elbadawi A, Yalla SV, Resnick NM: Structural basis of geriatric voiding dysfunction. III. Detrusor overactivity, *J Urol* 150:1668-1680, 1993.
25. Resnick NM, Yalla SV: Detrusor hyperactivity with impaired contractile function, *JAMA* 257:3076-3081, 1987.
26. Fujii K: Evidence for adenosine triphosphate as an excitatory transmitter in guinea-pig, rabbit and pig urinary bladder, *J Physiol* 404:39-52, 1985.
27. Kinder RB, Mundy AR: Pathophysiology of idiopathic detrusor instability and detrusor hyper-reflexia: an in vitro study of human detrusor muscle, *Br J Urol* 60:509-515, 1987.
28. German K, Bedwani J, Davies J, et al: What is the pathophysiology of detrusor hyperreflexia? *Neurourol Urodyn* 12:335-336, 1993.
29. Speakman MJ, Brading AF, Gilpin CJ, et al: Bladder outflow obstruction: a cause of denervation supersensitivity, *J Urol* 138:1461-1466, 1987.
30. Harrison SCW, Ferguson DR, Doyle PT: Effect of bladder outflow obstruction on the innervation of the rabbit urinary bladder, *Br J Urol* 66:372-379, 1990.
31. Gosling J, Gilpin SA, Dixon JS, Gilpin CJ: Decrease in the autonomic innervation of human detrusor muscle in outflow obstruction, *J Urol* 136:501-504, 1986.
32. Harrison SCW, Hunnam GR, Farman P, et al: Bladder instability and denervation in patients with bladder outflow obstruction, *Br J Urol* 60:519-522, 1987.
33. Cumming JA, Chisholm GD: Changes in detrusor innervation with relief of outflow tract obstruction, *Br J Urol* 69:7-11, 1992.
34. Brading AF, Turner WH: The unstable bladder: towards a common mechanism, *Br J Urol* 73:3-8, 1994.
35. Westfall DP, Lee TJF, Stitzel RE: Morphological and biochemical changes in supersensitive smooth muscle, *Fed Proc* 34:1985-1989, 1975.
36. Lee TJF, Westfall DP, Fleming WW: The correlation between spontaneous contractions and postjunctional supersensitivity of the smooth muscle of the rat vas deferens, *J Pharm Exp Ther* 192:136-148, 1975.
37. Sethia KK, Brading AF, Smith JC: An animal model of non-obstructive instability, *J Urol* 143:1243-1246, 1990.
38. Restorick JM, Mundy AR: The density of cholinergic and alpha and beta adrenergic receptors in the normal and hyper-reflexic human detrusor, *Br J Urol* 63:32-35, 1988.
39. Eaton AC, Bates CP: An in vitro study of normal and unstable human detrusor muscle, *Br J Urol* 54:653-657, 1982.
40. Sjögren C, Andersson K-E, Husted S, et al: Atropine resistance to transmurally stimulated isolated human bladder muscle, *J Urol* 128:1368-1371, 1982.
41. Edwards L, Malvern J: The urethral pressure profile: theoretical considerations and clinical application, *Br J Urol* 46:325-336, 1974.
42. Rekers H, Drogendijk AC, Valkenburg HA, et al: The menopause, urinary incontinence and other symptoms of the genito-urinary tract, *Maturitas* 15:101-111, 1992.
43. Zinner NR, Sterling AM, Ritter RC: Role of inner urethral softness in urinary incontinence, *Urology* 16:115-117, 1980.
44. Berkow SG: The corpus spongiosum of the urethra: its possible role in urinary control and stress incontinence in women, *Am J Obstet Gynecol* 65:346-351, 1953.
45. Enhorning G: Simultaneous recording of intravesical and intraurethral pressure, *Acta Chir Scand* 276(suppl):1-6, 1961.
46. Raz T, Caine H, Zeigler M: The vascular component in the production of intraurethral pressure, *J Urol* 108:93-96, 1972.
47. Greenland JE, Brading AF: *Urethral lamina propria blood flow changes during voiding,* Bristol, 1994, International Continence Society, U.K. Section.
48. Versi E, Cardozo LD: Urethral vascular pulsations, *Proc Int Cont Soc* 593-594, 1985.
49. Tsai CC, Semmens JP, Semmens EC, et al: Vaginal physiology in postmenopausal women, *South Med J* 80:987-990, 1987.
50. Versi E, Cardozo L, Brincat M, et al: Correlation of urethral physiology and skin collagen in postmenopausal women, *Br J Obstet Gynaecol* 95:147-152, 1988.
51. Ulmsten U, Ekman G, Giertz G, et al: Different biomechanical composition of connective tissue in continent and stress incontinent women, *Acta Obstet Gynecol Scand* 66:455, 1987.
52. Rechberger T, Donica H, Baranowski W, et al: Female urinary stress incontinence in terms of connective tissue biochemistry, *Eur J Obstet Gynecol Reprod Biol* 49:187-191, 1993.
53. Falconer C, Ekman G, Malmstrom A, et al: Decreased collagen synthesis in stress-incontinent women, *Obstet Gynaecol* 84:583-586, 1994.
54. Keane DP, Sims TJ, Bailey AJ, et al: Analysis of pelvic floor electromyography and collagen status in pre-menopausal nulliparous females with genuine stress incontinence, *Neurourol Urodyn* 11:308-309, 1992.
55. Jackson SR, Avery N, Jameson T, et al: Connective tissue analysis in genitourinary prolapse, *Proc R Soc Med,* 1995.
56. Brincat M, Moniz CJ, Studd JW, et al: Long-term effects of the menopause and sex hormones on skin thickness, *Br J Obstet Gynaecol* 92:256-259, 1985.
57. Brincat M, Versi E, Moniz CF, et al: Skin collagen changes in postmenopausal women receiving different regimens of estrogen therapy, *Obstet Gynecol* 70:123-127, 1987.
58. Savvas M, Bishop J, Laurent G, et al: Type III collagen content in the skin of postmenopausal women receiving oestradiol and testosterone implants, *Br J Obstet Gynaecol* 100:154-156, 1993.
59. Holland EF, Studd JW, Mansell JP, et al: Changes in collagen composition and cross-links in bone and skin of osteoporotic postmenopausal women treated with percutaneous estradiol implants, *Obstet Gynecol* 83:180-183, 1994.
60. Vereecken RL, De Meirsman G, Puers B: Sphincter electromyography in female incontinence. In *Advances in diagnostic urology,* Berlin, 1981, Springer-Verlag, pp 314-318.
61. Anderson RS: A neurogenic element to urinary genuine stress incontinence, *Br J Obstet Gynaecol* 91:41-45, 1984.
62. Snooks SJ, Badenoch D, Tiptaft R, et al: Perineal nerve damage in genuine stress urinary incontinence, *Br J Urol* 57:422-426, 1985.
63. Smith ARB, Hosker GL,Warrell DW: The role of pudendal nerve damage in the aetiology of genuine stress incontinence of urine: a neurophysiological study, *Br J Obstet Gynaecol* 96:29-32, 1989.
64. Smith ARB, Hosker GL, Warrell DW: The role of partial denervation of the pelvic floor in aetiology of genitourinary prolapse and stress incontinence of urine: a neurophysiological study, *Br J Obstet Gynaecol* 96:24-28, 1989.
65. Snooks SJ, Swash M, Setchell M, et al: Injury to the pelvic floor sphincter musculature in childbirth, *Lancet* 2:546-550, 1984.
66. Snooks SJ, Swash M, Mathers SE, et al: Effect of vaginal delivery on the pelvic floor: a 5 year follow-up, *Br J Surg* 77:1358-1360, 1990.
67. Allen RE, Hosker GL, Smith ARB, et al: Pelvic floor damage and childbirth: a neurophysiological study, *Br J Obstet Gynaecol* 97:770-779, 1990.
68. Burnett SJ, Spence-Jones C, Speakman CT, et al: Unsuspected sphincter damage following childbirth revealed by anal endosonography, *Br J Radiol* 64:225-227, 1991.
69. Kamm MA: Obstetric damage and faecal incontinence, *Lancet* 344(8924):730-733, 1994.
70. Gilpin SA, Gosling JA, Smith ARB, et al: The pathogenesis of genitourinary prolapse and stress incontinence of urine: a histopathological and histochemical study, *Br J Obstet Gynaecol* 96:15-23, 1989.

71. Christmas TJ, Chapple CR, Lees AJ, et al: Role of subcutaneous apomorphine in Parkinsonian voiding dysfunction, *Lancet* 2:1451-1453, 1988.
72. Malone Lee JG, Wiseman P: Detrusor function in Parkinson's disease, *Neurourol Urodyn* 10:355-356, 1991.
73. Buck AC, McRae CU, Chisholm GD: The diabetic bladder, *Proc R Soc Med* 67:81-83, 1974.
74. Brocklehurst JC, Bee P, Jones D, Palmer MK: Bacteriuria in geriatric hospital patients: its correlates and management, *Age Ageing* 6:240-245, 1977.
75. Beers MH, Ouslander JG, Fingold SF, et al: Inappropriate medication prescribing in skilled nursing facilities, *Ann Intern Med* 117:684-689, 1992.
76. Gormley EA, Griffiths DJ, McCracken PN, et al: Polypharmacy and its effects on urinary incontinence in a geriatric population, *Br J Urol* 71:265-269, 1993.
77. Walter S, Kjaergaard B, Lose G, et al: Stress urinary incontinence in postmenopausal women treated with oral estrogen (estriol) and an alpha adrenergic stimulating agar (phenylpropanolamine): a randomised double-blind placebo controlled study, *Int Urogynecol J* 1:74, 1990.
78. Stanton SL, Cardozo LD, Kerr-Wilson R: Treatment of delayed onset of spontaneous voiding after surgery for incontinence, *Urology* 13:494, 1979.
79. Isaacs B, Walkey FA: A survey of incontinence in elderly hospital patients, *Gerontologia Clinica* 6:367-376, 1964.
80. Brocklehurst JC, Dillane JB: Studies of the female bladder in old age. II. Cystometrograms in 100 incontinent women, *Gerontologia Clinica* 8:306-319, 1966.

Chapter 58 Behavior Therapy

Kathryn L. Burgio, Patricia S. Goode

Behavior therapies are a group of extremely important treatment options for older people that improve bladder control by changing the incontinent person's behavior or environment. Behavioral therapies involve learning new skills and strategies for preventing urine loss. Thus they are most appropriate for nondemented individuals who are both able and willing to take an active role in their own treatment by practicing these new skills and making some changes in their daily habits. The most widely used treatments for these patients are pelvic muscle training and exercise, biofeedback, behavioral strategies for dealing with urgency, and bladder training.

Behavior Therapy as a First-Line Therapy

In 1988 the National Institutes of Health Consensus Conference on Urinary Incontinence in Adults concluded that "in general, the least invasive or dangerous procedure should be tried first . . . for many types of incontinence, behavioral treatments meet this criterion."[1] Indeed for stress, urge, and mixed urinary incontinence, which are the most common forms of incontinence in community-dwelling older adults, behavior therapy is an appropriate, low-risk, first-line intervention. In addition, behavioral procedures are especially attractive for older men and women because they avoid the common side effects associated with medications prescribed for incontinence. Finally, for those older persons who have medical conditions that are relative contraindications to medications such as alpha-adrenergic or anticholinergic agents for incontinence, behavioral treatments provide a safe alternative.

Although it is still widely believed that behavioral treatments are minimally effective, several years of research on these methods now provide compelling evidence to the contrary.[2-19] With proper training, motivation, and time, most appropriately selected patients experience significant improvement or complete control with behavioral intervention. There is also growing evidence that significant reduction in the frequency of incontinent episodes, even in the absence of total cure, produces a high level of satisfaction in most older patients. This is not to say that behavior therapy is always the best solution, only that it is an effective, low-risk option that can be offered to patients as a first-line approach, an adjunct to another therapy, or when other therapies have failed.

The Bladder Diary

Before behavioral treatment is begun, an appropriate evaluation that includes a behavioral assessment of incontinence should be performed. This can be accomplished with a careful interview to explore the frequency, timing, and volume of urine loss with particular attention given to the antecedents or precipitants of urine loss. The bladder diary is an extremely useful tool for documenting voiding habits and patterns of incontinence on a daily basis (see Appendix C). The diary serves two purposes. First, it provides a picture of the patient's behavior that, together with the interview, can be used to identify preventable causes of incontinence and formulate an accurate diagnosis and treatment plan. Second, it can be used to evaluate progress and test the effectiveness of treatment. Self-recording eliminates an important source of error by circumventing the patient's verbal report. It can be difficult for patients to judge the frequency or patterns of incontinence retrospectively, especially if the patterns are irregular. Keeping a diary for a period of two weeks will often reveal patterns of variability that the patient finds difficult to communicate. Patients are sometimes surprised at the actual number of accidents once they are required to record them.

Patients may profess improvement, whereas their diaries showed no change in the volume or frequency of accidents. Thus the bladder diary can compensate for any tendencies patients may have to report positively on their progress for the purpose of pleasing the doctor. There are many different forms of bladder diaries. An example is displayed in Appendix I. Whatever form of bladder diary is selected, it should be small enough to be carried everywhere by the patient so that entries can be made in a timely fashion. It also should be simple enough that patients do not become burdened or confused by too many entries.

To assess the timing and severity of urine loss, patients should record the occurrence of every episode of urine loss large or small. When the time is noted, the therapist can examine the diary for clues in the temporal pattern of urine loss. For example, large accidents first thing in the morning might require a specific treatment plan different from that designed for small accidents throughout the day with no temporal pattern. It is also essential to have patients record the reasons for or circumstances of incontinent episodes. This helps to distinguish stress incontinence from urge incontinence, which is essential for understanding the mechanisms of urine loss and for the selection of a treatment plan. Further, the specific circumstances of urine loss for an individual patient yields invaluable information for designing and tailoring intervention.

It is the nature of behavior therapy that change or improvement occurs gradually over time. Learning takes time, and muscles require time to be strengthened. It is important that the patient be encouraged and supported during the early phases of treatment until therapeutic results are evident. Gradual changes that are often unnoticed by the patient can be measured by means of the bladder diary and demonstrated objectively. Objective feedback of such small changes can help to maintain the motivation and persistence needed for a successful outcome.

STRESS INCONTINENCE

The goal of behavior therapy for stress incontinence is to teach patients how to use voluntary contractions of the pelvic muscles to occlude the urethra and prevent urine loss during physical exertion. This involves helping the patient to identify, exercise, and then use the pelvic muscles actively in everyday life.

Biofeedback: Identifying the Pelvic Muscles

Traditionally, pelvic muscle exercises have been taught by brief verbal instructions to interrupt the urinary stream or lift the pelvic floor. Such verbal or written instructions are not widely effective because patients usually are not able to identify or isolate the pelvic muscles properly. It is more useful to provide immediate verbal feedback of attempted pelvic muscle contractions based on vaginal or anal palpation. Perhaps the best way to be sure that the patient acquires the proper pelvic muscle contraction is to actually measure muscle activity and provide immediate visual or auditory feedback of muscle responses using biofeedback. Biofeedback is a behavioral training technique that facilitates the acquisition of control over physiologic responses of which we are normally unaware, in this case, learning to contract and relax pelvic muscles. Biofeedback not only facilitates learning but also ensures proper muscle response and, when achieved, helps to sustain patient motivation. There is some evidence in the literature that patients taught with biofeedback have a better outcome than those who learn without biofeedback.[9,11] Several approaches have been developed to measure pelvic muscle activity and provide biofeedback.

Vaginal manometry. Originally, Arnold Kegel devised a biofeedback device he called a "perineometer" for this purpose.[2,3] It consisted of a pneumatic chamber placed into the vagina and a hand-held external pressure gauge that registered the strength of vaginal muscle contractions. This device provided immediate visual feedback of pelvic muscle contractions to help women identify the proper muscle group and to guide pelvic muscle exercise. Although Kegel advocated using the perineometer to teach and guide pelvic muscle exercises, until recently few clinicians adopted this method.

Vaginal electromyography. More recently techniques have been developed to measure electrical activity of circumvaginal muscles. Surface electrodes may be placed inside the vagina, but it is easier and has become more popular to use electrodes embedded in a vaginal probe.[13] Different types of probes are distinguished by their unique placement of electrodes as well as size and shape, and feedback is provided by an auditory signal, light display, or a variety of graphics displayed on a computer monitor. Vaginal probes are usually comfortable and easy to insert and remove, making it possible for most patients to do this themselves making portable models, or "home trainers," possible for daily biofeedback sessions at home. One drawback of the home trainer is that patients who depend on the device for correct practice may lose interest in its use when the novelty wears off but before they have achieved the ability to exercise independently. Nevertheless, there are reports that the home trainers might enhance the effectiveness of training for some patients.

Urethral sphincter pressure and electromyography. A pressure-sensitive catheter may be used to measure intraurethral pressure. Although many urodynamic laboratories have access to such equipment, these catheters are quite costly and fragile; therefore it is unlikely that this technique will have widespread use. Periurethral muscle activity can also be recorded by electromyography using needle electrodes or wire electrodes inserted into the area or by surface electrodes attached to a urinary catheter. Although these techniques offer proximity to motor units of interest, they tend to be the most difficult to implement because of problems with consistent electrode placement, pain, and the need for sterile technique. Needles and wires are commonly used as methods of evaluation, but there is limited potential for their use in providing biofeedback.

Anal sphincter manometry and electromyography. It is well known that the external anal sphincter and the external urinary sphincter have similar innervation by means of branches of the pudendal nerve.[20-22] Several studies indicate that the sphincters act in concert,[23-27] and there is evidence to indicate that training and controlling the anal sphincter results in urinary sphincter activity that corresponds in magnitude.[28] Therefore biofeedback of the external anal sphincter can be used for the treatment of urinary incontinence. Activity of the anal sphincter can be measured with ease and comfort using a small air-filled balloon placed at the anal opening or by means of surface electrodes placed in the perianal area or embedded in an anal probe. This is particularly helpful for women with inability to use intravaginal devices because of severe surgical narrowing or shortening of the vagina, as well as for men with postprostatectomy stress incontinence.

Abdominal Muscle Biofeedback

Regardless of the particular technique used to measure and train pelvic muscle responses, there is one difficulty that is encountered universally—the distinct tendency among most incontinent individuals to contract other muscle groups simultaneously with pelvic muscles. Contractions of other muscles is not only unhelpful but most often counterproductive as well. It is common, for example, to observe tightening of rectus abdominis muscles, buttocks, or thighs during attempts at maximal pelvic muscle contraction to avoid incontinence. Abdominal contraction increases intravesical pressure and consequently contributes to the pressure that expels urine from the bladder. To minimize inappropriate tensing of abdominal muscles, it is helpful to train patients to relax these muscles while contracting pelvic muscles. Some patients will accomplish this by means of simple instruction, deep breathing, and relaxation, or by feedback from placing a hand on the abdomen. However, for many patients these techniques are not adequate, and some form of simultaneous abdominal muscle biofeedback is required to acquire selective control. This may be accomplished by use of surface electrodes on the abdomen (measuring a rectus abdominis EMG) or with a rectal balloon (measuring intra-abdominal pressure).

Combined Pelvic Muscle and Abdominal Biofeedback

One convenient method uses a three-balloon anorectal probe developed by a gastroenterologist and used originally for manometric assessment of anorectal responses and to provide biofeedback in the treatment of fecal incontinence.[29,30] Subsequently, this method has been applied to the treatment of urinary incontinence. The anorectal assembly consists of a rectal tube with three small balloons attached, which are inserted and then inflated with air. The balloon positioned inside the rectum measures intra-abdominal pressure; the balloon positioned at the anal opening measures activity of the external anal sphincter; a third balloon positioned at the internal anal sphincter stabilizes the recording apparatus but provides no data when used for treatment of urinary incontinence. With this combined pelvic muscle and abdominal biofeedback training, it is possible for most patients to contract and relax pelvic floor muscles selectively while keeping intra-abdominal pressure and thus bladder pressure low.

Once selective contraction is acquired it is important to train patients how to sustain contractions for up to 10 seconds with equal periods of rest between contractions. At first most patients exhibit only brief muscle contractions. This can be an indication of muscle weakness, but it may also be a reflection of a skill deficit. With biofeedback many patients can learn in a matter of minutes to sustain their pelvic muscle contractions. In addition to strengthening pelvic muscles, patients with stress incontinence can be trained to use muscle contraction during coughing, lifting, or other physical activities known to produce incontinence. Although muscle exercise may improve resting tone, the goal of training is to learn a skill: active contraction of pelvic muscles to produce a momentary rise in intraurethral pressure that is adequate to prevent urine loss during physical exertion.

Daily Practice

Daily practice has two functions. First, daily exercise increases the *strength* of pelvic muscles so that they can occlude the urethra more effectively, Second, repeated practice improves voluntary control of the pelvic muscles and allows the patient to use them quickly to avoid urine loss. Sample instructions for daily practice are presented in Appendix K. One exercise is defined as one pelvic muscle contraction sustained for up to 10 seconds with an equal period of rest. Although the ideal number of exercises has yet to be established, 45 to 50 per day is widely recommended and has yielded good results in several studies.[10-16,18] Very frail patients may need to start with 10 exercises per day and gradually over several weeks to increase this number until they attain 45 to 50 per day. Also, if patients are unable to sustain contractions for 10 seconds during the training session, they should be started on a shorter duration depending on their ability and then gradually over several weeks should increase how long they sustain their contractions. For all patients, the exercises should be divided between two or more sessions across the day to help avoid problems with muscle fatigue and to encourage awareness and frequent use of muscles.

It is best to recommend to patients that they do exercises in various positions, for example, lying, sitting, and standing. Commonly, the sensations generated by exercising are different in different positions. Further, it may be necessary to prevent leakage in any of these positions, and practicing in various positions helps the patients to feel comfortable and control pelvic muscles in all positions. It is not unusual that a patient complains of being unable to feel the muscles contracting when standing. Usually patients are contracting properly but simply cannot feel the contraction in this position. Because it is especially important to be able to use muscles in the standing position, they need to be reassured that sensation during contraction will increase as the muscles strengthen.

Exercise alone can increase resting tone, but active, maximal contraction is usually needed to prevent stress incontinence. Thus patients should be instructed and reminded to use their muscles actively to prevent urine loss during coughing, lifting, or whatever activity causes incontinence. Many patients complain that they forget to squeeze their muscles during a cough or sneeze, or that it came on too suddenly and they did not have time. This kind of problem is common to treatments that rely on behavior change and is normal when changing habits or developing new ones. A useful way to handle the problem is to encourage patients to squeeze as soon as they remember. This does not prevent the accident, but it helps to develop the new habit. Once the new habit is firmly established, using muscles becomes more automatic and thus requires less effort on the patient's part.

Muscles need time to gain strength, and people need time to master skills. Perhaps the biggest mistake people make is to give up too soon, sometimes after only a few days of practice. Typical is the story of a patient who tries the exercises for less than a week, judges them to be ineffective, and stops. It is the challenge of behavior therapy to sustain patient compliance with treatment procedures for a period of time until results are noticeable. This is best accomplished by maintenance of frequent contact with patients in follow-up visits every 1 to 2 weeks. This gives the therapist the opportunity to answer questions, dispel misconceptions, facilitate compliance, buffer setbacks, and reinforce progress. Usually patients will observe improvement within 2 to 4 weeks of exercise. Then the positive effects of treatment reinforce their efforts and help sustain the new habits, which need to be continued indefinitely.

URGE INCONTINENCE

The goal of behavior therapy for urge incontinence is to improve the patient's ability to inhibit detrusor contraction voluntarily using pelvic muscle training, urge strategies, or temporal voiding schedules such as bladder training.

Pelvic Muscle Training

Pelvic muscle training and exercises, generally associated with the treatment of stress incontinence, are also highly effective in the treatment of urge incontinence because pelvic muscles play a critical role in the control of detrusor function. Deliberate, voluntary contraction of pelvic muscles in response to the sensation of urgency can inhibit or abort detrusor contractions. Even in the presence of detrusor spasm, a strong contraction of periurethral muscles can occlude the urethra, preventing urine loss until the detrusor relaxes. The training can be accomplished in the same way as that described for stress incontinence, and the same instructions can be used for home practice (see Appendix K). However, instead of instructing patients to contract their muscles actively with physical exertion, they are taught to use strong pelvic muscle contractions in response to urgency. When pelvic muscle training alone does not produce the desired results, it can be conducted simultaneously with bladder-pressure biofeedback using a pressure-sensitive urethral catheter. Such combined bladder and sphincter biofeedback allows patients to observe bladder pressure and coordinate pelvic muscle contractions with any increases in bladder pressure. Further, the bladder can be filled incrementally to reproduce urgency in the clinic and give the patients the opportunity to practice using their muscles with a full bladder. The act of watching the bladder-pressure tracing during a detrusor contraction and of observing the rapid drop in intravesical pressure in response to pelvic muscle contraction demonstrates the effectiveness of the technique and motivates continued practice of the new skill.

Urge Strategies

Most patients with urge incontinence have developed a maladaptive way of responding to urgency. When they feel the urge to void, they rush to the toilet believing that the faster they get there, the more likely it is that they can avoid leaking. Although intuitively it seems as though it were the best thing to do, this behavior is actually counterproductive because it increases abdominal pressure on the bladder and can increase the feeling of urgency and bladder fullness. It also can stimulate bladder contractions and interfere with the concentration needed to inhibit detrusor contraction. Further, the closer one comes to the bathroom, the more salient are the cues that trigger urination. Since leakage often starts just before they reach the toilet, patients conclude that if they had gotten to the bathroom a little sooner, they would have avoided leakage. However, it is no coincidence that urgency reaches its peak or leakage begins just as the patient reaches the toilet. For the person with urge incontinence, the cues of the bathroom itself enhance detrusor contraction and trigger incontinence, and approaching the toilet may be the final determinant of urge incontinence. From this perspective, the worst time to head for the bathroom is when the patient already has a strong urge to void. The best time is before the onset of the urge or after the urge has passed. Although many people believe that urination is the only way to relieve the strong sensation of urgency, most urges come in waves that will pass even if voiding does not occur.

Behavioral training provides a new response pattern for coping with the sensation of urgency. Instead of rushing to the toilet, patients are instructed to sit or stand quietly and to repeatedly contract pelvic muscles to inhibit detrusor spasm. They should practice suppressing urgency, wait for the urge to subside, and then walk at a normal pace to the toilet. Patient instructions are summarized in Appendix L. These instructions usually seem counterintuitive to the patient, but most skeptics can be convinced to try this new strategy based on the failure of their current habits. It is crucial for the patient to understand that the strategy is a new skill that needs to be practiced and that their initial attempts may be unsuccessful. To avoid failure, the therapist should make certain that the patient has identified the pelvic muscles and has completed at least a week of pelvic muscle exercises. This will help ensure that the patient is familiar with the active use of the muscles and is somewhat prepared to use them under the challenging conditions of having a full bladder. The patient might also be told to try the strategy first under conditions that are relatively safe from embarrassment such as at home. Usually the first successful use of the urge strategy helps to confirm the usefulness of the strategy in the patient's mind and reinforces compliance with the new behavior.

BLADDER TRAINING AND VOIDING SCHEDULES

The voiding schedule is the main component of treatment procedures such as habit training and bladder training. Habit training is generally used in patients who are unable to learn new skills. They are prescribed on a fixed or flexible voiding schedule that avoids incontinence by having the patient empty the bladder regularly and before it reaches a volume that triggers urgency and incontinence. In habit training, the goal of therapy is to avoid leakage by keeping the bladder from reaching fullness; there is no effort to change bladder capacity or function. Habit training is useful for demented patients with motivated caregivers and can greatly decrease the number of incontinent episodes.

Bladder training is different in that the aim is to increase bladder capacity by gradually increasing the interval between voids. This approach is based on the bladder drill originally described by Frewen and used in an intensive form on an inpatient basis.[6,7] Subsequently, it has been modified and used successfully with outpatients.[17] Instructions for the therapist appear in Appendix M. Perhaps the most difficult part of bladder training is postponing urination until the next scheduled voiding time. Some patients find that a distraction such as reading will take their minds off the bladder and help them cope during this period. Clearly this is also an opportunity to combine behavioral interventions. If patients have learned to do pelvic muscle exercises, they can be instructed to squeeze those muscles several times to reduce urgency and help them cope until it is time to void. If they have learned urge strategies, they can implement these strategies to relax and inhibit detrusor contractions. Both of these interventions will prepare patients to postpone urination in a bladder training program.

Conclusion

The behavioral treatments described in this chapter are easily applied in the outpatient urology practice as well as outpatient gynecology and primary care medicine practices. There is ample evidence that the procedures can be implemented successfully by nurses, nurse practitioners, physical therapists, and other nonphysician health providers in many outpatient settings. Behavioral procedures have been shown to be effective for both men and women with stress or urge incontinence secondary to stroke[15] or prostatectomy[14] or of unknown cause.

Perhaps the most common pitfall encountered by new therapists is to underestimate the complexity and richness of this apparently simple group of therapies. The treatments are based on a highly developed science of human behavior that itself is elegant and complex. Although the individual components of behavior are easily learned by most older adults, the selection of appropriate techniques, the timing of their introduction, the encouragement of practice, and the incorporation of their use into the patient's daily routine require considerable expertise on the part of the therapist. The therapist who acquires a knowledge of fundamental behavioral principles, and classical and operant conditioning will be best prepared to implement behavioral treatments for incontinence. Specific training with an experienced clinician is important, and after that, there is no substitute for experience in discovering the various ways of implementing these treatments based on the individual characteristics of the patient, the nature of their home environment, the type of urinary dysfunction, and their voiding habits, motivation, ability, and willingness to change behavior. A standardized behavioral protocol will yield some success, but optimal results will be obtained only when the treatments are individualized.

Behavior therapies are based on the learning process. The ability to remain continent is learned in childhood. The loss of bladder control can usually be partially or totally reversed through relearning old skills or by learning new skills and habits to compensate for deficits. Thus patients selected for behavior therapy should not only be *able* to learn but be *willing* to learn as well. They should be made aware that their progress and success in the program will depend mainly on their active participation and persistence. The patients who choose behavior therapy, whether as a first-line therapy, should understand the nature of the therapy, have reasonable expectations about its course, and be prepared for their critical role in achieving a successful outcome.

References

1. Consensus Conference: Urinary incontinence in adults, *JAMA* 261:2685-2690, 1989.
2. Kegel AH: Progressive resistance exercise in the functional restoration of the perineal muscles, *Am J Obstet Gyncol* 56:238-248, 1948.
3. Kegel AH: Stress incontinence of urine in woman: physiologic treatment, *J Int Coll Surg* 25:487-499, 1956.
4. Cardozo LD, Stanton SL, Hafner J, Allan V: Biofeedback in the treatment of detrusor instability, *Br J Urol* 50:250-254, 1978.
5. Cardozo LD, Abrams PD, Stanton SL, Feneley RCL: Idiopathic bladder instability treated by biofeedback, *Br J Urol* 50:27-30, 1978.
6. Frewen WK: An objective assessment of the unstable bladder of psychosomatic origin, *Br J Urol* 50:246-249, 1978.
7. Frewen WK: The management of urgency and frequency of micturition, *Br J Urol* 52:367-369, 1980.
8. Jarvis GJ, Miller DR: Controlled trial of bladder drill for detrusor instability, *Br Med J* 281:1322-1323, 1980.
9. Shepherd AM, Montgomery E, Anderson RS: Treatment of genuine stress incontinence with a new perineometer, *Physiotherapy* 69:113, 1983.
10. Burgio KL, Whitehead WE, Engel BT: Urinary incontinence in the elderly: Bladder-sphincter biofeedback and toileting skills training, *Ann Intern Med* 104:507-515, 1985.
11. Burgio KL, Robinson JC, Engel BT: The role of biofeedback in Kegel exercise training for stress urinary incontinence, *Am J Obstet Gynecol* 157:58-64, 1986.
12. Burton JR, Pearce KL, Burgio KL, et al: Behavioral training for urinary incontinence in elderly ambulatory patients, *J Am Geriatr Soc* 36:693-698, 1988.
13. Baigis-Smith J, Smith DAJ, Rose M, Newman DK: Managing urinary incontinence in community-residing elderly persons, *Gerontologist* 29:229-233, 1989.
14. Burgio KL, Stutzman RE, Engel BT: Behavioral training for post-prostatectomy urinary incontinence, *J Urol* 141:303-306, 1989.
15. Middaugh SJ, Whitehead WE, Burgio KL, Engel BT: Biofeedback in treatment of urinary incontinence ins troke patients, *Biofeedback Self Regul* 14:3-19, 1989.
16. Burns PA, Pranikoff K, Nochajski T, et al: Treatment of stress incontinence with pelvic floor exercises and biofeedback, *J Am Geriatr Soc* 38:341-344, 1990.
17. Fantl JA, Wyman JF, McClish DK, et al: Efficacy of bladder training in older women with urinary incontinence, *JAMA* 265:609-613, 1991.
18. Wells TJ, Brink CA, Diokno AD, et al: Pelvic muscle exercise for stress urinary incontinence in elderly women, *J Am Geriatr Soc* 39:785-791, 1991.
19. McDowell BJ, Burgio KL, Dombrowski M, et al: Interdisciplinary approach to the assessment and behavioral treatment of urinary incontinence in geriatric outpatients, *J Am Geriatr Soc* 40:370-374, 1992.
20. Bradley W, Timm GW, Scott FB: Innervation of the detrusor muscle and urethra. In *Symposium on neurogenic bladder, Urologic Clinics of North America,* 1:3-27 Philadelphia, 1974, Saunders.
21. Snooks SJ, Swash M: The innervation of the muscles of continence, *Ann R Coll Surg Engl* 68:45-49, 1986.
22. Schuster M: Motor action of rectum and anal sphincters in continence and defecation. In Code CF, editor: *Handbook of physiology: alimentary canal,* vol 4, Washington, D.C., 1968, American Physiological Society.
23. Sundin T, Petersen I: Cystometry and simultaneous electromyography for the striated urethral and anal sphincters and from levator ani, *Invest Urol* 13:40-46, 1975.

24. Rodriguez AA, Award E: Detrusor muscle and sphincteric response to anorectal stimulation in spinal cord injury, *Arch Phys Med Rehabil* 60:269-272, 1979.
25. Lose G, Tanko A, Colstrup H, Anderson JT: Urethral sphincter electromyography with vaginal surface electrodes: a comparison with sphincter electromyography recorded via periurethral coaxial, anal sphincter needle and perianal surface electrodes, *J Urol* 133:815-818, 1985.
26. Vereecken RL, Verduyn H: The electrical activity of the paraurethral and perineal muscles in normal and pathological conditions, *Br J Urol* 42:457, 1970.
27. Scott FB, Quesada EM, Cardus D: Studies on dynamics of micturition: observations on healthy men, *J Urol* 92:455-463, 1964.
28. Burgio KL, Engel BT, Quilter RE, Arena VC: The relationship between external anal and external urethral sphincter activity in continent women, *Neurourol Urodyn* 10:555-62, 1991.
29. Whitehead WE, Schuster MM: Manometric and electromyographic techniques for assessment of the anorectal mechanism for continence and defecation. In Hoelzl R, Whitehead WE, editors: *Psychophysiology of the gastrointestinal tract: experimental and clinical applications,* New York, 1983, Plenum.
30. Engel BT, Nikoomanesh P, Schuster MM: Operant conditioning of rectosphincteric responses in the treatment of fecal incontinence, *N Engl J Med* 290:646, 1974.

Chapter 59 Pharmacologic Management

Scott A. MacDiarmid

Urinary incontinence in older people occurs at a time in their life when physical impairments often restrict their daily activities and coexisting medical conditions frequently complicate the management of incontinence. The cause of incontinence in older people is more complex than in younger adults, which further complicates treatment of incontinence in this group. Because of the complexity of incontinence in older people and coexisting morbid conditions, conservative therapy is frequently the preferred initial treatment approach for older patients. Pharmacologic therapy of urinary incontinence in older people is an important initial conservative therapeutic approach for this group. However, pharmacologic therapy has many limitations in the elderly because of a lower tolerance for side effects and of frequently less effective clinical responses when compared with younger patients.

Although there are often problems with side effects and the efficacy of pharmacologic therapy of urinary incontinence in older patients, use of medications for treatment of incontinence should always be considered by the clinician in these patients. For example, when medications result in side effects in older patients, lower doses can be used in combination with other medications, which can also be used in lower doses. Often, multiple medications can be used at lower doses in older patients to achieve the desired pharmacologic effect on bladder function. Also, behavioral therapy is extremely effective in older people. Pharmacologic therapy and behavioral therapy can be combined to achieved the desired clinical response of improving the quality of life of the older person by decreasing the severity of incontinence without compromising the treatment outcome with intolerable side effects of medications.

Successful pharmacologic management of incontinence in older people is dependent on clinical information obtained from the history, physical exam, and urodynamic studies, which are extremely important for these patients. Although "trial-and-error" pharmacologic management of older patients can be done, without excellent urodynamic information the outcome often becomes an "error." The problem with older patients is the complexity of the bladder and urethral dysfunction. For example, elderly women who appear to have urge incontinence caused by detrusor hyperactivity by clinical history will often have coexisting sphincteric incompetence or significantly elevated residual urine. Likewise, in elderly men who appear to have urge incontinence caused by detrusor hyperactivity, coexisting outlet obstruction caused by benign prostate hyperplasia is often a factor in the detrusor hyperactivity. Unless these coexisting bladder dysfunctions that commonly exist in older patients have been identified, pharmacologic therapy will fail and combination drug therapy cannot be used in an informed and clinically successful manner by the clinician. Medical therapy can be used in treating older patients who suffer from either stress or urgency incontinence.[1-2] To maximize the efficacy of pharmacotherapy, the clinician needs to have a sound knowledge of the anatomy and physiology of the lower urinary tract and understand the underlying pathophysiology of urinary incontinence. The physician also needs to know the various drugs available within the therapeutic armamentarium.

ANATOMY OF THE LOWER URINARY TRACT

As people become older, there are significant changes that occur in the physiologic processes of the bladder and the central nervous system control of the bladder. The lower urinary tract consists of a smooth muscle detrusor and a sphincter-active urethra and should be considered as a single functional vesicourethral unit. In the female, the urethral sphincter mechanism consists of the proximal two thirds of the urethra blending imperceptibly with the bladder outlet. The wall of the female urethra consists primarily of an outer sleeve of slow-twitch striated muscle (the rhabdosphincter), a middle layer of smooth muscle, and an inner "seal" of mucosa and submucosa, all of which are responsible for maintaining passive urinary continence.[3] This sphincter mechanism is anatomically separate from the adjacent paraurethral striated muscle of the pelvic floor capable of voluntarily stopping and starting the urinary stream. In older women, there is a steady decline in urethral pressure with aging, which compromises the urethral mucosal seal and increases the likelihood of coexisting sphincteric incompetence as a component of urinary incontinence in this group.

In the male, the entire proximal urethra is sphincter active, consisting of a proximal (bladder neck) and distal (external) sphincter mechanism. Both sphincters are independently capable of maintaining passive continence. The proximal sphincter consists of a well-developed ring of smooth muscle. The distal sphincter comprises an outer layer of slow-twitch striated muscle fibers confined to the wall of the membranous urethra. Paraurethral striated pelvic floor musculature is located posteriorly and is capable of momentarily interrupting voiding. When outlet obstruction is a component of detrusor hyperactivity in older men, videourodynamic studies suggest that the bladder neck does not open normally in many of these patients.

The bladder smooth muscle is richly innervated by cholinergic parasympathetic fibers mediated by the pelvic nerve from S2 to S4. Acetycholine causes coordinated contraction of the detrusor resulting in bladder emptying. Cholinergic stimulation of the bladder neck and urethra produces less predictable effects and is probably not clinically relevant. The sympathetic nervous system via the hypogastric nerve from T11 to L2 is primarily involved with bladder storage. Adrenergic stimulation of alpha receptors primarily located at the bladder neck and proximal portion of the urethra result in smooth muscle contraction and increased sphincteric tone. Stimulation of beta-adrenergic receptors located in the bladder dome theoretically relax smooth muscle and improve bladder storage, but clinically these effects appear to be minimal.

A third component of the autonomic innervation of the bladder and urethra probably exists and is referred to as the nonadrenergic, noncholinergic nervous system. Stimulation of these nerves appear to cause bladder contraction, and their presence may help explain the relative refractoriness of anticholinergic medications in some patients.

The voluntarily controlled striated muscle of the paraurethral pelvic floor and urethra are innervated by the pudendal nerve. In theory, relaxation of them reduces outflow resistance favoring bladder emptying. During bladder filling the bladder wall accommodates to increasing volumes resulting in little or no rise in bladder pressure. Under normal conditions the urethral sphincter produces a urethral pressure that is greater than the intravesical pressure maintaining continence. Voluntary micturition is a complex coordinated event in which there is relaxation of the pelvic floor and urethral sphincter mechanism accompanied by a coordinated bladder contraction resulting in urination.

Stress Incontinence

Stress incontinence is the involuntary loss of urine associated with activities that increase intra-abdominal pressure such as coughing, sneezing, lifting, and physical exertion. It is often associated with loss of pelvic floor support resulting in descensus of the bladder neck and proximal portion of the urethra. When the bladder descends, increases in intra-abdominal pressure are no longer compensated for by the proximal portion of the urethra. This elevates intravesical pressure above the maximum pressure exerted by the urethral sphincter mechanism, resulting in stress incontinence.

Some patients with stress incontinence have a lesser degree of bladder descensus but have a weak urethral sphincter mechanism. This is referred to as intrinsic sphincter deficiency, and it occurs much more commonly in the elderly presumably because of tissue atrophy. The majority of male patients with postprostatectomy incontinence have urethral sphincter deficiency because of sphincteric injury at the time of surgery.

Medications used to facilitate bladder storage and decrease stress urinary incontinence do so by increasing bladder outlet resistance. For practical purposes, one might consider classifying the various medications into being either "clinically relevant" or "theoretical" (see box below).

Alpha-Adrenergic Agonists

Stimulation of the smooth muscle alpha-adrenergic receptors located at the bladder neck and proximal portion of the urethra can increase bladder-outlet resistance and improve stress urinary incontinence. In females, alpha-adrenergic stimulation has been shown to improve mild to moderate stress incontinence but produces little benefit in more severe cases.[4,5] To maximize efficacy, therapy should be combined with pelvic floor strengthening exercises and estrogen therapy when clinically indicated.[6] The agents often produce an improvement in symptoms but rarely total dryness. Alpha-adrenergic medications need to be utilized in older patients with extreme caution. Patients who have coexisting cardiac disease are at significantly increased risk for use of these medications. It is often advisable to consult with the geriatrician or internist who manages the patient before

Medical Management of Incontinence

STRESS INCONTINENCE
Increase outlet resistance
- Clinically relevant
  - Alpha-adrenergic agonists
  - Tricyclic antidepressants
  - Estrogens
- Theoretical
  - Beta-adrenergic antagonists

URGENCY INCONTINENCE
Inhibit bladder contractility, increase bladder compliance
- Clinically relevant
  - Anticholinergic agents
  - Musculotropic agents
  - Tricyclic antidepressants
- Theoretical
  - Calcium antagonists
  - Prostaglandin inhibitors
  - Beta-adrenergic agonists

Decreased sensory input
- Theoretical
  - Neurotoxic compounds

using alpha-adrenergic medications for treatment of incontinence in the elderly.

A trial of alpha-adrenergic stimulation before surgical intervention is reasonable in female patients with mild to moderate stress leakage. It also offers patients who decline surgery or who are at higher risk for an operation a noninvasive therapeutic alternative.

Similarly, male patients with mild stress incontinence after a prostatectomy may benefit from alpha-adrenergic stimulation, but in general its efficacy is limited.[7] The occasional excellent result in patients with mild symptoms justifies a therapeutic trial combined with Kegel exercises. If a therapeutic response is not obvious within the first few months of therapy, an alternative therapeutic regimen should be considered.

The most commonly prescribed alpha-adrenergic agonists are ephedrine sulfate and phenylpropanolamine hydrochloride. Ephedrine, 25 to 50 mg four times daily, is a sympathomimetic agent that causes the release of norepinephrine as well as directly stimulates alpha-adrenergic and beta-adrenergic receptors. Pseudoephedrine hydrochloride (Sudafed) is a stereoisomer with a similar mechanism of action. Ephedrine and pseudoephedrine should be used with extreme caution in older patients because of the potential risk of serious cardiac side effects. Phenylpropanolamine in doses of 50 to 75 mg two to three times daily can be prescribed in its pure form or in combination with chlorpheniramine maleate (Ornade) or with guaifenesin (Entex La). In older patients, the starting dose should be much lower (50 mg daily) with a gradual increase based on efficacy and side effects. The combined forms sometimes produce increased drowsiness. The comparative efficacies of these drugs have not been directly studied but appear to be similar.

Treatment with alpha-adrenergic stimulants may be accompanied by numerous side effects. These include weakness, insomnia, drowsiness, anxiety, elevation in blood pressure, and occasional tachyphylaxis. For this reason, they should be used with extreme caution in all elderly patients, especially those with hypertension, cardiovascular disease, and hyperthyroidism. It is an important practical consideration to use these medications after consultation with the patient's geriatrician or internist to assess potential risk for the patient.

Tricyclic Antidepressants

Imipramine is a tricyclic antidepressant that is clinically effective in treating mild stress incontinence.[8-9] It increases bladder outlet resistance by peripheral blockade of norepinephrine reuptake, potentiating the alpha-mediated smooth muscle tone of the bladder neck and proximal portion of the urethra. Imipramine also has anticholinergic and musculotropic properties. The "combined" effect of Impramine often proves useful in patients with mixed stress and urgency incontinence. The recommended dosage is 25 mg twice daily, though other investigators use dosages as high as 100 to 150 mg daily.[8-9] Imipramine should be used with caution in older people. Because of the alpha-adrenergic effects, a potential for serious cardiac side effects exists. In addition, any potential changes in mental function should be monitored closely, especially in older patients who drive automobiles or those who are at risk for falls. Imipramine is generally well tolerated by elderly patients. Side effects most frequently seen with imipramine are those attributable to its anticholinergic properties or occur with higher antidepressant dosages. Potential side effects include orthostatic hypotension, dry mouth, ataxia, tachycardia, restlessness, and hallucinations.

Estrogens

Several studies support the efficacy of estrogen in treating mild stress urinary incontinence in postmenopausal women.[10,11] Beneficial effects of estrogen have been attributed to numerous factors including enhancement of the alpha-mediated smooth muscle contractile response to sympathomimetics, mucosal proliferation, and improvement of the "mucosal seal" secondary to increased mucosal blood flow. Its exact mechanism of action remains speculative.[12]

Estrogen appears to enhance the effectiveness of alpha-adrenergic agonists, possibly by increasing the number of alpha-adrenergic receptors.[12-14] Postmenopausal patients with mild stress incontinence and atrophic changes on pelvic examination are most likely to benefit from a trial of estrogen therapy with or without alpha-adrenergic agonists. Patients who are not receiving oral conjugate estrogen can be treated topically with Premarin vaginal cream applicators 0.5 to 1.0 g three times weekly and reassessed in approximately 2 months. Similarly, women with frequency, urgency, and urge incontinence secondary to atrophic vaginitis and urethritis may benefit from estrogen therapy. Estrogen therapy in older women is an excellent medication to use in combination with behavioral therapies or other pharmacologic therapies. Patients receiving long-term therapy are at risk for endometrial carcinoma and should be followed closely.

Beta-Adrenergic Antagonists

Theoretically, beta-adrenergic antagonists increase urethral resistance by blocking beta-adrenergic stimulated relaxation of the proximal urethra. Indirectly this potentiates alpha-adrenergic mediated smooth muscle tone. Although moderate successes have been reported, its practical usage is limited by its modest effectiveness and potential cardiac side effects.[15-16]

URGE INCONTINENCE

Urge incontinence is the involuntary loss of urine associated with a strong desire or urge to urinate and is very common in the elderly. Patients affected may also complain of urinary frequency and nocturia. Urge incontinence is often associated with an involuntary rise in intravesical pressure during bladder filling referred to as an unstable bladder contraction or "bladder spasm." Urge incontinence is also seen in patients who have poor bladder compliance and in patients with a hypersensitive bladder resulting in a small functional bladder capacity.

In the majority of cases, the treatment of urge incontinence is primarily medical. Pharmacologic management of urge incontinence is directed toward inhibiting unstable bladder contractions, increasing bladder capacity, increasing bladder compliance, and decreasing sensory input to increase bladder capacity and decrease symptoms. Medications most commonly used are anticholinergics, musculotropic agents, and tricyclic antidepressants.

The potential of pharmacotherapy in treating patients with urge incontinence should not be underestimated. Expertise in patient and treatment selection will optimize treatment success. To maximize the benefit of medical therapy, patients should be simultaneously started on either a bladder drill or timed voiding. In addition, clinical response and tolerability to medication has enormous patient variability and is unpredictable. For this reason, consecutive trials with the different medications are recommended until an acceptable clinical response is achieved.

Anticholinergic Agents

Anticholinergics (antimuscarinics) competitively inhibit the effects of acetycholine at the level of the postganglionic autonomic receptors sites, thereby decreasing involuntary bladder contractility and improving bladder capacity.[17] Total inhibition of contractility cannot be achieved by anticholinergic agents presumably because of the presence of nonadrenergic noncholinergic bladder innervation. The clinical effects of anticholinergics are varying in part because of uneven and generally poor absorption from the gastrointestinal tract.

The therapeutic effect of anticholinergics is often accompanied by moderate systemic anticholinergic side effects, including dry mouth, blurred vision, increased heart rate, drowsiness and constipation. Careful dose titration is often necessary to maintain good compliance. Anticholinergic agents are contraindicated in patients with narrow-angle glaucoma, and they may precipitate urinary retention in patients with coincident bladder outlet obstruction.

Propantheline bromide (ProBanthine) is the most commonly prescribed anticholinergic agent given orally in dosages of 15 to 30 mg four times daily.[18] Anticholinergic side effects occur less often than with atropine possibly because ProBanthine is more selective for the lower urinary tract. Hyoscyamine sulfate (Levsin) is an anticholinergic agent available in capsule, in sublingual and elixir forms, and as an extended-release capsule (Levsinex). The dose of Levsinex using one tablet twice daily is usually adequate for urge incontinence, though little exists in the literature to document its clinical effects.

Musculotropic Agents

Musculotropic agents directly inhibit smooth muscle contractility by papaverine-like action and possess variable anticholinergic and local anesthetic properties as well.

Oxybutynin chloride (Ditropan) is the most commonly prescribed musculotropic agent for urinary incontinence.[19] It has moderate anticholinergic properties and hence the side effects. The usual dosage ranges from 2.5 to 5 mg three times daily and is titrated based on effectiveness and side effects. One should start elderly patients at much lower dosages (2.5 mg two to three times daily) and if necessary gradually increase the dosage every 5 to 7 days. If it is tolerated, refractory cases may respond to increasing the dosage or increasing the frequency to four times daily. Ditropan should be used with caution in the elderly because one of the potential side effects is confusion, which can be a serious side effect in older patients who drive automobiles or are at high risk for injury because of falls. Intravesical administration of oxybutynin in patients on clean intermittent catheterization has proved to be effective, especially in patients with neurogenic bladder dysfunction.[20,21]

Dicyclomine hydrochloride (Bentyl), 20 to 30 mg three times daily, and flavoxate hydrochloride (Urispas), 100 to 200 mg three times daily, both have musculotropic as well as anticholinergic and local analgesic activity.[22-24] Their side effects are primarily anticholinergic but occur less frequently than with oxybutynin. For this reason, these drugs are excellent choices to use in combination with other medications in an effort to manage older patients who have difficulty tolerating side effects of pharmacologic management.

Tricyclic Antidepressants

As previously mentioned, imipramine has musculotropic and anticholinergic effects on bladder smooth muscle and is clinically useful in treating patients with urgency incontinence. Similarly, doxepin (Sinequan) is another tricyclic antidepressant that has been shown to be clinically effective.[25]

Calcium Antagonists

Calcium antagonists have been shown to be effective in blocking detrusor smooth muscle contractility by either altering calcium inflow, intercellular calcium release, or calcium concentration. Their inhibitory effect on detrusor contractility has been well established in in vitro studies, but generally their usefulness in clinical practice has been limited by their potential to cause serious cardiac side effects.[26-27] These include hypotension, tachycardia, and heart block. Reports of adverse cardiac events are uncommon, and generally the side effects are related to its anticholinergic properties. More common side effects include headache, abdominal cramping, constipation, nausea, facial flushing, weakness, and dizziness.

Terodiline has combined calcium antagonistic and anticholinergic properties and has been used extensively in Europe in treating patients with bladder instability and urgency incontinence. It has been shown to have clinical beneficial effects in a large portion of patients treated but has been withdrawn from the market because of sporadic reports of cardiac adverse side effects.[28-30]

Prostaglandin Inhibitors

Prostaglandins appear to potentiate neurotransmission to the bladder, and their inhibition may decrease bladder contractility. Prostaglandin synthetase inhibitors have been shown to improve symptoms in patients with bladder instability, but the degree of improvement was limited, and side effects were significant.[31] At this point, prostaglandin inhibitors are not routinely prescribed as treatment for bladder instability and urge incontinence.

Beta-Adrenergic Agonists

In vitro studies with beta-adrenergic agents show a strong bladder-relaxant effect because of the stimulation of beta-adrenergic receptors primarily located within the body of the bladder.[32]

Clinical trials with terbutaline (Bricanyl), 5 mg three times daily, have shown it to be clinically useful in treating urge incontinence, but currently it is not routinely used in clinical practice.[33-34]

Neurotoxic Compounds

Many patients who complain of frequency, urgency, and urge incontinence do not have bladder instability but have bladder hypersensitivity with a small functional capacity. This is referred to as "sensory urgency," the most common example being frequency that accompanies a urinary tract infection. Defunctionalization of the afferent innervation of the bladder with medication theoretically could decrease sensory input, increasing bladder capacity and improving symptoms. Capsaicin, the pungent ingredient in red peppers, is a neurotoxic compound that desensitizes sensory neurons by depleting their content of certain neuropeptides. Capsaicin may prove clinically useful in the future.[35-36]

Pharmacologic therapy is an extremely important treatment option in the treatment of management of urinary incontinence in older people. The major reason for the role of pharmacologic therapy in older patients is the need for conservative management in this population when possible. However, pharmacologic therapy must be used with great care in older people. The side effects of medications can be serious in some patients. Combination pharmacologic therapy using low doses to avoid side effects can be effective in many older people. However, without a clear understanding of the underlying cause of incontinence for each patient, pharmacologic management cannot be done with confidence and success by the physician. It is extremely important to consider utilizing combined behavioral therapy with pharmacologic therapy in older people to achieve the best treatment outcome using conservative management with minimal side effects.

If conservative management using pharmacologic therapy and behavioral therapy is unsuccessful and the patient is a candidate for a surgical procedure, surgery can be successful in older people and should be considered a treatment option when feasible. Surgical treatment of incontinence in older people is associated with a higher incidence of postoperative problems related to the bladder than that in younger adults. Therefore pharmacologic therapy combined with behavioral therapy is often an important part of the postoperative management of patients who have elective surgery for treatment of urinary incontinence. Therefore the complexity of incontinence in older patients often requires a combination of treatment modalities that address the urethral dysfunction and the bladder dysfunction while coexisting medical conditions and the long-term effect on the quality of life of the patient are being considered.

REFERENCES

1. Wein AJ: Nonsurgical management of bladder dysfunction. In Webster GW et al, editors: *Reconstructive urology,* Boston, 1993, Blackwell Scientific Publications.
2. Bissada NK, Finkbeiner AE: Urologic manifestations of drug therapy, *Urol Clin North Am* 15:725, 1988.
3. Gozling JA: The structure of the female lower urinary tract and pelvic floor, *Urol Clin North Am* 12:207, 1985.
4. Stewart BH, Banowsky LHW, Montague DK: Stress incontinence: conservative therapy with sympathominetic drugs, *J Urol* 115:558, 1976.
5. Diokno AC, Taub M: Ephedrine in treatment of urinary incontinence, *Urology* 5:624, 1975.
6. Wells TJ: Pelvic (floor) muscle exercises, *J Am Geriatr Soc* 38:333, 1990.
7. Awad S, Downie, J, Kiruluta H: Alpha adrenergic agents in urinary disorders of the proximal urethra: stress incontinence, *Br J Urol* 50:332, 1978.
8. Castleden CM, George CF, Renwick AG, Asher MJ: Imipramine: possible alternative to current therapy for urinary incontinence in the elderly, *J Urol* 125:318, 1981.
9. Gilja I, Radej M, Kovacic M, Parazajder J: Conservative treatment of female stress incontinence with imipramine, *J Urol* 132:909, 1984.
10. Caine M, Raz S: The role of female hormones in stress incontinence, presented at the Sixth Congress of Société Internationale d'Urologie, Amsterdam, 1973.
11. Schreiter F, Fuchs P, Stockamp K: Estrogenic sensitivity of alpha receptors in the urethral musculature, *Urol Int* 31:13, 1976.
12. Batra SC, Losif CS: Female urethra: a target for estrogen action, *J Urol* 129:418, 1983.
13. Beisland HO, Fossberg E, Moer A, Sander S: Urethral sphincteric insufficiency in post-menopausal females: treatment with phenylpropanolamine and estriol separately and combination, *Urol Int* 39:211, 1984.
14. Walter S, et al: Stress urinary incontinence in post-menopausal women treated with oral estrogen (estriol) and alpha adrenoceptor stimulation agent (phenylpropanolamine): a randomized double blind placebo controlled study, *Int Urogynecol J* 1:74, 1990.
15. Gleason D, Reilly RJ, Bottaccini MR, et al: The urethral continence zone and its relation to stress incontinence, *J Urol* 112:81, 1974.
16. Kaisary AU: Beta adrenoceptor blockade in the treatment of female stress urinary incontinence, *J Urol* (Paris) 90:351, 1984.
17. Wein AJ, Levin RM, Barrett DM: Voiding function: relevant anatomy, physiology and pharmacology. In Gillenwater JY et al, editors: *Adult and pediatric urology,* St Louis, 1987, Mosby.
18. Holmes DM, Montz FJ, Stantion SL: Oxybutynin vs. propantheline in the management of detrusor instability: a patient regulated variable dose trial, *Br J Obstet Gynaecol* 96:607 1989.
19. Zorzitto ML, Holliday PJ, Jewett MA, et al: Oxybutynin chloride for geriatric urinary dysfunction, a double-blind placebo controlled study, *Age Ageing* 18:195, 1989.
20. Greenfield SP, Feram M: The use of intravesical oxybutynin chloride in children with neurogenic bladder, *J Urol* 146:532, 1991.
21. Madersbachers H, Jilg G: Control of detrusor hyperreflexia by intravesical instillation of oxybutynin hydrochloride, *Paraplegia* 29:84, 1991.
22. Fischer C, Diokno A, Lapides J: The anticholinergics effects of dicyclomine hydrochloride in uninhibited neurogenic bladder dysfunction, *J Urol* 120:328, 1978.
23. Jonas U, Petri E, Kissal J: The effect of flavoxate on hyperactive detrusor muscle, *Eur Urol* 5:106, 1979.
24. Briggs RS, Castleden CM, Asher MJ: The effect of flavoxate on uninhibited detrusor contraction and urinary incontinence in the elderly, *J Urol* 123:656, 1980.
25. Lose G, Jørgensen L, Thunedeborg P: Doxepin in the treatment of female detrusor overactivity: a randomized double-blind cross over trial, *J Urol* 142:1024, 1989.
26. Finkbeiner AE: Effect of extracellular calcium and calcium blocking agents on detrusor contractility: an in-vitro study, *Neurourol Urodyn* 2:245, 1983.
27. Malkowicz SB, Wein AJ, Brendler K, Levin RM: Effect of diltiazem on in-vitro rabbit bladder function, *Pharmacology* 31: 24, 1985.
28. Peters D: Multi-Center Study Group: Terodiline in the treatment of urinary frequency and motor urge incontinence, a controlled multicenter trial, *Scand J Urol Nephrol* 87(suppl):21, 1984.
29. Tapp A, Fall M, Norgaard J, et al: Terodiline: a dose titrated multicenter study of the treatment of ideopathic detrusor instability in women, *J Urol* 142:1027, 1989.

30. McCleod AA, Torogood S, Barnett S: Torsades de pointes complicating treatment with terodiline, *Br Med J* 302:1469, 1991.
31. Cardozo LD, Stanton SL, Robinson H, Hole D: Evaluation of flurbiprofen in detrusor instability, *Br Med J* 180: 281, 1980.
32. Norlén L, Sundin T, Waagastein F: Beta-adrenceptor simulation of a human urinary bladder in-vivo, *Acta Pharmacol Toxicol* 43:26, 1978.
33. Abrams P: Terodilene in clinical practice, *Urology* 4(suppl):50, 1990.
34. Lindholm P, Lose G: Terbutaline (Bricanyl) in the treatment of female urge incontinene, *Urol Int* 41:158, 1986.
35. Maggi CA, Barbanti G, Santicioli P, et al: Cystometric evidence that capsaicin sensitive nerves modulate the afferent branch of micturition reflex on humans, *J Urol* 142:150, 1989.
36. Maggi CA: Capsaicin and primary afferent neurons: from basic science to human therapy? *J Auton Nerve Syst* 33:1, 1991.

Chapter 60 Surgical Management Decisions in Geriatric Incontinence

Gopal H. Badlani

Incontinence is a common problem in the elderly, with tremendous social, medical, and economic implications. The cause of incontinence in the geriatric population can be extremely complex; however, patients who have been properly assessed and have failed conservative management may benefit from surgical intervention and should not be disqualified on the basis of age alone. Modern anesthetic techniques and perioperative care as well as innovations in minimally invasive surgery make it possible for the elderly to obtain results similar to those of younger patients without excessive risk of illness and death. However, it is important to focus on the preoperative evaluation necessary to identify good surgical candidates and to utilize the newer minimally invasive modifications of standard approaches to surgically treat incontinence whenever possible.

The geriatric population is a diverse group with a broad range of physical and cognitive abilities as well as varying requirements for social and health care support. Clearly the community-dwelling elderly have fewer functional impairments than the "frail elderly" in nursing homes. The chronic care elderly and the community-dwelling elderly are made up of a greater proportion of women. At any given age, mental status can vary widely and is likely to be more deteriorated in the nursing home population and the frail elderly.

Surgical decision-making in the elderly demands careful analysis of the risks versus benefits of the intended intervention. This requires a thorough understanding of the great effect of incontinence socially and medically, the individual's or family's expectations for treatment outcome, the relative indications for surgery, and the probability of successful outcome in a given patient. The adverse effect of incontinence obviously depends on the patient's status as a community or nursing home dweller and his or her quality of life. Similarly, expectations for treatment outcome may be higher in the independent, functional elderly than in the cognitively impaired or bed-ridden institutionalized elderly. In general, surgical treatment of incontinence is indicated to improve quality of life and to prevent or minimize complications of incontinence such as urosepsis, external skin changes, and bed sores. The probability of successful outcome is best determined from a thorough multidisciplinary evaluation of the patient's physical and cognitive abilities, mental status, available social support, and general medical condition.[1] Using this approach, patients who are at risk for unsatisfactory outcome or who are likely to encounter particular postoperative problems can be identified preoperatively. Timely interventions can then be instituted to optimize treatment outcome. For example, slower recovery may be anticipated in the elderly. Therefore social and health care support issues should be addressed preoperatively to ensure that the patient will obtain maximal benefit from the procedure.

Diagnosis

Accurate diagnosis of urinary incontinence is critical in selecting appropriate surgical candidates and ensuring optimal surgical results. Unfortunately, diagnosing the cause of incontinence is typically much more difficult in the elderly than in younger patients for several reasons. For example, incontinence is usually multifactorial in the elderly patient. The elderly are also notorious for underreporting symptoms and may be poor historians as well.[2] In addition, normal age-related changes in the lower urinary tract can predispose the elderly to incontinence. Such changes include the onset of uninhibited detrusor contractions in 10% of women and 25% to 35% of men, an increase in nocturnal fluid excretion, prostatic enlargement in men, urethral shortening and sphincter weakening in women, decreased bladder capacity, and possibly decreased bladder contractility in both sexes.[3,4] Reversible, nonurologic conditions often precipitate incontinence in an otherwise continent patient who may or may not have underlying lower urinary tract abnormality. Examples of such conditions include delirium, infection, atrophic vaginitis, pharmaceuticals, psychologic state, endocrine disorders, restricted mobility, and stool impaction.[5] Geriatric patients also have a greater prevalence of comorbid conditions such as cerebrovascular accident (CVA), Parkinsonism, and other central nervous system lesions, and bladder and prostate cancer, which can also produce incontinence, thus further complicating the diagnosis.

The complex nature of incontinence in the elderly demands a thorough, stepwise evaluation.[6] The focus of the initial evaluation in the geriatric patient is to identify and address reversible causes or more serious underlying conditions presenting as incontinence. A typical screening evaluation should include a history and physical examination (emphasizing neurologic function), a urine culture with sensitivity, and a urine cytologic examination (in those at risk for bladder cancer). When urodynamic evaluation is indicated, a simple cystometry and uroflowmetry with postvoid residual measurement should be performed initially. Complex urodynamic assessment may not be necessary based on the results of the initial studies. If a complex urodynamic assessment is required, it can be performed later with fluoroscopy and simultaneous pressure-flow analysis.

Depending on the findings, the initial management approach is usually conservative. Patients or their caregivers are given a voiding diary to document the amount and timing of their voiding and incontinent episodes in relation to fluid intake. Behavioral modifications such as fluid restriction, timed voiding, leg elevation (in patients with pedal edema), and pelvic floor training (relaxation or strengthening) can benefit up to 75% of the patients.[7] Once the reversible causes have been addressed, and more serious conditions excluded, the differential diagnosis of established urologic causes can be considered if incontinence persists.

Incontinence can originate from either bladder or urethral causes or a combination of both. Bladder causes can be divided into detrusor overactivity, detrusor underactivity, or outflow obstruction. Detrusor overactivity may produce urge incontinence, whereas detrusor underactivity may result in overflow incontinence. Both detrusor overactivity and underactivity may occur as result of outflow obstruction. Normal aging processes and upper motor neuropathic lesions may also cause detrusor overactivity. Urethral causes of incontinence include anatomical incontinence (hypermobile stress incontinence) and intrinsic sphincter deficiency (ISD).[8] Both conditions result in stress incontinence. ISD may cause passive incontinence.

Generally, unless patients present in retention (with overflow incontinence) or with clinically evident stress incontinence, the typical diagnostic challenge in the geriatric patient is to differentiate between detrusor overactivity and outflow obstruction in men, or between stress incontinence and detrusor overactivity in women. Multichannel urodynamic testing is particularly useful in establishing the correct diagnosis in the elderly population, where many confounding coexisting conditions exist. In incontinent geriatric men with detrusor overactivity and coexisting upper motor neuropathic conditions (CVA or parkinsonism) and benign prostatic hyperplasia (BPH), it is clinically important to know whether the detrusor overactivity is attributable to the central nervous system lesion or the outlet obstruction. Surgery is indicated in patients with significant bladder obstruction with or without detrusor overactivity. However, many of these patients (particularly those with CVA-related detrusor overactivity) will have persistent voiding symptoms, including incontinence, after prostatectomy.[8] Although the incontinence may result from intraoperative injury to the external sphincter, it is most likely attributable to persistent detrusor hyperactivity, which is present in 50% of incontinent elderly patients after prostatectomy.[9] Therefore it should be determined preoperatively whether the detrusor overactivity has a neurologic cause (CVA or parkinsonism) or is attributable to the bladder outlet obstruction. A history of voiding difficulty before the onset of the neurologic disease combined with sophisticated multichannel urodynamic evaluation, including a micturating urethral pressure profile,[10] can help differentiate between the two. Surgical candidates with detrusor overactivity should undergo a preoperative trial of anticholinergic medication to determine its effect on detrusor overactivity.[11] This should be done with a clear understanding by the patient and the family that the medication may precipitate urinary retention. Nonresponders are likely to experience worsening of symptoms (that is, incontinence) postoperatively because of decreased outlet resistance. Definitive surgery therefore is not indicated in these patients. Temporary treatment such as balloon dilatation of the prostate or prostatic stent placement (which preserve smooth sphincter function) may be beneficial in these patients.[8]

Multichannel urodynamic evaluation with simultaneous fluoroscopic imaging (videourodynamics) is also useful in determining the cause of de novo incontinence after prostatectomy (radical retropubic, perineal, or transurethral). The objective is to distinguish detrusor overactivity from intrinsic sphincter deficiency (related to anastomotic external sphincter fibrosis) by measuring Valsalva leak point pressures (LPP)[12] with and without the urethral catheter in place. Low leak point pressure is suggestive of intrinsic sphincter dysfunction (ISD), which often requires surgical intervention. High leak point pressures (even after removal of the urethral catheter) with detrusor overactivity may first be treated with an anticholinergic agent or with relief of the obstructing stricture.

In elderly women, symptoms of urge incontinence or stress incontinence are unreliable for predicting whether the incontinence is caused by detrusor overactivity, pure stress incontinence, or a combination of both.[13] The prevalence of both CVA and stress incontinence among elderly females further complicates the evaluation. Multichannel videourodynamic assessment can be helpful in clarifying the cause of incontinence in this situation. Also the specific type of stress incontinence (anatomic or ISD) can be determined by measurement of the Valsalva LPP. This distinction is clinically important because the surgical management is different for each condition. In patients with very low LPP, the urinary outlet should be occluded during filling cystometry to evaluate capacity, compliance, and detrusor activity. The presence of detrusor overactivity does not preclude surgery in candidates for stress incontinence surgery. However, patients who fail to respond to anticholinergic therapy for their detrusor overactivity may be at higher risk for persistent irritative voiding symptoms postoperatively. The likelihood of unsatisfactory long-term results in candidates for artificial urinary sphincter (AUS) implantation or periurethral collagen injection therapy is also greater among those with refractory detrusor overactivity.[14]

Detrusor hyperactivity with impaired contractility (DHIC) is a common cause of incontinence, afflicting both males and females, particularly in the frail elderly population (85 years and older).[15,16] Unfortunately, DHIC can imitate several lower urinary tract disorders including anatomic stress incontinence, bladder outlet obstruction, and detrusor underactivity.[16,17] Multichannel videourodynamic testing can be useful in differentiating DHIC from other lower urinary tract conditions. Since DHIC is not surgically treatable, it is important to distinguish it from other causes of incontinence that are amenable to surgical correction.

Once the surgical diagnosis has been firmly established and surgical intervention has been deemed necessary, it becomes the onus of the surgeon to select the appropriate procedure. In the geriatric population, this is best done on an individualized basis. The guiding principle is to select the procedure that can achieve the desired effect with minimal invasiveness, minimal morbidity, and the shortest hospital stay to avoid the associated problems such as nosocomial infection and disorientation. Choice of anesthetic technique is an important consideration as well. When possible, local or regional anesthesia should be selected over general anesthesia to minimize the anesthesia-related morbidity of the surgery. In my opinion, in the geriatric patient it is acceptable to compromise long-term results if an alternative technique (with less certain long-term results) can deliver immediate success with lower morbidity and reduced convalescence on a temporary basis. These principles, along with increasingly present economic pressures, have led to many modifications of standard surgical approaches that have valuable application in geriatric urology. Carefully planned elective surgery utilizing techniques aimed at minimizing invasiveness and decreasing hospitalization and convalescence usually does not pose a significantly elevated risk in the geriatric age group.[18] Both the patient and the family should have a clear understanding of the expectations for successful treatment as well as potential problems arising postoperatively.

Outlet Obstruction: Benign Prostate Hyperplasia

Detrusor hyperactivity is a common cause of incontinence in older men and often occurs as a result of bladder outlet obstruction. Transurethral resection of the prostate (TURP) remains the standard in the surgical treatment of BPH. However, there is a relatively high morbidity (18%) with prolonged duration of catheterization (3 days) and hospitalization (5 days) associated with TURP,[19] which has resulted in a multitude of alternative surgical approaches. There are numerous advances in the surgery of BPH that may be considered as a treatment option in the older man.

Intraurethral Stents

Intraurethral stents are self-expanding, woven-mesh devices made of surgical-grade alloy. They can be inserted relatively easily into the prostatic urethra by direct vision endoscopically or under ultrasound guidance with local anesthesia or light intravenous sedation. The devices can be used on a temporary or a permanent basis. Removable stents (Nessenkorn stent,[20] Urocoil[21]) can be used to temporarily treat urinary retention in surgically unfit elderly patients. Use of the stent instead of an indwelling Foley catheter avoids the septic complications associated with prolonged catheterization. The lifespan of the removable stent (depending on the type) is limited to 3 to 24 months, after which they become encrusted and may become displaced either proximally into the bladder or distally across the external sphincter causing passive incontinence. Permanent stents such as the Urolume Wall Stent[22] are capable of expanding to 42 French gauge and undergo complete epithelialization in 3 to 12 months.

The North American Study Group[23] reported considerable improvement in symptom score (15 to 6.3) and uroflow (8.6 ml/sec to 15.6 ml/sec), and postvoid residual volume with minimal morbidity at 1 year after insertion in 95 patients (mean age, 68). The intraurethral stents are not currently available in this country but are expected to be released into the United States market in 1997.

Laser Ablation of the Prostate

Laser ablation of the prostate is believed to provide significant improvement over standard TURP in terms of decreased recovery time, lower complication rate, and thus improved patient satisfaction. Several active trials of various laser ablation techniques are underway in the United States. Transurethral laser incision of the prostate (TULIP),[24] which uses intraurethral ultrasound positioning of the laser beam, has been evaluated in a multicenter trial.[25] Significant subjective and objective improvement was found, though peak flow rates did not increase to the same degree as with TURP. Unfortunately, many patients experienced exacerbated irritative and obstructive voiding symptoms immediately postoperatively. These symptoms may persist, necessitating bladder drainage (urethral or suprapubic catheter) for 1 to 2 weeks. Maximal benefit may not be seen for up to 6 to 8 weeks.

More recently, direct application of Nd:YAG laser energy utilizing side-firing fibers under direct transurethral endoscopic vision has been popularized. Two approaches have been used with this technique. In the noncontact technique, the fiber tip is positioned in the urethra a few millimeters from the prostatic tissue. Laser energy delivered into the prostatic tissue in this fashion produces tissue dehydration and coagulation necrosis. As the necrotic tissue sloughs off over several weeks, the bladder outlet opens. In the contact technique, laser energy is applied to the prostate by a fiber that is in direct contact with the prostate. This high-intensity energy delivery causes vaporization of the prostatic tissue, with only a thin rim of coagulated tissue left behind. Thus the complete effect of relieving obstruction is more immediate. Significant debate has taken place over which technique is better. Both techniques offer safety advantages over TURP in terms of minimal bleeding and fluid absorption. Laser prostatectomy can be performed in patients fully anticoagulated with warfarin therapy with no significant bleeding.[26,27] Convalescence time is reduced by laser prostatectomy.[28] Since there is no bleeding, no catheter irrigation or nursing care is required; therefore surgery can be performed on an outpatient basis.[27] Spinal or epidural anesthesia may be used to minimize the anesthesia-related risks. The indwelling catheter can be removed in the office on postoperative day 1 after contact vaporization. Clinical efficacy using subjective and objective evaluation has been demonstrated by numerous investigators.[28-31] Symptomatic and objective improvement equivalent to TURP has been maintained over 18 months of follow-up study.[32]

Our own experience with 32 patients treated with contact laser vaporization of the prostate has mirrored this success.[33] Analyzing subjective and objective data available on 23 men over a mean follow-up time of 9 months, we found peak uroflow rates increased from 5 to 16 ml/sec. Pressure flow analysis in 20 patients revealed decreased mean detrusor pressures from 89 to 56 cm H_2O. Minimal morbidity and no mortality were encountered. However, laser prostatectomy is not without drawbacks. Irritative voiding symptoms may persist for 4 to 8 weeks, and maximal improvement symptoms and stream flow may not be reached for several weeks using the noncontact method.

Other disadvantages of this modality include the immediate cost of the procedure (which is significantly higher than TURP), the length of operating time, and in some cases longer indwelling catheter duration than that with TURP. No tissue specimens are obtained for pathologic study, and so prostate specific antigen (PSA) levels must be monitored routinely to detect occult cancer.

Transurethral Electrovaporization of the Prostate

Transurethral electrovaporization of the prostate is a modification of the standard TURP using a modified rollerball cutting loop (Vaportrode) that vaporizes with high-intensity current (200 to 300 W). The technique is similar to TURP.[34] A similar resectoscope and the same power generator is used. Unlike TURP and similar to laser ablating techniques, electrovaporization leaves behind a zone of coagulated tissue 1 to 3 mm deep, which virtually eliminates bleeding and fluid absorption. This technique has the same potential benefits as laser ablation in terms of minimal morbidity, decreased hospitalization, and faster recovery time. Unlike the laser techniques, the procedure can be performed in the same amount of time as TURP, with no significant learning curve for the surgeon and with readily available equipment as compared to expensive laser generators and fibers. The procedure may be performed by use of intravenous sedation or local anesthesia with intraurethral lidocaine. The full benefit of the surgery is seen almost immediately because the prostatic tissue is vaporized. Preliminary results show considerable improvement in symptom score (17.8 to 4.2) and uroflow (7.4 to 17.3ml/sec) at 3 months of follow-up time. The mean duration of an indwelling Foley catheter was 14.6 hours. Minimal morbidity and no significant postoperative irritative symptoms (unlike those from the laser techniques) were encountered.[35] My experience shows similar subjective improvement. Objective evaluation with uroflow and pressure-flow analysis reveals greatly improved flow rates from 10 to 22 ml/sec and reduction in voiding detrusor pressures from 84 to 44 cm H_2O at the preliminary follow-up exam. Although the long-term results of electrovaporization and the full effects of high-intensity current on periprostatic tissue are unknown at this time, this technique appears quite promising.

URETHRAL STRICTURE IN MEN

Overflow incontinence in elderly men occasionally results from a urethral stricture. Urethral strictures are common in elderly men because of prior surgical procedures such as prostatectomy, urethral catheterization, and condom catheter usage. Traditional treatment involves repeated dilatation with metal dilators, filiform and followers, or coudé catheters, usually with considerable pain and bleeding. Often, iatrogenic manipulation may create false urethral passages, which make it difficult or impossible to place catheters in these patients. One is often left with a choice between performing a suprapubic punch cystotomy or leaving a follower in place. Using a modification of the standard Amplatz dilating system,[36] we have minimized the morbidity and improved the accuracy of treating this condition with the use of a flexible cystoscope and coaxial endoscopic dilatation. Under flexible cystoscopic guidance, a soft-tipped guidewire is worked through the stricture into the bladder. Subsequently, serial coaxial dilatation over a wire is performed achieving virtually atraumatic dilatation. An indwelling catheter with a council tip or generous tip incision can be threaded over the wire and left in place. This technique can be performed with topical anesthesia and may be used with minimal bleeding in patients who are using anticoagulants.

Recurrent bulbar urethral strictures may be effectively treated by the endoscopically placed Urolume wall stent. This is the same device used to relieve outflow obstruction caused by BPH. A multicenter prospective Food and Drug Administration trial of the Urolume endourethral prosthesis for the treatment of recurrent bulbar urethral strictures in 175 patients was recently completed.[37] Significant improvements in symptom score, peak urine flow rate, and mean urine flow rate were noted within 6 weeks and sustained over the 2-year follow-up period. The retreatment rate fell from 75.3% before insertion to 14.3% after insertion for at least 1 year. The device is deployed under local anesthesia or light intravenous sedation in the same fashion as that for the treatment of obstructive BPH, with minimal morbidity.

BLADDER OUTLET OBSTRUCTION IN WOMEN

True fixed bladder outlet obstruction is rare in women. More commonly, a functional obstruction is present, usually caused by a large cystocele, dry sterile dressing, or failure of pelvic floor relaxation. By far, the most common source of obstruction in geriatric women is a large cystocele that angulates the bladder neck. Correction of the cystocele typically results in relief of the outlet obstruction. Fixed bladder outlet obstruction in women can occur after surgical procedures to correct incontinence.

DETRUSOR OVERACTIVITY

Detrusor overactivity is not routinely treated surgically in the elderly unless it occurs in association with a small-capacity or poorly compliant bladder that has not responded to anticholinergic therapy. Evidence of upper urinary tract sequelae such as hydronephrosis or impaired renal function provides further impetus for surgical intervention. Surgical options for treating a small-capacity bladder in the elderly include hydrodistension,[38-40] bladder denervation procedures,[41,42] and urinary diversion or bladder augmentation procedures.[43] Hydrodistension and bladder denervation procedures have been shown to have limited long-term success.[46] Bladder augmentation has been found to be safe and efficacious in older patients[18] with excellent reported results.[45] If poor compliance is present in addition to small capacity, the choice becomes either urinary diversion or bladder augmentation. With any of these procedures, patients should be prepared for the prospect of lifelong intermittent catheterization. Adequate renal function is necessary to tolerate the metabolic derangements involved with the use of bowel segments.[48]

Detrusor overactivity may occur in one half to two thirds of elderly women with stress incontinence, producing a "mixed-incontinence" picture. This usually resolves with correction of the stress incontinence.[47] In elderly men, detrusor overactivity often occurs in association with outlet obstruction. With relief of the obstruction at least 50% will resolve.[48] Unfortunately those who do not resolve may have worsened symptoms, including passive incontinence, once the outlet resistance is decreased. Since there is no way preoperatively to identify those patients who will not resolve, surgery is recommended only for those who respond preoperatively to anticholinergic medication.

Detrusor Underactivity

In the geriatric population, detrusor underactivity presenting as overflow incontinence rarely requires surgical intervention. The mainstay of therapy in these patients is clean intermittent catheterization (CIC) either by oneself or by an aide. Surgery to create an easily catheterized abdominal stoma may be indicated in female patients who have difficulty catheterizing themselves because of reduced manual dexterity or poor mobility (such as paraplegia).

Sphincteric Causes

Anatomic Stress Incontinence

The surgical treatment of stress incontinence depends on the negative social effect of the incontinence on the patient, severity and type of incontinence (hypermobility alone, or in combination with ISD), degree of cystocele present, and presence of other anatomic abnormalities (uterine prolapse, enterocele, rectocele, or pelvic disorders). In general, surgical treatment of anatomic stress incontinence is the same in the geriatric patient as it is in younger patients. Age alone should not disqualify a patient from consideration for surgical treatment. In fact, elderly patients achieve cure rates equal to those of younger patients without a significantly higher complication rate.[49] Indeed, less active elderly woman may do better after bladder neck suspension than an active younger women because less stress is placed on the repair. Correct diagnosis and proper patient selection are the key factors in obtaining optimal outcome.

The list of surgical procedures used to treat anatomic stress incontinence is extensive, attesting to the difficulty of satisfactorily treating all patients. As in younger women, the goal of surgical correction in elderly women is to restore the normal position of the bladder neck within the pelvis and to prevent descent of the bladder neck during episodes of abdominal stress. Both retropubic abdominal and transvaginal approaches have been used with good overall success.[50-52] Retropubic abdominal bladder neck suspension procedures such as the Marshall-Marchetti-Krantz (MMK)[53,54] and the Burch[55] procedure have been used in the elderly population with similar success rates and morbidity as in younger women.[56,57] Successful vaginal approaches include various modified Pereyra[58] bladder neck needle suspension techniques described by Gittes,[59] Stamey,[60] and Raz.[61] All three techniques have been used with varying degrees of success and minimal morbidity in elderly women. Atrophic endopelvic fascia and poor urethral and bladder neck mobility in elderly women are believed to play a role in those failing the Gittes procedure or the Stamey procedure. For these reasons, we favor the Raz technique for geriatric patients undergoing simple bladder neck suspension. The Raz modification involves dissection of the fascia supporting the bladder neck and urethra, allowing adequate mobilization of those structures. Sutures are placed into the urethropelvic ligament and anterior vaginal wall (excluding epithelium) under direct vision, which allows the surgeon to identify and incorporate the strongest tissue into the repair while minimizing the risk of bladder or urethral injury. Follow-up comparisons of women over 65 years of age with women under 65 show no significant difference in cure rate or morbidity.[62]

We advocate transvaginal needle suspension procedures over retropubic approaches when possible in elderly patients. The transvaginal approach avoids the potential morbidity associated with abdominal approaches. The operative time is reduced as is the length of hospitalization and time of recovery.[63] Also, the vaginal approach permits an access to repair any associated vaginal disorder simultaneously. The retropubic approach is advocated if there is a concomitant pelvic disorder requiring surgery, or, if vaginal atresia, significant scarring and fibrosis or radiation changes are present.

Recent surgical innovations include laparoscopic modifications of standard retropubic approaches[64] and a percutaneous needle bladder neck suspension technique.[65] Initial results with these minimally invasive techniques are promising. We are currently involved in a prospective multicenter evaluation of a percutaneous needle bladder neck suspension system (Vesica). A multifunctional needle is used to place sutures in the pubocervical fascia and vaginal wall, which are then secured to the pubic tubercles with special bone anchors. Preliminary cure rates exceed 95% with minimal complications.[66] Long-term follow-up study awaits.

Regardless of the procedure used to correct the stress incontinence, both the patient and the family should be aware of the possible postoperative sequelae, including persistent or de novo urgency, urinary retention requiring indwelling or clean intermittent catheterization, and secondary genital prolapse (uterine, cystocele, enterocele, rectocele).

Intrinsic Sphincter Deficiency

Intrinsic sphincter deficiency or dysfunction (ISD) is a common component of the cause of incontinence in elderly women. Improper urethral coaptation in a correctly positioned bladder neck and urethra is known as intrinsic sphincter deficiency. The resulting passive incontinence is usually severe, often requiring surgical intervention. Preoperative evaluation with multichannel videourodynamics is advocated to confirm the ISD and identify coexistent bladder neck hypermobility (in women) or detrusor overactivity and to assess bladder contractility, compliance, and capacity.

The goal of surgery is to provide urethral coaptation without causing obstruction. Surgical treatment options in the elderly are the same as those for younger patients and include pubovaginal sling procedures, artificial urinary sphincter (AUS) implantation, and periurethral bioinjection therapy. Pubovaginal sling procedures[67] are used primarily in women and offer the advantage of suspending the bladder neck in addition to actively occluding the urethra. This is the procedure of choice in women with combined anatomic stress incontinence and ISD. I also favor this approach in women who have failed previous bladder neck suspension procedures. In the standard pubovaginal sling, a 20 cm strip of rectus fascia (harvested through a suprapubic incision) is tunneled under the urethra and sutured to the anterior abdominal wall. Various autologous and synthetic materials have been used as slings. Modifications of this technique involve the use of the anterior vaginal wall to compress the urethra (vaginal wall sling) and the use of needle suspension sutures to aid in sling placement. These modifications maintain the excellent cure rate of standard techniques[67-69] and offer decreased morbidity and hospital stay. Complications of pubovaginal sling procedures include de novo irritative voiding symptoms and urinary retention (up to 11%).[67]

The implantable AUS can be used in both men and women to provide a physiologic voiding pattern without increasing the risk of detrusor overactivity or urinary retention.[70] The device is also compatible with CIC.[71] The AUS is commonly used to treat postprostatectomy incontinence in men. Its use in women is limited by the fact that pubovaginal sling procedures are usually easier to perform. Candidates for the AUS must have adequate cognitive function and manual dexterity to operate the device. Although the AUS provides the highest cure rate of any therapy for ISD, it remains uncertain whether the device will survive for the duration of a younger patient's life.[72]

Periurethral injection of bulking agents such as Teflon, autologous fat, silicone, and collagen has been successfully used to treat ISD by passive urethral occlusion. Presently, collagen (that is, Contigen) is the only FDA-approved bioinjectable material. Success varies between 64% and 95%[73] and depends heavily on patient selection. In general, women do better than men. The ideal female patient should have ISD alone, with no associated hypermobility, detrusor overactivity, or periurethral scarring. Desirable male candidates are those who have postprostatectomy incontinence but are poor surgical candidates for AUS implantation.[14] Radiation therapy and bladder neck incision adversely affect outcome.[74] Patients should be aware that repeated injection may be required to achieve the desired effect. Bioinjection therapy can be performed transurethrally or periurethrally under cystoscopic guidance using local anesthesia, with minimal morbidity. Hence this is an attractive procedure for elderly patients with ISD who are poor surgical candidates for AUS implantation or pubovaginal sling procedure. The long-term effects of collagen injection are yet to be determined.

CONCLUSION

Urinary incontinence is a considerable problem in the elderly population, often with complex causes. With proper evaluation and systematic elimination of contributing factors, the correct diagnosis can usually be reached. Conservative management, including behavioral modification will benefit many patients. In carefully selected patients who fail conservative management, surgical therapy can be offered. Using modern minimally invasive techniques, the elderly can achieve similar results as younger patients do without excessive risk of increased morbidity. Elderly patients desiring surgery should not be denied the benefits of surgery on the basis of age alone.

REFERENCES

1. Resnick MI, Palmer RM: Surgical decisions. In O'Donnell P, editor: *Geriatric urology,* Boston, 1994, Little, Brown.
2. Badlani GH: *Urodynamics in the elderly: problems.* (Course handout) *Difficult problems in urodynamics,* AUA Post-Graduate Course No. 20, Las Vegas, April 1995, American Urological Association, Baltimore, Md.
3. Resnick NM: Voiding dysfunction in the elderly. In Yalla SV, McGuire EJ, Elbadawi A, Blaivas JG, editors: *Neurourology and urodynamics: principles and practice,* New York, 1988, Macmillan.
4. Diokno AC, Brown MB, Brock BM, et al: Clinical cystometric characteristics of continent and incontinent noninstitutionalized elderly, *J Urol* 140:567-571, 1988.
5. Pannill FC, Williams TF, Davis R: Evaluation and treatment of urinary incontinence in long-term care, *J Am Geriatr Soc* 36:902-910, 1988.
6. Resnick NM: Initial evaluation of the incontinent patient, *J Am Geriatr Soc* 38:311-315, 1995.
7. Payne CK: Stress urinary incontinence in females. In *Current therapy in urology,* ed 3, Philadelphia, 1994, Saunders.
8. Badlani GH: Application of surgical treatment to frail and functionally dependent incontinent male. Conference syllabus: *Managing incontinence in elderly dependent institutionalized and community dwelling persons: an agenda for research and care,* NIH Consensus Conference, Atlanta, Ga, March 1994, National Institutes of Health, Bethesda, Md.
9. Khan Z, Bhola A: Prostatism and male urinary incontinence, *Semin Urol* 5:108, 1987.
10. Yalla SV, Sharma GV, Barsamian EM: Micturitional static urethral pressure profile: a method of recording urethral pressure profile during voiding and its implications, *J Urol* 124:649, 1980.
11. Badlani GH: Incontinence associated with CVA. In O'Donnell P, editor: *Geriatric urology,* Boston, 1994, Little, Brown.
12. Badlani GH, Ravalli R, Moskowitz MO: A tool for the objective assessment of passive incontinence, *Contemp Urol* 5(7):29, 1993.
13. Ouslander J, Staskin D, Raz S, et al: Clinical versus urodynamic diagnosis in an incontinent geriatric female population, *J Urol* 137:68, 1987.
14. Press SM, Badlani GH: *Injection therapy for urinary incontinence,* AUA Update Series, vol 14, lesson 2, Baltimore, Md, 1995, American Urological Association.
15. Resnick NM, Yalla SV, Laurino E: The pathophysiology and clinical correlates of established urinary incontinence in frail elderly, *N Engl J Med* 320:1-7, 1989.
16. Resnick NM, Yalla SV: Detrusor hyperactivity with impaired contractile function: an unrecognized but common cause of incontinence in elderly patients, *JAMA* 257:3076-3081, 1987.
17. Resnick NM, Brandeis GH, Yalla SV: Detrusor hyperactivity with impaired contractility (DHIC) commonly mimics urethral causes of incontinence in elderly women, *Proc 20th annual meeting, International Continence Society,* pp 261-262, 1990.
18. Nitti VW, Bregg KJ, Raz S: Surgical management of incontinence in elderly women. In O'Donnell P, editor: *Geriatric urology,* Boston, 1994, Little, Brown.
19. Mebust WK, Holtgrewe HL, Cockett AT, Peters PC: Transurethral prostatectomy: immediate and postoperative complications: a cooperative study of 13 participating institutions evaluating 3,885 patients, *J Urol* 141:243-247, 1989.
20. Nissenkorn I, Slutzner D: The intraurethral catheter: long term follow-up in patients with urinary retention due to intravesical obstruction, *Br J Urol* 68:277, 1991.
21. Yachia D, et al: Minimally invasive treatment of penile, bulbomembranous and penile urethral strictures using tailored temporary coil stents, Urocoil, *J Endourol* 7(suppl 1):S112, 1993.
22. Sarramon JP, Joffre F, Rischmann P, et al: Use of the Wall stent endourethral prosthesis in the treatment of recurrent urethral strictures, *Eur Urol* 18(4):281, 1990.

23. Osterling JE: The North American Study Group: the North American experience with the Urolume endoprosthesis as a treatment for symptomatic BPH long term results, *J Urol* 149:216A, 1993.
24. Roth RA, Aretz HT: Transurethral ultrasound guided laser induced prostatectomy (TULIP Procedure): a canine prostate feasibility study, *J Urol* 146:1128, 1991.
25. McCullough DL, Roth RA, Babayan RK, et al: Transurethral ultrasound guided laser-induced prostatectomy: National Human Cooperative study results, *J Urol* 150:1607, 1993.
26. Bolton DM, Costello AJ: Management of benign prostatic hyperplasia by transurethral laser ablation in patients treated with warfarin anticoagulation, *J Urol* 151:79, 1994.
27. Kabalin JN, Gill HS. Urolase laser prostatectomy in patients on warfarin anticoagulation: a safe treatment alternative for bladder outlet obstruction, *Urology* 42(6):738, 1993.
28. Kabalin JN: Laser prostatectomy performed with a right angle firing neodymium:YAG laser fiber at 40 watts power setting, *J Urol* 150:95,1993.
29. Costello AJ, Bowsher WG, Bolton DM, et al: Laser ablation of the prostate in patients with benign prostatic hypertrophy, *Br J Urol* 69:603, 1992.
30. Norris JP, Norris DM, Lee RD, Rubenstein MA: Visual laser ablation of the prostate: clinical experience in 108 patients, *J Urol* 150:1612, 1993.
31. Narayan P, Fournier G, Indudhara R, et al: Transurethral evaporation of prostate (TUEP) with Nd:YAG laser using a contact free beam technique: results in 61 patients with benign prostatic hyperplasia, *Urology* 43(6):813, 1994.
32. Kabalin JN, Gill HS, Bite G, Wolfe V: Comparative study of laser versus electrocautery prostate resection: 18-month follow up with complex urodynamic assessment, *J Urol* 153:94, 1995.
33. Sonn DJ, Desautel MG, Badlani GH: Pressure flow analysis: a measure of successful outcome for benign prostatic hyperplasia by contact laser vaporization of the prostate, *Urology* (submitted).
34. Te AE, Reiss R, Kaplan SA: TVP: a new modification of TURP, *Contemp Urol* 7(5):74, 1995.
35. Kaplan SA, Te AE: Transurethral electrovaporization of the prostate: a novel method for treating men with benign prostatic hyperplasia, *Urology* 45(4):556, 1995.
36. Badlani GH, Smith AD: Intraoperative endourological urethral manipulation, *Urol Clin North Am* 17:25, 1990.
37. Badlani GH, Press SM, Defalco A, et al: Urolume endourethral prosthesis for the treatment of urethral stricture disease: long-term results of the North American Multicenter Urolume Trial, *Urology* 45(5):846, 1995.
38. Whitfield HN, Mayo ME: Prolonged bladder distension in the treatment of the unstable bladder, *Br J Urol* 47:635, 1975.
39. Ramsden PD, Smith JC, Dunn M, et al: Distension therapy for the unstable bladder: later results including an assessment of repeat distension, *Br J Urol* 46:645, 1976.
40. Smith JC, Higson RH: Cystodistension. In Stanton SL, Tanagho EA, editors: *Surgery of female incontinence,* London, 1980, Springer.
41. Ingleman-Sundberg A: Urge incontinence in women, *Acta Obstet Gynecol Scand* 54:153, 1975.
42. Blackford HN, Murray K, Stephenson TP, Mundy AR: Results of transvesical infiltration of the pelvic plexuses with phenol in 116 patients, *Br J Urol* 56:647, 1984.
43. Kreder KJ: Bladder augmentation: treatment of the low compliance bladder, *Prob Urol* 5:669, 1992.
44. Appell RA: Surgical approaches in females including periurethral injections. Conference syllabus: *Managing incontinence in elderly dependent institutionalized and community dwelling persons: an agenda for research and care,* NIH Consensus Conference, Atlanta, Ga., March 1994, National Institutes of Health, Bethesda, Md.
45. Linder A, Leach GE, Raz S: Augmentation cystoplasty in the treatment of neurogenic bladder dysfunction, *J Urol* 129:491, 1983.
46. Golomb J, Klutke CG, Raz S: Complications of bladder substitution and continent urinary diversion, *Urology* 34:329, 1989.
47. McGuire EJ: Clinical evaluation of the female lower urinary tract, *Urol Clin North Am* 12:225-229, 1985.
48. Blaivas JG, Berger Y: Surgical treatment for male geriatric incontinence, *Clin Geriatr Med* 2(4):777, 1986.
49. Nitti VW, Bregg KJ, Sussman EM, Raz S: The Raz bladder neck suspension in patients 65 years old and older, *J Urol* 149:802, 1993.
50. McDuffie RW, Litin RB, Blundun KE: Urethrovesical suspension (Marshall-Marchetti-Krantz), *Am J Surg* 141:297, 1981.
51. Kelly MJ, Leach GE: Long term results of bladder neck suspension procedures, *Prob Urol* 5(1):94, 1991
52. Nielsen E, Lundvall F: Urethrovaginal fixation to Cooper's ligament in the treatment of incontinence, *Acta Chir Scand* 433(suppl):118, 1973.
53. Marshall VF, Marchetti AA, Krantz KE:. The correction of stress incontinence by simple vesicourethral suspension, *Surg Gynecol Obstet* 88:509, 1949.
54. Marshall VF, Vaughn ED, Parnell JP: Suprapubic vesicourethral suspension (Marshall-Marchetti-Krantz) for stress incontinence. In Walsh PC, Gittes R, Perlmutter A, Stamey T, editors: *Campbell's urology,* ed 5, Philadelphia, 1986, Saunders.
55. Burch JC: Urethrovaginal fixation to Cooper's ligament for correction of stress incontinence, cystocele and prolapse, *Am J Obstet Gynecol* 81:281, 1961.
56. Stanton SL, Cardozo LD: Surgical treatment of incontinence in elderly women, *Surg Gynecol Obstet* 150:55, 1980.
57. Gillon G, Stanton SL: Long-term follow up of surgery for urinary incontinence in elderly women, *Br J Urol* 56:478-481, 1984.
58. Peryera AJ, Lebherz TB: The revised Peryera procedure. In Buchsbaum HJ, Schmidt JD, editors: *Gynecologic and obstetric urology,* Philadelphia, 1978, Saunders.
59. Gittes RF, Loughlin KR: No-incision pubovaginal suspension for stress incontinence, *J Urol* 138:568, 1987.
60. Stamey TA: Endoscopic suspension of vesical neck for urinary incontinence, *Surg Gynecol Obstet* 136:547, 1973.
61. Raz S: Surgical therapy for urinary incontinence. In *Atlas of transvaginal surgery,* Philadelphia, 1992, Saunders.
62. Golomb J, Goldwasser B, Mashiach S: Raz bladder neck suspension in women younger than sixty-five years compared with elderly women: three years' experience, *Urology* 43(1):40, 1994.
63. Payne CK, Babiarz JW, Raz S: Genitourinary problems in the elderly patient, *Surg Clin North Am* 74(2):401, 1994.
64. Liu CY: Laparoscopic retropubic colposuspension (Burch procedure): a review of 58 cases, *J Reprod Med* 38(7):526, 1993.
65. Benderev TV: A modified percutaneous outpatient bladder neck suspension system, *J Urol* 152:2316-2320, 1994.
66. Rackley RR, Appel RA: Use of a bone anchoring needle suspension for genuine stress urinary incontinence (GSUI) (Abstract), Presented at American Urogynecology Society Meeting, Sept 1994, Toronto, Canada.
67. Blaivas JG: Pubovaginal sling, AUA Update Series, vol 2, lesson 36, Baltimore, Md., 1992, American Urological Association.
68. Juma S, et al: Vaginal wall sling for intrinsic sphincteric deficiency, *World J Urol* 8:198, 1990.
69. Couillard DR, Deckard-Janatpour KA, Stone AR: The vaginal wall sling: a compressive suspension procedure for recurrent incontinence in elderly patients, *Urology* 43(2):302, 1994.
70. Webster GD, Perez LM, Khoury JM, Timmons SL: Management of type III stress urinary incontinence using artificial urinary sphincter, *Urology* 39(6):499-503, 1992.
71. Diokno AC, Sonda LP: Compatibility of genitourinary prostheses and intermittent self catheterization, *J Urol* 125:659, 1990.
72. Scott FB: The artificial urinary sphincter: experience in adults, *Urol Clin North Am* 16:105, 1989.
73. Appell RA: Injectables for urethral incompetence, *World J Urol* 8:208, 1990.
74. McGuire EJ, et al: Collagen injection therapy in treatment of incontinence secondary to radical retropubic prostatectomy (Abstract), AUA annual convention, Las Vegas, Nevada, April 1995, American Urological Association, Baltimore, Md.

Chapter

61 Containment of Involuntary Urine Loss

Carol A. Brink

There will always be some patients who have residual incontinence after treatment, who do not respond at all to any form of therapy, or who are not candidates for any kind of current treatment. In these patients, their quality of life is dependent on the long-term management of the problem of incontinence that involves the best possible containment methods. Urinary incontinence (UI) makes ordinary life difficult to manage for significant numbers of older individuals, including their care providers who often lack precise knowledge of what to do to help.[1] Many manage to contain their urine by using a variety of products—some homemade and others designed by manufacturers—to reduce the unpleasant effects of involuntary wetting. Adequate and reliable methods of containing urine include the use of absorbent products, collecting systems, and occluding devices.

Absorbent Pads and Garments

Absorbent products consist of pads and underwear designed to soak up and contain urine to protect clothes, bedding, furniture, and floors from soiling, as well as preserve the dignity and comfort of the individual.[2] All products can be classified as either disposable or reusable (washable) except for pant or pad systems, which combine a disposable pad with a carefully styled washable pant.

Pad Construction

Both reusable and disposable pads are designed with a surface area next to the skin that must receive the urine and transmit it quickly to an absorbent inner core. This inner core facilitates the spread of urine to unsaturated areas and requires sufficient absorption capacity to prevent leakage. A waterproof plastic outer layer is often incorporated for extra protection.

The absorbent layer in disposable pads usually contains fluffed wood pulp with or without the addition of superabsorbent polymers that gel with the urine. The use of polymers in the construction of diapers, pant liners, and pads improves the absorption efficiency. Reusables, on the other hand, are made of cloth material with the absorbent core composed of rayon or polyester fibers. The size and arrangement of these fibers influence their absorption potential. Philips and her colleagues describe the choice of materials used for the inner surface layer of reusable products in relation to a consumer preference for good wet or dry comfort.[3] Good wet comfort is facilitated by the use of a hydrophobic material, such as polyester, that allows the urine to pass through to the absorbent layer yet maintains a dry surface next to the skin. Cotton, on the other hand, is good in absorbing body moisture and provides "dry comfort" before voiding. Once wet, however, the comfort level is quickly reversed. Hence the length of time between wet-pad changes becomes an important comfort and skin care issue.

Further Classification

Absorbent products include those that are worn on the body and those that cover or protect furniture from soiling.

Body-worn pads. Body-worn products include diapers, undergarments, liners, and pant or pad systems. Here, the terminology used to identify products for advertising and marketing purposes is often confusing. The adult diaper is marketed as a disposable or reusable brief. Adult disposable diapers are made for roll-on bed application and are suitable for both fecal and moderate to heavy urinary incontinence. Styles include elastic leg gathers, self-adhesive tapes, and an outer plastic cover. Most are sized by waist and hip measurement and are sold as small, medium, or large. The undergarment is similar in concept to a disposable diaper and consists of a waterproof-backed large pad that extends to the waist and is held in place by reusable elastic side straps. This one-piece, form-fitting product seems to be acceptable to ambulatory individuals with large urine loss. One size fits all with hip and waist measurements up to 54 inches.

Alternative terms for pant liners include pads, guards, shields, and inserts.[2] These pads, similar conceptually to menstrual pads, are designed to soak up urine and provide protection for light to moderately heavy incontinence. In fact, menstrual pads were found to be the most commonly used pant liner (63%) in one study of community-living incontinent women and the pad of choice of women in a later study who attributed their preference to lower cost and less bulk.[4,5] Women simply substituted the pads for a different purpose. Today, however, incontinent-specific liners are designed with a feminine appeal. Many contain a dry gel polymer and also material to reduce odor. Newer designs have a soft, contour shape and have added a wide adhesive strip to hold the pad in place. Popular, well advertised brand names, such as Serenity (guards) and Poise (pads) are becoming common household words among women with UI. Drip collectors for men are designed as a sheathlike pouch with absorbent material to envelope the penis.[6] These have waterproof backing and are held in place by a stretch-mesh brief or snug-fitting underwear.

Pant or pad systems vary in composition and design. Although most are unisex, a few are specific to either the male or the female. Some systems, such as Promise, are useful for the doubly incontinent because its pad is designed to be next to the patient's skin. Dignity, on the other hand, is designed to contain only urine, since its pad is held in an inside waterproof pouch with pant or crotch material next to the patient's skin surface. The Tranquility system claims its new high-capacity pads have a degradable core that can be flushed down the toilet. A new washable pant with a paper-thin liner by Undercare claims to hold up to 11 ounces of urine. Further, the liners are reported to dissolve and disappear as the pants are laundered. All pants are usually fitted according to waist and hip circumference or body weight. The pads are styled and sized for a specific pant.

Underpads. Washable and disposable underpads designed to protect beds and chairs are useful and often found in combination with a body-worn pant or pad system.[2] Underpads are alternatively called bed pads, bed sheets, draw sheets, or chair pads. The cheap, disposable blue pads have, for the most part, been replaced by superior products. The high absorption capacity pads feature a stay-dry surface next to the patient's skin. The PatientGuard underpad also features a broad-spectrum antimicrobial fiber claimed to be effective against ammonia-producing bacteria responsible for odors, as well as other fungi and viruses.

Discussion and Issues

The quality and performance of absorbent products have been shown to vary and are influenced by cost. The choice of which products to use or recommend varies widely depending on the severity of wetting. Attends, for example, has a range of pads that provide protection from "very light" to "maximum" depending on the volume lost during any one episode or over time. Further, mobility and manual dexterity must be considered. An ambulatory person is likely to prefer a pant or pad system or undergarment over a diaper, and Velcro straps on clothing rather than buttons are easier for arthritic hands to manipulate.

Key factors related to pad selection and satisfaction have been identified[7] (see box). Leakage occurs if the pad is saturated beyond its absorption capacity or if the garment has been improperly fitted so that it is too loose, especially around the leg. Slippage occurs when the pad is improperly applied or secured. Convenience is associated with ease of application, removal, storage, and disposal. Skin is sensitive and can react to certain materials, producing itchiness or a rash, or both. Some products have been found to be more comfortable and to eliminate unpleasant urine odor. Pads are discreet if they are not visible or noticeable under clothing and durable if they do not disintegrate when wet. Cost varies and is related to the design and construction of the product.

In summary, absorbent pads and garments continue to be widely used, as reflected by the growth of the market of disposable pads and adult diapers from $99 million in 1972 to $173 million in 1982 to $496 million in 1987.[8] The growth spurt in the 1980s resulted from pressure placed by large companies on the Federal Communications Commission to lift the taboo against national televised advertising of absorbent products.[9] As a result, products are now being advertised on television and radio and are available, without prescription, in drug, grocery, and other retail stores.

Factors in Pad Selection and Satisfaction

- Leakage
- Slippage
- Convenience
- Skin sensitivity
- Comfort
- Odor
- Discretion
- Durability
- Cost

There is concern that people will use these as a first response to UI and not seek proper diagnostic evaluation and treatment.[10] The product industry has expanded to the point where it is difficult to keep up with design and cost differences. The Help for Incontinent People Resource Guide of products and services for incontinence is available at minimal cost and has been a major source of information and support to the public in this country.[6]

COLLECTING DEVICES

A device is a "mechanical invention or contrivance for some specific purpose," and in this context it would be to collect and store the urine until it can be suitably emptied.[11] Collection devices, such as bedpans and urinals, have received little attention as aids to containing urine. Bedpans are of ancient origin, come in multiple designs, each of which offers different advantages, and, in general, serve individuals confined to bed.[12] Urinals, on the other hand, can be useful in both sitting and standing positions and have been designed for women as well as men. For males, a retracted penis prohibits their use. These hand-held, bottle-shaped receptacles vary by the degree of neck curvature, the handle design, and the shape and size of the opening. Neck curvature needs to be angled sufficiently to prevent runback leakage, and the handles must be large enough to provide an easy, secure grip. Some have a snap-closing lid with visual measurement of contents in ounces or milliliters (equivalent to cubic centimeters).

Newer styles offer more management options. The female and male Para Quad urinals are designed for wheelchair use with the opening extending to a horizontal collector that meets at right angles with a holding tank. The opening for the female is designed to cup over the urethral area and funnel the urine inside. In contrast, a bedside urinal, with a handle designed to hook over the side rail, allows urine to drain into an attached collecting bag.[6] Although simple conceptually, these devices can offer relief for select individuals. Other available styles of urinals are shown in the Active Living Catalogue.[13] These include the male, millie female, and a guaranteed no-spill urinal—ideal again for men who insist on keeping their urinals next to them in bed. A variety of designs offer choices to people with different body shapes and functional needs.

External Collecting Devices

External collecting devices are attached to the body and can provide a comfortable and satisfactory means of catching and storing urine. In the male these devices usually consist of a formed latex cone or sheath worn over the penis with tubing that leads to a leg bag. Often, some type of encircling device or adhering tape is used to seal the top of the sheath around the penis to prevent leakage. Problems of detachment, twisting, and pooling of urine within the condom have been identified in cheaper products, as well as circulatory disruption to the penis secondary to improper application. Therefore professional guidance is recommended in selecting, sizing, applying, and removing the condom. A variety of styles are available including ones with adhesive for self-application requiring no strip or pants, others requiring adhering tape, and a reusable condom that is secured by filling an inflation ring with air.[6]

Female collecting devices have attempted to encompass the external urinary opening using a variety of methods to stabilize and hold the device in place, including a vaginal locator, adhesive fixative, suction, and special snug-fitting elasticized pants reminiscent of a girdle. With these devices, urine is funneled via tubing to a leg bag designed to prevent urine backflow. Major problems with female devices relate to skin irritation and leakage. Nonetheless, both men and women can choose to wear an external collecting device for special outings or events, and alternate with absorbent pads or garments when at home.

Occluding Devices

Occluding devices are used to obstruct the flow of urine by compressing the urethra.

For men. The penile clamp, a V-shaped frame with a foam cushion, fits over and under the penis. When closed, it should pinch off the urine flow without discomfort. Another type of compression device that is size adjustable encircles the penis and stops the flow of urine when it is inflated with air.[6] These devices are useful for men who are, first, mentally capable of remembering to release the clamp on a regular 2- to 3- hour schedule and then manually able to manipulate it.

For women. Although there is no specially designed female counterpart currently available in this country, a pessary can stop the flow of urine. Pessaries are cube, ring, or doughnut-shaped devices made of rubber or silicone materials designed to be inserted into the vagina to reduce pelvic prolapse. They have, however, been inserted for the purpose of compressing the urethra, thus acting as an occluding device. Although this is *not* a recommended use of the pessary, in these instances women need to be informed about the obstructive purpose and taught when and how to remove and clean the device. Contraceptive diaphragms may have the same occluding effect in younger women.

A recent report showed that an intraurethral insert was a highly effective means of controlling urine loss associated with stress and mild urge incontinence in women.[14] Although this occluding device remains under investigation and is not currently available, it has promise as an option for the future.

SUMMARY

In summary, absorbent products and collecting and occluding devices for urine containment continue to be developed and improved upon, as manufacturers respond to consumer needs and competition within the marketplace. Issues of cost, quality, and reimbursement remain problematic. Costs vary greatly, as do third-party reimbursement practices, which for the most part fail to cover expenses incurred in the home. Thus, for those required to pay out of pocket, items such as diapers or pads become financially inaccessible. Devices, if medically prescribed and justified, remain covered by Medicare. For the institutionalized, the cost of pads and diapers are often hidden, that is, included as part of a room rate inflated to cover these materials. Cheaper products of inferior make are often used by a facility in an effort to reduce expenses.

Finally, videotapes produced by manufacturers to promote their products are a new education and marketing vehicle. More teaching materials aimed at professionals need to be developed.

REFERENCES

1. Brink C: Keeping dry: aids to coping with incontinence, *The Southwestern* 6(2):57-67, 1990.
2. Brink C: Absorbent pads, garments, and management strategies, *J Am Geriatr Soc* 38(3):368-373, 1990.
3. Philips J, Cottended A, Ledger D: A testing time, *Nurs Times* 89:59-62, 1993.
4. Brink C, Wells T, Diokno A: Urinary incontinence in women, *Public Health Nurs* 4(2):114-119, 1987.
5. Skoner M: Self-management of urinary incontinence among women 31-50 years of age, *Rehab Nurs* 19(6)339-343, 347, 1994.
6. Verdel L, editor: *Help for Incontinent People, resource guide*, ed 6, Union, SC, 1994, Help for Incontinent People, PO Box 544, Union, SC 29379.
7. Brink C: Absorbent products and collection devices for the patient with intractable incontinence. Presented at conference: Managing incontinence in elderly dependent institutionalized and community dwelling persons: an agenda for research and care, NIH Consensus Conference, Atlanta, Ga., March 1994, National Institutes of Health, Bethesda, Md.
8. Urinary incontinence in adults, clinical practice guideline, AHCPR Pub No 92-0038, Rockville, Md., 1992, Agency for Health Care Policy and Research, Public Health Service Deptartment of Health and Human Services.
9. Wells T: Conquering incontinence, *Geriatr Nurs* 13(3):133-135.
10. Ouslander J: Geriatric urinary incontinence. In Bone R, editor: *Disease-a-Month* 38(2), 1992.
11. Neufeldt V, editor: *Webster's New World Dictionary,* ed 3, New York, 1994, Warner Books.
12. Wells T, Brink C: Elimination: urinary. In Burnside IM, editor: *Nursing and the aged*, ed 3, New York, 1988, McGraw-Hill.
13. *Active Living™ Catalogue*, South Burlington, Vt., 1993, Laborie Medical Technologies Corp.
14. *Multicenter experience using an expandable urethral insert for management of urinary stress incontinence.* Data presented at the American Urological Association, Las Vegas, Nev., April 27, 1995, AUA, Baltimore, Md.

Chapter 62

Nursing Management

Thelma J. Wells

Nursing management of urinary incontinence in older people has changed radically in the last 15 years. Over those years relevant literature has grown from one or two articles to an extensive information base. National Institutes of Health–funded research with nurse principal or coinvestigators has yielded important findings in assessment, diagnoses, and treatment of urinary incontinence. The issue today is separating what is known from what is not known and, equally difficult, utilizing new knowledge in practice.[1]

Registered nurses in direct care roles may be prepared as generalists (baccalaureate, associate, or diploma) or specialists (advanced degrees and roles of nurse practitioner or clinical nurse specialists). Pearce has distinguished levels of urinary incontinence care in outpatient settings.[2] Level I is basic assessment and management, appropriate for both generalist and specialist nurses, and Level II is focused assessment and management, more appropriate for those with special training. In this chapter the focus will be on basic management to reduce or resolve transient urinary incontinence. Topics include communication, environment, fluid management, drugs, constipation or impaction, urinary tract infections, and health factors. Other chapters in this text address the aspects of focused assessment and management.

Communication

Goldstein et al. report a study of 136 participants at a senior citizen center.[3] Thirty-six percent had experienced urinary incontinence, and of these more than half (59%) had not sought treatment. The most common reasons given for not seeking help were the belief that incontinence is a normal part of aging (62%), followed by lack of knowledge about available treatments (38%) and belief that incontinence is a normal sequela of childbirth (27%).

There is a major need for public education in urinary incontinence. A recent report of urinary incontinence knowledge among community-dwelling people 65 years and older supports the need for such education, particularly for men, those 85 and over, and those less educated.[4] Appendix N displays the incontinence quiz developed by the investigators primarily from the 1992 AHCPR guidelines for urinary incontinence in adults.[5] In the study subjects commonly agreed incorrectly that most people with urinary incontinence talk to their doctors about it (71%), urine loss is a result of normal aging (58%), most physicians ask older patients about urine control (47%), and by 85 years of age most people have regular urinary incontinence (42%). In addition, 53% of subjects were uncertain if over-the-counter medications cause urine loss when it is well established that selected over-the-counter medications can cause or contribute to urinary incontinence. Overall, no one in the 1140 subject sample correctly answered all items. The mode was six correct responses, with 26% having eight or more correct and 5% being wrong on all 14 items. Disseminating knowledge about urine control and urinary incontinence is essential. The nonprofit organizations listed provide a variety of educational materials including media, guides, booklets, and newsletters. In addition, selected drug and product companies produce a range of patient teaching material, some very helpful. Primary care settings should have selected brochures available, resource lists posted, and perhaps a loan library of books. The incontinence quiz with answers provided might be a meaningful waiting-room teaching opportunity. Community outreach is often appropriate with presentations to senior groups or articles in local senior newspapers.

Urinary incontinence in older women was explored in a qualitative study by Dowd.[6] Seven women, 58 to 79 years of age and having urinary incontinence from 1½ to 50 years, described their experience. Analysis revealed that the basic social problem was preventing threats to self-esteem. Major threats were a visible wetting accident in public, nonvisible wetting accidents, odor, and revealing a wetting problem in conversation. Sequential life-adjustment phases were evident: (1) being in charge through effective self-care management strategies, (2) accepting urinary incontinence through self-care confidence and minimizing the problem, and (3) normalizing through acceptable adjustment and routine.

Gender may play a role in patient comfort regarding the sensitive topic of urine control; for instance, woman-to-woman discussion may be less threatening to self-esteem. Provider emphasis on patient self-care, distinguishing research-based practice from common belief, should help in teaching basic management techniques. Determining the patient's lifestyle and personal agenda, providing choices, and building on routine should facilitate management programs.

A scale that has potential to monitor the effectiveness of patient urinary incontinence management has been developed. The Coping with Urinary Incontinence Scale has been refined to 39 items in 10 subscales such as rearranging physical environment, concealing attempts, and managing in social situations.[7] An item example within the subscale rearranging physical environment is "to prevent loss of urine in public places, I stay at home near the toilet." Responses are graded on a four-point Likert-like scale. Initial psychometric testing has focused on internal consistency, stability, and construct validity in samples of community-living elderly incontinent individuals.

ENVIRONMENT

Patients come from diverse settings and may, over time, move or be transferred to different settings. But the key environmental question remains the same: What is toilet access for this individual? Toilet access combines toilet location and design with patient functional ability in terms of mobility, clothes manipulation, and cognitive status. In older private homes toilet access may require climbing stairs or, in some rural areas, going to the outside privy. Toilet availability in congregate living settings varies greatly across the range of resources from single-occupancy residential hotel rooms to skilled nursing units. Apart from the living-situation toilet access, questions arise about lifestyle and toilet access during required or desired activity. Urine control problems can be helped or resolved though selection of a commode, toilet adaptation, mobility aid, or clothing adaptation. Physical and occupational therapists have special expertise in those areas.

FLUID MANAGEMENT

Amount of Fluid

Individuals with urine control problems may subscribe to either a restrictive or an excessive fluid intake behavior. In one study of community-living women with urinary incontinence (N = 338, age 55 to 90 with a mean of 67.5 years), 313 completed fluid-intake diaries for an average of four consecutive 24-hour periods. Fluid intake ranged from an average of 585 to 3852 ml per day, with a mean of 1748 (SD 564). Thirty-four percent of these women drank on average less than 1500 ml per day; of these, 21 drank less than 1000 ml daily. Fewer women were at the high-volume intake, with only 10 exceeding 3000 ml on average.[8] Certainly there is an appealing logic that restrictive fluid intake might yield less urine. Diminished urine might mean less incontinence or, at least, easier management of urine control. This reasoning is commonly expressed by those with urinary incontinence.

However, of two studies reporting the relationship of fluid intake to voluntary voiding and urinary incontinence, both found only modest relationships between diurnal voiding, nocturnal voiding, and incontinence episodes.[9,10] The study with community-living incontinent women concluded that the association of fluid intake to bladder behavior was complex, hypothesized that fluid manipulation might play a minor role in urine control, and cautioned against fluid intake restrictions.[9] The other study focused on frail elders of both sexes who were institutionalized and being evaluated for potential discharge or transfer to sheltered housing. In this study a subgroup of more cognitively impaired patients with severe incontinence and urge incontinence by urodynamic evaluation were identified as potential candidates for a fluid manipulation and nocturnal toileting program.[10]

In general the state of knowledge indicates that fluid intake in individuals with urine control problems should not differ from the accepted norm. There is a basic formula to calculate fluid maintenance requirements per 24 hours in adults. The formula is based on body weight in kilograms (kg) and implies a positive health status, modest activity, and stable environmental temperature. There are three steps in calculation: (1) for the first 10 kg the fluid requirement is 100 ml/kg, or 1000 ml; (2) for the second 10 kg the fluid requirement is 50 ml/kg, or 500 ml; and (3) for weight over 20 kg the fluid requirement is 20 ml/kg, with ideal weight used for obese individuals.[11] Thus, a 95-pound (43.2 kg) woman would need 1964 ml of fluid for maintenance per 24 hours, whereas a 180-pound (81.8 kg) man would need 2736 ml. Of course health status, activity level, and environmental temperature variance would make specific individual requirements different.

In addition, liquid fluid intake is only one of three methods by which water is added to body fluids. There is water in food, estimated for the average American adult diet to be 800 to 1000 ml per day. And lastly, oxidative processes in food metabolism within the body produce about 300 to 400 ml of water daily.[12] Although food intake and its metabolism can produce significant amounts of fluid, the general recommendation for liquid fluid intake in adults is 1500 to 2500 ml, or 6 to 10 cups of liquid per day.

Type of Fluid

Caffeine, a xanthine derivative, is a natural diuretic. It acts similar to thiazide diuretics and thus may contribute to urinary frequency. In addition, the effect of caffeine on bladder muscle was studied in 20 women with confirmed bladder instability and 10 normal volunteers. Both groups were given 200 mg of caffeine citrate to drink, followed in 30 minutes by urodynamic evaluation. The normal group had no response to the caffeine. But the women with bladder instability, all of whom had precaffeine and postcaffeine measures, had a significant increase in bladder pressure on filling in response to caffeine. The researchers hypothesize that caffeine has a direct excitatory effect on bladder smooth muscle, which may be compensated in normal bladders and is symptomatic in those with an underlying disorder.[13]

The exact amount of caffeine in a liquid is subject to brand and consumer taste variance. Table 62-1 displays the approximate caffeine dose in common beverages.[14] Methods to help individuals decrease caffeine intake start with awareness through careful label reading and keeping a daily diary. In addition to the fluids shown in the table, caffeine is commonly found in many over-the-counter medications. Persons with large caffeine intake should decrease slowly to avoid significant withdrawal responses such as headache and depression. Alcohol also causes a diuretic effect by inhibiting a release of antidiuretic hormone from the posterior pituitary.[15] Thus evaluation of alcohol use and counseling if necessary are useful in urine control management.

Table 62-1 Approximate Caffeine per 8* Ounces in Common Beverages

BEVERAGE	CAFFEINE (MG)
Drip coffee	179
Percolated coffee	133
Instant coffee	96
Leaf or bag tea	66
Instant tea	45
Regular colas	40
Cocoa or hot chocolate	8
Chocolate milk	5
Decaffeinated coffee	5

*Except for regular colas, which is for a 12-ounce can.

DRUGS

Polypharmacy, use of more medications than are clinically indicated for a specific patient, and drug misuse are areas of concern in geriatrics.[16] Thus assessment of both prescribed and over-the-counter medication is critical. Many types of drugs have been implicated in drug-induced urinary incontinence, as noted in the box.[17,18] In one study of drugs affecting urine control in the elderly, 62% of patients were receiving up to four drugs each for other medical conditions that could potentially alter urine control.[19] For example, a commonly used antihypertensive, prazosin hydrochloride (Minipres), is an alpha-adrenergic blocking agent that reduces urethral closure pressure and decreases functional urethral length. In one report 29% of women taking prazosin and having urinary incontinence were cured when prazosin was stopped, with an additional 29% much improved.[20] All these women had been diagnosed as having stress incontinence by urodynamic evaluation.

Diuretics have often been implicated in urine control problems. Two studies of community-living incontinent older women found nocturia greater for those on diuretics.[21,22] In addition, one study found significantly more incontinent episodes, diurnal frequency, and greater fluid loss in testing (bladder instability subjects only) for those receiving diuretics.[22] Another study used an epidemiologic survey to examine diuretic use and urine control in a sample of continent and incontinent individuals 60 years of age and older living in the community.[23] They found no significant difference in the prevalence of incontinence for either men or women receiving diuretics compared to those not receiving diuretics. But in males with uninhibited bladder contractions during cystometrics, diuretic users had a significantly higher prevalence of urinary incontinence compared to nonusers. These authors postulate that diuretics could cause a bladder-filling surge effect to trigger uninhibited contractions.

Diuretic use should be carefully monitored for the lowest dose necessary for physiologic effect. Some elderly may prefer taking diuretics in the late afternoon because they would rather be housebound for toileting needs in the evening. Trials with alternative diuretics should be explored for those having significant wetting.

Drug-Induced Urinary Incontinence

- Diuretics
- Antidepressants
- Antihistamines
- Neuroleptics
- Antiparkinsonians
- Alpha-adrenergic agonists
- Alpha-adrenergic antagonists
- Psychotropics

CONSTIPATION AND IMPACTION

Constipation in the elderly can lead to fecal impaction especially in those who are frail and immobile. Dehydration and drug side effects also contribute to this problem. A hard mass of feces can exert pressure through the soft tissue of the perineal area to create an outflow obstruction at the bladder neck.

One study has shown that elderly people living in the community are more likely to describe a complaint of constipation as straining with bowel movement rather than the more common medical criterion of stool frequency less than three times per week.[24] Within this framework 30% of males and 29% of females reported that they were constipated more than once per month. Constipation was significantly associated with taking more medications (excluding laxatives) but not associated with self-reported food fiber or fluid intake. This latter finding was supported in a study comparing constipated elderly with controls.[25] However, in both studies fiber and fluid intake were low in comparison to what is recommended. The Nutrition Screening Initiative has focused on the elderly and, although it recommends further study of dietary and fluid management of constipation, it supports fluid interventions of eight or more cups per day with half of these water and at least 6 to 10 g of dietary fiber daily.[26]

Impaction presents with symptoms of abdominal pain, distension, and a history of a lack of bowel movement, though overflow fecal incontinence is common. Physical signs include abdominal tenderness, noticeable abdominal distension, and a mass in the left lower quadrant. Hard stool is usually felt in the rectum but is not always present as a sign of impaction. Enemas are a first choice for clearing the rectum. If necessary, hard fecal masses can be broken up with digital manipulation. Care must always be taken in this procedure to avoid damage to the anal sphincter and pain and discomfort to the patient. Lidocaine 5%, applied to the anus 5 to 10 minutes before the procedure, and gentle dilatation of the anal sphincter, are helpful approaches.[27,28]

URINARY TRACT INFECTION

It is agreed that bacteriuria is common in the elderly and that those who are asymptomatic should be treated.[29] Health care providers usually counsel patients in behaviors to avoid urinary tract infections. Leiner reviewed the research base for common preventive advice and found conflicting findings for such behavior as drinking cranberry juice, directing women to wipe differently in perineal cleaning after defecation, and type of underwear.[30] However, there are many design issues and few elderly samples in these studies. Encouraging fluid management as discussed earlier and recommending daytime toileting frequency on a 2 to 3 hour pattern are simple empiric preventive measures.

HEALTH FACTORS

Cough

A cough increases intra-abdominal pressure and is a stimulus to leakage in both overflow and stress urinary incontinence. In a large epidemiologic study of continent and incontinent community-living elderly, a larger proportion of incontinent men and women reported that they cough or sneeze often compared to continent individuals.[31] The most obvious source of preventable cough is cigarette smoking. Bump and McClish report a study of 606 women, 13 to 87 years of age (mean, 46 years), in which 322 were incontinent and 284 were not.[32] They examined the relationship between current, former, and never smokers on incontinence, reporting a 28% attributable risk of incontinence caused by smoking. Women who currently smoked had a 2.5-fold increase in the risk of stress incontinence, whereas former smokers' risk was a 2.2-fold increase. The authors postulate that a smoker's deep and frequent cough damages urethral sphincteric mechanisms. They also note that nicotine action on bladder muscle, antiestrogen effects of smoking, products of tobacco smoke, or other processes associated with smoking may also contribute.

Health teaching to prevent the start of cigarette smoking, especially among school-age children and young adults, might be enhanced by knowledge of the risk of urinary incontinence in later years. Although urethral mechanism damage may not be reversible, smoking cessation will improve or resolve cough and reduce the frequency of that stimulus for urine leakage.

Other sources of cough are worth exploring for resolution or reduction. Allergies may be a source of frequent cough or sneeze. Respiratory disorders need to be evaluated and managed to reduce cough.

Obesity

Obesity is defined as an accumulation of excess body fat such that one is 20% or more over desirable body weight. Body Mass Index (BMI) is a weight (kg)-to-height (meters) ratio (weight divided by height squared) most often used as the criterion for obesity or severe overweight. It is recommended that individuals over 65 years of age have a BMI of 24 to 29.[33] Values above 29 indicate obesity, with a high risk for such starting at 27. Survey data estimate 28.2% of female and 26.3% of males 65 years of age and over are obese.[34]

Obesity is commonly considered a factor in severity of leakage in both overflow and stress incontinence, with the belief being that increased abdominal adipose tissue increases intra-abdominal pressure. Bump et al. reviewed previous studies of obesity and urinary incontinence, noting conflicting findings and design limitations. These authors then report a study of 13 women, 22 to 65 years of age (mean, 41), with BMIs of 38.6 to 62.2 (mean, 49.4), 12 of whom complained of urinary incontinence. These morbidly obese women had urodynamic evaluation before and after gastric bypass surgery. The aftermeasure was done when their weight stabilized (11 to 24 months after surgery) with postsurgery BMIs of 21.2 to 38.6 (mean, 33.1). Significant differences were seen in urodynamic evaluation before and after weight loss in all intravesical pressure measurements and in all cough-related parameters with before–weight loss measures greater than those after weight loss. It was determined that changes were attributable to weight loss decreases in abdominal pressure. Further, there was a significant reduction in incontinence episodes and pad use after weight loss, with 11 of the 12 previously incontinent women satisfied with their new urine control.[35]

Obesity is not usually so extreme as in these study women. However, typical obese individuals may deter providers from evaluating urinary incontinence because of a range of factors from difficulty in perineal examination to negative beliefs about obesity and treatment adherence. Obese individuals may have low self-esteem and be very reluctant to acknowledge urine loss problems. Obesity may be a risk factor for incontinence or urine loss severity. For these and other important health care reasons, obese individuals should trigger sensitive urine control evaluation and weight reduction programs.

SUMMARY

Health care providers should be a source of education in urine control and urinary incontinence problems through office material distribution and display as well as outreach activities. Individuals with urinary incontinence cope through a variety of self-care management strategies that need to be recognized and supported if appropriate. The most critical environmental issue is toilet access with problem resolution possible through various adaptations. In general fluid intake recommendations for incontinent individuals should be based on normal adult requirements, averaging 6 to 10 cups of liquid per day. Caffeine and alcohol have diuresing effects and should be limited. Medications must be carefully evaluated for urine control side effects with special attention given to diuretic management. Recommended prevention measures for constipation and impaction are fluid intake of at least 8 cups and 6 to 10 g of dietary fiber daily. Fluid intake as noted and a pattern of 2- to 3-hour daytime toileting may be helpful in preventing symptomatic bacteriuria. Reducing cough and obesity are likely to reduce overflow and stress incontinence leakage.

REFERENCES

1. Wells TJ: Nursing research on urinary incontinence, *Urol Nurs* 14(3):109-112, 1994.
2. Pearce KL: Levels I and II: care in the outpatient setting, *Nurs Pract Forum* 5(3):146-151, 1994.
3. Goldstein M, Hawthorne ME, Engeberg S, et al: Urinary incontinence: why people do not seek help? *J Gerontol Nurs* 18(4):15-20, 1992.
4. Branch LG, Walker LA, Wetle TT, et al: Urinary incontinence knowledge among community-dwelling people 65 years of age and older, *J Am Geriatr Soc* 42:1257-1262, 1994.
5. Urinary Incontinence Guideline Panel: *Urinary incontinence in adults: clinical practice guideline,* AHCPR Pub No 92-0038, Rockville, Md., 1992, Agency for Health Care Policy and Research, Public Health Service, U.S. Department of Health and Human Services.
6. Dowd TT: Discovering older women's experience of urinary incontinence, *Res Nurs Health* 14:179-186, 1991.
7. Talbot LA: Coping with urinary incontinence: development and testing a scale, *Nurs Diag* 5(3):127-132.
8. Wells TJ, Brink CM, Diokno AC: R01 AG03542 (1982-1987), unpublished data.
9. Wyman JF, Elswick RK, Wilson MS, et al: Relationship of fluid intake to voluntary micturitions and urinary incontinence in women, *Neurourol Urodyn* 10:463-473, 1991.
10. Griffiths DJ, McCracken PM, Harrison GM, et al: Relationship of fluid intake to voluntary micturition and urinary incontinence in geriatric patients, *Neurourol Urodyn* 12:1-7, 1993.
11. Herfindal ET, Gourley DR, Hart LL, editors: *Clinical pharmacy and therapeutics,* ed 5, Philadelphia, 1992, Williams & Wilkins.
12. West JB, editor: *Best and Taylor's physiological basis of medical practice,* ed 12, Baltimore, 1991, Williams & Wilkins.
13. Creighton SM, Stanton SL: Caffeine: does it affect your bladder? *Br J Urol* 66:613-614, 1990.
14. Continence Program of the University of Rochester: *Caffeine reduction program monograph,* Rochester, N.Y., 1992, University of Rochester.

15. Martin PR, Lovinger DM, Breese GR: Alcohol and other substances abuse. In Munson PL, editor: *Principles of pharmacology,* New York, 1995, Chapman & Hall.
16. Montamet SC, Cusack B: Overcoming problems with polypharmacy and drug misuse in the elderly, *Clin Geriatr Med* 8(1):143-158, 1992.
17. Shimp LA: Influence of drug therapy on urinary incontinence, *Top Geriatr Rehabil* 3(2):30-41, 1988.
18. Ruiz JG, Lowenthal DT: Geriatric pharmacology. In Munson PL, editor: *Principles of pharmacology,* New York, 1995, Chapman & Hall.
19. Gormley EA, Griffiths DJ, McCracken PM, et al: Polypharmacy and its effect on urinary incontinence in a geriatric population, *Br J Urol* 71:265-269, 1993.
20. Dwyer PL, Teele JS: Prazosin: A neglected cause of genuine stress incontinence, *Obstet Gynecol* 79(1):117-121, 1992.
21. Shimp LA, Wells TJ, Brink CA, et al: Relationship between drug use and urinary incontinence in elderly women, *Drug Intell Clin Pharm* 22:786-787, 1988.
22. Fentl JA, Wyman JF, Wilson M, et al: Diuretics and urinary incontinence in community-dwelling women, *Neurourol Urodyn* 9:25-34, 1990.
23. Diokno AC, Brown MB, Herzog AR: Relationship between use of diuretics and continence status in the elderly, *Urology* 38(1):39-42, 1991.
24. Whitehead UE, Drinkwater D, Cheskin LJ, et al: Constipation in the elderly living at home, *J Am Geriatr Soc* 37:423-429, 1989.
25. Towers AL, Burgio KL, Locker JL: Constipation in the elderly: influence of dietary, psychological, and physiological factors, *J Am Geriatr Soc* 42:701-706, 1994.
26. Dwyer JT: *Screening older Americans' nutritional health: current practices and future possibilities,* Washington, D.C., 1991, Nutrition Screening Initiative.
27. Brocklehurst JC: Constipation in the elderly. In Kamm MA, Lennard-Jones JE, editors: *Constipation,* Bristol, Penn., 1994, Wrightson Biomedical Publishing.
28. Stone JT: Managing bowel function. In Chenitz WC, Stone JT, Salisbury SA, editors: *Clinical gerontological nursing,* Philadelphia, 1991, Saunders.
29. Nicolle LE: Urinary infection in the elderly. In Oreopoulos DG, Michelis MF, Herschorn S, editors: *Nephrology and urology in the aged patient,* Boston, Mass., 1993, Kluwer Academic Publisher.
30. Leiner S: Recurrent urinary tract infections in otherwise healthy adult women, *Nurs Pract* 20(2):48-56, 1995.
31. Diokno AC, Brock BM, Herzog AR, et al: Medical correlates of urinary incontinence in the elderly, *Urology* 36(2):129-138, 1990.
32. Bump RC, McClish DR: Cigarette smoking and urinary incontinence in women, *Am J Obstet Gynecol* 167(5):1213-1218, 1992.
33. American Academy of Family Physicians, The American Dietetic Association, National Council on the Aging, Inc: *Nutrition screening manual for professionals caring for older Americans,* Washington, D.C., 1991, Greer, Margolis, Mitchell, Grunwald & Associates, Inc.
34. Danney AJ, editor: *Statistical record of older Americans,* Detroit, 1994, Gale Research.
35. Bump RC, Sugerman HJ, Fantl JA, et al: Obesity and lower urinary tract function in women: effect of surgically induced weight loss, *Am J Obstet Gynecol* 167(2):392-399, 1992.

PATIENT EDUCATION MATERIALS

Monographs/pamphlets

Urinary Incontinence Guideline Panel: *Urinary incontinence in adults: a patient's guide,* AHCPR Pub. No. 92-0040. Rockville, Md. 1992, Agency for Health Care Policy and Research.

Books

Bruning N: *What you can do about bladder control,* New York, 1992, Lynn Sonberg Book, Dell Medical Library.

Burgio RL, Pearce RL, Lucco AJ: *Staying dry: a practical guide to bladder control,* Baltimore, Md. 1989, Johns Hopkins University Press.

Chalker R, Whitemore KE: *Overcoming bladder disorders,* New York, 1991, Harper Perennial.

Gartley CB, editor: *Managing incontinence: a guide to living with loss of bladder control,* Ottawa, Ill., 1985, Jameson Books.

Nonprofit organizations

Continence Restored, Inc.
785 Park Avenue
New York, NY 10021

Help for Incontinent People
PO Box 544
Union, SC 29379

The Simon Foundation
Box 815
Wilmette, IL 60091

Urinary Incontinence Quality of Life Questionnaire

APPENDIX A

1. I worry about wetting myself.
2. I worry about coughing or sneezing because of my incontinence.
3. I have to be careful standing up after I've been sitting down because of my incontinence.
4. I worry about where toilets are in new places.
5. I feel depressed because of my incontinence.
6. Because of my incontinence, I don't feel free to leave my home for long periods of time.
7. I feel frustrated because my incontinence prevents me from doing what I want.
8. I worry about others smelling urine on me.
9. Incontinence is always on my mind.
10. It's important for me to make frequent trips to the toilet.
11. Because of my incontinence, it's important to plan every detail in advance.
12. I worry about my incontinence getting worse as I grow older.
13. I have a hard time getting a good night of sleep because of my incontinence.
14. I worry about being embarrassed or humiliated because of my incontinence.
15. My incontinence makes me feel as if I am not a healthy person.
16. My incontinence makes me feel helpless.
17. I get less enjoyment out of life because of my incontinence.
18. I worry about not being able to get to the toilet on time.
19. I feel as if I have no control over my bladder.
20. I have to watch what I drink because of my incontinence.
21. My incontinence limits my choice of clothing.
22. I worry about having sex because of my incontinence.

APPENDIX

B

Incontinence Questionnaire

Name: ______________________________

Patient #: ____________________________

1. Do you ever leak urine or lose control of urination? ____________________

2. If you lose control, do you know when it happens or do you just find yourself wet?

   ❍ Know when it happens ❍ Find myself wet

3. How often do you lose control of urination and wet yourself or your pads because you feel a strong urge and can't stop it?

   ❍ Never ❍ Few times/year ❍ Few times/month ❍ Few times/week ❍ Daily

4. How often do you lose control and wet yourself or your pads when you cough or sneeze?

   ❍ Never ❍ Few times/year ❍ Few times/month ❍ Few times/week ❍ Daily

5. How often do you lose control and wet yourself or your pads when you engage in physical activity (running, jumping, lifting, sports, etc.)?

   ❍ Never ❍ Few times/year ❍ Few times/month ❍ Few times/week ❍ Daily

6. How often do you lose control and wet yourself or your pads when you raise yourself from a sitting to a standing position?

   ❍ Never ❍ Few times/year ❍ Few times/month ❍ Few times/week ❍ Daily

7. How often do you wear pads or other forms of protection because of the wetting?

   ❍ Never ❍ Few times/year ❍ Few times/month ❍ Few times/week ❍ Daily

8. On average, how many pads do you use a day? __________

9. On average, how wet are they when you change them?

   ❍ Dry ❍ Moist ❍ Damp ❍ Wet ❍ Soaked

10. On a scale of 0-10 (0 is not at all; 10 is intolerable), how badly does loss of urinary control bother you? __________

11. How often must you push or strain to start urination?

    ❍ Never ❍ Few times/year ❍ Few times/month ❍ Few times/week ❍ Daily

12. How would you describe the usual force of the stream?

    ❍ Strong ❍ Not as strong as it used to be ❍ Weak ❍ Interrupted ❍ Dribbling

APPENDIX B *is for* CHAPTER 7

Voiding Diary

Name: ______________________________ Date: ____________________

Time of urge to void	Strength of pain or urge	Time of actual void	Voided volume	Incontinence (S, U, or W) see below	Amount of leakage (Large = L, Medium = M, Small = S)

Urgency is the feeling that you have to urinate badly.

Incontinence is the loss of urine control before reaching the bathroom.

S = Stress incontinence is wetting or leaking or leakage at times of coughing, sneezing, or with physical activity, etc.

U = Urge incontinence is wetting or leakage because of urgency

W = Unaware incontinence is wetting without conscious awareness of when it happens.

APPENDIX D

Micturition Record

Micturition Record

Name: ______________________

Age: __________ Date of Birth: __________ Today's Date: __________

Voiding history:

Daytime wetting: Yes/No Days per week: ______

Nighttime wetting: Yes/No Nights per week: ______

Age of toilet training: ______

Number of times child voids/24 hrs: 1-3 4-6 6-8 more

History of urinary infection: Yes/No

Other problems:

Bowel history:

Number of bowel movements/week: ______________________

Soiling underwear (skid mark, formed stool): ______________________

Number of bowel accidents/week: ______________________

Other bowel problems: ______________________

Please record if volume of urine is measured. Also record if the child has any symptoms such as burning on urination, or straining to void.

Record events as follows:

void = void, **wet** = urinary accident, **BM** = bowel movement, **ENC** = bowel accident

	Day 1	Day 2	Day 3
7 AM			
8 AM			
9 AM			
10 AM			
11 AM			
12 NOON			
1 PM			
2 PM			
3 PM			
4 PM			
5 PM			
6 PM			
7 PM			
8 PM			
9 PM			
10 PM			
11 PM			
12 MIDNIGHT			
MIDNIGHT - 7 AM			

Comments:

APPENDIX D *is for* CHAPTER 19

American Urological Association (AUA) Symptom Index (range from 0 to 35 points)

APPENDIX E

	Not at all	Less than 1 time in 5	Less than half the time	About half the time	More than half the time	Almost always
1. Over the last month, how often have you had a sensation of not emptying your bladder completely after you finished urinating?	0	1	2	3	4	5
2. Over the last month, how often have you had to urinate again less than 2 hours after you finished urinating?	0	1	2	3	4	5
3. Over the last month, how often have you found you stopped and started again several times while urinating?	0	1	2	3	4	5
4. Over the last month, how often have you found it difficult to postpone urination?	0	1	2	3	4	5
5. Over the last month, how often have you had a weak stream while urinating?	0	1	2	3	4	5
6. Over the last month, how often have you had to push or strain to begin urinating?	0	1	2	3	4	5
7. Over the last month, how many times did you most typically get up to urinate from the time you went to bed until the time you got up in the morning?	0 None	1 Time	2 Times	3 Times	4 Times	5 Or more times

AUA SI Score (0-7 mild; 8-18 moderate; 19-35 severe symptoms) ☐

APPENDIX E *is for* CHAPTER 24

APPENDIX F

SEAPI Incontinence Score—Subjective

(From Raz S: *Female urology,* Philadelphia, Saunders, publication pending)

SEAPI Incontinence Score—Subjective
(From Raz S: *Female urology,* Philadelphia, Saunders, publication pending)

S	Stress-Related Leakage	0 = No urine loss
		1 = Loss with strenuous activity
		2 = Loss with moderate activity
		3 = Loss with minimal activity, or gravitational incontinence
E	Emptying Ability	0 = No obstructive symptoms
		1 = Minimal symptoms
		2 = Significant symptoms
		3 = Voiding only in dribbles, or urinary retention
A	Anatomy	0 = No descent during strain
		1 = Descent, not to introitus
		2 = Descent through introitus with strain
		3 = Through introitus without strain
P	Protection	0 = Never used
		1 = Used only for certain occasions
		2 = Used daily for occasional accidents
		3 = Used continually for frequent accidents or constant leaking
I	Inhibition	0 = No urgency incontinence
		1 = Rare urgency incontinence
		2 = Urgency incontinence once a week
		3 = Urgency incontinence at least once a day

APPENDIX F
is for
CHAPTER 33

SEAPI Incontinence Score—Objective Measures

(Modified from Raz S: *Female urology,* Philadelphia, Saunders, publication pending)

S	Stress-Related Leakage	Observe for leak during Valsalva and cough 0 = No leak 1 = Leak at >80 cm water 2 = Leak at 30-80 cm water 3 = Leak at <30 cm water
E	Emptying Ability	Postvoid residual should be verified by repeat measurement 0 = 0-60 ml 1 = 61-100 ml 2 = 101-200 ml 3 = >200 ml or unable to void
A	Anatomy	Position of bladder neck relative to symphysis during cough or Valsalva seen on lateral cystogram 0 = Above symphysis with strain 1 = <2 cm below symphysis with strain 2 = >2 cm below symphysis with strain 3 = >2 cm below symphysis at rest
P	Protection	0 = Never used 1 = Used only for certain occasions 2 = Used daily for occasional accidents 3 = Used continually for frequent accidents or constant leaking
I	Inhibition	Involuntary rise in pressure during cystometry 0 = No pressure rise 1 = Rise late in filling >500 ml) 2 = Medium fill rise (150-500 ml) 3 = Early rise <150 ml)

SEAPI Incontinence Score—Objective Measures
(Modified from Raz S: *Female urology,* Philadelphia, Saunders, publication pending)

APPENDIX G *is for* CHAPTER 33

APPENDIX

H

Instructions for Biofeedback

Electromyography (EMG) is the observation and recording of electrical activity within your pubococcygeus muscle. This activity is picked up by a sensor. The sensor transfers the electrical activity into a line graph on the instrument screen.

Biofeedback specifically refers to the use of electronic instruments to monitor, amplify, and display (or feed back) information about a specific event—in this situation, the activity of the pelvic muscles.

The *biofeedback procedure* begins with:

Relaxing the pelvic muscle and watching the electrical recordings as they appear as a dotted graph on the computer monitor. We will begin with helping you to relax your pelvic muscles.

The therapist will coach you in the different types of muscle contractions to perform:

- Contract your pelvic muscle as if you were performing a quick muscle exercise.
- Now relax the muscle and try to return the line graph to the relaxed state.
- Contract the pelvic muscle and hold as long as you can.
- Again relax your pelvic muscle and try to return the reading to the original relaxed state.

The above procedure is repeated several times during each biofeedback session. At the completion of each session we will compare your EMG readings to previous sessions and discuss your progress.

APPENDIX H
is for
CHAPTER 38

Sample Voiding Diary

Time	Amount Urinated In Toilet	Small Accident	Large Accident	Reason For Accident	Fluid Intake
______	______	______	______	______	______
______	______	______	______	______	______
______	______	______	______	______	______
______	______	______	______	______	______

Type of pads used____

Number of pads used today____

Comments____

____

____

____

____

____

APPENDIX I *is for* CHAPTER 55

APPENDIX J

Quality of Life Instruments

Urogenital Distress Inventory Short Form (UDI-6)

Do you experience and, if so, how much are you bothered by:

	0 = not at all	1 = slightly	2 = moderately	3 = greatly
1. Frequent urination	❑	❑	❑	❑
2. Urine leakage related to feeling of urgency	❑	❑	❑	❑
3. Urine leakage related to activity, coughing, or sneezing	❑	❑	❑	❑
4. Small amounts of urine leakage (drops)	❑	❑	❑	❑
5. Difficulty emptying your bladder	❑	❑	❑	❑
6. Pain or discomfort in lower abdominal or genital area	❑	❑	❑	❑

Incontinence Impact Questionnaire Short Form (IIQ-7)

Has urine leakage affected your:

1. Ability to do household chores (cooking, housecleaning, laundry)?	❑	❑	❑	❑
2. Physical recreation such as walking, swimming, or other exercise?	❑	❑	❑	❑
3. Entertainment activities (movies, concerts, etc.)?	❑	❑	❑	❑
4. Ability to travel by car or bus more than 30 minutes from home?	❑	❑	❑	❑
5. Participating in social activities outside your home?	❑	❑	❑	❑
6. Emotional health (nervousness, depression, anger)?	❑	❑	❑	❑
7. Feeling frustrated?	❑	❑	❑	❑

Both instruments are scored: 0 = not at all, 1 = slightly, 2 = moderately, 3 = greatly. Scores are summed and multiplied by 33⅓ to put scores on a scale of 0 to 100. High scores indicate greater symptom distress or life impact. Items from the longer versions[10] may be added if the clinician desires.

APPENDIX J *is for* CHAPTER 55

Pelvic Muscle Exercises

- Do 45 pelvic muscle exercises *every* day, 15 at a time, 3 times a day
  - Do 15 lying down in the morning
  - Do 15 standing up in the afternoon
  - Do 15 sitting in the evening

For each exercise:

- Squeeze for __________ seconds
- Relax for __________ seconds

Remember to *relax* all the muscles in your abdomen when you do these exercises and continue to breathe normally.

Once a day, practice slowing or stopping the stream of urine when you void.

APPENDIX

L

The Urge Strategy in 6 Steps

(From Burgio KL, Pearce KL, Lucco AJ: *Staying dry: a practical guide to bladder control,* Baltimore, 1989, The Johns Hopkins University Press, p. 81.)

1. Stop what you are doing and stay put. Sit down when possible, or stand quietly. Remain very still. When you are still, it is easier to control your urge.
2. Squeeze your pelvic floor muscles quickly several times. Do not relax fully in between.
3. Relax the rest of your body. Take a few deep breaths to help you relax and let go of your tension.
4. Concentrate on suppressing the urge feeling.
5. Wait until the urge subsides.
6. Walk to the bathroom at a normal pace. Do not rush. Continue squeezing your pelvic floor muscles quickly while you walk.

The Urge Strategy in 6 Steps

(From Burgio KL, Pearce KL, Lucco AJ: *Staying dry: a practical guide to bladder control,* Baltimore, 1989, The Johns Hopkins University Press, p. 81.)

APPENDIX L

is for

CHAPTER 58

Bladder Training Instructions

Step 1 Review the patient's bladder diary and identify a voiding interval that the patient can adopt with comfort during the daytime.

Step 2 Instruct the patient to void:

- Soon after rising in the morning
- Every time the voiding interval passes during the day
- At bedtime

If the patient has an urge to void before the interval has passed, he or she should suppress it and wait until the interval has passed. If the interval has passed and still there is no urge to void, the patient should void anyway. This places the patient in control of both initiating and inhibiting the micturition reflex.

Step 3 Once the patient feels comfortable on a voiding schedule for at least three days, the interval should be increased. Typically 30-minute increases are used, but the increases can be smaller or larger depending on the judgement of the therapist or the confidence of the patient.

Step 4 Continue to increase the interval until an acceptable voiding interval is achieved, usually every three or four hours.

APPENDIX N

Incontinence Quiz

(Modified from Branch LG, Walker LA, Wetle TT, et al: Urinary incontinence knowledge among community-dwelling people 65 years of age and older, *J Am Geriatr Soc* 42:1257-1262, 1994.)

Incontinence Quiz

(Modified from Branch LG, Walker LA, Wetle TT, et al: Urinary incontinence knowledge among community-dwelling people 65 years of age and older, *J Am Geriatr Soc* 42:1257-1262, 1994.)

Next, I'll read some general statements about urinary incontinence. Please tell me whether you agree or disagree with each statement. The (first/next) statement is (READ ITEM). Do you agree or disagree with this statement?

	Agree	Disagree	Refused	Don't Know	Professional Consensus Response
1. Involuntary loss of urine, often called a leaky bladder or urinary incontinence, is one of the results of normal aging.	1	2	7	8	DISAGREE
2. Most people will involuntarily or accidentally lose control of their urine on a regular basis by the time they reach 85.	1	2	7	8	DISAGREE
3. Many common over-the-counter medications can cause involuntary urine loss.	1	2	7	8	AGREE
4. Other than pads, diapers, and catheters, little can be done to treat or cure involuntary urine loss.	1	2	7	8	DISAGREE
5. Once people start to lose control of their urine on a regular basis, they usually can never regain complete control over it again.	1	2	7	8	DISAGREE
6. Most people who currently have involuntary urine loss live normal lives.	1	2	7	8	AGREE
7. Most physicians ask their older patients whether they have bladder control problems.	1	2	7	8	DISAGREE
8. Women are more likely than men to develop urinary incontinence.	1	2	7	8	AGREE
9. Most people with involuntary urine loss talk to their doctors about it.	1	2	7	8	DISAGREE
10. Involuntary urine loss is caused by only one or two conditions.	1	2	7	8	DISAGREE
11. Many people with involuntary urine loss can be cured and almost everyone can experience significant improvement.	1	2	7	8	AGREE
12. Involuntary loss of urine can be caused by several easily treatable medical conditions.	1	2	7	8	AGREE
13. The best treatment for involuntary urine loss is usually surgery.	1	2	7	8	DISAGREE
14. There are exercises that can help control urine if one leaks when one coughs, sneezes, or laughs.	1	2	7	8	AGREE

APPENDIX N *is for* CHAPTER 62

INDEX

C

T

U

V

W

Y